Acknowledgments

We thank the Demos team of Diana M. Schneider, Ph.D., Publisher, and Joan Wolk, Managing Editor, as well as Julayne Campbell, Shannon White, Jean Cunningham, Dori Taylor, RMA, and Mary Rose for their administrative support and persistence during the writing of this book.

Multiple Sclerosis

Diagnosis, Medical Management, and Rehabilitation

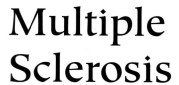

Multiple
Sclerosis

Diagnosis, Medical Management,
and Rehabilitation

EDITED BY

JACK S. BURKS, M.D., AND
KENNETH P. JOHNSON, M.D.

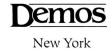

New York

Demos Medical Publishing, Inc., 386 Park Avenue South, New York, New York 10016

Library of Congress Cataloging-in-Publication Data

Multiple sclerosis : diagnosis, medical management, and rehabilitation /
edited by Jack S. Burks and Kenneth P. Johnson.
     p. cm.
Includes bibliographical references and index.
   ISBN 1-888799-35-8
  1. Multiple sclerosis. I. Burks, Jack S. II. Johnson, Kenneth P.,
1932–
   RC377 .M847 2000
   616.8'34—dc21   00-035858

Made in the United States of America

Dedication

This book is dedicated to a courageous group of patients who have emerged as the true heroes in the long battle against MS and to two individuals whose lives and contributions have made an enduring difference. The MS patients who have willingly consented to participate in numerous clinical trials of experimental therapies have been centrally responsible for the improved quality of life now available to most MS patients, especially those in the early stages of their disease.

Over the past two and a half decades, as the immunologic basis for MS has become better understood, numerous apparently logical treatments have been proposed. Experience has shown that the usefulness of these agents cannot be determined in the laboratory or in animals, but must be tested in carefully designed experimental trials in consenting humans with MS. Many trial participants have been assigned to placebo groups, at times for three to four years, so that comparisons between treatment and placebo can be made. Some recently conducted MS trials have shown that the treatment being investigated was useless or even made the disease worse. In a few trials, serious, life-threatening side effects due to the treatment were observed. In all, several thousand dedicated patients have been inconvenienced at least, and have been exposed to real risk, providing the evidence for the FDA-approved treatments that are now available to reduce relapses and disability. The task in unfinished. The available treatments do not cure or totally control MS. Further clinical trials enlisting other groups of patients will be required before this battle is won. We honor the future as well as the past participants in MS treatment trials.

This book is also dedicated to Nancy Cobble, M.D., and Linda Coulthard-Morris, MA. Both made extraordinary contributions to improve the lives of people with multiple sclerosis. Both died as young adults, but will not be forgotten.

Dr. Cobble was a rehabilitation medicine physician who helped introduce the tenets of rehabilitation of multiple sclerosis to the world. Her concept of integrating clinical care teams for MS patients in the 1970s was a cornerstone of the current comprehensive care approach to the disease. She wrote the guidelines for multiple sclerosis training of rehabilitation residents. Her faith in God and her love for her young family transcended her wonderful clinical skills by adding spirituality to the care of people with MS. At a time before disease-modifying agents were available, she connected with the healing process and provided much comfort to her patients and set an example for the rest of us who struggled with this disease of unknown cause and no cure. Even today, the combination of knowledge, wisdom, caring, and faith she displayed is a role model for the rest of us.

Linda Coulthard-Morris was a psychological counselor who led the development of stress management techniques for MS patients. Her kind, gentle, and reassuring manner helped many people with MS face their difficult situation with new strategies to achieve a better quality of life. At the same time, she began developing an interest and subsequent expertise in neurologic scales to measure the function of MS patients. She died at age 36, just after completing the MS scales chapter for our book. Her last, uncompleted, project was to design a strategy for testing complementary and alternative medicine therapies for people with MS that would be scientifically sound and acceptable for publication in Western medicine journals.

Contents

VII   SOCIETAL ISSUES

VIII   MULTIPLE SCLEROSIS IN THE COMMUNITY

Preface

Multiple sclerosis (MS) is a common neurologic disease displaying great variability and, unfortunately, tragic consequences for many patients. Its predilection to appear in young adult women, its poorly understood pathogenesis, its often progressive course, and the tremendous human and economic cost of the disease, present immense challenges to patients and their families, their health care providers, the payers of health care, and the community in general.

While the recently approved immunomodulating treatments have made dramatic inroads into lessening the impact of the disease, no cure is in sight. Most patients still progress. In fact, imaging and MRI spectroscopy shows a picture of significant early central nervous system (CNS) damage of a magnitude not previously appreciated. Axonal and neuronal loss further complicates the consequences of demyelination and may be the primary reason for fixed disability. Cognitive problems, often unrecognized early in the disease course, frustrate patients, their families, employers, and health care providers. Dealing with the many subtle and not so subtle but complex issues requires many different levels of care. Expertise by multiple health professionals is needed, and the best MS physician cannot alone adequately deal with the numerous patient issues.

The first portion of this text is a state of the art description of the history and epidemiology of MS, the current knowledge of the pathogenesis of the disease, important differential considerations, and the rationale for and results of studies on immunomodulating therapies. The individual chapter authors combine their research expertise with their substantial clinical experience to present a readable text for the scientist and the clinician. Useful treatment programs and options are clearly stated. The various chapters have been written to aid both the experienced neurologist and the increasing number of generalists who care for MS patients.

The second and largest section of the book covers in-depth the treatment of specific problems encountered by the MS patients. Most MS textbooks cover these topics in a few paragraphs or pages. In contrast, this book devotes chapters to each individual topic, recognizing that successful disease management requires more than targeted drug therapy. Each chapter author focuses on the practical aspects of the treatments, based on the available clinical data combined with their long clinical expertise. While providing details of symptom management, the chapters are written with an easy-to-follow sequential reasoning, often with useful algorithms.

The chapters are designed to provide practical management strategies when encountering these specific symptoms in the health care professional's office. While new drugs will undoubtedly be available for specific symptoms, the approach to symptom management detailed in this section should remain useful.

The rehabilitation chapters describe the keys to maintaining best possible function in spite of worsening neurologic impairment. Quality of life for the MS patient is affected by much more than neurologic impairment. The rehabilitation chapters emphasize safety as well as improvement of quality of life concerns.

The last section of the book covers areas that are nonmedical in a strict sense but that are important to help patients to better integrate into their communities and remain productive and creative.

The underlying theme in this book is comprehensive information in a practical format. While designed for the neurologist or other MS health care specialist, it will be a useful reference for all health care professionals.

We are honored to have chapter contributions from many of the best minds in the field of MS management. Each of the authors has made original contributions to this field and they must be awarded the thanks of the reader who learns from this book.

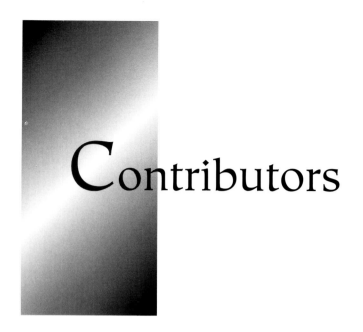

Contributors

James Ahearn, CSW, ACSW
President, National Multiple Sclerosis Society
Rochester Area Chapter
Rochester, New York

Mindy L. Aisen, M.D.
Veterans Health Administration
Department of Veterans Affairs
Rehabilitation Research
Washington, D.C.

Catherine W. Britell, M.D.
Department of Rehabilitation Medicine
University of Washington
Seattle, Washington

Jack S. Burks, M.D.
Clinical Professor of Medicine (Neurology)
University of Nevada
School of Mediine
    and
President, Multiple Sclerosis Alliance
Reno, Nevada

Jeffrey A. Cohen, M.D.
Mellen Center for MS Treatment and Research
Department of Neurology
Cleveland Clinic Foundation
Cleveland, Ohio

Suhayl Dhib-Jalbut, M.D.
Professor of Neurology of
University of Maryland School of Medicine
    and
Baltimore VA Medical Center
Baltimore, Maryland

P. K. Coyle, M.D.
Professor of Neurology
Director, Stony Brook MS Comprehensive Care Center
School of Medicine
State University of New York at Stony Brook
Stony Brook, New York

Mary Dierich, RN, MSN, C-NP, CURN
University of Minnesota
Urologic Surgery Department

Benjamin H. Eidelman, M.D., Ph.D.
Professor and Vice Chairman for Clinical Affairs
Department of Neurology
University of Pittsburgh
Pittsburgh, Pennsylvania

Robert M. Elfont, M.D., Ph.D.
Department of Neurology
MCP Hahnemann University
Philadelphia, Pennsylvania

Leigh E. Elkins, Ph.D.
Assistant Professor of Neurology
School of Medicine
State University of New York at Stony Brook
Stony Brook, New York

Elliot M. Frohman, M.D., Ph.D.
Department of Neurology
Department of Ophthalmology
University of Texas Southwestern Medical Center
    at Dallas
Dallas, Texas

Teresa C. Frohman, B.A.
Department of Neurology
University of Texas Southwestern Medical Center at
 Dallas
Dallas, Texas

Donald E. Goodkin, M.D.
Medical Director, The UCSF/MT Zion
 Multiple Sclerosis Center
Associate Professor of Neurology
The University of California at San Francisco
San Francisco, California

Jacqueline A. Hall, M.S., O.T.R./L.
Department of Rehabilitation Medicine
University of Washington
Seattle, Washington

June Halper, MSN, ANP, FAAN
Executive Director
Gimbel MS Center
MS Network of New Jersey
Executive Director
Consortium of MS Centers
Teaneck, New Jersey

Jodie K. Haselkorn, M.D., M.P.H.
Director, Multiple Sclerosis Clinic
Puget Sound Health Care System
Department of Veterans Affairs
Associate Professor, Rehabilitation Medicine
University of Washington
Seattle, Washington

Robert M. Herndon, M.D.
Department of Neurology
G. V. Montgomery Veterans Affairs Medical Center
Jackson, Mississippi
 and the
University of Mississippi Medical Center

Fay Horak, Ph.D.
Oregon Health Sciences University
Portland, Oregon

Karen Hunter, RN,C
Program Specialist and Clinical Supervisor
Fairview Home Care and Hospice
Minneapolis, Minnesota

Bruce Idelkope, M.D.
Medical Director Rehabilitative Services
Healthsystem Minnesota
Associate Clinical Professor
Department of Neurology
University of Minnesota
Vice President, Minneapolis Clinic of Neurology
Saint Louis Park, Minnesota

Douglas R. Jeffery, M.D., Ph.D.
Wake Forest University School of Medicine
Department of Neurology
Winston-Salem, North Carolina

Kenneth P. Johnson, M.D.
Professor and Chair, Department of Neurology
University of Maryland Medical Center
Baltimore, Maryland

Rosalind C. Kalb, Ph.D.
Clinical Psychologist
MS Care Center, St. Agnes Hospital
New York Medical College
 and
Special Projects Consultant
National Multiple Sclerosis Society
New York, New York

Lauren B. Krupp, M.D.
Professor of Neurology
School of Medicine
State University of New York at Stony Brook
Stony Brook, New York

John F. Kurtzke, M.D.
Professor of Neurology
Georgetown University School of Medicine
Chief, Neuroepidemiology Section
Veterans Affairs Medical Center
Washington, D.C.
 and
Distinguished Professor of Neurology
Uniformed Services University of the Health Sciences
Bethesda, Maryland

Nicholas G, LaRocca, Ph.D.
Director, Health Care Delivery and Policy Research
National MS Society
New York, New York

Shayla E. Leer, M.P.T.
Department of Rehabilitation Medicine
University of Washington
Seattle, Washington

Jeri A. Logemann, Ph.D.
Ralph and Jean Sundin Professor
Communication Sciences and Disorders
Department of Neurology, Otolaryngology, and Dental
 Prosthetics
Northwestern University
Chicago, Illinois

Fred D. Lublin, M.D.
Department of Neurology
MCP Hahnemann University

Roland Martin, M.D.
Acting Chief, Cellular Immunology Section
Neuroimmunology Branch
National Institute of Neurological Disorders and
    Stroke
National Institutes of Health
Bethesda, Maryland

Aaron Miller, M.D.
Director, Division of Neurology and MS Center
Maimonides Medical Center
Brooklyn, New York
    and
Professor of Clinical Neurology
State University of New York—Health Science Center
    at Brooklyn
Brooklyn, New York

Linda Coulthard-Morris, MA, LPC
Rocky Mountain Multiple Sclerosis Center
Englewood, Colorado

T. Jock Murray, OC, MS, FRCPC, MACP, LLD, DSc
Professor of Medical Humanities
Director, Dalhousie MS Research Unit
Dalhousie University
Halifax, Nova Scotia B3H 4H7
Canada

Marie Namey, RN, MSN
Advanced Practice Nurse
Mellen Center for Multiple Sclerosis Treatment and
    Research
Cleveland Clinic Foundation
Cleveland, Ohio

R. Joan Oshinsky, M.D., Ph.D.
Department of Neurology
MCP Hahnemann University
Philadelphia, Pennsylvania

Debra J. Pate, M.S., C.T.R.S.
University of Washington
Department of Rehabilitation Medicine
Seattle, Washington

Donald W. Paty, M.D., F.R.C.P.C., F.A.C.P.
Professor, Division of Neurology
Vancouver Hospital and University of British Columbia
Vancouver, British Columbia
Canada

Jack H. Petajan, M.D., Ph.D.
Department of Neurology
University of Utah School of Medicine
Salt Lake City, Utah

Nancy Popp, RN
Home Care Liaison
Fairview University Medical Center
Minneapolis, Minnesota

Mary R. Rensel, M.D.
Mellen Center for MS Treatment and Research
Department of Neurology
Cleveland Clinic Foundation
Cleveland, Ohio

Phillip D. Rumrill, Jr., Ph.D., CRC
Associate Professor and Coordinator, Rehabilitation
    Counseling Program
Director, Center for Disability Studies
Kent State University
Kent, Ohio

Audrey Sorgen Saunders, M.A.
Yeshiva University
Ferkauf Graduate School of Psychology
Bronx, New York

Jack H. Simon, M.D., Ph.D.
Professor of Radiology and Neurology
Department of Radiology
University of Colorado Health Sciences Center
Denver, Colorado

Randall T. Schapiro, M.D.
Director, Fairview MS Center
Clinical Professor of Neurology
University of Minnesota
Minneapolis, MN

Pamela Miller Sorensen, M.A., C.C.C.-S.L.P.
2843 South Uinta Street
Denver, CO 80231-4173

Kenneth M. Viste, Jr., M.D.
Lakeside NEUROCARE
Oshkosh, Wisconsin

Mitchell T. Wallin, M.D., M.P.H.
Instructor of Neurology
Georgetown University School of Medicine
Assistant Chief, Neuroepidemiology Section
Veterans Affairs Medical Center
Washington, D.C.

Karen Wenzel, M.A., CTRS/CLP
Rocky Mountain Multiple Sclerosis Center
Englewood, Colorado

Robert R. Young, M.D.
Department of Neurology
University of Southern California
Irvine, California

Carol F. Zimmerman, M.D.
Department of Ophthalmology
University of Texas Southwestern Medical Center at
   Dallas
Dallas, Texas

I

HISTORY

1

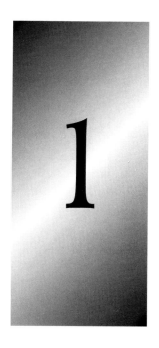

The History of Multiple Sclerosis

T. Jock Murray, M.D.

"The story of knowledge of multiple sclerosis is like a history of medicine in miniature."

Tracy J. Putnam 1938 (1)

Multiple sclerosis (MS) is known to the general public as a common, debilitating neurologic disease that affects young adults. It is now well known because it is common, because research on the disease has been a major thrust in neurosciences in recent decades, and because the MS Societies have increased public awareness of the disorder.

In an era when patients often suspect their own diagnosis when a neurologic symptom appears, it may seem surprising that the disorder was only clearly delineated in the latter half of the nineteenth century and that it was initially regarded as rare. Over the next century and a half, theories about the disease changed with major advances in medical science.

Multiple sclerosis has been known by many names during the last century and a half. Robert Carswell referred to it as a "peculiar disease state," and Jean Cruveilhier commented on "gray degeneration of the cord" (2). William Moxon (3) referred to "insular sclerosis," which was also used by the English and by William Osler

(4) for many decades. "Disseminated sclerosis" was a common term in England in the earlier part of this century, but the more widely used "multiple sclerosis," a derivation from the German *multiple sklerose*, has become widespread. The French use the term *sclérose en plaque*. In this brief history of the disease, I use the term *multiple sclerosis* when discussing contributions by physicians who may have used another term.

THE EARLIEST CASES

Multiple sclerosis has been with us for many centuries, but we are not sure if its frequency is increasing or if its patterns are changing. Examination of the earliest cases that resemble MS can be instructive by revealing how chronic neurologic disease was viewed and managed when illness was systemic rather than having a disease focus. Many cases in the medical literature that may be early examples of MS are so sketchy in their details that the disease can be suggested only as a possibility.

Saint Lidwina van Schiedam

One early but uncertain report, often put forward as the earliest recorded case of MS, relates to the "strange disease of the Virgin Lidwina." Confounding issues of religious fervor surround the reports of her illness, causing me to hesitate to conclude that she had MS, but the story has been told so often that it bears repeating.

The first document commenting on Lidwina van Schiedam (1380–1433) was an official document dated August 4, 1421, in which Jan van Beieren, Count of Holland, acknowledges a letter of the Schiedam local authorities about her disease and states that he personally had seen the young woman (5). Details of her illness came from her biographer, the Franciscan Priest Johannes Brugman (1400–1473), who obtained information from relatives, her priest and confessor, local clerics, and other "reliable persons," as well as from Thomas à Kempis, who wrote "Vita Lidewigis Virginis" some 15 years after her death, based on the information published by Brugman.

Lidwina was born on April 18, 1380, in Schiedam, Holland, the daughter of a laborer, and one of nine children. She was healthy and active as a child and teenager. On February 2, 1396, she fell while skating and broke ribs on the right side. An abscess formed in the area of the fracture, after which she had difficulty walking. She was described as having violent lancinating pain in her teeth, which could have been trigeminal neuralgia. Many physicians were consulted, including the famous Godfried Sonderdank, court physician to Duke Albrecht of Holland and Duchess Margaretha of Burgundy. He somberly reported that this disease was incurable as it came directly from God and that any attempt to cure her would impoverish her father and do no good, and that even Hippocrates and Galen could do little in this situation.

By the time she was 19 years old, walking was more difficult and she developed paralysis in her right arm as well as more sporadic pains. There is mention of a split face and hanging lip, which probably indicate facial weakness. Soon she was unable to walk, had some loss of sensation, and eventually developed pressure sores.

From 1407 onward a number of visions of God and angels appeared to Lidwina. During these "extases" her sight improved and she was more mobile. She became increasingly weak, had difficulty swallowing—first solid food and later liquids—and had more pain. The disease progressed slowly over 37 years with occasional periods of improvement. She bore her increasing disability and pain as reparation for the sins of others. Beginning in 1407 she began to experience supernatural gifts, ecstasies, and visions in which she participated in the Passion of Christ, saw purgatory and heaven, and visited with saints. In the last years of her life, she was going blind and was said to take little sustenance but Communion, and to sleep little if at all, both of which are difficult to credit.

Her suffering attracted wide attention, and when a new parish priest accused her of hypocrisy, the townspeople threatened to drive him away. She died on April 14, 1433, and as early as 1434 a chapel was built over her grave (6). A cult developed around her memory and eventually led to her canonization. An ecclesiastical commission declared her experiences to be valid (7). She was said to be a "prodigy of human suffering and heroic patience" (8).

Lidwina's bones were found in 1947 and analyzed at the Laboratory of Anatomy and Embryology at the University of Leiden in 1957. There were changes in keeping with paralysis of the legs and probably of the right arm (5).

Halla, the Drummer Bock, and the Hudson Bay Official

A less credible case, because of a paucity of information, is that of Halla in the Icelandic saga of St. Thorlakr. This information was found by Dr. Margaret Cormack while studying as a fellow at the Ukrainian Research Institute of Harvard. A woman named Halla developed an acute illness with loss of the sight of both eyes, and on the next day she lost her speech. She made a vow to Almighty God and to the Holy Bishop Thorlakr for intercession, that if cured she would walk to Skalholt fasting and saying prayers. On the third day a candlewick was put around her head and her sight began to return; she later recovered her speech on the feast of St. Michael. The miracle was said to have occurred somewhere between 1293 and 1323, but no other information is known about this young woman. There is flimsy evidence for the diagnosis of MS in an era when powerful emotions were associated with religious belief, but I mention it because it is in the literature of MS (9).

Another case with incomplete information is that of a drummer named Bock, described in a paper by C. J. T. de Meza in 1810 and reported by Stenager (10). When describing the beneficial effects of electricity on seven conditions, de Meza outlined Bock's course of illness. It began in 1789 with "arthritic seizures" and paralysis of the right arm and leg; recovery occurred within six weeks after electrical therapy. There is little clue to substantiate a suggestion of MS.

William Brown, born in Ayrshire, Scotland, in 1790, became a Hudson Bay trader at York Factory in the Canadian West. In 1811 he began to develop leg weakness and vision problems. He found it too difficult to carry out some of his duties and was censured by Governor Simpson when he sent a replacement out on a survey. He had a remitting and progressive disorder, with visual symptoms, weakness, and gait difficulty, and eventually had to leave his post and return to Scotland to the care of his family. He died a few years later. (Maria Aguayo, personal communication)

Sir Augustus d'Esté

In the case of Augustus d'Esté (1794–1848), the grandson of George III, there is no doubt of the diagnosis because he kept a detailed diary of his progressive disease for decades (11). The Regent did not approve of the marriage of his son, Prince Augustus Frederick, Duke of Sussex, to Lady Augusta Murray, and had the marriage annulled (the marriage of a Royal descendent required the monarch's consent). Although he was later given a knighthood, the young Augustus was made illegitimate and was frustrated for the rest of his life by rebuffs in his attempt to reestablish his links with the royal family. His progressive and puzzling illness would be even more frustrating.

Augustus began to keep a diary in 1822, when he was age 28. The first page describes blurring of vision after leaving the funeral of a beloved relative. His vision deteriorated so much that he had to have others read to him, but it gradually cleared without treatment. Visual blurring recurred twice during the next few years. Dr. Spanganberg sent him to a spa at Driburg, where he "drank steel-water, bathed in it and douched my Eyes with it:—my Eyes again recovered." In the next few years he developed numbness in his legs and difficulty walking. He consulted Dr. Kent, who completely changed his medical regimen and recommended that he "eat beef steaks twice a day, drink London Porter and sherry and Madeira wines." His legs were to be rubbed twice a day with brushes and his back with a liniment made of camphorated alcohol, opium, and Florence oil. He was pleased to write in his diary: "This new system succeeded completely. Every day I found strength returning." This was the hopeful observation of many patients taking many different treatments for MS, a disease that waxes and wanes. Later he continued to have his legs rubbed with flesh brushes but discontinued the back rubs, replacing them with slaps on the back by the open hand of a servant. He also took up horseback riding as therapy.

A Milan physician treated him for pain in the area of his kidneys with a counterirritant plaster to produce an eruption of the skin over the area. This was of no help, so he switched to flannel bandages as hot as he could tolerate. He took baths and a wash of sulfate of zinc and aqua plantaginis. He was treated with herbs and flowers and daily shower baths. He took 20 to 30 drops of valerian twice a day.

On the recommendation of his father, he consulted a number of prominent physicians, including Sir Astley Cooper, Dr. W. C. Mattin, physician to the Westminster Hospital, Dr. Kent, and Mr. Pettigrew. He followed their prescriptions and also took up sea bathing. At the seaside he developed a liaison with a young woman but noticed that his "acts of Connection" lacked a "wholesome vigor," and some medicines and pills provided by Dr. Courtenay proved of some benefit. He later underwent a course of electricity, took tepid douches to the loins and sacrum, and was subjected to a course of galvanism, with disappointing results. He derived more benefit from a trip to Scotland, where he was "much braced and invigorated by the Highland air." He found the horseback riding and walking to be helpful, and he continued the waters, warm baths and douches, and visits to various spas .

By 1840, 18 years after the onset of his disease, he made a note in his diary indicating that he was no longer using any measures for the improvement of his health or for the restoration of his vigor and strength, presumably because of disappointment with all the previous treatments. At this point he read a book on hydropathy and decided to visit the celebrated Dr. Priesznitz, who thought his infirmity originated in the nerves. He was treated five times over two days with the application of wet sheets and friction and walked around wearing a wet cincture around his waist. He next consulted Sir Benjamin Brodie and a surgeon, Mr. John Scott, who prescribed tincture of Lytta or Spanish fly, which seemed to have little effect. His prescriptions over the next few years included zinc sulfate, Spanish fly, strychnine, quinine, silver nitrate, and stramonium. Later he developed vertigo and—other than a little brandy with water—he took no medicines. John Scott recommended that he ride a horse and walk every day as long as he could. Mercury was added to the regimen and later another course of electricity, which he believed was making him worse. He was seen in consultation by Sir Richard Bright, who agreed to an increase in the amount of iron in his medicine.

His diary is a remarkable saga of medicine and therapy as practiced on the upper classes in the early nineteenth century and is a moving story of a young man trying to understand and cope with a relentless disease.

Heinrich Heine, Poet

Although many people may think they do not know the poetry of Heinrich Heine (1797–1856), his work is familiar through the music of composers such as Schubert, Wagner, and Strauss. His disabling illness continues to baffle historical diagnosticians. Putnam (1938) and others thought that he had multiple sclerosis but also considered neurosyphilis, amyotrophic lateral sclerosis, sarcoidosis, encephalomyelitis, porphyria, spinal muscular atrophy, chronic polyneuropathy, and tuberculosis (12).

Heine's illness began with a transient palsy of both hands in 1832. Five years later he had sudden bilateral loss of vision with some dilation of the left pupil. This gradually improved but visual loss progressed until the end of his life. In 1843 he developed ptosis of the left lid and hyperesthesia of the left side of his face. In 1846 he developed symptoms of bulbar involvement, which disappeared by 1850. About 1846 he developed ataxic paraplegia, which progressed until his death in 1856.

Much of the information about his illness comes from correspondence with his brother Max, a physician.

During the course of his progressive disease, he had increasing weakness, fatigue, paralysis, visual difficulty, double vision, and many other symptoms, with periods of improvement. He was treated by numerous physicians with a number of therapies, including sulfur baths, morphine, leeches, iodine mixtures, laxatives, diets, enemas, and cutaneous ointments applied over an incision that was kept open on the nape of his neck. These had little effect and he became progressively weaker and paralyzed and spent his life in what he called his "Mattress Grave." Stenager (12) suggests that it was unfortunate that he did not live long enough to consult Charcot. However, Charcot had a negative view of therapy in diseases such as multiple sclerosis, so it is unlikely that he would have had much to offer, although we would have been delighted to have had his thoughtful assessment of the poet.

Did Heine have MS? The recurrent nature of the symptoms with its later relentless progression and the constellation of symptoms over 22 years makes it very likely. Perhaps the one unusual feature is the unilateral ptosis, which would be very unusual in MS unless he were closing the eye to prevent diplopia.

Margaret Gatty, Victorian Writer

Mrs. Margaret Gatty (1809–1873) was a popular author of children's books during the Victorian era. At age 41 she talked about having a nervous disorder, and a year later noted that her hand was "losing its cunning" and had a tremor. Her progressive neurologic illness may have been MS but, like so many of these early cases, the clinical details are sparse. Her illness had a variable course that moved from one arm to the other and then affected her legs. She developed a "tic" in her face and some speech difficulty. Ten years after the onset she was dead (Personal communication from Dr. Susan Drain of Mount Saint Vincent University in Halifax, who is writing the life of Mrs. Gatty).

W. N. P. Barbellion

Dealing with a longstanding and disabling medical condition that alters one's feelings and attitudes about life, self, and the future is a struggle known to many MS patients. One who endured the battles, winning some and losing others to this relentless foe, was B. F. Cummings (1889–1919). In his diary he documented a progressive form of MS and died in 1919 at age 28, 10 years after the onset of his first symptoms (13,14).

Cummings, who wrote under the pseudonym W. N. P. Barbellion, thought his adopted initials "concealed the bravado" of Wilhelm Nero Pilate. He took the name Barbellion from a confectionery shop sign and thought this to also be "appropriately inflated." By the time he started writing his diary in 1903, at age 13, it was apparent that he had talents for mathematics and essay writing and had a great appreciation of nature and the outdoors. Initially he wished to become a naturalist and eventually obtained a position on the staff of the Natural History Museum in London. By age 18 he was experiencing the early symptoms of MS but was determined to deal with the disease and live his life as planned. "I am not going to be beaten. If I develop all the disease in the doctors' index, I mean to do what I set out to do if it has to be done in a Bath-chair."

He had recurrent numbness and weakness in his limbs, vertigo, depression, decreased sight in one eye, and numbness on the side of his face. He gradually became blind and said that men looked like trees walking and that print was hopelessly blurred. He continued to see physicians, taking their medicine without any sense of optimism, and realized that he was worsening. He thought of suicide and recognized that he was taking medicines that included arsenic and strychnine.

He mentioned going to a Christian Science church but makes no further mention about whether he attended or used their approaches to his illness. He consulted a homeopathic therapist in Finsbury Circus with disappointing results. He had no better luck with the many physicians he consulted. He commented, "I could write a book on the doctors I have known and the blunders they have known about me." He still did not understand what was happening and saw other physicians in hope of an answer. The next physician thought he was quite young to have such a neurologic disease and suggested that he should travel and continue to take arsenic. He was referred to a well-known neurologist, "Dr. H.," undoubtedly Sir Henry Head, who asked him suspiciously if he had ever been with women and then ordered two months complete rest in the country. He said Dr. H. "chased me around his consulting room with a drumstick tapping my tendons and cunningly working my reflexes."

Perhaps it was not so unusual in that era that his physicians would inform his fiancée of the diagnosis but not him. He thought the physicians would advise against marriage, but when his doctor made light of his paralysis and suggested that it was related to a recent fall, he married Eleanor Benger in September 1915. Only after their marriage did he discover the truth by looking at the report that indicated why he would not be accepted for service in World War I. Although he read a lot about the disease after that, he always left a blank when writing about it and could not bring himself to use the words *multiple sclerosis*. He thought he could sense his body deteriorating and he always wanted music playing, or he would lie in bed whistling so he would not hear the paralysis creeping. He repeatedly visualized his illness as bacteria gnawing away at his spinal cord producing a creeping paralysis, and he thought he could hear the sound of the gnawing.

As so often happens, the specter of a serious illness and impending death helped him put life in a proper context. He became frustrated by the artificial nature of much of life, and he wanted to strip away the walls, the partitions and "walk about with my clothes off, to make a large ventral incision and expose my heart." From this quotation one can see why his diary was originally entitled "A Study in the Nude."

We have a record of his incredible course because of two of his publications. His journal, *The Journal of a Disappointed Man* (13), is still in print and is widely read. *Last Diary* (14) was published after his death. The saga of his progressive illness and his approach to it made him famous but limited his writing so that the only other publication was *Enjoying Life,* which was published in 1919. His published journal was well received and brought pleasure to his last months. "The kindness everyone has shown the journal and the fact that so many have understood its meaning have entirely changed my outlook. My horizon has cleared, my thoughts are tinged with sweetness, and I am content." At age 28 he made a false diary entry "Barbellion died on December 32 (1917)," but in fact he died two years later. His brother, A. J. Cummings, said of his last days, "Never was a half-dead man more alive."

He wrote the hidden dream of most MS patients: "It would be nice if a physician from London, one of these days, were to gallop up hotspur, tether his horse to the gait post and dash in waving a reprieve—the discovery of a cure!" Alas, the cure did not arrive and his failing strength caused him to resign his position at the museum in 1917. He died on October 22, 1919, in a cottage at Gerrard's Cross.

A. F. Pollard, the editor of *History,* suggested that H. G. Wells was the real author of this remarkable diary. Wells, who is often said to be critical of Barbellion as an egotist who was seeking immortality, responded that he was not that clever. Some believed the brother may have written it, and they pointed to discrepancies in the text. However, it is clear that Barbellion put in material later and rewrote sections, which would explain errors of dates and weather in the diary.

W. N. P. Barbellion, a young man who fought a long and losing battle with multiple sclerosis, is remembered for his open and honest documentation of his illness. In the words of Peter Clifford, he "embodied that rare fusion of scientific and literary genius which can observe nature and self with equal sensitivity, analyzing with scientific detachment, yet feeling with poetic intensity."

THE EARLY MEDICAL REPORTS

In the late eighteenth and early nineteenth centuries, interest in the classification of medical diseases was following the lead of botanists, who had made spectacular advances in organizing the plant and animal kingdoms. Cullen and others recommended the careful classification of all diseases. Although the earliest attempts often mixed diseases and symptoms, the development of better techniques for clinical examination made the classification of diseases into more specific categories a rapidly advancing and exciting aspect of medicine. No group was more in the forefront of differentiating neurologic disease in that era than the French school of neurology, with the English school lagging behind. In the Croonian lectures in London on hemiplegia, paraplegia, paralysis partialis, and epilepsy (1819), Dr. John Cooke relied on the writings of Galen as well as the more recent ones by Bichet and Legallois to explain the function and dysfunction of the spinal cord. He noted that different things can affect the spinal cord, but he did not differentiate the various types of disease as they were not "sufficiently interesting." As interest in assessing the syndromes of the spinal cord developed, the concept of a separate syndrome of MS gradually evolved.

Charles Prosper Ollivier

Spillane has suggested that the first reported case of unmistakable relapsing-remitting MS in the medical literature can be found in *Maladies de la moelle epiniére* by Charles Prosper Ollivier d'Angers (15). Ollivier first published a monograph on disorders of the spinal cord in Paris in 1824 and included a case that seems to be MS in three editions of this work (16,17).

Ollivier said his monograph was merely an "outline" review of the diseases of the spinal cord, but it was actually a major study of the anatomy, physiology, and pathology of the cord. He made remarkable original observations in this work, particularly in the area of congenital malformations. He described the association of hydrocephalus with spina bifida; the cervical cord anomalies in anencephaly, such as bifidity, cyst formation, and absent or fused vertebrae; elongation of the fourth ventricle into the cervical cord; stenosis of the foramen magnum; and absence and faults in the cord itself. He described cavitation of the cord in spina bifida, gave the earliest and most accurate description of syringomyelia, and included a case that is probably multiple sclerosis.

The patient was a 20-year-old man who developed a transient weakness of his right foot in 1808. By age 29 he had weakness of both legs, but this later improved so that he was able to walk with a cane. He noted that hot spa waters would induce a loss of feeling in his right leg and numbness and clumsiness of his hands, undoubtedly the earliest positive "hot bath test" (18). This young man had urinary retention, which was relieved by pressing on his abdomen, and progressive deterioration of his motor function and speech. His intellect was said to remain intact and he retained the "gaiety of his character" despite advanced disability, reminiscent of the surprising cheerfulness of MS patients that would be noted by later authors. Ollivier called this *myelitis*, which could be due to an infection, and suggested that the treatment should be bleeding and liberal application of leeches over the thoracic area.

Robert Carswell

The first pathologic demonstration of MS was by Robert Carswell in an atlas of pathologic conditions published in 1838 (19). One of his drawings (plate 4) was of the spinal cord, pons, and medulla under the title "Brown transparent discoloration without softening of the spinal chord," demonstrating a condition he described as "a peculiar diseased state of the cord and pons Varolii accompanied by atrophy of the discolored portions, all of them occupying the medullary substance which was hard, semitransparent and atrophied. It begins on the surface of the white and extends to the gray substance." The patient was paralyzed but no other clinical details are given and Carswell only saw the patient in the pathology laboratory. The nervous system was found to have fresh lesions as well as old scars, and Carswell believed these changes were probably due to a deficiency of the blood supply.

In the associated text, Carswell wrote, "I have met with two cases of a remarkable lesion of the spinal cord accompanied with atrophy. One of the patients was under the care of M. Chomel at the Hospital of La Charité, both of them affected with paralysis. I did not see either of the patients but I could not ascertain that there was anything in the character of the paralysis or the history of the cases to throw any light on the nature of the lesion found in the region of the spinal cord. I have represented the appearances observed in one case in plate 4, figure 4." The beautiful drawings are signed by Carswell and some are annotated that they were drawn directly on the lithographic stone. Some, including the two plates on MS, are indicated as printed by "lithographers to the King," indicating that they were likely completed in 1836 and printed before June 1837, thus after the date that Victoria ascended the throne in June 1837.

Carswell was later appointed to the Inaugural Chair of Pathology at London University but was allowed to remain in Paris after his appointment and studied with Louis while he completed his atlas of drawings. He resigned his London post in 1840 because of failing health from respiratory problems. He changed careers to become physician to King Leopold of Belgium, believing the air of Belgium would be cleaner than the smog and fog of London. He died in 1857. We know of no other contributions to medicine by Carswell.

Although the first case in the medical literature would seem to be the case described by Ollivier, Lawrence McHenry (20) suggested that Robert Hooper might have published an earlier case of MS in his *Morbid Anatomy of the Human Brain* (21), which contains lithographs based on 4,000 necropsies carried out at St. Marylebone Infirmary in London over a 30-year period. McHenry refers to his plate 4 as MS, but his description is of plate 4 from Carswell's work, and a search of Hooper's drawings and lithographs at McGill University by Compston showed no convincing illustrations suggestive of multiple sclerosis (22,23).

Jean Cruveilhier

Credit for the first illustration of MS is given to Carswell (19), but his was followed shortly by similar beautiful illustrations by Jean Cruveilhier (1835–1842), who reported four patients in his atlas under the heading "Diseases of the Spinal Cord" in whom autopsy demonstrated gray degeneration in patches though the nervous system (2,24). These have been well described by Compston (22).

There was controversy for many years over which of the illustrators was first, and for some time this was accorded to Cruveilhier because Charcot in his famous lesson gave credit to Cruveilhier, mistakenly giving the publication date as 1835 (25).

One of the patients had patches in the cerebellar peduncles, optic thalami, the corpus callosum, and the fornix. Cruveilhier had seen this patient daily until her death and noted her progressive disease, but her mental state was said to have been perfect throughout the course.

Compston (22) clarified the controversy about whether Cruveilhier or Carswell should be credited with the first published pathologic description of MS. Cruveilhier's atlas was published in two volumes bearing the dates 1835 and 1842, respectively. The separate Livraisons began to appear in 1829. Volume I, which was published in 1835, contained Livraisons 1–20 and Volume 2 contained numbers 21–40. The illustrations of MS are in Livraisons 32, plate 2 and Livraisons 38, plate 5, both of which were included in Volume 2, which was published after 1841 (22).

Jean Cruveilhier was born in Limoges in 1791 and studied medicine under Dupuytren in Paris soon after entering the priesthood, graduating in 1811 (22). He was unsuccessful in two applications to be a surgeon to the City Hospital in Limoges, but obtained the Chair of Operative Surgery in Montpellier. He was later appointed to the Professorship of Anatomy in Paris in 1825 and was the first to hold the Chair of Pathology in the Faculty of Medicine, secured by a provision made in Dupuytren's will. After the siege of Paris he moved to his country estate at Succac near Limoges and died at age 83 in 1874.

Compston (22) indicates that surviving copies of Cruveilhier's atlas exist with the Livraisons bound sequentially by number, a heterogeneous collection of plates and clinical descriptions, or in copies rearranged by subjects, with the plates interleaved in varying order, presumably at the whim of individual collators, or as a separate volume. Some of the patients described in Livraisons 32 were alive in the late months of 1838, and the publication date of the Livraisons is 1839. In Livraisons 38 there is the case of Josephine Paget who was blind and paraplegic and had severe proprioceptive sensory loss mimicking locomotor ataxia. She was in bed 16 of St. Joseph Ward at La Charité on May 4, 1840, and died on March 20, 1841. Another patient in this Livraison was also alive in August 1841, and there is reference to Marshall Hall's *Diseases and Derangements of the Nervous System,* which was published in 1841 (26). Thus, if we accept Josephine Paget as a case of MS, the text could not have been published before 1841. M. Paget would later appear in the case discussions of Charcot.

Due credit must be given to Cruveilheir for giving the first clinical and pathologic correlation. He outlined the history of the cook, Darges, aged 37, who had a progressive disease over six years, with increasing gait difficulty, falls in the street, weakness and tremulousness, speech difficulty, visual loss, involuntary laughing and crying, and spasms of the limbs. Cruveilheir believed this condition was due to a similar cause as rheumatic diseases, a general suppression of sweat (1).

He also described a woman, aged 54, who had had her progressive neurologic disease many years before being admitted to the Salpêtrière, where she had been for 10 years. "There seems to be a very incomplete controlling power of the will over the muscles which seemed to obey imperiously some involuntary cause; and this conflict between the will and some involuntary cause produces incoordinate movements similar to those seen in Chorea. If the patient is carried from bed to bed, the most violent reactions take place in the legs, and the attendants must exercise care not to be struck by them. These contractions take place when the patient is asked to move the limbs voluntarily. The only thing she can use moderately well is snuff tobacco. To this she makes a sudden violent effort with the hand in which she holds the snuff, at the same time moving her head towards it; by the sudden combined movement of the head and hand the snuff reaches the nostrils." He described the toes as "being strongly flexed." Compston believes that some of the other cases are not convincing for multiple sclerosis (22).

Because Carswell and Cruveilhier were working in Paris in the years 1826–1831, carrying out the same kind of project in the same city, it is highly likely that they met and knew of each other's work. Compston notes that there is a striking similarity in the lesions in the pons illustrated by Carswell and Cruveilhier, but Josephine Paget was still alive when Carswell's atlas was published, so it could not have been the same case.

Marx

Keppel Hesselink (23,27) put forward the suggestion that the first clinical pathologic description of MS was in a Latin monograph presented by Marx to the Royal Scientific Society in Göttingen in December 1833 and subsequently published in German in 1838 by Richardson. The patient had a progressive paralysis and, although she stayed mentally clear and cheerful until her death, Marx noted at autopsy that the spinal pathology could be consistent with other diagnoses such as arteriovenous malformation or multilocular tumors.

Marshall Hall

Charcot and Vulpian were interested in the differentiation of paralysis agitans and multiple sclerosis. The confusion in their era can be shown by the case in Marshall Hall's text, *Lectures on the Nervous System and its Diseases* (1836) (26), which has a case referred to as paralysis agitans (Parkinson's disease) but who probably had MS and manifested what would later be known as Charcot's triad of nystagmus, intention tremor, and scanning speech. This 28-year-old man had weakness of his right arm and leg, and a tremor of his arm that was worse with movement. He had a "peculiar rocking motion of the eyes" and speech difficulty described as stammering and defective articulation.

Friedrich Theodore von Frerichs

In the early nineteenth century the clinicians in Germany and France often followed their cases to the autopsy room and examined the brains and spinal cords to try to understand the nature of the neurologic affliction. As the approach of medicine was moving from a general concept of illness to an understanding of specific diseases, these observations were revealing the nature of many different ways the nervous system could be affected. It is not surprising that it can be difficult to see if MS is being reported by these early writers, who were just beginning to define different illnesses.

Putnam examined many of the volumes that described neurologic disease in that era (1). Romberg's outstanding *Textbook on Nervous Disease* (1846) contains a case of a young woman with hemiplegia, first on one side and then the other, who was noted on autopsy to have "yellow softenings" about the lateral ventricles (1,28). No cases were found by Putnam in the great pathologic collections of Bonet or Morgagni nor in the Treatises of Haslem, Pinel, and Calmeil (1).

In 1849 Friedrich Theodore von Frerichs (1819–1895), a German clinician-pathologist, made the first clinical diagnosis in a living patient of the myelitis that would become known as multiple sclerosis (29). His clinical skills allowed him not only to diagnose the patient in life but also to recognize certain features of the disease such as spontaneous remissions and the usual presence of nystagmus, which was later incorporated into Charcot's triad. Although there was great interest in differentiating this sclerosis from cases of tabes and syringomyelia in the years that followed, there was "much adverse comment" on these diagnoses by Frerichs. In 1856, however, his pupil Valentiner was able to publish the subsequent history and autopsy reports on these cases with pathologic findings, demonstrating "the brilliant correctness of the diagnosis" (30).

Frerichs carefully examined the spinal cords of the patients with this disease and noted "an abnormal firmness of leathery consistency in irregularly circumscribed parts of the white, rarely involving the gray matter of the cord, with a poverty of blood-vessels. The patches are almost normal in color or milky white, dull and occasionally grayish red. There is a loss of nerve elements" (29). He said that clinically the disease had the following characteristics: (1) The condition is gradual with exacerbations and remissions; (2) One side of the body is involved, then the other; (3) Paralysis of the legs occurs early and gets much worse; (4) Motor changes are greater than sensory changes; (5) The seat of the disease is in the medulla with disturbances of the ninth, tenth, and eleventh cranial nerves; (6) There are frequent psychic episodes and mental changes; (7) Sclerosis of the nervous system is more frequent in the young; and (8) General health remains normal for a long time.

Ludwig Turck

When he referred to previous cases of MS in his lesson, Charcot mentioned Ludwig Turck (1810–1868), a quiet and modest physician who made a number of contributions to neurology and neuroanatomy and had a particular interest in the spinal cord. He noted that the direction of tract degeneration corresponded to the direction of conduction, which led to a number of clinical observations based on this principle. He outlined six tracts in the spinal cord, and the anterior corticospinal tract bears his name. He described the syndrome of hemisection of the cord, now attributed to Brown-Sequard, and Charcot referred to his description of a case of MS (31). His observations on the spinal cord were one of the major medical contributions of the nineteenth century, but they were essentially ignored while others were applauded when they later made the same observations. His last years of life were devoted to studies of laryngology, and there is some indication that he may have been the inventor of the laryngoscope (32).

Carl Rokitansky

Carl Rokitansky (1804–1878) carried out careful investigations of neurologic diseases by microscopic examination while working at the Institute of Pathology in Vienna. He was one of the first to carefully examine MS lesions microscopically. In 1856 Rokitansky published his *Pathological Anatomy* with a description of the connective tissue proliferations within the spinal cord that cause paraplegias in normal gray matter. He confused some aspects with tabes dorsalis. He observed in 1857 that there were "fatty corpuscles" in the MS lesions, which Charcot later described as "the wreck and detritus resulting from the disintegration of the nerve-tubes" (33).

Eduard Rindfleisch

In 1863 Eduard Rindfleisch (1836–1908) noted the consistent location of a blood vessel in the center of MS plaques (34). He showed changes in the blood vessels and nerve elements secondary to inflammation combined with hyperemia. He recognized perivascular cell infiltrations and fatty changes in the neuroglia He then postulated that we should search for a primary cause of the disease in an alteration of individual blood vessels and their ramifications, a suggestion that would be taken up in 1940 when anticoagulants became widely available and were used to treat the apparent vascular lesion in the center of MS plaques, which some felt was a thrombosis or vasospasm.

E. Leyden

E. Leyden in the same year summarized the then-current understanding of the disease and showed that multiple sclerosis and the so-called chronic myelitis were the same condition (35). He indicated that women were attacked more often than men, and gave the proportion as 25:9. The onset was noted to be between ages 20 and 25 years. He noted that only one of his cases was hereditary. He believed that the cause was related to exposure to dampness and cold and to concussions of the body, but that psychic effects were important in producing the disease, as any sudden fright or prolonged worry might cause it. In fact, he believed that many associated acute diseases could bring on the disorder. The prognosis was unfavorable although in some acute cases moderate or complete restoration could occur.

Edme Felix Alfred Vulpian

Although the long shadow of Charcot was prominent in French neurology of the day and he is accorded appropriate credit in elucidating the nature of MS, an important figure in this story—and one important to Charcot—was Edme Felix Alfred Vulpian (1826–1887).

Vulpian was a friend and contemporary of Charcot; they were both appointed the same year to the Salpêtrière. Vulpian worked more in the area of neuropathology, particularly in relation to the physiology and pharmacology of his patients' problems. He replaced Cruveilhier in the Chair of Pathological Anatomy, an appointment that was made over violent opposition because of a tract he wrote on the higher functions of the brain that was criticized by clerics and conservatives. He was a careful experimenter and recognized that microscopy was not given as much attention in France as it was in Germany. He was a very influential clinician-scientist and published 225 papers. His stone statue in the rue Antoine Dubois, next to the École de Medecine in Paris notes his contributions, including his contribution to the description of multiple sclerosis (32).

Vulpian first used the term *sclérose en plaque disseminé* for the disorder in 1866 (36). He had presented three cases before the Societé Medical of the Paris hospitals. One of the patients, Mme. V., was later presented by Charcot in his 1868 clinical lessons. Vulpian had "bequeathed" the patient along with the detailed notes to Charcot when Vulpian left the Salpêtrière.

THE FRAMING OF THE DISEASE: THE DESCRIPTION BY CHARCOT

Jean-Martin Charcot was born in Paris in November 1825, the son of a coach builder. We know little of his childhood except that he preferred to be alone to read and draw pictures (48,49). Many of these early caricatures were donated to the Salpêtrière by Jean Charcot, his son (1867–1936), who later was an intern at the Salpêtrière. Charcot was educated at the Lycée Bonaparte and the University of Paris. He was influenced by Professor Rayer, the Dean of Medical Studies and Instructor in Pathology, who taught him the admonition that a clinician's skill is only as good as his skill as a pathologist (48,49). While an intern at the Salpêtrière in 1853, he wrote his doctoral thesis on the differentiation between rheumatoid arthritis and gouty arthritis (50). Charcot married Augustine-Victoire Durvis, a young and wealthy widow who continually supported Charcot and often fended off the many students and visitors who continually sought him out. Charcot's character has been seen differently by different individuals. Leon Daudet considered him timid and emotional (51), but others saw him as solemn and withdrawn. Charcot died at age 68 in 1893 of pulmonary edema.

Charcot brought to the forefront the elegant combination of clinical science and pathologic correlation. He added to the understanding of hyperthyroidism, heredity amyloidosis, multiple sclerosis, amyotrophic lateral sclerosis, intermittent claudication, diabetic gangrene, and diseases characteristic in the elderly. He contributed to the localization of cortical functions. Along with Bouchard, he published early papers on aphasia and important contributions to the understanding of hysteria. This collaboration is remembered today by the interest in Charcot-Bouchard aneurysms.

It remained for Charcot in 1868 to pull together all the clinical and pathologic information that had been accumulated by Vulpian and his predecessor. He would turn on the clinical light that would allow all clinicians to see the pattern presented by their patients. That was his great contribution, to take the experiences of the patients and the patterns described by the clinicians, to recognize that they represented a unified clinical concept, and to put a name to the result. The picture was that of *sclérose en plaque*—disseminated sclerosis—later to be called *multiple sclerosis*. Although many others described and knew well the features of the disease and its pathology, it was Charcot who defined it more clearly and made it known so that other clinicians from then onward recognized what they were seeing in their offices, wards, and clinics.

In May 1866 Vulpian and Charcot reported the clinical features and autopsy findings in multiple sclerosis to the *Societé Medicale des Hopitaux*. Vulpian described one case and Charcot presented two. Vulpian managed most of the discussion. When the presentation was published, only Vulpian was listed as an author (36). In 1868 Charcot gave a lecture before the *Societé des Biologie* on the characteristics of disseminated sclerosis and indicated that, although it was not usually recognized clinically, the disease had distinct neurologic and pathologic features that could be clearly differentiated from Parkinson's disease. He published this lecture and another report on the histology of MS the same year (37,38). In these important presentations, Charcot clearly defined the clinical features of this disorder. Naturally, these patients all had advanced signs of the disease, but over the next few years Charcot would also begin to study less severe cases and their symptoms (39). In his lectures and later in his publications he gave credit to the many earlier observations by others, making it clear that he was clarifying further what others had observed before him (25,40).

Initially Charcot was attempting to differentiate Parkinson's tremor from the tremor seen in other neurologic diseases, but he soon pursued additional studies of the disease, recognizing the clinical features, variations of the disorder, and pathologic changes, which he drew by his own hand. He recognized the nature of transient symptoms in the disease and the possibility of remissions. He commented on variations in the disease, including spinal forms and the late appearance of amyotrophy.

Perhaps the most important step in addressing any disease is its clear delineation, separating it from other similar sounding conditions, so that it can be more clearly recognized, understood, and researched, and hopefully managed, cured, or prevented.

In the first lesson Charcot described lesions in three categories: spinal, cephalic or bulbar, and combined cerebrospinal. He thought that lesions in different areas of the nervous system would produce different symptoms. In his second lecture he discussed the tremor of MS, cephalic symptoms, and the state of the legs in the disease. He described the visual findings of nystagmus, diplopia, and amblyopia; difficulty with speech; and intellectual changes, which constituted cephalic symptoms. He noted memory change, including slowness in forming concepts and the blunting of intellectual and emotional faculties. Patients might be indifferent, but they also might demonstrate unexpected laughter or crying for no reason. He outlined the clinical appearance of intention tremor, nystagmus, and scanning speech as three realizable indicators of multiple sclerosis (Charcot's triad).

Charcot commented that he and Vulpian had studied the pathology of MS in the 1860s, using a carmine stain that showed that myelin was specifically destroyed, whereas axons were preserved. He noted that the plaques, which could be seen by the naked eye, looked gray initially but took on a rosy hue when left open to the air. Charcot did his own drawings of the microscopic anatomy of the plaques and the disruption of myelin. Despite his major contribution to MS, he thought the disease was a rare curiosity.

In his Tuesday clinics and Friday lectures Charcot made many contributions to clinical neurology and medicine and attracted admirers and students from abroad, enhancing the reputation of the Salpêtrière and French neurology (41–43). Charcot displayed marvelous clinical skill and knowledge and used numerous audiovisual methods, including drawing, photographs, slide projections, and plaster casts. Along with Albert Londe, he created a photographic studio, which was annexed to the Anatomy and Pathology Museum (44,45). Charcot's observations became even more widely known when his *Leçons* were published in 1872–1873 and in translation in London and Philadelphia in 1877 (under the title *Lectures on the Diseases of the Nervous System*) (25).

Charcot wrote little else on MS, but his thinking and teaching were purveyed through the writings of his pupils Bourneville and Guerard (46) and by Ordenstein (47). Charcot's original interest in the disorder was in differentiating the tremor of MS from that of Parkinson's disease, but in defining the nature of MS he was able to note that it occurred in younger people, often with fleeting symptoms and sometimes complete remission. The woodcuts from his classic 1868 paper were published up into this century and, as stated by Putnam (1), the pathologic observations of Charcot served as "the textbooks of a generation" and little was added to his pathologic observations for 50 years.

Jean-Martin Charcot was said to resemble an English gentlemen. He spoke slowly and carefully and, although his Tuesday clinics and Friday lectures were very popular, he was not a great orator. His seemingly effortless teaching manner was the result of hard work and study. He prepared for his sessions all week and memorized his carefully made notes.

According to D. M. Bourneville and I. Guerard, students of Charcot and the authors of the first book on MS, Charcot first became aware of the disease by asking a woman who had some motor problems to serve as his housemaid (46). He was able to follow the course of disseminated sclerosis by watching her symptoms over the years. When she became too ill to function on her own, he arranged for her to be admitted to the Salpêtrière and later examined her brain and spinal cord. Although he had originally suspected her of having syphilis, the postmortem changes showed the plaques of MS and not tabes dorsalis (46).

The Early Monographs

Although Charcot did not publish a great deal on MS—perhaps only 34 cases (52)—his great contribution was to clarify the clinical and pathologic picture so that others could recognize the disease and build on his description and understanding. Ebers has pointed out that he probably had additional thoughts and views on the disease that were expressed through the writings of his pupils Bourneville and Guerard (46) in the first monograph on the disease and by Ordenstein (47) in his monograph. Both monographs contain Charcot's beautiful woodcuts showing the pathologic changes and his descriptions of the pathology in MS, which were described by Putnam as "the textbooks of a generation to which the next 70 years added little" (1).

Ordenstein published the first monograph on MS as an aggregation thesis in 1867 (47). Following the interest of his teacher, Charcot, the thesis was half devoted to MS and half to Parkinson's disease and contained the first publication of Charcot's chromolithography of gross MS plaques. As noted by Ebers, the text is repetitious, limited in its critical analysis, erroneous on some facts, and neglectful of previous contributors (18). Bourneville and Guerard's monograph described more cases and reviewed previous contributions more fully (46). This monograph contains the woodcuts from the 1868 Gazette Hopitaux article and clinical descriptions of two of the cases in Cruveilhier's atlas.

Pierre Marie

Pierre Marie presented 25 cases of MS in his monograph "Insular Sclerosis and the Infectious Diseases" (53). Some of the cases were from a monograph by Kahler and Pick (1879), who noted that the onset often followed acute illness. Carrying this even further, Marie said the causes are well known—overwork, exposure to cold, injury, and excess of every kind. But although these are common precipitants, he said he knew of another cause that is even more common—infection, "or rather *infections.*" He then listed the most common infections he had seen precipitate the disease—typhoid, malaria, smallpox, diphtheria, erysipelas, pneumonia, measles, scarlatina, whooping cough, dysentery, cholera, and other fevers.

Marie confessed that the evidence was not yet conclusive and prudent reserve was reasonable from a purely scientific approach. Although this seems open-minded, in a footnote he indicates that his infectious theory is acknowledged by most, and it would be ungracious of him to find fault with those who disagreed, even though some had been very hostile. He went on to say that some even disagreed with his theory that most epilepsy had an infectious origin, but until that was proven he would just repeat that his opinion on this remained unchanged. Since his first publication of the infectious origin of MS, Marie believed he had accumulated more facts that made the case more convincing. He outlined the usual scenario—a person aged 20 to 30 years old contracts an infectious disease, and during the disease, or in the months that follow, symptoms of a neurologic disease begin.

He mentioned that the question of the microorganism that might be involved was embarrassing because so little is known. He added that some colleagues, who had obviously not read his papers, concluded that he had found the organism of MS, and he assured them that he never said so and believed that many organisms may initiate the disease, or more likely combined infections. He concludes, "These, gentlemen, are suppositions, and I put them before you without unreasonably insisting upon them. The one point in this discussion which I would fix in your minds is the following fact, a fact which, thank God, has been well established, viz., that the cause of insular sclerosis is intimately connected with infectious diseases."

In his later writings Marie mused that he was uncertain about how common the disease was but noted that Uhthoff had seen 100 cases of ocular disorder due to MS over six to seven years in the hospitals and polyclinics of Berlin, so it was not rare (54). He thought the sexes were equally affected, the onset was usually between 20 and 30, and if a patient presents with a neurologic disease after age 40, MS has scarcely to be considered. Although rare in children, he had collected 13 cases from others, although he questioned some of these diagnoses.

EARLY REPORTS OF MULTIPLE SCLEROSIS IN THE MEDICAL LITERATURE

J. C. Morris

The first American report of what would now be recognized as MS was presented by Dr. J. C. Morris in 1867 and published the next year, with the pathology by S. Weir Mitchell (55). The patient was a young physician, Dr. Pennock, a graduate of the University of Philadelphia who later studied in Paris. He noted symptoms of heaviness and numbness of his left and later his right leg in 1843, and his weakness became so progressive that he had to cease the practice of medicine six years later. During the course of his disease he noted that his symptoms would always worsen when the weather was warm. By 1853 he was unable to walk and then developed progressive weakness of his left and then right arms and hands to the point that he was unable to feed himself. He was noted to be alert and positive throughout the course of his disease, and this happy state of mind continued to the end. He developed urinary retention and died in 1867.

S. Weir Mitchell, often referred to as the father of American neurology, commented on the irregular gray translucent spots in the cervical and dorsal spinal cord, mainly in the white matter, and mainly in the lateral columns. Under the microscope he saw a total absence of the nerve tubes and nerve cells in these lesions, and small globules of fat and numerous degenerated fibers.

Morris and Mitchell were not aware that they were describing the same disease reported by the French clinicians and classified by Charcot that same year, and they suggested no cause for the disease and had no references to other literature on similar conditions. They were merely reporting a puzzling case, well-described.

William Moxon

The first English description of MS appeared in four brief reports in *Lancet* between 1873 and 1875 (3). These were case reports from Guy's Hospital, and, although they were anonymous, three of the four were said to be under the care of Dr. William Moxon. These same patients appeared in a later report by Moxon when he reported eight cases (56). This report was the first major description of MS, which he called *insular sclerosis,* in the English language. He described eight features of MS, including paralytic weakness, nystagmus, speech abnormalities, and changes in mental status. He also clearly described cases of involuntary laughter.

He noted the placebo response of MS patients, particularly to their physician. He stated:

"The patients, who, as a rule, are cheerful and thankful for what is done on their behalf, are apt to declare themselves generally rather better, so that the report of the clinical clerk putting down their answers may read like a statement of continual good progress toward recovery. But the general result has been that, after many months stay in hospital, the poor people are found to have grown steadily though slowly worse" (56).

William A. Hammond

Mitchell's colleague from the Civil War, William A. Hammond, published a textbook in 1871 that contained chapters on "Multiple Cerebral Sclerosis" and "Multiple Cerebro-spinal Sclerosis" with descriptions of the pathology and referred to the many French authors on the subject. In his discussion he mentioned that he had cared for 11 cases (57).

Allan McLane Hamilton

In 1878 Allan McLane Hamilton of New York City published a textbook on neurologic conditions describing the picture of cerebrospinal sclerosis, referring to both the title, *Sclérose en Plaques Disséminées* and the insular sclerosis of Moxon (58). He described three states, the first with episodic symptoms of weakness, poor balance, tremor, and speech disorder. In the second stage rigidity of the limbs, contractures, and tremor were characteristic. In the third stage the patient had a rapid decline, bladder and bowel incontinence, bed sores, and dementia.

With the clear reports of Morris, Hammond, and Hamilton, it is surprising that the credit for the first report of MS in the United States was for many years given to Sequin (59).

Samuel Wilks

Dr. Samuel Wilks (1824–1911), publishing his lectures on the nervous system delivered at Guy's Hospital, noted that he had seen the disorder of patches throughout the nervous system but did not know what he was seeing until Charcot clarified the disorder (60). Wilks went on to illustrate the disease process with two cases, one of whom had the brain and spinal cord examined by Dr. Moxon. The first was a veterinary surgeon aged 33 who had a recurrent neurologic disease over the last two years. The second was a woman of 25 who had the onset of neurologic symptoms after some febrile illnesses and eventually died, and the examination by Moxon revealed scattered gray insular patches throughout the cord and brain. Wilks noted that the patients had intellectual impairment but were not depressed, and indeed they often had a happy emotional outlook and were ready to laugh or cry when spoken to, more often to laugh. He had no comment on cause or treatment.

Samuel Wilks was said by the *Times* of London to be "the most philosophical of English physicians," and in the notes accompanying his caricature in *Vanity Fair* it was said that he "has done much to rid ladies of sickheadache" and that "he thinks the most wonderful thing in the world is a woman's nervous system."

Australian Reports

The first description in Australia was by MacLauren (61), who published an elegant clinical description of retrobulbar neuritis. This was followed in 1875 by a dissertation on MS by Alfred K. Newman (62) in the *Australasian Medical Journal* and in 1886 a report by Dr. James Jamieson (63).

Canadian Report

The earliest Canadian reports were by William Osler, presented to the Medical and Chirgical Society of Montreal in 1879 and published 1880 (4). Osler presented careful clinical and pathologic observations but speculated little on the etiology or the treatment of such cases. Osler was busy doing pathologic correlations during his Montreal years, and, in a clever approach to epidemiology, Ebers looked at over 800 autopsies by Osler during those years and found one definite case and two possible cases of MS and concluded that the prevalence of MS may not be much different than today (64).

Sir William Gowers

In his small 1884 monograph on *Symptoms and Diagnosis of Diseases of the Spinal Cord*, William Gowers does not discuss MS specifically, but case 3 (pages 84–85), a man aged 28 with a progressive cord lesion was thought to have slow progression due to a local sclerosis (65). He indicated that he did not like the term *sclerosis* because the term implies connective tissue overgrowth and hardening, whereas the lesions might be softer than normal. He was equally unhappy about nonspecific terms such as *chronic myelitis, degeneration,* and *sclerosis,* as they did not differentiate between a pathologic process and a disease. When he used the terms, he would mean a process, and he was resistant to prematurely classifying diseases when only the process is apparent, although he recognized that the clinical history was helpful in formulating the processes into categories. (66)

THREE LANDMARK OVERVIEWS OF MULTIPLE SCLEROSIS

Most advances in medicine are recorded by the date of publication of the discovery and remembered in association with the discoverer, but we normally do not recognize that the field can advance by an intelligent review of the state of the art by an expert or by a pivotal meeting. The understanding of MS was advanced significantly by the 1921 meeting of the Association for Research in Nervous and Mental Disease (ARNMD) (67) and by the reviews by Russell Brain in 1930 (68) and the monograph by McAlpine, Compston, and Lumsden in 1955 (69). These clinicians had tremendous impact, and each clarified what was becoming a confusing state of affairs. Each stood back and looked at the array of ideas and observations and intelligently tried to put them in a reasonable context, emphasizing some views, questioning or discarding others.

The ARNMD Report of 1922 was a landmark in the understanding of MS (67). It brought together individuals who summarized the state of knowledge at the time and consolidated views. The published report came from a meeting held in New York City, December 27–28, 1921. The many papers, some now classics, would review the pathology, epidemiology, etiology, and clinical features of the disease. In writing the conclusions to the meeting, the commissioners emphasized that MS was among the most common organic disease affecting the nervous system. They deemphasized the importance of the Charcot triad but agreed on the importance of the abdominal reflexes, which was lost in 83.7 percent of patients, and on the value of temporal pallor of the optic disc as a sign. They concluded that there was no particular psychic disorder characteristic of the disease. They did not think that euphoria was very characteristic and found mental deterioration often to be absent. They could not confirm Dr. Jelliffe's belief that MS was "schizophrenia of the spinal axis" with repressed tensions causing plaques (70). Impressed by the negative transmission studies, they concluded that there was no solid evidence for a bacteriologic cause but expected further experiments on this. In answer to the question posed throughout the meeting, whether MS was an inflammatory disease or a degenerative disease, the commission took the middle road and thought that it might be initially inflammatory and later degenerative.

Russell Brain's remarkable review of the state of understanding of the disease in 1930 brought clarity to an increasingly confused field (68). This was not a consensus; this was the personal conclusion and perception of an outstanding physician about an increasingly confusing field. Compston (71) assessed the impact of the 1930 review and the changing information and views in the many editions of Brain's textbook *Diseases of the Nervous System* from 1933 to the present, with editions since 1969 under the editorship of Lord Walton.

Equally influential in summarizing the state of understanding of MS was the review textbook of the disease, *Multiple Sclerosis* by McAlpine, Compston, and Lumsden in 1955 (69). Alastair Compston, the son of Nigel Compston, recently wrote that the review was based on 1,072 cases accumulated by McAlpine, collated painstakingly by Compston, who wrote the first draft. Lumsden wrote the pathology section. Up to the present, with its 1998 third edition (72), this has been the major single reference about the disease. Although terms such as *disseminated sclerosis* were still in vogue in England up to the 1950s, when this classic work appeared with *multiple sclerosis* as the title of their book, this became the accepted term in the English-speaking world.

THEORIES OF CAUSATION

"The most difficult things to explain are those which are not true."

A. S. Wiener, 1956

In the initial descriptions of this disease by Ollivier, Frerichs, Turck, and others, there was limited speculation as to cause, other than that it was sometimes associated with acute fevers or exposure to dampness and cold. Pierre Marie, as we have noted, was adamant that this was due to infections or more likely many infections, and he listed many that he had seen associated with the onset or worsening of the disorder. Lewellys F. Barker (73) discussed the exogenous causes of multiple sclerosis at the 1921 ARNMD meeting and indicated it was accepted clinically that infections could produce an exacerbation of MS, but a specific infection was unlikely, and there was not much support for Oppenheim's belief in an environmental toxin (74). Again separating a causative agent from an aggravating one, he noted that thermic injury occurred in 40 percent of cases but was likely an aggravating factor, not a cause. A relationship to trauma was suggested by some investigators, but Barker was skeptical and noted that patients easily incriminate trauma, and "neurologists, who see many patients suffering from epilepsy, brain tumor, mental deterioration, and other organic processes, are very familiar with the prevalence of this conception." He pointed out that no one had been able to reproduce multiple sclerosis in animals by trauma. Barker concluded that "if multiple sclerosis is a disease entity due to a single cause that acts in early life, it may be due to some specific infection, but the evidence available is strongly against its being caused by any of our well-known infections, by any ordinary intoxication (organic or inorganic), or by electrical, thermal or traumatic influences" (73). Oppenheim believed that all MS begins in infancy and only manifests later in life. He reviews many reports and adds some of his own cases (74).

Charles Dana believed that MS patients are more of the linear dolichocephalic type (75). He indicated that people were beginning to agree that there were two types of morphology, with humans either thin with high basal metabolism, mentally nervous but self-controlled, and the more broadly built, brachycephalic, who tend to be stout, variable in weight, and emotional. He added the odd comment that, "I have never seen multiple sclerosis in a fat man or a woman even when long bedridden." He had some other unusual ideas, including the fact that it was more common in males than females (3:2) and that the duration of the disease was eight years but could be as short as a year or more than 30 years. He thought it occurred in persons who did skilled manual work more often than in ordinary laborers or in "brain workers." He believed it was not a familial disease and not inherited even though there might be rare and doubtful exceptions. He thought that in the ancestry of MS patients there was often evidence of a "neuropathic stock."

By 1950 the list of possible etiologic factors was narrowing. There was no longer a strong belief in factors such as stress, cold and dampness, trauma, heavy metal poisoning, or other external toxins. Reese summarized the thought in the mid century by stating that there were two possibilities: a transmissible agent, either a virus or a chemical agent; or a particular reaction of the nervous system to many causes (76).

THE SEARCH FOR AN INFECTION

"It is a tragedy that some problems of multiple sclerosis, not only pathologicaoanatomical, but clinical, give rise to so many controversies."

Dr. George B. Hassin, 1952

At the end of the nineteenth century a belief in an infectious etiology of MS was widely held, with strong proponents such as Pierre Marie. Marie believed that the advances of Pasteur and Koch would eventually lead to a vaccine for the disease, and it would be a logical step to use their techniques to try to transmit the disease. Because there were limited specific medicines or therapies for infection at that time, general approaches to treatment were used. When the advances in therapy of syphilis were announced by Erlich, these approaches were applied to MS, not because physicians thought MS was syphilis (they would repeatedly point out that it was not) but both diseases affected wide areas of the central nervous system (CNS) with devastating and progressive disability, so it seemed logical to apply therapy for one to the other. Antisyphilitic therapies would be used until World War II (77).

Great discoveries were being made in the area of infectious disease around the turn of the century and many of the approaches were applied to MS. The first apparent discovery was by Bullock, who announced that he had transmitted MS from man to rabbits (78). The importance of this observation was supported by Kuhn and Steiner (79), who took cerebrospinal fluid (CSF) from MS patients and claimed that they had produced typical MS in guinea pigs and rabbits; this was confirmed by others, and spirochetes were reported in autopsy material. Others could not confirm the transmission experiments and the neurologic community was uncertain about the importance of the claims. In 1921 Bullock, now publishing under his new name of Gye taken from his wife, again published experiments showing that the disease could be transmitted to two out of ten rabbits (80). Gye would later claim transmission to rabbits from blood and CSF but not if the CSF was filtered through a Berkefeld filter; this suggested that it was a filterable agent, probably a virus.

Between 1913 and 1923 many still argued the spirochete theory, notably Kuhn and Steiner, Siemerling, Marinesco, and Petit, but others continued to fail in their attempts to do the same transmission experiments. Dr. Oscar Teague of the New York Neurological Institute summarized this work at the 1921 ARNMD meeting on MS (81). At this point five investigators concluded that it was an infectious transmissible disease, and four opposed this view on the basis of their negative findings. Teague obtained a grant from the Commonwealth Foundation to study this question and presented his results at this meeting. He had used spinal fluid from acute chronic progressive and stable cases of MS. He used a variety of routes but injected 220 animals. No fluids showed spirochetes. No animals developed a paralytic disease. In the discussion Dr. Tilney indicated that rabbits often developed a paralytic disease, so its presence was not good evidence for the transmission of MS. The controversy did not end, however, and at the same meeting Charles L. Dana stated, "I am assuming that there is an infecting organism at the bottom of the multiple sclerosis lesions. I even assume it is an animal type, i.e. some variant of spirochaetae, hence I place the problem of multiple sclerosis in the domain of animal ecology" (75).

Interest grew in a viral cause when two articles appeared in *Lancet*. Kathleen Chevassut, working under the supervision of Sir James Purves-Stewart, claimed that she could recover a virus from 90 percent of MS patients (82). A companion paper by her mentor, Purves-Stewart, named the virus *Spherula insularis* and he announced the production of an autogenous vaccine that he had already given to 128 people with MS, 70 of whom were followed up long enough to yield results. Of the 70 cases, 40 had demonstrated improvement (83). It would seem that they had not only discovered the cause of MS but also had developed a vaccine that produced clinical improvement. There was widespread quiet skepticism by the neurologic community, and it became more vocal as they presented their work at medical meetings. Carmichael (84) was asked to investigate the research methods and results in their laboratory. When he presented his conclusions that there was nothing of merit in this, Miss Chevassut left the room in tears and Purves-Stewart later retired to a lighthouse at Beachy Head, where he wrote a long autobiography. Purves Stewart's biography was titled *Sands of Time* and discussed his early life and his enjoyable period in training at Queen Square (85). He dwelled on current world events and was very concerned about the impending shadows of war and the dangers of dictators. Nowhere did he mention the *Spherula insularis* research, nor did he refer to multiple sclerosis or to Miss Chevassut.

The story did not end there. Steiner and Kuhn (86) again reported finding spirochetes in the brains and spinal cords of people who had died of MS. Adams (87) found spirochetes when looking at the CSF from monkeys injected with MS tissue, and the spirochete looked similar to that of Steiner and Kuhn. No one could culture the spirochete, however, and there was general skepticism in neurologic circles despite the enthusiasm of the proponents of this theory and observations. Attempts to culture the spirochete from patients' CSF failed, but reports of a spirochete would continue to appear. Rose Ichelson of Philadelphia reported in 1957 that six years previously she had devised a culture medium that grew a few spirochetes from MS CSF, but modification of the culture resulted in a heavy growth of spirochetes in a few days (88). She reported that 59 of her 76 cases (78 percent) had positive cultures, whereas 100 percent of the normal controls were negative. The organism was a spiral organism with a loop at one end, or sometimes resembled a tennis racquet. She said it was similar in appearance to that of the *Spirocheta myelophthora* of Steiner. It was the careful work of Kurtzke that showed these results to be invalid (89). Even in the last decade the "discovery" of a spirochete in MS would make the pages of the popular press.

When Gajdusek (91) and others formulated the concept of a slow virus in neurologic disease, one that could infect cells and after a very long incubation period of years cause disease, MS was considered a prime suspect. Transmission experiments all failed, however. Currently many believe, as did Gowers a century earlier, that the virus, if present, is probably a triggering agent rather than the cause.

The neurologic community was disturbed to read in 1994 that a prominent German neurologist had carried out unethical experiments involving the transmission of MS materials to humans during World War II (the Schaltenbrand experiments) (90).

EPIDEMIOLOGY

There were many reports in the late nineteenth century looking at the characteristics of groups of MS patients. It was becoming apparent that the disease was not as rare as Charcot and others thought, as larger and larger numbers of patients were being accumulated in hospitals and clinics in Germany, France, Austria, and the United States. There was confusing information about gender distribution, as some investigators were reporting many more men, others equal numbers, and some more women. It is puzzling that a 1922 review of 26 studies of MS showed a consistent male predominance of 58 percent to 42 percent female (92). Six of the studies did show a slight female predominance but most showed a male predominance. Although there had been suggestions of MS occurring more in some occupations, Morawitz disagreed, indicating that every occupation and social class was involved. By mid century Kurland would conclude after reviewing the studies that the numbers of men and women with MS were equal (93–95). Currently we understand that the female to male ratio is 2.5:1.

The frequency of the disease was also debated. Although Charcot and others believed it to be a rare neurologic curiosity, others found many cases in their clinics and wards. There were reports of a low rate in Boston of one case per thousand "nervous cases," a slightly higher rate in New York City among "nervous cases," a rate of 2 to 7 per thousand (97), but higher rates of 18 per thousand among the Jewish patients at Montefiore Home. Van Wart in 1905 found a rate of 44 per thousand among 500 cases of neurologic disease and concluded that in Louisiana and surrounding states the disease was frequent (97).

The Bramwells (98,99) found a rate of 20 and later 32 in neurologic cases in Scotland. Rates varied from 27 per thousand patients in Manchester to 60 per thousand in a more rigidly selected group of neurologic patients at the National Hospital for Paralyzed and Epileptics in London. Repeatedly it was commented that MS was much less frequent in the United States than in Europe. It was clear that Scandinavians had a higher incidence in many of the studies and that blacks had a low rate, although they were not immune, and the disease was less common in Japan.

Charles B. Davenport gave an important review of geographic distribution in 1921 (97). He noted high rates in adjacent northern U.S. states, particularly around the Great Lakes, and wondered if that could be related to other diseases that had a similar distribution such as goiter or to a particular group of people, such as Swedes and Finns who live in that part of the country. He found higher rates in urban communities and in those with higher white to black populations, and in those who lived near the sea rather than the mountains.

Poser indicated that the earliest reports of epidemiology of MS commented on the increased prevalence in persons of Scandinavian decent (100). Percival Bailey (101) noted this in his survey of U.S. troops after World War I. Davenport (97), Brain (68), and McAlpine (102) also commented on the higher incidence in northern European countries. This was also noted in northern U.S. studies by Steiner (103), Ulett (104), and Limburg (105). Bulman and Ebers (106) believed that the higher prevalence rate in northern United States and in Canada was related to individuals of Scandinavian decent, and that might also explain the high incidence in Olmsted County, Minnesota, where 25.7 percent of the population are of Scandinavian decent, in contrast to 4.7 percent for the United States in general (107). Poser speculated that this may relate to the Viking raids over 1,000 years ago (100). They raided most European countries, settled in Normandy and Sicily, and engaged in trade with widespread lands. They migrated to the east and established the Russian state, and under the name Varangians became part of the Byzantine Army that saw action across the Byzantine Empire. They participated in the Crusades. He mentions that the habit of capturing, keeping, or selling women and children was widespread in the Middle Ages and, along with the slave trade in men, could be important factors in genetic dissemination.

Since the 1950s it has been known that MS has an unusual geographic distribution (95,105,108). Multiple sclerosis increases in frequency with geographic latitude both in the Northern (109) and Southern Hemispheres (110). Alter (108) noted that the geographic distribution above and below the equator had a parabolic gradient that increased sharply with latitude, and that although the curve dramatically increased at increasing latitudes, it appeared to be lower or absent in very far north and south latitudes. In Europe the incidence of MS was highest in the central European areas and lower both north and south of that.

Limberg (105) in 1948 noted that death rates were higher in countries that are farther away from the equator, and that after corrections were made in some of the classifications of cases, the same observation was present. This observation has been confirmed in many studies over the next 50 years. Allison (111) and Steiner (103) noted that there were more cases in rural groups than in urban groups, but this would not stand the test of time and other studies.

In 1952 Kurland (93,94,95) reviewed the epidemiologic evidence and noted that most comments had been based on personal observations rather than convincing studies, until Limburg (105) noted an increase in the number of MS-related deaths farther away from the equator. In looking for an etiologic factor or factors, Kurland warned that diagnosis may be uncertain and that the disorder may be a syndrome rather than a disease. The difficulty was illustrated by the study in 15 New York and New Jersey hospitals in 1930–1939, which found 33 cases of MS in 25,000 deaths, but at autopsy one third were found to have other conditions. Also there were 11 other cases found at autopsy that were not diagnosed clinically as MS before death (112). Kurland thought the incidence was not increasing (95).

Sutherland (113) in Scotland confirmed Davenport's observation (97) that there was a higher risk in those of Nordic descendants than in Celts. The highest rates have been recorded in the Shetland and Orkney Islands off the coast of Scotland. Skegg in New Zealand (114) used the novel technique of assessing the number of Mc/Mac's in the telephone book to show that the incidence of MS was higher in communities that had a higher number with Scottish ancestry. Perhaps the geographic distribution of MS in the world and the increasing prevalence farther away from the equator is related to where those with Nordic ancestry migrated. Those migrating from Northern and Central Europe were more likely to go to more temperate climes than warm or equatorial areas.

Dean found 10 cases of MS in South Africa in 1958, but 42 cases over the period from 1959 to 1968 and believed that this suggested an increase in frequency (115). He thought that most factors had stayed the same, suggesting that an infective agent had been introduced from high-risk European countries by immigrants and by South Africans who used air travel to go abroad. By 1985 Rosman and colleagues were suggesting that there was an epidemic, as they had found five new cases in Pretoria and Wonderboom (population 319,868), an eightfold increase since Dean conducted his study, but these numbers were small and may simply have represented better case finding (116).

In all the studies there was surprising uniformity in the clinical features of MS, regardless of the geography or the incidence of the area. Some variations were noticed, with a higher incidence of Devic's disease in India and Japan and higher rates of transverse myelopathy and optic neuropathy in Orientals. Some factors that were proposed to explain the geographic difference were later excluded, including amounts of solar radiation, annual temperature, and the number of neurologists in these regions (108). That the geographic distribution was not an artifact, however, was convincingly demonstrated by the Israeli study by Alter and colleagues (117), which showed a difference in the prevalence in Jews in Israel depending on their region of origin. Alter reviewed the possibilities that might explain the geographic and migration study differences, looking at solar radiation, temperature, diet toxins and deficiencies, sanitation, and diet. He noted that many did not seem to apply, but that it was interesting that the distribution of animal fat in the diet followed the same parabolic curve north and south of the equator that MS followed (108).

Kuroiwa defined the study of MS in Japan in three periods: (1) the period of neglect (1910–1950), in which it was thought that MS was nonexistent, including the view of Professor Miura, who was a pupil of Charcot; (2) the period of recognition (1950–1970), in which cases of MS were increasingly recognized; and (3) the period of development (1972–1975 and beyond), when the incidence, epidemiology, and characteristics were better defined (118). The prevalence rate was initially calculated as 2–4 per 100,000 population, lower than in most western countries, but with no north/south gradient within Japan.

Whenever there are groups or clusters of MS cases, it is tempting to look for an association that might explain the occurrence. Four people doing work on sheep swayback developed an MS-like disease (119), which sparked great interest as swayback is an animal demyelinating disease related to copper deficiency. However, swayback did not occur in some of the high incidence areas for MS, and copper studies in MS patients were negative. Lead was suspected in the six cases living within 600 years of each other in Berkshire County, England, in 1950, but again there was no evidence of increased MS in lead workers or high lead areas (120). Many other heavy metals were suspected, such as lead, mercury, zinc, and magnesium, but these were all negative. Such ideas recur, however, and in recent years discussions about mercury from dental fillings being a factor in MS have led many patients to have costly and painful dental work based on no evidence of cause or benefit.

The Faroes are a small number of Danish islands between Iceland and Norway, settled by the Norse Vikings over a millennium ago. Intensive search for all cases on the Faroe Islands in the 1970s revealed 25 cases among native-born residents up to 1977 (121–125). All had the onset between 1943 and 1960 except for one case that had an onset in 1970. They excluded four cases in Faroese who had prolonged residence in foreign countries and five among Danish-born Faroese. The 24 cases met the criteria for a point-source epidemic. The median year of onset was 1949, and the cumulative risk of MS for Faroese in 1940 was 87 per 100,000. British troops had occupied the Faroe Islands in large numbers beginning in April 1940 and continuing throughout World War II. During the war all but three patients resided in locations where troops were stationed, and those three were also in direct contact with the British. Kurtzke in 1979 (122) suggested that this constituted an epidemic related to the introduction of British troops (or their baggage) and wondered if this were so, then MS was a transmissible disease and infection, with only 1 in 500 of the exposed individuals being affected (123).

Cluster studies are often reported to MS clinicians (three students in the same class who later develop MS; four people living on the same street, and so on), but the investigation of such events is challenging. Presumably, if there had been some external factor, it would have occurred many years before; a "fishing expedition" often led to some potential and intriguing observation, some common factor they shared, but often was not translatable to other situations or MS in general, and likely coincidental.

THE GENETICS OF MS

Virtually all the early authors on MS, including Leydon, Charcot Marie, Gowers, and Russell, noted familial cases but thought it was rare, and each downplayed the importance of these occasional cases. McKay surveyed all such reports from 1896 to 1948 and demonstrated that this was not an occasional or unimportant factor (126). He documented all familial cases reported from Eichdorst's report from 1896 to 1948. He later showed a concordance rate of 23 percent in monozygotic twins, clearly indicating a genetic factor, that was later confirmed by Canadian and British studies (127). Other cases were added by Pratt, Compston, and McAlpine (128), and a collection of 4,500 cases from the literature showed a familial rate of 1.8 percent.

Convincing evidence of a genetic factor had been noted by Curtius in Germany in 1933, showing that MS was 10 times more common in families with MS than in the general population (129). His studies were not given much attention, as they came at a time when information about genetic impurity was a very sensitive issue in Germany. Curtius believed that any nervous disease in the family indicated a constitutional predisposition, and he noted greater numbers of people with neurologic psychiatric disease and developmental defects than in a comparison group with fractures. Thus MS patients come from families that are predisposed to CNS disorders.

Davenport emphasized heredity and internal conditions and constitution as predisposing conditions but thought that most but not all patients have no family history of MS (97). The most famous family was described by Pelizaeus (1885) and reported 24 years later by Merzbacher (1909) with 12 cases, 10 of them males. After presenting some accounts of hereditary MS, Davenport concluded with the following insightful comment, "In conclusion, may I be permitted the suggestion that, whatever may be eventually proven to be the endogenous cause of multiple sclerosis, the factor of heredity cannot be left out of account? Just as tumors inoculated into a mouse will, or will not, grow, according to the racial constitution of the mouse, and just as the bacillius tuberculosis that inhabits the body of all of us does or does not flourish there depending upon the constitution and condition of the individual, so there are probably internal conditions that inhibit, and others that facilitate the development of this disease or the endogenous factors upon which it depends" (97).

VASCULAR THEORY

Very early in the descriptions of the pathology of MS there was comment on the vascular change in the area of the plaque and the presence of a vessel near the center of the plaque. Marie believed that the vascular change was secondary to an infection, but others speculated that a thrombotic or vasospastic change might be the primary cause of the plaque. Following the discovery of effective anticoagulants a few years earlier, anticoagulants were used in clinical trial in MS but interest in this approach rapidly declined. Speculation on a vascular basis for MS would again arise when Swank and others developed a theory and approach that stated that there was a dietary factor in MS related to high fat intake affecting vascular flow (130). The treatment would logically be a diet low in animal fat (Swank diet), and Swank continues to treat patients with this approach half a century after he originally proposed it. Putnam proposed anticoagulants for the treatment of MS based on the possibility that there was a thrombosis in the vessel found in the center of a plaque (131). This was soon abandoned.

THE IMMUNOLOGIC THEORY

The possibility that MS could be due to a hypersensitivity reaction dates back to the observation of Glanzmann (1932), who noted postinfectious CNS involvement in chickenpox, smallpox, and vaccinations (132). The creation of a model of experimental allergic encephalomyelitis (EAE) in 1933 by Rivers, Sprunt, and Berry seemed to strongly support the possibility that a similar process could be operating in MS. Variations on the EAE model are still used to assess possible changes and effects in MS and to assess the likelihood that drugs might be effective in the disease (133,134). For years there were arguments that this was not MS, but it has been an important and lasting model for study of processes that probably occur in the human disease as well. In 1946 McAlpine suggested that MS was an immune reaction following an infection, setting up a process that might be recurrent (102).

Research on the immunology of MS has been extensive over the years. Ebers, who recently reviewed the background and theory of immunology in MS (135), reported a comment of Helmut Bauer that more than 7,000 papers have been written on this topic. Much of the current therapy is based on modifying the immune system (136, 137).

THE NATURE OF THE MULTIPLE SCLEROSIS PLAQUE

Early writers speculated little on the nature of the gray softenings they saw and felt in the spinal cords of their patients and did not examine these areas with a microscope. Charcot (1877) believed that an overgrowth of glia was the specific abnormality and that the glia damaged the myelin sheaths and sometimes the axons. Local vascular changes were presumed to be secondary to the glial overgrowth and the breakdown of nerve tissue that was followed by macrophage removal of lipid products of myelin. His student Joseph Babinski (138,139) also thought it was a demyelinating process, even though Compston (140) pointed out that one of the illustrations to his thesis showed the appearance of remyelination, with thin layers of myelin surrounding the axon and fat granule cells removing the myelin debris. Marburg (141), Dawson (142), and Hassin (143) also believed that the process occurring in the shadow plaques was demyelination, but Dawson thought that the vascular change shown by Rindfleisch (34) was the primary change. Marie (54) admitted the importance of the vascular element but believed the cause to be infection or, as he emphasized, infections. Early on there was a significant focus on the glia; even Charcot considered the glia feature at first, with everything else being secondary to it. Rindfleisch (34) thought that the principal abnormality was a vascular abnormality, although he did acknowledge that the glia were involved in the process.

Dr. William G. Spiller (144) initially wondered whether the change was in the "noble tissues" using the French term referring to the nerve fibers, or whether it was primarily in the neuroglia; he concluded it to be the latter. He concluded that MS was probably an acute and partly inflammatory disease, and that it probably was dependent on the vascular supply to the area of the plaques, possibly caused by some circulating toxin. Joshua H. Leiner indicated that the axis cylinder could be involved in the lesion, although it may survive (145).

Studies on the proliferative progenitor oligodendrocyte are summarized by Compston (140). Professor Ian McDonald and his colleagues at Queens Square would show over the next decade that the remyelinated axon had distinct morphologic features and that these nerves had slowed conduction with a reduced safety factor (146,147). Later diagnostic tests would be developed that capitalized on the slowing of remyelinated central nerve fibers.

Once it was understood that nerves could demyelinate in MS, but could remyelinate again, it begged the question of why the disease progressed. Even if nerves had thin myelin and conducted slowly, reasonable function should continue. There must be some other factor that limits the process and causes the disease to eventually, and sometimes primarily, progress. Evidence now is accumulating that the key is in observations, made over and over by even the earliest workers such as Charcot, that axons are often damaged. Even if this were a minor part of an acute demyelinated plaque, repeated events in the area and in other connecting areas meant that more unrepairable axonal damage would accumulate. It is conceivable that the axon requires the presence of myelin to continue to be viable. However, understanding the processes of axonal degeneration is crucial in understanding the nature of the progression of this disease and may allow us to more effectively focus our therapeutic efforts.

INVESTIGATIONS

Despite the development of elegant investigative techniques for the confirmation of MS, the clinical history and examination continue to be the gold standard for the diagnosis. Early on, however, efforts were made to complement the clinical assessment. The first important advance was the identification of increased gamma globulin in the CSF of MS patients. It was noted by Hinton that the CSF was often abnormal in MS (148). The most characteristic change was the gold chloride test, with 50 percent of the fluids showing a paretic curve and 20 percent a luetic curve.

Dr. Elvin Kabat of Columbia University studied the immunologic response in the CSF of MS patients and used the new technique of electrophoresis to look at MS CSF (149). He noticed that the CSF of MS patients contained an increased proportion of gamma globulin. This supported the suggestion that there was an immunologic process occurring in MS. This also sparked an increasing interest in the immunologic basis for the development of the MS plaque and also directed the therapeutic approach with drugs that modified or suppressed the immune system, an approach that continues to the present day.

The development of imaging techniques in MS were reviewed by Ormerod, du Boulay, and McDonald (150), showing the remarkable advances made from the era of pneumoencephalography to the time of magnetic resonance imaging (MRI). The earliest evidence of MS on imaging was the demonstration of ventricular enlargement and cortical atrophy (151). Myelography could demonstrate expansion of the cord in an area of transverse myelitis (152). Radionuclide scans occasionally showed evidence of breakdown in the blood-brain barrier (153). PET scanning showed some variations from a normal group, not a helpful diagnostic method in MS.

With the advent of CT scanning in the 1970s, efforts were made to use this technique in MS (154). Studies showed from 9 percent to 75 percent enhancing lesions,

depending on how selective the cases were. Another helpful aspect was the effectiveness of eliminating other diagnoses that could produce the same symptoms manifested by MS patients.

A few years ago it would have been difficult to accept that there would be a test that would have people lie inside a machine, and without any injections, any X-rays, or any other invasion, we would spin the molecules in the body and use a computer to print out remarkable pictures of the nervous system, equivalent to the black and white photographs of early anatomy atlases. But, in fact, within a short period of time we moved from the impressive technology of the CT scan to the remarkable technology of the MRI, which soon became the most effective confirmatory diagnostic test in MS.

In a previous century innovators were remembered as heroes of medicine, often with a technique or disease named after them, but who remembers the amazing scientific feat of Isidor Rabi, Norman F. Ramsey, Edward M. Purcell, Felix Bloch, Nicholas Blomembergen, Richard R. Ernst, Raymond V. Damadian, or Paul C. Lauterbur? These men were the pioneers of MRI, the last two of whom were the pioneers who particularly made the technology applicable to the diagnosis of human disease. Although arguments continue about who made the major contributions and who was the foremost pioneer, in the end it is the nature of modern innovations to be made by many individuals from many disciplines who ultimately remain anonymous (155).

In 1981 Ian Young and his colleagues at the Hammersmith Postgraduate Hospital published the striking pictures of MS lesions demonstrated by the new technique of MRI (156). They showed the striking difference between the picture of CT and MRI in the same patient, with a normal CT scan but five lesions demonstrable on the MRI. He accurately predicted "The technique may also prove a measure of the severity of disease . . . and thus be used to monitor the effectiveness of therapeutic regimens." They then compared the lesions seen in 10 patients (eight definite and two possible MS patients) and saw 19 lesions on CT but these and 112 more on MRI. Since then the characteristics of the lesions in MS have been better defined and the technology of MRI has improved year by year (157).

In 1986 Robert Grossman showed that the enhancing agent gadolinium-DPTA caused some lesions to enhance while others did not (158). He indicated that the enhancement identified breakdown of the blood-brain barrier, indicating areas of inflammation. It then became an important technique to demonstrate new and active MS lesions, effectively monitoring the disease activity, which became important in subsequent clinical trials of new drugs for MS. The technology of MRI continues to improve and the next few years will see further advances.

Based on the increasing knowledge of the slower conduction in demyelinated and remyelinated nerves, the evoked potential technology was developed for the visual system, the auditory–brainstem system and the sensory-cortical system (159,160). These are useful, especially when they can demonstrate another area of involvement and confirm that there are lesions in different areas of the nervous system.

COGNITIVE CHANGES IN MS

Until recent times there was a tendency to suggest to MS patients that mental changes were not a feature of the disease, but cognitive and emotional changes have in fact been noted throughout the known history of the disease. There was controversy about how common this was and whether it was a reaction to the emotional stress of the disease, due to the demyelinating lesions in the nervous system, or perhaps both were involved (161).

The cook Darges, briefly described by Cruveilhier, had normal intelligence but demonstrated pathologic laughing and crying. He said, "she became seized with an emotion difficult to describe. She blushed, laughed and cried" (2,24). Mental changes were also noted in the cases of Vulpian, (36) and Frerichs (29), Valentiner (30), Morris (55), Moxon (3), Seguin (59), Wilks (60), and Osler (4). In the second lecture on MS, Charcot (25) described mental changes, memory difficulty, slow learning, blunting of emotions, indifference, pathologic laughing and crying, and occasional transition to classic forms of mental illness. He commented:

"There is marked enfeeblement of the memory; conceptions are formed slowly; the intellectual and emotional faculties are blunted in their totality. The dominant feeling in the patients appears to b a sort of almost stupid indifference in reference to all things. It is not rare to see them give way to foolish laughter for no cause, and sometimes, on the contrary, to melt into tears for no reason. Nor is it rare, amid this state of mental depression, to find psychic disorders arise which assume one or other of the classic forms of mental alienation" (25).

Gowers, in his text *Diseases of the Nervous System* (1893), said slight mental changes were common and characteristic in MS (66). He said there may be memory failure, and alternating complacency and contentment, often a happy personality in spite of grave disability. Rarely, there may be a form of mental disturbance bordering on chronic insanity.

Eduard Muller in 1904 reviewed the literature on MS in Germany and noted that euphoria was more common than depression and that lack of insight was common (162). He commented that pathologic crying and laughing was an organic change, not a psychological one, but that the cause of the other emotional changes and the euphoria was uncertain. The impact of such changes in the patient are well described by W. N. P. Barbellion (B. F. Cummings) in *The Journal of a Disappointed Man* (1923) (13,14). He noted the "kaleidoscopic changes" in his emotions at periods of his disease and described well the roller coaster of his emotions from deep depression to pleasure and exultation.

Sachs and Freedman (163) indicated that mental changes occurred in 15.6 percent of MS cases. Sanger Brown and Thomas Davis (164) argued that the mental and emotional changes in MS were due to the organic cerebral changes in MS, whereas Smith Ely Jelliffe (70) believed they were psychologically based. Brown and Davis published an expanded version of their 1921 ARNMD paper a year later, dividing their discussion into sections on euphoria, depression, mental deterioration, hallucinations, schizophrenia-like states, personality change, and the course of the mental symptoms. They suggested that the mental changes were organic because the patients were not abnormal before getting the disease, but allowed that stress and personality factors could alter reactions to the disease. Jelliffe put forward the alternative view that these mental changes were due to emotional and psychodynamic factors and even suggested that psychological factors could be involved in the development of some forms of MS. In the conclusion of the ARNMD report it was stated that there was no specific psychic disorder characteristic of the disease.

A further "stocktaking" meeting occurred in Paris three years after the New York ARNMD meeting. Henri Claude, a promising young psychiatrist, did not agree that mental changes were common in this disease. He thought that many of the suggested cases were misdiagnoses, even though he allowed that some minor symptoms could occur, such as puerilism, attention difficulties, depression, and apathy, but usually only in the advanced cases (165). In fact, he believed that the serious mental changes reported were in *forme frustes* and other related diseases.

S. A. Kinnear Wilson and S. S. Cottrel (1926) attempted to carefully evaluate the mental and emotional changes in MS and believed that they were more specific of the disease than the Charcot triad (166). Cottrel was a young American psychiatrist working with the more senior and prominent Wilson. Their work was important for another reason—it was one of the first to address the methodology of performing such studies and used representative samples, successive cases, operational definitions, reliable data collection techniques, such as semi-structured interviews, and data analysis. They did not specifically measure cognitive changes, although they discussed these features in their patients. They discussed "spes sclerotica," "eutonia sclerotica," "euphoria sclerotica," and emotional lability as characteristic of MS.

They believed that 70 percent had some degree of euphoria due to organic changes, but cognitive change was said to be rare. Russell Brain, in an influential overview of MS (1930), believed that Wilson and Cottrel overlooked the common hysterical manifestations of MS patients (68). However, he also noted that the mental changes had received too little attention in studies of the disease

Omberdane (1929) attempted a systematic assessment of MS patients in Paris hospitals (167). His MD thesis, later published a book in 1929, was on 50 cases studied by a systematic psychometric evaluation, plus 10 from the literature. He separated mental changes into (1) sclerotic mental state, which included mood (74 percent) and cognitive change (72 percent); and (2) dementia and psychosis. He concluded that affective disorders and euphoria were associated with intellectual deterioration. An additional conclusion is puzzling, as he said that the intellectual deterioration was more related to a diffuse toxic state than to plaques. Although widely quoted and influential, his report is hard to evaluate because he rated fatigue as cognitive impairment and fatalism as a form of depression. His work, the only MS research of his career, was thoroughly reviewed by Berrios and Quemada (168), who analyzed the data by current statistical techniques (1990) and concluded that there were too many hidden factors in his data to make any conclusions of correlation of emotional change and intellectual change. However, that did not stop it from being influential for many years. They suggest that the direction of the neuropsychiatry of MS would have been different if it were not for this flawed study 70 years ago.

In 1938 David Arbuse reviewed the literature on psychiatric aspects of MS and concluded that mild euphoria was present in most people with MS and that inappropriate laughter and crying was not infrequent (169). Sugar and Nadell (170) agreed with Wilson and Cotrell, and Arbuse, but could not decide if the changes were psychological or the result of organic changes. Borberg and Zahle (171) agreed that in their series of 330 patients "light euphoria" was the most common psychological symptom. Pratt compared MS with muscular dystrophy and confirmed that the MS patients were more cheerful, with more mood swings and euphoria (172).

A number of reviews of euphoria have suggested that it is a reflection of organic change. Rabins used pre-MRI studies to show that euphoria was associated with greater brain involvement with MS, particularly in the periventricular areas, but occurred in fewer than 10 percent of patients (173). Current MRI correlations show that the cognitive and emotional changes have specific neuroanatomic correlations.

Once better neuropsychometric techniques were developed in the postwar period, cognitive and psychological changes were separated but were difficult to compare because they reflected different approaches and different schools of thought, and often were not based on a solid epidemiologic approach. Stenager argues that in the 150 years since Charcot's descriptions, the observations about cognitive and emotional change have moved from broad case-based generalizations about the MS patient to detailed, specific studies of emotional trauma, memory, and depression (161,174). More recently MRI has allowed speculation about the localization of specific mental changes (175).

Only in the last three decades have psychometric techniques clarified the definitions, the approaches, and the results in MS. In addition, there have been approaches that recognized that subtle changes required specific tools and that changes had to be isolated from other phenomena such as depression and fatigue and also had to be correlated with these. Paradoxically, as we are learning to separate and more effectively measure the cognitive changes and the affective changes, the separation has made it possible to learn how they are linked.

THERAPY

"When more is known of the causes and essential pathology of the disease in different cases, more rational methods may brighten the therapeutic prospect."

Sir William Gowers, 1898

In a disease that fluctuates spontaneously, that often recovers after an acute worsening, and that may go into long remission, whatever therapy that was taken may appear to be responsible for the improvement. In addition, there is a strong placebo effect in any chronic, distressing, unpredictable disease. In this situation all ineffective therapies appear to work.

Even in the earliest recognized cases treatment was attempted, both to treat the symptoms, the acute worsening, and to try to affect the underlying disease. Treatment was often the current therapies applied to any illness, or based on the theory of what the cause of the disease might be at the time. To a great extent the belief changed with the major scientific medical interest at the time. In the late nineteenth century it centered around the possibility of infection. Although this concept did not disappear, suspicion of a vascular cause, and later an immunologic cause, and our current interest in a genetic cause, all reflect the major interest in medical science of their times.

The physician to St. Lidwina in the fifteenth century was more pragmatic and announced that the disease was heaven-sent and that attempts at therapy would accomplish nothing except to impoverish her father:

"Believe me there is no cure for this illness, it comes directly from God. Even Hippocrates and Gallenus would not be able to be of any help here. Let us admit this in all honesty rather than to bereave the poor father from his last means. The Lord's hand has touched this woman."

Although his physicians were puzzled by his nervous condition, Augustus d'Esté was treated by many physicians with a continuing array of therapies. Sometimes his symptoms would clear without therapy, but as his disease progressed he was subjected to leeches, purges, venesection, liniments, spa waters, and a long list of medications, including prescriptions containing mercury, silver, arsenic, iron, antimony, and quinine, to mention just a few.

Charcot was similarly negative about the results of treating this disease. At the end of his lecture, when he came to the point of discussing therapy of multiple sclerosis, Charcot said: "After what precedes need I detain you long . . . the time has not yet come when such a subject can be seriously considered" (25).

Marie strongly believed that infection was the cause of MS and predicted that a vaccine like those of Pasteur or the lymph of Koch would be discovered for MS in the future and eliminate the disease (54). In the meantime he prescribed therapies that were suitable for sclerotics, such as iodide of potassium or sodium, and for infections, such as mercury.

The late nineteenth century was an era of polypharmacy and enthusiastic empiric therapies, and such empiric therapies were often widely used for most serious illnesses, so it is not surprising that a wide variety of treatments were aimed at improving people with MS. In the 1890s mercury was the predominant medication applied to MS.

Sir William Gowers in 1893 said, ". . . even less can be done than for other degenerative diseases of the nervous system" (66). However, he recommended nerve tonics such as arsenic, nitrate of silver, and quinine. He recommended hydrotherapy, electricity, maintenance of general health, avoidance of depressing influences, and avoidance of pregnancy.

Beevor (1898) believed that worry and overwork could cause the disease, so his therapy included rest and avoidance of worry (176). He was unsure what other therapies would work, but advocated nerve tonics, strychnine, quinine, iron, cod liver oil, and increasing doses of liquor arsenacalis. He doubted that electrical therapy and baths were of any help. Risien Russell believed infection could worsen the disease but was not its cause. He advocated silver and arsenic, avoidance of stress, cold, and mental and physical fatigue, and limitation of indulgence in "wine and venery" (177).

One of the continuing themes in the writings of the nineteenth century was the similarities but differences between MS and syphilis. Even though Marie, Gowers, Beevor, Russell, and others would state that MS was not a form of syphilis, the syphilis therapies were repeatedly used. Arsenic, silver, and potassium iodide were used for syphilis and were also often used for MS and other neurologic diseases. New therapies developed for syphilis were soon used in MS, and this continued until the antibiotic era (77). By 1911, because of the conceptual relationship between the neurologic features of neurosyphilis and MS, salvarsan was used and other luetic therapies were tried, even the fever therapies that would undoubtedly cause great distress to the MS patient.

In 1911 Buzzard suggested that a spirochete might be the cause and recommended salvarsan therapy (178). The transmission experiments of Bullock (Gye) and Steiner and others over the next decade increased the interest in this theory, so it was logical to turn to all the therapies of the other spirochete disease that affects the nervous system, syphilis. At Queens Square intravenous (IV) typhoid vaccine was given three times a week. If there were severe reactions, intramuscular mild injections were given. Denny-Brown said the results were poor and sometimes disastrous, which is not surprising (179).

Oppenheim argued that the cause of MS was a toxin (74) such as lead, copper, and zinc, and some unknown factor. For therapy he recommended silver nitrate and potassium iodide, mild galvanic current to the back of the head, spa baths at Oeynhausen or Nauheim, and leeches. Even up to the present some clinicians use detoxification methods to treat MS even though they have never been shown to be helpful. Recognizing that there were no specific treatments, iodides were said by some to be helpful, as were colloidal silver preparations either by inunction or IV (141), and intramuscular injections of fibrolysin every five to seven days.

In the 1930s infection continued to be a primary concern, so tonsillectomy, adenoidectomy, and tooth extraction were commonly used. In the 1930s and 1940s treatments applied to tuberculosis were also applied to MS. In the 1940s immune globulins were used, and in the 1950s antibiotics, Russian vaccine (which appears to be rabies vaccine), plasma and blood transfusions, and dietary changes (130) were used in MS. In the 1970s antiviral agents and in the 1980s interferons were assessed as treatments, all on the basis that MS might be an infection.

As well as recommended therapies, there were things to avoid. The ARNMD (1922) rejected Oppenheim's view of a toxic cause and detoxification therapies and expressed caution about therapies aimed at spirochetes (74). Reviewing therapy, Sachs and Friedman (163) listed helpful approaches and things to avoid. They recommended avoidance of extreme temperatures; iodides in silver, mercury, and neoarsphenamine. Farradic stimulation should be avoided. Multiple sclerosis patients were implored to avoid pregnancy, heavy exertion, and extremes of temperature. Tremor was treated with veronal and hyoscin. The most beneficial treatment, however, was arsenic given either by mouth or through injections of cacodylate of soda. Sodium nucleinate was considered helpful. Various spas were recommended, and warm baths, moderate and skillful massage, and methodic exercises "are in order." They suggested that for spastic contractures the Foerster operation is recommended, even though Foerster himself was not enthusiastic about it. Constipation was treated with enemas, and incontinence with tincture of belladonna. Spasticity was treated with passive motion, warm baths, and baking, whereas ataxia was treated with Fraenkel exercises.

Despite the array of possible treatments, Russell Brain came to one sobering conclusion after reviewing the following list of therapies in 1930: malarial therapy, typhoid vaccine, milk injections, phlogitan, Sulfosian, African relapsing fever spirochete inoculation, staphylococcal vaccine, neoarsphenamine, Chevassut vaccine, arsenic, sodium encodylate, neoarsenobillon, silver salvarsan, IV colloidal silver, antimony, Bayer 205, sodium salicylate, intramuscular urotropin, intramuscular quinine, intramuscular mercury, oral iodides, intramuscular sodium nucleinate, diathermy, and X-ray irradiation (68). His conclusion?—"No mode of therapy is successful enough to achieve, at the most, a greater improvement than might have occurred spontaneously."

In the 1930s Putnam referred to the observation of vascular change within the plaques and suggested that thrombosis might be the cause of the scattered pathology. He had initially proposed psychotherapy as an approach to the treatment of MS but later abandoned this and suggested the use of anticoagulants (131). Denny-Brown said he was more impressed with the dangers of anticoagulants than with its benefits (179).

It is interesting to contemplate the approach to therapy of MS through the years. Therapy might be governed by the concept of etiology, the concept of pathology, the nature of the symptoms, or just the need to offer some kind of help. We also see intertwined the enthusiasm for anything new and the common and sometimes useful phenomenon of extrapolating from a beneficial therapy in another disease.

Adrenocorticotropic Hormone (ACTH)

When steroids became available, they were tried in MS with unconvincing results, but the popularity of these wonder drugs caused them to persist as a therapy up to the present day. Oral steroids have been studied in repeated trials, without convincing results, since the early 1960s and still are frequently used. Those who argue that IV steroids achieve better results only because of dosage find support from recent evidence that oral methylprednisolone in very high doses may be beneficial. One of the early proponents of ACTH therapy was Dr. Leo Alexander of New York (180). Alexander was a prominent and widely published neurologist who had investigated Nazi medical experiments and helped draft the Nuremburg Code (181). The "Alexander Regimen" was widely used even though the prolonged use of ACTH caused many steroid side effects.

ACTH was used extensively for acute attacks. One of the early well-controlled trials of this agent in MS was conducted in 1969 and demonstrated a positive but very modest improvement over placebo. Despite the marginal results, ACTH treatment became the standard for many years but has been replaced since the mid-1980s with high-dose IV methylprednisolone.

Immunosuppressant Therapy

It would seem logical in a disease that seems to be immunologically mediated to try to improve patients using drugs that suppress the immune system. Knowledge of the intricacies of the immune mechanisms in MS is imperfect, as it is for how many of these agents work, so attempts were necessarily empiric. Therapies that have been tried include azathioprine (182), cyclophosphamide (183), cyclosporine (184), sulphinpyrizone (185), total lymphoid irradiation (186), and plasmapheresis (187); studies with bone marrow transplantation are planned. Although there is still wide use of azathioprine in Europe, most of the immune suppressants have faded from the clinical scene because of lack of effect or marginal effect in the face of serious side effects and long-term concerns.

Interferons

The interferons were described by Isaacs and Lindenmann in 1957 (188). It had been noted that, during a viral infection in tissue culture, a soluble substance was released into the surrounding milieu, and that this tissue culture fluid could be harvested and used to protect other cells. Because this protection "interfered" with the process of the viral infection of the cells, the substance was named *interferon*. Soon after, it was noted that the interferon had other biologic effects, such as antiproliferative and immunomodulatory properties. Three types were recognized, named for the primary cells of their origin, leukocyte interferon, fibroblast interferon, and immune interferon. The first two shared many properties and were later classified as type 1, and the distinct immune interferon was classified as type 2. Later the type 1 was renamed alpha and beta interferon, whereas type 2 was named gamma interferon. A number of other interferons have subsequently been identified.

The interferons were independently discovered by two groups in the 1950s, Issacs and Lindenmann (188), and Negano and Kojima (189). The interferons are proteins that are capable of interfering with viral infection in cells. The study of viral interferons over many years resulted in this discovery, but it was noted that these cytokines have diverse biologic actions, which include inhibition of the proliferation of normal and transformed cells, regulation of differentiation, host responses to various pathogens, and modulation of the immune system, including activation of natural killer cells and macrophages (190).

The antiproliferative property of the interferons led to interest in them as a potential anticancer agent. Efforts were made to develop variations by cloning and development of recombinant forms of interferons in the 1970s and early 1980s. The initial promise did not play out, but the work continues and interest in its use in diseases such as MS developed at the same time.

In the early 1980s Fog, Knobler and his associates, and Jacobs and his associates began to use interferons in the treatment of patients with MS. The early studies were with the Cantell preparation of interferon alpha made from human leukocytes prepared from the Finnish Red Cross Blood Donor Program. The popular press began to talk about a "breakthrough" when word got out that MS treatment trials studies were beginning at the Scripps Clinic in La Jolla, California, and the University of California, San Francisco. The first reports were disappointing because they did not reach statistical significance even though some patients reported feeling better. A third study was carried out by Jacobs and his colleagues in Buffalo, New York, using intrathecal injections of interferon-beta. Although there were only 10 patients who received and 10 placebo patients, there was a statistically significant reduction in exacerbations and disease severity. Jacobs used intrathecal natural interferon beta because the interferon did not appear to cross the blood-brain barrier in appreciable concentrations (191,192). He carried out weekly intrathecal injections for four weeks and then monthly intrathecal injections for five months. Over a two-year period, the attack rate was reduced from 1.79 to 0.76 per year in the treated patients compared with a drop of 1.98 to 1.48 per year in the placebo group. It was recognized that there were major practical disadvantages associated with intrathecal injections and the flulike reactions that occurred in the treated group. Also, a chemical meningitis appeared to occur, with an elevation of white blood cell counts and protein in the CSF.

Despite some criticisms of the small study and differences between the number of lumbar punctures in the treated and placebo groups, it raised interest in the use of interferons in the long-term treatment of MS. As Knobler (193) points out, a number of important lessons were learned from these three pioneering studies. The interferons were not useful in treating acute attacks but seemed to be of benefit for patients with relapsing-remitting disease in the longer term. Also, the natural interferon had a number of side effects that might be reduced by more purified recombinant variations. Finally, the drug could be administered by subcutaneous injection, which was an acceptable form of long-term therapy. Studies of different interferons demonstrated that interferon gamma worsened the disease, but evidence accumulated that interferon beta-1a and interferon beta-1b were beneficial.

When sufficient supplies of beta-interferons became available, a multiple sclerosis collaborative research group (MSCRG) was formed by Lawrence Jacobs to study its effect in MS patients (194). Were the positive results due to a suppression of a virus involved in the etiology of MS or to a suppression of other viral infections that might aggravate or exacerbate MS, or was there an independent action on the immune system because of its immunomodulatory effects?

To study the effects of interferon beta-1b, 30 patients were enrolled in 1986 and received doses varying from 0.8 to 16 MIU of Betaseron. The patients showed a dose-related trend for a reduction of acute attacks and for the number of patients free of attacks. Side effects, particularly flulike symptoms and injection site reactions, were significant but manageable. The results were sufficiently positive to develop a large multicenter trial, involving seven centers in the United States and four in Canada from the summer of 1988 to early 1993. This pivotal trial showed that Betaseron in a dose of 8 MIU every second day injected subcutaneously led to a 30 percent reduction in the frequency of acute attacks and a 50 percent reduction in moderate and severe attacks over a period of almost five years. The study was not adequately powered to demonstrate measures of disability, but the placebo group trended toward clinical worsening, an important observation because placebo groups in trials do better than expected, for a number of reasons that include selection, care, improvement of their attitudes and expectations, and other factors. Aside from the important clinical information, perhaps the most persuasive data came from the MRI data on these patients. There was a dramatic reduction both in new lesions and in the accumulated lesion burden, as confirmed by the frequent MRI subset analyses of 52 patients at the University of British Columbia under the direction of Donald Paty. A not unexpected but puzzling feature was the development of neutralizing IgG antibody against the interferon beta-1b. Although the titers were quite high in some patients, there was no clear correlation with exacerbation rates, side effect, or other measures. To add to the confusion, antibody titers often fell as treatment continued. Subsequently observations have indicated that the presence of antibody is not consistently related to outcome, that the antibodies can disappear during treatment, and that antibodies occasionally are found in the placebo groups, indicating that the assays are problematic.

A major event in the treatment of MS occurred on Friday, March 11, 1993, in the hearing at the U.S. Food and Drug Administration to review the Betaseron trial for approval for marketing in the treatment of MS. Even though the clinical data were impressive, demonstrating for the first time a significant alteration of the underlying disease in MS, the MRI data were the most persuasive. Betaseron was approved in August 1993 by a very rapid process.

The excitement was understandable, but the expectations in the MS community were out of proportion to the sober and objective results of the trial. It is always difficult to extrapolate a highly focused controlled trial to the realities of individual patients, but appropriate expectations would be that patients would experience two thirds of their attacks on this drug, but that the attacks would be less severe and that their MRIs would improve in appearance. This was not a normal clinical assessment long term, and the MRI improvement was out of proportion to the clinical improvement. There was worldwide publicity, and the demands for the drug led to concerns about its supply and availability. Although the criteria for approval of the drug tended to comply with the criteria for the clinical trial, which is not always a very realistic or rational approach, patients with more progressive or more severe disease than allowed in a trial also wanted the drug.

Berlex Laboratories, the company that produced Betaseron, decided to use a lottery to distribute the drug to those who wanted the new therapy because they initially could not meet the demand. This created a public relations disaster even though it did focus the therapy toward those who were expected to benefit from it. Treatment was initiated if patients had insurance to cover the high cost, or could afford it, and were selected by the lottery to receive it.

As commonly occurs in pharmacologic research, clinical results were obtained only after more than four decades of painstaking laboratory and then clinical steps over four decades, from the development of interferons to its current demonstration of use in relapsing-progressive MS. The drug is now available in the form of three preparations from three companies (two in the United States) (195).

Copaxone (Cop-I)

Ruth Arnon (1996) recently related the long saga of 27 years of "persistent research effort, perseverance,

and tenacity of purpose" that brought Copolymer I, later named Copaxone, to the market (196). Following the production of random copolymers that resembled myelin basic protein in the laboratory of Professor Ephraim Katchalski at the Weitzman Institute in Israel, the team expected these agents to produce encephalitogenic activity. Surprisingly, they had the capacity to protect against EAE. Dr. Oded Abramsky carried out the first clinical trial in MS patients, and Drs. Helmut Bauer and Murray Bornstein planned others. Bornstein carried out three trials that showed the copolymer, called Copolymer I, reduced the number of exacerbations of MS with remarkably few side effects. Production problems delayed the movement of the drug from laboratory studies to the marketplace, but it was released for MS patients in the United States almost a quarter of a century after the drug was produced, a "designer drug" for MS patients.

Diet

Diet was part of the general treatment of disease in past centuries, and patients were often put on strict regimens. For instance, Augustus d'Esté was treated with beefsteaks and Madeira wines.

Roy Swank was probably the first to systematically study the relationship of diet and MS and to suggest that a diet low in animal fat was a specific therapy for MS (130). He had assessed the incidence of MS from 1935 to 1948 in 18 counties in Norway and found considerable variation between different regions and between farming dairying areas versus fishing districts and between inland and coastal areas (197). He assessed diet by a seven-day recording of food intake and compared these with incidence rates and suggested a strong association between the risk of MS and both butterfat consumption and fish consumption. Over a 50-year period (and Swank continues to follow his loyal patients who are faithful to the Swank diet to this day), he reported less progression in his cases, but these were compared with published reports and were not convincing to the neurologic community. Despite that, many diets have appeared, some of which are very complex, combining gluten-free and antimigraine diets, as well as various supplements; most have as their central factor a lowering of the amount of animal fat and an increase in the amount of vegetable oils.

Not all believed the theory of animal fat and in 1950 Crane suggested a treatment with fat-soluble vitamins, animal fat, and ammonium chloride (198). Agranoff and Goldberg looked at MS-related deaths between 1949 and 1967 and compared them with food consumption data for the United States, concluding that there were high correlation coefficients, in the range 0.8–0.9, with latitude, low temperature, and per capita milk consumption (199). All three variables seemed to be independently related to

MS risk, but fish and vegetable fat intake were inversely related. They also studied data on 20 countries belonging to the Organization for Economic Cooperation and Development (OECD) and again found correlation with fat intake, animal fat, butterfat, and meat fat, and a negative association with vegetable and fish consumption. Knox found the same kind of relationship from World Health Organization data and showed a correlation with intake of meat, eggs, butter, sugar, and milk. The correlation was particularly related to intake of total fat. Butcher emphasized the correlation between MS prevalence and milk consumption. He showed differences in the intensity of diary cow breeding between Nordic and Celtic populations in Scotland: an MS gradient parallel to milk consumption in Norway, Australia, and South Africa, as well as in Japan.

Alter and colleagues correlated food consumption data from the UN with MS prevalence in various countries and showed a correlation coefficient of approximately 0.7 with total fat and animal calories, but much less with total protein and total calories (117,200). He discussed the harmful role of lipids in MS and the possible influence of early cow milk–feeding on the later development of MS and pointed out that both the distribution of MS and the distribution of animal fat in diets follow a parabolic curve. Nangi and Narod (201) looked at dietary factors in 23 countries and again showed a correlation with total fat, all meat and pork, but not with beef consumption. Most of these studies did not correct for a possible confounding affluence factor in many of these countries.

Malosse and coworkers studied 29 countries and again suggested a correlation with milk consumption (202). Similarly, Lauer studied data from 21 countries on three continents and found that of 76 commodities in diet, 16 passed their three-part steps for possible correlation, and these included animal fat, total fat, calcium, riboflavin, total meat, pork, margarine, coffee, and beer (203–207). Lauer's review of studies in the United States comparing the dietary patterns with MS suggests a relationship with meat, diary food, and low temperature.

Alternative Therapies: The Parallel System

Alternative medicine has always been with us and experiences waves of acceptance. Therapies that were once in the forefront of medical approaches to symptoms and diseases are now in the list of alternative or complementary therapies, and alternative therapies that are eventually shown to be beneficial enter the realm of medical therapy. Alternative medicine is a different system, based on belief and sometimes longstanding historical and cultural practices rather than science. Physicians often forget that science is a relative newcomer to the philosophy of medicine, and for thousands of years medical practice looked very much like current-day alternative medicine.

Any chronic disease for which there is not an effective treatment tends to have a lot of alternative approaches to treatment, and MS is a good example. One need only consult the frequently updated *Therapeutic Claims in Multiple Sclerosis* (207a) book to see the long but incomplete list of the most frequently used medical and alternative approaches to MS. Speaking in 1930 about the wide range of medical therapies, Russell Brain concluded, "the multiplication of remedies is eloquent of their inefficacy" (68).

Many of these have a long history in conditions other than MS. For example, spa therapy, herbal preparations, stimulants, minerals, detoxification, and rest therapies have been used for over a century and a half in MS and wax and wane in popularity. Other therapies appear as advances in medicine, and changes in theories occur, as we saw with antisyphilitic therapy, antimicrobials and antibiotics, anticoagulants, immunosuppressants, and antioxidants.

This is not a small or peripheral issue. More people use alternative therapies and go to alternative therapists than take medications or consult physicians. Some will see their neurologist once every 6 to 12 months but see an alternative therapist many times a month or even many times a week.

Richard Thomas wrote a holistic guide that suggests a long list of forms of natural therapies, including acupuncture, cupping, acupressure, healing or faith healing, therapeutic touch, homeopathy, flower remedies, (olive for exhaustion, crab apple for shame about the disease, mustard for depression—and a rescue therapy that combines five of these), reflexology, crystal and gem therapy, aura-soma oils, and aromatherapy (208).

Therapy with hyperbaric oxygen was suggested by some early anecdotal reports and uncontrolled use of hyperbaric chambers occurred in many communities, supported by ARMS in Britain. Following this, Fischer and his colleagues in 1983 published a randomized double-blind control study in the *New England Journal of Medicine* suggesting benefit from this treatment (209). The first ARMS center was formed in Dundee in 1982 and many centers then sprang up around the country as enthusiasm increased, despite unimpressive follow-up studies by Barnes and others (1985) (210). The treatment then became very controversial, and ARMS would discount the negative reports, releasing another report on 147 cases treated in Glasgow and concluding that the treatment was beneficial and safe (211).

In 1983 Jane Clarke published a book that suggested a new theory for the cause of MS—that overheating caused the disease, and lack of repair of myelin was caused by a deficiency of copper and/or molybdenum in their diet, leading to therapy based on this concept. Most recently, interest has been sparked in the media about bee venom therapy and the Cari Loder diet, but such alternative approaches occur frequently, fading slowly as the next one comes to the fore (212).

MULTIPLE SCLEROSIS SOCIETY

"It is possible that the cause of the disease lies buried somewhere in these lengthy protocols waiting to be found by anyone ingenious enough to unearth it."

Dr. Henry Miller, 1972

An important impetus for change and encouragement for research in MS in the last half century has been the formation of MS societies in each country. By the end of World War II Putnam and others complained that the public, who knew so well the problem of polio, had little inkling of the MS that afflicted young adults. The public needed to be made aware of this illness and contribute to the efforts to find its cause and a cure.

The first step was taken by Miss Sylvia Lawry, who was distressed about her brother who had been diagnosed with MS and placed an advertisement in the *New York Times* on May 1, 1945 which stated: " Multiple Sclerosis. Will anyone recovered from it please communicate with the patient. T272 Times."

From the responses it was apparent to Miss Lawry that there should be an organization to foster research into the cause, treatment, and eventual cure of MS. The organization was named the Association for the Advancement of Research into Multiple Sclerosis (AARMS) but a few months later it was changed to the Multiple Sclerosis Society (213).

Shortly afterward, Evelyn Opal, a Montreal housewife who had MS, heard of the New York group and began to raise funds, forming a chapter of the American group named for her physician, Dr. Colin Russel of the Montreal Neurological Institute. Another Montreal patient, Harry Bell, an engineer, also formed a group, the Canadian MS Research Organization. Lawry brought them together and in 1948 the Multiple Sclerosis Society of Canada was formed with Dr. Wilder Penfield as honorary chairman of the scientific advisory committee. The first grant went to Dr. Roy Swank and Dr. Donald McEachern for work on lipids and diet in MS. One grant per year was given for the first two decades, and then the support of research expanded each year.

In 1952 the Multiple Sclerosis Society of Great Britain and Northern Ireland was formed, with Dr. Douglas McAlpine as chairman of the medical advisors. Each of these national organizations was formed with the encouragement and enthusiastic support of Miss Lawry. Each appointed society leading clinicians in MS to sit on the advisory committees that awarded the results of the first fund-raising efforts, and year by year these grants increased and encouraged more clinicians and later basic scientists to enter the field of MS research.

Sylvia Lawry was not finished organizing for MS. At the 8th International Conference of Neurology in September 1965 in Vienna, she proposed the formation of an international organization, supported by Dr. William Breed and Dr. Houston Merritt, which was formed the next year.

From a few thousand dollars to many million dollars per year these societies supported research into basic science, clinical research, epidemiology, psychosocial research, and clinical care. There is little question that the current vibrant research effort in all aspects of MS developed because an MS society in each country supported and funded the best efforts in research.

As I conclude this selective review of the early contributors to the understanding of MS, I acknowledge their pioneer efforts and vision and that of the MS societies of the world that support their work and introduce the reader to the coming chapters of this book, written by their worthy successors, the clinicians and researchers who are currently addressing the remaining questions about MS.

"The story of multiple sclerosis is not yet closed, but neither is the history of medicine."

Tracey Putnam, 1938

*A*cknowledgments

I am indebted to many people for information, assistance, and inspiration in this work. Dr. Andrea Rideout began a lot of the background library work when working with me as an elective student a decade ago. I relied on the excellent historical work of Alistair Compston, Ian McDonald, and George Ebers, three of the greatest contributors to the knowledge of MS, as well as the history of the disease. My tireless secretary, Roxy Pelham, suffered through many drafts, and my wife, Janet Murray, assisted in some of the library work at the Wellcome Institute for the History of Medicine in London and helped with the referencing.

*R*eferences

1. Putnam TJ. The centenary of multiple sclerosis. *Arch Neurol Psychiatry* 1938; 40(4):806–813.
2. Cruveilhier J. *Anatomie pathologique du corps humain.* Paris: JB Bailière, 1829–42. (Individual livraisons in this

work appeared separately but Livraisons 32 and 38, both of which deal with MS, also can be found in Volume 2, published in 1842.

3. Moxon W. Eight cases of insular sclerosis of the brain and spinal cord. *Guy's Hosp Rep* 1875; 20:437–478.

4. Osler W. Cases of insular sclerosis. *Can Med Surg J* 1880; 1–11.

5. Medaer R. Does the history of multiple sclerosis go back as far as the 14th century? *Acta Neurol Scand* 1979; 60:189–192.

6. Albers P. St. Lidwina. *Catholic encyclopedia.* London: Encyclopedia Press, 1913.

7. Delaney, John J. *Dictionary of saints.* New York: Doubleday, 1980.

8. *The book of saints.* London: Adams and Charles Black, 1966.

9. Anonymous. Thorlaks saga. C. In: *Byskua Sogur,* Editiones Armagnaenae Series A, Vol. 13.2. Copenhagen: John Helgason, 1978.

10. Stenager E. A note on the treatment of Drummer Bock: An early Danish account of multiple sclerosis? *J History Neurosciences* 1996; 5(2):197–199.

11. Firth D. *The case of Augustus d'Esté.* Cambridge, UK: Cambridge University Press, 1948.

12. Stenager E. The course of Heinrich Heine's illness: Diagnostic considerations. *J Med Biog* 1996; 4(1):28–32.

13. Barbellion WNP (pseudonym for Cummings BF). *The journal of a disappointed man.* London: Chatto & Windus, 1919.

14. Barbellion WPN. *Journal of a disappointed man* and *The last diary.* Gloucester: Allan Sutton Publishing Ltd., 1984 (with bibliographical notes by Peter Clifford).

15. Spillane JD. *The doctrine of the nerves.* New York: Oxford University Press, 1981.

16. Ollivier CP. *De La Moelle Epiniére et de ses maladies.* Paris: Crevot, 1824.

17. Ollivier CP. *Traité De La Moelle Epinière et de Ses Maladies, Contenant L'Historie Anatomique, Physiologique et Pathologique de Centre Nerveau Chez L'Homme.* Paris: Crevot, 1827.

18. Ebers G. A historical overview. In: Paty DW, Ebers GC (eds.). *Multiple sclerosis.* Philadelphia: FA Davis, 1998:1–4.

19. Carswell R. *Pathological anatomy: Illustrations of the elementary forms of disease.* London: Longman, Orme, Brown, Green and Longman, 1938.

20. McHenry L. *Garrison's history of neurology.* Springfield: Charles C Thomas, 1969:253–254.

21. Hooper R. *Illustrated by colored engravings of the most frequent and important organic diseases to which that viscus is the subject.* London: Longman, Rees, Orme, Brown and Longman, 1828.

22. Compston A. The 150th anniversary of the first depiction of the lesions of multiple sclerosis. *J Neurol Neurosurg Psychiatry* 1988; 51:1249–1252.

23. Keppel Hesselink JM. *Beeldon in de mist: de geschiedenis van de neurologie in capita selecta.* Rotterdam: Erasmus, 1994.

24. Cruveilhier J. *Anatomie pathologique du corps humain, ou descriptions avec figures lithographiees et coloriees, des diverses alterations morbides dout le corps humain est suceptible.* Paris: J. B. Ballière, 1835–1842, Vol. 2.

25. Charcot JM. *Lectures on diseases of the nervous system.* Translated by G. Sigerson. London: The New Sydenham Society, 1877:158–222 (p. 221).

26. Hall M. *On diseases and derangements of the nervous system in their primary forms and in their modifications by age, sex, constitution, hereditary predisposition, excesses, general disorder and organic disease.* London: Ballière, 1841.

27. Keppel Hesselink JM. Een Monografie van KFH Marx uit, 1938: Mogelijk de eerste Klinisch-Pathologische Beschrijving van Multipele Sclerose. *Ned Tijdschr Geneeskd* 1991; 135:2439–2443.

28. Romberg MH. *Lehrbuch der Nervenkrankheiten des Menschen.* Berlin: A. Duncker, 1846.

29. Frerich FT. Ueber Hirnsklerose. *Arch für die Gesamte Medizin* 1849; 10:334–350.

30. Valentiner W. Ueber die Sklerose des Gehirns und Rückenmarks. *Deutsche Klin* 1856:147–151, 158–162, 167–169.

31. Türch L. Quoted by Kinnier Willson (1940).

32. Haymaker, Webb. *The founders of neurology.* Springfield: Charles C Thomas, 1953:92–95.

33. Rokitansky. Bericht der Akadmie der Wissenschaft zu Wien 24. 1857. (Cited by Charcot 1868, 1877).

34. Rindfleisch E. Histologische Detail zu der Grauen Degeneration von Gehirn und Rückenmark. *Virchow Arch Path Anat* 1863; 26:474–483.

35. Leyden E. Ueber graue Degeneration des Rückenmarks. *Deutsche Klin* 1863; 15:121–128.

36. Vulpian EFA. Note sur la sclérose en plaques de la moelle épinière. *Union Méd* 1866; 30:459–465, 475–482, 541–548.

37. Charcot M. Histologie de le sclérose en plaques. *Gaz Hôp Paris* 1868; 141:554–555, 557–558.

38. Charcot JM. Histologie de la sclérose en plaques. *Gaz Hôp Civils Milit (Paris)* 1868a; 41:554–555, 557–558, 566.

39. Charcot JM. Diagnostic des formes frustes de la sclérose en plaques. *Prog Méd* 1879; 7:97–99.

40. Charcot JM. Séance du 14 mars: Un cas de sclérose en plaques généralisée du cerveau et de la moelle épinière. *Comp Rend Soc Biol* 1986b; 20:13–14.

41. Goetz CG. Visual art in the neurological career of Jean-Martin Charcot. *Arch Neurol* 1991; 48:421–425.

42. Goetz CG, Bonduelle M. Charcot as therapeutic interventionist and treating neurologist. *Neurology* 1995; 45:2102–2106.

43. Goetz CG, Bonduelle M, Gelfand T. *Charcot: Constructing neurology.* New York: Oxford University Press, 1995.

44. Londe A. *Le service photograpique de la Salpêtrière.* Paris: Doin, 1892.

45. Didi-Huberman G. *Invention de l'hystérie: Charcot et l'iconographie photographique de la Salpêtrière.* Paris: Editions Macula, 1982.

46. Bourneville DM, Guérard L. *De la sclérose en plaques disseminées.* Paris: Delahayne, 1869.

47. Ordenstein L. *Sur la paralysie agitante et la sclérose en plaques generalisées.* Paris: Delahaye, 1868.

48. Guillain GJM. *Charcot (1825–1893): Sa vie—son oeuvre.* Paris: Masson, 1955.

49. Guillain G. *JM Charcot 1825–1893: His life—his work.* Edited and translated by P. Bailey. London: Pitman Medical, 1959.

50. Lellouch A. Charcot, Découvreur de Maladies. *Rev Neurol (Paris)* 1994; 150:506–510.

51. Daudet L. *Les oeuvres dans les Hommes.* Paris: Nouvelle Librairie Nationale, 1992.

52. Sherwin AL. Multiple sclerosis in historical perspective. *McGill Med J* 1957; 26:39–48.

53. Marie P. La sclérose en plaques et maladies infectieuses. *La Progres Medicale* 1884; 12:287–289.

54. Marie P. *Lectures on diseases of the spinal cord.* Lubbock M (Trans). London: New Sydenham Society, 1895, 153:134–136.

55. Morris JC. Case of the late Dr. CW Pennock. *Am J Med Sci* 1868; 56:138–144.

56. Moxon D. Case of insular sclerosis of brain and spinal cord. *Lancet* 1873; 1:236.

56a. Anon. Guy's Hospital. Case of insular sclerosis of the brain and spinal cord (under the care of Dr. Moxon). *Lancet* 1873; i:236.

56b. Anon. Guy's Hospital. Two cases of insular sclerosis of the brain and spinal cord (under the care of Dr. Moxon). *Lancet* 1875; i:471–473.

56c. Anon. Report on Clinical Society of London. *Lancet* 1875; i:545.

56d. Anon. Guy's Hospital. Two cases of insular sclerosis of the brain and spinal cord (under the care of Dr. Moxon). *Lancet* 1875; i:609.

57. Hammond WA. A treatise on diseases of the nervous system. Ch. VII, *Multiple cerebro-spinal sclerosis.* New York: D. Appleton and Co., 1871:637–653.

58. Hamilton AM. *Nervous diseases: Their description and treatment.* London: J & A Churchill, 1878:346–351.

59. Sequin EC, Shaw JC, Van Derveer A. A contribution to the pathological anatomy of disseminated cerebro-spinal sclerosis. *J Nerv Ment Dis* 1878; 5:281–293.

60. Wilks S. *Lectures on diseases of the nervous system, delivered at Guy's Hospital.* London: J & A Churchill, 1878:282–284.

61. MacLaurin H. Case of amblyopia from partial neuritis, treated with subcutaneous injection of strychnia. *NSW Med Gazette* 1873; 3:214.

62. Newman AK. On insular sclerosis of the brain and spinal cord. *Aust Med J* 1875; 20:369–374.

63. Jamieson J. Cases of multiple neuritis. *Aust Med J* 1886; 8:295–302.

64. Ebers GC. Osler and neurology. *Can J Neurol Sci* 1985b; 12:236–242.

65. Gowers WR. *A manual and atlas of medical ophthalmoscopy.* ed 3. Edited with the assistance of Marcus Gunn. London: J & A Churchill, 1890.

66. Gowers WR. *A manual of diseases of the nervous system.* 2nd ed. London: J & A Churchill, 1893, Vol. 2:544, 557–558.

67. Association for Research in Nervous and Mental Disease: *Multiple sclerosis (disseminated sclerosis).* New York: Paul B Hoeber, 1922.

68. Brain WR. Critical review: Disseminated sclerosis. *Q J Med* 1930; 23:343–391.

69. McAlpine D, Compston ND, Lumsden CE. *Multiple sclerosis.* Edinburgh: E & S Livingstone, 1955.

70. Jelliffe SE. Emotional and psychological factors in multiple sclerosis. In: *Multiple sclerosis: An investigation by the Association for Research in Nervous and Mental Disease.* New York: Paul B Hoeber, 1921:82–90.

71. Compston A. Reviewing multiple sclerosis. *Postgrad Med J* 1992; 68(801):507–515.

72. Compston A, et al. *McAlpine's multiple sclerosis.* 3rd ed. London: Churchill Livingstone, 1998.

73. Barker LF. Comment in *Multiple sclerosis: Association for Research in Nervous and Mental Diseases.* Vol. 2. New York: Paul B Hoeber, 1922:62.

74. Oppenheim H. *Textbook of nervous diseases for physicians and students.* Bruce A (trans). Edinburgh: Otto Schulze & Co., 1911:350 (translation of 1908 German edition).

75. Dana CL. Multiple sclerosis and the methods of ecology. In: *Multiple sclerosis: Association for Research in Nervous and Mental Diseases.* Vol. 2. New York: Paul B Hoeber. 1922:43–47.

76. Reese HH. Multiple sclerosis and the demyelinating diseases. Critique of theories concerning multiple sclerosis. *JAMA* 1950; 143:1470–1473.

77. MacDonald WI. Attitudes to the treatment of multiple sclerosis. *Arch Neurol* 1983; 40:667–670.

78. Bullock WE. The experimental transmission of disseminated sclerosis to rabbits. *Lancet* 1913; Oct 25:1185–1186.

79. Khun P, Steiner G. Uber die Ursache der multiplen Sklerose. *Medicinizinische Klinik* 1917; 13:1007–1014.

80. Gye NE. The experimental study of disseminated sclerosis. *Brain* 1921; 44:213–222.

81. Teague O. Bacteriological investigation of multiple sclerosis. In: *Multiple sclerosis: Association for Research in Nervous and Mental Diseases.* Vol. 2. New York: Paul B Hoeber, 1922:121–131.

82. Chevassut K. Aetiology of disseminated sclerosis. *Lancet* 1930; 1:522–560.

83. Purves-Stewart J. A specific vaccine treatment in disseminated sclerosis. *Lancet* 1930; 1:560–564.

84. Carmichael EA. The aetiology of disseminate sclerosis: Some criticisms of recent work especially with regard to the 'Spherula insularis'. *Proc R Soc Med* 1931; 34:591–599.

85. Purves-Stewart, Sir James. *Sands of time: Recollections of a physician in peace and war.* London: Hutchinson and Co. 1939.

86. Steiner G, Kuhn L. Acute plaques in multiple sclerosis, their pathogenic significance and the role of spirochetes as etiological factors. *J Neuropath Exp Neurol* 1952; 11:343–373.

87. Adams DK, Blacklock JWS, Dunlop EM, et al. An investigation into the pathogenesis of disseminated sclerosis. *Q J Med* 1924; 17:129–150.

88. Ichelson RR. Cultivation of spirochetes from spinal fluids of multiple sclerosis cases and negative controls. *Proc Soc Exp Biol (NY)* 1957; 95:57–58.

89. Kurtzke JF, Martin A, Myerson RM, Lewis JI. Microbiology in multiple sclerosis: Evaluation of Ichelson's organism. *Neurology* 1962; 12:915–922.

90. Shevell M, Evans BK. The "Schaltenbrand experiment"—Würzburg, 1940: Scientific, historical, and ethical perspectives. *Neurology* 1994; 44:350–356.

91. Gajdusek DC, Gibbs CJ Jr, Alpers M (eds). Slow latent and temperature virus infections. Washington, DC: U.S. Dept. of Health, Education and Welfare, 1965.

92. Morawitz P. Zurkenntnis der multiplen sklerose. *Deutsches Arch F klin Med Leipz* 1904; 151–166.

93. Kurland LT. The frequency and geographic distribution of multiple sclerosis as indicated by mortality statistics and morbidity surveys in the United States and Canada. (Thesis submitted to School of Hygiene and Public Health, The Johns Hopkins University, in conformity with requirements for the degree of Doctor of Public Health, May 1951).

94. Kurland LT, Epidemiologic characteristics of multiple sclerosis. *Am J Med* 1952; 21:561–571.

95. Kurland LT, Westlund KB. Epidemiologic factors in the etiology and prognosis of multiple sclerosis. *Ann NY Acad Sci* 1954; 58:682

96. Kurland LT. The evolution of multiple sclerosis epidemiology. *Ann Neurol* 1994; 36:S2–S5.

97. Davenport C. Multiple sclerosis: From the standpoint of geographic distribution and race. *Arch Neurol Psychiatry* 1922; 8:51–58.

98. Bramwell B. Disseminated sclerosis with special reference to the frequency and etiology of the disease. *Clin Stud* 1904; 2:193–210.

99. Bramwell B. The prognosis in disseminated sclerosis: Duration in two hundred cases of disseminated sclerosis. *Edin Med J* 1917; 18:15–23.

100. Poser CM. The dissemination of multiple sclerosis: A Viking saga? A historical essay. *Ann Neurol* 1994; 36:S231–S243.

101. Bailey P. Incidence of multiple sclerosis in United States troops. *Arch Neurol Psychiatry* 1922; 7:582–583.

102. McAlpine D. The problem of disseminated sclerosis. *Brain* 1946; 69:233–250.

103. Steiner G. Multiple sclerosis. I. The etiological significance of the regional and occupational incidence. *J Nerv Ment Dis* 1938; 88:42–66.

104. Ulett G. Geographic distribution of multiple sclerosis. *Dis Nerv Syst* 1946; 9:342–346.

105. Limburg C. The geographic distribution of multiple sclerosis and its estimated prevalence in the United States. *Res Publ Assoc Res Nerv Ment Dis* 1950; 28:15–24.

106. Bulman D, Ebers G. The geography of multiple sclerosis reflects genetic susceptibility. *J Trop Geog Neurol* 1992; 2:66–72.

107. Wynn D, Rodriguez M, O'Fallon W, Kurland L. A reappraisal of the epidemiology of multiple sclerosis in Olmsted County, Minnesota. *Neurology* 1992; 40:780–786.

108. Alter M. Clues to the cause based on the epidemiology of multiple sclerosis. In: Field EJ (ed.). *Multiple sclerosis: A clinical conspectus*. Baltimore: University Park Press, 1977:35–82.

109. Behrend RC. Multiple sclerosis in Europe. *Eur Neurol* 1969; 2:129.

110. McCall MG, Brereton, TL, Dawson A, et al. Frequency of multiple sclerosis in three Australian cities—Perth, Newcastle, and Hobart. *J Neurol Neurosurg Psychiatry* 1968; 31:I.

111. Allison RS. Disseminated sclerosis in North Wales. *Brain* 1931; 53:391–430.

112. Pohlen K. Statistics of clinical and pathological statements on causes of death. Health and statistics. *Statistical Bulletin* II: Nos. 4/5 (November) 1942. Battle Creek, Michigan: W.K. Kellogg Foundation.

113. Sutherland JM. Observations on the prevalence of multiple sclerosis in Northern Scotland. *Brain* 1956; 79:635–654.

114. Skegg DCG, Corwin PA, Craven RS, Malloch JA, Pollock M. Occurrence of multiple sclerosis at the north and south of New Zealand. *J Neurol Neurosurg Psychiatry* 1987; 50:134–139.

115. Dean, G. Annual incidence, prevalence and mortality of multiple sclerosis in white South African–born and in white immigrants to South Africa. *Brit Med J* 1967, 2:724–730.

116. Rosman KD, Jacobs HA, VanDerMerwe CA. A new multiple sclerosis epidemic? A pilot survey. *S Africa Med J* 1985: 68:162–163.

117. Alter M, Hallpern L, Kurland LT, et al. Multiple sclerosis in Israel. Prevalence among immigrants and native-born inhabitants. *Arch Neurol* 1962; 7:253.

118. Kuroiwa Y. History of multiple sclerosis studies in Japan. In: Yoshigoro Kuroiwa (ed.). *Multiple Sclerosis in Asia: Proceedings of the Asian Multiple Sclerosis Workshop.* Tokyo: University of Tokyo Press, 1977:3–5.

119. Campbell AMG, Daniel P, Porter RJ, et al. Disease of the nervous system occurring among research workers on swayback in lambs. *Brain* 1947; 70:50–59.

120. Campbell AMG, Herdan G, Tatlow WFT, Whittle EG. Lead in relation to disseminated sclerosis. *Brain* 1950; 73:52–71.

121. Kurtzke JF. A reassessment of the distribution of multiple sclerosis. *Acta Neurol Scand* 1975; 51:110.

122. Kurtzke JF, Hyllested K, Multiple sclerosis in the Faroe Islands. 1. Clinical and epidemiological features. *Ann Neurol* 1979; 5:6–21.

123. Kurtzke JF, Hyllested K. Multiple sclerosis in the Faroe Islands. 2. Clinical update, transmission, and the nature of MS. *Neurology* 1986; 36:307–328.

124. Kurtzke JF, Hyllested K. Multiple sclerosis in the Faroe Islands. 3. An alternative assessment of the three epidemics. *Acta Neurol Scand* 1987; 76:317–339.

125. Kurtzke JF, Hyllested K, Heltberg A, Olsen A. Multiple sclerosis in the Faroe Islands. 5. The occurrence of the fourth epidemic as validation of transmission. *Acta Neurol Scand* 1993; 88:161–173.

126. MacKay RP. *Multiple sclerosis and the demyelinating diseases. The familial occurrence of multiple sclerosis and its implications.* Baltimore: Williams & Wilkins, 1950.

127. McKay RP, Myrianthropoulos NC. Multiple sclerosis in twins and their relatives: Preliminary report on a genetic and clinical study. *Arch Neurol Psychiatry* 1958; 80:667–674.

128. Pratt TRC, Compston ND, McAlpine D. The familial incidence of disseminated sclerosis and its significance. *Brain* 1951; 74:191–232.

129. Curtius F. *Multiple sklerose and erbanlage*. Leipzig: G. Thieme, 1933.

130. Swank RL. Multiple sclerosis: A correlation of its incidence with dietary fat. *Am J M Sc* 1950; 220:421–430.

131. Putnam TJ, Chiavacci LV, Hoff H, et al. Results of treatment of multiple sclerosis with dicoumarin. *Arch Neurol* 1947; 57:1–13.

132. Glaszmann FL. Die nervosen komplikationen von varizellen, Variole Vakzine. *Schweiz med Wschr* 1927; 57:145.

133. Rivers TM, Schwentker F. Encephalomyelitis accompanied by myelin destruction experimentally produced in monkeys. *J Exp Med* 1935; 61:698–702.

134. Rivers TM, Sprunt DH, Berry GP. Observations on attempts to produce acute disseminated encephalomyelitis in monkeys. *J Exp Med* 1933; 58:39–53.

135. Ebers G. Immunology of MS. In: Paty DW, Ebers GC (eds.). *Multiple sclerosis*. Philadelphia. FA Davis, 1999: 403–426.

136. Paty DW, Hashimoto SA, Ebers GC. Management of multiple sclerosis and interpretation of clinical trials. In: Paty DW, Ebers GC (eds.). *Multiple sclerosis*. Philadelphia. FA Davis, 1999:427–545.

137. Noseworthy JH, Seland TP, Ebers GC. Therapeutic trials in multiple sclerosis. *Can J Neurol Sci* 1984; 11:355–362.

138. Babinski J. *Étude anatomique et clinique sur la sclérose en plaques*. Paris: G. Masson, 1885 (Paris: A. Parent).

139. Babinski J. Recherches sur l'anatomie pathologique de la sclérose en plaques et étude comparative des diverses variétés de scléroses de la moelle. *Arch Physiol Norm Pathol* 1985; 5 (series 3):186–207.

140. Compston A. Remyelination in multiple sclerosis: A challenge for therapy. The 1996 European Charcot Foundation Lecture. *Multiple Sclerosis* 1997; 3:51–70.

141. Marburg O. Die sogenannte akute multiple Sklerose (Encephalomyelitis periaxialis scleroticans). *Jahrb f Psychiat U Neurol* 1906; 27:1.

142. Dawson J. The history of disseminated sclerosis. Transactions of the Royal Society of Edinburgh, 1916; 50:517–740.

143. Hassin GB. Pathological studies in the pathogenesis of multiple sclerosis. In: *Multiple sclerosis: Association for Research in Nervous and Mental Diseases*. Vol. 2. New York: Paul B Hoeber, 1922:144–175.

144. Spiller WG, Camp CD. Multiple sclerosis, with a report of two additional cases with necropsy. *J Nerv Ment Dis* 1904; 31:433–445.

145. Leiner JH. An investigation of the axis cylinder in its relation to multiple sclerosis. In: *Multiple sclerosis: Association for Research in Nervous and Mental Diseases*. Vol. 2. New York: Paul B Hoeber, 1922:197–208.

146. McDonald WI. The mystery of the origin of multiple sclerosis. *J Neurol Neurosurg Psychiatry* 1986; 49:113–123.

147. McDonald WI. The dynamics of multiple sclerosis: The Charcot lecture. *J Neurol* 1993; 240(1):28–36.

148. Hinton WA. CSF in MS. In: Ayer, JB, Foster HE. Studies in the cerebrospinal fluid and blood in multiple sclerosis. In: *Multiple sclerosis: Association for Research in Nervous and Mental Diseases*. Vol. 2. New York: Paul B Hoeber, 1922:113–121.

149. Kabat EA, Moore DH, Landow H. An electrophoretic study of the protein components in cerebrospinal fluid and their relationship to the serum proteins. *J Clin Invest* 1942; 21:571–577.

150. Ormerod IEC, du Boulay GH, McDonald WI, Imaging in multiple sclerosis. In: McDonald WI, Silberg DH (eds.). *Multiple sclerosis*. London: Butterworth, 1986: 11–36.

151. Freedman W, Cohen R. Electroencephalographic and pneumoencephalographic studies of multiple sclerosis. *Arch Neurol Psychiatry* 1945; 53:246–247.

152. Haughton VM, Ho KC, Boe-Decker RA. The contracting cord sign of multiple sclerosis. *Neuroradiology* 1979; 17:207–209.

153. Antunes JL, Schlesinger EB, Michelsen WJ. The abnormal brain scan in demyelinating diseases. *Arch Neurol* 1974; 30:269–271.

154. Cala LA, Mastaglia FL, Computerized axial tomography in multiple sclerosis. *Lancet* 1976; 1:689.

155. Mattson J, Merrill S. *The Pioneers of NMR and magnetic resonance in medicine. The story of MRI.* Jericho, NJ: Bar-Ilan University Press/Dean Books Company, 1996.

156. Young IR, Hall AS, Pallis CA, et al. Nuclear magnetic resonance imaging of the brain in multiple sclerosis. *Lancet* 1981; 2:1063–1066.

157. Ormerod IEC, Miller DH, McDonald WI, et al. The role of NMR imaging in the assessment of multiple sclerosis and isolated neurological lesions. A quantitative study. *Brain* 1987; 110:1579–1616.

158. Grossman RI, Conzales-Scarano F, Atlas SW, Galetta S, Silberberg DH. Multiple sclerosis: Gadolinium enhancement in MR imaging. *Radiology* 1986; 161:721–725.

159. Halliday AM, McDonald WI, Mushin J. Delayed visual evoked response in optic neuritis. *Lancet* 1972, I:982–985.

160. Halliday AM, McDonald WI, Mushin J. Delayed pattern-evoked responses in optic neuritis in relation to visual acuity. *Trans Opthalmol Soc UK* 1973; 93:315–324.

161. Stenager E, Knudsen L, Jensen K. Historical notes on mental aspects of multiple sclerosis. In: Jensen K, Knudsen L, Stenager E, Grant I (eds.). *Mental disorders and cognitive deficits in multiple sclerosis*. London: John Libbey, 1989:1–7

162. Müller E. Die multiple sclerose des Gehirns and Rückenmarks. Ihre Pathologie and Behandlung. Jena: Gustav Fischer, 1904.

163. Sachs B, Friedman ED. General symptomatology and differential diagnoses of disseminated sclerosis. *Arch Neurol Psychiatry* 1922; 7:551–560.

164. Brown S, Davis TK. The mental symptoms of multiple sclerosis. *Arch Neurol Psychiatry* 1922; 7:629–634.

165. Claude H. Quelques remarques sur le diagnostic de la sclérose en plaques. *Rev Neurol* 1924; 31:727–730.

166. Cottrell SS, Wilson SAK. The affective symptomatology of disseminated sclerosis. *J Neurol Psychopath* 1926; 7:1–30.

167. Ombredane A. Sue les troubles mentaux de la sclérose en plaques. Thesis. Paris: Les Presses Universitaires de France, 1929.

168. Berrios GE, Quemada JI, Andre G. Ombredane and the psychiatry of multiple sclerosis: a conceptual and statistical history. *Comp Psychiat* 1990; 31(5):438–446.

169. Arbuse DI. Psychotic manifestations in disseminated sclerosis. *J Mt Sinai Hosp* 1938; Nov/Dec:403–410.

170. Sugar C, Nadell R. Mental symptoms in multiple sclerosis. *J Nerv Ment Dis* 1943; 98:267–280

171. Borberg NC, Zahle V. On the psychopathology of disseminated sclerosis. *Acta Psychol Neurol* 1946; 21:75–89.

172. Pratt RTC. An investigation of the psychiatric aspects of disseminated sclerosis. *J Neurol Neurosurg Psychiatry* 1951; 14:326–335.

173. Rabins PV. Euphoria in multiple sclerosis. In: Jensen K, Knudsen L, Stenager LE, Grant I (eds.). *Mental disorders and cognitive deficits in multiple sclerosis*. London: John Libbey, 1989:119–120.

174. Stenager E. Historical and psychiatric aspects of multiple sclerosis. *Acta Psychiat Scand* 1991; 84:398

175. Rao SM, Leo GJ, Ellington I, et al. Cognitive dysfunction in MS. *Neurology* 1991; 41:I, 692–696; II, 685–691.

176. Beevor CE. *Diseases of the nervous system.* London: H. K. Lewis, 1898:272–278.

177. Russell JSR. Disseminate sclerosis. In: Albutt TC (ed.). *A system of medicine.* London: Macmillan & Co., 1899:7:52–53, 90.

178. Buzzard EF. The treatment of disseminated sclerosis: A Suggestion. *Lancet* 1911; 1:98.

179. Denny-Brown D. Multiple sclerosis: The clinical problem. *Am J Med* 1952; 12:501–509.

180. Alexander L. Minutes of the Medical Advisory Board, National Multiple Sclerosis Society, 1949.

181. Shevell MI. Neurology's witness to history: Part II. Leo Alexander's contributions to the Nuremberg Code (1946 to 1947). *Neurology* 1998; 50:274–278.

182. Yudkin PL, Ellison GW, Ghezzi A, et al. Overview of azathioprine treatment in multiple sclerosis. *Lancet* 1991; 338:1051–1055.

183. Hauser SL, Dawson DM, Lehrich JR, et al. Intensive immunosuppression in progressive multiple sclerosis. *N Engl J Med* 1983; 308:173–180.

184. Kappos L, Patzold U, Dommasch D, et al. Cyclosporine versus azathioprine in the long term treatment of multi-

ple sclerosis: Results of the German multi-centre study. *Ann Neurol* 1988; 23:56–63.

185. Noseworthy JH, Ebers GC, Vandervoort MK, et al. The impact of binding on the results of a randomized, placebo-controlled multiple sclerosis clinical trial. *Neurology* 1994; 44:16–20.

186. Devereux C, Troiano R, Zito G, et al. Effect of total lymphoid irradiation on functional status in chronic multiple sclerosis: importance of lymphopenia early after treatment—the pros. *Neurology* 1988; 38(2):32–37.

187. Noseworthy JH, Ebers GC, Gent M. The Canadian cooperative trial of cyclophosphamide and plasma-exchange in progressive multiple sclerosis. *Lancet* 1991; 337:441–446.

188. Issacs A, Lindenmann J. Virus interference I: The interferon. *Proc Roy Soc Lond* 1957; 147:258–267.

189. Nagano Y, Kojima Y. Inhibition de l'infection vaccinale par un facteur liquide dans le tissu infect par le virus homologue. *C R Soc Biol* 1958; 152:1627–1627.

190. Pfeffer LM, Constantinescu SN. The molecular biology of interferon-ß from receptor binding to transmembrane signalling. In: Reder AT (ed.). *Interferon therapy of multiple sclerosis.* New York: Marcel Dekker, 1997:1–39.

191. Jacobs L, O'Malley J, Freedman A, Ekes R. Intrathecal interferon reduces exacerbations of multiple sclerosis. *Science* 1981; 214:1026–1028.

192. Jacobs L, O'Malley J, Freedman A, Ekes R. Intrathecal interferon in multiple sclerosis. *Arch Neurol* 1982; 39:609–615.

193. Knobler RL. Interferon beta-1b (Betaseron) treatment of multiple sclerosis. In: Reder AT (ed.). *Interferon therapy of multiple sclerosis.* New York: Marcel Dekker, 1997:353–413.

194. Jacobs L, Cookfair DL, Rudick RA, et al. A phase III trial of intramuscular recombinant interferon beta for exacerbating-remitting multiple sclerosis: design and conduct of study; baseline characteristics of patients. *Multiple Sclerosis* 1995; 1:118–135.

195. Johnson KP. The historical development of interferons as multiple sclerosis therapies. *J Mol Med* 1997; 75(2):89–94.

196. Arnon R. The development of Cop I (Copaxone), an innovative drug for the treatment of multiple sclerosis: Personal reflections. *Immunol Lett* 1996; 50:1–15.

197. Swank R, Lerstad O, Ström A, Backer J. Multiple sclerosis in rural Norway: Its geographic and occupational incidence in relation to nutrition. *N Engl J Med* 1952; 246:721–728.

198. Crane JE. Treatment of multiple sclerosis with fat-soluble vitamins, animal fat and ammonium chloride. *Connecticut State Med J* 1950; 14:40.

199. Agranoff BWA, Goldberg D. Diet and the geographical distribution of multiple sclerosis. *Lancet* 1974; 2:1061–1066.

200. Alter M, Yamoor M, Harshe M. Multiple sclerosis and nutrition. *Arch Neurol* 1974; 31:267–272.

201. Nanji AA, Narod S. Multiple sclerosis, latitude and dietary fat: Is pork the missing link? *Med Hypotheses* 1986; 20:279–282.

202. Malosse D, Perron H, Sasco A, Seigneurin JM. Correlation between milk and dairy product consumption and multiple sclerosis prevalence: a worldwide study. *Neuroepidemiology* 1992; 11:304–312.

203. Lauer K. A factor-analytical study of the multiple-sclerosis mortality in Hesse and Baden-Wuerttemberg, Germany. *J Public Health (Weinheim)* 1993; 1:319–327.

204. Lauer K. Multiple sclerosis in relation to meat preservation in France and Switzerland. *Neuroepidemiology* 1989; 8:308–315.

205. Lauer K. The Fennoscandian focus of multiple sclerosis and dietary factors: An ecological comparison. *L'Arcispedale S. Anna* 1996; 46(Suppl):S17–S18.

206. Lauer K. A possible paradox in the immunology of multiple sclerosis: Its apparent lack of "specificity" might provide clues to the etiology. *Med Hypotheses* 1993; 40:368–374.

207. Lauer K. Diet and multiple sclerosis. *Neurology* 1997; 49:(Suppl 2)S55–S61.

207a. Sibley WA. *Therapeutic claims in multiple sclerosis.* 4th ed. New York: Demos, 1996.

208. Thomas, Richard. *Multiple sclerosis: A comprehensive guide to effective treatment.* Brisbane: Element Books Ltd., 1996 (holistic).

209. Fischer BH, Marks M, Reich T. Hyperbaric-oxygen treatment of multiple sclerosis: A Randomized, placebo-controlled, double-blind study. *N Engl J Med* 1983; 308:181–186.

210. Barnes MP, Bates D, Cartlidge NEF, et al. Hyperbaric oxygen and multiple sclerosis: Short term results of a placebo-controlled, double-blind trial. *Lancet* 1985; i:297–300.

211. Webster C, McIver C, et al. Long-term hyperbaric oxygen therapy for multiple sclerosis patients: Two year results in 128 patients. ARMS Education Service, Stanstead, UK, 1992.

II

PATHOLOGY AND PATHOPHYSIOLOGY

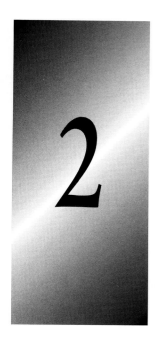

2 Pathology and Pathophysiology

Robert M. Herndon, M.D.

Multiple sclerosis (MS) is a chronic relapsing inflammatory disease of the central nervous system (CNS) of unknown etiology. Central myelin and the cells that form central myelin, the oligodendrocytes, appear to be the primary targets of attack. The disease usually does not affect peripheral myelin although there are rare cases of a disease clinically and pathologically indistinguishable from MS in which there also is peripheral demyelination in a pattern indistinguishable from chronic inflammatory demyelinating polyneuropathy. Correlation between the clinical picture and the pathologic processes in MS is far from perfect, but understanding of the pathology and pathophysiology of the disease helps to explain many of its clinical features and provides the rationale for current approaches to disease management.

ETIOLOGY

The etiology of MS is not known. The most widely believed hypothesis is that it is a virus-induced autoimmune disease, but the possibility of its being a primary infectious process with an associated immune reaction has not been entirely ruled out despite repeated failure to identify a causative agent. Over the past four decades there have been repeated reports of virus-like particles

in brain tissue from MS patients and of virus isolation from the brains of MS patients, but it has never been possible to clearly demonstrate a connection between any of these agents and the disease process. The demonstration of herpesviruses, particularly 1, 2, and 6, in a significant proportion of MS plaques over the past few years (1,2,3), evidence that the antiherpes drug acyclovir will reduce the number of attacks of MS (4), and more recently evidence for chlamydial infection (5) have renewed interest in infectious hypotheses. Only time will tell if any of these agents play a role in disease causation. The report of a patient with MS developing acute optic neuritis two months after an allogenic bone marrow transplant for chronic myelogenous leukemia suggests that it is not purely an autoimmune disease (6).

Extensive effort has gone into the attempt to understand the role of the immune system in MS. Much of this effort has been directed at understanding the immunology of experimental autoimmune encephalomyelitis (EAE). This work has taught us an enormous amount regarding immunology in general and immunology as it applies to the human CNS. A good deal of effort has gone into attempts to apply what has been learned about EAE in MS, but most attempts have been unsuccessful making it clear that MS is not simply EAE. On the other hand, it is also clear that autoimmunity is involved in the disease and immunomodulaters such as the beta interferons, glatiramer acetate, and immunosuppressant drugs such as methotrexate can slow the disease process.

STRUCTURE OF CENTRAL MYELIN

Knowledge of the structure of CNS myelin and identification of the oligodendrocyte as the myelin-forming cell is a rather recent development. The layered structure of myelin was identified through X-ray diffraction in the 1930s, and there was conjecture that oligodendrocytes were responsible for forming myelin. It was not until the late 1950s that it was shown to be a spirally wrapped membrane. Arguments over the nature of the spiral wrapping and whether more than one oligodendrocyte contributed to a given internode, or indeed which cell was the myelin-forming cell, continued into the 1960s. It was finally clearly established by Peters (7) that each central myelin internode is a continuously wrapped membrane arising from a single oligodendrocyte process. The structure of central myelin is shown schematically in Figure 2-1.

A central myelin internodal segment is produced by an oligodendrocyte in contact with and in cooperation with

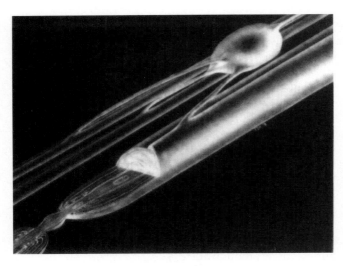

FIGURE 2-1

Artist's illustration of the relationship of an oligodendrocyte to the central myelin sheath and central node. Given the angle of the connection between the oligodendrocyte process and the sheath, it would be impossible to show by electron microscopy in a cross section of the sheath. This explains the historical difficulty in demonstrating that oligodendrocytes were the myelin-forming cell. In larger fibers, there is a marked constriction at the paranode, not seen in small fibers. The slight bulge of nodal membrane shown is common but is not always seen. Not shown is the astrocyte process, which typically abuts the nodal area.

an axon. Peripheral myelin is produced by Schwann cells interacting with peripheral axons. Myelin forms a sheath around most CNS axons with a diameter greater than 2.5μ. Occasionally smaller axons down to 1 diameter are myelinated. The central myelin sheath is a cytoplasmic extension of an oligodendrocyte in an obligatory anatomic, physiologic, and metabolic relationship with an axon. The nature of the signaling between the axon and the myelin-forming cell that leads to myelin formation is poorly understood, but myelin membranes do not normally form in the absence of axons. If the axon is severed, Wallerian degeneration ensues and the myelin disintegrates.

For normal fibers of a given diameter, the myelin sheath has uniform thickness and myelin segments between nodes of Ranvier (internodal segments) are of uniform length except near the end of the fiber, where internodes become progressively shorter. Each internodal segment ends in a complex specialized paranodal structure, which is separated from the next paranode by a very short segment of highly specialized nodal membrane. The internodes range in length from a few tens of microns in the smallest fibers to up to 1–2 mm in the largest fibers. One oligodendrocyte usually forms internodal segments on a number of different fibers. In the rat a single oligodendrocyte may form 20 to 40 internodal segments in the optic nerve (8) and 18 to 60 internodal segments in the spinal cord (9). This differs markedly from the peripheral nervous system, where one Schwann cell contributes myelin to only one internodal segment. This difference may, in part, account for the greater efficiency of regeneration in peripheral myelin.

If unrolled, myelin would appear as a thin oligodendrocyte process terminating in a large, flat, trapezoidal, membranous expansion with the cytoplasm of the expansion squeezed out to the edges to form a narrow rim and the cytoplasmic surfaces of the two membranes fused over most of their surface (10,11). This fused area in cross section appears as the major dense line of compact myelin. When wrapped around an axon, the outer surfaces of the oligodendrocyte plasmalemma come into contact, forming the minor period (intra- or interperiod) line. In the paranodal region, the oligodendrocyte cytoplasm forms a continuous spiral connecting the outer loop of the myelin sheath to the innermost loop, thus maintaining cytoplasmic continuity between the oligodendrocyte soma and the innermost layer of myelin. The paranodal loops are bound to each other and to the axon by tight junctions (transverse bands), which limit diffusion of extracellular material into the periaxonal space.

The nodes of Ranvier are composed of a short segment of specialized axonal or "nodal" membrane between the paranodal loops of two adjacent internodal segments of myelin. In large fibers, the fiber diameter is constricted by as much as 50 percent in the paranodal and nodal regions (11). In small fibers, there may be no change in fiber diameter at the node. When examined at high magnifications under the electron microscope, the nodal membrane is seen to have a dense undercoating (12) that has a tripartite structure (13) and specific staining characteristics (14). This region has a high concentration of sodium channels, and on freeze-fracture preparations they appear to correspond to E-face particles that are concentrated in the nodal membrane (15). Early estimates of sodium channel numbers in peripheral axons based on saxitoxin binding studies and the assumption that sodium channels were confined to axons ranged from less than $1,000/\mu2$ to $18,000/\mu2$ in mammalian axons (16,17,18). More recently it has been shown that there are significant numbers of sodium channels in Schwann cells, and the assumption that sodium channels were not present in the Schwann cells had caused these erroneously high estimates. Current estimates for sodium channels in nodal membrane are $1,000–2,000/\mu2$ (19). The high concentration of voltage-sensitive sodium channels is needed for the relatively high sodium currents required for saltatory conduction. Astrocytic processes are located adjacent to central nodes and appear to play an important role in controlling the extracellular ionic milieu (20).

There is a strong correlation between axon size and sheath thickness and between fiber thickness and internodal length (11,21). The matching of internodal length and myelin thickness to axon diameter requires local control of myelin thickness by the axon, particularly because different sized axons supplied by a single oligodendrocyte will have different myelin thickness (15). In the early stages of myelination, the oligodendrocyte processes in contact with the axon to be myelinated contain ribosomes and granular endoplasmic reticulum, but as the myelin matures, these elements decrease and virtually disappear. The region of myelin formation is at a distance from the oligodendrocyte soma. As a result, myelin synthesis in the more mature sheaths must involve transport along the oligodendroglial process analogous to axonal transport, local synthesis in the oligodendroglial process (15), local uptake of myelin constituents, or a combination of these processes.

MYELIN CHEMISTRY

Central myelin is composed of highly modified oligodendrocyte plasmalemma. Lipids make up 80 percent of the dry weight of myelin, with proteins constituting most of the remainder. Many of these proteins and lipids are peculiar to central myelin. Inborn errors of both protein and lipid metabolism can affect myelin formation and degradation and account for a number of hereditary myelin disorders, including adrenoleukodystrophy, a peroxisomal disorder that affects fatty acid metabolism; Pelizaeus-Merzbacher disease, a disorder of proteolipid protein metabolism; and metachromatic leukodystrophy, a disorder of sulfatide metabolism. There is no convincing evidence that metabolic abnormalities contribute to MS.

Myelin Proteins

Proteolipid protein (PLP), myelin basic protein (MBP), and their isoforms make up 80 percent to 90 percent of the protein, with relatively minor proteins, including 2',3' cyclic nucleotide 3' phosphohydrolase (CNPase), myelin associated glycoprotein (MAG), myelin oligodendrocyte protein (MOG), and the Wolfgram proteins, making up most of the rest. Neither PLP nor CNPase is present in significant quantities in peripheral myelin. Myelin basic protein is much less abundant in peripheral myelin, constituting only about 10 percent of peripheral myelin protein (22). MAG and MOG constitute approximately 1 percent of the total of CNS myelin protein. CNPase appears near the onset of myelination and is associated with myelin, so it is generally considered a "myelin protein" but is found primarily in uncompacted oligodendrocyte processes.

Proteolipid protein is a phylogenetically highly conserved, acylated, transmembrane protein with two alternative forms. It mediates compaction of the intraperiod line. It has two forms with molecular weights of 25 kD and 20 kD. The former is known as proteolipid protein and the latter as DM20. Proteolipid protein is acylated with fatty acids. Palmitic, oleic, and stearic acids make up approximately 2 percent of its weight. It is synthesized by the granular endoplasmic reticulum and subsequently acylated near its site of insertion into the myelin membrane (24). Defects in the PLP gene are responsible for Pelizaeus-Merzbacher disease. Both MBP and PLP can be used to induce EAE, a commonly used experimental animal model used to study immunologic demyelination.

Myelin basic protein is actually a family of proteins constituting 20 percent to 30 percent of central myelin protein. They arise from seven axons, with several alternative splicings resulting in at least six isoforms, which differ in internal deletions and range from 14 to 21 kD in size. Myelin basic protein is found on the cytoplasmic surface of the myelin membrane and mediates compaction of the major dense line (22,24). Additionally, some of the isoforms appear to localize within the sheath with 17 kDa and 21.5 kDa isoforms concentrated in the interlamellar junctions (radial component). Thus the isoforms are probably not interchangeable (25).

Despite its enzymatic capabilities, CNPase appears to function in central myelin as a structural protein. It is found in the noncompacted regions of the oligodendrocyte membrane. There is no substrate for the enzyme in myelin, and it makes up too high a proportion of the total myelin protein to be there for enzymatic purposes. It is thought possibly to serve as an anchor for cytoskeletal elements (26).

Myelin Lipids

Lipids, including some unique lipids, constitute 80 percent of the dry weight of myelin. Some of these lipids are supplied by the oligodendrocyte, but some appear to come from the axon. During the early development of neurochemistry it was widely held that the major lipids in neurons and axons consisted of gangliosides, whereas cholesterol, sphingomyelin, and cerebrosides (including sulfatides) were characteristic of myelin. DeVries and colleagues demonstrated that phospholipids, cholesterol, and galactolipids (both cerebrosides and sulfatides) constitute 13 percent of the dry weight of axonal content (27). Neurons have been shown by Benjamins and coworkers to be able to synthesize sulfatide (28). What had originally been thought to be characteristic myelin lipids exist in the axon as well. Neurons and axons are known to contain large amounts of gangliosides, so their possible role in myelinogenesis has been closely examined. Brady and Quarles noted that ganglioside turnover is maximal just before myelination and the concentration of gangliosides is highly enriched in the plasma cell membrane, suggesting that these compounds may be involved in cell-to-cell interactions (29). They also suggested that the ganglioside pattern of the oligodendroglia is modified when myelination occurs.

When myelin is first deposited and during remyelination, it has a shorter chain fatty acid pattern different from that of mature adult myelin. During maturation the fatty acids of both nonmyelin and myelin lipids undergo various changes in composition, one of which is an increase in the average chain length. Thus it is possible that the shorter chain fatty acids present in gangliosides become incorporated into cerebrosides and sulfatides very early, even before myelination begins, and that the longer chains found in the sulfatides represent maturation. When 14C-fatty acids are injected into brain, they are rapidly transformed into long chain, more highly unsaturated derivatives (30). Cholesterol esters containing a high proportion of C16-fatty acids accumulate in human premyelinating cells. These esters may serve as intermediaries as well as donors in the intracellular transport of fatty acids when lipogenesis is maximal. The onset of myelination is linked to an increase in cholesterol esterase activity; thus cholesterol esters may be an important source of fatty acid for the synthesis of a variety of complex lipids (31). Cholesterol esters appear before the onset of active myelination, and, because they also occur during the breakdown of nervous tissues, they are presumably carriers of fatty acids during myelin biosynthesis and degradation.

Traditionally oligodendroglia were believed to be entirely responsible for the synthesis of myelin lipids, and cerebrosides and sulfatides in particular. It is now clear that neuronal elements have an important role in galactosphingolipid metabolism. Isolated neuronal perikarya and axons can synthesize both galactocerebroside and glucocerebroside from ceramide and UDP-galactose. Cerebroside sulfotransferase is present in cat neurons, its activity increases during myelination, and sulfatide synthesis has been demonstrated in mouse brain neurons.

Many important steps in the biochemical sequences of myelinogenesis remain unknown. What have been considered the characteristic lipids of myelin—cerebrosides and sulfatides—can be found in and synthesized by neurons and axons. The richness of the gangliosides in the axonal membrane coming directly in contact with the myelin sheath has lead to the hypothesis that axons make direct biochemical contributions to the formation of myelin, and it is likely that this applies to remyelination as well as the initial process of myelination.

Nerve Conduction

Axoplasm has a high potassium and low sodium ion concentration relative to extracellular fluid. The different ion concentrations are maintained by the sodium-potassium pump, which exchanges intracellular sodium for extracellular potassium. The axonal membrane in the resting state is permeable to potassium but relatively impermeable to sodium ions, allowing potassium to leak out of the axon down its concentration gradient. The leakage of positively charged potassium ions out of the axon results in a net negative charge in the axoplasm relative to the extracellular fluid. At equilibrium, the tendency of potassium to diffuse out of the nerve fiber because of the concentration gradient is just balanced by the negative charge in the axoplasm, which attracts the positively charged potassium ions. The electrical potential at equilibrium is approximately −70 mV. The ionic gradients between the intracellular and extracellular fluid are the immediate source of energy for the action potential. The difference in ion concentration is adequate to allow continued conduction of hundreds or even thousands of impulses in the absence of active metabolism. Poisoning of the sodium-potassium pump will cause conduction failure only after repeated impulse conduction has decreased ionic gradients to a point at which they are insufficient to repolarize the membrane.

In unmyelinated fibers, sodium channels are distributed over the surface of the axon with a density of approximately 110 per $5\mu^2$ (32). The voltage-sensitive sodium channels open when the membrane potential drops from its resting level of −70 mV to approximately −30 mV, permitting a rapid influx of sodium ions with further depolarization of the membrane. This depolarizes adjacent membrane, opening additional sodium channels and allowing a wave of depolarization to move along the fiber. A fraction of a millisecond after the channel opens, a second gate in the channel closes, which blocks further sodium influx. The membrane is repolarized by continuing movement of potassium out of the axoplasm. With repolarization, the gates in the sodium channels reset, preparing the axon for another impulse. Thus the action potential is a wave of depolarization and repolarization passing down the axon. Conduction velocity in mammalian unmyelinated fibers is approximately 0.5–2 meters per second. There is a brief period of inexcitability following an impulse, the absolute refractory period. This is followed by a period of decreased excitability, the relative refractory period, as the membrane completes the process of repolarization.

In myelinated fibers the sodium channels are largely restricted to the nodal membrane, the concentration in internodal membrane being orders of magnitude lower. Aside from their distribution, the sodium channels have characteristics similar to those in unmyelinated fibers and open as depolarization approaches –30 mV. The sodium current passing inward through the nodal membrane during depolarization flows down the axon to depolarize and activate the next node, which in large axons may be up to 2 mm away. The current from the node can accomplish this because, as a result of the myelin, little current needs to be expended in discharging capacitative charge on the internodal membrane. The rate of conduction is much faster because little time is required to discharge the small membrane capacitance in the myelinated fiber and the current passes down the axon much more rapidly. The longitudinal resistance of the axoplasm, which is proportional to axonal cross-sectional area, thus becomes the main limiting factor in conduction velocity (20).

PATHOLOGY OF MULTIPLE SCLEROSIS

The pathology of MS consists of lesions disseminated in location and varying in age, as would be expected from the clinical features. Lesions are present in both white matter and gray matter, but the gray matter lesions are less evident on casual inspection because of the relatively small amount of myelin present. The lesions occur in different parts of the CNS and are in different stages of activity or maturity. Lesions range from acute plaques with active inflammatory infiltrates and macrophages loaded with lipid and myelin degeneration products through various degrees of lesser activity to chronic, inactive, demyelinated glial scars.

There appear to be two very different patterns of pathology, both of which may occur in the same individual (33). The first and best-known consists of multifocal discrete inflammatory demyelinating lesions. These occur in both white matter and gray matter and often involve both. When small, a perivenular distribution is usually apparent, and they have a predilection for periventricular white matter. The second pattern of demyelination is less dramatic but more common. It consists of diffusely scattered demyelination involving individual fibers or small groups of fibers interspersed with normal appearing myelinated fibers. This type of demyelination is accompanied by much more limited, diffuse inflammatory infiltrates. The former pattern is typical of relapsing-remitting MS and is more common in younger patients; the latter is characteristic of the chronic progressive pattern typically seen in older patients. A combination of both patterns is characteristic of secondary progressive MS. In these patients, old, inactive, scarred, multifocal lesions coexist with progressive diffuse demyelination.

The MS plaque appears to begin with margination and diapedesis of lymphocytes and macrophages forming perivascular cuffs about capillaries and venules. This is followed by diffuse parenchymal infiltration by inflammatory cells, edema, astrocytic hyperplasia, macrophage activity stripping myelin from axons, and the appearance of increased numbers of lipid-laden macrophages and demyelinated axons (34). As plaques enlarge and coalesce, the initial perivenular distribution of the lesions becomes less apparent. The inflammatory reaction usually is less pronounced in gray matter, probably because of the smaller amount of myelin in these areas and correspondingly fewer macrophages needed to remove it.

The extent of axonal loss in the demyelinated areas is highly variable but is usually substantial (35). The sparing of axons is relative and some axonal loss occurs in almost all lesions (Figure 2-2). Cumulative axonal loss from long tracts where there may be several plaques along their course can be substantial. It is important to recognize that axonal loss is an important factor in MS and experimental efforts to improve conduction in surviving fibers will not affect those symptoms that are caused by axonal loss, even though they may produce dramatic improvement in symptoms that result from conduction failure in surviving axons.

Immunocytochemical studies have shown the inflammatory cells in the actively demyelinating central area of acute plaques to be mainly Ia-positive cells. The Ia-positive cells are mostly macrophages with few T cells and antibody-producing plasma cells. The T cells in the acute plaque are a mixture of T4+ (helper-inducer) and T8+ (suppressor/cytotoxic) lymphocytes and are more numerous near the center of the plaque, diminishing in numbers peripherally. As the lesion enlarges, T cells become relatively more numerous peripherally, whereas macrophages take their place centrally. T4+ cells invade

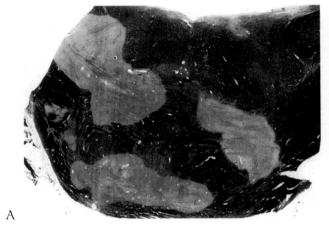

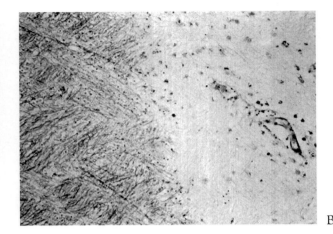

FIGURE 2-2

Pathology of MS. A. Myelin-stained section of pons showing three large plaques of demyelination. B, C. Photomicrographs of the edge of an MS plaque. B. Luxol fast blue myelin stain, note the loss of myelin in the right half of the section. C. Adjacent section with a nerve fiber (Bodian) stain. Note the decrease in the density of the nerve fibers in the demyelinated area indicating significant fiber loss in addition to the loss of myelin.

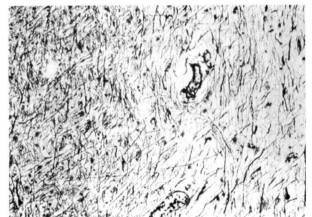

the normal appearing white matter around the lesion, whereas the T8+ cells are largely confined to the plaque margins and perivascular cuffs. The plaque margins contain increased numbers of oligodendrocytes as well as astrocytes and inflammatory cells (36–38). As the lesions become more mature, myelin remnants and macrophages progressively disappear from the central part of the plaque, which eventually becomes a gliotic scar. At the plaque margin, a hypercellular "glial wall" contains lymphocytes, oligodendrocytes, and a few macrophages and astrocytes. In many instances the disease process appears to continue, with low-grade activity at the plaque margins, manifested by lipid-laden macrophages and lymphocytes, often accompanied by a few thin perivascular cuffs. In chronically active MS, inflammatory cells are scattered in small numbers throughout much of the normal appearing white matter. These include T4+, T8+, and Ia+ cells. They probably are involved in the diffuse, slowly progressive demyelination described by Lumsden (33).

Chronic inactive MS plaques have a sharply demarcated border with little if any hypercellularity. Occasional

T4+ and Ia+ cells are scattered through the lesions. At the edges a few T4+, T8+, and Ia+ cells, including macrophages and B-lymphocytes, may be seen and these also occur in small numbers throughout the otherwise normal appearing white matter.

Plaquelike areas of very pale myelin staining are a frequent occurrence in many cases of MS. On examination these areas have increased cellularity and abnormally thin myelin sheaths of relatively uniform thickness. The thickness of the myelin about individual axons in these "shadow plaques" bears no relationship to fiber diameter as it does in normally myelinated areas. Some investigators have regarded these "shadow plaques" as evidence of partial demyelination, but it is now clear that they represent areas of remyelination (34). Until the late 1950s it was believed that remyelination did not occur and that oligodendroglia, like neurons, were end-stage cells incapable of regeneration. Since Bunge and coworkers (39) first unequivocally demonstrated central remyelination in the cat in 1958, remyelination has been shown to occur in the CNS in essentially every species tested, including tadpole, mouse, rat, guinea pig, rabbit, cat, and dog (40). The characteristics of the shadow plaque are virtually identical to those of remyelinated areas in experimental animals. They include (1) an increased number of oligodendrocytes, which, contrary to traditional views, are capable of proliferation (41,42); (2) thin myelin sheaths of relatively uniform thickness; and (3) short internodes. The alternative possibility that shadow plaques arise from partial demyelination seems unlikely because partial demyelination has been convincingly demonstrated only during the acute phase of the demyelinating process or when mechanical pressure is continually present. There is abundant evidence for remyelination in experimental animals and man, and the appearance of shadow plaques strongly suggests that they represent areas of remyelination (40).

Regeneration of central myelin is often accompanied by Schwann cell invasion of the CNS and consequently the presence of peripheral myelin within the demyelinated area (43). Schwann cells occur in small numbers in normal spinal cord, but it is uncertain whether they come from peripheral nerves innervating CNS blood vessels or occur independent of blood vessels. In pathologic conditions most of the Schwann cell remyelination within CNS occurs near root entry or exit zones. Breaches in the glial limitans caused by the demyelinating process allow Schwann cells in the nerve roots or in autonomic nerves accompanying cerebral blood vessels to migrate to the central white matter, where they retain their capability to form myelin.

With progression of the pathologic process, demyelination at the plaque margins causes slow enlargement of the plaques. Over time, demyelination of newly remyelinated areas may result in scarring so that further remyelination cannot occur and the plaque becomes a hypocellular glial scar. Shadow plaques are thus more likely to be seen on autopsy examination of younger patients with continued active remitting disease (44) and are much less common in older patients with inactive disease or with chronically active, indolent disease progression. In most cases the end result is a nervous system riddled with chronically scarred, relatively inactive plaques and a considerable amount of Wallerian degeneration resulting in pallor of long tracts in myelin-stained preparations.

Despite a number of reports of "virus-like particles" seen by electron microscopy of MS biopsy and postmortem material (45,46,47), credible morphologic evidence for the presence of true virions has not been reported. Dense bodies surrounded by a membrane have been seen intracellularly, mainly in macrophages, in proximity to actively demyelinating areas. These are of variable size, do not closely resemble any particular virus or class of viruses, and are generally regarded as myelin breakdown products. A number of other investigators beginning with Prineas (45) reported "paramyxovirus-like" tubules in the nuclei of inflammatory cells in MS plaques. These consist of strands of 18–20 nm intranuclear filaments or tubules. In size and appearance, they bear a resemblance to the nucleocapsid of paramyxoviruses. They have been seen in a variety of conditions, including normal tissues fixed under acidic conditions, and appear to be chromatin strands, which have an altered appearance due to the metabolic state of the cell or conditions of tissue fixation (48).

Using newer techniques of polymerase chain reaction (PCR), representational difference analysis, in situ hybridization, and immunocytochemical techniques, viruses are frequently found in MS plaques. The effort to tie viruses found in brain to the disease process has failed thus far. The viruses of greatest interest are the herpesviruses. These viruses are found latent in nervous tissue, are activated by other viral infections, just as new attacks of MS frequently follow viral infection, and could theoretically activate an inflammatory process in the nervous system, resulting in a new attack of MS. Challoner and colleagues (1) reported the detection of human herpesvirus 6 (HHV-6) in MS brain using PCR and representational difference analysis followed by localization in plaques using immunocytochemistry. Subsequently Sanders and coworkers (2) detected several herpesviruses in brain tissue (Table 2-1). Although several were more common in MS brains and more common in MS plaques, the differences did not reach statistical significance. Nothing in this work indicates an etiologic relationship to MS but the presence of latent viruses, which are easily activated in plaques, suggests that they could contribute to the pathology.

CONDUCTION IN DEMYELINATED AND REMYELINATED FIBERS

The occurrence of conduction in demyelinated fibers was inferred by Charcot in 1877 from the fact that patients with considerable residual vision just before death were found on postmortem examination to have completely demyelinated optic nerves. During the process of demyelination, conduction failure is probably invariable in the affected fibers. Clinically silent lesions probably occur when demyelination affects a minority of fibers in a pathway at any one time, leaving intact conduction in other fibers. The causes of conduction failure during demyelination are not completely understood but may include (1) damage to the nodal sodium channel (49,50), (2) virtual absence of sodium channels from the internodal membrane (16), and (3) increased membrane capacitance in the demyelinated region (20). The role if any of alterations in the extracellular fluid composition in the inflamed area is unclear.

TABLE 2-1
Viruses in MS Brain Detected by Polymerase Chain Reaction

Virus	MS Brain Plaque	Active Plaque	Inactive Brain	Control
Herpes simplex	37%	41%	20%	28%
HHV-6	57%	32%	17%	43%
Varicella zoster	43%	14%	10%	32%
Epstein-Barr	27%	5%	10%	38%
Cytomegalovirus	16%	9%	10%	22%

There is reasonably good evidence that the nodal membrane is damaged by lysolipids generated from myelin by enzymes present in the inflammatory exudate. Various enzymes are released by inflammatory cells, including a variety of proteases, lipases, neuraminidase, phosphatases, and glycosidases. Of these, phospholipase appears to produce the most rapid and extensive damage to myelin. Phospholipase also specifically destroys sodium channels, as measured by saxitoxin binding (49,50). Proteases alone appear to cause relatively little damage, probably because membrane proteins are inaccessible to the enzyme; however, in the presence of lipases, membrane proteins may become accessible to proteases, which can then further damage the membrane.

The internodal membrane normally contains very few sodium channels (11,51). Indeed, if sodium channels of a myelinated fiber were evenly distributed over the length of the fiber, the density would be much less than half that in most unmyelinated fibers and would be too few to support conduction (18). For continuous conduction to develop in a demyelinated axon, additional sodium channels must be inserted into the axonal membrane. This is a prerequisite for the restoration of continuous conduction along a demyelinated fiber but alone will not ensure that conduction will occur. Whether the newly inserted sodium channels in the demyelinated membrane are identical to those normally present or have altered kinetics has not been determined but clearly they are able to support continuous conduction.

Increased membrane capacitance and the resulting increase in capacitive charge on the demyelinated axolemma results in an increase in the amount of current required to depolarize the membrane to threshold. The current, which must pass down the axon from the myelinated region, is normally insufficient to discharge the demyelinated membrane to threshold. This can be most easily understood if you regard the axolemma and myelin as the dielectric of a tubular capacitor, with the extracellular fluid and axoplasm serving as the plates (Figure 2-3). Because capacitance is inversely proportional to the distance between the two plates of a capacitor, the capacitance of a demyelinated fiber is many times that of a myelinated fiber, where numerous layers of myelin membrane separate the axoplasm and the extracellular space.

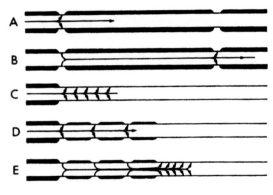

FIGURE 2-3

Diagram illustrating the problem with nerve conduction in demyelinated fibers. A. Impulse coming from the left depolarizes the first node. B. Sodium channels have opened and the inward sodium current is passing down the fiber to depolarize the next node. C. The current passing down the fiber reaches a demyelinated segment. The large capacitative charge on the relatively large area of unmyelinated membrane of the demyelinated fiber prevents the small current from bringing the membrane to threshold. Additionally, in the acute stage, there would be too few sodium channels in the demyelinated segment to support continuous conduction. D. Remyelination has occurred at the plaque margin. This allows several closely spaced nodes to depolarize almost simultaneously. E. The current from the closely spaced nodes summates to bring the demyelinated membrane to threshold. During the recovery period additional sodium channels have been added to the demyelinated membrane, and once it reaches threshold continuous conduction can now occur but at a much reduced velocity and with a much reduced safety margin for conduction.

The current passing along the last myelinated segment to a demyelinated segment comes mainly from the last node, which is as much as 1–2 mm away. This is normally insufficient to depolarize the demyelinated membrane to threshold. Thus conduction fails at the junction of the myelinated and demyelinated segments even if the number of sodium channels in the demyelinated membrane has increased enough to support continuous conduction. In the electrophysiologic literature, this conduction problem is termed *impedance mismatch*.

Conduction block caused by impedance mismatch can be overcome in two ways. First, membrane capacitance can be decreased by increasing the distance between the two "plates" of the capacitor. This is accomplished by remyelination and is an effective and important mechanism both in experimental animals and in humans. Additionally, the sodium current can be increased enough to discharge the additional capacitative charge on the demyelinated membrane. This is also an important mechanism and is also dependent on remyelination.

In preterminal axons there is a need to increase the sodium current to depolarize the rather large unmyelinated membrane area of the terminal. This is accomplished by an anatomic arrangement in which the last few internodes are much shorter than normal, allowing a summation of current from several adjacent nodes (52). Similarly, in demyelinated fibers the sodium current can be increased by decreasing the distance between nodes just proximal to the area of demyelination. New myelin regenerated at the plaque margins has such very short internodes. This allows summation of current from several nodes, which may discharge the added capacitance of the demyelinated membrane, permitting continuous conduction in the demyelinated segment. This results in considerable energy expenditure because the increased intracellular sodium that enters through the additional channels must eventually be pumped out by the sodium-potassium pump. Nevertheless, this will restore conduction through the demyelinated segment, albeit with markedly decreased safety margin for conduction, prolonged refractory period, and conduction failure with heavy impulse traffic.

Conduction in demyelinated central fibers is suboptimal (52). Experimental studies of demyelinated fibers show temperature sensitivity such that a rise in temperature of as little as 0.5°C above normal will cause conduction failure in some fibers (53). The increased influx of sodium that occurs as a result of increased number of nodes and sodium channels at the plaque margin and in the demyelinated segments is another important factor that leads to rapid nerve fiber fatigue with conduction failure. Demyelinated fibers have a poor ability to conduct trains of impulses, in part because of an increased refractory period in the demyelinated segment. In addition, studies in experimentally demyelinated fibers have

demonstrated a progressive reduction in longitudinal current amplitude followed by conduction block, which Sears and Bostock (54) attribute to an increase in intracellular sodium. The capacity of the sodium pump is soon saturated by the increased sodium influx. These and other features of demyelinated and partially remyelinated fibers help explain some of the features of motor fatigability and activity-related failure of neurologic function that are clinically prominent in MS.

Slowed conduction and conduction failure in demyelinated fibers have been well demonstrated in MS in the form of delays in and loss of evoked potentials. This has important clinical consequences. Delayed and degraded feedback from proprioceptors accounts for much of the imbalance and tremor in MS. In some patients this results in an inability to monitor arm or leg position concurrently with the movement so that force cannot be adjusted to the demand of the task. This results in inaccurate movement and terminal tremor, often described as cerebellar but actually caused by problems related to delayed proprioceptive feedback. Conduction failure that is due to nerve fiber fatigue or to an increase in body temperature, or both, accounts for many of the limitations in activity, such as walking, that MS patients experience.

SUMMARY

Multiple sclerosis is an inflammatory demyelinating disorder of unknown but most likely infectious and/or autoimmune origin. Much of the permanent disability results from axonal destruction, which falls most heavily on very long pathways such as the pyramidal tract supplying the legs and the dorsal columns carrying sensory information from the legs. These long pathways take multiple hits over the years, with increasing axonal destruction leading to the loss of lower extremity function that is so common in advanced MS. Other aspects of the disease, such as incoordination and imbalance, are due to delayed and degraded information resulting from slowed conduction of proprioceptive information and the inability to monitor, on line, motor processes caused by conduction delays and signal dispersion occurring as the signals pass through demyelinated areas. Transient loss of function with fever and with fatigue, including Uhthoff's phenomenon (recurrence of scotoma during exercise), is attributable to conduction failure in demyelinated fibers, which fatigue rapidly and fail with an increase in temperature. Every attack, even subclinical attacks, cause some permanent damage, and it is the accumulation of damage from repeated demyelinating episodes that accounts for most of the long-term disability. It is this progressive accumulation of damage that provides the best rationale for early use of disease-altering therapies.

References

1. Challoner PB, Smith KT, Parker JD, et al. Plaque-associated expression of human herpesvirus 6 in multiple sclerosis. *Proc Nat Acad Sci USA* 1995; 92:7440–7444.

2. Sanders VJ, Felisan S, Waddell A, Tourtellotte WW. Detection of herpesvirdae in postmortem multiple sclerosis brain tissue and controls by polymerase chain reaction. *J Neurovirol* 1996; 2:249–258.

3. Weiner LP, Shubin RA, Fleming JO. Mechanisms of virus-induced demyelination and the relationship to multiple sclerosis. In: Herndon RM, Seil FJ (eds.). *Multiple sclerosis: Current status of research and treatment.* New York: Demos, 1994:67–78

4. Lycke J, Svennerholm B, Hjelmquist E, et al. Acyclovir treatment of relapsing-remitting multiple sclerosis. A randomized, placebo-controlled, double blind study. *J Neurol* 1996; 243:214–224.

5. Yao S, Sriram S, Mitchell W, Stratton C, Tharp A. CNS infection with *C. pneumoniae* in MS. *Neurology* 1998; 50(Suppl 4):A423

6. Jeffery DR, Alshami E. Allogenic bone marrow transplantation in multiple sclerosis. *Neurology* 1998; 50(Suppl 4):A147

7. Peters A. Observations on the connexions between myelin sheaths and glial cells in the optic nerves of young rats. *J Anat* 1964; 98:125–134.

8. Peters A, Proskauer CC. The ratio between myelin segments and oligodendrocytes in the optic nerve of the adult rat. *Anat Rec* 1969; 163:243.

9. Mathews MA, Duncan D. A quantitative study of the morphological changes accompanying the initiation and progress of myelin production in the dorsal funiculus of the rat spinal cord. *J Comp Neurol* 1971; 142:1–22.

10. Hirano A, Dembitzer HM: A structural analysis of the myelin sheath in the central nervous system. *J Cell Biol* 1967; 34:555–567.

11. Hirano A, Llena JF. Morphology of central nervous system axons. In: Waxman SG, Kocsis JD, Stys PK (eds.). *The axon.* New York: Oxford University Press, 1995:49–67

12. Peters A. The node of Ranvier in the central nervous system. *Q J Exp Physiol* 1966; 51:229–236.

13. Chan-Palay V. The tripartite structure of the undercoat in the initial segments of Purkinje cell axons. *Z Anat Entwicklungsgesch* 1972; 141:125–150.

14. Waxman SG, Bradley WG, Hartveig EA. Organization of axolemma in amyelinated axons: A cytochemical study in dy/dy dystrophic mice. *Proc Roy Soc Lond* (Biol) 1978; 201:301–308.

15. Black JA, Sontheimer H, Youngsuk O, Waxman SG. The oligodendrocyte, the perinodal astrocyte, and the central node of Ranvier. In: Waxman SG, Kocsis JD, Stys PK (eds.). *The axon.* New York: Oxford University Press, 1995:116–143

16. Ritchie JM, Rogart RB. Density of sodium channels in mammalian myelinated nerve fibers and nature of the axonal membrane under the myelin sheath. *Proc Natl Acad Sci* 1977; 74:211–215.

17. Neumcke B, Stampfli R. Conductance and number of Na+ channels in rat myelinated nerve fibers. *Physiol Soc Proc* 1982:69.

18. Querfurth HW, Armstrong R, Herndon RM. Sodium channels in normal and regenerated feline ventral spinal roots. *J Neurosci* 1987; 7:1705–1716.

19. Howe JR, Ritchie JM. Sodium currents in Schwann cells from myelinated and non-myelinated nerves of neonatal and adult rabbits. *J Physiol* 1990; 425:169–210.

20. Waxman SG. Voltage-gated ion channels in axons: Localization, function and development. In: Waxman SG, Kocsis JD, Stys PK (eds.). *The axon.* New York: Oxford University Press, 1995:218–243

21. Berthold C-H, Rydmark M. Morphology of normal peripheral axons. In: Waxman SG, Kocsis JD, Stys PK (eds.). *The axon.* New York: Oxford University Press, 1995:13–48.

22. Monuki ES, Lemke G. Molecular biology of myelination. In: Waxman SG, Kocsis JD, Stys PK (eds.). *The axon.* New York: Oxford University Press, 1995:144–163.

23. Lees MB, Bizzozero OA. Structure and acylation of proteolipid protein. In: Martenson RE (ed.). *Myelin biology and chemistry.* Boca Raton: CRC Press, 1992:237–255

24. Herndon RM, Rauch HL, Einstein ER. Immuno-electron microscopic localization of the encephalitogenic basic protein in myelin. *Immunol Comm* 1973; 2:163–172.

25. Karthigasan J, Garvey JS, Ramamurthy GV, Kirschner DA. Immunolocalization of 17 and 21.5 kDa MBP isoforms in compact myelin and radial component. *J Neurocytol* 1996; 26:1–7.

26. Sprinkle TJ. 2',3'-cyclic nucleotide 3'-phosphodiesterase, an oligodendrocyte—Schwann cell and myelin-associated enzyme of the nervous system. *Crit Rev Neurobiol* 1989; 4:235–301.

27. DeVries G, Norton W. The fatty acid composition of sphingolipids from bovine CNS axons and myelin. *J Neurochem* 1974; 22:251.

28. Benjamins J, Guarnieri M, Miller K, Sonneborn M, McKhann G. Sulphatide synthesis in isolated oligodendroglial and neuronal cells. *J Neurochem* 1974; 23:751–757.

29. Brady R, Quarles R. The enzymology of myelination. *Mol Cell Biochem* 1973; 2:23–29.

30. Mead J, Dhopeshwarkar G. Types of fatty acids in brain lipids: Their derivation and function. *Proceedings of the Ciba Foundation Symposium on Lipids, Malnutrition and the Developing Brain.* Amsterdam: Associated Scientific Publishers, 1972

31. Sweasey D, Patterson D, Glancy E. Biphasic myelination and the fatty acid composition of cerebrosides and cholesterol esters in the developing central nervous system of the domestic pig. *J Neurochem* 1976; 27:375.

32. Ritchie JM, Rogart RB, Strichartz ER. A new method for labeling saxitoxin and its binding to non-myelinated fibers of the rabbit vagus, lobster walking leg and garfish olfactory nerves. *J Physiol* (London) 1976; 271:477–494.

33. Lumsden CE: The neuropathology of multiple sclerosis. In: Vinken PJ, Bruyn GW (eds.). *Handbook of clinical neurology. Vol. 9. Multiple sclerosis and other demyelinating diseases.* New York: American Elsevier, 1970:217–309.

34. Prineas JW. Pathology of the early lesions of multiple sclerosis. *Hum Pathol* 1975; 6:531–535.

35. Trapp BD, Peterson J, Ransohoff RM, et al. Axonal transection in the lesions of multiple sclerosis. *N Engl J Med* 1998; 338:278–285.

36. Traugott U, Reinherz EL, Raine CS. Multiple sclerosis: Distribution of T cells, T cell subsets and Ia positive macrophages in lesions of different ages. *J Neuroimmunol* 1983; 4:201–221.

37. Traugott U. On the role of astrocytes for lesion pathogenesis. In: Herndon RM, Seil FJ (eds.). *Multiple sclerosis: Current status of research and treatment.* New York: Demos, 1994:13–31.

38. Traugott U, Raine CS. Further lymphocyte characterization in the central nervous system in multiple sclerosis. *Ann NY Acad Sci* 1984; 436:163.

39. Bunge MB, Bunge RP, Ris H. Ultrastructural study of remyelination in an experimental lesion in adult cat spinal cord. *J Biophys Biochem Cytol* 1961; 10:67–94.

40. Hommes OR. Remyelination in human CNS lesions. *Prog Brain Res* 1980; 53:39–63.

41. Arenella L, Herndon RM. Mature oligodendrocytes: Division following experimental demyelination in adult animals. *Arch Neurol* 1984; 41:1162–65.

42. Ludwin SK. Proliferation of mature oligodendrocytes after trauma to the central nervous system. *Nature* 1984; 308:274–76.

43. Itoyama Y, Webster H deF, Richardson EP, Trapp BD. Schwann cell remyelination of demyelinated axons in spinal cord multiple sclerosis lesions. *Ann Neurol* 1983; 14:339–346.

44. Prineas JW, Connel F. Remyelination in multiple sclerosis. *Ann Neurol* 1979; 5:22–31.

45. Prineas J. Paramyxovirus like particles associated with acute demyelination in chronic relapsing multiple sclerosis. *Science* 1972; 178:760.

46. Raine CS, Powers JM, Suzuki K. Acute multiple sclerosis—confirmation of "paramyxovirus-like" tubules. *Arch Neurol* 1974; 30:39–46.

47. Field EJ, Cowshall S, Narang HK, Bell TM. Viruses in multiple sclerosis? *Lancet* 1972; ii:280–281.

48. Raine CS, Schaumberg HH, Snyder DK, Suzuki K. Intranuclear "paramyxovirus-like" material in multiple sclerosis, adreno-leukodystrophy and Kuf's disease. *J Neurol Sci* 1975; 25:29–41.

49. Kasckow J, Abood LG, Hoss W, Herndon RM. Mechanism of phospholipase A2-induced conduction block in bullfrog sciatic nerve I. Electrophysiology and morphology. *Brain Res* 1986a; 373:384–391.

50. Kasckow J, Abood LG, Hoss W, Herndon RM. Mechanism of phospholipase A2-induced conduction block in bullfrog sciatic nerve II. Biochemistry. *Brain Res* 1986b; 373:392–398.

51. Ritchie M. Physiology of axons. In: Waxman SG, Kocsis JD, Stys PK (eds.). *The axon.* New York: Oxford University Press, 1995:68–96

52. Waxman SG. Conduction in myelinated, unmyelinated and demyelinated fibers. *Arch Neurol* 1977; 34:585–589.

53. Rasminsky M. The effects of temperature on conduction in demyelinated single nerve fibres. *Arch Neurol* 1972; 28:287–292.

54. Sears TA, Bostock H. Conduction failure in demyelination: Is it inevitable? *Adv Neurol* 1981; 31:357–375.

III

RISK FACTORS AND THEORIES OF CAUSATION

3 Epidemiology

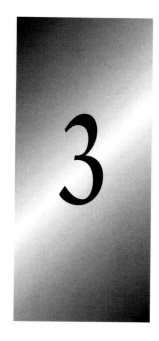

John F. Kurtzke, M.D., and Mitchell T. Wallin, M.D., M.P.H.

Research into multiple sclerosis (MS) has included many epidemiologic inquiries. One definition of this field is that epidemiology is the study of the natural history of disease. Its content and uses are described in Figure 3-1. The epidemiologic unit is a person with a diagnosed disorder. The basic question, after diagnosis, is how common is the disease, and this in turn is delineated by measures of the number of cases (numerator) within defined populations (denominator). These ratios, with the addition of the time factor to which they pertain, are referred to as rates (2).

RATES

The population-based rates in common use are the incidence rate, the mortality rate, and the prevalence "rate." All are ordinarily expressed in unit-population values. For example, 10 cases among a community of 20,000 inhabitants represent a rate of 50 per 100,000 population or 0.5 per 1,000 population.

The *incidence* or *attack rate* is defined as the number of new cases of the disease beginning in a unit of time within the specified population. This is usually given as an annual incidence rate in cases per 100,000 population per year. The date of onset of clinical symptoms ordinarily decides the time of accession, although occasionally the date of first diagnosis is used. The *mortality* or *death rate* refers to the number of deaths with the disease as the underlying cause of death occurring within a unit of time and population, and thus an annual death rate per 100,000 population. The *case fatality ratio* refers to the proportion of those affected who die of the disease. When this is high, as in glioblastoma multiforme, accurate death rates reflect the disease well. When it is low, as in epilepsy, death rate data may be strongly biased. The *point prevalence "rate"* is more properly called a ratio, and it refers to the number with the diagnosis within the community at one point in time, again expressed per unit of population. If over time there is no change in case fatality ratios or annual incidence rates, and no migration, the average annual incidence rate times the average duration of illness in years equals the point prevalence rate. Both incidence and prevalence rates of diseases are derived from specific surveys within a circumscribed population. When both numerator and denominator for the rates refer to the entirety of a community, their quotient provides a *crude rate, all ages*. When both terms of the ratio are delimited by age or sex or race or other criteria, we are speaking of *age-specific* or *sex-specific* or similar rates.

Because different communities differ in their age distributions, the proper comparisons among communities are those for the age-specific (and sex-specific) rates. Such

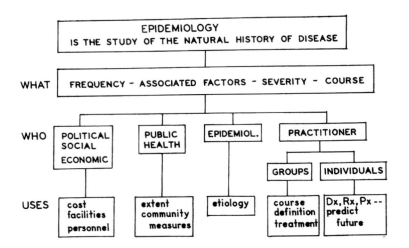

FIGURE 3-1

Epidemiology. Content and uses. *From Kurtzke, 1974 (1).*

comparisons become unwieldy when more than a few surveys are considered, and the proper step then is the calculation of age-adjusted rates. One method of age adjustment is to take the age-specific rate for each age group from birth on and multiply it by a factor representing that proportion of a standard population that this same age group contains. The sum of these individual adjusted figures provides an *age-adjusted rate, all ages,* or a *rate all ages, adjusted to a standard population.* One standard population often used is that of the United States for a census year. Different standards, of course, give different results, so the base used must always be explicit. Age adjustment is especially important when dealing with common disorders that primarily affect either end of the age spectrum.

COMMENT ON EPIDEMIOLOGY IN MULTIPLE SCLEROSIS

In virtually all studies of MS we are dealing with a clinical diagnosis without recourse to a pathognomonic diagnostic test or to pathologic verification. Several schemes for diagnostic criteria have been put forth, none with universal acceptance. In almost all of these, there are several grades relating to the degree of confidence in the correctness of the label. If we limit attention to the classes considered the better ones, and discard "possible MS" and "uncertain MS," we have defined groups that are quite similar in time and space. Thus the assessments of morbidity data that follow are based on series of cases variously labeled "definite," "clinically definite," and "probable" MS.

The major clinical criteria in current use for a diagnosis of MS are those of Poser and coworkers (3) and Schumacher and colleagues (4). An earlier categorization still used in some surveys is that of Allison and Millar (5): probable, early probable or latent, and possible.

The geographic distribution of MS has been the subject of many mortality and morbidity surveys as well as the topic of several symposia (6). Recent reviews of the epidemiology of MS are those of Acheson (7), Dean (8), Ebers and Sadovnick (9), Firnhaber and Lauer (10), Gonzales-Scarano and coworkers (11), Kesselring (12), Koch-Henriksen (13), Kurtzke (14–16), Martyn (17), Pryse-Phillips (18), Weinshenker and Rodriguez (19), and Wynn and colleagues (20). This listing is provided here so that the reader may seek interpretations that may differ—often drastically—from the views in this chapter. The most penetrating analyses to 1985 are those of Acheson. His final summation was:

In the summary of the epidemiological chapters in the last edition [of McAlpine's *Multiple Sclerosis*] I concluded that the principal result of work using this approach had been to demonstrate that there are crucial environmental factors which determine whether or not an individual acquires multiple sclerosis. Subsequent work has reinforced that conclusion with all the grounds for optimism which stem from it (7, p. 40).

MORTALITY DATA

International Comparisons

The earliest analysis of MS mortality rates from many countries was made by Limburg (21), who found that death rates were higher in temperate zones than in the tropics or subtropics. He also noted higher rates in the northern United States and northern Italy than in the southern parts of those countries. Goldberg and Kurland (22) presented death rates for a number of neurologic diseases from all countries responding to their request for data. For most lands the deaths were those for five years within the period from 1951 to 1958. All rates were age adjusted to the 1950 population of the United States and referred to diseases coded as the underlying cause of death. These death rates from MS are shown in Figure 3-2. The rates in most of Western Europe were on the order of 2 or more per 100,000 population per year. The northernmost lands of Europe were closer to 1 per 100,000, as too were Canada and U.S. whites, and New Zealand. Deaths from the disease would then appear overall to be notably less common in these groups of countries. In Iceland the rate was only 0.3 per 100,000. This low rate apparently contrasts with the high prevalence of MS in Iceland (described subsequently) even

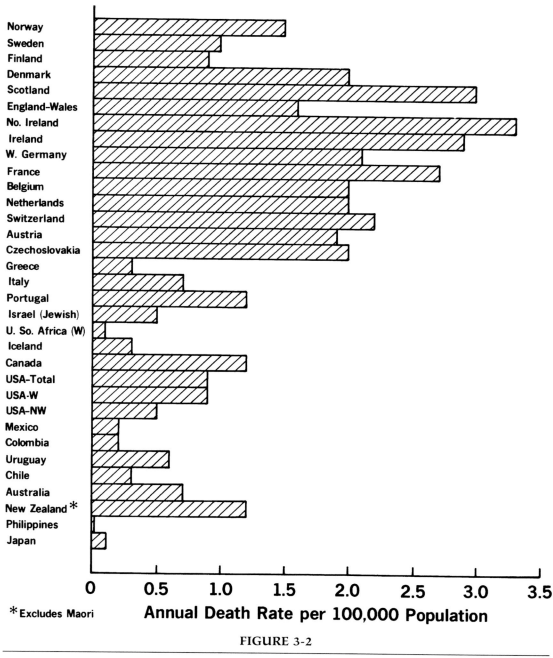

FIGURE 3-2

Average annual death rates per 100,000 population for MS by country, 1951–1958, with rates adjusted for age to the 1950 U.S. population. W = Whites, NW = Nonwhites. *Modified from data of Goldberg and Kurland, 1962 (22); from Kurtzke, 1977 (2).*

though the upper 95 percent confidence limit on this rate is approximately 0.9. Actually, MS in Iceland appears to have changed in frequency (see below). Similar age-adjusted international death rates for 1967 to 1973 were presented by Massey and Schoenberg (23). Most rates were the same or lower than those in Figure 3-2, but the overall ranking was quite similar. The Portuguese rate was 1.1, in agreement with the earlier rate of 1.2. Iceland, however, then had a rate of 1.0 per 100,000 population, and, again, morbidity data give support for this change.

Within Europe there seemed to be a sharp drop between the rates in the north and those for the Mediterranean basin. South American rates were rather low, as were those for U.S. nonwhites (of whom more than 90 percent are African Americans). The Asian and African rates were clearly the lowest recorded.

United States Death Rates

From special tabulations of deaths in the United States from 1959 to 1961, the average annual age-adjusted death rate for MS was found to be 0.8 per 100,000 population, with a slight female and marked white preponderance. The male:female ratio on the rates was 0.9; the white:nonwhite ratio was 1.6. Both findings were consistent by geographic (census) region of the United States. Geographically, all states south of the 37° parallel of north latitude showed low death rates (mostly 0.3 to 0.5), whereas almost all states to the north of this line were well in excess of the national mean. This held true for residence at birth as well as at death, and for whites alone as well as for all residents. There was little consistent difference in MS death rates between urban and rural counties, although for whites the urban rates tended to be somewhat higher (2,6). Later data support these findings; by the 1970s the death rates for whites had declined (6).

DISTRIBUTION FROM PREVALENCE SURVEYS

Prevalence studies provide our best information on the distribution of disease but are expensive in time, people, and money. Despite this, there are now well over 300 such surveys for MS. Almost all of them have been performed since World War II. To epitomize distributions, prevalence rates of 30 or more per 100,000 population were considered high frequency, those of 5 to 29 were called medium frequency, and rates under 5 per 100,000 were classed as low frequency MS regions. This trichotomy, made in the early 1960s, still seems to provide a valid overview (6,25).

Prevalence in Europe

Prevalence rates for Europe and the Mediterranean basin as of 1980 are shown in Figure 3-3, correlated with geographic latitude. The distribution then comprised two clusters, one for prevalence rates of 30 and over, and one for rates below 30 but above 4 per 100,000. Taking only the best studies, the high prevalence zone extended from 44° to 64° north latitude. The medium zone extended from 32° to 47° north, plus two sites (numbers 11 and 12) from the west coast of southern Norway. The only high rate below 44° was that for a small survey of Enna, Sicily (no. 51j).

However, southern Europe and western Norway are now high-frequency regions (6). Figure 3-4 from Lauer (27) summarizes the recent situation. Both Portugal and Greece are also now high, with prevalence rates in the 40's (25).

Boiko of Moscow University has recently summarized a large literature on the distribution of MS in the former Soviet Union, which was unavailable in the west (28). Much of northwestern Russia down past Kiev and Moscow appears to be high prevalence (over 30 per 100,000), surrounded to the north, east, and south by medium prevalence areas. Overall, the Ukraine and the Caucasus seemed to average in the medium prevalence range. The Asian part of his work will be discussed in a subsequent section.

Prevalence in the Americas

Prevalence surveys from the Americas as of 1974 are denoted in Figure 3-5. Here we see all three risk zones: high frequency from 37° to 52°, medium frequency from 30° to 33°, and low frequency (prevalence less than 5 per 100,000) from 12° to 19° and from 63° to 67° north latitude. The coterminous United States and southern Canada are represented by all the surveys from numbers 88 to 119a, except for numbers 106 (Greenland), 109 (Jamaica), 113 (Alaska), 117 (Netherlands Antilles), and 118 (Mexico City). The Alaskan rate of zero referred to natives of that state. The prevalence rates for the northern United States and Canada then are quite similar to the high frequency rates of Western Europe. There were no studies from South America. There are now several MS/ALS ratio estimates for Argentina and Uruguay, and for Lima, Peru, which indicate that these are medium frequency areas. Similar material for Venezuela and Brazil apparently allots these regions to the low frequency zone (26). Studies from the 1997 World Congress of Neurology in Argentina provide additional materials for Latin America, with evidence that Mexico, Costa Rica, and Cuba are medium prevalence areas. Recent works confirm all of Canada and the northern United States as

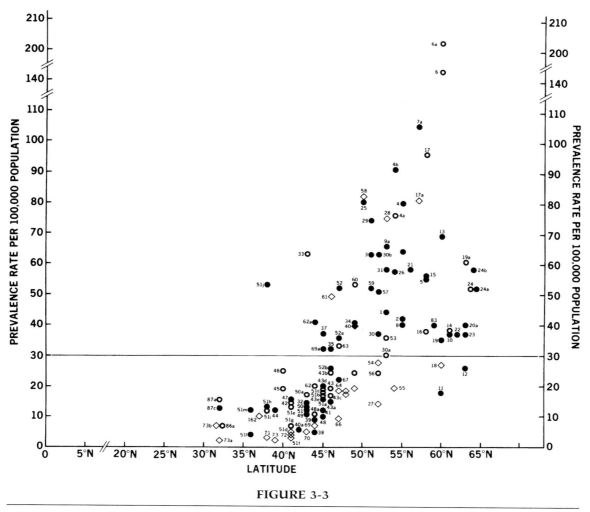

FIGURE 3-3

Prevalence rates per 100,000 population as of 1980 for probable MS in Europe and the Mediterranean area, correlated with geographic latitude. Numbers identify studies as indicated in Kurtzke, 1980 (26). Solid circles represent best (class A) surveys; open circles good (class B); open diamonds poor (class C); and solid diamonds estimates from ALS: MS case ratios (class E). *From Kurtzke, 1980 (26).*

clearly high frequency regions, with prevalence rates mostly in the range of 60 to 120 or so (6). (Figure 3-5)

U.S. Veteran Series

The modest number of studies noted in Figure 3-5 and cited elsewhere (6) for the United States leaves the distribution of MS poorly defined. However, our recent history has provided us with a truly unique series. This consists of 5,305 veterans of World War II or the Korean Conflict who were "service-connected" for MS according to U.S. legislation. They were matched with military peers on the basis of age, date of service entry, branch of service, and survival of the war (30). Figure 3-6 shows the distribution of MS by state of residence at entry into

active duty. Case control ratios under 0.75 would be equivalent to prevalence rates under 30 per 100,000 population. All states (and northern California) above the 37° parallel fall into the high frequency zone, except Virginia (0.69 for 51 MS vs. 74 controls) and Kentucky (0.60 for 37 vs. 62). In the east, then, the high-to-medium dividing line passes the 39° parallel.

Prevalence Elsewhere

Australia and New Zealand comprise, in general, high prevalence areas for 44°–34° south latitude and medium frequency for 33°–13° south. This high zone includes all of New Zealand and southeastern Australia with Tasmania (6,26,29).

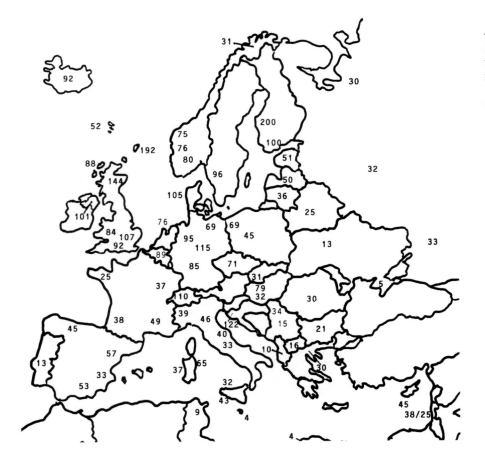

FIGURE 3-4

Prevalence rates per 100,000 population for MS in Europe and the Mediterranean basin from publications 1980–1994, modified from Lauer 1994 (27), with permission. *From Kurtzke, 1997 (6).*

In Asia and Africa earlier assessments provided low prevalence rates throughout, except English-speaking whites of South Africa (29). Rates are still low in Japan, Korea, China, and Southeast Asia (6) but not in the former Soviet Union.

Boiko (28) has summarized prevalence studies from Russia and other parts of the former Soviet Union. In the southern regions of the Ukraine, the Volga area, the Caucasus, and into Novosibirsk and Kazakhstan, rates were generally in the medium prevalence range (5 to 29 per 100,000), whereas Uzbekistan, Samarkand, Turkistan, and Turkmenistan areas were low. In the Far East medium prevalence once again appeared, and rates were indeed in the high range in the central and western parts of the Amur region, which abuts the Pacific Ocean above China and includes Vladivostok. In all these areas, rates were higher for Russian-born or those of Russian parentage than for the indigenous population.

The northern African shores of the Mediterranean are now of medium prevalence, and this extends into the Near East, with Israel in fact of high frequency. South Africa is now of medium prevalence for all whites (6,25).

Worldwide Distribution

The general worldwide distribution of MS thus seems well described by a division into high prevalence (30+ per 100,000), medium prevalence (5 to 29 per 100,000), and low prevalence (under 5 per 100,000) regions, as proposed years ago. A "super high" class for prevalence of, say, 90+ seems not yet indicated. Figure 3-4 shows how scattered such regions would be in Europe. The most recent distribution is shown in Figure 3-7.

Sex and Race

Death rates in the United States indicate that nonwhites have MS recorded as a cause of death only half as often as whites, and both mortality and morbidity data demonstrate low frequencies of the disease in Asia. In fact, all the high-risk and medium-risk areas for MS have predominantly white populations. Regardless of residence in the United States, in the veteran series blacks or African Americans have only half the risk of white males (Table 3-1). Young white females have nearly twice the risk of MS as white males. The group consisting of the "Other" races suggests a paucity as well in Native Americans and

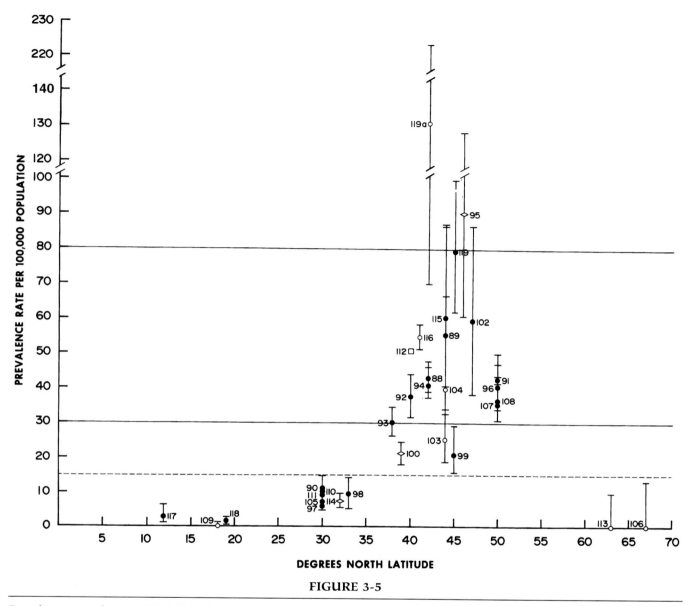

FIGURE 3-5

Prevalence rates for probable MS in the Americas as of 1974 with 95 percent confidence intervals on the rates, as in Figure 3-3; solid circles are class A surveys, open circles class B, open diamonds class C, open squares class E. *From Kurtzke, 1975 (29).*

in Asians (Table 3-2). The apparent deficit found among Hispanics would seem more a reflection of geography than of race. This is borne out when comparisons by race are made among the foreign-born cases (Table 3-3). The deficit in the first two groups is equal by race. Japanese and possibly Polynesians in Hawaii are low, as are Filipinos in the Philippines.

Multiple sclerosis then is predominantly the white person's disease. However, it is clear that, where there are good data, the less susceptible racial groups do share the geographic gradients of the whites, with higher frequencies in high-risk areas than in low-risk areas.

MIGRATION

The fate of migrants who move into regions of differing risk of MS is critical to our understanding of the nature of the disease. If migrants retain the risk of their birthplace, then either the disease is innate or it is acquired early in life. However, if upon moving they do change their risk, then clearly there is a major environmental cause or precipitant active in this disorder. If such altered risk is also dependent on age at migration, we can define not only external cause but also internal (personal) susceptibility. Furthermore, if an age of susceptibility can be

TABLE 3-1

*Multiple sclerosis: Case control ratios by tier of residence at entry into active duty (EAD)
for major sex and race groups, United States veteran series*

SEX AND RACE	TIER OF RESIDENCE AT EAD[a]			TOTAL[b]
	NORTH	MIDDLE	SOUTH	
MS/CONTROL RATIO				
White male	1.41	1.02	0.58	1.04
White female	2.77	1.71	0.80	1.86
Black male	0.61	0.59	0.31	0.45
TOTAL[c]	1.41	1.00	0.53	1.00
MS/CONTROL CASES				
White males	2195/1544	2059/2022	688/1161	4922/4737
White females	97/35	65/38	20/25	182/98
Black males	28/46	88/150	61/194	177/390
TOTAL[c]	2323/1647	2213/2219	62/1425	5298/5291[b]

[a]States north of 41°–42° comprised the North tier, and those south of 37° comprised the South tier.
[b]Excludes 1 male case and 11 male controls inducted in foreign countries.
[c]Includes black females and other (nonwhite, nonblack) persons.
Data of Kurtzke et al., 1979 (30).

TABLE 3-2

*Multiple sclerosis: Case/control ratios for "other" (nonwhite, nonblack)
males by birthplace and race, United States veteran series*

BIRTHPLACE AND RACE	RATIO	CASE/CONTROL[a]		
		TOTAL	NORTH	SOUTH
Coterminous United States	0.48	11/23[b]	6/12	5/11
Native American	0.38	3/8	3/6	0/2
Mexican–Spanish American	0.60	6/10	1/1	5/9
Japanese	0.50	2/4	2/4	0/0
Mexico and Latin America	0.29	6/21		
Mexican–Spanish American	0.00	0/5		
Puerto Rican	0.38	6/16		
Hawaii	0.00	0/15		
Japanese	0.00	0/10		
Other	0.00	0/5		
Asia	0.00	0/14		
Chinese	0.00	0/4		
Filipino	0.00	0/9		
Other	0.00	0/1		
TOTAL	0.23	17/73		

[a]North = Northern plus Middle tier of birth, South = Southern tier. For white males the MS/control ratios are 1.2 North and 0.6 South.
[b]Includes 1 Filipino control.
From Kurtzke et al., 1979 (30).

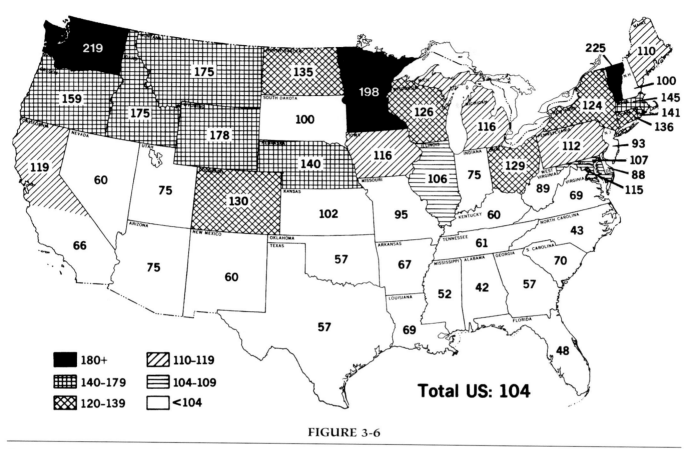

FIGURE 3-6

Case control ratios expressed as percentages for U.S. white male veterans of World War II according to state of residence at entry into active duty. *Modified from Kurtzke et al., 1979 (30).*

delineated in this manner, there may also be found a duration of exposure needed for acquisition.

An essential feature of epidemiology is that the investigators are totally dependent on the experiments of nature. Nowhere is this more true than in the assessment of diseases in migrants. For this to be meaningful in studying MS we need: (1) regions with distinctly different disease frequency based on accurate incidence or prevalence rates; (2) MS cases with appropriately defined diagnostic criteria; (3) appropriate—or at least unselected—case ascertainment; (4) a populace who moved from one risk area to another for reasons unrelated to disease; and (5) sufficient numbers to distinguish changes in rates.

There is considerable evidence that migrants do change their risk for MS (6). Martyn agrees that risk is clearly reduced by moves from high-risk to low-risk areas, but he believes that the reverse is not well established (17, pp. 22,23).

Figure 3-6 shows state of residence at entry into military service for the U.S. veteran case control series. In Table 3-1 these residences were allocated within three horizontal tiers for the coterminous United States: a northern tier of states above 41–42° north latitude; a middle tier; and a southern tier below 37°, including California from Fresno south. Migrants would be those born in one tier who entered service from another tier. In Table 3-4 the marginal totals provide the ratios for birthplace and residence at service entry for whites of World War II or Korean service. The major diagonal (north–north, middle–middle, south–south) gives the case control ratios for nonmigrants and cells off this diagonal define the ratios for the migrants (31).

All ratios decrease as we go from north to south. The nonmigrant ratios are 1.48 north, 1.03 middle, and 0.56 south. For the migrants, those born north and entering service from the middle tier have a ratio of 1.27; if they enter from the south, their ratio is 0.74, only half that of the nonmigrants. Birth in the middle tier is marked by an increase in the MS/C ratio for northern entrants to 1.40 and a decrease to 0.73 for the southern ones. Migration after birth in the south seems to raise the ratios to 0.65 (middle) and 0.70 (north). The migrant risk ratios

TABLE 3-3

*Multiple sclerosis: Case/control ratios according to race and birthplace for
foreign-born service men in selected regions, United States veteran series.*

		CASE/CONTROL			
REGION	RATIO	TOTAL	WHITE	BLACK	OTHER
Mexico, Central America	0.14	2/14	1/9	1/0	0/15
Puerto Rico	0.42	14/33	6/14	2/3	6/16
Hawaii	0.06	1/16	1/1	0/0	0/15
Japan, Korea	—	4/0	4/0	0/0	0/0
China	0.00	0/4	0/0	0/0	0/4
Philippines, Southeast Asia	0.00	0/12	0/2	0/0	0/10

From Kurtzke et al., 1979 (30).

are intermediate between those characteristics of their birthplace and their residence at entry.

From the marginal totals of Table 3-4, residence at birth has approximately the same gradient of risk as does residence at service entry—and therefore about age 23 for the World War II veterans. For the migrants, there is no clear difference in risk for moves from high to low regions versus low to high. If the disease is acquired over a short interval, the point midway between birth and age 23 would seem the most reasonable to account for our findings. This would indicate age 10 to 15 years, which would be in accord with other data on migrants (6), suggesting disease acquisition by age 15 in high-risk areas (see also below). These data would thus minimize the effect of high to low moves because only under age 15 or so would southward moves be expected to lower the rate of MS. Still, the northern U.S. veterans reduced their ratios of MS by half by moving south before service entry, although this was still above the southern-born ratios.

This would also be an incomplete reflection of south to north alterations of risk because it would include persons who had already defined their MS risk (i.e., already acquired the disease) while in the south. For the southern-born veterans, migration under age 10 to 15 years would increase their risk, and migration between that age and service entry (average 23 years) also would increase risk in

TABLE 3-4

*Multiple sclerosis: Case/control ratios for all white veterans of World War II or the Korean Conflict
by tier of residence at birth and at entry into active duty (EAD), coterminous United States only.*

	ENTRY INTO ACTIVE DUTY (EAD) TIER			
BIRTH TIER	NORTH	MIDDLE	SOUTH	BIRTH TOTAL
CASE/CONTROL RATIOS				
North	1.48	1.27	0.74	1.44
Middle	1.40	1.03	0.73	1.04
South	0.70	0.65	0.56	0.57
EAD TOTAL	1.46	1.03	0.58	1.06
CASE/CONTROL NUMBERS				
North	2033/1377	133/105	39/53	2205/1535
Middle	160/114	1899/1836	80/110	2139/2060
South	21/30	50/77	565/1007	636/1114
EAD TOTAL	2214/1521	2082/2018	684/1170	4980/4709

From Kurtzke et al., 1985 (31).

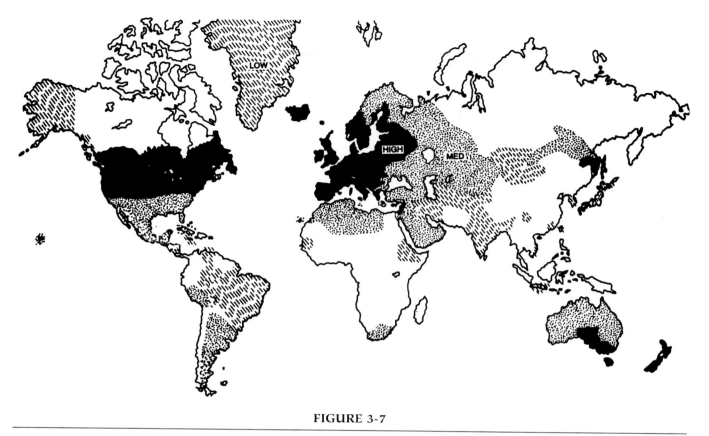

FIGURE 3-7

Worldwide distribution of MS as of 1998 with high (prevalence 30+; solid), medium (prevalence 5–29; dotted), and low (prevalence 0–4; dashed) regions defined. Blank areas are regions without data or people.

that unknown proportion not already affected in the south. However, the veteran series is limited to a 9- or 10-year incidence cohort of MS by laws defining service-connection: onset in service (average 39 months for World War II, 24 months for Korean Conflict) or within seven years after discharge (30). Thus the southern-born migrant veterans would likely have expressed well under half their true risk of MS after moves to the north. Input is limited to residence by age 23, and output by disease symptoms by age 32 or 33 on the average. The fact that these veterans did not exceed the rate from their northern-born peers is thus readily explained; they did show significant increase, however, over their southern brethren who stayed home.

In a study of European immigrants to South Africa, the MS prevalence rate, adjusted to a population of all ages, was 13 per 100,000 for immigration under age 15, which is the same medium prevalence rate as for the native-born English-speaking white South Africans (Table 3-5). But for age groups older at immigration, the prevalence was some 30 to 80 per 100,000, the same as expected from their high-risk homelands (32). This change was sharp and occurred exactly at age 15 (Figure

3-8). This indicates that natives of high-risk areas are not susceptible to MS acquisition much before age 15 and that there is a long incubation period between acquisition and onset of symptoms.

Inferences as to the opposite migration, low to high, were afforded by North African migrants to France (33). Among some 7,500 respondents with known place of birth who had completed a nationwide questionnaire survey for MS in France in 1986, there were 260 born in former French North Africa (Morocco, Algeria, Tunisia). They had migrated to France between 1923 and 1986, but 66 percent came between 1956 and 1964. Two thirds were from Algeria, where virtually the entire European population had emigrated in 1962 at the end of the Algerian war for independence (Figure 3-9). The 225 migrants with onset more than one year after immigration presumably acquired their MS in France. They provided an age-adjusted (U.S. 1960) MS prevalence rate 1.54 times that for all France (Table 3-6). If the latter is taken at 50 per 100,000 population, their estimated adjusted rate is 76.8, with 95 percent confidence interval (CI) of 67.1 to 87.5. The other 27 with presumed acquisition in North

TABLE 3-5

Adjusted MS prevalence rates per 100,000 immigrants to South Africa, 1960, all ages, according to age at immigration (AAI) in northern European immigrants [all and those from UK (revised)]*

AAI	UK MS	UK Rate	ALL MS	ALL Rate
0–14	4	12.8	7	12.9
15–19	7	66.1	15	81.1
20–24	7	31.8	13	31.3
25–29	14	59.4	26	58.4
(20–29)	(21)	(45.7)	(39)	(44.9)
30–39	21	58.2	34	52.4
40–49	} 12 {	57.7	} 23 {	62.4
50+		70.5		80.8
Total	65	47.5	118	49.4

*Adapted from S Afr Med J 1970; 44:663–669 (32).

Africa gave an estimated adjusted prevalence of 16.6 per 100,000 (95 percent CI 10.9–24.1). For those migrants with acquisition in France there was a mean interval of 13 years between immigration or age 11 and clinical onset, with a minimum of three years. The oldest patient at immigration was the only one to enter France in the fifth decade of life. This series provides further support for the theses: (1) that MS is due to an environmental factor acquired after childhood; and (2) that acquisition requires prolonged or repeated exposure (here three years for these medium to high MS risk migrants) followed by a prolonged latent or incubation period between acquisition and symptom onset (here 10 years).

EPIDEMICS

In the past there has been little reason to consider that MS occurred in the form of epidemics. All known geographic areas that had been surveyed at repeated intervals up to 1980 provided either stable or increasing prevalence rates, the latter compatible with both better case-ascertainment and perhaps improved survival. Epidemics of MS would

TABLE 3-6

Rates per 100,000 population for multiple sclerosis by age in 1986 vs. 1982 population of France: A. North African migrants with (1) presumed acquisition of MS in North Africa[a], and (2) presumed acquisition in France; B. All French MS

	A. Migrant MS[b]					B. All MS		
			(CALCULATED RATES)					
AGE	POPULATION[c]	N (1)	RATE (1)	N (2)	RATE (2)	POPULATION (K)	N	RATE
0–14	124,612	0	—	0	—	11232.80	20	0.18
15–24	132,097	0	—	1	0.76	8593.52	138	1.61
25–34	236,732	2	0.84	53	22.39	8568.20	1104	12.88
35–54	401,748	9	2.24	132	32.86	12798.82	4177	32.64
55+	78140	16	20.48	39	49.91	13079.68	2068	15.81
Total	973,329	27	2.77	225	23.12	54273.20	7507	13.83
Age adj.[d]			4.33		20.06			12.854
Age adj.[e]								13.067
			(estimated rates per 100,000 population)					
Est. rate			16.57		76.76			50.00
95% CI[f]			(10.92–24.10)		(67.06–87.47)			

[a]Clinical onset before, at, or one year after immigration
[b]Excludes cases and population of undefined age
[c]*Source:* Table 3, Nationalité RP 1982, INSEE Paris (10)
[d]Age adjusted to U.S. 1960 population
[e]Age adjusted (U.S. 1960) from five-year age-specific rates
[f]95% confidence interval (Poisson)
From Kurtzke et al., 1998 (33).

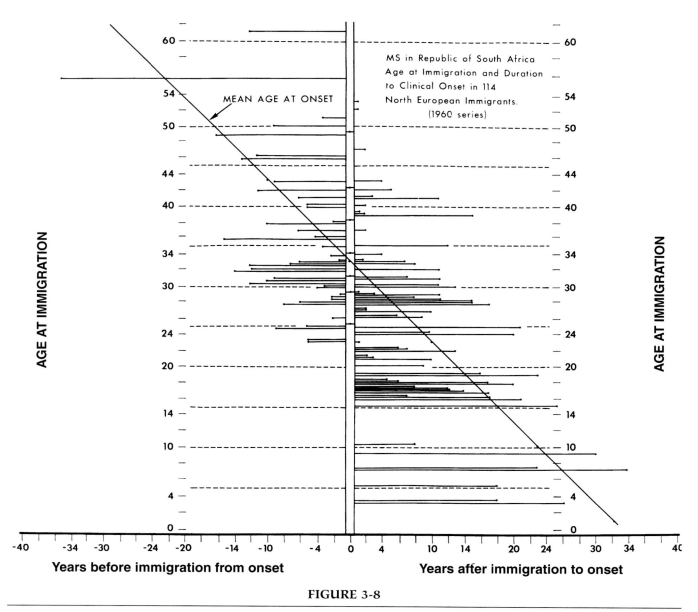

FIGURE 3-8

Multiple sclerosis in migrants from northern Europe to South Africa by age at immigration (Y-axis) and years between immigration and clinical onset (X-axis) who were ascertained in 1960 MS prevalence survey of South Africa. Each patient is represented by a bar whose locus on Y-axis ± years from immigration on X-axis indicates age at clinical onset. Diagonal reflects mean age at onset for this series. *Modified from Kurtzke et al., 1970 (32).*

serve to define the disease as not only an acquired one but also perhaps a transmittable one. We seem to have encountered separate epidemics of MS, which in fact may have common precipitants, and which have occurred in the ethnically similar lands of the Faroe Islands, the Shetland-Orkney Islands, and Iceland.

An epidemic may be defined as disease occurrence clearly in excess of normal expectancy and derived from a common or propagated source. Epidemics are divisible

into two types: type 1 epidemics occur in susceptible populations, exposed for the first time to a virulent infectious agent. Type 2 epidemics occur in populations within which the organism is already established (6, p. 124). If the entire populace is exposed to a type 1 epidemic, the ages of those affected clinically will define the age range of susceptibility to the infection. Type 2 epidemics will tend to have a young age at onset, as the effective exposure of the patients will then begin when they first reach

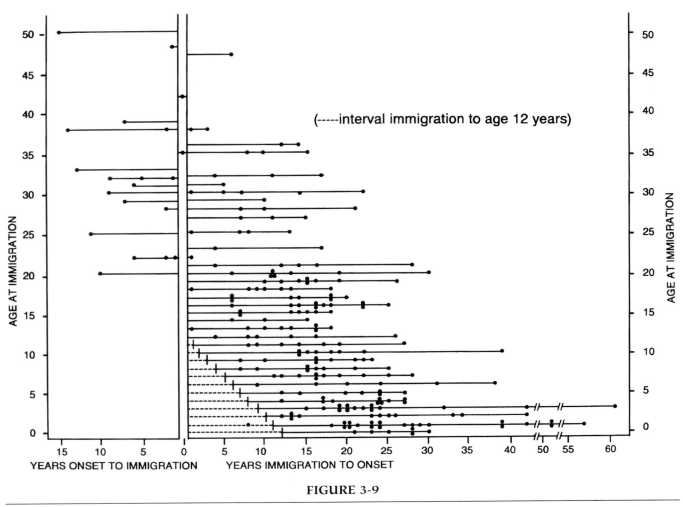

FIGURE 3-9

Multiple sclerosis in migrants from French North Africa (two thirds from Algeria) by age at immigration (Y-axis) and years between immigration and clinical onset of MS (X-axis). Each patient is represented by a solid circle whose locus reflects age at onset as the algebraic sum of age at immigration and years from immigration to onset. *From Kurtzke et al., 1998 (33).*

the age of susceptibility. Epidemics may, of course, be due to toxins and deficiency states as well as infections and allegorically may describe any sudden increase in adverse health effects (automobile accidents, myocardial infarction). If the causative agent of a "true" epidemic is persistent in an area, the epidemic will generally end when the number of susceptibles within the populace is exhausted. Any further cases would then be dependent on the arrival of new susceptibles—by birth, age, or immigration. If the agent is transient in occurrence, new cases can arise after its disappearance only by transmission from those affected to new cohorts of the unaffected, so that successive epidemics in such an instance are limited de facto to the action of infectious agents. We described the occurrence of an MS epidemic in the Faroe Islands in the middle of this century (34).

Iceland

After our earlier work on the Faroes, an obvious next question was what had happened with MS in Iceland. The same Norse Vikings had settled Iceland at about the same time as the Faroes. Like the Faroes, Iceland had been a county of Denmark, but it had attained semi-independence in 1918. Also like the Faroes, it was occupied in World War II—not only by the British, but also by Canadians and Americans. Iceland declared its independence as a nation during that war. With Sverrir Bergmann and the late Kjartan Gudmundsson, we had collected between 1974 and 1979 all MS cases known in Iceland with onset from 1900 to 1975 (35). They numbered 168 among native-born resident Icelanders. Annual incidence rates reveal that there has been at least one definite type

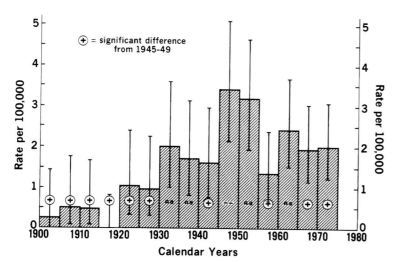

FIGURE 3-10

Multiple sclerosis in Iceland: average annual incidence rates per 100,000 population with 95 percent confidence intervals on the rates for consecutive five-year periods 1900–1974. A "+" indicates significant differences at the 5 percent level for rates vs that for 1945–1949; "ns" indicates no significant difference. *From Kurtzke et al., 1982 (35).*

2 epidemic of MS in Iceland beginning in 1945. The average annual incidence rate from 1923 to 1944 was 1.6 per 100,000. For 1945 to 1954 it was significantly higher at 3.2, and then it declined significantly to 1.9 for 1955 to 1974. Most of the individual five-year intervals from 1900 on had incidence rates significantly below those of 1945 to 1949 or 1950 to 1954 (Figure 3-10), and by 10-year intervals all showed the significant difference. Furthermore, age at onset in the 1945 to 1949 interval (23 years) was significantly lower than for any other quinquennium 1900 to 1974.

The Shetland-Orkney Islands

The Shetland-Orkney Islands off northern Scotland were once possessions of Denmark, and in the Viking era had considerable occupations from Norway, as with Iceland and the Faroes. Earlier we had pointed out that the Shetland-Orkneys, taken together, had at the time of study the highest prevalence rates for MS known (numbers 6 and 6a in Figure 3-3). These islands have been formally surveyed as to the occurrence of MS five times (6). The fifth set of surveys was that of Cook and coworkers, who reported a decline in incidence in the Shetland Islands "beginning between 1951 and 1968" (36), similar to that they had previously noted for the Orkneys. Incidence rates for each of Shetland and the Orkneys for 1911 to 1985 have been presented and are summarized in Figure 3-11 for both combined; the period from 1981 to 1985 was incomplete for the Orkneys. The occurrence after 1970 is significantly lower than that for the prior 30 or 35 years. The individual annual incidence rates show considerable fluctuations and do apparently differ in peaks and valleys somewhat between the islands, but the overall impression of at least one epidemic between 1941 and 1970 seems valid, as does the clear decline after 1970—at least up to 1983 or 1986.

The Faroe Islands

The Faroe Islands comprise a group of 18 major volcanic islands lying in the North Atlantic Ocean at 7° west longitude and 62° north latitude. First settled by Norse Vikings in the ninth century, they had long been a standard county *(amt)* of Denmark. In 1948 the Faroes achieved semi-independence, although they remained part of the Kingdom of Denmark, which is still responsible for their health and welfare services. The population numbered some 48,000 in 1989.

Critical to our findings and interpretations of epidemic status is the requirement that we have found *all* cases of MS that have occurred among Faroese in the twentieth century. We are limited by the fact that the person must have been seen medically and neurologic symptoms recorded. But two points argue for completeness: MS clinically is a disorder with repeated or progressive symptomatology over time; and medical care for Faroese, not constrained by financial factors, is of high quality and well documented. Furthermore, MS is usually the first consideration for unexplained neurologic symptoms in young adults—suspects will be overreported rather than the reverse. Ascertainment of potential cases of MS has been ongoing since 1972 using all available resources (37,38).

We subdivided cases of MS among the Faroese according to their residence history, based on criteria first defined in 1974 (35). In order to avoid attributing to the Faroes the occurrence of disease that had in fact been acquired elsewhere, we then decided to exclude from the resident series those we had *a priori* decided had lived "too long" off the islands before clinical onset: Persons off the Faroes for three plus years before onset were thus to be excluded (Group C); those not off (Group A) or off less than two years (Group B) were to be included. In the

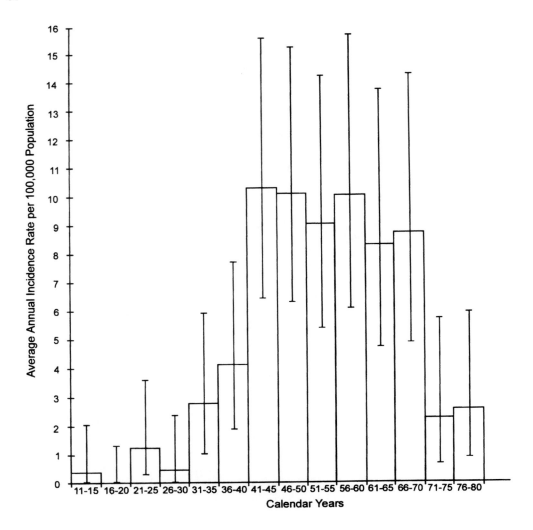

FIGURE 3-11

Multiple sclerosis in the Shetland and Orkney Islands: average annual incidence rates per 100,000 population with 95 percent confidence intervals, for 1911–1980.

recent analysis requirements for new exclusions (Group C') have been made more stringent because of the potential for exposure to this disease in both Denmark and the Faroes. Validation of the exclusion criteria was provided by the findings for the migrants (37–39).

The Excluded "Migrant" Multiple Sclerosis

The patients with foreign residence were not only potential "rejects" but also comprised two groups of immigrants from a low-risk MS area (Faroes) to a high-risk area (Denmark). Figure 3-12 provides for each patient the ages and durations of foreign residence. For Group C, C', ignoring short childhood visits for one of them, all patients had at least two years of their stay off the Faroes between age 11 and age 36, and two years was the minimum period for such stays.

The foreign residences for Group B showed little consistency in time to MS onset. On the other hand, the Group C residences clustered within 10 years or so before clinical onset. Subtracting the two years "exposure" that is common to all from each patient's overseas residence interval gave an "incubation" period of 7.2 years (range 5–13).

From this we concluded that residence in a high-risk MS area by a susceptible but virgin (as to MS) population, for a period of two years from age 11 on, could result in clinical MS beginning after a further period of some seven years. Additionally, residence need not have been maintained in that endemic area for the entire interval. Thus seven years is a true incubation or latent interval between disease acquisition and symptom onset. Furthermore, short periods of residence in the same place and at the same age did not result in MS.

The Resident Series

By 1991 we had ascertained 42 cases of MS among native-born resident Faroese. We could not find one single resident patient with clinical onset of MS in this cen-

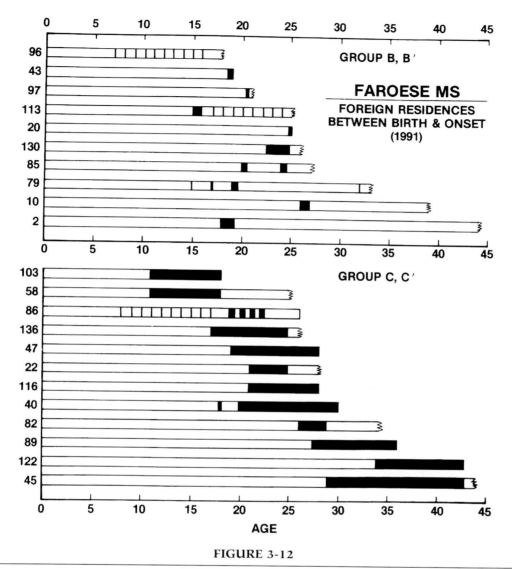

FIGURE 3-12

Faroese MS. Ages and durations of foreign residences (black segment of bars) for Groups B, B' and C, C' patients as of 1991. Clinical onset of MS is the terminus of each patient's bar with its origin at birth; a straight terminal line indicates symptom onset while overseas, a jagged line while in the Faroes. Numbers identify the patients in Kurtzke and Hyllested 1986 (37) and Kurtzke et al. (38). *From Kurtzke, 1993 (16).*

tury until July 1943. Then there were 16 patients with onset between 1943 and 1949 and another 26 with onset thereafter.

Annual incidence rates per 100,000 population showed an early and dramatic rise and fall, followed by three irregular secondary peaks (Figure 3-13, top). The rate exceeded 10 per 100,000 in 1945. The first question was whether this was a single epidemic with a very irregular tail or whether the incidence rate curve in fact reflected separate epidemics. The migrant series suggested that MS was acquired by Faroese only if they were at least 11 years of age at first exposure and only if the exposure

was then for at least two years duration. Hence, we classified the resident series according to the calendar time when the patients had attained age 11, whether by 1941 (two years before first clinical onset) or thereafter. Figure 3-14 shows the results as of 1986; there clearly seemed to be a separation into discrete subsets—or epidemics. The 1991 update of this material provides the annual incidence rates by epidemic shown in Figure 3-13, bottom. Epidemic I then comprised all patients age 11+ in 1941 plus one (see below) age 11 by 1943 (n = 20). Epidemic I accounted for all cases contributing to the first MS incidence rate peak. Epidemic II comprised the

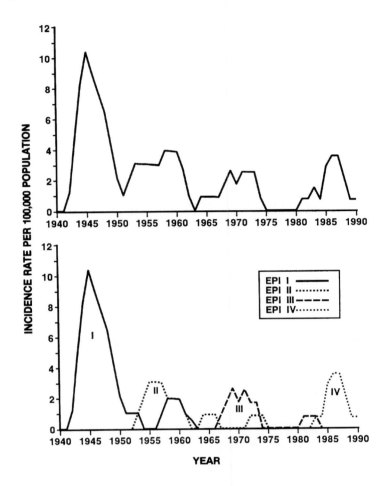

FIGURE 3-13

Multiple sclerosis in native resident Faroese. Annual incidence rates per 100,000 population calculated as three-year centered moving averages as of June 1991. Upper panel: total series; Lower panel: incidence rates by epidemic. *From Kurtzke et al., 1993 (38).*

patients age 11 in 1946–1951; they accounted for the second incidence rate peak (n = 9). Epidemic III included the patients age 11 in 1956–1967; they accounted for the third incidence rate peak (n = 6). Epidemic IV patients achieved age at first effective exposure in 1973–1980; thus the fourth incidence rate peak (n = 7). Age at clinical onset was similar, near age 21, for epidemics II, III, and IV patients, but all were significantly lower than age at onset for epidemic I cases, age 30. Incubation averaged some six years from 1943 or age 13, whichever came later (five, eight, eight, and seven years for epidemics I, II, III, and IV, respectively) (38).

The median year of symptom onset was 1947 for epidemic I and 1986 for epidemic IV (38). If the four epidemics are equidistant, there would be an average interval of some 13 years ([1986–1947 = 39]/3) between each epidemic's onset or end. Thus, if there are four such epidemics, they would have begun about 1943, 1956, 1969, and 1982, respectively, and the few years before these respective dates would be the "valleys" of virtually no cases. Results are given for seven years "on" (high case expectation) followed by six years "off" (low) for each epidemic (eight- and five-year division results were quite similar) (Table 3-7).

The hypothesis of three epidemics after the first within *population cohorts,* each defined by the calendar time age 11 occurred, can also be tested with the same *a priori* division of 13-year intervals (seven "on," six "off") used previously, beginning in 1945. Thus, if this is a valid criterion, age 11 "on" intervals should start near 1945, 1958, and 1971. Even with these very small numbers, the findings are still statistically significant (Table 3-8). Consolidating the three "high" periods and comparing them with the three "low" gives risk ratios of 1.21 and 0.30 per 1,000, respectively, with $\chi^2_c = 6.24$, $0.02 > p > 0.01$. The relative risk is 4.00 for high versus low intervals.

Geographic Distribution and British Troops

The pertinence of residence location within the Faroes has to do with our assessment of the British occupation in World War II. The Faroes were occupied by British troops for five years from April 1940. From 1941 to 1944 there were at least 1,500 troops stationed on the islands. The most rigid and unbiased criterion for exposure of Faroese to British troops is that Faroese MS patients lived where the troops were billeted (Figure 3-15). It was clear that

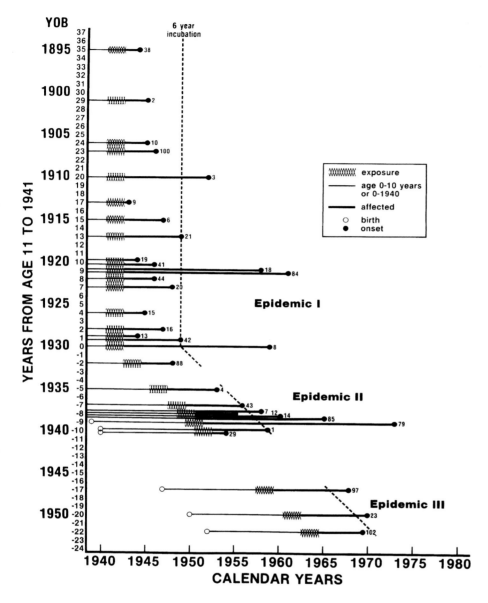

FIGURE 3-14

Multiple sclerosis in native resident Faroese as of 1986. Each patient is represented by a bar with the thin portion the time and ages *before* exposure to PMSA (the primary MS affection; see text) and the two years of cross-hatching the period of PMSA exposure, following which (heavy portion of bar) the patient is affected but neurologically asymptomatic (the incubation period). Solid circles at terminus of each bar represent time and age of clinical onset, with the numbers identifying the patient in Kurtzke and Hyllested 1987 (39). Open circles for lower bars define time of birth. Location of each bar on the Y-axis is specified by the number of years from 1941 at which time the patient attained age 11; calendar year of birth (YOB) is also identified. Dashed line represents a six-year incubation time of acquisition of PMSA after the two-year exposure. *From Kurtzke and Hyllested, 1987 (39).*

the locations of troop encampments were strongly correlated with the place of residence of all MS patients, regardless of epidemic (37–39).

Our conclusion was that British troops brought MS to the Faroese in the Faroe Islands during 1941–1944 (this was why we included in epidemic I one patient age 11 in 1943).

It was also clear that the disease had not spread throughout the islands. In formal testing of troop locations versus residence of patients of epidemics I–IV an odds ratio (OR) of 20.43 was calculated (p < 0.001); versus epidemics II–IV the OR was 9.00 (p < 0.01). There is also a highly significant association between residence of patients of epidemics II–IV and that of epidemic I: OR = 32.63 (p < 0.001) (38). Therefore, this disease has

remained geographically stable on the Faroes for half a century, and the MS risk areas remain in essence those defined by the British troop occupation sites of World War II.

Transmission of Multiple Sclerosis in the Faroe Islands

The principal conclusion from the Faroes work, and one compatible with other epidemiologic evidence (6,16), is that clinical neurologic MS (CNMS) is the rare late manifestation of infection with what we call PMSA—the primary MS affection. In this concept PMSA is transmissible; CNMS is not. Evidence as to the characteristics of PMSA derives entirely from the epidemiologic features of

TABLE 3-7

Faroese CNMS cases: Average annual incidence rates per 100,000 population, divided into four epidemic periods of 13 years with each period expected to comprise seven "high" followed by six "low" years.

PERIOD	PERSON-YEARS	MS-O	MS-E	χ^2A	RATE[a]	95% CL
1943–49	205,033	16	4.888	25.261	7.80	4.46–12.67
1950–55	192,711	4	4.594	0.077	2.08	0.57–5.31
1956–62	239,155	7	5.702	0.295	2.93	1.17–6.03
1963–68	221,324	2	5.276	2.034	0.90	0.11–3.26
1969–75	277,106	5	6.606	0.390	1.80	0.58–4.21
1976–81	257,194	0	6.132	6.132	0.00	0.00–1.43
1982–89[b]	369,205	8	8.802	0.369	2.17	0.93–4.27
TOTAL	1,761,728	42	42.000	34.558	2.38	1.72–3.22

[a]Rate per 100,000 person-years. $\chi^2_6 = 34.558$, $p < 0.00001$
[b]Results similar for 1982–88.
From Kurtzke et al., 1993 (38).

CNMS. Among Faroese, these indicate that some two years of exposure to PMSA are necessary before its acquisition; Faroese under age 11 are not susceptible; and once PMSA is acquired, those Faroese who develop CNMS do so after an average incubation period of some six or seven years (38,39).

Transmission models were devised to explain separate consecutive epidemics of CNMS: there must have been separate consecutive cohorts of the population who acquired PMSA. The first cohort (F1) would have acquired PMSA from the British troops during the occupation of World War II. However, since the troops had left the islands by then, the second (F2) cohort must have

acquired the disease from the F1 cohort and then in turn transmitted PMSA to a third (F3) population cohort (39). If this were true, the expectation was that the F3 cohort would transmit PMSA to a fourth cohort, and this would be demonstrated by the occurrence of a fourth epidemic of CNMS—which is what happened (38).

The way in which we were able to construct separate cohorts out of the continuum, which is the Faroese population over time, was to define an *age* beyond which PMSA would not be transmissible, and we took this age to be the average age of symptom onset of CNMS in general, age 27. This permitted new cohorts over time for Faroese: age 11–12 susceptible to PMSA; age 13–26

TABLE 3-8

Risk of CNMS per 1,000 population age 11, for three epidemics after epidemic I divided into periods of 13 years with each period expected to comprise seven "high" followed by six "low" years. O = observed, E = expected

PERIOD	PERSONS AGE 11	PATIENTS AGE 11 O	PATIENTS AGE 11 E	χ^2A	RISK[a]	95%CI
1945–51	3,963.6	9	3.112	11.140	2.27	1.04–4.31
1952–57	3,994.5	1	3.137	1.456	0.25	0.01–1.39
1958–64	5,070.5	4	3.981	0.000	0.79	0.21–2.02
1965–70	4,465.5	1	3.506	1.791	0.22	0.01–1.25
1971–77	5,804.4	5	4.558	0.043	0.86	0.28–2.01
1978–83[b]	4,719.1	2	3.706	0.785	0.42	0.05–1.53
TOTAL	28,017.6	22	22.000	15.215	0.79	0.49–1.19

[a]Per 1,000 persons age 11. $\chi^2_5 = 15.215$, $0.02 > p > 0.01$.
From Kurtzke et al., 1993 (38).

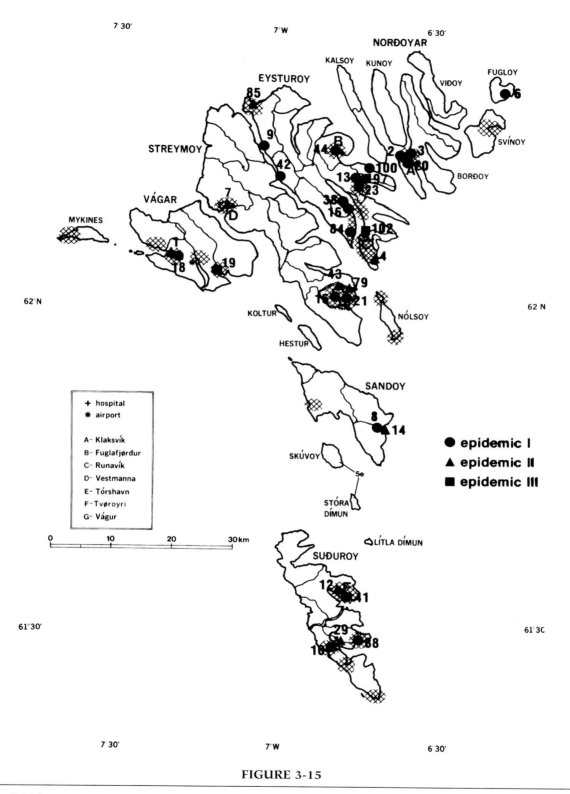

FIGURE 3-15

British troop encampments in the Faroes in World War II (cross-hatched areas) and residence of Faroese MS patients in 1943 or at age 11 if then younger for patients known as of 1986, subdivided by epidemic: I (solid circles), II (triangles), III (squares). Numbers identify the patients in Kurtzke and Hyllested 1987 (39). *From Kurtzke and Hyllested, 1987 (39).*

affected and transmissible. The models are fully detailed elsewhere (37–39), but they do give reasonable explanations for PMSA in consecutive Faroese population cohorts (F1–F4), which provide the denominators for the four consecutive epidemics of CNMS in Faroese.

EPITOME

Epidemiology is the study of the natural history of disease. Measures of disease frequency involve a numerator (cases) and a denominator (population at risk). Incidence and death rates refer to new cases and to deaths per unit time and population; prevalence rates to cases present at one time per unit population. Incidence and prevalence rates arise from specific surveys for the disease within circumscribed populations; death rates come from standard published governmental sources.

As to MS, the best measures of geographic distribution come from prevalence studies, of which there are now more than 300. These works indicate that, geographically, MS is distributed throughout the world within three zones of high, medium, and low frequency. High frequency areas, with prevalence rates of 30 and above per 100,000 population, include most of Europe into the former Soviet Union, Israel, Canada and northern United States, New Zealand, and southeastern Australia. This also seems to include the easternmost part of Russia.

These high regions are bounded by areas of medium frequency with prevalence rates of 5 to 29 and mostly 15 to 25 per 100,000, which then include most of Australia, southern United States, southwestern Norway and northern Scandinavia, the southern Mediterranean basin, probably Russia from the Urals into Siberia as well as the Ukraine, South Africa, and perhaps much of the Caribbean region and parts of South America. All other known areas of Asia and Africa and possibly northern South America are low, with prevalence rates under 5 per 100,000 population. A number of nationwide prevalence studies in Europe provide evidence for geographic clustering of the disease, which is stable over time, but with evidence of diffusion over time. This last seems also likely on an international basis as well.

In MS there is a female preponderance, which appears to be increasing. There is also a clear predilection for whites, but other racial groups share the geographic distributions of the whites though at lower levels. Thus, location, sex, and race are independent risk factors for this disease.

Prevalence studies for migrants from high-risk to low-risk areas indicate the age of adolescence to be critical for risk retention: those migrating beyond age 15 retain the MS risk of their birthplace; those migrating under age 15 acquire the lower risk of their new residence. Several low-to-high studies show that those migrating in childhood or adolescence do in fact increase their risk of MS. In one such study the prevalence among the migrants exceeded that for the native-born and suggested a susceptible period from approximately age 11 to age 40 or so with a three-year exposure period required. The migrant data support the idea that MS is ordinarily acquired in early adolescence, with a lengthy "incubation" or "latent" period between disease onset and symptom onset, and with young children not susceptible to this illness. But susceptibility extends to approximately age 45.

Recently epidemics of MS have been described, one (definite) in the Faroe Islands; the others (probable) in Iceland and the Shetland-Orkneys. To 1991 we have been able to identify on the Faroe Islands 42 cases of MS among native-born resident Faroese. They comprised four successive epidemics with peaks at 13-year intervals and the first case in 1943. The 20 cases included as the first epidemic met all criteria for a type 1 point-source epidemic. Present evidence as to a source for the epidemic points to the British troops, who occupied the Faroes in large numbers for five years from April 1940 and were stationed where the patients lived. The later epidemics were the result of transmission from and to successive cohorts of the Faroese population, all cases occurring in residents of the same locations as the British and the first epidemic patients.

If these findings are valid, these studies would indicate the definition of MS as not only an acquired disease but also a transmissible one. What we believe is transmissible is a widespread, specific (but unknown) persistent infection of adolescents and young adults, which we call PMSA (the primary multiple sclerosis affection), and which only rarely leads to clinical neurologic MS after years of incubation. In this context PMSA is transmissible, CNMS is not. Furthermore, prolonged exposure (at least two years) is required to acquire PMSA. The best place to seek an MS transmissible agent may be in the Faroes, because there is in those islands a unique control group: there are parts of the Faroes that are still free of CNMS, even after 50 years of presence of the disease on the islands.

References

1. Kurtzke JF. Neurologic needs of the community. In: Kurtzke JF (ed.). Neuroepidemiology. American Academy of Neurology Special Course 1974. Minneapolis, MN, Education Marketing Corp., 1974: 61–65 + tape cassette.
2. Kurtzke JF. Multiple sclerosis from an epidemiological viewpoint. In: Field EJ (ed.). *Multiple sclerosis: A critical conspectus.* Lancaster, England: Medical and Technical Publishing Press, 1977:83–142.

3. Poser CM, Paty DW, Scheinberg L, et al. New diagnostic criteria for multiple sclerosis: Guidelines for research protocols. *Ann Neurol* 1983; 13:227–231.

4. Schumacher GA, Beebe GW, Kibler RF, et al. Problems of experimental trials of therapy in multiple sclerosis: Report by the panel on the evaluation of experimental trials of therapy in multiple sclerosis. *Ann NY Acad Sci* 1965; 122:552–568.

5. Allison RS, Millar JHD. Prevalence and familial incidence of disseminated sclerosis (a report to the Northern Ireland Hospitals Authority on the results of a three-year study). Prevalence of disseminated sclerosis in Northern Ireland. *Ulster Med J* 1954; 23(Suppl 2):5–27.

6. Kurtzke JF. The epidemiology of multiple sclerosis. In: Raine CS, McFarland H, Tourtellotte WW (eds.). *Multiple sclerosis: Clinical and pathogenetic basis.* London: Chapman & Hall, 1997:91–139.

7. Acheson ED. The epidemiology of multiple sclerosis. 1. The pattern of disease. 2. What does this pattern mean? In: Matthews WB, Acheson ED, Batchelor JR, Weller RO. *McAlpine's multiple sclerosis.* Edinburgh: Churchill Livingstone 1985:3–46.

8. Dean G. Epidemiology of multiple sclerosis. *Neuroepidemiology* 1984; 3:58–73.

9. Ebers GC, Sadovnick AD. Epidemiology. In: Paty DW, Ebers GC (eds.). *Multiple sclerosis.* Philadelphia: FA Davis, 1998:5–28.

10. Firnhaber W, Lauer K (eds.). *Multiple sclerosis in Europe. An epidemiological update.* Darmstadt: LTV Press, 1994.

11. Gonzalez-Scarano F, Spielman RS, Nathanson N. Neuroepidemiology. In: McDonald WI, Silberberg DH (eds.). *Multiple sclerosis.* Boston: Butterworth, 1986:37–55.

12. Kesselring J. Epidemiology. In: Kesselring J (ed.). *Multiple sclerosis.* Cambridge, England: Cambridge University Press, 1997:49–53.

13. Koch-Henriksen N. An epidemiological study of multiple sclerosis. Familial aggregation, social determinants, and exogenic factors. *Acta Neurol Scand* 1989; 80 (Suppl 124):1–123.

14. Kurtzke JF. Epidemiology of multiple sclerosis. In: Vinken PJ, Bruyn GW, Klawans HL (eds.). *Handbook of clinical neurology. Vol. 3 (rev.). Demyelinating diseases.* Amsterdam: Elsevier, 1985:Chapter 9, 259–287.

15. Kurtzke JF. Risk factors, course and prognosis of multiple sclerosis. In: Cazzullo CL, Caputo D, Ghezzi A, Zaffaroni M (eds.). *Virology and immunology of multiple sclerosis: Rationale for therapy.* Berlin: Springer-Verlag, 1988:87–109.

16. Kurtzke JF. Epidemiologic evidence for multiple sclerosis as an infection. *Clin Microbiol Rev* 1993; 6:382–427.

17. Martyn C. The epidemiology of multiple sclerosis. In: Matthews WB, Compston A, Allen IV, Martyn CN. *McAlpine's multiple sclerosis.* 2nd ed. Edinburgh: Churchill Livingstone, 1991:3–40.

18. Pryse-Phillips W. The epidemiology of multiple sclerosis. In: Cook SD (ed.). *Handbook of multiple sclerosis.* New York: Marcel Dekker, 1990:1–24.

19. Weinshenker BG, Rodriguez M. Epidemiology of multiple sclerosis. In: Gorelick PB, Alter M (eds.). *Handbook of neuroepidemiology.* New York: Marcel Dekker, 1994:553–564.

20. Wynn DR, Rodriguez M, O'Fallon WM, Kurland LT. Update on the epidemiology of multiple sclerosis. *Mayo Clin Proc* 1989; 64:808–817.

21. Limburg CC. The geographic distribution of multiple sclerosis and its estimated prevalence in the United States. *Proc Assoc Res Nerv Ment Dis* 1950; 28:15–24.

22. Goldberg ID, Kurland LT. Mortality in 33 countries from disease of the nervous system. *World Neurol* 1962; 3:444–465.

23. Massey EW, Schoenberg BS. International patterns of mortality from multiple sclerosis. *Neuroepidemiology* 1982; 1:189–196.

24. Kurland LT, Kurtzke JF, Goldberg ID. *Epidemiology of neurologic and sense organ disorders.* Cambridge: Harvard University Press, 1973:64-107.

25. Kurtzke JF, Wallin MT. A further assessment of the geographic distribution of multiple sclerosis from prevalence rates into the 1990s (in preparation).

26. Kurtzke JF. The geographic distribution of multiple sclerosis: An update with special reference to Europe and the Mediterranean region. *Acta Neurol Scand* 1980; 62:65–80.

27. Lauer K. Multiple sclerosis in the old world: The new old map. In: Firnhaber W, Lauer K (eds.). *Multiple sclerosis in Europe. An epidemiological update.* Darmstadt: LTV Press, 1994:14–27.

28. Boiko AN. Multiple sclerosis prevalence in Russia and other countries of the USSR. In: Firnhaber W, Lauer K, (eds.): *Multiple sclerosis in Europe. An epidemiological update.* Darmstadt: LTV Press, 1994:219-230.

29. Kurtzke JF. A reassessment of the distribution of multiple sclerosis. Part One, Part Two. *Acta Neurol Scand* 1975; 51:110–136, 137–157.

30. Kurtzke JF, Beebe GW, Norman JE Jr. Epidemiology of multiple sclerosis in United States veterans: I. Race, sex, and geographic distribution. *Neurology* 1979; 29:1228–1235.

31. Kurtzke JF, Beebe GW, Norman JE Jr. Epidemiology of multiple sclerosis in United States veterans: III. Migration and the risk of MS. *Neurology* 1985; 35:672-678.

32. Kurtzke JF, Dean G, Botha DPJ. A method of estimating age at immigration of white immigrants to South Africa, with an example of its importance. *S Afr Med J* 1970; 44:663–669.

33. Kurtzke JF, Delasnerie-Lauprêtre N, Wallin MT. Multiple sclerosis in North African migrants to France. *Acta Neurol Scand* 1998; 98:302–309.

34. Kurtzke JF, Hyllested K. Multiple sclerosis. An epidemic disease in the Faeroes. *Trans Am Neurol Assoc* 1975; 100:213–215.

35. Kurtzke JF, Gudmundsson KR, Bergmann S. Multiple sclerosis in Iceland: I. Evidence of a postwar epidemic. *Neurology* 1982; 32:143–150.

36. Cook SD, MacDonald J, Tapp W, Poskanzer D, Dowling PC. Multiple sclerosis in Shetland Islands: An update. *Acta Neurol Scand* 1988; 77:148–151.

37. Kurtzke JF, Hyllested K. Multiple sclerosis in the Faroe Islands: II. Clinical update, transmission, and the nature of MS. *Neurology* 1986; 36:307–328.

38. Kurtzke JF, Hyllested K, Heltberg A, Olsen A. Multiple sclerosis in the Faroe Islands. V. The occurrence of the fourth epidemic as validation of transmission. *Acta Neurol Scand* 1993; 88:161–173.

39. Kurtzke JF, Hyllested K. Multiple sclerosis in the Faroe Islands. III. An alternative assessment of the three epidemics. *Acta Neurol Scand* 1987; 76:317–339.

IV

DIAGNOSIS, SIGNS AND SYMPTOMS, AND CLASSIFICATION

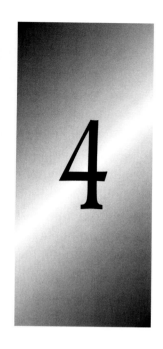

4 Initial Symptoms

Donald W. Paty, M.D., F.R.C.P.C, F.A.C.P.

The initial symptoms of multiple sclerosis (MS) may be the result of new lesions in any portion of the white matter of the central nervous system (CNS). In our experience at the University of British Columbia (UBC), we have determined the initial symptoms in 1,721 patients with clinically definite MS seen at our MS Clinic (1). Table 4-1 lists the most common symptoms and the percentage at which they are seen. In this study, the average age for the initial symptoms to appear was 30 years, with the exception of a slowly developing motor deficit that appeared, on average, at age 40. Some initial neurologic events are more likely to announce the onset of MS than others (Table 4-2).

SENSORY SYMPTOMS IN THE LIMBS

The most frequent initial MS symptom is an acute or subacute onset of numbness or tingling in one or more limbs. The symptoms usually begin distally in the limbs and expand proximally. The symptoms occasionally will migrate from one side to the other, probably as a result of lesions expanding transversely across the spinal cord to involve multiple limbs.

New sensory symptoms usually reach their maximum extent in less than a week. In some patients a parox-ysmal sensory symptom in the back or lower limbs brought on by flexing the head forward (Lhermitte's symptom) may precede the persistent sensory symptoms or may occur in isolation. Many times the sensory disturbances are not associated with any functional abnormality in the involved limb. The majority of these symptoms usually will resolve spontaneously before the patient has been seen by a physician or neurologist. Therefore at the time of examination there may be neither continued symptoms nor neurologic signs.

Occasionally sensory symptoms may occur in a radicular distribution associated with pain, itching, numbness, or dyesthesia. These symptoms probably are due to an acute lesion at the sensory root entry zone in the spinal cord or brainstem. These radicular syndromes occasionally may mimic spinal root compression caused by disk herniation. In our experience it is not unusual to find MS patients who have had prior spinal surgery to relieve radicular symptoms that later were found to be caused by MS.

A very specific and characteristic sensory symptom seen in MS is the useless hand syndrome (2). The useless hand is one that is functionally impaired by proprioceptive sensory loss. The sensory loss is usually confined to discriminatory sensation such as vibration, two-point discrimination, position sense, or, more grossly, joint position. One or both hands usually become functionally use-

TABLE 4-1
Symptoms Seen at Onset of MS (UBC Data)

	PERCENT
Sensory symptoms in arms/legs	33
Unilateral visual loss	16
Slowly progressive motor deficit	9
Acute motor deficit	5
Diplopia	7
Polysymptomatic onset	14
Others	16

less because of the sensory loss, even though one can demonstrate on physical examination that under visual control, with concentration, motor function is normal. The lesion responsible for the useless hand syndrome is probably in the posterior column of the spinal cord. A characteristic complaint is that the patient cannot recognize coins or other objects in the pocket or purse.

Another characteristic sensory MS symptom is Lhermitte's sign, which was first described by Babinski and Dubois in 1891 (3). It is usually described as an electric current–like shock sensation traveling down the back or the legs brought on by neck flexion. When originally described, it was seen in patients with traumatic diseases of the cervical spinal cord. Later Lhermitte and his colleagues (4) pointed out that the symptom was most frequently seen in MS. The symptom was described as a "clinical sign." It is indeed a sign of cervical spinal cord pathology, but it is not specific to MS and therefore it probably is best to be indicated as a symptom rather than a sign. Lhermitte's symptom occasionally can be brought

TABLE 4-2
Follow-Up on Single Symptoms in Prediction of Onset of Clinically Definite MS

	RISK FOR MS 5 YEARS	RISK FOR MS 10 YEARS
Unilateral Optic Neuritis	High	High
Bilateral Optic Neuritis	Low	Low
Complete Acute Transverse Myelopathy (ATM)	Low	Low
Incomplete ATM	High	High
Chronic Progressive Myelopathy	High	High
Acute Brainstem Episode	High	High

on by lateral flexion of the neck or even by walking over uneven ground. As in other paroxysmal symptoms caused by MS, Lhermitte's symptom can usually be reduced by low doses of anticonvulsants or benzodiazepines.

VISUAL LOSS (OPTIC NEURITIS)

Optic neuritis (ON) has a close relationship with MS. It was the initial symptom in 16 percent of patients in this series and is a common condition throughout the course of MS. There have been a number of excellent reviews of visual loss in MS (5,6). The visual loss produced by ON usually begins with acute or subacute loss of monocular vision, with the central vision being most affected. Optic neuritis is almost always associated with diminished visual acuity. The maximum loss of vision usually develops within the first week, although chronically progressive visual loss may be seen. Other visual symptoms such as flashes of light or color are also described, particularly in association with eye movements.

The visual loss occasionally may be temporal, peripheral, or hemionoptic. Altitudinal defects may also be experienced.

The Optic Neuritis Treatment Trial (ONTT) (7,8) has shown clearly that in patients with ON, if a magnetic resonance imaging (MRI) scan has four or more lesions, the likelihood of developing MS in the first two to four years of follow-up is high. Additionally, in patients with multiple cerebral MRI lesions at the onset of ON, the second episode that allows the diagnosis of clinically definite multiple sclerosis (CDMS) could possibly be delayed by several months if the ON is treated early (within one week) with high-dose intravenous methylprednisolone.

With acute ON, most patients also have pain on eye movement. The pain is not necessarily specific for ON, so acute ON should always be investigated by a knowledgeable ophthalmologist or neurologist. The pain of ON usually resolves before the recovery of visual acuity. The severity and duration of the pain probably has no effect on visual outcome. Magnetic resonance imaging and computed tomography (CT) studies can visualize the lesions in the optic nerve during acute ON. Miller and coworkers (9) found that the visual loss in ON was proportional to the length of the involved segment of the optic nerve as detected by enhanced MRI.

Another interesting aspect of ON is the loss of the retinal nerve fiber layer (RNFL) that may occur. Approximately half of MS patients have defects in the RNFL (10). The functional and pathologic significance of this axonal loss is not known. However, the frequency of the finding suggests that loss of the nerve fiber layer could be diagnostically and pathologically important. Because the optic nerve is the only place in the body in which nerves can be directly visualized in a noninvasive fashion, systematic study and follow-up of the phenomenon should be informative concerning the axonal loss component of MS pathology.

An aspect of the physical examination associated with ON is the afferent pupillary defect (APD) or Marcus Gunn pupil (11). The APD may be the only hard evidence present on physical examination other than the visual loss. A subtle APD may be demonstrated by using the ophthalmoscope in dim room light. One can focus on the magnified pupil and reveal a enlarged red reflex. After the red reflex has been seen, the light can be moved from eye to eye and the pupillary reflex can be clearly identified by the change in the size of the red reflex. In APD the pupil of the involved eye will not constrict or will actually dilate in spite of the light, showing that the consensual reflex is stronger than the direct reflex in the involved eye.

If one plots time versus diagnosis of CDMS after an episode of ON, 50 percent of the people who develop CDMS will do so within five years. However, the curve is not linear and gradually flattens out so that the second symptom of MS may not occur for as long as 30 years after the initial ON. Overall, the risk for MS is between 60 percent and 70 percent within 10 years following unilateral ON.

The implication for MS is quite different after bilateral ON. Very few adults with simultaneous bilateral ON go on to develop MS (12). Bilateral sequential ON, however, has the same high risk for developing MS as unilateral ON.

SLOWLY DEVELOPING MOTOR ONSET

Multiple sclerosis patients with slowly developing motor onset belong to a diagnostically heterogeneous group with what is referred to as chronic progressive myelopathy (CPM). The typical patient is older than the average MS patient at onset. When the motor deficit is slowly progressive, there is usually no clinical evidence for dissemination in anatomic space on initial physical examination. It is in these patients that reliable paraclinical evidence for dissemination in space and probably dissemination in time is most useful (13,14). Even though a slow onset may occur with any of the anatomic categories of MS (spinal, brainstem, cerebellar, and so forth), the majority of such chronically progressive patients show spinal cord involvement. All such patients should have a spinal MRI to exclude structural and/or compressive causes of spinal cord dysfunction. A head MRI can easily show dissemination of lesions in space. Visual evoked potentials are particularly important if there is no clinical evidence of a lesion above the level of foramen magnum on MRI scan. However, because these patients are usually older, one

must be careful about nonspecific MRI changes that develop with age (15).

Additionally, if oligoclonal banding (OB) is found in the cerebrospinal fluid (CSF) in addition to paraclinical evidence for dissemination in space (MRI or evoked potentials), laboratory-supported definite MS (LSDMS) can be diagnosed. A diagnosis of LSDMS is probably as reliable as a diagnosis of CDMS (14).

A number of conditions can mimic spinal MS with slow onset, including arteriovenous malformations, herniated thoracic disks, intramedullary tumors, Arnold-Chiari malformations, or syringomyelia. Human T cell lymphotrophic virus type 1 (HTLV-1)–associated myelopathy (HAM) or tropical spastic paraplegia (TSP) must also be considered in patients who come from or have sexual exposure to individuals from the Caribbean, Japan, or other endemic areas. Combined system disease secondary to vitamin B12 deficiency is another consideration.

Eighty percent of patients with chronic progressive myelopathy who do not have a compressive or structural lesion will eventually be diagnosed as LSDMS or CDMS with adequate follow-up (13).

DIPLOPIA

Eye movement disorders are very common in MS (16), but diplopia is seen in only 7 percent of patients at onset. Because the diplopia may disappear by the time the patient is seen by a neurologist, the history is particularly important. An observant patient usually can identify whether the diplopia is vertical, horizontal, or diagonal. Six-nerve palsies, fourth-nerve palsies, or non-pupil–involved third-nerve palsies may be the initial presentation. The most frequent cause of horizontal bilateral double vision on lateral gaze is a bilateral intranuclear ophthalmoplegia (INO). A fully developed bilateral INO in a young person is almost pathognomonic for MS, but metastases to the brainstem and vascular abnormalities also may cause bilateral INO. The diplopia in INO usually, but not always, is horizontal. Careful examination will usually pick up a lag in the abducting eye on lateral gaze associated with an irregular (ataxic) nystagmus in the abducting eye. After resolution of the diplopia, the only physical finding may be loss of smooth pursuit.

ACUTELY EVOLVING MOTOR DYSFUNCTION

Acutely developing motor symptoms in one or more extremity are less common than sensory symptoms initially. The onset occasionally is very dramatic, with complete paralysis below the level of the lesion.

Acute complete transverse myelopathy (ATM), however, just like bilateral simultaneous ON, does not usually

(14 percent) lead to CDMS (17) (Table 4-2). Acute partial transverse myelopathies, often with a partial or complete Brown-Séquard syndrome, are most typical of the acute onset of MS (18). In these patients MRI may be particularly helpful in the diagnosis. On physical examination, one occasionally finds hyperactive reflexes below the level of acute lesion. Rarely, if the acute transverse lesion occurs in the midcervical cord, one of the cervical deep tendon reflexes will be abolished when there are hyperactive reflexes below that level on the involved side.

VERTIGO

Vertigo is a common symptom in general neurologic practice. Most patients with vertigo have a peripheral vestibular disturbance rather than MS. Patients with MS occasionally present with vertigo, and when it occurs by itself, it is indistinguishable from the paroxysmal vertigo that accompanies acute inner ear disturbances. Vertigo may also occur during the course of MS, and it is difficult to be sure whether the vertigo is directly due to MS or to a superimposed vestibular disturbance. Brainstem lesions are occasionally seen in patients with acute vertigo, raising the possibility of the diagnosis of MS.

BLADDER SYMPTOMS

Bladder disturbances may occasionally occur at the onset of MS. They become very common during the subsequent course of the disease. Symptoms are usually urgency, frequency, and urinary incontinence. Hesitancy or actual obstruction may also occur. The most difficult set of symptoms to manage are urgency, frequency, and hesitancy.

TABLE 4-3

*Uncommon Symptoms Seen at Onset of MS
(all seen at less than 5 percent)*

- Bladder symptoms
- Heat intolerance
- Paroxysmal symptoms
- Pain
- Movement disorders
- Higher cortical function disorders
- Dementia

After Table 4-3, Paty DW, Ebers GC (eds.), *Multiple Sclerosis*. Philadelphia: FA Davis, 1998.

TABLE 4-4

Symptoms and Signs at Onset Most Characteristic of Multiple Sclerosis

- Bilateral intranuclear ophthalmoplegia
- Unilateral useless hand syndrome

HEAT AND EXERCISE INTOLERANCE

One characteristic but uncommon symptom of early MS is seen in the patient who develops a neurologic symptom or frank deficit after exercise or exposure to heat. When it occurs with visual loss, it is called Uhthoff's phenomenon (19). These heat- or exercise-related symptoms may be brought on by activity, sunbathing, hot baths, emotion, fatigue, fever, or other factors associated with an increase in body temperature. Patients typically complain of blurring of vision or sensory symptoms after exercise or of weakness in one or both legs. These symptoms usually disappear with rest and cooling but may be quite confusing to both patients and physicians. The phenomenon has a neurophysiologic explanation. The demyelinated nerve fiber is very sensitive to heat and local changes in microchemistry (20) (see Chapter 2).

OTHER SYMPTOMS

There are a number of other symptoms that are rarely seen at the onset of MS (Table 4-3). These include paroxysmal sensory or motor symptoms, pain, dementia, fatigue, movement disorders, seizures, and higher cortical function disturbances such as aphasia in addition to autonomic abnormalities. Dementia in a young person is a significant but rare initial event in MS. A young person occasionally will have presenting symptoms of cognitive difficulties, including poor memory, speech hesitancy, and slowed information processing. Cognitive deficits produce a very distressing situation and require immediate MRI investigation to determine if MS-like lesions in the cerebral hemispheres are the underlying

---

TABLE 4-5

Strong Predictors for the Diagnosis of Clinically Definite MS

- Multiple MRI lesions
- Presence of oligoclonal IgG bands in CSF
- Multiple neurologic episodes

cause. Neuropsychological evaluation is also useful. These unusual symptoms are rarely observed at the onset of MS but unfortunately are seen more frequently during the course of the disease.

In summary, in our experience the two symptom complexes most likely to characterize MS at the onset are bilateral intranuclear ophthalmoplegia and unilateral useless hand syndrome (Table 4-4). When combining clinical signs and symptoms with laboratory indicators, Table 4-5 shows the best correlated predictors of clinically definite MS.

References

1. Paty DW, Noseworthy JH, Ebers GC. Diagnosis of multiple sclerosis. In: Paty DW, Ebers GC (eds.). *Multiple sclerosis. Contemporary neurology series.* Philadelphia: FA Davis, 1997.
2. Lu CS, Tsai CH, Chiu HC, Yip PK. Pseudoathetosis as a presenting symptom of spinal multiple sclerosis. *J Formosan Med Assoc* 1992; 91(1):106–109.
3. Babinski J, Dubois R. Douleurs a forme de decharge electrique, consecutive aux tramatismes de la nuque. *Press Med* 1891: 26:64.
4. Lhermitte J, Bollak G, Nicholas M. Les doleurs a type de decharge electrique consecutives a la flexion cephalique dans la sclerose en plaques. *Rev Neurol* 1924; 42:56–62.
5. McDonald WI, Barnes D. The ocular manifestations of multiple sclerosis. I. Abnormalities of the afferent visual system. *J Neurol Neurosurg Psychiatry* 1992; 55:747–752.
6. Perkin GD, Rose FC. *Optic neuritis and its differential diagnosis.* New York: Oxford University Press, 1979.
7. Beck RW, Cleary PA, Trobe JD, et al. The effect of corticosteroids for acute optic neuritis on the subsequent development of multiple sclerosis. The Optic Neuritis Study Group. *N Engl J Med* 1993; 329:1764–1769.
8. Beck RW, Arrington J, Murtagh FR, Cleary PA, Kaufman DI, and the Optic Neuritis Study Group. Brain MRI in acute optic neuritis experience of the Optic Neuritis Study Group. *Arch Neurol* 1993; 50:841–846.
9. Miller DH, Youl BD, Turano G, et al. Acute optic neuritis: Relationship between clinical, electrophysiological, and MRI abnormalities. *Neurology* 1991; 41(Suppl):168.
10. MacFadyen DJ, Drance SM, Douglas G, et al. The retinal nerve fiber layer, neuroretinal rim area, and visual evoked potentials in MS. *Neurology* 1988; 38:1353–1358.
11. Anderson DP, Cox TA. Visual signs and symptoms. In: Paty DW, Ebers GC (eds.). *Multiple sclerosis. Contemporary neurology series.* Philadelphia: FA Davis, 1997.
12. Parkin PJ, Hierons R, McDonald WI. Bilateral optic neuritis: A long-term follow-up. *Brain* 1984; 107:951–964.
13. Paty DW, Blume WT, Brown WF, Jaatoul N, Kertesz A, McInnis W. Chronic progressive myelopathy: Investigation with CSF electrophoresis, evoked potentials and CT scan. *Ann Neurol* 1979; 6(5):419–424.
14. Lee KH, Hashimoto SA, Hooge JP, et al. Magnetic resonance imaging of the head in the diagnosis of multiple sclerosis. A prospective 2-year follow-up with comparison of clinical evaluation, evoked potentials, oligoclonal banding, and CT. *Neurology* 1991; 41:657–660.
15. Fazekas F, Offenbacher H, Fuchs S, et al. Criteria for an increased specificity of MRI interpretation in elderly subjects with suspected multiple sclerosis. *Neurology* 1988; 388:1822–1825.
16. Barnes D, McDonald WI. The ocular manifestations of multiple sclerosis. II. Abnormalities of eye movements: Review. *J Neurol Neurosurg Psychiatry* 1992; 55:863–868.
17. Altrocchi PH. Acute transverse myelopathy. *Arch Neurol* 1963; 9:21–29.
18. Ford B, Tampieri D, Francis G. Long-term follow-up of acute partial transverse myelopathy. *Neurology* 1992; 42:250–252.
19. Uhtoff W. Untersuchungen uer bei multiplen Hersklerose vorkommenden Augenstorungen. *Archiv Fur Psychiatrie und Nervenkrankheiten* 1890; 21:55–116, 303–410.
20. Waxman SG. Clinical course and electrophysiology of multiple sclerosis. In: Waxman SG (ed.). *Advances in neurology: Functional recovery in neurological disease.* New York: Raven Press, 1988:157–184.

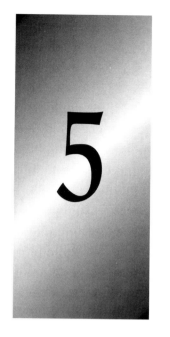

5

Diagnosis and Classification of Inflammatory Demyelinating Disorders

P. K. Coyle, M.D.

Multiple sclerosis (MS) is the major inflammatory and demyelinating disease of the central nervous system (CNS). It is the prototype in a spectrum of acquired disorders characterized by similar white matter damage accompanied by varying degrees of inflammation (Table 5-1). The ability to make a precise and correct diagnosis, and to differentiate MS from these other conditions, is essential because each disease course, prognosis, pathogenesis, and treatment are not necessarily the same. Multiple sclerosis itself is quite variable and heterogeneous, and a number of genotypes are associated with the MS phenotype (1). With the development of partially effective disease-modifying therapies, MS is now treatable (2–10). The recent appreciation that there is early, ongoing, and potentially irreversible damage to axons (11), accompanied by progressive brain atrophy (12), highlights the need for early and aggressive treatment (13). Similar approaches are being applied to autoimmune and immune-mediated diseases in general.

In this context early accurate diagnosis is critical. It guides optimal therapy, removes uncertainty, allows informed planning, and improves the patient's sense of well-being by providing an explanation for their problems. Unfortunately, the misdiagnosis rate for MS approximates 5 percent to 10 percent, even by experienced health care providers (14). Misdiagnosis should be minimized by a thoughtful analysis of the history and examination, supplemented by appropriate data collection and analysis. This chapter first covers basic diagnostic principles for MS and then discusses characteristics that distinguish the other disorders within the MS spectrum.

MULTIPLE SCLEROSIS

Basic Diagnostic Principles

Multiple sclerosis is ultimately a clinical diagnosis because there is no definitive laboratory test. It is common practice, however, to perform a battery of pertinent investigations as part of the diagnostic process. This helps to exclude other conditions and co-diagnoses, to provide objective evidence that MS is the correct diagnosis, and to create a prognostic profile to guide therapeutic choices.

Certain basic principles apply for a diagnosis of MS (Table 5-2). There is a characteristic demographic profile. Most patients are young women whose presenting symptoms are episodic neurologic problems that spontaneously improve. The less common presentation is an older man or woman who has gradual development of neurologic deficit. This most often takes the form of a progressive myelopathy. Multiple sclerosis is clearly a gender preference disease, and overall 70 percent to 75 percent of MS patients are female. The only exception is the

TABLE 5-1
The Spectrum of Inflammatory and Demyelinating CNS Disorders

Multiple Sclerosis
- Asymptomatic
- Symptomatic

Multiple Sclerosis Variants
- Marburg variant (acute/fulminant course)
- Balo's concentric sclerosis
- Concentric lacunar leukoencephalopathy
- Myelinoclastic diffuse sclerosis (Schilder disease)
- Disseminated subpial demyelination
- Unilateral mass lesion

Other Disorders
- Neuromyelitic optica (Devic syndrome)
- Monophasic syndrome
  - Postinfectious encephalomyelitis
  - Clinically isolated syndromes
- Optic neuritis
- Transverse myelitis/myelopathy
- Other syndromes

TABLE 5-2
Basic Principles for the Diagnosis of MS

Demographic Profile
- Female gender preference
- Caucasian race preference
- Young age at onset
- Geographic residence

Clinical Profile
- Symptomatic disease
- Abnormal examination
- White matter involvement
- Consistent pattern (relapsing or progressive)

Laboratory Profile
- No alternative diagnosis
- Consistent pattern of abnormalities

primary progressive subtype (see subsequent section), which shows an equal sex ratio. Most MS patients are Caucasian (> 90 percent), with a Western European/Scandinavian racial background. Multiple sclerosis is rare among Africans, Asians, and Native Americans. African Americans, presumably as a result of mixing of the gene pool, show a frequency in between that of Caucasians and Africans (15). Asians are more likely to express clinical spinal cord–optic nerve disease, almost consistent with neuromyelitis optica (see subsequent section) (16). This so-called Asian type MS has an older age onset, fewer brain lesions on magnetic resonance imaging (MRI) but more contrast-enhancing spinal cord lesions, and distinct human leukocyte antigen (HLA) haplotype associations.

The average onset of MS is at 28 to 30 years of age. Fewer than 1 percent of patients have disease that begins under the age of 10 years (0.15 percent to 0.7 percent) or over age 60. Most patients (90 percent) develop disease between the ages of 15 and 50. The incidence of MS starting before age 16 has ranged from 1.2 percent to 6 percent (17). Multiple sclerosis cases are not evenly distributed. Most geographic distribution studies report little MS at the equator and in tropical zones, with increasing patient numbers as one moves north and south of the equator (18). There may even be a west–east gradient in the United States, although ethnic and genetic factors may play some role (19). There are recognized low (<5/100,000), medium (5 to 30/100,000), and high risk (>30/100,000) zones for MS (20). There are also areas of very high frequency, such as the Shetland and Orkney

Islands. This geographic risk involves age-related (childhood) exposure and has been interpreted to indicate that ubiquitous environmental pathogens may play a role in disease development. Multiple sclerosis is much less likely for those who grow up in a very low risk area, such as Central America or the Caribbean.

The clinical profile for MS requires symptomatic disease over time, confirmed by objective abnormalities. Symptomatic disease means neurologic worsening in the form of episodic attacks or slow progression. The most common neurologic manifestations are sensory disturbances (numbness, paresthesias, pain, Lhermitte's sign), motor abnormalities, and visual problems (optic neuritis). Laboratory testing is used to help document that there are no alternative disorders to explain the neurologic picture, and that there is a pattern of CNS lesion involvement and immune disturbances consistent with MS. With currently accepted criteria, a diagnosis of definite MS cannot be made at the first clinical attack. This may soon change. When such an attack is characteristic of MS, and when it is accompanied by MRI and/or cerebrospinal fluid (CSF) abnormalities, there is a reliable predictive value for the development of MS over the subsequent 10 years. A recent study of clinically isolated syndromes (CISs) involving optic nerve, brainstem, or spinal cord found that initial total lesion volume on MRI predicted 100 percent conversion to MS by 10 years (21). There is now discussion that neuroimaging criteria should be used in cases of characteristic CISs to allow an MRI-supported definite diagnosis (22). It is likely that the diagnostic criteria for MS will be revised in the near future to use modern MRI-based data.

Although MRI is recognized as an invaluable laboratory test for MS, it is not appropriate to use it in isolation to make a diagnosis. Many currently misdiagnosed cases reflect overinterpretation of lesions visualized on

---

TABLE 5-3
*Schumacher Criteria for the
Clinical Diagnosis of MS (27)*

- Appropriate age
  - 10–50 years
- CNS white matter disease
- Lesions disseminated in time and space
  - Two or more separate lesions
- Objective abnormalities
- Consistent time course
  - Attacks lasting ≥ 24 hours; spaced one month apart
  - Slow/stepwise progression ≥ 6 months
- No better explanation
  - Minimum routine laboratory investigation
- Diagnosis by a physician competent in clinical neurology

---

do not distinguish between pathologies, it is important to be cautious about interpretation of MRI lesions even in the setting of clinical disease. Interpretation of MRI lesions will be improved now that specific lesion features have been identified, which increase the probability that they are due to MS (see subsequent section).

Formal Classification Criteria

A number of formal criteria have been proposed over the years to allow diagnostic categorization into possible, probable, and definite MS based on clinical parameters. The criteria include those of Allison and Miller (23), McAlpine, Lumsden, and Acheson (24), McDonald and Holliday (25), and Rose and coworkers (26). The most widely accepted criteria, however, have been those proposed by Schumacher and colleagues in 1965 (27). They outline the major requirements for a clinically definite diagnosis (Table 5-3). If these requirements are not met, it may be that a single category of suspected MS is more reasonable than trying to distinguish between probable and possible categories (28). The Schumacher criteria recognize the importance of an appropriate age of onset (10 to 50 years), the concept of lesions disseminated in time and space, the need to document objective abnormalities

brain MRI. There should always be an appropriate clinical context before making a diagnosis of MS. Because MRI is a sensitive tool that detects subclinical changes, because many conditions produce similar lesions on MRI, and because current standard neuroimaging techniques

---

TABLE 5-4
Poser Committee Criteria for the Diagnosis of MS (30)

CLINICAL DIAGNOSIS

CATEGORY		CLINICAL ATTACKS	CLINICAL EVIDENCE		PARACLINICAL EVIDENCE
Definite	1	2	2		—
	2	2	1	and	1
Probable	1	2	1		—
	2	1	2		—
	3	1	1	and	1

LABORATORY-SUPPORTED DIAGNOSIS

CATEGORY		CLINICAL ATTACKS	CLINICAL EVIDENCE		PARACLINICAL EVIDENCE	CSF
Definite	1	2	1	or	1	+
	2	1	2		—	+
	3	1	1		—	+
Probable	1	2	—		—	+

(although not required, ideally at the time of diagnosis), and diagnosis by a competent clinician. The requirement that there be no better explanation for the problems requires formulation of a differential diagnosis with appropriate laboratory investigation. Schumacher also recognized that relapses of MS should last at least 24 hours and that distinct MS attacks had to be spaced at least a month apart. To ensure progression, slow worsening had to be observed for a minimum of six months.

Bauer first proposed that diagnostic criteria formally include laboratory testing (29). The subsequent Poser Committee criteria, which were published in 1983, are now the most widely accepted formal MS diagnostic criteria (30). They are routinely used in research studies. The Poser criteria involve definite and probable diagnoses, which are clinically or laboratory supported (Table 5-4). Poser broadened the acceptable age of disease onset (10 to 59 years). He also broadened the definition of relapse to include brief symptoms, such as Lhermitte's sign or paroxysmal attacks, provided they recurred multiple times over a period of days to weeks. Clinical evidence requires documented abnormalities on examination (this can include historical documentation in the medical records). Paraclinical evidence involves lesions demonstrated by neuroimaging, evoked potential studies, urologic testing, or other modalities. Laboratory-supported diagnosis requires one of two possible immune disturbances in CSF: IgG oligoclonal bands or intrathecal IgG production. Certain clarifications address some confusing aspects of the Poser Committee criteria. In general, a definite diagnosis requires two separate disease attacks to document dissemination in time consistent with a multiphasic disease process. Primary progressive MS, which involves slow worsening from onset, is considered a single attack. Therefore, a distinct new event and/or lesion is needed for definite diagnosis. Such patients often must be observed for two or more years before that requirement is met. When there is one attack, clinical or paraclinical evidence must develop at a later and clearly separate time point to be considered a second attack (28).

Clinical Subtypes

Multiple sclerosis is characterized by great variability. It can be divided into asymptomatic (subclinical or pathologic disease) and symptomatic disease. In the past a number of different terms were used to describe symptomatic forms of MS, including the terms *chronic progressive* and *relapsing progressive*. These two terms are no longer used. International expert consensus recently defined four major clinical subtypes based on disease patterns (Table 5-5) (31). Multiple sclerosis involves either a relapsing course or a more severe progressive course. Approximately 85 percent of MS patients begin with the relaps-

TABLE 5-5
Classification of Multiple Sclerosis

Asymptomatic
- Pathologic diagnosis

Symptomatic
- Relapsing (85% at onset)
  – benign/mild (10%–20%)
- Primary progressive (10%)
- Secondary progressive (up to 80% of untreated relapsing MS)
- Progressive relapsing (5%)
- ? Transitional

ing clinical subtype. They experience neurologic attacks with variable recovery but are clinically stable in between attacks. Among this group are a minority of patients who will have minimal disease activity and little to no disability 25 years into their course. These patients have benign or mild MS and may make up 10 percent to 20 percent of symptomatic MS patients. There are three progressive subtypes. Approximately 15 percent of MS patients have a progressive course from onset. They have either primary progressive MS (10 percent) and never experience acute attacks, or progressive relapsing MS (5 percent), with later attacks superimposed on a progressive course. The third progressive subtype, secondary progressive, is the major progressive form and accounts for approximately 30 percent of all MS patients (32). All secondary progressive patients start out with relapsing disease, but 5–15 years into disease they begin to slowly worsen. By 10 years 50 percent and by 20 to 25 years at least 80 percent of untreated relapsing patients will become secondary progressive (33,34).

An additional term in the literature, *transitional MS,* was not recognized in the recent subtype revision. It has been used variably to refer to relapsing patients who are evolving into the secondary progressive stage (35), relapsing MS patients with accelerating disease activity (36), or patients who progress years after a single attack (transitional progressive MS) (37).

Laboratory Evaluation

Certain basic principles also apply to the laboratory investigation for suspected MS. Blood tests are used to exclude appropriate alternative diagnoses or co-diagnoses. Magnetic resonance imaging studies, supplemented by CSF analysis, are the main laboratory tests for MS. All other tests are ancillary, but additional tests are helpful in certain circumstances (nonsupportive MRI/CSF to document disease involvement and/or extent of disease and to guide therapy). The laboratory evaluation for MS is outlined in Table 5-6. Blood studies are selected based on the differential diagnosis formulated after a careful history and examination. Antibodies to human T cell lymphotrophic virus type 1 (HTLV-1), for example, are not routinely indicated but would be appropriate in patients with progressive myelopathy and a history of blood transfusion, intravenous drug use, or birth in an endemic (tropical) region. Lyme serology is not appropriate unless patients have endemic area exposure and a typical neurologic Lyme disease syndrome, onset of illness after tick bite or summer flu, or suggestive extraneural disease.

Magnetic resonance imaging is the major diagnostic test for MS. Brain MRI with contrast is the standard for diagnosis, whereas spinal MRI is reserved for patients with nonsupportive brain studies, for older individuals, or when it is important to rule out spinal cord pathology. Features that increase the probability that lesions are due to MS include multiplicity, large diameter, ovoid shape perpendicular to the ventricles, white matter predominance, suggestive localization (periventricular white matter, brainstem/infratentorial, corpus callosum, juxtacortical), enhancement, and open ring enhancement. Neuroimaging is discussed further in Chapter 6.

Compared with neuroimaging, CSF analysis is somewhat invasive and is not used as often to establish the diagnosis of MS. It provides important complementary information. Cerebrospinal fluid studies also have predictive value for development of MS in CISs. Cerebrospinal fluid analysis is particularly valuable with equivocal or normal MRI or when the history and examination features are atypical. The critical abnormalities involve intrathecal immune disturbances (either detection of oligoclonal bands or intrathecal IgG production) and are discussed further in Chapter 8. Oligoclonal bands are the most specific CSF test for MS (38), although the false-positive rate is said to be 4 percent (28). They may occur with any chronic infectious or inflammatory CNS condition. The test is run as a paired sample along with serum. Oligoclonal bands in serum will produce CSF bands due to leakage rather than true intrathecal production. Oligoclonal bands correlate with plasma cell infiltration of meninges (39) and once positive remain detectable. A single (monoclonal) band is abnormal but not oligoclonal. Monoclonal bands often reflect a transition stage with subsequent development of oligoclonal bands. Oligoclonal bands involve the presence of two or more distinct IgG bands in the gamma region of the electrophoresis. Techniques to measure oligoclonal bands include agarose gel electrophoresis and isoelectric focusing. Although isoelectric focusing is more sensitive, it is also more likely to produce a false-positive result and needs to be interpreted by experienced personnel. When CSF IgG is used to diagnose MS, intrathecal IgG production is more valuable than a simple CSF IgG measurement. It adjusts for elevated serum IgG levels, and for

---

TABLE 5-6
Laboratory Evaluation for the Diagnosis of MS

Blood Work (to exclude other conditions)
- Autoantibodies (antinuclear antibodies, antiphospholipid antibodies, etc.) to rule out collagen vascular disease, antiphospholipid syndrome
- Antibodies to *Borrelia burgdorferi*, *Brucella* sp., *Chlamydia pneumoniae*, *Treponema pallidum*, retroviruses, herpesviruses; polymerase chain reaction for selected agents to rule out infection
- Thyroid functions, cortisol, glucose
- Vitamins B12, E, B6, folate (nutritional deficiency)
- Angiotensin converting enzyme, calcium, IgG levels (sarcoidosis)
- ESR, C reactive protein, ANCA (vasculitis)
- Very long chain fatty acids (adrenoleukodystrophy)
- Anti-acetylcholine receptor antibodies (myasthenia gravis)

Neuroimaging
- Cranial MRI with contrast, including foramen magnum views
- Spinal MRI (in selected cases)

Cerebrospinal Fluid
- Oligoclonal bands (with paired serum)
- Intrathecal IgG production (IgG index or 24-hour synthesis rate) (with paired serum)
- Other tests (cell count, protein and glucose, VDRL, selected studies including myelin basic protein)

Evoked Potential Tests
- Somatosensory evoked potentials
- Visual evoked potentials
- Brainstem auditory evoked potentials

Ancillary Tests
- Urologic testing (for neurogenic bladder)
- Skin biopsy (CADASIL, vasculitis)
- Electrophysiologic tests (to exclude other diseases)
- Neurocognitive testing

---

blood–brain barrier and blood–CSF barrier damage. Cerebrospinal fluid myelin basic protein has limited diagnostic utility. Unlike oligoclonal bands or intrathecal IgG production, which remain positive, myelin basic protein levels fluctuate over time. They are most likely to be elevated in the setting of acute relapses with sufficient tissue damage to release myelin debris into the CSF. Any disorder that damages CNS tissue, such as head trauma, stroke (especially posterior), or hypoxic encephalopathy, may produce detectable CSF myelin basic protein.

Cerebrospinal fluid studies are used not only to support the diagnosis of MS but also to suggest a misdiagnosis. In particular, a CSF cell count above 50 white blood cells per mm, or a CSF protein level above 100 mg percent, are very atypical in MS and should suggest an alternative diagnosis. Disappearance of oligoclonal bands, or clearance of intrathecal IgG production, should also suggest an alternative diagnosis. Both MRI and CSF abnormalities increase over time, so that the sensitivity rates improve with disease duration. The majority (over 90 percent to 95 percent) of MS patients ultimately have supportive MRI and CSF changes.

Evoked potential tests are used to document lesions disseminated in space, to provide objective evidence for a subjective complaint, or to confirm a pattern of CNS involvement consistent with MS. They are not necessary when the clinical diagnosis of MS is supported by consistent MRI and/or CSF findings. Latency prolongation is more helpful than decreased amplitude and wave dispersion because it suggests a demyelinating process. For somatosensory evoked potentials, lower extremity testing is more valuable than upper extremity testing because it evaluates the entire spinal cord. The addition of sympathetic skin responses increases the yield for abnormalities by 14 percent (40). With visual evoked potentials, a latency of greater than 10 milliseconds between the eyes is abnormal even when the absolute values are within normal range. However, factors such as drowsiness, inattention, inability to focus, or visual problems can all impair responses. Brainstem auditory evoked potentials are less likely to be abnormal than visual or somatosensory potentials. At least one major MS center has stopped using them for the diagnosis of MS (41).

In unusual circumstances a number of other diagnostic procedures may be indicated for MS. Additional ancillary laboratory testing might include urodynamics to document neurogenic bladder, neurocognitive tests to document cognitive abnormalities, electrophysiologic tests to rule out peripheral nerve involvement, or skin biopsy to diagnose cerebral autosomal dominant arteriopathy with subcortical infarctions and leukoencephalopathy (CADASIL) (42,43).

Diagnostic Pitfalls

Approximately 5 percent to 10 percent of people who are told they have MS do not have the disease (14,44). Incorrect diagnosis may lead to inappropriate treatments, failure to recognize other conditions, and unnecessary emotional stress. It is worth highlighting major diagnostic pitfalls to avoid in order to minimize wrong diagnoses (Table 5-7). The topic of MS misdiagnosis is discussed in depth in Chapter 7.

TABLE 5-7

Pitfalls to Avoid in Order to Prevent a Misdiagnosis of MS

- Failure to perform any laboratory tests
- Make the diagnosis despite a normal neurologic examination
- Failure to consider the possibility of a genetic disorder
- Make the diagnosis in the setting of normal or atypical brain MRI and CSF
- Make the diagnosis when there are atypical clinical features
  - Progressive disease starting before age 35
  - Prominent gray matter symptoms
  - Extraneural disease
  - Peripheral nervous system involvement
  - Disease onset at a very early or very late age

VARIANTS OF MULTIPLE SCLEROSIS

There are a number of disorders that are sufficiently similar to MS that they are considered to be variants.

Marburg Variant

As noted previously, MS is a variable disease. At the far end of the clinical spectrum is an acute fulminant form called Marburg variant disease. This is most often a monophasic illness that occurs in young people and results in death within weeks to months. The first case in the literature, recorded in 1906, was a 30-year-old woman who died within a month of presentation (45). There have been a handful of other case reports, and in most instances the course has been rapidly progressive (46–48). Death generally occurs from brainstem involvement. The pathology is consistent with an acute MS process. It involves intense inflammation with diffuse infiltration by macrophages and to a lesser extent T cells (49). There is widespread often confluent demyelination, axonal damage, and edema, although multiple discrete lesions may also be found. Axon involvement is often extensive and more severe than in typical MS with actual necrosis. In one recent biopsy study the infiltrating macrophages showed a marked upregulation of messenger RNA coding for tumor necrosis factor α (TNF-α) and inducible nitric oxide synthase (iNOS), two factors that are known to damage myelin and oligodendrocytes as well as to cause conduction block (49). Infiltrating cells show marked expression of HLA class II antigens (50). In another recent autopsy study of a 27-year-old woman with a six-week course, CNS myelin basic protein was found to be developmentally immature and much less cationic, with extensive citrullination and poor phosphorylation (51). The authors postulated that a genetic factor, leading to unstable myelin, might be implicated in acute Marburg variant MS.

In general, Marburg variant MS occurs in a previously healthy young person. There have also been a few cases in which a patient with documented MS subsequently went on to a fulminant terminal course. Cerebrospinal fluid findings are variable, and oligoclonal bands may be lacking because illness is so acute. There are reports that rapid glucocorticoid therapy may ameliorate disease, and a recent patient with presumed Marburg variant had a good response to glucocorticoid and mannitol therapy (52). This was quite an atypical case, however, with disappearance of oligoclonal bands and a relapsing, steroid-responsive course over four-year follow-up.

Balo's Concentric Sclerosis

Balo's concentric sclerosis is a rare variant of MS first reported by Marburg in 1906 (53) but named after Balo, who described the characteristic pathology in a 23-year-old man who came to autopsy after an eight-month illness (54). This variant is characterized pathologically by alternating concentric bands of myelination, separated by bands of demyelination (55,56). In two dimensions they appear as rings, but in three dimensions they form globular spheres. Lesions usually center around blood vessels. The clinical course is severe and often monophasic, leading to death within weeks to months from herniation sequelae or complicating pneumonia. Patients often show progressive encephalopathy and features of increased intracranial pressure syndrome, with headache, drowsiness, seizures, and cognitive deficits. The youngest documented case is in a four-year-old boy, but the typical age of onset ranges from 20 to 50 years (57). Balo's concentric sclerosis is said to be more common in China and the Philippines (58). Cerebrospinal fluid changes are those of MS, with oligoclonal bands and intrathecal IgG production. Although the diagnosis is generally made post mortem, in recent cases MRI has allowed antemortem diagnosis (59–64). There are reports of individual patients who have responded to a variety of treatments. These have included glucocorticoids, immunosuppressives, and plasma exchange in a steroid nonresponder (58,65,66). The responses to a spectrum of immunomodulatory approaches was interpreted to suggest that both humoral and cellular immune abnormalities might contribute to disease pathogenesis (58). It is clear that patients may not respond to glucocorticoids (67). Based on very limited data, early aggressive therapy appears to be associated with the best outcome. One characteristic feature of Balo's concentric sclerosis, in contrast to MS, is that demyelination is largely supratentorial. It is unusual to have involvement of spinal cord, cerebellum, brainstem, or optic chiasm. The pathologic pattern of demyelination is quite distinct from that of patients with Marburg variant disease. Cerebrospinal fluid often shows detectable oligoclonal bands. In one concentric sclerosis patient, high CSF levels of TNF-α and interleukin-6 (IL-6) were noted, consistent with blood–brain barrier disruption. It is unclear whether the myelinated rings represent remyelination or relatively intact areas with early demyelination (56,68). Some patients have shown both characteristic concentric lesions and more typical plaque areas. It has been postulated that Balo's concentric sclerosis may represent an intermediary stage between Marburg variant and typical MS, but this does not explain the unusual demyelinating pattern (56).

Concentric Lacunar Leukoencephalopathy

Concentric lacunar leukoencephalopathy involves extensive axon damage in addition to demyelination, with zones of cavitation separated by bands of gliosis (69,70). This rare entity is similar to Balo's concentric sclerosis. It is not known whether this variant is differentiated solely by extensive axon involvement.

Myelinoclastic Diffuse Sclerosis (Schilder Disease)

Myelinoclastic diffuse sclerosis, previously called Schilder disease, has also been referred to as juvenile or childhood MS because it mainly affects children. The initial case report in 1912 described a 14-year-old girl who died after an illness that lasted 19 weeks (71). Subsequent reports mistakenly described cases of adrenoleukodystrophy, subacute sclerosing panencephalitis, and Canavan's spongy degeneration of infancy as Schilder disease, contributing to early diagnostic confusion (72–74). In retrospect, it is now appreciated that most cases in the literature actually represent adrenoleukodystrophy. True myelinoclastic diffuse sclerosis is a very rare disorder characterized by bilateral symmetric hemispheral demyelinating lesions, typically larger than 3 x 2 cm (75). Although lesions are primarily demyelinating, they may also involve axons with tissue necrosis and cavitation. There is involvement of subcortical fibers in addition to adjacent vertex. Gliosis tends to be prominent and may take the form of multinucleated giant astrocytes (50). The clinical presentation frequently involves headache, vomiting, seizures, and visual problems including cortical blindness (76). In 1986 Poser suggested diagnostic criteria (Table 5-8) (77), which required that other conditions (in particular adrenoleukodystrophy) be ruled out.

Some patients show a dramatic response to glucocorticoids (78). This is an extremely unusual condition,

---

TABLE 5-8

Diagnostic Criteria for Myelinoclastic Diffuse Sclerosis (77)

- Atypical symptoms and signs for early MS
  - Bilateral optic neuritis
  - Increased intracranial pressure
  - Disturbed level of consciousness
  - Headache and vomiting
  - Psychiatric manifestations
- No prior fever, infection, vaccination
- Normal very long chain fatty acids in serum
- Bilateral large areas of hemispheral demyelination
- CSF normal or atypical for MS

---

and only a handful of cases meet rigorous diagnostic criteria (77,79).

Disseminated Subpial Demyelination

There are two case reports in the literature of undiagnosed neurologic disease associated with subpial demyelination (80,81). The first case involved a 66-year-old man with progressive neurologic deterioration over eight months (80). Disseminated subpial demyelinating foci of different ages were found throughout the forebrain and brainstem. In this case CSF was never examined. The second case involved a 34-year-old woman with a history of intravenous drug use and congenital heart disease, who had a 14-month course involving relapsing psychiatric episodes (81). No evidence for immunodeficiency or infection was noted. Cerebrospinal fluid showed low-grade pleocytosis, oligoclonal bands, and elevated IgG levels. The multiple subpial demyelinating foci showed a striking predilection for brainstem. The authors postulated that these cases were an unusual variant of MS.

Mass Lesion

Multiple sclerosis rarely presents as unifocal or multifocal mass lesions. This presentation mimics brain tumor or abscess (82–91). There are even case reports of MS misdiagnosed as butterfly glioma of the corpus callosum (84,87). These patients often present with atypical features such as headache, confusion, seizures, and aphasias, and may undergo biopsy before the correct diagnosis is realized. Biopsy specimens typically contain large numbers of infiltrating macrophages, with variable myelin loss. In their subsequent course these patients go on to show more typical clinical and lesion features, which are otherwise indistinguishable from MS.

OTHER DISORDERS

There is another set of disorders that are considered as distinct from MS rather than variants. This division is somewhat artificial because a definable proportion of patients who present with these disorders do go on to develop MS.

Neuromyelitis Optica (Devic Syndrome)

Neuromyelitis optica (Devic syndrome) is a rare disorder that involves the spinal cord and optic nerves. The first case report in the literature was by Eugene Devic in 1894 (92). There are no uniformly accepted criteria for definition, but central to the syndrome is the temporally linked development of lesions affecting the spinal cord and one or both optic nerves. In more than 80 percent of cases both optic nerves are involved (48). These areas may be involved simultaneously, within days to weeks of each other, or separated by months to years.

Neuromyelitis optica was originally believed to be an inflammatory and demyelinating process, within the spectrum of MS. An optic-spinal form of MS is known to be more common among Asian, Indian, and African American patients (48,93,94). In Asians this optic-spinal MS is associated with antithyroid antibodies (95). However, it has now become clear that most patients with neuromyelitis optica do not have MS (96). Neuromyelitis optica may occur as a postinfectious syndrome and may also occur in the setting of collagen vascular disease and pulmonary tuberculosis (96,97). There are clear-cut clinical, MRI, and CSF differences from MS (Table 5-9) (98–103). Only 10 percent of people with neuromyelitis optica actually go on to develop typical MS (48).

The cause of neuromyelitis optica is not known. It does appear to be more common in Asians and as opposed to MS is associated with a decreased frequency of the HLA-DR2 haplotype. In a study of patients from the Mayo Clinic, those with a monophasic course were equally divided between men and women (101). They had a younger age of onset (mean 27 years). Most patients made an excellent recovery, although there were occasional individuals with a relentlessly progressive course to death. In contrast, those with a relapsing course were more likely to be women (by a ratio of almost 4:1). They had a worse outcome, with frequent and severe relapses. Respiratory failure develops in 22 percent of cases and may be a cause of death. Neuromyelitis optica in children has a particularly good prognosis; most children make an excellent recovery (104).

The neuroimaging pattern of neuromyelitis optica is distinct from that of MS. Spinal MRI typically shows dramatic lesions, often over several segments. In contrast, brain MRI generally is normal. In the relapsing form of the disease, 50 percent of patients ultimately show lesions on MRI. Cerebrospinal fluid is also quite distinct from that of MS, including lower levels of matrix metalloproteinase 9 (Table 5-9) (105). It is worth noting that experimental allergic encephalomyelitis induced with myelin oligodendrocyte glycoprotein (MOG) shows a topographic distribution of lesions similar to neuromyelitis optica (106). It is not known if anti-MOG antibodies play any role in this disorder.

Optimal treatment for neuromyelitis optica is not clear. There are anecdotal reports of response to glucocorticoids, azathioprine, intravenous immune globulin, and plasma exchange (105,107–110). In contrast, cyclophosphamide, methotrexate, and interferon beta are not effective. Poorer outcome has been associated with older age, marked CSF pleocytosis, and severe myelitis (98).

A variant of neuromyelitis optica has been described in a handful of Antillian females from Martinique and Guadaloupe. This new syndrome has been called recurrent optic neuromyelitis with endocrinopathies because it is associated with hypothalamic-hypophyseal dysfunction. Patients may manifest with variable galactorrhea-amenorrhea, hypothyroidism, and hyperphagia (111). The spinal cord shows cavitation-like changes, and most patients have a syringomyelia syndrome. Recurrent attacks generally result in death within five years of disease onset.

Monophasic Syndromes

There are a series of disorders that present as acute monophasic neurologic syndromes. They may be polyregional or monoregional, but all carry a risk for development of MS.

Postinfectious Encephalomyelitis

Postinfectious encephalitis/encephalomyelitis is also referred to as postvaccinal encephalomyelitis and acute disseminated encephalomyelitis. There is also a fulminant, hyperacute form called acute hemorrhagic leukoencephalitis (112). Postinfectious encephalomyelitis is a monophasic polyregional syndrome that usually is temporally related to infection or vaccination and is most common in children. At least 70 percent of patients report a precipitating event in the weeks before onset of their illness. However, there are examples of the disorder developing without any sentinel event (113–116). The major

TABLE 5-9
Distinguishing Features of Neuromyelitis Optica vs. MS

FEATURES	NEUROMYELITIS OPTICA	MS
Clinical		
Course	Relapsing (55%), monophasic (35%), or development of MS (10%)	Relapsing (85%), or progressive (15% initially, ≥ 80% ultimately)
Therapeutic response	Glucocorticoids, azathioprine	Glucocorticoids, disease-modifying therapy
Imaging Features		
Brain MRI	Normal	Abnormal
Spinal MRI	Acute swelling; three or more segments involved	Rare swelling; ≤ 2 segments involved
Optic nerve	Chiasmal signal changes	Optic nerve changes
CSF		
Cell count	Often ↑, generally >100 WBC neutrophils common	Often normal, neutrophils rare
Protein	Often ↑	Often normal
Oligoclonal bands, intrathecal IgG production	Uncommon	Common
Matrix metalloproteinase 9	↓	↑
Pathology	Necrosis, vascular proliferation, variable perivascular inflammation	Perivascular inflammation and demyelination, variable axonal damage

triggers are viruses and to a much lesser extent bacteria and nonpathogens. Ubiquitous viruses that cause exanthematous illness (measles, varicella zoster virus, rubella) have been the major identified precipitants, whereas nonspecific upper respiratory tract pathogens (such as influenza virus and respiratory syncytial virus) are associated with the more fulminant form. Other viruses associated with postinfectious encephalomyelitis include mumps, Epstein-Barr, and hepatitis A. The major bacterial trigger has been *Mycoplasma*, but *Bordetella pertussis*, *Borrelia burgdorferi*, and *Campylobacter jejuni* are also implicated. *Campylobacter* has been associated with an unusual pattern of gray matter involvement with an immune-mediated vasculitis (117). Noninfectious triggers include inoculations such as the semple rabies vaccine, serum treatments, and certain drugs. In fact, the only epidemiologically proven association is with semple rabies vaccine (48). Approximately one in 220 vaccinees is affected, presumably because the semple vaccine contains brain tissue (118), unlike the tissue culture rabies vaccine currently used in the United States.

Postinfectious encephalomyelitis is estimated to account for approximately 20 percent of acute encephalitis cases. It does not represent direct infection of CNS tissue. Pathologic and immunologic data support that this disorder is an immune-mediated process, perhaps directed against myelin antigens. The classic pathologic changes are perivascular mononuclear cell infiltration with adjacent demyelination (119,120). The hyperacute form causes necrosis of small blood vessels, intense inflammation, severe edema, and multiple small hemorrhages superimposed on demyelination. This syndrome most often follows influenza or upper respiratory tract infection.

A number of features help to distinguish postinfectious encephalomyelitis from a first attack of MS (Table 5-10), but there are no absolute criteria. Even the requirement of a monophasic attack is not absolute. In rare instances postinfectious encephalomyelitis has taken a recurrent multiphasic course, with relapses reported out to 18 months and clinical deterioration or progression over several months (121–126). It has been suggested that a time frame of six months be used before considering that postinfectious encephalomyelitis is no longer monophasic.

Postinfectious encephalomyelitis tends to be clinically more severe than a first attack of MS. There is abrupt onset of symptoms, which may include fever and decreased level of consciousness. Seizures occur in 50 percent of patients. As opposed to MS, there is multifocal involvement with polyregional abnormalities. Lesions on MRI tend to be extensive and fairly symmetric, with widespread enhancement. However, patients may have enhancing and nonenhancing lesions on the same scan. Basal ganglia and/or deep gray matter involvement is common (127,128). A key feature to support postinfectious encephalomyelitis over MS is improvement of lesions, without new lesions, on subsequent MRI performed months later. Cerebrospinal fluid is abnormal in at least 67 percent of patients, with low-grade mononuclear pleocytosis (27 percent) and increased protein (44 percent). Although oligoclonal bands and intrathecal IgG production may occur in postinfectious encephalomyelitis, these immune disturbances are seen much less frequently than in MS. If positive, they are transient and clear over time. More severe cases may show neutrophilic predominance.

The HLA haplotype pattern appears to differ between MS and postinfectious encephalomyelitis. A recent study of rabies postvaccinal encephalomyelitis found an association with HLA haplotypes (DR9, DR17) that was distinct from MS (118). This suggests that a unique genetic susceptibility may play a role in the development of at least some forms of postinfectious encephalomyelitis. Another recent report suggests that detection of serum antibodies to arrestin, a family of brain and retinal proteins that help to inactivate G-protein coupled receptors, may distinguish a first attack of MS from a monophasic postinfectious process (129). This finding awaits confirmation.

There is no proven therapy for postinfectious encephalomyelitis, although glucocorticoids are commonly used. Anecdotal cases with response to intravenous immune globulin, plasma exchange, cyclophosphamide, polyinosinic-polycytidylic acid-polylysine, and glatiramer acetate (130–135) have been reported. Supportive therapy is critical because most survivors make an excellent recovery.

Clinically Isolated Syndromes

As discussed previously, CISs are monoregional acute monophasic syndromes that classically encompass optic neuritis, transverse myelitis, and isolated brainstem or cerebellar syndromes. They carry a high risk of MS based on whether they are associated with multiple brain MRI lesions and CSF immune (oligoclonal bands, intrathecal IgG production) abnormalities. Recent studies indicate that T2-weighted MRI lesions predict a greater than 80 percent conversion to MS by 10 years, that initial contrast lesions predict early (within three years) risk of MS, and that the quantified lesion load and number correlate with long-term risk of MS, clinical subtype, and disability (21,136).

Optic Neuritis

The incidence rate of optic neuritis is reported in the range of 0.56 to 5.15 per 100,000 population (137). It is a frequent feature of MS. Optic neuritis is the initial monore-

TABLE 5-10
Factors That Distinguish Postinfectious Encephalomyelitis from MS

FACTOR	POSTINFECTIOUS ENCEPHALOMYELITIS	MS
Time course	• Monophasic (rarely relapsing/multiphasic)	• Multiphasic
Preceding event	• Common (70%)	• Uncommon
Demographics	• Most common in children	• Most common in young adults
	• Equal gender ratio	• Female predominance
Clinical features	• Abrupt onset	• Subacute onset
	• Seizures common (50%)	• Seizures very unusual (< 5%)
	• ↓Level of consciousness common	• ↓Level of consciousness very unusual
	• Polyregional	• Monoregional > polyregional
	• Bilateral optic neuritis	• Unilateral optic neuritis
	• Complete transverse myelitis with areflexia	• Incomplete transverse myelitis with hyperreflexia
	• Mortality 25%	• No mortality
Neuroimaging	• Lesions are bilateral, symmetric, and extensive	• Lesions are bilateral, asymmetric, and limited in size
	• Nonperiventricular lesions	• Periventricular lesions
	• Multiple enhancing lesions	• No or several enhancing lesions
	• Basal ganglia lesions common	• Basal ganglia lesions uncommon
	• Serial MRI shows partial resolution, no new lesions	• Serial MRI shows new lesions
CSF	• Moderately↑ cell count	• Normal or minimally↑ cell count
	• ↑ Protein	• Normal protein
	• Oligoclonal bands and intrathecal IgG production uncommon, transient	• Oligoclonal bands and intrathecal IgG production common, persistent

gional attack of MS in 14 percent to 18 percent of MS patients and is part of a polyregional presentation in 22 percent to 41 percent (138). In one German series, isolated optic neuritis made up 16.6 percent of first relapses, whereas optic neuritis combined with other neurologic problems made up 34.7 percent of first relapses (139). Optic neuritis ultimately occurs in 27 percent to 66 percent of all MS patients.

Optic neuritis, to be considered a CIS, must be idiopathic and not the result of toxic, vascular, systemic, retinal, or compressive causes. A number of studies have examined the overall risk for development of MS after idiopathic optic neuritis. Development of MS ranged from 1.5 percent to 85 percent (140,141). This wide variability in large part reflects variable follow-up periods. In extended follow-up, ranging from 15 to 40 years, 60 percent to 75 percent of

patients develop MS (137,140,142,143). The risk for development of MS after isolated optic neuritis increased steadily in the first 10 years, and then more gradually over time (140). Not all idiopathic optic neuritis turns out to be MS, and it may also be a postinfectious syndrome.

In addition to MRI and CSF studies, a number of other factors help to predict the likelihood of development of MS (Table 5-11). In a partially retrospective and longitudinal study of 165 patients seen over a seven-year period, ocular pain and visual evoked potential abnormalities were less common in those who went on to develop MS, whereas CSF, MRI, and sedimentation rate abnormalities were more common in those who went on to develop MS (141). This study is in contrast to the general finding that ocular pain is present in most cases of optic neuritis that are due to MS (144).

TABLE 5-11

Factors That Affect the Risk for Development of MS After Isolated Optic Neuritis

---

↑ *Risk*
- Young adult (26–40 years) (±)
- Female gender (±)
- History of minor neurologic symptoms
- Unilateral optic neuritis
- Retrobulbar optic neuritis
- Pain
- Normal disc
- Venous sheathing
- Recurrent optic neuritis
- Brain MRI lesions
- Abnormal CSF (oligoclonal bands, intrathecal IgG production, cell count, protein)
- Abnormal multimodality evoked potentials

↓ *Risk*
- Children (< 10 years)
- No history of minor neurologic symptoms
- Bilateral optic neuritis
- Papillitis
- Mild vision loss
- Absence of pain
- Macular star/exudates
- Retinal or disc hemorrhage
- Severe disc edema
- Normal brain MRI
- Normal CSF

(±) Indicates conflicting data

The North American Optic Neuritis Treatment Trial was a multicenter study that initially entered 457 patients (145). They were randomized to intravenous high-dose methylprednisolone, followed by oral prednisone taper, intermediate-dose oral prednisone, or oral placebo. The final outcome was that intravenous glucocorticoids increased the early rate of recovery, but by two years there was no treatment difference. An unexpected finding was that patients who received intravenous high-dose steroids were less likely to develop a second and MS-defining attack over the next two years, although by three years any group differences had disappeared. The validity of this puzzling observation has been criticized (146). In a five-year follow-up of 388 of these patients, the overall risk of developing MS was 30 percent, and treatment had no effect on this risk (145). In this multicenter study, the most important predictor for the development of MS was the number of lesions on the initial brain MRI. Forty-two percent of those with an abnormal MRI developed clin-ically definite MS, compared with only 16 percent of those with normal brain MRI. Higher numbers of MRI lesions were associated with greater risk of MS. Other factors that increased risk of MS were prior nonspecific neurologic symptoms (most often brief paresthesias), viral syndrome in the month before the optic neuritis, female gender, and Caucasian race. Factors that decreased risk for MS were absence of pain and mild vision loss. Multiple sclerosis did not develop in patients with certain fundus characteristics (severe disc edema, disc or peripapillary hemorrhage, vascular exudates). Of those who developed MS by five years, disability was unusual. Others have found increased risk for MS with pain and normal disc (147,148). Reports on female gender and early age of onset as risk factors are conflicting (145). In a recent Scandinavian study of 147 consecutive patients with optic neuritis seen during a five-year period, the risk factors that were most strongly associated with the development of clinically definite MS were the presence of three or more MS-like lesions on MRI and CSF oligoclonal bands. HLA haplotype Dw2 was also associated with increased MS risks (149). Cerebrospinal fluid abnormalities (IgG disturbances, antiviral immunoglobulin, cell count, protein) also increase MS risk (141,144,150–152).

Onset of optic neuritis in childhood carries a much lower risk for MS. In a Mayo Clinic study of 94 cases under the age of 16 years seen between 1950 and 1988, detailed follow-up was available in 79, with a median follow-up of 19.4 years (153). Multiple sclerosis developed in 13 percent at 10 years, 19 percent at 20 years, 22 percent by 30 years, and 26 percent by 40 years.

Early optic nerve involvement with significant vision loss may occur in patients with Leber's hereditary optic neuropathy (LHON). This disorder involves a mutation in mitochondrial DNA (154). Women with LHON caused by the 11778 mutation may go on to have subsequent relapses or progressive disease consistent with MS (155–157). They show characteristic MRI, CSF, and evoked potential abnormalities. It has been estimated that 45 percent of British women with LHON have an MS-like disorder (158).

Transverse Myelitis/Myelopathy

Transverse myelitis is another CIS with risk for development of MS (159,160). As an MS feature, it is more common in Asians than in Caucasians (161). Certain features are quite helpful to predict the likelihood of MS (Table 5-12) (160,162–165). Among the most important is whether the transverse myelitis is complete or incomplete. A complete syndrome carries low risk under 14 percent (28), whereas the risk can approximate 70 percent with incomplete syndromes (166). Children have a low risk, and most cases are believed to be parainfectious

TABLE 5-12

Factors That Affect the Risk for Development of MS After Isolated Transverse Myelitis

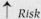 *Risk*

- Incomplete transverse myelitis
- Asymmetric motor/sensory findings
- Abnormal brain MRI
- Abnormal CSF
- Abnormal multimodality evoked potentials
- Spinal MRI showing limited, nonconfluent intramedullary lesion(s)

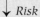 *Risk*

- Complete transverse myelitis
- Symmetric motor/sensory findings
- Normal brain MRI
- Normal CSF
- Spinal MRI showing swollen cord or large, multi-level confluent intramedullary lesions

(167,168). Certain spinal MRI findings are helpful (large cross-sectional area, multisegment length, cord expansion, central isointensity surrounded by hyperintensity, peripheral enhancement, slow T2 lesion regression with enhancing nodule) to distinguish non-MS cases (169). Episodes that affect complete segments may represent localized forms of postinfectious encephalomyelitis (170). The presence of CSF oligoclonal bands favors MS rather than a parainfectious etiology (171). Transverse myelitis may be recurrent (172,173). Patients do not appear to have classic MS because disease remains confined to the spinal cord.

Other Syndromes

Clinically isolated syndromes include acute monophasic brainstem and cerebellar syndromes. Similar to lesions affecting optic nerve and spinal cord, the risk for MS is affected by evidence of more diffuse neuroimaging and CSF abnormalities at onset, consistent with MS (166).

SUMMARY

Early and accurate diagnosis of MS is now essential. This mandates that the approach to patients with possible MS be deliberate, thoughtful, and thorough. With advances in immunology, neurobiology, and MS, there is an increased understanding of the spectrum of diseases related to MS. As further information becomes available on their etiology and pathogenesis, it is expected that diagnostic and therapeutic advances will follow. In turn, these advances will result in a better understanding and management of MS.

References

1. Ebers GC, Dyment DA. Genetics of multiple sclerosis. *Semin Neurol* 1998; 18:295–299.
2. The IFNβ Multiple Sclerosis Study Group. Interferon beta-1b is effective in relapsing-remitting multiple sclerosis: I. Clinical results of a multicenter, randomized, double-blind, placebo-controlled trial. *Neurology* 1993; 43:655–661.
3. Paty DW, Li DKB, UBC, MS/MRI Study Group and the IFNβ Multiple Sclerosis Study Group. Interferon beta-1b is effective in relapsing-remitting multiple sclerosis: II. MRI analysis of results of a multicenter, randomized, double-blind, placebo-controlled trial. *Neurology* 1993; 43:662–667.
4. The IFN(Multiple Sclerosis Study Group and the University of British Columbia MS/MR Analysis Group. Interferon beta-1b in the treatment of multiple sclerosis: final outcome of the randomized controlled trial. *Neurology* 1995; 45:1277–1285.
5. Jacobs LD, Cookfair DL, Rudick RA, et al. Intramuscular interferon beta-1a for disease progression in relapsing multiple sclerosis. *Ann Neurol* 1996; 39:285–294.
6. Simon JH, Jacobs LD, Campion M. Magnetic resonance studies of intramuscular interferon β-1a for relapsing multiple sclerosis. *Ann Neurol* 1998; 43:79–87.
7. Johnson KP, Brooks BR, Cohen JA, et al. Copolymer 1 reduces relapse rate and improves disability in relapsing remitting multiple sclerosis: results of a phase III multicenter, double-blind, placebo-controlled trial. *Neurology* 1995; 45:1268–1276.
8. Johnson KP, Brooks BR, Cohen JA, Ford CC, Goldstein J, Lisak RP, Myers LW, Panitch HS, Rose JW, Schiffer RB, Vollmer T, Weiner LP, Wolinsky JS, Copolymer 1 Multiple Sclerosis Study Group. Extended use of glatiramer acetate (Copaxone) is well tolerated and maintains its clinical effect on multiple sclerosis relapse rate and degree of disability. *Neurology* 1998; 50:701–708.
9. PRISMS (Prevention of Relapses and Disability by Interferon (-1a Subcutaneously in Multiple Sclerosis) Study Group. Randomized double-blind placebo-controlled study of interferon (-1a in relapsing/remitting multiple sclerosis. *Lancet* 1998; 352:1498–1504.
10. European Study Group on Interferon β-1b in Secondary Progressive MS. Placebo-controlled multicentre randomized trial of interferon β-1b in treatment of secondary progressive multiple sclerosis. *Lancet* 1998; 352: 1491–1497.
11. Trapp BD, Peterson J, Ransohoff RM, et al. Axonal transection in the lesions of multiple sclerosis. *N Engl J Med* 1998; 338:278–285.
12. Simon JH, Jacobs LD, Campion MK, et al. A longitudinal study of brain atrophy in relapsing multiple sclerosis. *Neurology* 1999; 53:139–148.
13. National Multiple Sclerosis Society. Early intervention: National Multiple Sclerosis Society (NMSS) disease management consensus statement. In: *Compendium of multiple sclerosis information 1997 (updated 1998).* New York: National Multiple Sclerosis Society.

14. Herndon RM, Brooks B. Misdiagnosis of multiple sclerosis. *Semin Neurol* 1985; 5:94–98.

15. Dupont B, Lisak RP, Jersild C. HLA antigens in black American patients with multiple sclerosis. *Transplant Proc* 1976; 91:181–185.

16. Kira J-I, Kanai T, Nishimura Y, et al. Western versus Asian types of multiple sclerosis: immunogenetically and clinically distinct disorders. *Ann Neurol* 1996; 40:569–574.

17. Eraksoy M. Multiple sclerosis in children: A review. In: Siva A, Kesselring J, Thompson RJ (eds.). *Frontiers in multiple sclerosis*, Vol. 2. London: Martin Dunitz, 1999:67–73.

18. Martyn CN, Gale CR. The epidemiology of multiple sclerosis. *Acta Neurol Scand* 1997; 169S:3–7.

19. Kurtzke JF. A reassessment of the distribution of multiple sclerosis: Pts I and II. *Acta Neurol Scand* 1975; 51:110–136, 137–157.

20. Kurtzke JF, Beebe GW, Norman JE. Epidemiology of multiple sclerosis in US veterans. I. Race, sex, and geographic distribution. *Neurology* 1979; 29:1228–1235.

21. Sailer M, O'Riordan JI, Thomas AJ, et al. Quantitative MRI in patients with clinically isolated syndromes suggestive of demyelination. *Neurology* 1999; 52:599–606.

22. Paty DW, Li DKB. Diagnosis of multiple sclerosis 1998: Do we need new diagnostic criteria? In: Siva A, Kesselring J, Thompson AJ (eds.). *Frontiers in multiple sclerosis*, Vol. 2. London: Martin Dunitz, 1999:47–50.

23. Allison RS, Millar JHD. Prevalence and familial incidence of disseminated sclerosis (a report to the Northern Ireland Hospitals Authority on the results of a three-year survey): Prevalence of disseminated sclerosis in Northern Ireland. *Ulster Med J* 1954; 23:5–27.

24. McAlpine D, Lumsden CE, Acheson ED. *Multiple sclerosis: A reappraisal.* Edinburgh: Churchill Livingstone, 1972.

25. McDonald WI, Halliday AM. Diagnosis and classification of multiple sclerosis (review). *Br Med Bull* 1977; 33:4–9.

26. Rose AS, Ellison GW, Myers LW, Tourtellotte WW. Criteria for the clinical diagnosis of multiple sclerosis. *Neurology* 1976; 26:20–22.

27. Schumacher GA, Beebe G, Kibler RF et al. Problems of experimental trials of therapy in multiple sclerosis. Report by the panel on the evaluation of experimental trials of therapy in multiple sclerosis. *Ann NY Acad Sci* 1965; 122:552–568.

28. Paty DW, Noteworthy JH, Ebers GC. Diagnosis of multiple sclerosis. In: Paty DW, Ebers GC (eds.). *Multiple sclerosis*. Philadelphia: FA Davis, 1998:48–134.

29. Bauer J. IMAB-enquete concerning the diagnostic criteria for multiple sclerosis. In: Bauer HJ, Poser S, Ritter G (eds.). *Progress in multiple sclerosis research*. Berlin: Springer, 1980:555–563.

30. Poser CM, Paty DW, Scheinberg L, et al. New diagnostic criteria for multiple sclerosis: Guidelines for research protocols. *Ann Neurol* 1983; 13:227–231.

31. Lublin FD, Reingold SC. Defining the clinical course of multiple sclerosis: Results of an international survey. *Neurology* 1996; 46:907–911.

32. Jacobs LD, Wende KE, Brownscheidle CM, et al. A profile of multiple sclerosis: The New York State Multiple Sclerosis Consortium. *Multiple Sclerosis* 1999 (in press).

33. Weinshenker BG, Bass B, Rice GP, et al. The natural history of multiple sclerosis: A geographically based study. I. Clinical course and disability. *Brain* 1989; 112:133–146.

34. Runmarker B, Anderson O. Prognostic factors in a multiple sclerosis incident cohort with twenty-five years of follow-up. *Brain* 1993; 116:117–134.

35. Paty DW, Blumhardt LD, PRISMS study group. High-dose subcutaneous interferon β-1a is efficacious in transitional multiple sclerosis, a group at high risk of progression in disability. (Abstract), 123rd Annual Meeting of the American Neurological Association, October 18–21, 1989, Montreal, Quebec, Canada.

36. Weinstock-Guttman B, Kinkel RP, Cohen JA, et al. Treatment of multiple sclerosis with intravenous cyclophosphamide. *Neurologist* 1997; 3:178–185.

37. Gayou A, Brochet B, Dousset V. Transitional progressive multiple sclerosis: A clinical and imaging study. *J Neurol Neurosurg Psychiatry* 1997; 63:396–398.

38. Andersson M, Alvarez-Carmeno J, Bernardi G, et al. Cerebrospinal fluid in the diagnosis of multiple sclerosis: A consensus report. *J Neurol Neurosurg Psychiatry* 1994; 57:897–902.

39. Farrell MA, Kaufmann JCE, Gilbert JJ, et al. Oligoclonal bands in multiple sclerosis: Clinically pathologic correlation. *Neurology* 1985; 35:212–218.

40. Yokota T, Matsunaga T, Okiyama R, et al. Sympathetic skin response in patients with multiple sclerosis compared with patients with spinal cord transection and normal controls. *Brain* 1991; 114:1381–1394.

41. Paty DW, Ogar JJF, Kastrukoff LF et al. Magnetic resonance imaging in the diagnosis of multiple sclerosis (MS): A prospective study with comparison of clinical evaluation, evoked potentials, oligoclonal banding and CT. *Neurology* 1988; 38:180–184.

42. Chabriat H, Vahedi K, Joutel A, et al. Cerebral autosomal dominant arteriopathy with subcortical infarcts and leukoencephalopathy (CADASIL). *Neurologist* 1997; 3:137–145.

43. Dichgans M, Mayer M, Uttner I, et al. The phenotypic spectrum of CADASIL: Clinical findings in 102 cases. *Ann Neurol* 1998; 44:731–739.

44. Engell T. A clinico-pathoanatomical study of multiple sclerosis diagnosis. *Acta Neurol Scand* 1998; 78:39–44.

45. Marburg O. Die sogenannte "akute Multiple Sklerose." *Jahrb Neurol Psychiatr* 1906; 27:211–312.

46. Johnson MD, Lavin P. Whetsell WO Jr. Fulminant monophasic multiple sclerosis, Marburg's type. *J Neurol Neurosurg Psychiatry* 1990; 53:918–921.

47. Mendez MF, Pogacar S. Malignant monophasic multiple sclerosis or "Marburg's disease." *Neurology* 1998; 38:1153–1155.

48. Weinshenker BG, Lucchinetti CF. Acute leukoencephalopathies: Differential diagnosis and investigation. *Neurologist* 1998; 4:148–166.

49. Bitsch A, Wegener C, da Costa C, et al. Lesion development in Marburg's type of acute multiple sclerosis: from inflammation to demyelination. *Multiple Sclerosis* 1999; 5:138–146.

50. Moore GRW. Neuropathology and pathophysiology of multiple sclerosis. In: Paty DW, Ebers GC (eds.). *Multiple sclerosis*. Philadelphia: FA Davis, 1998:257–327.

51. Wood DD, Bibao JM, O'Connors P, Moscarello MA. Acute multiple sclerosis (Marburg type) is associated with developmentally immature myelin basic protein. *Ann Neurol* 1996; 40:18–24.

52. Giubilei F, Sarrantonio A, Tisei P, Gasperini C, Salvetti M. Four year follow-up of a case of acute multiple sclerosis of the Marburg type. *Ital J Neurol Sci* 1997; 18:163–166.

53. Marburg O. Die Sogenannte "akute multiple sklerose" (Encephalomyelitis periaxialis scleroticans). *Jahrb neurol Psychiatr* 1906; 27:213–312.

54. Balo J. Encephalitis periaxialis concentrica. *Arch Neurol Psychiatry* 1928; 19:242–264.

55. Itoyama Y, Tateishi J, Kuroiwa Y. Atypical multiple sclerosis with concentric or lamellar demyelination lesions: Two Japanese patients studied post mortem. *Ann Neurol* 1985; 17:481–487.

56. Moore GRW, Neumann PE, Suzuki K, et al. Balo's concentric sclerosis: New observations on lesion development. *Ann Neurol* 1985; 17:604–611.

57. Murakami Y, Matsuishi T, Shimizu T, et al. Balo's concentric sclerosis in a 4-year old Japanese infant. *Brain Develop* 1998; 20:250–252.

58. Sekijima Y, Tokuda T, Hashimoto T, et al. Serial magnetic resonance imaging (MRI) study of a patient with Balo's concentric sclerosis treated with immunadsorption plasmapheresis. *Multiple Sclerosis* 1997; 2:291–294.

59. Garbern J, Spence AM, Alvord EC Jr. Balo's concentric demyelination diagnosed premortem. *Neurology* 1986; 36:1610–1614.

60. Hanemann CO, Kleinschmidt A, Reifenberger G, Freund H-J, Seitz RJ. Balo's concentric sclerosis followed by MRI and positron emission tomography. *Neuroradiology* 1993; 35:578–580.

61. Nandini M, Gourie-Devi M, Shankar SK, Mustare VB, Ravi V. Balo's concentric sclerosis diagnosed intravitum on brain biopsy. *Clin Neurol Neurosurg* 1993; 95:303–309.

62. Gharagozloo A, Poe L, Collins G. Antemortem diagnosis of Balo concentric sclerosis: Corrective neuroimaging and pathologic features. *Radiology* 1994; 191:817–819.

63. Korte J, Born EP, Vos LD, Breuer TJ, Wondergem JH. Balo's concentric sclerosis: MR diagnosis. *Am J Neuroradiol* 1994; 15:1284–1288.

64. Chen C, Ro LS, Chang CN, Ho YS, Lu CS. Serial MRI studies in pathologically verified Balo's concentric sclerosis. *J Comput Assist Tomogr* 1996; 20:732–735.

65. Spiegel M, Kruger H, Hoffmann E, Kappos L. MRI Study of Balo's concentric sclerosis before and after immunosuppressant therapy. *J Neurol* 1989; 236:487–488.

66. Louboutin J, Elie B. Treatment of Balo's concentric sclerosis with immunosuppressant drugs followed by multimodality evoked potentials and MRI. *Muscle Nerve* 1995; 18:1478–1480.

67. Castaigne P, Escourolle R, Chain F, et al. Balo's concentric sclerosis. *Rev Neurol* (Paris) 1984; 140:479–487.

68. Yao D, Webster HD, Hudson LD, Brenner M, Liu DS, Escobar AI. Concentric sclerosis (Balo): Morphometric and in situ hybridization study of lesions in six patients. *Ann Neurol* 1994; 5:18–30.

69. Currie S, Roberts AH, Urich H. The nosological position of concentric lacunar leukoencephalopathy. *J Neurol Neurosurg Psychiatry* 1970; 33:131–137.

70. Grcevic N. Concentric lacunar leukoencephalopathy. *Arch Neurol* 1960; 2:266–273.

71. Schilder P. Zur Kenntnis der sogenannten diffusen sklerose (Uber encephalitis periaxialis diffusa). *Z Gesamte Neurol Psychiat* 1912; 10:1–60.

72. Schilder P. Zur Frage der encephalitis periaxialis diffusa. *Z Gesamte Neurol Psychiat* 1913; 15:359–376

73. Schilder P. Die encephalitis periaxialis diffusa. *Arch Psychiat* 1924; 71:327–356.

74. Canavan NM. Schilder's encephalitis periaxialis diffusa. Report of a case in a child aged sixteen and one half months. *Arch Neurol* 1931; 25:229–308.

75. Eblen F, Poremba M, Grodd W, et al. Myelinoclastic diffuse sclerosis (Schilder's disease): Cliniconeuroradiologic correlations. *Neurology* 1991; 41:589–591.

76. Sedwick LA, Klingele TG, Burde RM, Fulling KH, Gado MH. Schilder's (1912) disease. Total cerebral blindness due to acute demyelination. *Arch Neurol* 1986; 43:85–87.

77. Poser CM, Goutieres F, Carpentier MA, Aicardi J. Schilder's myelinoclastic diffuse sclerosis. *Pediatrics* 1986; 77:107–112.

78. Pretorius M-L, Looke DB, Ravenscroft A, Schoeman JF. Demyelinating disease of Schilder type in three young South African children: Dramatic response to corticosteroids. *J Child Neurol* 1998; 13:197–201.

79. Mehler MF, Rabinowich L. Inflammatory myelinoclastic diffuse sclerosis. *Ann Neurol* 1988; 23:413–415.

80. Galaburda AM, Waxman SG, Kemper TL, Jones HR. Progressive multifocal neurologic deficit with disseminated subpial demyelination. *J Neuropathol Exp Neurol* 1976; 35:481–494.

81. Neumann PE, Mehler MF, Horoupian DS, Merriam AE. Atypical psychosis with disseminated subpial demyelination. *Arch Neurol* 1988; 45:634–636.

82. Van der Velden M, Bots G, Endtz L. Cranial CT in multiple sclerosis showing mass effect. *Surg Neurol* 1979; 12:307–310.

83. Nelson MJ, Miller SL, McLain LW Jr, Gold LHA. Multiple sclerosis: Large plaque causing mass effect and ring sign. *J Comput Assist Tomogr* 1981; 5:892–894.

84. Rieth K, Di Chiro G, Cromwell L. Primary demyelinating disease simulating glioma of the corpus callosum: Report of three cases. *Neurosurgery* 1981; 55:620–624.

85. Sagar H, Warlow CP, Sheldon PW, Esiri MM. Multiple sclerosis with clinical and radiological features of cerebral tumor. *J Neurol Neurosurg Psychiatry* 1982; 45:802–808.

86. Hunter S, Ballinger W, Rubin J. Multiple sclerosis mimicking primary brain tumor. *Arch Pathol Lab Med* 1987; 111:464–468.

87. Kalyan-Raman UP, Garwacki DJ, Elwood PW. Demyelinating disease of corpus callosum presenting as glioma on magnetic resonance scan: a case documented with pathological findings. *Neurosurgery* 1987; 21; 247–250.

88. Mastrostefano R, Occhipinti E, Bigotti G, Pompili A. Multiple sclerosis plaque simulating cerebral tumor: case report and review of the literature. *Neurosurgery* 1987; 21:244–246.

89. Giang DW, Poduri KR, Eskin TA, et al. Multiple sclerosis masquerading as a mass lesion. *Neuroradiology* 1992; 34:150–154.

90. Kepes J. Large focal tumor-like demyelinating lesions of the brain: Intermediate entity between multiple sclerosis and acute disseminated encephalomyelitis—a study of 31 patients. *Ann Neurol* 1993; 33:18–27.

91. Dagher A. Smirniotopoulos J. Tumefactive demyelinating lesions. *Diagn Neuroradiol* 1996; 38:560–565.

92. Devic E. Myelite subaigue compliquee de neurite optique. *Bull Med* 1894; 5:18–30.

93. Jain S, Maheshwari MC. Multiple sclerosis: Indian experience in the last thirty years. *Neuroepidemiology* 1985; 4:96–107.

94. Phillips PH, Newman NJ, Lynn MJ. Optic neuritis in African Americans. *Arch Neurol* 1998; 55:186–192.

95. Sakuma R, Fujihara K, Sato N, Mochizuki H, Itoyama Y. Optic-spinal form of multiple sclerosis and anti-thyroid antibodies. *J Neurol* 1999; 246:449–453.

96. O'Riordan JI, Gallagher HL, Thomson AJ, et al. Clinical, CSF, and MRI findings in Devic's neuromyelitis optica. *J Neurol Neurosurg Psychiatry* 1996; 60:382–387.

97. Silber MH, Willcox PA, Bowen RM, Unger A. Neuromyelitis optica (Devic's syndrome) and pulmonary tuberculosis. *Neurology* 1990; 40:934–938.

98. Whitham RH, Brey RL. Neuromyelitis optica: Two new cases and review of the literature. *J Clin Neurol-ophthalmol* 1985; 5:263–269.

99. Leonardi A, Arata L, Farinelli M, et al. Cerebrospinal fluid and neuropathological study in Devic's syndrome. Evidence of intrathecal immune activation. *J Neurol Sci* 1987; 82:281–290.

100. Mandler R, Davis LE, Jeffery DR, Kornfeld M. Devic's neuromyelitis optica: A clinicopathological study of 8 patients. *Ann Neurol* 1993; 34:162–168.

101. Hogancamp W, Weinshenker B. The spectrum of Devic's syndrome (abstr). *Neurology* 1996; 46(Suppl):254.

102. O'Riordan JI. Central nervous system white matter diseases other than multiple sclerosis. *Curr Opin Neurol* 1997; 10:211–214.

103. Piccolo G, Franciotta DM, Camana C, et al. Devic's neuromyelitis optica: long-term follow-up and serial CSF finding in two cases. *J Neurol* 1990; 237:262–264.

104. Jeffery AR, Buncic JR. Pediatric Devic's neuromyelitis optica. *J Ped Ophthalmol Strabismus* 1996; 33(Suppl): 223–229.

105. Mandler RN, Ahmed W, Agius M, Dencoff J, Rosenberg G. Devic's neuromyelitis optica. Pathogenic characteristics and favorable response to immunotherapy in six acute patients (abstr). *Multiple Sclerosis* 1997; 3:407.

106. Storch MK, Stefferl A, Brehm U, et al. Autoimmunity to myelin oligodendrocyte glycoprotein in rats mimics the spectrum of multiple sclerosis pathology. *Brain Pathol* 1998; 8:681–694.

107. Aguilera AJ, Carlow TJ, Smith KJ, Simon TL. Lymphocytoplasmapheresis in Devic's syndrome. *Transfusion* 1985; 25:54–56.

108. Arnold TW, Myers GJ. Neuromyelitis optica (Devic's syndrome) in a 12-year-old male with complete recovery following steroids. *Pediatr Neurol* 1987; 3:313–315.

109. Mandler RN, Ahmed W, Dencoff JE. Devic's neuromyelitis optica: A progressive study of seven patients treated with prednisone and azathioprine. *Neurology* 1998; 51:1219–1220.

110. Rensel MR, Weinstock-Guttman B, Rudick R. Devic's disease: Diagnostic and therapeutic challenge. *Multiple Sclerosis* 1997; 3(Suppl):408.

111. Vernant JC, Cabre P, Smadja D, et al. Recurrent optic neuromyelitis with endocrinopathies: A new syndrome. *Neurology* 1997; 48:58–64.

112. Hurst E. Acute haemorrhagic leucoencephalitis: A previous undefined entity. *Med J Aust* 1941; 2:1–6.

113. Saito H, Endo M, Takase S, Itahara K. Acute disseminated encephalomyelitis after influenza vaccination. *Arch Neurol* 1980; 37:564–566.

114. Lukes S, Norman D. Computed tomography in acute disseminated encephalomyelitis. *Ann Neurol* 1983; 13:567–572.

115. Atlas SW, Grossman RI, Goldberg HI, et al. MR diagnosis of acute disseminated encephalomyelitis. *J Comput Assist Tomogr* 1986; 10:798–801.

116. Kesselring J, Beer S. Clinical data bank at the University Department of Neurology, Bern, Switzerland: Basis for an epidemiological study of multiple sclerosis in a high prevalence area. *Ital J Neurol Sci* 1987; (Suppl 6):29–34.

117. Nasralla CAW, Pay N, Goodpasture HC, Lin JJ, Svoboda WB. Postinfectious encephalopathy in a child following *Campylobacter jejuni* enteritis. *Amer J Neurol* 1993; 14:444–448.

118. Piyasirisilp S, Schmeckpeper BJ, Chandanayingyong, D, Hemachudha T, Griffin DE. Association of HLA and T-cell receptor gene polymorphisms with semple rabies vaccine-induced autoimmune encephalomyelitis. *Ann Neurol* 1999; 45:595–600.

119. Hart M, Earle K. Haemorrhagic and perivenous encephalitis: A clinical-pathological review of 38 cases. *J Neurol Neurosurg Psychiatry* 1975; 38:585–591.

120. Tolly T, Wells R, Sty J. MR features of fleeting CNS lesions associated with Epstein-Barr virus infection. *J Comput Assist Tomogr* 1989; 13:665–668.

121. Alcock N, Hoffman H. Recurrent encephalomyelitis in childhood. *Arch Dis Child* 1962; 37:40–44.

122. Kesselring J, Miller DH, Robb SA, et al. Acute disseminated encephalomyelitis: MRI findings and the distinction from multiple sclerosis. *Brain* 1990; 113:291–302.

123. Mizutani K, Atsuta J, Shibata T, Azuma E, Ito M, Sakurai M. Consecutive cerebral MRI findings of acute relapsing disseminated encephalomyelitis. *Acta Paediatr Jpn* 1994; 36:709–712.

124. Khan S, Yaqub BA, Posner CM, Al Deeb SM, Bohlega S. Multiphasic disseminated encephalomyelitis presenting as alternating hemiplegia. *J Neurol Neurosurg Psychiatry* 1995; 58:467–470.

125. Orrell RW, Shakir R, Lane RJM. Distinguishing acute disseminated encephalomyelitis from multiple sclerosis. *Br Med J* 1996; 313:802–804.

126. Tsai M-L, Hung K-L. Multiphasic disseminated encephalomyelitis mimicking multiple sclerosis. *Brain Develop* 1996; 18:412–414.

127. Donovan M, Lenn N. Postinfectious encephalomyelitis with localized basal ganglia involvement. *Pediatr Neurol* 1962; 5:311–313.

128. Baum, PA, Barkovich J, Koch TK, Berg BO. Deep gray matter involvement in children with acute disseminated encephalomyelitis. *Am J Neurol* 1994; 15:1275–1283.

129. Ikeda Y, Sudoh A, Chiba S, et al. Detection of serum antibody against Arrestin from patients with acute disseminated encephalomyelitis. *Tohoku J Exp Med* 1999; 187:65–70.

130. Abramsky O, Teitelbaum D, Arnon R. Effect of a synthetic polypeptide (cop-1) on patients with multiple sclerosis and with acute disseminated encephalomyelitis. *J Neurol Sci* 1977; 31:433–438.

131. Salazar AM, Engel WK, Levy HB. Poly ICLC in the treatment of postinfectious demyelinating encephalomyelitis. *Arch Neurol* 1981; 38:382–383.

132. Kleiman M, Brunquell P. Acute disseminated encephalomyelitis: Response to intravenous immunoglobulin? *J Child Neurol* 1995; 10:481–483.

133. Hahn JS, Siegler DJ, Enzmann D. Intravenous gammaglobulin therapy in recurrent acute disseminated encephalomyelitis. *Neurology* 1996; 46:1173–1174.

134. Tselis AC, Lisak RP. Acute disseminated encephalomyelitis. In: Antel J, Birnbaum G, Hartung H-P (eds.). *Clinical neuroimmunology.* Malden, Mass.: Blackwell Science, 1998:16–147.

135. Haase CG, Faustmann PM, Diener HC. Acute disseminated encephalomyelitis (ADEM). *Aktuelle Neurologie* 1999; 26(2):68–71.

136. O'Riordan JI, Thompson AJ, Kingsley DPE, et al. The prognostic value of brain MRI in clinically isolated syndromes of the CNS. A 10-year follow-up. *Brain* 1998; 121:495–503.

137. Jin Y-P, de Pedro-Cuesta J, Soderstrom M, Strawiarz L, Link H. Incidence of optic neuritis in Stockholm, Sweden 1990-1995: I. Age, sex, birth and ethnic-group related patterns. *J Neurol Sci* 1998; 159:107–114.

138. Matthews WB. Symptoms and signs. In: Matthews WB, Compston A, Allen IV, Martyn CN (eds.). *McAlpine's multiple sclerosis*, 2nd ed. New York: Churchill Livingstone, 1991:43–77.

139. Wikstrom J, Poser S, Ritter G. Optic neuritis as an initial symptom on multiple sclerosis. *Acta Neurol Scand* 1980; 61:178–185.

140. Rodriguez M, Siva A, Cross SA, O'Brien PC, Kurland LT. Optic neuritis: A population-based study in Olmsted County, Minnesota. *Neurology* 1995; 45:244–250.

141. Corona-Vazquez T, Ruiz-Sandoval J, Arriada-Mendicoa N. Optic neuritis progressing to multiple sclerosis. *Acta Neurol Scand* 1997; 95:85–89.

142. Francis DA, Compston DAS, Batchelor JR, McDonald WI. A reassessment of the risk of multiple sclerosis developing in patients with optic neuritis after extended follow-up. *J Neurol Neurosurg Psychiatry* 1987; 50:758–765.

143. Hutchinson WM. Acute optic neuritis and the prognosis for multiple sclerosis. *J Neurol Neurosurg Psychiatry* 1976; 39:283–289.

144. Anderson D, Cox J. Visual signs and symptoms. In: Paty DW, Ebers GC (eds.). *Multiple sclerosis*. Philadelphia: FA Davis, 1998:229–256.

145. Optic Neuritis Study Group. The 5-year risk of MS after optic neuritis. Experience of the Optic Neuritis Treatment Trial. *Neurology* 1997; 49:1404–1413.

146. Goodin DS. Perils and pitfalls in the interpretation of clinical trials: A reflection on the recent experience in multiple sclerosis. *Neuroepidemiology* 1999; 18:53–63.

147. Bradley WG, Whitty CWM. Acute optic neuritis: Prognosis for development of multiple sclerosis. *J Neurol Neurosurg Psychiatry* 1968; 31:10–18.

148. Kahana E, Alter M, Feldman S. Optic neuritis in relation to multiple sclerosis. *J Neurol* 1976; 213:87–95.

149. Soderstrom M, Ya-Ping J, Hillert J, Link H. Optic neuritis: Prognosis for multiple sclerosis from MRI, CSF, and HLA findings. *Neurology* 1998; 50(3):708–714.

150. Jacobs LD, Kaba SE, Miller CM, Priore RL, Brownscheidle CM. Correlation of clinical, magnetic resonance imaging, and cerebrospinal fluid findings in optic neuritis. *Ann Neurol* 1997; 41:392–398.

151. Frederikson JL, Sindic CJ. Intrathecal synthesis of virus-specific oligoclonal IgG, and of free lambda oligoclonal bands in acute monosymptomatic optic neuritis. Comparison with brain MRI. *Multiple Sclerosis* 1998; 4:22–26.

152. Cole SR, Beck RW, Moke PS, Kaufmann DI, Tourtellotte WW. The predictive value of CSF oligoclonal bands for MS 5 years after optic neuritis. Optic Neuritis Study Group. *Neurology* 1998; 51: 885–887.

153. Lucchinetti CF, Kiers L, O'Duffy A, et al. Risk factors for developing multiple sclerosis after childhood optic neuritis. *Neurology* 1997; 49(5):1413–1418.

154. Chalmer RM, Schapira AHV. Clinical, biochemical and molecular genetic features of Leber's hereditary optic neuropathy. *Biochimica et Biophysica Acta* 1999; 1410:147–158.

155. Harding AE, Sweeney MG, Miller DH, et al. Occurrence of a multiple sclerosis-like illness in women who have a Leber's hereditary optic neuropathy mitochondrial DNA mutation. *Brain* 1992; 115:979–989.

156. Flanigan KM, Johns DR. Association of the 11778 mitochondrial DNA mutation and demyelinating disease. *Neurology* 1993; 43:2720–2722.

157. Nikoskelainen EK, Marttila RJ, Huoponen, et al. Leber's "plus": Neurologic abnormalities in patients with Leber's hereditary optic neuropathy. *J Neurol Neurosurg Psychiatry* 1995; 59:160–164.

158. Riordan-Eva P, Sanders MD, Govan GG, et al. The clinical features of Leber's hereditary optic neuropathy defined by the presence of a pathogenic mitochondrial mutation. *Brain* 1995; 118:319–337.

159. Simnad VI, Pisani DE, Rose JW. Multiple Sclerosis presenting as transverse myelopathy. Clinical and MRI features. *Neurology* 1997; 48:65–73.

160. Scott TF, Bhagavatula K, Snyder PJ, Chieffe C. Transverse myelitis. Comparison with spinal cord presentations of multiple sclerosis. *Neurology* 1998; 50:429–433.

161. Toshiyuki F, Hamada T, Tashiro K, Moriwaka F, Yanagihara T. Acute transverse myelopathy in multiple sclerosis. *J Neurol Sci* 1990; 100:217–222.

162. Altrocchi PH. Acute transverse myelopathy. *Arch Neurol* 1963; 9:21–29.

163. Lipton HL, Teasdall RD. Acute transverse myelopathy in adults: A follow-up study. *Arch Neurol* 1973; 28: 252–257.

164. Ropper AH, Poskanzer DC. The prognosis of acute and subacute transverse myelopathy based on early signs and symptoms. *Ann Neurol* 1978; 4:51–59.

165. Tippett DS, Fishman PS, Panitch HS. Relapsing transverse myelitis. *Neurology* 1991; 41:703–706.

166. Miller DH, Ormerod IEC, Rudge P, et al. The early risk of multiple sclerosis following isolated acute syndromes of the brainstem and spinal cord. *Neurology* 1989; 26:635–639.

167. Adams C, Armstrong D. Acute transverse myelopathy in children. *Can J Neurol Sci* 1990; 17:40–45.

168. Knebusch M, Strassburg HM, Reiners K. Acute transverse myelitis in childhood: nine cases and review of the literature. *Develop Med Child Neurol* 1998; 40:631–639.

169. Choi KH, Lee KS, Chung SO, et al. Idiopathic transverse myelitis: MR characteristics. *Am J Neurol* 1996; 17:1151–1160.

170. Al Deeb SM, Yaqub BA, Bruyn GW, Biary NM. Acute transverse myelitis. A localized form of postinfectious encephalitis. *Brain* 1997; 120:1115–1122.

171. Jeffery DR, Mandler RN, Davis LE. Transverse myelitis. Retrospective analysis of 33 cases, with differentiation of cases associated with multiple sclerosis and parainfectious events. *Arch Neurol* 1993; 50:532–535.

172. Pandit L, Rao S. Recurrent myelitis. *J Neurol Neurosurg Psychiatry* 1996; 60:336–338.

173. Ungurean A, Palfi S, Dibo G, Tiszlavicz L, Vecsei L. Chronic recurrent transverse myelitis or multiple sclerosis. *Functional Neurol* 1996; 11:209–214.

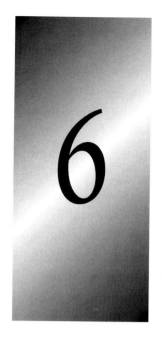

Magnetic Resonance Imaging in the Diagnosis of Multiple Sclerosis, Elucidation of Disease Course, and Determining Prognosis

Jack H. Simon, M.D., Ph.D.

Multiple sclerosis (MS) traditionally has been characterized based on its clinical features, including exacerbations, which on average are infrequent (<1 year), and by disability progression, which often occurs slowly and/or stepwise over periods of years (1,2). However, in vivo imaging, particularly magnetic resonance (MR) imaging, has shown that the pathologic changes in MS are in fact more frequent and dynamic than is appreciable by clinical means. Magnetic resonance imaging already has had a direct impact on how we diagnose MS in the clinic, and in the early preclinical stages it provides important prognostic information. Magnetic resonance imaging is providing new conceptual models for disease progression and classification and has driven development, testing, and approval of new therapies. The practical use of MR imaging in these four general areas is the subject of this chapter.

BASIC OVERVIEW OF MAGNETIC RESONANCE IMAGING IN MULTIPLE SCLEROSIS

Human MR imaging instruments are capable of acquiring various types of quantitative information in vivo. Most relevant to MS, MR provides measures related to the con-

centration of water in the central nervous system (CNS) and is sensitive to the various compartments and physical states of water in healthy and pathologic conditions. Although the dry content of brain is approximately 70 percent fat, this structured fat is largely MR invisible. However, most of the water protons, which are present at a concentration of approximately 110 molar in the brain, are readily detected (3). If this water signal is suppressed, whole body human MR instruments may be used to characterize and quantitate far less abundant chemical species, present in millimolar concentrations, such as the neuronal marker N-acetylaspartate (NAA) (4). With specialized magnetization transfer imaging (MTI) pulse sequences, additional information about water-macromolecule interactions can be presented (5), and diffusion-sensitive pulse sequences can provide information about the influence of microscopic structure on the diffusion of water molecules (6). The application of these advanced MR capabilities in MS studies are discussed in subsequent sections.

Independent of greater chemical characterization, what sets MR imaging apart from earlier methods such as computed tomography (CT) imaging is the use of MR techniques to create images that emphasize differences in the relaxation properties of the water in tissues (7). Both CT and MR imaging provide information proportionate to the concentration of water protons, but in addition, MR is sensitive to the T1 (longitudinal) and

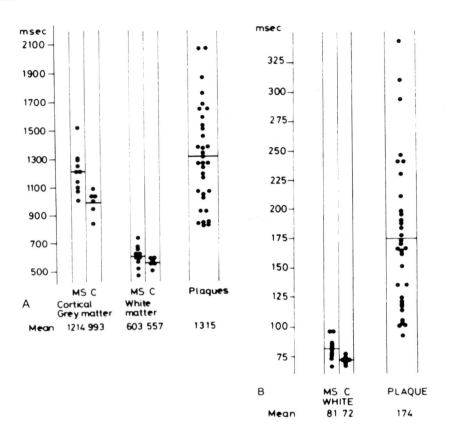

FIGURE 6-1

Distribution of T1- and T2-relaxation times in MS lesions and normal brain. Lesions (plaques) have elevated T1- (A) and T2- (B) relaxation times. C = values from control tissue. From Larsson HBW, Frederiksen J, Kjaer L, et al. In vivo determination of T1 and T2 in the brain of patients with severe but stable multiple sclerosis. *Magn Reson Med* 1988; 7:43–55; with permission.

T2 (transverse) relaxation rates of protons (8). These relaxation rates (the inverse of the relaxation times) are two independent and fundamental MR properties that influence the signal characteristics that make up an MR image and fortuitously provide a very sensitive measure of pathology. Most MS lesions are characterized by both increased T1- and increased T2-relaxation times (Figure 6-1). Images that emphasize the T1-relaxation differences of normal and pathologic tissues are called T1-weighted images (Figure 6-2a). This set of images is used to define anatomy, is the basis for detecting abnormalities of the blood–brain barrier when acquired after intravenous injection of an MR contrast media (Figure 6-2b), and defines a subset of MS lesions—the T1-hypointense lesions (T1-holes), which are focal areas of severe tissue disruption (9) (Figure 6-2a). Multiple sclerosis lesions appear hyperintense (bright) relative to normal white matter on T2-weighted MR imaging series (Figure 6-2c).

THE NATURAL HISTORY OF AN MS LESION BASED ON MR IMAGING

The development and evolution of MS in the CNS in patients with relapsing and secondary progressive dis-

ease follows a characteristic course that is most conveniently viewed from the perspective of the individual acute lesion, including its evolution into a chronic lesion (Figure 6-3).

The Early Lesion Stages

The acute inflammatory lesion in relapsing MS reaching the critical size necessary for detection by MR imaging almost always is accompanied by a local disturbance in the blood–brain barrier, which may be detected by MR imaging with gadolinium enhancement or with less sensitivity by CT imaging using iodinated contrast agents (10,11). Normally, compounds such as the gadolinium-chelates (molecular weight approximately 600 daltons) are effectively excluded from the CNS, primarily by the tight junctions of the endothelial cells making up the blood–brain barrier (12). The inflammatory events basic to MS either primarily or secondarily disrupt the endothelial tight junctions, making gadolinium enhancement a convenient marker for many of the early events in the inflammatory-demyelination cascade (13–15). As acute MS lesions may also be the site of significant axonal transection or injury (16,17), enhancing lesions may likewise mark the initial events ultimately responsible for irreversible CNS damage.

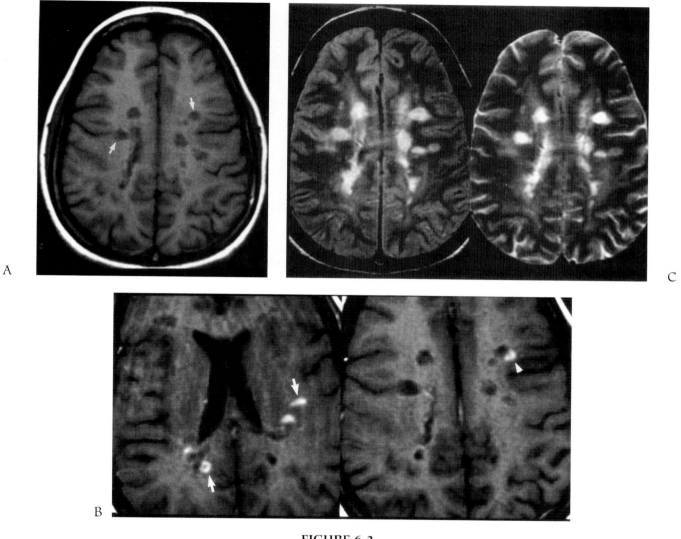

FIGURE 6-2

Characteristic appearance of MS lesions. On T1-weighted images (A) a fraction of the MS lesions in an individual may have a low signal relative to normal white matter (T1-holes; arrows). Chronic T1-hypointense lesions are thought to be regions of relatively severe local destructive change. Most chronic MS lesions will be inconspicuous on T1-weighted images, as they are isointense to normal white matter. (B) T1-weighted images are used for detection of acute, enhancing lesions *(arrows in b)*. Enhancing lesions correspond to the early inflammatory stages of lesion development. Most acute lesions enhance homogeneously, some evolve to ringlike enhancement, and many recurrent lesions may enhance along their borders *(arrowhead in B)*. (C) T2-weighted images are sensitive for longstanding lesions, but nonspecific, as mild pathology (edema), demyelination and severe destructive changes all appear equally hyperintense (bright).

The correspondence between MR-detected enhancing lesions and the acute inflammatory stages of MS lesions has been suggested based on several studies that correlated specimens at autopsy or biopsy with prior gadolinium enhancement by MR imaging (18–20). Further support for this correlation in the early stages of demyelination comes from studies of experimental allergic encephalomyelitis (EAE), an induced autoimmune animal model for MS (Figure 6-4). In EAE, the MR detectable enhancement temporally correlates with inflammatory events within lesions (21–23).

Gadolinium enhancement is observed in acute MS lesions for a period of only two to eight weeks in most cases (24,25), but enhancement may last from less than one to two weeks (25) to as long as 16 weeks. Most lesions tend to start as small (2–10 mm) homogeneously

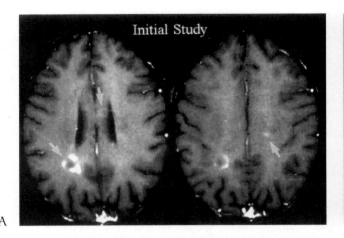

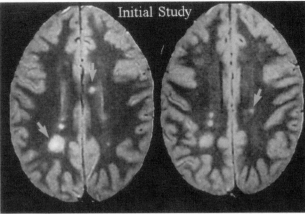

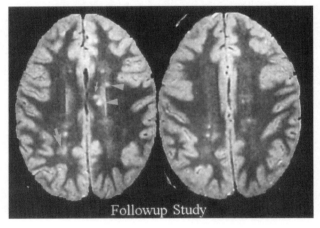

FIGURE 6-3

Evolution of the acute MS lesion. (A) Multiple acute enhancing lesions on consecutive T1-weighted MR images on an initial study *(arrows)*. Corresponding proton density weighted series. (B) shows these same *(arrows)* and addition T2-hyperintense lesions. The follow-up proton density weighted study (C) shows that the initial lesions have left smaller "footprints" *(arrows)*. Additional T2-hyperintense lesions have developed between studies *(arrowheads)*.

enhancing areas, some of which progress to ringlike enhancing areas after approximately four weeks (26) (Figure 6-2b).

In contrast to relapsing and secondary progressive MS, the acute lesions of primary progressive MS appear to be less intensely inflammatory based on histopathology and the lower numbers of enhancing lesions observed on MR imaging studies (27,28).

On T2-weighted images, the acute MS lesion is bright compared with normal white matter (T2-hyperintense), the T2-hyperintense area often extending beyond the borders of the enhancing part of the lesion. The more peripheral areas of T2-hyperintensity most likely represent reversible perilesional edema. Overall, the T2-hyperintense lesion is a relatively nonspecific manifestation of a locally disturbed water environment and, as such, has many potential etiologies. Contributing factors are thought to include an increased local water concentration within the core of the lesion and changes in the environment of this water, which result in increases in the T1- and T2-relaxation times (decreased relaxation rates). In some cases a rim of T2-hypointensity may be seen (Figure 6-5), possibly related to zones of

macrophage infiltration in actively demyelinating areas along the lesion's border (20,29).

On T1-weighted images, acute MS lesions are frequently isointense to normal white matter (same signal as) or may be hypointense (less bright). The latter transient finding may be related to more severe lesion edema at the time of the imaging study (20) or may occur in larger acute lesions in which the hypointensity is simply more conspicuous.

Lesion Regression Stages

After reaching a maximal T2-hyperintense lesion size over a period of approximately four to eight weeks, both the T2 hyperintensity (26,30,31) and the underlying gadolinium-enhancing areas decrease over a period of weeks (32,33). Visually, MR enhancement becomes completely unapparent during these late subacute stages of lesion evolution. Although this finding suggests that the blood–brain barrier damage is returning to normal, in fact the barrier is likely to continue to be partially damaged, as indicated by the serum protein leakage detected in most lesions on biopsy, irrespective of activity, and as seen in

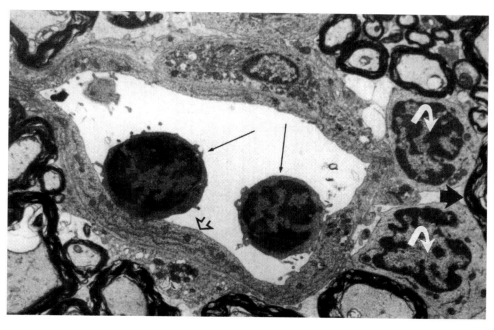

FIGURE 6-4

Migration of lymphocytes through the blood–brain barrier in experimental allergic encephalomyelitis. Electron micrograph from mouse spinal cord. Two intraluminal lymphocytes *(long arrows)* are attached to the postcapillary endothelium *(short open arrow)*. Other lymphocytes have already migrated through the endothelium *(curved arrows)* and abut myelinated nerve fibers *(short closed arrow)*. Figure from Raine CS. The Dale E. McFarlin Memorial Lecture: The immunology of the multiple sclerosis lesion. *Ann Neurol* 1994; 36(Suppl):S61–S72; with permission.

longstanding MS plaques (20,34). In the future, dynamic contrast-enhanced MR imaging studies may provide a more objective measure of these chronic areas of damaged blood–brain barrier (35).

After several months, the MS lesion becomes a chronic, smaller residual area of abnormality as seen on T2-weighted images (Figure 6-3c). This T2-hyperintense area is the "footprint" of the prior acute event. The footprint typically is approximately one third to one half the size of the initial lesion (30,31), and most of these lesions will not change over a period of many years (Figure 6-6).

The acute lesions, whether initially T1-hypointense or isointense, evolve on T1-weighted imaging over a period of weeks to become in most cases indistinguishable from normal white matter, or may later become areas of persistent hypointensity (T1-holes) (9). Some lesions in the subacute stages have a T1-hyperintense rim, which may be visible for more than a year (26).

The Chronic MS Lesion

The chronic MS lesion typically is seen as a focal area of elevated signal intensity on T2-weighted MR images (Fig-ure 6-2c). With extensive accumulation of disease over time, these T2-lesions may appear confluent (Figure 6-7). Despite a highly variable underlying histopathology, the chronic T2-hyperintense lesion has a relatively uniform appearance and signal characteristics. The underlying histopathology ranges from near normal to severe pathology, with variable degrees of myelin loss, astrogliosis, and axonal loss (36,37).

In contrast to the appearance of lesions by T2-weighted imaging, by T1-weighted imaging chronic lesions tend to separate into two distinct groups. Most MS lesions are isointense to normal white matter, but a smaller fraction of lesions appear hypointense (lower signal) compared with normal white matter (Figures 6-2 and 6-7). Preliminary studies based on autopsy material suggest that these T1-hypointense lesions do in fact correspond to regions with reduced axonal density (38). The hypointense lesions (9,39) also seem to correspond to MS lesions with abnormal (reduced) magnetization transfer (MT) indexes (40) and are considered potential markers for more destructive MS (see subsequent discussion).

Although the major areas of involvement represented by T2-hyperintense lesions are stable from month

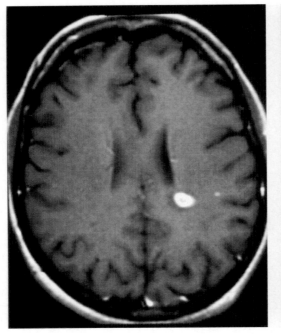 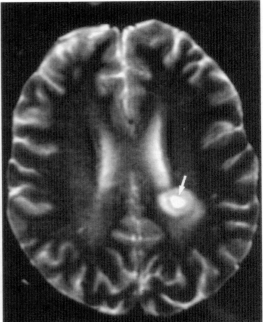

A   B

FIGURE 6-5

An acute, enhancing MS lesion showing a bullseye appearance. (A) The corresponding lesion on a T2-weighted series (B) shows several different zones, including a centrally hyperintense area with a peripheral rim of hypointensity *(arrows),* and surrounding hyperintensity, the latter probably reversible perilesional edema.

to month, and in many cases over periods of years (Figure 6-6), the natural history of the disease is one of a gradual accumulation of T2-hyperintense lesions by the addition of new lesions and expansion of preexisting lesions (Figure 6-8). In patients enrolled in research studies in the relapsing stages of disease, an increment in T2-lesion area or volume is seen on the order of 5 percent to 12 percent (41–43) or approximately 0.45 to 0.7 cc per year (41). The variation in T2-hyperintense lesion changes in individuals is far greater. Some patients show no change on annual evaluations. But for patients with only a few lesions, increases on the order of 100 percent of their initial lesion volume are not uncommon. Similarly, large volume decreases may occur as acute lesions shrink (Figure 6-3). Consequently, a patient may appear to improve based on total T2-lesion load over time, largely due to regression in the reversible component of the acute insult (edema), yet the number of new lesions may be increasing, suggesting ongoing disease activity. Lesion load increases over time and the addition of new or enlarging lesions have become the basis for measuring an individual patient's cumulative CNS event-history in clinical trials and natural history studies (Figure 6-8) (31,33,44,45).

THE TYPICAL APPEARANCE OF MS BY IMAGING

X-Ray Studies

Although the dynamic changes in MS lesions over time were first shown by CT imaging (30), CT of the brain is no longer used today in the evaluation of known or suspected MS, because its sensitivity and specificity are unacceptably poor compared with MR imaging (46,47). When lesions are identified, they appear hypodense to normal white matter, and if acute, enhancement may be detected, particularly using high doses of contrast agent (10,11). Additional findings include cerebral atrophy (ventriculomegaly, enlarged sulci) or, rarely, masslike lesions.

Myelography and CT-myelography also have no current role in the diagnosis or evaluation of MS, as these methods can only detect, with low sensitivity, late findings (atrophy), or rare mass lesions, and offer relatively little specificity in diagnosis. The exception is in patients with safety (e.g., pacemakers) or other contraindications to MR imaging such as patients with severe metal-induced artifacts, who occasionally may benefit from a CT or myelographic evaluation.

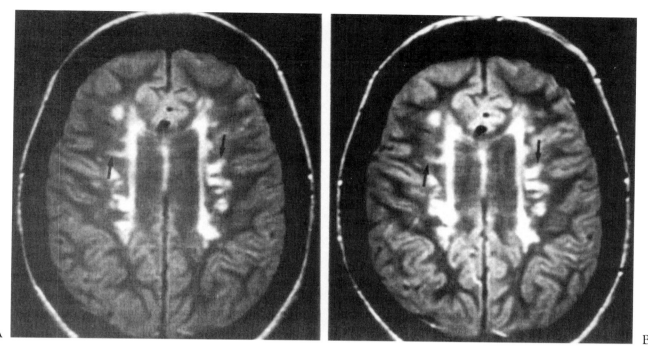

A
B

FIGURE 6-6

Stable T2-hyperintense lesions. (A) Intermediate T2-weighted image shows multiple white matter lesions, many of which are ovoid and oriented at right angles to the ventricular surface *(arrows)*. (B) A study one year later shows that the majority of these periventricular lesions are stable. From Simon JH. Neuroimaging of multiple sclerosis. *Neuroimag Clin North Am* 1993; 3:229–246; with permission.

Magnetic Resonance Imaging

In contrast to CT scanning, most patients with a diagnosis of definite MS by clinical criteria will have a brain MR study with findings suggestive of MS. Using strict Poser criteria and only clinical features to classify cases, one or more focal brain lesions were seen in 113 of 114 (99 percent) of the patients in one series and 197 of 200 (98.5 percent) in a second series (48,49). However, there are patients with well-characterized MS who have lesions only in the spinal cord (50), so a negative brain MR imaging cannot independently exclude a diagnosis of MS. The common appearance of MS lesions in the brain in established relapsing and progressive MS are summarized in Table 6-1.

Distribution and Appearance of Lesions

In most cases MS is characterized by the majority of lesions being located in the periventricular white matter (abutting the ventricle surface) rather than within the more peripheral white matter or juxtacortical white matter (touching gray matter). Many periventricular lesions are ovoid and seem to project at right angles away from the ventricular surface (51) (Figure 6-9). Ovoid lesions

are not specific for MS, but they are common, even in the early stages of disease, and their absence in patients with abundant T2-hyperintense lesions would be unusual in established disease. Multiple sclerosis with greater peripheral as opposed to periventricular lesions would be unusual.

Periventricular lesions by pathology and MR imaging most commonly are located along the trigones and body of the lateral ventricle, but occur in all regions abutting a deep CSF surface, including the occipital and frontal and temporal horns, the floor of the fourth ventricle, and around the third ventricle (48,52). Lesions abutting the temporal horns are frequent in MS, but rare by other common etiologies such as normal aging or small vessel disease. Multiple sclerosis lesions are very common in the centrum ovale, corpus callosum, and other white matter tracts (fornix, optic chiasm, and optic nerves), and not infrequently seen in or adjacent to the internal capsules.

Lesions in the brain that are more peripherally located, such as those that are juxtacortical, within or abutting U-fibers, can be seen using conventional sequences, sometimes with difficulty (53), but are becoming increasingly appreciated as T2-weighted inver-

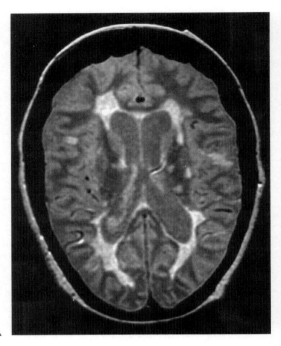 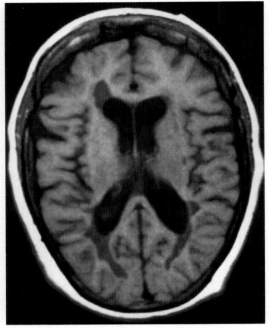

A   B

FIGURE 6-7

Confluent MS lesions in a patient with secondary progressive MS. Although there are several isolated lesions, most of the lesions in this patient appear confluent on the T2-weighted (A) and T1-weighted (B) series.

TABLE 6-1
Classic Magnetic Resonance Imaging Features and Red Flags

CLASSIC FEATURES OF RELAPSING OR SECONDARY PROGRESSIVE MS	RED FLAGS SUGGESTING POSSIBLE ALTERNATE DIAGNOSIS
BRAIN	
• Asymmetric involvement	• Symmetry
• Periventricular >> peripheral	• Mostly peripheral white matter lesions
• Brainstem surface >>> deep brainstem	• Mostly deep lesion (no CSF contact)
• Lesions abut inner surface of corpus callosum	• Outer or full thickness of callosum
• Ovoid (right-angle) lesions	• No ovoid lesions present when many lesions seen
• Cerebellar peduncle and cerebellum	
• T1-hypointense lesions	
• Enhancing lesions (ring, rim, or solid)	
• Mixed, enhancing and nonenhancing	• Synchronous enhancement (ADEM)
• Generalized atrophy, but central atrophy > peripheral atrophy	• Predominantly cortical or cerebellar atrophy
• Minority of lesions show mass effect	• Multiple mass lesions
SPINAL CORD	
• Partial thickness of cord involvement	• Full thickness T2 hyperintense or enhancing lesions
• Asymmetric involvement	• Symmetric involvement
• Lateral and dorsal surfaces common	• Central cord only
• Short vertical segments, with gaps	• Continuous long lesions
• Multiple segments	
• Enhancing lesions	
• Focally swollen cord	• Long segment swelling
• Focal atrophy	

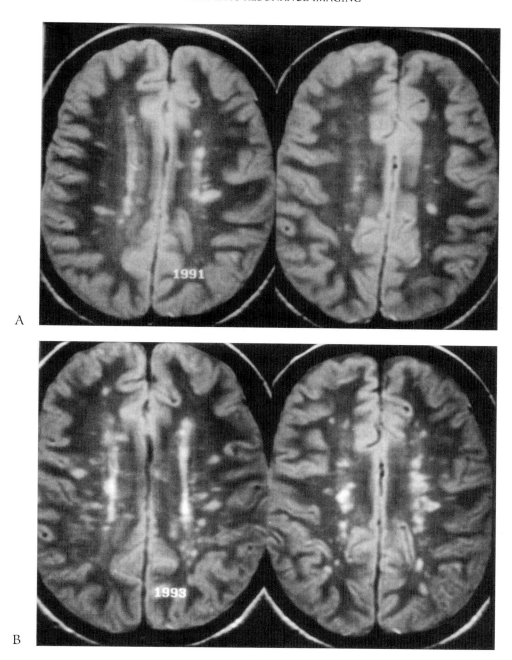

FIGURE 6-8

Accumulating T2-hyperintense lesion load over time. (A) Initial T2-weighted study in a patient with relapsing MS. (B) Study two years later shows major increase in lesion load. This patient had consistently active disease with more than 10 enhancing lesions on the baseline, year one and year two series (not shown).

sion recovery pulse sequences are used in clinical practice (Figure 6-9). In particular, the fluid attenuated inversion recovery (FLAIR) sequence eliminates (nulls) the usual intense and confounding signal of normal CSF (54).

Gray Matter Lesions

Macroscopic, MR-detected, pure gray matter lesions are relatively rare in MS, even with optimized pulse sequences, although gray matter MS lesions are com-

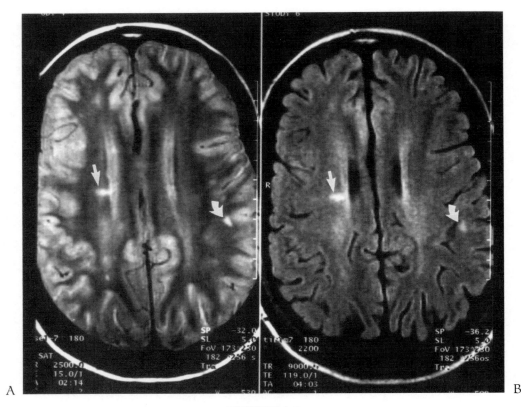

A   B

FIGURE 6-9

Proton density-weighted fast spin-echo (A) compared with a fast (turbo) FLAIR image (B). The right periventricular and ovoid lesion *(arrow)* and the left subcortical lesion *(curved arrow)* can be seen by both techniques, although the contrast-noise ratio and lesion conspicuity is greater on the fast FLAIR series, primarily due to suppression of adjacent CSF signal.

monly seen by the pathologist (52). In Ormerod's series (48), lesions were seen in the basal ganglia in 25 percent of patients.

Masslike and Unusual Multiple Sclerosis

These lesions occur frequently enough to cause diagnostic confusion and unnecessary biopsy (55). Particularly in the setting of masslike lesions in the spinal cord, if primary demyelination is entertained as a diagnosis based on clinical or laboratory findings, a brain MR study suggestive of MS may prevent an unnecessary biopsy.

Corpus Callosum

The frequent involvement of the corpus callosum in MS as seen by MR imaging and at autopsy (56–62) is thought to be due to lesions "spreading" from the ventricular surface along the ependymal veins that project into the adjacent white matter. Multiple sclerosis may result in focal

or diffuse T2-hyperintense lesions of the corpus callosum and/or focal or diffuse atrophy of the corpus callosum (56,57) (Figure 6-10). There are two important characteristic features of these lesions that are helpful as imaging signs of MS. First, T2-hyperintense lesions of the corpus callosum almost always are located along the inner callosum (56,59) and almost never along the outer fiber surfaces unless they also abut the inner surface. Second, inner callosal lesions often penetrate the more peripheral (outer) fibers in an irregular pattern in contrast to edema, small vessel-related disease and aging changes that are more often observed as smooth inner callosal or ependymal-based processes (63) (Figure 6-11). Unfortunately, corpus callosal lesions are not 100 percent specific for MS (59,60). Absence of T2-hyperintense inner callosal lesions in established MS makes the diagnosis of MS much less likely but does not exclude the diagnosis. Their presence in a characteristic pattern makes the diagnosis of MS more likely, but these lesions may occur with other pathologies.

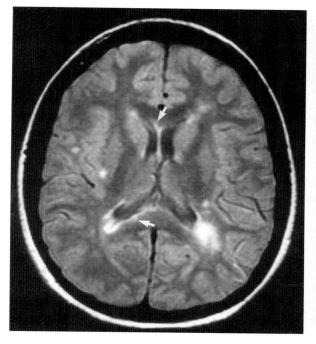

A

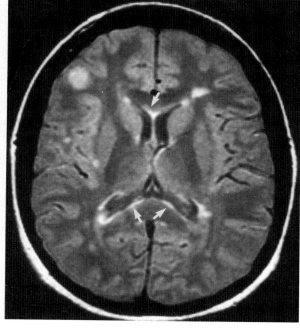

B

FIGURE 6-10

Lesions of the corpus callosum. Corpus callosum lesions *(arrows)* occur along the inner (deep) callosal surfaces and have irregular outer borders, which do not follow the expected contours of the nerve fibers. Axial (A and B) and sagittal projections (C).

C

Visual Pathways

Direct imaging of the optic nerve usually is not required in patients who present with clinically typical optic neuritis. Optic nerve imaging is, however, useful in research studies (64–69) and in patients who have atypical clinical presentations. Magnetic resonance imaging is sensitive to lesions of the optic nerve in the acute stages. Findings include a T2-hyperintense, enhancing nerve, the signal abnormalities often extending into the perineural tissues. The optimal methodology includes coronal, T1-weighted contrast enhanced (64) and/or high resolution T2-weighted studies combined with frequency-selective fat-suppression imaging sequences (3,67).

Brainstem and Cerebellum

Brainstem, cerebellar peduncle and cerebellar involvement is very common in established MS (70). In the brainstem the lesions most frequently abut the external (cisternal) or internal (ventricular or aqueductal) CSF surfaces (Figure 6-12). As brainstem surface and deep cerebellar lesions are uncommon in aging and small vessel disease, the presence of these lesions may be used as an aid in differential diagnosis (71,72).

Spinal Cord

Most patients with established MS will have lesions detectable within the spinal cord if optimal methodolo-

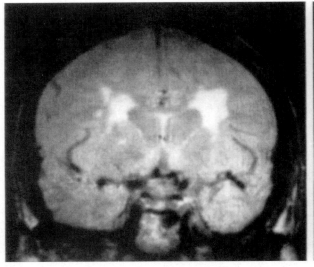
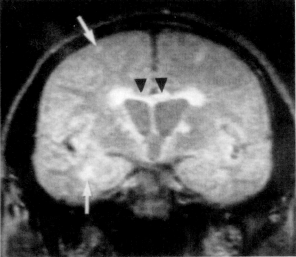

A   B

FIGURE 6-11

Binswanger disease versus demyelination. In A, a study from a demented elderly hypertensive patient with Binswanger disease, T2-hyperintense lesions are seen in the periventricular white matter and basal ganglia/internal capsule, which are areas supplied by long penetrating medullary arteries and arterioles. Areas supplied by the short arterioles, including corpus callosum, cortex, and subcortical U bundles are spared. In MS (B), note the extensive corpus callosum lesions *(arrowheads)* and subcortical lesions *(best shown by upper arrows)*. From: Moody DM, Bell MA, Challa VR: The corpus callosum, a unique white matter tract: Anatomic features that may explain sparing in Binswanger disease and resistance to flow of fluid masses. *AJNR* 1988; 9:1051-1058; with permission.

gies are used (73). The total volume of spinal cord lesions will be relatively small compared with that seen in the brain, even in patients with predominantly spinal manifestations and disability (73). Although spinal cord lesions are not a specific sign, they are relatively rarely seen

related to normal aging, even in the greater than 50-year-old age range, where nonspecific T2-hyperintense lesions frequently are seen in the brain.

Multiple sclerosis lesions are found at all levels of the spinal cord, with the majority observed in the cervical

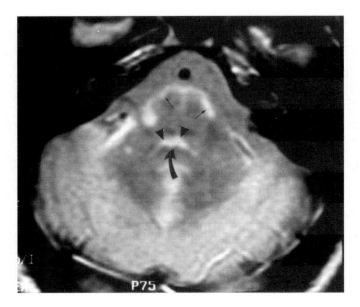

FIGURE 6-12

Brainstem lesions. MS lesions of the brainstem *(arrows)* are most frequently located along the superficial *(arrows)* and deep surfaces *(arrowheads)* adjacent to CSF, in comparison to aging and small vessel changes, which occur most frequently deeper within the brainstem. Curved arrow shows fourth ventricle.

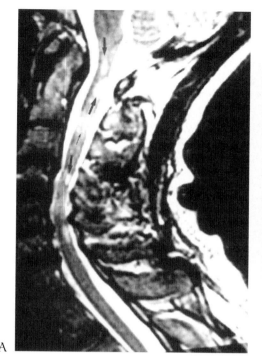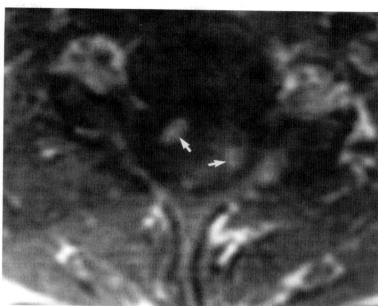

FIGURE 6-13

Spinal cord MS lesions. (A) Sagittal and (B) axial images. MS lesions *(arrows)* tend to be vertically elongated and lie along the spinal cord surface. On axial images, the lesions are typically asymmetric.

region by autopsy (74) and by MR imaging (74). Although T2-hyperintense lesions are commonly observed in the spinal cord, T1-hypointensities are rare. Most T2-hyperintense MS lesions in the spinal cord are less than 10–15 mm in length (75), and multiple, gapped lesions are commonly seen (Figure 6-13a). Lesions typically are asymmetric, the majority located along the surface of the spinal cord, most frequently along the dorsal or lateral surfaces (75–77) (Figure 6-13). Similar to brain lesions, spinal cord lesions usually enhance during their active stages (78), although for technical reasons (image quality) enhancement detection may be lower than in the brain. Current versions of FLAIR imaging fail to detect many MS lesions in the spinal cord (79). More rarely, acute lesions may result in a swollen spinal cord. Secondary changes in the spinal cord include focal and diffuse volume loss (73,80,81).

DIFFERENTIAL DIAGNOSIS

Irrespective of the contributions made through MRI to the description of the appearance and course of MS in the brain and spinal cord, the diagnosis of MS still requires clinical confirmation. For patients beyond approximately 50 years of age, nonspecific T2-hyperintensities may be mistaken for MS (82–84), as may small vessel pathology secondary to atherosclerosis, hypertension, and diabetes. Neurosarcoidosis (85,86), the vasculitides (87), and Lyme disease (88) usually do not appear similar to MS on imaging studies but rarely may be indistinguishable by both MR and clinical features.

Fortunately, many conditions that mimic MS by MR imaging present with clinical features that are not characteristic of MS (89). Differential diagnosis has been reviewed recently (89). Some potentially helpful differential points are highlighted here.

Nonspecific Aging and Small Vessel Disease–Related Changes

The classic findings in MS were described previously, but in patients older than 50 years overlap with aging and small vessel disease may present a confusing picture. Non-MS patients less than 50 years may also be found to have one to two small (< 3–4 mm) T2-hyperintensities. The Fazekas criteria (71,72) are helpful in this group, as cerebellar and/or brainstem lesions greater than 6 mm, frequent in MS, are uncommon as nonspecific findings. Small artery and arteriolar disease generally spare the deep substance of the corpus callosum and the subcortical U fibers (Figure 6-11), which commonly are affected in MS (63). T2-hyperintensities in the brainstem frequently are seen in the elderly, presumably from small vessel disease. These tend to be central rather than surface-based, as is typical for MS. Hypertensive disease, unlike MS, may result in focal destructive lesions (lacunes) in the basal ganglia. Although lesions of the basal ganglia may occur in MS, in most cases they should be only a small percent of the total observed lesion volume. Acute hemorrhagic lesions or lesions rimmed by hemosiderin (T2-hypointense surfaces) are for practical purposes never seen in MS. Not infrequently, the rim of a subacute MS lesion may be hyperintense (bright) on T1-weighted images. This should not be misinterpreted as hemorrhage.

The vasculitides such as systemic lupus erythematosus (SLE) (87) and more rarely Behçet disease (90) may resemble MS clinically and by their white matter lesional pattern in the brain and spinal cord. The brain lesions of the vasculitides tend to be more numerous in the peripheral compared with the periventricular white matter and are more likely to have resulted in focal areas of cortical damage and cortical atrophy. Behçet disease, as compared with MS, is more commonly centralized within the brainstem, basal ganglia, and thalamus (90). Migraine-associated lesions may result in focal areas of gray matter damage and a peripheral white matter distribution (91,92).

Acute disseminated encephalomyelitis (ADEM) is an acute inflammatory demyelinating disease of the CNS that has many features in common with MS. It usually is distinguished from MS by its clinical course, characteristically a single episode with acute onset, accompanied by fever and headache. A history of a recent viral infection or vaccination may be helpful. The MR appearance of individual lesions in ADEM are indistinguishable from those in MS (93,94). The major distinguishing feature is that in ADEM lesions most frequently are synchronously enhancing, a finding that is very rare in MS. However, cases of ADEM may evolve into an MS-like pattern, and MS rarely may present with synchronous enhancing lesions. Long-term serial follow-up, for example at six months and one year, in theory should differentiate the monophasic pattern of ADEM from the multiphasic pattern of MS but may not be definitive for MS cases that may become relatively inactive after the initial presentation (95).

Infection

The scattered, asymmetric lesions characteristic of progressive multifocal leukoencephalopathy (PML) may appear MS-like, but they are only rarely enhancing and usually are seen in patients with known risk factors (severe immunocompromise), who then show rapid deterioration. Whipple's disease, which is treatable with antibiotics, may in its early stages appear MS-like (89). Lyme disease (neuroberylliosis) may mimic MS by clinical criteria and may present with optic neuritis and a relapsing course. As a treatable, often underdiagnosed entity, it is important to consider Lyme disease in endemic regions. Enhancement of the leptomeninges may be seen in Lyme disease (89) but is not seen in MS.

Malignancies, including metastases, and lymphomatosis (96) rarely produce lesional patterns similar to MS.

Spinal Cord Disease

Differentiation of the various acute non-MS myelopathies often is a difficult and frustrating task when based on MR imaging alone (97–100). The classic features of MS in the spinal cord have been outlined previously. Involvement of white matter, asymmetry, and short lesions favor MS. Symmetric, full-thickness, long lesions are more likely the result of non-MS etiologies.

Pediatric Multiple Sclerosis

Multiple sclerosis does occur in childhood, but it is relatively rare (101). Computed tomography and MR imaging features are similar to those seen in adult MS (102–104), although many reports emphasize a more severe presentation. This may be the result of a selection bias, as subclinical and minimally clinical cases may not present until early adulthood, whereas cases with brainstem and spinal cord disease may present earlier. Postinfectious and postvaccination ADEM are likely more common in childhood and should not be mistaken for MS. Long-term follow-up may be helpful. It is interesting that childhood optic neuritis has a lower risk of progression to MS compared with optic neuritis in adults (105), and many cases are associated with systemic infection.

MR-BASED RESEARCH CRITERIA FOR MULTIPLE SCLEROSIS

Criteria for the diagnosis of MS have been developed for research purposes. These criteria increase the sensitivity and/or specificity of the MR imaging study. Objective MR imaging criteria for MS were established by Fazekas and others (71). Final criteria with a specificity of 100 percent could be achieved when at least two of three of the following were observed: (1) lesions at least 6 mm or larger, (2) lesions abutting the ventricle body, or (3) an infratentorial location. These criteria were subsequently evaluated (72) in 1,500 consecutive brain MRI studies, including 134 cases with a clinical diagnosis of MS. In that analysis, the specificity and sensitivity of the Fazekas criteria were 96 percent and 81 percent, compared with the Paty criteria (106; see subsequent section), which had a specificity and sensitivity rate of 92 percent and 87 percent, respectively. Beyond age 50 years, there is a marked decrease in specificity for the diagnosis of MS, using any MR imaging criteria alone (72).

THE RELATIONSHIP BETWEEN MR IMAGING AND THE CLINICAL CATEGORIES OF MS

Multiple sclerosis typically is classified as relapsing-remitting, secondary progressive, primary progressive, or relapsing-progressive disease (107). Relapsing-remitting disease, with complete or near complete recovery from each acute event tends to evolve over 5–10 years into a secondary progressive phase of disease that is dominated by disability accumulation in the face of less dramatic or unapparent exacerbations. Magnetic resonance imaging studies in these two groups of patients suggest more similarities than differences (Table 6-2). Quantitative evaluations show a greater average T2 lesion load in secondary progressive MS (9,108–112), in most but not all studies, and greater T1-hypointense lesion volumes in secondary progressive MS (9,110) (Figure 6-7).

Several studies also suggest a greater accumulation of brain tissue with abnormal magnetization transfer imaging (MTI) indexes in secondary progressive MS (113) and lower levels of NAA relative to abnormal tissue as determined by magnetic resonance spectroscopy (112,114). As secondary progressive MS follows relapsing MS, these findings are not entirely unexpected.

Several but not all series suggest a decrease in the probability of enhancing lesions in secondary progressive MS. From 24 percent to 57 percent of patients with secondary progressive MS have one or more enhancing lesions, compared with 40 percent to 72 percent of patients characterized as having relapsing MS (27,112,116–118). In one large trial of patients with mild to modest disability relapsing MS, 53 percent of the patients had enhancing lesions (118) despite a study requirement of no clinical exacerbations in the two months preceding the entry MR imaging study. Although the reduced number of enhancing lesions in secondary progressive MS likely correlates with the reduction in apparent relapses in the latter stages of disease, and immunologic changes, another possibility is that the reduction in enhancing lesions may be a technical issue; for example, contrast enhancement may be less conspicuous in the more severely damaged tissue that is frequently seen in the later stages of disease.

Insight into the earliest stages of MS and the earliest stages of relapsing disease comes from studies in patients whose presenting symptom is an isolated, monosymptomatic neurologic syndrome affecting the spinal cord, brainstem, or optic nerve(s). A positive MR imaging study at this clinical presentation increases the risk for the subsequent development of MS (see subsequent section). Consequently, many of these patients are likely to be early MS or first onset MS patients.

TABLE 6-2
Magnetic Resonance Findings in Multiple Sclerosis by Disease Classification

CLASSIFICATION	ENHANCING LESION ACTIVITY (% PATIENTS WITH ≥ 1 ENHANCING LESION)	T2-HYPERINTENSE LESION VOLUME	COMMENTS
First Onset*	About 25%–50%	Mean about 2 cc	MR lesion load at onset predicts probability for developing CDMS
Relapsing MS	40%–72%	Mean 10–25 cc, most series	
Secondary Progressive MS	24%–57%	Mean typically greater than for relapsing MS	Much overlap in appearance with relapsing MS
Primary Progressive MS	Low	Mean typically less than for relapsing MS	Fewer inflammatory lesions compared with relapsing and progressive MS

* Isolated, monosymptomatic attack (brainstem, spinal cord, optic nerve), resembling demyelination, not meeting criteria for diagnosis of clinically definite MS (CDMS)

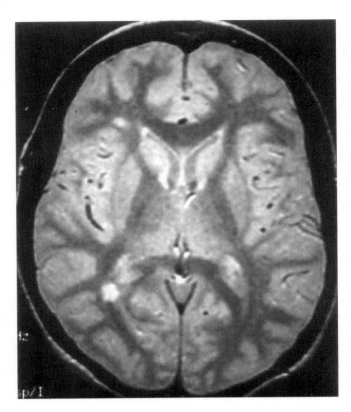

FIGURE 6-14

Brain MR imaging in "first onset MS." Patients with a first (monosymptomatic) neurologic event resembling demyelination and a positive brain MR imaging study are at increased risk for a subsequent second attack and a diagnosis of clinically definite MS. On average, the brain lesion load is small, as shown, although some patients have surprising large numbers of subclinical lesions.

Multiple sclerosis lesions at the time of first presentation are qualitatively similar to those seen in relapsing MS (Figure 6-14). T2-hyperintense lesion location, lesion size, and signal intensity characteristics on multiple pulse sequences are indistinguishable from relapsing MS. The major difference appears to be the smaller number and volume of lesions in these early stage patients. In addition, first onset patients rarely show visible signs of cerebral atrophy. T1-hypointense lesions are not rare, but their overall volume is small compared with patients who have relapsing or secondary progressive MS.

Until only recently, primary progressive MS patients frequently were considered together with secondary progressive patients in MS studies and clinical trials, but based on clinical and immunologic grounds, this group is thought to be either a distinct clinical entity or one that lies at the end of the spectrum of MS (28). Primary progressive MS patients typically have few enhancing lesions

(119,120,28). This finding may correspond to the lesser degree of inflammation seen by histopathology (28). The basis for the severe disability that may accompany primary progressive MS has not yet been determined by standard imaging tests. For example, although primary progressive MS patients may have severe and progressive disability localized to the spinal cord, the number or volume of T2-hyperintense spinal cord lesions is not elevated compared with other MS groups (73). The presence of enhancing lesions does not exclude the diagnosis of primary progressive MS, and there are no distinct MR imaging features that may be used as selection criteria in clinical trials, although one study suggests that some primary progressive patients may have more diffuse abnormalities of the spinal cord on MR imaging (121).

PROGNOSIS FOR MULTIPLE SCLEROSIS BASED ON MAGNETIC RESONANCE IMAGING AT FIRST ONSET

The majority of MS patients experience their first neurologic event, which typically is transient, with involvement commonly traced in retrospect to the spinal cord, brainstem, or optic nerve (122). Unfortunately, by clinical criteria alone, it is difficult to predict the likelihood of progression to clinically definite MS (CDMS) in these patients. Estimates for development of CDMS after optic neuritis range from as low as 13 percent to as high as 88 percent after variable periods of follow-up (123–129).

Several early MR studies established that at the time of the first onset of a neurologic event resembling demyelination, many patients have multiple, previously unsuspected, and widely distributed lesions in the brain and/or spinal cord, primarily in clinically silent areas of the white matter (130,131). Subsequent studies have shown that a positive MR at first presentation increases the likelihood of a subsequent diagnosis of CDMS. Morissey and coworkers (132) found that for spinal cord, brainstem, or optic nerve presentations, the risk for CDMS was greater in patients with larger numbers of T2-hyperintense lesions on their initial MR imaging study. Further studies after a five-year follow-up by Filippi and coworkers (133) established that the volume of T2-hyperintense lesions predicted both time to CDMS and disability. After 10 years, 83 percent of the patients with an initially abnormal MR imaging study from this original study population converted to CDMS, compared with only 11 percent of the patients with an initially normal brain MR study (134).

The relationship between MR imaging findings and CDMS also was shown by the results of the Optic Neuritis Treatment Trial (135,128). Conversion to CDMS occurred in only 16 percent of the 202 patients who had a negative brain MR imaging study (lesions < 3 mm diameter) at presentation. This same risk rate was seen for the 202 patients with a negative MR study followed by Jacobs and coworkers (136). The conversion to CDMS in some patients despite a negative brain MR study is to be expected, as some MS patients with an established diagnosis of MS and a positive spinal cord MR examination may not have any brain MR lesions. In the Optic Neuritis Treatment Trial, there was a 51 percent conversion rate to CDMS after five years in the 89 patients who had a positive MR study (128).

Overall, more than 10 series support the initial observations that a negative brain MR study at presentation predicts a low—but not zero—probability for subsequent CDMS, whereas a positive MR predicts a greater likelihood, but not 100 percent for a second attack and CDMS within three to five years (137).

Imaging Criteria for Prediction of Clinically Definite Multiple Sclerosis After First Presentation

Several imaging criteria to predict CDMS have been established and tested in research studies that provide some guidance that may be helpful in making clinical judgments as well. The Paty Criteria (106) are based on four or more T2-hyperintense lesions or only three T2-hyperintense lesions provided one is in a periventricular location. In two independent studies, the sensitivity and specificity by these criteria were 94 percent and 57 percent (106), and 88 percent and 54 percent (138), respectively. Tas and colleagues (139) found that requiring a minimum of one enhancing lesion and one nonenhancing lesion increases the specificity to approximately 80 percent, whereas sensitivity decreases to 59 percent. This is likely because not all MS patients will have enhancing lesions at all observations. In addition, enhancing lesions probably serve to predict, to some extent, more active patients who are likely to develop a second event over a shorter observation interval, assuming parallels with relapsing and progressive MS (41,140–143). A four Parameter Model based on enhancing lesions, juxtacortical lesions, infratentorial lesions, and periventricular lesions was developed by Barkoff and colleagues (138). The sensitivity and specificity by these criteria were 82 percent and 78 percent, respectively.

An important confounding factor with any predictor based on MR imaging criteria is the effect of age. Most patients at first onset are likely younger than 50 years, but for older patients, nonspecific T2-hyperintensities (144) are likely to decrease specificity based on imaging criteria (72).

Finally, it is important to note that there is some evidence that these selection and prediction algorithms may be improved by combining additional independent criteria, such as those provided by CSF analyses. Some studies find a stronger relationship between abnormal factors such as IgG in the CSF and subsequent CDMS as compared with MR (136), whereas others have not (139). In a large prospective study of patients presenting with optic neuritis (145), oligoclonal bands were strongly associated with subsequent conversion to MS and had a greater sensitivity, lower specificity, and a stronger positive predictive value compared with MR imaging. The combination of two or fewer MR lesions and absent oligoclonal bands was a powerful predictor against CDMS in that study.

THE CLINICAL SIGNIFICANCE OF MAGNETIC RESONANCE ABNORMALITIES (TABLE 6-3)

Because of the location of the majority of MS lesions, most acute activity in the CNS is clinically silent. At presentation and early in the course of disease, patients commonly have multiple lesions scattered throughout the white matter (dissemination in space), and many have MR evidence of dissemination in time (several but not all lesions enhancing). The greater sensitivity of MR imaging compared with clinical measures for acute events in relapsing MS is well established. Magnetic resonance will detect approximately 5 to 10 independent cerebral events for every clinical event (31,33,78,146–149). Completely unsuspected MS is detected at autopsy (88,89) and as an incidental finding on imaging.

Magnetic Resonance as a Measure of Acute Events

Although most MS insults to the CNS events are clinically silent, the minority that occur in functionally sensitive areas are likely to elicit acute, important symptoms and signs. For this group of lesions, the time course for symptoms usually parallels the time course for the lesion's evolution as seen by MR imaging. The strong correspondence between a clinical event and an MR lesion is best shown in the case of optic neuritis, where the time course for optic nerve enhancement parallels that of clinical dysfunction (150). Lesions of other cranial nerve nuclei and sensitive tracts also are likely to be symptomatic (151,152).

Clinical attacks occur in relapsing-remitting MS with a frequency of approximately 0.4 to one event per year on average and more rarely up to two times per year (1), and the clinical attack rate is modestly correlated with the MR attack rate (41). Because MR imaging provides a simple, sensitive method to detect acute cerebral events, compared with the clinical evaluation (Figure 6-15), serial

TABLE 6-3

Summary of Magnetic Resonance Imaging Compared with Clinical Measures of Disease

Category	Description
Diagnostic	Clinical criteria for diagnosis of CDMS always required
Specificity	MR data supports diagnosis of CDMS for two attacks, but clinical evidence of only one lesion
	Brain MR can be negative in CDMS with spinal cord involvement
Prognosis: First Onset	After monosymptomatic presentation, negative brain MR strongly predictive against progression to CDMS (but rate not zero)
	After monosymptomatic attack, a positive brain MR moderately predictive for progression to CDMS (but some patients do not progress)
Prognosis: Relapsing and Secondary Progressive Disease	Enhancing lesions on MR correlated with increased risk for subsequent new lesions and lesion accumulation by MR
	Probable relationship between enhancing lesions and subsequent increased clinical activity
Extent of Disease	MR almost always shows widely scattered lesions unsuspected by clinical examination
Activity Correlations	For functionally sensitive areas (e.g., optic nerve), strong correlation between MR and onset and resolution of acute clinical symptoms
	Modest correlation between acute clinical events and new MR events over time
Attack Rate	MR events exceed clinical events by factor of 5–10:1
Disability	T2-hyperintense lesion load only poorly correlated with clinical disability in population studies and no correlation in individuals
	Better correlations between tissue damage measures and clinical disability in populations
MS Disease Classification	MR shows much overlap between relapsing and secondary progressive MS on average (Greater lesion volume but fewer active lesions in secondary progressive MS). Rare enhancing lesions in primary progressive MS

CDMS=clinically definite MS

imaging at monthly intervals has become the standard approach to monitoring therapy in Phase II treatment trials (137,149,153). However, in the individual patient, interpretation of change in MS status based on a single MR study would be hazardous because of the likelihood of typical month-to-month changes (up or down), and one could not determine if activity is stable, increasing, or decreasing from a study at a single point in time. McFarland and coworkers (154) have shown that three monthly MR studies provide a reasonably good assessment of an individual's activity rate, but again the practical implementation for individual patient assessments awaits further formal evaluation as a therapy monitoring strategy.

The Relationship Between Magnetic Resonance Abnormalities and Clinical Disability

For an individual, the T2-lesion load in the brain or spinal cord does not correlate with disability. It is not uncommon to observe a minimally disabled MS patient in the clinic with a large T2 lesion load, whereas another patient with minimal T2-lesions of the brain or spinal cord may be severely disabled. This MR-disability discrepancy also has been seen in larger studies in relapsing MS, where the correlation between T2-lesion load and Expanded Disability Status Scale (EDSS) score is only poor, with correlation coefficients typically in the range 0.2 to 0.3 (41,43,155).

The MR-disability discrepancy in individuals and in populations is most likely multifactorial:

1. T2-lesions are known to reflect many pathologies. Areas of the brain or spinal cord with minimal damage (e.g., edema with minimal demyelination) will appear on T2-weighted imaging sequences to be as severely affected as regions with complete tissue disruption (e.g., severe axonal loss and astrogliosis).
2. Disability scoring methods are imperfect (156).
3. Long observation periods may be required to observe a stronger MR imaging–disability correlation.
4. Small lesions in functionally sensitive locations are more disabling.
5. Global CNS MR measures are too simplistic.

One of the often cited problems with the EDSS is its emphasis on ambulation. It was therefore surprising that studies of T2-lesion load in the spinal cord also showed poor correlations with disability (73).

Alternative measures of clinical dysfunction include those based on neuropsychological testing. Multiple studies suggest that these generally correlate more strongly with T2-lesion load and cerebral atrophy in the brain than do the standard disability measures (157–162). A functional composite scoring system combining neuropsychological measures (PASAT), ambulation (timed walk),

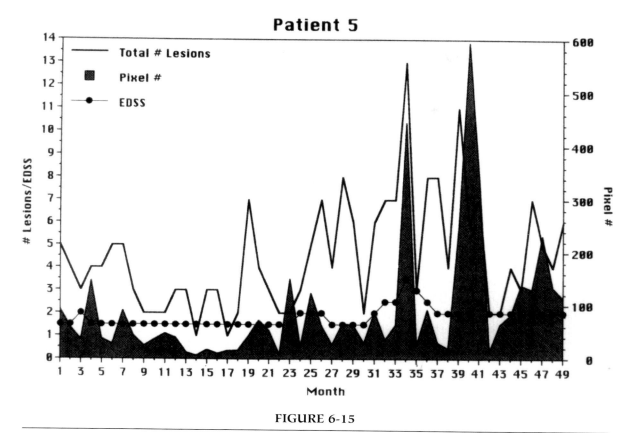

FIGURE 6-15

Variations in gadolinium-enhancing lesions on monthly MR imaging studies in one patient. Large month-to-month intraindividual changes in the number or volume of enhancing lesions are the norm in patients with active disease. The majority of new lesions are not detected clinically and over a short interval are not strongly reflected by changes in disability. From Frank JA, Stone LA, Smith ME, et al. Serial contrast-enhanced magnetic resonance imaging in patients with early relapsing-remitting multiple sclerosis: Implications for treatment trials. *Ann Neurol* 1994; 26(Suppl)S86–S90; with permission.

and fine motor, upper extremity testing (nine-hole peg test) has been developed (163) but has not yet been formally tested against MR outcome measures.

Several studies suggest that the more damage-specific measures, including N-acetylaspartate (4, 164–166), T1-hypointense lesion volume (9), MTI (113), and measures of atrophy of the brain or spinal cord (80,167), may be more strongly correlated with disability and neuropsychological impairment than is T2-hyperintense lesion volume. In particular, volume loss occurs in the spinal cord (80,81), cerebellum (165), corpus callosum (57,60), and tissues surrounding the ventricles based on the ex vacuo expansion of the third and lateral ventricles, and nearly all correlative studies have shown associations between atrophy and disturbances in neuropsychological and clinical function (140,158–162).

Despite weak correlations between the global conventional MR measures and disability, there do appear to be important MR relationships that can be seen in large

clinical trials that suggest that the direct view of MS pathology afforded by MR imaging is important to the patient. The gadolinium-enhancing lesion activity appears to be the best predictor of subsequent new and enlarging T2-lesions and T2-lesion volume increments in relapsing (41) and progressive MS (142), over periods of months and years (140–143). Enhancing lesions also predict cerebral atrophy in patients with mild to modest disability relapsing MS (140). Enhancing lesions predict subsequent enhancing lesions, which suggests that the activity pattern by MR imaging is relatively stable, over a period of at least one to two years, despite the known month-to-month fluctuations that are seen on monthly MRI studies (24,154).

MONITORING THERAPY BY MRI

There are no standardized rules for the use of MR imaging to monitor clinical trials, but guidelines have been

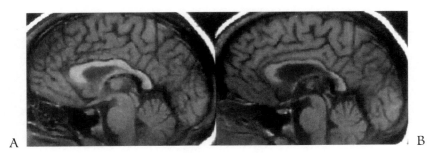

FIGURE 6-16

Brain atrophy in MS. Near-normal thickness corpus callosum is seen at baseline (A). After a two-year interval, the callosum in this patient with interval active disease (many enhancing lesions) has shrunk to one half its original size (B).

A   B

published (137,168). To date, phase I (safety and toxicity) trials have not used MR imaging as an outcome measure, although in theory development of more than the predicted number of enhancing lesions could become one of several objective measures of toxicity.

Phase II trials (efficacy, extended safety) typically are based on monthly MR imaging studies for periods of approximately 4–12 months. Phase II trials are designed to screen for promising therapies, which may then be studied more formally by a phase III clinical outcome–based trial. The primary outcome measure is based on enhancing lesions or alternatively on new T2-hyperintense lesion counts (137,149,153). One popular approach is a crossover design, with each patient undergoing a pretreatment period (1–6 months) followed by a treatment period (3–6 months). This design allows for a relatively small sample size. However, interpretation may be confounded with this trial design because decreased clinical and MR activity may occur naturally, rather than as a treatment effect, in any population selected for active disease or recent disease activity ("regression toward the mean effect"). Alternatively, a phase II trial may be based on a parallel groups design with independent treatment and placebo arms, provided there is an adequate sample size.

In phase III (definitive) clinical trials, which typically are based on 300 to 800 patients, MR measures are used as important secondary outcome assessments. A typical trial would include annual or every six monthly assessments of lesion load or accumulation of new and enlarging T2-hyperintense lesions for a period of two to three years. Annual measures of enhancing lesions may be used or, alternatively, a smaller cohort may be followed more intensely (e.g., monthly) for new enhancing or new T2-hyperintense lesions.

THE EFFECT OF TREATMENT ON THE MAGNETIC RESONANCE IMAGING STUDY

Corticosteroids

Corticosteroids remain the principal therapy for acute, symptomatic MS exacerbations (169) to decrease the severity and duration of symptoms. A clinical response to corticosteroids may occur within hours of administration. Corticosteroids have a strong effect on the damaged blood–brain barrier, as closure of leakage of CT or MR contrast occurs within minutes to hours (170–172). Unfortunately, this practical effect on the blood–brain barrier is transient because lesions may reenhance after several days, and over a period of weeks lesion enhancement may return to expected, untreated levels (172). The effect of corticosteroids on the size of the T2-hyperintense lesion is less predictable (171).

High-dose intravenous corticosteroid therapy may also have some long-range effects. For example, a decrease in time to CDMS (a second attack) was detected in the two-year follow-up from the optic neuritis treatment trial for the subgroup of patients with a positive MR imaging study at presentation (135). This effect could not be demonstrated beyond two years (128). Further studies are required to determine whether multiple administrations of corticosteroids may result in a long-term therapeutic benefit, either as a delay in CDMS or as a reduction in accumulating damage as indicated by MR detectable activity.

Beta-Interferons

Interferon beta-1a (Avonex, Biogen, Inc.) and interferon beta-1b (Betaseron, Berlex, Inc.) have been approved in North America for relapsing MS and are widely used in Europe as well (118,173). The beta-interferons decrease the relapse rate and progression of disability, presumably through their immunomodulatory effects (169). On MR the beta-interferons decrease the number of new and/or enhancing lesions (13,41–43,118,174–176), suggesting an effect on factors that disturb the blood–brain barrier. This effect occurs rapidly, within one week to two months after treatment is initiated (176). The beta-interferons also decrease the accumulated volume of T2-hyperintense lesions in relapsing MS (41–43). This is likely primarily to their inhibiting new lesion development.

Copolymer-1

Positive clinical results have been reported for relapsing MS treated with copolymer-1 (177), but results for defin-

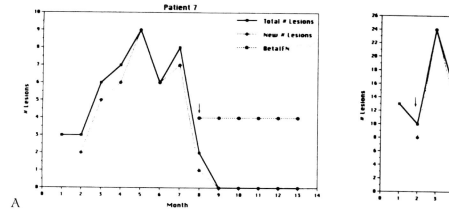
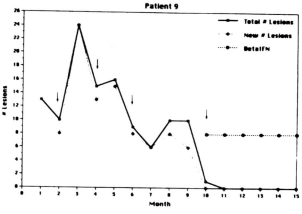

FIGURE 6-17

Magnetic resonance imaging to measure treatment responses in an individual patient. This graph shows the total and new enhancing lesion numbers on monthly MR imaging studies in two relapsing-remitting MS patients (A, B). Note that after treatment with interferon beta-1b, the number of enhancing lesions decreases. Arrows indicate data most affected by pulse cortocosteroid administration. From Stone LA, Frank JA, Albert PS, et al. The effect of interferon-ß on blood–brain barrier disruptions demonstrated by contrast enhanced magnetic resonance imaging in relapsing-remitting multiple sclerosis. *Ann Neurol* 1995; 37:611–619; with permission.

itive MR imaging–based trials are not yet reported. A small study involving 10 patients with relapsing-remitting MS using a crossover design suggested a reduction in new enhancing lesions (178).

Other Immunomodulatory Agents

Many new treatments have been tested with MRI-based phase II strategies (179–184). Studies with cladribine, a cytotoxic purine analogue, for example, have shown that this agent may halt the development of enhancing lesions (184).

CLINICAL AND ADVANCED MAGNETIC RESONANCE PROCEDURES

Gadolinium-Enhanced Magnetic Resonance Imaging

Gadolinium-enhanced MR imaging is used in the clinic to provide evidence for dissemination of disease in time, is helpful with differential diagnosis, and is used by some clinicians as a measure of active disease. Standard doses (0.1 millimolar per kg) of any of the approved MR contrast agents (gadolinium-chelates) are acceptable and appropriate for clinical imaging. Although cost-prohibitive in most cases, improved lesion detection and lesion conspicuity may be achieved using triple (0.3 mmole per kg) rather than single doses. Higher doses of MR contrast agents will in many cases increase the number of lesions detected by 50 percent to 100 percent, on average (27,185–187). Another approach to increase enhancing lesion detection is through T1-weighted MTI sequences (185,188). The magnetization transfer pulse can be used to decrease the signal of normal brain tissue but has minimal effect on enhancing lesions, thereby increasing enhancing lesion contrast and conspicuity.

Detection of T2-Hyperintense Lesions

The dual-echo classic spin-echo sequence has been gradually replaced by imaging series based on a proton-density and more T2-weighted fast spin-echo (turbo spin-echo) sequence for clinical imaging of MS (189) in many centers. More recently, a fast FLAIR sequence has been used to replace the fast spin-echo proton density–weighted series and can be combined with a T2-weighted FSE series. The major benefit of the fast FLAIR sequence is improved conspicuity of subcortical and cortical lesions, but fast FLAIR is less optimal for lesion detection in the posterior fossa (190,191) and detection of spinal cord pathology (192).

The field strength of the MR instrument does not appear to be an important factor for MS diagnosis in the clinic (193). In our experience, low field (0.3–0.5 T), including open magnet architecture, instruments provide reliable diagnostic information in cooperative patients.

Magnetization transfer imaging takes advantage of the fact that a conventional MR instrument can be used to probe macromolecular structure, including aspects thought to be related to myelin membrane integrity (5,40,113,194–196). In MTI, the fraction of MR invisible water molecules that are associated with macromolecules are irradiated with radio frequency pulses. An exchange of magnetization between these protons and the MR visible mobile water protons results in image signal intensity changes that are readily measured.

Using a simple MTI measure, strong magnetization transfer effects are seen for normal white matter (for example, a 30 percent to 50 percent decrease in signal may be seen, depending on technique), whereas progressively less MTI effect is seen for areas with greater tissue damage. For the most severely damaged tissues, MTI values approach those for CSF (no decrease in signal). The MTI ratio in MS correlates modestly with loss of signal on T1-weighted imaging in a subset of lesions (T1-holes) (40) and, most important, clinical disability (113). Global MTI scores may someday become important outcome measures in clinical trials but require further validation in prospective and longitudinal studies. Magnetization transfer imaging is not used in individuals as a measure of disease.

Magnetic Resonance Spectroscopy (MRS)

Most 1.5 Tesla whole body clinical MR imaging instruments are capable of acquiring good quality proton spectra provided they are well maintained and include the appropriate pulse sequence and processing software. Fully automated methods for shimming and processing are already on some commercial products but not all MR systems. Additional expertise is required to acquire and process spectra if these products are not provided.

There is no current role for MRS in the clinical evaluation of MS. However, proton (1H) MRS is an important research tool because it provides information about brain neuron and axonal density or neurochemical integrity, in contrast to the relatively nonspecific information provided by standard MR imaging methods. The dominant peak from a proton MR spectrum is from N-acetylaspartate (NAA). The NAA peak is a pool of N-acetylated moieties, most likely precursor molecules as they are relatively abundant in brain (approximately 10 millimolar). N-acetylaspartate is considered to be a neuronal marker in the mature brain as this group of resonances is not detected outside neurons or axons (197,198). N-acetylaspartate is often reported as a ratio relative to creatine-phosphocreatine, the latter relatively stable in a variety of pathologies, or may be reported as an absolute concentration, after corrections for the effects of relaxation. Decreased NAA, implying neuronal or axonal damage or loss is seen in MS lesions, either transiently in acute-subacute lesions or persistently in chronic lesions (4). Decreased NAA-creatine ratios have been

reported in normal appearing white matter, presumably related to microscopic lesions). Elevated creatine (200,201) and/or decreased NAA (199) may account for these changes. Elevated creatine is a potential marker for abnormally increased levels of non-neuronal cells (astrocytes, microglia) (201). Several reports suggest stronger correlations between NAA and disability or dysfunction (4,165), compared with T2-lesion load measures and disability, and as such, NAA is being evaluated as a potentially more informative marker in clinical trials and natural history studies. Other resonances detectable by MR spectroscopy relevant to MS include choline, which may be acutely elevated in MS, and lipids, which are thought to be early markers in lesion development (202,203).

Quantitative Relaxation

Magnetic resonance images can be synthesized based on a quantitative representation of the T1- or T2-relaxation times or proton density for each image pixel (7). Unfortunately, simple (monoexponential) relaxation maps do not separate new and mature lesions because of large overlapping values of T1 and T2 (33) and provide little specific information. Another approach attempts to sort out the various water compartments in cells, tissues, and other spaces by generating multiexponential-based relaxation maps of the various water components (204). This approach may someday contribute to a finer biophysical and chemical characterization of the demyelination process in vivo.

Diffusion Magnetic Resonance Imaging

Diffusion MR imaging is another experimental procedure that may become useful to increase the specific characterization of normal and abnormal white matter, by providing quantitative information about the composition, shape, and orientation of water compartments in the CNS (205). The diffusion coefficient is abnormal in acute and chronic MS lesions (206), and based on animal demyelination models, diffusion MR imaging may be sensitive to early changes in an MS lesion (207,208).

Quantitation of Burden of Disease

Several recent studies and reviews have addressed the various methodologies that may be used in the setting of a clinical trial to quantitate the T2-hyperintense or T1-hypointense lesion load (137,168). In individuals, a simple practical quantitation scheme is determination of the number of new or enlarging MS lesions. Change in new and enlarging lesions correlates modestly with change in total T2-lesion burden (41) and, provided slice locations are well aligned or thin slice imaging is used, is an accurate, reproducible methodology that may be used to assess progressive changes over long intervals.

References

1. Weinshenker BG. The natural history of multiple sclerosis. *Neurol Clin* 1995; 13(1):119–146.
2. Ebers GC, Paty DW. Natural history studies and applications to clinical trials. In: Paty DW, Ebers GC (eds.). *Multiple sclerosis*. Philadelphia: FA Davis, 1998:192–228.
3. Szumowski J, Simon JH. Proton chemical shift imaging. In: Stark DD, Bradley WG (eds.). *Magnetic resonance imaging*. 2nd ed. St. Louis: Mosby–Yearbook, 1992:479–521.
4. Arnold DL, Wolinsky JS, Matthews PM, Falini A. The use of magnetic resonance spectroscopy in the evaluation of the natural history of multiple sclerosis. *J Neurol Neurosurg Psychiatry* 1998; 64:S94–S101.
5. Wolff SD, Balaban RS. Magnetization transfer contrast (MTC) and tissue water proton relaxation in vivo. *Magn Reson Med* 1989; 10:135–144.
6. Horsfield MA, Larsson HBW, Jones DK, Gass A. Diffusion magnetic resonance imaging in multiple sclerosis. *J Neurol Neurosurg Psychiatry* 1998; 64:S80–S84.
7. Hendrick RE, Raff U. Image contrast and noise. In: Stark DD, Bradley WG (eds.). *Magnetic resonance imaging*. 2nd ed. St. Louis: Mosby–Yearbook, 1992: 1:109–144.
8. Larsson HBW, Frederiksen J, Kjaer L, et al. In vivo determination of T1 and T2 in the brain of patients with severe but stable multiple sclerosis. *Magn Reson Med* 1988; 7:43–55.
9. Truyen L, van Waesberghe JHTM, van Walderveen MAA, et al. Accumulation of hypointense lesions ("black holes") on T1 spin echo MRI correlates with disease progression in multiple sclerosis. *Neurology* 1996; 47: 1469–1476.
10. Sears ES, McCammon A, Bigelow R, Hayman LA. Maximizing the harvest of contrast enhancing lesions in multiple sclerosis. *Neurology* 1982; 32:815–820.
11. Spiegel SM, Viñuela F, Fox AJ, Pelz DM. CT of multiple sclerosis: Reassessment of delayed scanning with high doses of contrast material. *AJNR* 1985; 6:533–536.
12. Hirano A, Kawanami T, Llena JF. Electron microscopy of the blood-brain barrier in disease. *Microsc Res Tech* 1994; 27:543–556.
13. Calabresi PA, Tranquill LR, Dambrosia JM, et al. Increase in soluble VCAM-1 correlate with a decrease in MRI lesions in multiple sclerosis treated with interferon ß-1b. *Ann Neurol* 1997; 41:669–674.
14. Giovannoni G, Lai M, Thorpe J, et al. Longitudinal study of soluble adhesion molecules in multiple sclerosis: Correlation with gadolinium enhanced magnetic resonance imaging. *Neurology* 1997; 48:1557–1565.
15. Trojano M, Avoilio C, Simone IL, et al. Soluble intercellular adhesion molecule-1 in serum and cerebrospinal fluid of clinically active relapsing-remitting multiple sclerosis. *Neurology* 1996; 47:1535–1541.
16. Ferguson B, Matyszak MK, Esiri MM, Perry VH. Axonal damage in acute multiple sclerosis lesions. *Brain* 1997; 120:393–399.
17. Trapp BD, Peterson J, Pansohoff RM, et. al. Axonal transection in the lesions of multiple sclerosis. *N Engl J Med* 1998; 338:278–285.
18. Katz D, Taubenberger JK, Cannella B, et al. Correlation between magnetic resonance imaging findings and lesion development in chronic, active multiple sclerosis. *Ann Neurol* 1993; 34:661–669.
19. Nesbit GM, Forbes GS, Scheithauer BW, et al. Multiple sclerosis: Histopathologic and and/or CT correlation in 37 cases at biopsy and three cases at autopsy. *Radiology* 1991; 180(2):467–474.
20. Bruck W, Bitsch A, Kolenda H, et al. Inflammatory central nervous system demyelination: Correlation of magnetic resonance imaging findings with lesion pathology. *Ann Neurol* 1997; 42:783–793.
21. Hawkins CP, Munro PMG, Mackenzie F, et al. Duration and selectivity of blood-brain barrier breakdown in chronic relapsing experimental allergic encephalomyelitis studied by gadolinium-DTPA and protein markers. *Brain* 1990; 113:365–378.
22. Seeldrayers PA, Syha J, Morrisey SP, et al. Magnetic resonance imaging investigation of blood-brain barrier damage in adoptive transfer experimental autoimmune encephalomyelitis. *J Neuroimmunol* 1993; 46:199–206.
23. Namer IJ, Steibel J, Piddlesden SJ, et al. Magnetic resonance imaging of antibody-mediated demyelinating experimental allergic encephalomyelitis. *J Neuroimmunol* 1994; 54:41–50.
24. Harris JO, Frank JA, Patronas N, et al. Serial gadolinium-enhanced magnetic resonance imaging scans in patients with early, relapsing-remitting multiple sclerosis: Implications for clinical trials and natural history. *Ann Neurol* 1991; 29:548–555.
25. Lai HM, Hodgson T, Gawne-Cain M, et al. A preliminary study into the sensitivity of disease activity detection by serial weekly magnetic resonance imaging in multiple sclerosis. *J Neurol Neurosurg Psychiatry* 1996; 60:339–341.
26. Guttmann CRG, Ahn SS, Hsu L, et al. The evolution of multiple sclerosis lesions on serial MR. *AJNR* 1995; 16:1481–1491.
27. Silver NC, Good CD, Barker GJ, et al. Sensitivity of contrast enhanced MRI in multiple sclerosis. Effects of gadolinium dose, magnetization transfer contrast and delayed imaging. *Brain* 1997; 120:1149–1161.
28. Thompson AJ, Polman CH, Miller DH, et al. Primary progressive multiple sclerosis. *Brain* 1997; 120:1085–1096.
29. Powell T, Sussman JG, Davies-Jones GAB. MR imaging in acute multiple sclerosis: Ringlike appearance in plaques suggesting the presence of paramagnetic free radicals. *AJNR* 1992; 13:1544–1546.
30. Koopsmans RA, Li DKB, Oger JJF, et al. The lesion of multiple sclerosis: Imaging of acute and chronic stages. *Neurology* 1989; 39:959–963.
31. Wiebe S, Lee DH, Karlik SJ, et al. Serial cranial and spinal cord magnetic resonance imaging in multiple sclerosis. *Ann Neurol* 1992; 32:643–650.
32. Kermode AG, Tofts PS, Thompson AJ, et al. Heterogeneity of blood-brain barrier changes in multiple sclerosis: An MRI study with gadolinium- DTPA enhancement. *Neurology* 1990; 40(2):229–235.
33. Miller DH, Rudge P, Johnson G, et al. Serial gadolinium enhanced magnetic resonance imaging in multiple sclerosis. *Brain* 1988; 111:927–939.
34. Kwon EE, Prineas JW. Blood-brain barrier abnormalities in longstanding multiple sclerosis lesions. An immuno-histochemical study. *J Neuropathol Exp Neurol* 1994; 53:625–636.
35. Tofts PS, Kermode AG. Measurement of the blood-brain barrier permeability and leakage space using dynamic

MR imaging.1. Fundamental concepts. *Magn Reson Med* 1991; 17:357–367.

36. Barnes D, Munro PMG, Youl BD, et al. The long-standing MS lesion. A quantitative MRI and electron microscopic study. *Brain* 1991; 114:1271–1280.

37. Newcombe J, Hawkins CP, Henderson CL, et al. Histopathology of multiple sclerosis lesions detected by magnetic resonance imaging in unfixed postmortem central nervous system tissue. *Brain* 1991; 114:1013–1023.

38. van Walderveen MAA, Kamphorst W, Scheltens P, et al. Histopathologic correlate of hypointense lesions on T1-weighted spin-echo MRI in multiple sclerosis. *Neurology* 1998; 50:1282–1288.

39. van Waesberghe JHTM, Castelijns JA, Scheltens P, et al. Comparison of four potential MR parameters for severe tissue destruction in multiple sclerosis lesions. *Magn Reson Imaging* 1997; 15:155–162.

40. Loevner LA, Grossman RI, McGowan JC, et al. Characterization of multiple sclerosis plaques with T1-weighted MR and quantitative magnetization transfer. *AJNR* 1995; 16:1473–1479.

41. Simon JH, Jacobs LD, Campion M, et al. Magnetic resonance studies of intramuscular interferon ß-1a for relapsing multiple sclerosis. *Ann Neurol* 1998; 43:79–87.

42. Paty DW, Li DKB, the UBC MS/MRI Study Group, IFNB Multiple Sclerosis Study Group. Interferon beta-1b is effective in relapsing-remitting multiple sclerosis. II. MRI analysis results of a multicenter, randomized, double-blind, placebo-controlled trial. *Neurology* 1993; 43:662–667.

43. The IFNB Multiple Sclerosis Study Group and the University of British Columbia MS/MRI Analysis Group. Interferon beta-1b in the treatment of multiple sclerosis: Final outcome of the randomized controlled trial. *Neurology* 1995; 45:1277–1285.

44. Simon JH. Magnetic resonance imaging of multiple sclerosis lesions. Measuring outcome in treatment trials. *West J Med* 1996; 164:502-509

45. Simon JH. Contrast-enhanced MR imaging in the evaluation of treatment response and prediction of outcome in multiple sclerosis. *JMRI* 1997; 7:29–37.

46. Jacobs L, Kinkel WR, Polachini I, Kinkel RP. Correlations of nuclear magnetic resonance imaging, computerized tomography, and clinical profiles in multiple sclerosis. *Neurology* 1986; 36:27–34.

47. Sheldon JJ, Siddharthan R, Tobias J, et al. MR imaging of multiple sclerosis: Comparison with clinical and CT examinations in 74 patients. *AJR* 1985; 145:957–964.

48. Ormerod IEC, Miller DH, McDonald WI, et al. The role of NMR imaging in the assessment of multiple sclerosis and isolated neurological lesions: a quantitative study. *Brain* 1987; 110:1579–1616.

49. Miller DH. Spectrum of abnormalities in multiple sclerosis. In: Miller DH, Kesselring J, McDonald W I, Paty DW, Thompson AJ (eds.). *Magnetic resonance in multiple sclerosis*. New York: Cambridge University Press, 1997:31–62.

50. Thorpe JW, Kidd D, Moseley IF, et al. Spinal MRI in patients with suspected multiple sclerosis and negative brain MRI. *Brain* 1996; 119:709–714.

51. Horowitz AL, Kaplan RD, Grewe G, et al. The ovoid lesion: A new MR observation in patients with multiple sclerosis. *AJNR* 1989; 10(2):303–305.

52. Brownell B, Hughes JT. The distribution of plaques in the cerebrum in multiple sclerosis. *J Neurol Neurosurg Psychiatry* 1962; 25:315–320

53. Miki Y, Grossman RI, Udupa JK, et al. Isolated U-fiber involvement in MS. *Neurology* 1998; 50:1301–1306.

54. Hajnal JV, Bryant DJ, Kasuboski L, et al. Use of fluid attenuated inversion recovery (FLAIR) pulse sequences in MRI of the brain. *JCAT* 1992; 16:841–844.

55. Giang DW, Poduri KR, Eskin TA, et al. Multiple sclerosis masquerading as a mass lesion. *Neuroradiology* 1992:150–154

56. Simon JH, Holtas SL, Schiffer RB, et al. Corpus callosum and subcallosal-periventricular lesions in multiple sclerosis: Detection with MR. *Radiology* 1986; 160:363–367.

57. Simon JH, Schiffer RB, Rudick RA, Herndon RM. Quantitative determination of MS-induced corpus callosum atrophy in vivo using MR imaging. *AJNR* 1987; 8:599–604.

58. Wilms G, Marchal G, Kersschot E, et al. Axial vs. sagittal T2-weighted brain MR imaging in the evaluation of multiple sclerosis. *JCAT* 1991; 15(3):359–364.

59. Gean-Marton AD, Vezina LG, Marton KI, et al. Abnormal corpus callosum: A sensitive and specific indicator of multiple sclerosis. *Radiology* 1991; 180:215–221.

60. Offenbacher H, Poltrum B, Strasser-Fuchs, et al. The contribution of corpus callosum lesions to the MRI diagnosis of multiple sclerosis. Presented at the 12th European Congress on Multiple Sclerosis, Copenhagen, Denmark, September 1996.

61. Barnard RO, Triggs M. Corpus callosum in multiple sclerosis. *J Neurol Neurosurg Psychiatry* 1974; 37:1259–1264.

62. Lumsden CE. The neuropathology of multiple sclerosis. In: Vinken PJ, Bruyn GW (eds.). *Handbook of clinical neurology. Vol. 9. Multiple sclerosis and other demyelinating diseases*. Amsterdam, North Holland: Elsevier, 1970:217–309.

63. Moody DM, Bell MA, Challa VR. The corpus callosum, a unique white matter tract: Anatomic features that may explain sparing in Binswanger disease and resistance to flow of fluid masses. *AJNR* 1988; 9:1051–1059.

64. Simon JH, Rubinstein D, Brown M, et al. Quantitative contrast-enhanced MR imaging of the optic nerve. *Acta Radiologica* 1994; 35(6):526–531.

65. Lee DH, Simon JH, Szumowski J, et al. Optic neuritis and orbital lesions: Lipid-suppressed chemical shift MR imaging. *Radiology* 1991; 179:543–546.

66. Miller DH, Newton MR, van der Poel JC, et al. Magnetic resonance imaging of the optic nerve in optic neuritis. *Neurology* 1988; 38:175–179.

67. Gass A, Barker GJ, MacManus DG, et al. High resolution magnetic resonance imaging of the anterior visual pathway in patients with optic neuropathies using fast spin echo and phased array local coils. *J Neurol Neurosurg Psychiatry* 1995; 58:562–569

68. Kapoor R, Miller DH, Jones SJ, et al. Effect of intravenous methylprednisolone on outcome in MRI-based prognostic subgroups in acute optic neuritis. *Neurology* 1998; 50:230–237.

69. Tien RD, Hesselink JR, Szumowski J. MR fat suppression combined with GD-DTPA enhancement in optic neuritis and perineuritis. *JCAT* 1991; 15(2):223–227.

70. Brainin M, Reisner T, Neuhold A, et al. Topographical characteristics of brainstem lesions in clinically definite and clinically probable cases of multiple sclerosis. *Neuroradiology* 1987; 29:530–536.

71. Fazekas F, Offenbacher H, Fuchs S, et al. Criteria for an increased specificity of MRI interpretation in elderly subjects with suspected multiple sclerosis. *Neurology* 1988; 38:1822–1825.

72. Offenbacher H, Fazekas F, Schmidt R, et al. Assessment of MRI criteria for a diagnosis of MS. *Neurology* 1993; 43:905–909.

73. Kidd D, Thorpe JW, Thompson AJ, et al. Spinal cord MRI using multi-array coils and fast spin echo. II. Findings in multiple sclerosis. *Neurology* 1993; 43:2632–2637.

74. Oppenheimer DR. The cervical cord in multiple sclerosis. *Neuropath Appl Neurobiol* 1978; 4:151–162.

75. Thielen KR, Miller GM. Multiple sclerosis of the spinal cord: magnetic resonance appearance. *JCAT* 1996; 20(3):434–438.

76. Honig LS, Sheremata WA. Magnetic resonance imaging of spinal cord lesions in multiple sclerosis. *J Neurol Neurosurg Psychiatry* 1989; 52(4):459–466.

77. Tartaglino LM, Friedman DP, Flanders AE, et al. Multiple sclerosis in the spinal cord: MR appearance and correlation with clinical parameters. *Radiology* 1995; 195:725–732.

78. Thorpe JW, Kidd D, Moseley IF, et al. Serial gadolinium-enhanced MRI of the brain and spinal cord in early relapsing-remitting multiple sclerosis. *Neurology* 1996; 46:373–378.

79. Keiper MD, Grossman RI, Brunson JC, Schnall MD. The low sensitivity of fluid-attenuated inversion recovery MR in the detection of multiple sclerosis of the spinal cord. *AJNR* 1997; 18:1035–1039.

80. Losseff NA, Webb SL, O'Riordan JI, et al. Spinal cord atrophy and disability in multiple sclerosis. A new reproducible and sensitive MRI method with potential to monitor disease progression. *Brain* 1996; 119:701–708.

81. Filippi M, Campi A, Colombo B, et al. A spinal cord MRI study of benign and secondary progressive multiple sclerosis. *J Neurol* 1996; 243(7):502–505.

82. Fazekas F, Kleinert R, Offenbacher H, et al. Pathologic correlates of incidental MRI white matter signal hyperintensities. *Neurology* 1993; 43:1683–1689.

83. Munoz DG, Hastak SM, Harper B, et al. Pathologic correlates of increased signals of the centrum ovale on magnetic resonance imaging. *Arch Neurol* 1993; 50:492–497.

84. Kirkpatrick JB, Hayman LA. White-matter lesions in MR imaging of clinically healthy brains of elderly subjects: Possible pathologic basis. *Radiology* 1987; 162:509–511.

85. Smith AS, Meisler DM, Weinstein MA, et al. High-signal periventricular lesions in patients with sarcoidosis: Neurosarcoidosis or multiple sclerosis? *AJNR* 1989; 10:485–490.

86. Sherman JL, Stern BJ. Sarcoidosis of the CNS. *AJNR* 1990; 11:915–923.

87. Miller DH, Ormerod IEC, Gibson A, et al. MR brain scanning in patients with vasculitis: Differentiation from multiple sclerosis. *Neuroradiology* 1987; 29:226–231.

88. Fernandez RE, Rothberg M, Ferencz G, et al. Lyme disease of the CNS: MR findings in 14 cases. *AJNR* 1990; 11:479–481

89. Kesselring J, Miller DH. Differential diagnosis. In: Miller DH, Kesselring J, McDonald WI, Paty DW, Thompson AJ (eds.). *Magnetic resonance in multiple sclerosis.* New York: Cambridge University Press, 1997:63–107.

90. Wechsler B, Dell'Isola B, Vidaihet M, et al. MRI in 31 patients with Behçet's disease and neurological involvement: prospective study with clinical correlation. *J Neurol Neurosurg Psychiatry* 1993; 56:793–798.

91. Soges, LJ, Cacayorin ED, Petro GR, et al. Migraine: Evaluation by MR. *AJNR* 1988; 9:425–429.

92. Bernasconi V, DE Benedittis G, Lorenzetti A, et al. Magnetic resonance imaging in migraine and tension-type headache. *Headache* 1995; 35: 264–268

93. Epperson LW, Whitaker JN, Kapila A. Cranial MRI in acute disseminated encephalomyelitis. *Neurology* 1988; 38:332–333.

94. Andreula CF, Luciani ANMR, Milella D. Magnetic resonance imaging in diagnosis of acute disseminated encephalomyelitis (ADEM). *Int J Neuroradiol* 1997; 3:21–34.

95. Mader I, Stock KW, Ettlin T, Probst A, et al. Acute disseminated encephalomyelitis: MR and CT features. *AJNR* 1996; 17:104–109

96. Scully RE, Mark EJ, McNeely WF, McNeely BU. Case records of the Masachusetts General Hospital, Case report 31-1995. *N Engl J Med* 1995; 333(15):992–999.

97. Simnad VI, Pisani DE, Rose JW. Multiple sclerosis presenting as transverse myelopathy: Clinical and MRI features. *Neurology* 1997; 48:65–73.

98. Campi A, Filippi M, Comi G, et al. Acute transverse myelopathy: Spinal and cranial MR study with clinical follow-up. *AJNR* 1995; 16:115–23.

99. Scott TF, Bhagavatula K, Snyder PJ, Chieffe C. Transverse myelitis. Comparison with spinal cord presentations of multiple sclerosis. *Neurology* 1998; 50:429–433.

100. Bakshi R, Kinkel RP, Mechtler LL, et al. Magnetic resonance imaging findings in 22 cases of myelitis: Comparison between patients with and without multiple sclerosis. *Eur J Neurol* 1998; 5:35–48.

101. Duquette P, Murray TJ, Pleines J, et al. Multiple sclerosis in childhood:clinical profile in 125 patients. *J Pediatr* 1987; 111:359–363.

102. Glasier CM, Robbins MB, Davis PC, et al. Clinical, neurodiagnostic, and MR findings in children with spinal and brainstem multiple sclerosis. *AJNR* 1995; 16:87–95.

103. Osborn AG, Harnsberger HR, Smoker WRK, Boyer RS. Multiple sclerosis in adolescents: CT and MR findings. *AJNR* 1990; 11:489–494.

104. Ebner F, Millner MM, Justich E. Multiple sclerosis in children: Value of serial MR studies to monitor patients. *AJNR* 1990; 11:1023–1027.

105. Lucchinetti CF, Kiers L, O'Duffy A, et al. Risk factors for developing multiple sclerosis after childhood optic neuritis. *Neurology* 1997; 49:1413–1418.

106. Paty DW, Oger JJF, Kastrukoff LF, et al. MRI in the diagnosis of MS: A prospective study with comparison of clinical evaluation, evoked potentials, oligoclonal banding, and CT. *Neurology* 1988; 38:180–185.

107. Lublin FD, Reingold SC. Defining the clinical cause of multiple sclerosis: Results of an international survey. *Neurology* 1996; 46:907–911.

108. Filippi M, Yoursy T, Campi A, et al. Comparison of triple dose versus standard dose gadolinium-DTPA for detection of MRI enhancing lesions in patients with MS. *Neurology* 1996; 46:379–384.

109. Hohol M, Guttmann CR, Orav J, et al. Serial neuropsychological assessment and magnetic resonance imaging analysis in multiple sclerosis. *Arch Neurol* 1997; 54: 1018–1025.

110. Giugni E, Pozzilli C, Bastianello S, et al. MRI measures and their relations with clinical disability in relapsing-remitting and secondary progressive multiple sclerosis. *Multiple Sclerosis* 1997; 3:221–225.

111. Filippi M, Rossi P, Campi A, et al. Serial contrast-enhanced MR in patients with multiple sclerosis and varying levels of disability. *AJNR* 1997; 18:1549–1556.

112. Matthews PM, Pioro E, Narayanan S, et al. Assessment of lesion pathology in multiple sclerosis using quantitative MRI morphometry and magnetic resonance spectroscopy. *Brain* 1996; 119:715–722.

113. Gass A, Barker GJ, Kidd D, et al. Correlation of magnetization transfer ratio with clinical disability in multiple sclerosis. *Ann Neurol* 1994; 36:62–67.

114. Falini A, Calabrese G, Filippi M, et al. Benign versus secondary-progressive multiple sclerosis: The potential role of proton MR spectroscopy in defining the nature of disability. *AJNR* 1998; 19:223–229.

115. Arnold DL, Matthews PM, Francis G, et al. Proton MR spectroscopy of human brain in vivo in the evaluation of multiple sclerosis: Assessment of the total lesion load of disease. *Magn Reson Med* 1990; 14:154–159.

116. Miki Y, Grossman RI, Udupa J, et al. Computer-assisted quantitation of enhancing lesions in multiple sclerosis: Correlation with clinical classification. *AJNR* 1997; 18:705–710.

117. Goodkin DE, Rudick RA, VanderBrug Medendorp S, et al. Low-dose oral methotrexate in chronic progressive multiple sclerosis: Analyses of serial MRIs. *Neurology* 1996; 47:1153–1157.

118. Jacobs LD, Cookfair DL, Rudick RA, et al. Intramuscular interferon beta-1a for disease progression in relapsing multiple sclerosis. *Ann Neurol* 1996; 39:285–294.

119. Kappos L, Stadt D, Rohrbach E, Keil W. Gadolinium-DTPA-enhanced magnetic resonance imaging in the evaluation of different disease course and disease activity in MS (abstract). *Neurology* 1988; 38(Suppl):225.

120. Losseff NA, Kingsley DPE, McDonald WI, et al. Clinical and magnetic resonance imaging predictors of disability in primary and secondary progressive multiple sclerosis. *Multiple Sclerosis* 1996; 1:218–222.

121. Lycklama a Nijeholt GJ, Barkhof F, Scheltens P, et al. MR of the spinal cord in multiple sclerosis: Relations to clinical subtype and disability. *AJNR* 1997; 18:1041–1048.

122. Matthews WB. Clinical symptoms and signs. In: Matthews WB, Acheson ED, Batchelor JR, Weller RO (eds.). *McAlpine's multiple sclerosis*. New York: Churchill Livingstone, 1985:96–118.

123. Perkin G-D, Rose FC. *Optic neuritis and its differential diagnosis*. Oxford: Oxford University Press, 1979: 246–248.

124. Sandberg-Wollheim M, Bynke H, Cronqvist S, et al. A long term prospective study of optic neuritis: Evaluation of risk factors. *Ann Neurol* 1990; 27:386–393.

125. Rizzo JF, Lessell S. Risk of developing multiple sclerosis after uncomplicated optic neuritis. A long term prospective study. *Neurology* 1988; 38:185–190.

126. Francis DA, Compston DAS, Batchelor JR, McDonald WI. A reassessment of the risk of multiple sclerosis developing in patients with optic neuritis after extended follow up. *J Neurol Neurosurg Psychiatry* 1987; 50: 758–765.

127. Hely MA, McManis PG, Doran TJ, et al. Acute optic neuritis: A prospective study of risk factors for multiple sclerosis. *J Neurol Neurosurg Psychiatry* 1986; 49:1125–1130.

128. Optic Neuritis Study Group. The 5-year risk of MS after optic neuritis. Experience of the optic neuritis treatment trial. *Neurology* 1997; 49:1404–1413.

129. Frederiksen JL, Larsson HBW, Henriksen O, Olesen J. Magnetic resonance imaging of the brain in patients with acute monosymptomatic optic neuritis. *Acta Neurol Scand* 1989; 80:512–517.

130. Jacobs L, Kinkel PR, Kinkel WR. Silent brain lesions in patients with isolated idiopathic optic neuritis: A clinical and nuclear magnetic resonance imaging study. *Arch Neurol* 1986; 43:452–455.

131. Ormerod IEC, Bronstein A, Rudge P, et al. Magnetic resonance imaging in clinically isolated lesions of the brain stem. *J Neurol Neurosurg Psychiatry* 1986; 49:737–743.

132. Morissey SP, Miller DH, Kendall BE, et al. The significance of brain magnetic resonance imaging abnormalities at presentation with clinically isolated syndromes suggestive of MS. A five year follow-up study. *Brain* 1993; 116:135–146.

133. Filippi M, Horsfield MA, Morrissey SP, et al. Quantitative brain MRI lesion load predicts the course of clinically isolated syndromes suggestive of multiple sclerosis. *Neurology* 1994; 44:635–641.

134. O'Riordan JI, Thompson AJ, Kingsley DPE, et al. The prognostic value of brain MRI in clinically isolated syndromes of the CNS. A 10 year follow-up. *Brain* 1998; 121:495–503.

135. Beck RW, Cleary PA, Trobe JD, et al. The effect of corticosteroids for acute optic neuritis on the subsequent development of multiple sclerosis. *N Engl J Med* 1993; 329:1764–1769.

136. Jacobs LD, Kaba SE, Miller CM, et al. Correlation of clinical, magnetic resonance imaging, and cerebrospinal fluid findings in optic neuritis. *Ann Neurol* 1997; 41:392–398.

137. Miller DH, Albert PS, Barkhof F, et al. Guidelines for the use of magnetic resonance techniques in monitoring the treatment of multiple sclerosis. *Ann Neurol* 1996; 39:6–16.

138. Barkhof F, Filippi M, Miller DH, et al. Comparison of MRI criteria at first presentation to predict conversion to clinically definite multiple sclerosis. *Brain* 1997; 120:2059–2069.

139. Tas MW, Barkhof F, van Walderveen MAA, et al. The effect of gadolinium on the sensitivity and specificity of MR in the initial diagnosis of multiple sclerosis. *AJNR* 1995; 16:259–264.

140. Simon JH. From enhancing lesions to brain atrophy in relapsing MS. *J Neuroimmunol* 1998, 98:7–15.

141. Tubridy N, Coles AJ, Molyneux P, et al. Secondary progressive multiple sclerosis: The relationship between short-term MRI activity and clinical features. *Brain* 1998; 121:225–231.

142. Molyneux PD, Filippi M, Barkhof F, et al. Correlations between monthly enhanced MRI lesion rate and changes in T2 lesion volume in multiple sclerosis. *Ann Neurol* 1998; 43:332–339.

143. Koudriavtseva T, Thompson AJ, Fiorelli M, et al. Gadolinium enhanced MRI predicts clinical and MRI disease activity in relapsing-remitting multiple sclerosis. *J Neurol Neurosurg Psychiatry* 1997; 62(3):285–287.

144. Christiansen P, Larsson HB, Thomsen C, et al. Age dependant white matter lesions and brain volume changes in healthy volunteers. *Acta Radiol* 1994; 35:117–122.

145. Soderstrom M, Ya-Ping J, Hillert J, Link H. Optic neuritis. Prognosis for multiple sclerosis from MRI, CSF, and HLA findings. *Neurology* 1998; 50:708–714.

146. Smith ME, Stone LA, Albert PS, et al. Clinical worsening in multiple sclerosis is associated with increased frequency and area of gadopenetate dimeglumine-enhancing magnetic resonance imaging lesions. *Ann Neurol* 1993; 33:480–489.

147. Isaac C, Li DKB, Genton M, et al. Multiple sclerosis: A serial study using MRI in relapsing patients. *Neurology* 1988; 38:1511–1515.

148. Willoughby EW, Grochowski E, Li DKB, et al. Serial magnetic resonance scanning in multiple sclerosis: A second prospective study in relapsing patients. *Ann Neurol* 1989; 25:43–49.

149. McFarland HF, Frank JA, Albert PS, et al. Using gadolinium-enhanced magnetic resonance imaging lesions to monitor disease activity in multiple sclerosis. *Ann Neurol* 1992; 32(6):758–766.

150. Youl BD, Turano G, Miller DH, et al. The pathophysiology of acute optic neuritis. *Brain* 1991; 114:2437–2450.

151. Gass A, Kitchen N, MacManus DG, et al. Trigeminal neuralgia in patients with multiple sclerosis: Lesion localization with magnetic resonance imaging. *Neurology* 1997; 49:1142–1144.

152. Atlas SW, Grossman RI, Savino PJ, et al. Internuclear opthalmoplegia: MR-anatomic correlation. *AJNR* 1987; 8:243–247

153. Nauta JJP, Thompson AJ, Barkhof F, Miller DH. Magnetic resonance imaging in monitoring the treatment of multiple sclerosis patients: Statistical power of parallel-groups and crossover designs. *J Neurol Sci* 1994; 122:6–14.

154. McFarland HF, Stone LA, Calabresi PA, et al. MRI studies of multiple sclerosis: Implications for the natural history of the disease and for monitoring effectiveness of experimental therapies. *Multiple Sclerosis* 1996; 2:198–205.

155. Filippi M, Paty DW, Kappos L, et al. Correlations between changes in disability and T2-weighted brain MRI activity in multiple sclerosis: A follow-up study. *Neurology* 1995; 45:255–260.

156. Whitaker JN, McFarland HF, Rudge P, Reingold SC. Outcomes assessment in multiple sclerosis clinical trials: A critical analysis. *Multiple Sclerosis* 1995; 1:37–47.

157. Rao SM, Leo GJ, Bernardin L, et al. Cognitive dysfunction in multiple sclerosis. 1: frequency, patterns and prediction. *Neurology* 1991; 41:685–691.

158. Rao SM, Leo GJ, Haughton VM, et al. Correlation of magnetic resonance imaging with neuropsychological testing in multiple sclerosis. *Neurology* 1989; 39:161–166.

159. Swirsky-Sacchetti T, Mitchell DR, Seward J, et al. Neuropsychological and structural brain lesions in multiple sclerosis: A regional analysis. *Neurology* 1992: 42:1291–1295.

160. Huber SJ, Paulson GW, Shuttleworth EC, et al. Magnetic resonance imaging correlates of dementia in multiple sclerosis. *Arch Neurol* 1987; 44:732–736.

161. Comi G, Filippi M, Martinelli V, et al. Brain MRI correlates of cognitive impairment in primary and secondary progressive multiple sclerosis. *J Neurol Sci* 1995; 132: 222–227.

162. Hohol MJ, Guttmann CRG, Orav J, et al. Serial neurophysiological assessment and magnetic resonance imaging analysis in multiple sclerosis. *Arch Neurol* 1997; 54:1018–1025.

163. Rudick R, Antel J, Confavreux C, et al. Recommendations from the National Multiple Sclerosis Society Clinical Outcomes Assessment Task Force. *Ann Neurol* 1997; 42:379–382.

164. DeStefano N, Matthews PM, Antel JP, et al. Chemical pathology of acute demyelinating lesions and its correlation with disability. *Ann Neurol* 1995; 38:901–909.

165. Davie CA, Barker GJ, Webb S, et al. Persistent functional deficit in multiple sclerosis and autosomal dominant cerebellar ataxia is associated with axonal loss. *Brain* 1995; 118:1583–1592.

166. Fu L, Matthews PM, De Stefano N, et al. Imaging axonal damage of normal appearing white matter in multiple sclerosis. *Brain* 1998; 121:103–113.

167. Losseff NA, Wang L, Lai HM, et al. Progressive cerebral atrophy in multiple sclerosis: A serial MRI study. *Brain* 1996; 119:2009–2019.

168. Filippi M, Horsfield MA, Ader HJ, et al. Guidelines for using quantitative measures of brain magnetic resonance imaging abnormalities in monitoring the treatment of multiple sclerosis. *Ann Neurol* 1998; 43:499–506.

169. Rudick R, Cohen JA, Weinstock-Guttman B, et al. Management of multiple sclerosis. *N Engl J Med* 1997; 337:1604–1611.

170. Barkhof F, Hommes OR, Scheltens P, et al. Quantitative MRI changes in gadolinium-DTPA enhancement after high-dose intravenous methylprednisolone in multiple sclerosis. *Neurology* 1991; 41(8):1219–1222.

171. Burnham JA, Wright RR, Dreisbach J, et al. The effect of high-dose steroids on MRI gadolinium enhancement in acute demyelinating lesions. *Neurology* 1991; 41(9): 1349–1354.

172. Miller DH, Thompson AJ, Morrissey SP, et al. High dose steroids in acute relapses of multiple sclerosis: MRI evidence for a possible mechanism of therapeutic effect. *J Neurol Neurosurg Psychiatry* 1992; 55:450–453.

173. IFNB Multiple Sclerosis Study Group. Interferon beta-1b is effective in relapsing-remitting multiple sclerosis. I. Clinical results of a multicenter, randomized, double-blind, placebo-controlled trial. *Neurology* 1993; 43:655–661.

174. Pozzilli C, Bastianello S, Koudriavtseva T, et al. Magnetic resonance imaging changes with recombinant human interferon-ß-1a: A short term study in relapsing-remitting multiple sclerosis. *J Neurol Neurosurg Psychiatry* 1996; 61:251–258.

175. Stone LA, Frank JA, Albert PS, et al. Characterization of MRI response to treatment with interferon beta-1b: Contrast enhancing MRI lesion frequency as a primary outcome measure. *Neurology* 1997; 49:862–869.

176. Calabresi PA, Stone LA, Bash CN, et al. Interferon beta results in immediate reduction of contrast-enhanced MRI lesions in multiple sclerosis patients followed by weekly MRI. *Neurology* 1997; 48:1446–1448.

177. Johnson KP, Brooks BR, Cohen JA, et al. Copolymer 1 reduces relapse rate amnd improves disability in relapsing remitting multiple sclerosis: results of a phase III multicenter, double-blind, placebo-controlled trial. *Neurology* 1995; 45:1268–1276.

178. Mancardi GL, Sardanelli F, Parodi RC, et al. Effect of copolymer-1 on serial gadolinium-enhanced MRI in relapsing remitting multiple sclerosis. *Neurology* 1998; 50:1127–1133.

179. Edan G, and the French and British Multiple Sclerosis Mitoxantrone Trial Group (1995). Demonstration of the efficacy of mitoxantrone (MTX) usiung MRI in MS patients with very active disease. *J Neuroimmunol* 1995; (Suppl 1):16.

180. Karussis DM, Meiner Z, Lehmann D, et al. Treatment of secondary progressive multiple sclerosis with the immunomodulator linomide: A double-blind, placebo-controlled pilot study with monthly magnetic resonance imaging evaluation. *Neurology* 1996; 47:341–346.

181. Durelli L, Bongioanni MR, Cavallo R, et al. Interferon alpha treatment of relapsing-remitting multiple sclero-

sis: Long term study of the correlations between clinical and magnetic resonance imaging results and effects on the immune function. *Multiple Sclerosis* 1995; 1:S32–S37.

182. Moreau T, Thorpe J, Miller D, et al. Preliminary evidence from magnetic resonance imaging for reduction in disease activity after lymphocyte depletion in multiple sclerosis. *Lancet* 1994; 344:298–301.

183. van Oosten BW, Lai M, Hodgkinson S, et al. Treatment of multiple sclerosis with the monoclonal anti-CD4 antibody cM-T412. *Neurology* 1997; 49:351–357.

184. Wagner S, Sipe JC, Romine JS, et al. Baseline disability measured by hypodense lesions on MRI in relapsing remitting multiple sclerosis—results of a cladribine study. Presented at the Academy of Neurology, Minneapolis, MN, 1998:S17.003.

185. van Waesberghe JHTM, Castelijns JA, Roser W, et al. Single-dose gadolinium with magnetization transfer versus triple-dose gadolinium in the MR detection of multiple sclerosis lesions. *AJNR* 1997; 18:1279–1285.

186. Wolansky LJ, Bardini JA, Cook SD, et al. Triple-dose versus single dose gadoteridol in multiple sclerosis patients. *J Neuroimag* 1994; 4(3):141–145

187. Filippi M, Yousry T, Campi A, et al. Comparison of triple dose versus standard dose gadolinium-DTPA for detection of MRI enhancing lesions in patients with MS. *Neurology* 1996; 46:379–384.

188. Mehta RC, Pike GB, Enzmann DR. Improved detection of enhancing and nonenhancing lesions of multiple sclerosis with magnetization transfer. *AJNR* 16:1771–1778.

189. Thorpe JW, Halpin S, MacManus DG, et al. A comparison between fast spin echo and conventional spin echo in the detection of multiple sclerosis lesions. *Neuroradiology* 1994; 36:388–392.

190. Yousry TA, Filippi M, Becker C, et al. Comparison of MR pulse sequences in the detection of multiple sclerosis lesions. *AJNR* 1997; 18:959–963.

191. Gawne-Cain ML, O'Riordan JI, Thompson AJ, et al. Multiple sclerosis lesion detection in the brain: A comparison of fast fluid-attenuated inversion recovery and conventional T2-weighted dual spin echo. *Neurology* 1997; 49:364–370.

192. Keiper MD, Grossman RI, Brunson JC, Schnall MD. The low sensitivity of fluid-attenuated inversion recovery MR in the detection of multiple sclerosis of the spinal cord. *AJNR* 1997; 18:1035–1039.

193. Lee DH, Vellet AD, Eliasziw, et al. MR imaging field strength: Prospective evaluation of the diagnostic accuracy of MR for diagnosis of multiple sclerosis at 0.5 and 1.5 T1. *Radiology* 1995; 194:257–262.

194. Lexa FJ, Grossman RI, Rosenquist AC. MR of wallerian degeneration in the feline visual system: characterization by magnetization transfer rate with histopathologic correlation. *AJNR* 1994; 15:201-212.

195. Dousset V, Grossman RI, Ramer KN, et al. Experimental allergic encephalomyelitis and multiple sclerosis: Lesion characterization with magnetization transfer imaging. *Radiology* 1992; 182:483–491.

196. Kimura H, Grossman RI, Lenkinski RE, Gonzalez-Scarano F. Proton MR spectroscopy and magnetization transfer ratio in multiple sclerosis: Correlative findings of active versus irreversible plaque disease. *AJNR* 1996; 17:1539–1547.

197. Moffett JR, Namboodiri MAA, Cangro CB, Neale JH. Immunohistochemical localization of N-acetylaspartate in rat brain. *NeuroReport* 1991; 2:131–134.

198. Urenjak EJ, Williams SR, Gadian DG, Noble M. Proton nuclear magnetic resonance spectroscopy unambiguously identifies different neural cell types. *J Neurosci* 1993; 13: 981–989.

199. Narayanan S, Fu L, Pioro E, et al. Imaging of axonal damage in multiple sclerosis: Spatial distribution of magnetic resonance imaging lesions. *Ann Neurol* 1997; 41:385-391.

200. Husted CA, Goodin DS, Hugg JW, et al. Biochemical alterations in multiple sclerosis lesions and normal appearing white matter detected by in vivo 31P and 1H spectroscopic imaging. *Ann Neurol* 1994; 36:157–165.

201. Rooney WD, Goodkin DE, Schuff N, et al. 1H MRSI of normal appearing white matter in multiple sclerosis. *Multiple Sclerosis* 1997; 3:231–237.

202. Davie CA, Hawkins CP, Barker GJ, et al. Serial proton magnetic resonance spectroscopy in acute multiple sclerosis lesions. *Brain* 1994; 117:49–58.

203. Narayana PA, Doyle TJ, Lai D, Wolinsky JS. Serial proton magnetic resonance spectroscopic imaging, contrast enhanced magnetic resonance imaging and quantitative lesion volumetry in multiple sclerosis. *Ann Neurol* 1988; 43:56–71.

204. Whittall KP, MacKay AL, Graeb DA, et al. In vivo measurements of T2 distributions and contents in normal human brain. *Magn Reson Med* 1997; 37:34–43.

205. Horsfield MA, Larsson HBW, Jones DK, Gass A. Diffusion magnetic resonance imaging in multiple sclerosis. *J Neurol Neurosurg Psychiatry* 1998; 64:S80–S84.

206. Christiansen P, Gideon P, Thomsen C, et al. Increased water self-diffusion in chronic plaques and in apparently normal white matter in patients with multiple sclerosis. *Acta Neurol Scand* 1993; 87:195–199.

207. Richards TL, Alvord EC, He Y, et al. Experimental allergic encephalomyelitis in non-human primates: diffusion imaging of acute and chronic brain lesions. *Multiple Sclerosis* 1995; 1:109–117.

208. Heide AC, Richards TL, Alvord EC, et al. Diffusion imaging of experimental encephalomyelitis. *Magn Reson Med* 1993; 29:478–484.

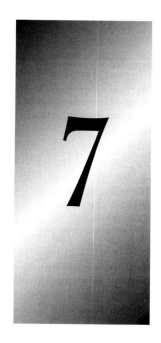

7 The Differential Diagnosis and Clues to Misdiagnosis

Jeffrey A. Cohen, M.D., and Mary R. Rensel, M.D.

In the absence of pathognomonic clinical features or a definitive laboratory test, multiple sclerosis (MS) remains ultimately a diagnosis of exclusion. Because of its heterogeneous manifestations, incorrect diagnosis is not uncommon. This factor is becoming more of an issue as effective therapies emerge and there is increased impetus to make the diagnosis as early as possible. The diagnosis of MS requires certain features, which are well outlined conceptually in the Schumacher criteria (1). These criteria can be restated as:

1. A clinical picture (history and examination) consistent with MS, with relapsing or progressive neurologic manifestations indicating multifocal involvement of the central nervous system (CNS) initially developing in a young adult.
2. Tests that support the diagnosis of MS, including magnetic resonance imaging (MRI), cerebrospinal fluid (CSF) examination, and evoked potentials.
3. Elimination of other potential diagnoses, i.e., the absence of manifestations pointing to an another disease process in the history, examination, or laboratory testing.

Evaluation for MS includes several diagnostic scenarios (Table 7-1). When the clinical features and MRI findings are typical of MS, the likelihood of finding another disorder is small. Further workup may be limited to screening blood work to rule out diseases that rarely mimic "classic" MS (Table 7-2). Magnetic resonance imaging sequences should include standard long TR images (T2-weighted and proton density), fluid attenuated inversion recovery (FLAIR), T1-weighted images, and T1-weighted images following administration of gadolinium (Gd). FLAIR generates images that are heavily T2-weighted with signal from CSF in the ventricles nulled, increasing sensitivity to MS lesions as compared with standard long TR images (2). Administration of Gd is useful for several reasons. First, it occasionally demonstrates pathology in areas where plaques not well seen on standard long TR images, such as the cerebral cortex, deep gray structures, or spinal cord. Second, the extent of Gd-enhancement provides an indication of disease activity that may not be apparent clinically (3). This factor has ramifications for prognosis and the need to consider disease-modifying therapy. Finally, in some patients the findings on long TR images may be compatible with MS but may be nonspecific. An atypical pattern of Gd-enhancement may be a red flag pointing to an alternative diagnosis.

When there is strong evidence of MS based on history, examination, and cranial MRI, CSF examination frequently is unnecessary. Evidence of intrathecal immunoglobulin G (IgG) synthesis probably does not

---

TABLE. 7-1
Diagnostic Scenarios

- Clinical picture and laboratory testing typical of MS
- Known MS plus a potential additional condition
- Clinical picture and laboratory testing consistent with MS but with atypical features

---

change the diagnostic certainty in such cases. That is, the presence of intrathecal IgG synthesis in a case with classic clinical and MRI features does not further increase diagnostic certainty. Conversely, the absence of intrathecal antibody synthesis does not eliminate MS as a possibility. In this situation, it is extremely rare to obtain findings on routine CSF studies that would point to an alternative diagnosis. Cerebrospinal fluid examination is useful when clinical features and MRI either fail to support the diagnosis of MS sufficiently or demonstrate atypical features. Nevertheless, clinicians should consider CSF examination in cases that lack convincing support for the diagnosis of MS from history, examination, and MRI, or where there are atypical features. There may be greater impetus in the future for CSF examination in typical cases of MS if studies identify specific findings that have prognostic value.

The second diagnostic scenario is an additional disease process superimposed on MS. In patients with worsening disability, the principal anatomic site of neurologic involvement needs to be evaluated so as not to miss a treatable cause.

Finally, the clinician must be vigilant for features atypical of MS, suggesting an alternative diagnosis. These "red flags" are outlined in Table 7-3. Although these features do not rule out the diagnosis of MS, they indicate caution in making that diagnosis. An exhaustive differ-

---

TABLE 7-2
Suggested Workup for "Classic" Multiple Sclerosis

- Comprehensive medical and neurologic history and examination
- Cranial MRI including long TR images, T1-weighted images, T1-weighted images with gadolinium
- CSF examination (optional in some cases)
- Screening blood studies including CBC, thyroid studies, ANA, syphilis serology, vitamin B12 level, Lyme titer (in some geographic areas)

TABLE 7-3
Red Flags for the Potential Misdiagnosis of Multiple Sclerosis

- Onset of symptoms before age 20 or after 50
- Very prominent family history
- Course
- Gradually progressive course from onset, particularly in a young patient or with manifestations other than a myelopathy
- Abrupt development of symptoms
- Unifocal manifestations (even if relapsing)
- Prominent neurologic manifestations unusual for MS (e.g., aphasia, deafness)
- Associated systemic manifestations
- Missing features, particularly in longstanding or severe disease
- Lack of oculomotor, optic nerve, sensory, or bladder involvement
- Normal MRI, CSF, and evoked potential studies
- Atypical response to treatment
- Lack of any response to corticosteroids
- Exceptionally rapid or dramatic response to corticosteroids or disease-modifying treatments

---

ential diagnosis for all potential manifestations of MS is extensive. This review focuses on the disorders that pose the greatest diagnostic difficulty or are most frequently considered when MS is being considered (Table 7-4).

INFECTION

Lyme Disease

Lyme disease is caused by infection with the tick-borne spirochete *Borrelia burgdorferi* (Bb). Neurologic involvement is common and varied: meningitis, cranial neuropathy, radiculoneuritis, peripheral neuropathy, encephalomyelitis, and encephalopathy. Numerous other manifestations have been described, some with unconvincing data. Neuroborreliosis-associated encephalomyelitis may be confused with MS. There have been many reports of encephalomyelitis causing a clinical picture similar to MS, with relapsing or progressive multifocal CNS symptoms and signs, similar CSF findings, and similar MRI changes (4–9). Cerebrospinal fluid examination usually demonstrates lymphocytic pleocytosis, mild elevation of protein, and typically normal glucose. Evidence of increased intrathecal IgG synthesis, including oligoclonal bands, may be present. T2-weighted MRI may demonstrate foci of abnormal signal in the cerebral white matter radiographically identical to lesions of MS.

TABLE 7-4
Principle Differential Diagnosis
of Multiple Sclerosis

Infection	Lyme disease, syphilis, progressive multifocal leukoencephalopathy, HIV, HTLV-1
Inflammatory	Systemic lupus erythematosus, Sjögren's syndrome, vasculitis, sarcoidosis, Behçet's disease
Metabolic	Vitamin B12 deficiency, lysosomal disorders, adrenoleukodystrophy, mitochondrial disorders, other genetic disorders
Neoplasm	CNS lymphoma
Spine disease	Vascular malformation, degenerative spine disease

TABLE 7-5
Distinguishing MRI Features of Diseases
That Can Mimic Multiple Sclerosis

PML	Confluent posterior T2-lesions with decreased signal on T1-weighted images without Gd-enhancement
HTLV-1-associated myelopathy	Thoracic spinal cord atrophy Sparse cerebral lesions
SLE and SS	Predominantly subcortical cerebral white matter lesions Gray matter involvement
Vasculitis	Ischemic lesions or cerebral infarcts Gray matter involvement Vascular or meningeal Gd-enhancement
Sarcoidosis	Parenchymal masses with persistent Gd-enhancement Vascular or meningeal Gd-enhancement
Behçets disease	Predominately brainstem involvement
Lymphoma	May be unifocal or multifocal Gray matter involvement Persistent Gd-enhancement Vascular enhancement
Vitamin B12 deficiency	Abnormal signal in cervical spinal cord or cerebral white matter possible
Adrenomyelo-neuropathy	Symmetric lesions in posterior cerebral white matter
Leukodystrophies	Diffuse white matter abnormality
Mitochondrial disorders	Multifocal gray or white matter lesions Basal ganglia calcification
Spinocerebellar degenerations	Brainstem or cerebellar atrophy Absence of signal abnormality
Spinal vascular malformation	Patchy increased T2 signal in spinal cord with faint Gd-enhancement or cord enlargement Draining veins may be visible Absence of cranial lesions
Motor neuron disease	Typically normal MRI Symmetric increased T2 signal in pyramidal tracts

The relationship between Lyme disease and MS remains uncertain and somewhat contentious. This issue becomes particularly difficult in areas in which Lyme disease is endemic. In a survey of patients referred to the MS clinic at State University of New York (SUNY)–Stony Brook, a Lyme endemic area, only 1 of 89 patients with definite MS demonstrated serum antibodies to Bb (10). However, the rate of Lyme seropositivity in unselected patients may be as high as 10 percent in some endemic areas (11). In a follow-up study at the SUNY–Stony Brook MS clinic, 19 of 283 consecutive patients had borderline or positive Bb serology (12). Only 10 of 19 patients were positive on repeat serologic testing. None of the 10 demonstrated intrathecal anti-Bb antibody production, and none exhibited decreased relapse rate after antibiotic treatment. These findings suggest that Bb infection rarely causes an MS-like illness.

Neurologic manifestations of Lyme disease usually occur in association with other systemic manifestations, i.e., preceding erythema migrans plus concomitant arthritis or cardiac manifestations, but numerous examples of isolated neurologic involvement with serologic evidence of Lyme disease exist. Many of these reports linking Lyme disease to a variety of neurologic manifestations should be viewed with skepticism. Compounding the diagnostic problem are reports of seronegative Lyme disease and recurrent or progressive symptoms of Lyme disease despite repeated or prolonged courses of high-dose parenteral antibiotics (13).

Thus, when trying to determine whether an MS-like illness is a consequence of Bb infection, diagnostic uncertainty arises from both potentially false-positive and false-negative serologies. As summarized in the report of the Quality Standards Subcommittee of the AAN (14), Lyme

encephalomyelitis masquerading as MS should be considered in those patients with neurologic disease suggesting MS plus systemic manifestations suggesting Lyme disease. Serum testing positive for anti-Bb IgG by enzyme-linked immunosorbent assay (ELISA) should be confirmed with Western blot.

Evidence of systemic Bb infection, however, does not prove it as the cause of the MS-like illness. *Borrelia burgdorferi* infection and MS may be coincident and not causally linked. Also, there is evidence that Bb infection may be capable of eliciting both humoral (15,16) and cell-mediated (17) autoimmune responses. It is likely that in only a very few patients is otherwise clinically typical MS due to CNS Bb infection. Intrathecal production of anti-Bb antibodies (elevated CSF Lyme antibody index) remains the most useful test to confirm active CNS Bb infection. Other CSF analyses show promise, including complexed anti-Bb antibodies, free Bb antigen, and Bb nucleic acid by polymerase chain reaction (PCR) (9,13,18), but the utility of these tests remains to be validated. The diagnosis of Lyme disease as the cause of an MS-like neurologic picture should be reserved for those patients who have unequivocal evidence of Bb infection in the nervous system, either by the demonstration of intrathecal anti-Bb antibody production or of the Bb organism by antigen or nucleic acid assays. In those patients, high-dose parenteral antibiotic therapy for Lyme disease is appropriate. Prolonged or repeated courses should be reserved for those patients who have evidence of ongoing or recurrent infection.

Syphilis

Syphilis continues to be an important consideration in the differential diagnosis of an MS-like illness. Increasingly, syphilis is exhibiting atypical presentations as a result of partial treatment or underlying immunocompromise, such as autoimmune deficiency syndrome (AIDS). Syphilis has been reported to cause acute monocular loss of vision with seroconversion during secondary syphilis with vasculitis (19). Meningovascular syphilis may produce an angiopathy with multifocal clinical and radiographic manifestations. Through a variety of pathogenic mechanisms, tertiary syphilis may produce a large number of progressive, multifocal manifestations, including cognitive impairment, chronic optic neuropathy, long tract motor signs, sensory loss, ataxia, and progressive myelopathy. The clinician may be misled by the presence of prominent CSF oligoclonal bands representing antibodies reactive with treponemal antigens (20). The diagnosis of neurosyphilis can be confirmed in most cases by the demonstration of a positive CSF VDRL.

Progressive Multifocal Leukoencephalopathy

Progressive multifocal leukoencephalopathy (PML) is an opportunistic viral infection of the brain caused by JC virus (JCV) that occurs virtually exclusively in patients with impaired cellular immunity due to immunosuppressive therapy, lymphoid neoplasms, or AIDS. Neurologic manifestations progress subacutely and include visual field defects or cortical blindness, motor abnormalities, cognitive impairment, altered personality, ataxia, or dysarthria. Magnetic resonance imaging findings demonstrate a characteristic picture (21) with white matter lesions that are high intensity on long TR images and low intensity on T1-weighted images. There is no enhancement following gadolinium administration. Single, multiple, or diffuse abnormal signal intensities may be seen in the periventricular white matter, corpus callosum, gray–white junction, and gray matter regions. Some but not all reports describe a parietal-occipital predominance. The CSF usually is normal. In rare cases there has been a mild pleocytosis or increased protein. At present, definitive diagnosis requires brain biopsy, including pathologic examination demonstrating the characteristic findings of PML, electron microscopy to demonstrate papova-like viral particles, in situ hybridization to demonstrate JCV nucleic acid, and immunohistochemistry to demonstrate JCV antigens (22). The detection of JCV nucleic acid in brain specimens, CSF, or peripheral blood lymphocytes by PCR (23–26) has the advantage of simplicity, greatly increased sensitivity, and the requirement for very small samples.

Human Immunodeficiency Virus (HIV)

The myriad neurologic manifestations of AIDS, including subacute vacuolar myelopathy, rarely are difficult to distinguish from MS. A neurologic disorder clinically and pathologically indistinguishable from MS may be the presenting manifestation of HIV-1 infection and may develop before immunocompromise (27–29). The course may follow a typical relapsing pattern (27,28) or may be fulminant with abrupt onset (29). Although the chance occurrence of both MS and HIV infection cannot be ruled out, in several reported cases the development of the MS-like illness occurred at the time of seroconversion.

Human T-Cell Lymphotrophic Virus-1 (HTLV-1)

The characteristic neurologic manifestation of HTLV-1 infection is a progressive thoracic myelopathy with predominantly upper motor neuron manifestations in the legs, mild sensory disturbance, and bowel and bladder dysfunction—termed *HTLV-1–associated myelopathy* (HAM). The other characteristic neurologic manifestations include an inflammatory myopathy that resembles polymyositis and axonal sensorimotor polyneuropathy (30,31). These manifestations often are steroid-responsive.

In HAM, MRI typically demonstrates atrophy of the thoracic spinal cord with or without abnormal increased signal and faint gadolinium enhancement (32,33). Cranial MRI is normal or more often shows scattered punctate foci of increased signal in the peripheral white matter (32–34). More extensive patchy and ovoid lesions in cerebral white matter have been described (31,32,34). Clinical expression of cerebral lesions on MRI is rare. However, we have seen a patient with prominent cognitive impairment out of proportion to myelopathy in the setting of HTLV-1 infection. Cerebrospinal fluid often shows increased protein and mild mononuclear cell pleocytosis. Oligoclonal bands and other indicators of intrathecal immunoglobulin synthesis may be prominent (32,33,35,36). The CSF immunoglobulins react with antigens of HTLV-1 virion.

Risk factors include those for AIDS, blood transfusion, therapeutic immunosuppression, and origin from the Caribbean or Japan, but in some cases the source of infection is unclear. An HTLV-1 titer should be included in the laboratory workup of progressive myelopathy, especially when primary progressive MS is a consideration.

INFLAMMATORY CONDITIONS

Systemic Lupus Erythematosus

The neurologic manifestations of systemic lupus erythematosus (SLE) are protean, with the most common being neuropsychiatric syndromes, seizures, aseptic meningitis, vascular events, movement disorders, headache, and cranial and peripheral neuropathy. Systemic lupus erythematosus is well recognized as a potential cause of transverse myelitis (37). Optic nerve involvement in SLE may take the form of acute optic neuritis, ischemic optic neuropathy, or chronic gradually progressive visual loss (38). Rarely, SLE also may produce relapsing, multifocal neurologic manifestations consistent with those of MS (39).

Cranial MRI in SLE often demonstrates atrophy and white matter lesions, although these more often are subcortical. They are relatively nonspecific, often more consistent with small-vessel ischemia than inflammatory foci. Periventricular lesions typical of MS are much less common (40,41). Also, involvement of the cortex and deep gray structures distinguishes the MRI findings of SLE from MS. Cerebrospinal fluid examination often is not helpful because the most common features in SLE, modest increase in protein and pleocytosis, are also found with MS. Furthermore, in one series, a high proportion (42 percent) of patients with SLE and CNS manifestations had CSF oligoclonal bands usually associated with increased IgG index (42). In our experience, the frequency of intrathecal antibody synthesis is not common in SLE but does occur occasionally.

Ultimately, the diagnosis of SLE requires positive serology and clinical features of systemic involvement.

The antinuclear antibody (ANA) must be interpreted with caution in MS. Dore-Duffy and coworkers reported low titer ANAs in 81 percent of patients with MS (43). In another series, the ANA was positive in 27 percent of cases of otherwise typical relapsing MS and 30 percent of progressive MS (44). These ANAs were believed to be false-positives because of their low titer and lack of other manifestations suggesting connective tissue disease. They probably reflect systemic immune dysregulation in MS. A very high ANA titer and the presence of other autoantibodies are more indicative of SLE.

Because of overlapping clinical, laboratory, and imaging features, it is difficult to confirm the diagnosis of MS in the setting of known SLE. A more common diagnostic issue is the finding of a modestly positive ANA in a patient with otherwise typical MS, possibly with vague rheumatic complaints but no other serologic abnormalities. In this setting, the separate diagnosis of SLE probably is unwarranted. These patients, however, should be monitored for the development of systemic manifestations of SLE.

Sjögren's Syndrome

Sjögren's syndrome (SS) is characterized by xerostomia, keratoconjunctivitis, and rheumatic symptoms. The most frequent neurologic complications of SS are peripheral neuropathy (axonal sensorimotor polyneuropathy, mononeuritis multiplex, or sensory ganglionopathy), cerebral vasculitis, aseptic meningitis, and myopathy. Acute transverse myelitis (45) and acute optic neuropathy (46) have been reported. Central nervous system involvement with clinical, CSF, and MRI features suggesting those of MS may occur in SS. In one series, approximately 20 percent of patients with SS had relapsing manifestations that reflected multifocal involvement of the cerebrum and spinal cord, suggesting MS (47). Cerebrospinal fluid examination demonstrated mild pleocytosis with intrathecal antibody synthesis manifested as increased IgG index and oligoclonal bands. Magnetic resonance imaging demonstrated multiple foci of increased signal in the cerebral white matter (48). The rate of overlap between MS and SS has been much lower in other series (49–51). Sjögren's syndrome is distinguished from MS by additional clinical features (sicca syndrome and rheumatic manifestations), serology (abnormal ANA, SS-A, SS-B), and the demonstration of inflammatory foci on minor salivary gland biopsy.

Vasculitis

Systemic vasculitides such as polyarteritis nodosa or Wegener's granulomatosis are rarely difficult to distinguish from MS. A more difficult diagnostic distinction is between MS and isolated angiitis of the CNS (IANS). IANS often produces relapsing or progressive clinical features, including focal or multifocal cerebral manifestations, brainstem manifestations, or cognitive impairment suggestive of those of MS (52,53). Relapsing or progressive myelopathy as the sole or predominant feature of IANS has been reported (54–56). Headache and meningeal signs are common but not always present. Strokelike episodes are uncommon.

When predominantly small vessels are involved in IANS, cranial MRI findings reflect small-vessel ischemia with patchy foci of increased signal in periventricular, deep, and subcortical white matter (57,58) and involvement of gray matter structures out of proportion to white matter. When larger vessels are involved, infarcts point to cerebral vasculitis. Prominent vascular or meningeal enhancement also points to IANS. Cerebrospinal fluid may be normal but more characteristically shows increased protein and prominent pleocytosis (52,53). Increased gamma globulin and oligoclonal bands rarely have been reported.

Confirmation of the diagnosis of IANS often is difficult and requires a high index of suspicion. Blood study abnormalities that are usually present with a systemic inflammatory reaction are normal. Cerebral angiography showing characteristic multifocal segmental narrowing of medium-sized arteries strongly suggests the diagnosis in the appropriate clinical setting, but angiography is relatively insensitive as a screening test, as vessels below the resolution of angiography may be involved (52,59). In most cases, the definitive diagnosis requires parenchymal and/or meningeal biopsy (52,53).

Pathologically, IANS comprises a spectrum from severe disease with marked vascular involvement by a granulomatous inflammatory reaction and vascular compromise to milder inflammatory reaction with neurologic symptoms caused by vasospasm (52,53,60). The more severe cases require aggressive immunosuppression with cyclophosphamide, whereas the benign cases can be treated with calcium channel blockers with or without less aggressive immunotherapy with oral corticosteroids. Thus, the distinction from MS is important.

Sarcoidosis

Sarcoidosis is a chronic, relapsing inflammatory disorder characterized by noncaseating granulomata in multiple organs, particularly the lungs. Neurologic involvement is common and may be the presenting manifestation or may occur out of proportion to systemic involvement. Most of the neurologic manifestations of sarcoidosis, such as cranial neuropathies, aseptic meningitis, meningovascular involvement, hypothalamic dysfunction, intracranial mass lesions, or mononeuropathy multiplex, do not

suggest MS. However, inflammatory optic neuropathy, abnormalities of eye movements, myelopathy, and multifocal cerebral or brainstem involvement may resemble MS clinically.

Magnetic resonance imaging findings (61) that point to sarcoidosis include prominent meningeal enhancement, hypothalamic involvement, hydrocephalus, and enhancing mass lesions. Sarcoidosis may produce multifocal white matter lesions that resemble those of MS. They may appear in the periventricular white matter. In a case of sarcoidosis involving the cervical spinal cord (62), MRI demonstrated a focal area of increased signal within the spinal cord with gadolinium enhancement and focal swelling. Cerebrospinal fluid findings of marked increase in protein, marked pleocytosis, and hypoglycorrhachia distinguish sarcoidosis from MS. However, the CSF picture in sarcoidosis may overlap that of MS, with modest increased protein, moderate pleocytosis, and evidence of intrathecal antibody synthesis (63).

For patients with manifestations that strongly suggest MS and in whom the level of suspicion of sarcoidosis is low or moderate, sedimentation rate, serum angiotensin-converting enzyme (ACE), and possibly a chest radiograph are all that is necessary to screen for sarcoidosis. Of note, increased serum ACE is not specific for sarcoidosis and may be seen in any chronic inflammatory condition. Modest elevation of serum ACE was seen in 23 percent of patients with otherwise typical MS and no evidence of sarcoidosis on further testing or follow-up (64). When the level of suspicion for sarcoidosis is high, further testing is required. Pulmonary function evaluation with diffusion capacity, gallium scan, chest CT to detect hilar adenopathy, and ophthalmologic evaluation looking for retinal/uveal/conjunctival involvement among others may be helpful. Ultimately, the diagnosis of sarcoidosis requires pathologic confirmation by biopsy of an involved tissue.

Behçets Disease

Behçets disease is a chronic inflammatory disorder characterized by oral and genital ulceration, skin lesions, aseptic meningitis, and uveitis. The most common neurologic manifestation is a focal meningoencephalitis involving the brainstem. Other neurologic manifestations include cerebrovascular syndromes, seizures, acute encephalopathy, and cranial neuropathies. Optic neuritis, myelopathy, long tract motor signs, and ataxia following a relapsing or progressive course may suggest MS.

Magnetic resonance imaging in Behçets disease (40,65) demonstrates multiple patchy foci of increased signal predominantly in the brainstem but also in cerebral white matter, deep gray matter structures, cerebellum, optic nerves, and spinal cord. Acute lesions enhance with gadolinium. Lack of predilection for the periventricular white matter and the more prominent involvement of the brainstem and basal ganglia distinguishes the MRI picture of Behçets disease from that of MS. Cerebrospinal fluid typically shows lymphocytic pleocytosis and increased protein but also may have oligoclonal bands (66)

When neurologic manifestations develop in the setting of systemic constitutional symptoms, mucocutaneous involvement, and clinical and CSF manifestations of aseptic meningitis, distinguishing Behçets disease from MS is not difficult. However, the clinical picture may closely resemble that of MS when these additional features are not present (67). Making the appropriate diagnosis of Behçets disease is important so that aggressive immunosuppression, which improves the prognosis, may be instituted (67,68).

METABOLIC DISORDERS

Vitamin B12 Deficiency and Nitrous Oxide Intoxication

The most common cause of vitamin B12 (cobalamin) deficiency is pernicious anemia (an antibody-mediated autoimmune disorder of gastric parietal cells, which leads to deficiency of intrinsic factor and decreased ability to absorb vitamin B12 in the terminal ileum). Other causes of decreased ileal absorption include intrinsic factor deficiency from gastric resection, blind loop syndrome with bacterial overgrowth, and ileal resection. Reduced dietary intake from a strict vegetarian diet may produce B12 deficiency, but that would take many years. Finally, there are very rare deficiencies of vitamin B12 binding and carrier proteins. The manifestations of vitamin B12 deficiency usually develop gradually. However, vitamin B12 deficiency may present more acutely in settings in which there is preexisting marginal vitamin B12 stores and the demand for vitamin B12 increases, such as following iron repletion for iron-deficiency anemia or in pregnancy.

Nitrous oxide inactivates cobalamin by irreversibly oxidizing the cobalt core of methylcobalamin, preventing it from functioning as a required cofactor for methionine synthase. Repeated nitrous oxide exposure leads to myeloneuropathy with gradual onset (69). An acute vitamin B12 deficiency syndrome may occur when nitrous oxide is used as anesthetic in patients with preexisting subclinical vitamin B12 deficiency (70–74).

The classic clinical picture of vitamin B12 deficiency consists of a combination of cervical myelopathy (initially predominantly involving the posterior columns and later the lateral columns) and peripheral neuropathy, so-called myeloneuropathy. Other neurologic manifestations include optic neuropathy, cognitive impairment, and fatigue. Neurologic manifestations typically occur in association with a macrocytic anemia and megaloblastic changes in leukocytes. When the complete syndrome occurs, vitamin B12 deficiency should not be mistaken for typical MS. However, partial syndromes often occur and neurologic and hematologic manifestations may occur separately (75). The neurologic symptoms of pernicious anemia may respond modestly to corticosteroids, presumably because of decreased antibody levels (76). Abnormalities in cerebral white matter suggesting those of MS have been reported in a patient with vitamin B12 deficiency and reversible cognitive dysfunction (77). Thus, in rare cases MS may be difficult to distinguish from vitamin B12 deficiency.

Direct measurement of serum B12 may be unreliable. The complete blood count (CBC) may be normal in vitamin B12 deficiency, but the demonstration of a macrocytic anemia or hypersegmented polymorphonuclear leukocytes is useful. Increased serum methylmalonic acid and homocysteine levels are useful metabolic indicators of cobalamin deficiency (75,78).

It is important to identify the cause of the vitamin B12 deficiency and to begin vitamin B12 replacement therapy as early as possible. We typically administer vitamin B12 at a dose of 1 mg intramuscularly weekly for four weeks, then monthly. Replenishment of tissue stores occurs rapidly, which prevents further damage and allows the initiation of central and peripheral axonal regeneration. To the extent that sensory loss results from degeneration of the peripheral projections of dorsal root ganglia neurons (i.e., peripheral neuropathy), return of sensation will parallel the extent of axonal regeneration. However, to the extent that sensory loss results from the degeneration of the CNS projections in the dorsal columns, restoration of sensory function will not occur until synapses of the first-order ascending sensory axons onto second-order neurons in nuclei gracilis and cuneatus are reestablished in the medulla.

Lysosomal Disorders

Metachromatic leukodystrophy (MLD) is an autosomal recessive disorder resulting from a defect in the lysosomal enzyme arylsulfatase A (79). Metachromatic leukodystrophy may begin at any age, including late-onset or adult forms. Typical manifestations of adult-onset MLD include prominent cognitive decline, optic atrophy, nystagmus, spastic weakness, gait disturbance, and urinary dysfunction (80–83). Key features that differentiate MLD from MS include peripheral neuropathy and symmetric diffuse abnormality of cerebral white matter on MRI. The definitive diagnosis of MLD is by demonstration of deficient arylsulfatase A activity in leukocytes or cultured fibroblasts (79).

Fabry disease is an X-linked recessive disorder caused by defective activity of the lysosomal enzyme alpha-galactosidase (79). Females usually are asymptomatic. The onset of symptoms in males usually occurs before adolescence, but onset in the second or third decade has been reported. Central nervous system manifestations result from multifocal small vessel occlusion, leading to ischemia or recurrent strokes, which in a young adult conceivably could be mistaken for MS. The presence of angiokeratomas and corneal dystrophy should suggest Fabry disease. The definitive diagnosis is made by the demonstration of deficient leukocyte alpha-galactosidase activity (79).

Krabbe disease is an autosomal recessive disorder resulting from deficient activity of galactocerebrosidase (79). Atypical and late-onset forms have been reported. Typical manifestations in adults include cognitive dysfunction, weakness, tremor, ataxia, dysarthria, and nystagmus (84–87). Peripheral nerve manifestations usually are present but not prominent. The definitive diagnosis is based on determination of leukocyte or fibroblast galactocerebrosidase activity (79).

Adrenoleukodystrophy

X-linked adrenoleukodystrophy (ALD) is a peroxisomal disorder characterized by abnormalities of CNS myelin, adrenal dysfunction, and accumulation of very long chain fatty acids in the blood and tissues (79). Adrenomyeloneuropathy is the most common form of ALD in adults and presents as a slowly progressing myelopathy in males beginning in the third decade of life and associated with depression, impotence, and sometimes adrenal insufficiency (88). A 43-year-old man with adult-onset ALD has been reported with progressive intellectual decline and normal adrenal function (89). Serial MRI demonstrated evidence of cerebral demyelination starting in the frontal white matter and spreading to the occipital white matter over several months. Symptoms and MRI findings resolved without therapy. Approximately 10 percent to 15 percent of female heterozygotes have symptoms similar to those described for males and frequently are misdiagnosed as MS (90). The diagnosis of ALD is by demonstration of increased serum very long chain fatty acid level (79).

Mitochondrial Disorders

The mitochondrial cytopathies are a clinically heterogeneous group of multisystem disorders caused by a variety of genetic defects affecting mitochondrial metabolism (91). These disorders demonstrate a maternal inheritance pattern and for the most part bear little resemblance to MS. However, because the mitochondrial disorders frequently cause incomplete syndromes with some manifestations that are relatively nonspecific, the inheritance pattern may be obscured, and the potential diagnosis of a mitochon-

drial disorder may be overlooked. The diagnostic confusion with MS may be increased by the presence of similar abnormalities in the cerebral white matter on MRI (92–94). Recognition of the characteristic combination of neurologic and systemic features atypical for MS usually serves to make the distinction. Clues pointing to the presence of a mitochondrial disorder include combined central and peripheral neurologic manifestations (neuropathy or myopathy), recurrent encephalopathy, vascular-type headaches, strokelike episodes with good recovery, sensorineural hearing loss, myoclonus, episodic nausea and vomiting, pigmentary retinopathy in combination with optic atrophy, basal ganglia calcification, cardiomyopathy or cardiac conduction abnormalities, diabetes, and increased serum lactate levels.

Leber's hereditary optic neuropathy (LHON) is the mitochondrial disorder that is most often mistaken clinically for MS. It is characterized by acute or subacute optic neuropathy in males with onset typically between the ages of 10 and 30 years. In affected males, involvement outside the optic nerves has been reported, including ataxia and spastic weakness (93,95–97). Neurologic symptoms and cranial MRI findings in female carriers of LHON, which may lead to the misdiagnosis as MS, also have been reported (93,95–97).

Clinically Defined Genetic Disorders

Hereditary degenerative disorders such as Friedreich ataxia, other hereditary ataxias, olivopontocerebellar atrophies, and hereditary spastic paraparesis sometimes may be mistaken for MS, particularly the primary progressive form. The prominent family history (particularly for the autosomal dominant disorders), lack of MRI findings, and normal CSF exam distinguish them from MS.

CENTRAL NERVOUS SYSTEM LYMPHOMA

Rarely, MS may present as a cerebral mass lesion with clinical features and findings on imaging studies suggesting a neoplasm. Biopsy then leads to the surprising finding of inflammatory demyelination (98–100). The converse situation, namely, the mistaken diagnosis of a neoplastic process as MS, also rarely occurs. The most common neoplasm to be mistaken for MS is CNS lymphoma (101,102). The prevalence of this disorder is increasing, largely in the setting of immunocompromise from AIDS and therapeutic immunosuppression, such as following organ transplantation.

Central nervous system lymphoma usually is unifocal but often may be multicentric. Cerebrospinal fluid examination may demonstrate cytologically abnormal lymphocytes but usually is normal or demonstrates only nonspecific abnormalities of protein or pleocytosis. Magnetic resonance imaging findings may look similar to those of MS, with T2-hyperintense lesions in the cerebral white matter extending into the corpus callosum and variable Gd-enhancement. Both the clinical and the radiographic manifestations of CNS lymphoma may respond to corticosteroid therapy, leading to further confusion. The radiographic distinction may be made by the demonstration of involvement of gray matter structures out of proportion to white matter; lesion behavior over time is more helpful. Enhancement of MS lesions rarely persists for longer than four to six weeks. Thus, persistent Gd-enhancement (particularly if there is a prominent component of enhancement along blood vessels) and continued enlargement of lesions strongly suggest a lymphocytic neoplasm. Ultimately, biopsy is necessary to make the correct diagnosis.

SPINE DISEASE

Spinal Vascular Malformations

The spinal vascular malformations most often mistaken for MS are dural arteriovenous fistulas and true malformations. Neurologic manifestations are thought to be due to venous hypertension with secondary edema and ischemia. Histologic findings on biopsy support this mechanism (103). The clinical features (103–108) are those of a thoracic myelopathy, with an acute, relapsing, or progressive course. Local pain is an inconsistent feature. Other than features of a myelopathy, examination usually is normal. A spinal bruit rarely is present but if present is pathognomonic.

Cerebrospinal fluid examination findings usually are nonspecific and consistent with although not diagnostic of MS (104–107). There may be no cells or a mild pleocytosis. Protein may be normal, mildly elevated, or rarely markedly increased. There are no findings of intrathecal antibody production. Magnetic resonance imaging usually demonstrates patchy increased signal within the spinal cord on long TR images (103,108). The spinal cord may be focally enlarged. There may be no Gd-enhancement or mild heterogeneous enhancement. One rarely can detect flow voids of enlarged draining veins. Myelography looking for vermiform filling defects from dilated draining veins remains a useful screening test when a vascular malformation is suspected. Both supine and prone myelographic examinations need to be performed so as not to miss dorsal vascular malformations. The definitive test for diagnosis and localization is selective spinal angiography. Because the clinical features and MRI findings are poor indicators of the level of the malformation, all pairs of radicular arteries need to injected until the feeder(s) of the malformation is (are) identified.

The clinical features and MRI findings of dural spinal vascular malformation often raise the question of an inflammatory demyelinating process in the spinal cord. In older individuals, nonspecific white matter lesions on cranial MRI may suggest those of MS. Myelopathic symptoms may demonstrate a transient response to corticosteroids as a result of reduced edema. Thus, it is easy to misdiagnose these malformations as MS. A high index of suspicion is necessary, as appropriate therapy by angiographic embolization or surgical repair may be curative in some cases.

Degenerative Spine Disease

Severe cervical spondylosis may mimic MS by producing a polyradiculopathy with motor and sensory symptoms in the arms and myelopathic manifestations in the legs. A relapsing or progressive course, nonspecific changes in the periventricular white matter on MRI, and increased protein on CSF examination may further confuse the diagnostic picture. This situation illustrates the importance of investigating the principle site of neurologic manifestations.

CONCLUSIONS

There is increasing emphasis on early diagnosis of MS to allow early initiation of disease-modifying treatment. This trend potentially increases the risk of misdiagnosis. The key to the accurate diagnosis of MS is vigilance for atypical features, which suggest the possibility of an alternative diagnosis. The appropriate diagnostic workup is determined by the clinical picture.

References

1. Schumacher GA, Beebe GW, Kibler RF, et al. Problems of experimental trials of therapy in multiple sclerosis: Report by the panel on the evaluation of experimental trials of therapy in multiple sclerosis. *Ann NY Acad Sci* 1965; 122:552–568.
2. Gawne-Cain ML, O'Riordan JI, Thompson AJ, Moseley IF, Miller DH. Multiple sclerosis lesion detection in the brain: A comparison of fast fluid-attenuated inversion recovery and conventional T2-weighted dual spin echo. *Neurology* 1997; 49:364–370.
3. Harris JO, Frank JA, Patronas N, McFarlin DE, McFarland HF. Serial gadolinium-enhanced magnetic resonance imaging scans in patients with early, relapsing-remitting multiple sclerosis: Implications for clinical trials and natural history. *Ann Neurol* 1991; 29:548–555.
4. Pachner AR. *Borrelia burgdorferi* in the nervous system: The new great imitator. *Ann NY Acad Sci* 1988; 539:56–64.
5. Kohler J, Kern U, Kasper J, Rhese-Kupper B, Thoden U. Chronic central nervous system involvement in Lyme borreliosis. *Neurology* 1988; 38:863–867.

6. Halperin JJ, Luft BJ, Anand AK, et al. Lyme neuroborreliosis: Central nervous system manifestations. *Neurology* 1989; 39:753–759.

7. Pachner AR, Duray P, Steere AC. Central nervous system manifestations of Lyme disease. *Arch Neurol* 1989; 46:790–795.

8. Logigian EL, Kaplan RF, Steere AC. Chronic neurologic manifestations of Lyme disease. *N Engl J Med* 1990; 323:1438–1444.

9. Halperin JJ, Volkman DJ, Wu P. Central nervous system abnormalities in Lyme neuroborreliosis. *Neurology* 1991; 41:1571–1582.

10. Coyle PK. *Borrelia burgdorferi* antibodies in multiple sclerosis patients. *Neurology* 1989; 39:760–761.

11. Steere AC, Taylor E, Wilson ML, Levine JF, Spielman A. Longitudinal assessment of the clinical and epidemiologic features of Lyme disease in a defined population. *J Infect Dis* 1986; 154:295–300.

12. Coyle PK, Krupp LB, Doscher C. Significance of reactive Lyme serology in multiple sclerosis. *Ann Neurol* 1993; 34:745–747.

13. Lawrence C, Lipton RB, Lowy FD, Coyle PK. Seronegative chronic relpasing neuroborreliosis. *Eur Neurol* 1995; 35:113–117.

14. Halperin JJ, Logigian EL, Finkel MF, Pearl RA. Practice parameters for the diagnosis of patients with nervous system Lyme borreliosis (Lyme disease). *Neurology* 1996; 46:619–627.

15. Sigal LH, Tatum AH. Lyme disease patients' serum contains IgM antibodies to *Borrelia burgdorferi* that cross-react with neuronal antigens. *Neurology* 1988; 38:1439–1442.

16. Aberer E, Brunner C, Suchanek G, et al. Molecular mimicry and Lyme borreliosis: A shared antigenic determinant between *Borrelia burgdorferi* and human tissue. *Ann Neurol* 1989; 26:732–737.

17. Baig S, Olsson T, Hojeberg B, Link H. Cells secreting antibodies to myelin basic protein in cerebrospinal fluid of patients with Lyme neuroborreliosis. *Neurology* 1991; 41:581–587.

18. Coyle PK, Schutzer SE, Deng Z, et al. Detection of *Borrelia burgdorferi*–specific antigen in antibody-negative cerebrospinal fluid in neurologic Lyme disease. *Neurology* 1995; 45:2010–2015.

19. Smith JL. Acute blindness in early syphilis. *Arch Ophthalmol* 1973; 90:256–258.

20. Vartdal F, Vandvik B, Michaelsen TE, Loe K, Norrby E. Neurosyphilis: Intrathecal synthesis of oligoclonal antibodies to *Treponema pallidum*. *Ann Neurol* 1982; 11:35–40.

21. Mark AS, Atlas SW. Progressive multifocal leukoencephalopathy in patients with AIDS: Appearance on MR images. *Radiology* 1989; 173:517–520.

22. Aksamit AJ, Sever JL, Major EO. Progressive multifocal leukoencephalopathy: JC virus detection by in situ hybridization compared with immunohistochemistry. *Neurology* 1986; 36:499–504.

23. Henson J, Rosenblum M, Armstrong D, Furneaux H. Amplification of JC virus DNA from brain and cerebrospinal fluid of patients with progressive multifocal leukoencephalopathy. *Neurology* 1991; 41:1967–1971.

24. Major EO, Amemiya K, Tornatore CS, Houff SA, Berger JR. Pathogenesis and molecular biology of progressive multifocal leukoencephalopathy, the JC virus-induced demyelinating disease of human brain. *Clin Microbiol Rev* 1992; 5:49–73.

25. Telenti A, Marshall WF, Aksamit AJ, Smilack JD, Smith TF. Detection of JC virus by polymerase chain reaction in cerebrospinal fluid from two patients with progressive multifocal leukoencephalopathy. *Eur J Clin Microbiol Infect Dis* 1992; 11:253–254.

26. White FA, Ishaq M, Stoner GL, Frisque RJ. JC virus DNA is present in many human brain samples from patients without progressive multifocal leukoencephalopathy. *J Virol* 1992; 66:5726–5734.

27. Berger J, Sheremata W, Resnick L, et al. Multiple sclerosis-like illness occurring with human immunodeficiency virus infection. *Neurology* 1989; 39:324–329.

28. Berger JR, Tornatore C, Major EO, et al. Relapsing and remitting human immunodeficiency virus-associated leukoencephalomyelopathy. *Ann Neurol* 1992; 31:34–38.

29. Gray F, Chimelli L, Mohr M, et al. Fulminating multiple sclerosis-like leukoencephalopathy revealing human immunodeficiency virus infection. *Neurology* 1991; 41:105–109.

30. Wiley CA, Nerenberg M, Cros D, Soto-Aguilar MC. HTLV-1 polymyositis in a patient also infected with the human immunodeficiency virus. *N Engl J Med* 1989; 320:992–995.

31. Douen A, Pringle CE, Guberman A. Human T-cell lymphotropic virus type 1 myositis, peripheral neuropathy, and cerebral white matter lesions in the absence of spastic paraparesis. *Arch Neurol* 1997; 54:896–900.

32. Bhagavati S, Ehrlich G, Kula RW, et al. Detection of human T-cell lymphoma/leukemia virus type 1 DNA and antigen in spinal fluid and blood of patients with chronic progressive myelopathy. *N Engl J Med* 1988; 318:1141–1147.

33. Sheramata WA, Berger JR, Harrington WJ, et al. Human T lymphotrophic virus type 1–associated myelopathy. A report of 10 patients born in the United States. *Arch Neurol* 1992; 49:1113–1118.

34. Kuroda Y, Matsui M, Yukitake M, et al. Assessment of MRI criteria for MS in Japanese MS and HAM/TSP. *Neurology* 1995; 45:30–33.

35. Grimaldi LME, Roos RP, Devare SG, et al. HTLV-1-associated myelopathy: Oligoclonal immunoglobyulin G bands contain anti-HTLV-1 p24 antibody. *Ann Neurol* 1988; 24:727–731.

36. Link H, Cruz M, Gessain A, et al. Chronic progressive myelopathy associated with HTLV-1: Oligoclonal banding and anti-HTLV-1 IgG antibodies in cerebrospinal fluid and serum. *Neurology* 1989; 39:1566–1572.

37. Andrianakos AA, Duffy J, Suzuki M, Sharp JT. Transverse myelopathy in systemic lupus erythematosus. Report of three cases and review of the literature. *Ann Intern Med* 1975; 83:616–624.

38. Jabs DA, Miller NR, Newman SA, Johnson MA, Stevens MB. Optic neuropathy in systemic lupus erythermatosus. *Arch Ophthalmol* 1986; 104:564–568.

39. Fulford KWM, Catterall RD, Delhanty JJ, Doniach D, Kremer M. A collagen disorder of the nervous system presenting as multiple sclerosis. *Brain* 1972; 95:373–386.

40. Miller DH, Ormerod IEC, Gibson A, et al. MR brain scanning in patients with vasculitis: differentiation from multiple sclerosis. *Neuroradiology* 1987; 29:226–231.

41. Miller DH, Buchanan N, Barker G, et al. Gadolinium-enhanced magnetic resonance imaging of the central nervous system in sytemic lupus erythematosus. *J Neurol* 1992; 239:460–464.

42. Winfield JB, Shaw M, Silverman LM, Eisenberg RA, Wilson HA. Intrathecal IgG synthesis and blood-brain bar-

rier impairment in patients with systemic lupus erythematosus and central nervous system dysfunction. *Am J Med* 1983; 74:837–844.

43. Dore-Duffy P, Donaldson JO, Rothman BL, Zurier RB. Antinuclear antibodies in multiple sclerosis. *Arch Neurol* 1982; 39:504–506.

44. Barned S, Goodman AD, Mattson DH. Frequency of anti-nuclear antibodies in multiple sclerosis. *Neurology* 1995; 45:384–385.

45. Konttinen YT, Kinnunen E, von Bonsdorff M, et al. Acute transverse myelopathy successfully treated with plasmapheresis and prednisone in a patient with primary Sjögren's syndrome. *Arthritis Rheum* 1987; 30:339–344.

46. Wise CM, Agudelo CA. Optic neuropathy as an initial manifestation of Sjögren's syndrome. *J Rheumatol* 1988; 15:799–802.

47. Alexander EL, Malinow K, Lejewski JE, et al. Primary Sjögren's syndrome with central nervous system disease mimicking multiple sclerosis. *Ann Intern Med* 1986; 104:323–330.

48. Alexander EL, Beall SS, Gordon B, et al. Magnetic resonance imaging of cerebral lesions in patients with the Sjögren syndrome. *Ann Intern Med* 1988; 108:815–823.

49. Miro J, Pena-Sagredo JL, Berciano J, et al. Prevalence of primary Sjögren's syndrome in patients with multiple sclerosis. *Ann Neurol* 1990; 27:582–584.

50. Noseworthy JH, Bass BH, Vandervoort MK, et al. The prevalance of primary Sjögren's syndrome in a multiple sclerosis population. *Ann Neurol* 1989; 25:95–98.

51. Sandberg-Wollheim M, Axell T, Hansen BU, et al. Primary Sjögren's syndrome in patients with multiple sclerosis. *Neurology* 1992; 42:845–847.

52. Moore PM. Diagnosis and management of isolated angiitis of the central nervous system. *Neurology* 1989; 39:167–173.

53. Calabrese LH, Furlan AJ, Gragg LA, Ropos TJ. Primary angiitis of the central nervous system: diagnositic criteria and clinical approach. *Cleve Clin J Med* 1992; 59:293–306.

54. Caccamo DV, Garcia JH, Ho KL. Isolated granulomatous aggiitis of the spincal cord. *Ann Neurol* 1992; 32:580–582.

55. Feasby TE, Ferguson GG, Kaufmann JCE. Isolated spinal cord arteritis. *Can J Neurol Sci* 1975; 2:143–146.

56. Rawlinson DG, Braun CW. Granulomatous angiitis of the nervous system first seen as relapsing myelopathy. *Arch Neurol* 1981; 38:129–131.

57. Ehsan T, Hasan S, Powers JM, Heiserman JE. Serial magnetic resonance imaging in isolated angiitis of the central nervous system. *Neurology* 1995; 45:1462–1465.

58. Greenan TJ, Grossman RI, Goldberg HI. Cerebral vasculitis: MR imaging and angiographic correlation. *Radiology* 1992; 182:65–72.

59. Vollmer TL, Guarnaccia J, Harrington W, Pacia SV, Petroff OA. Idiopathic granulomatous angiitis of the central nervous system. *Arch Neurol* 1993; 50:925–930.

60. Berger JR, Romano J, Menkin M, Norenberg M. Benign focal cerebral vasculitis. *Neurology* 1995; 45:1731–1734.

61. Miller DH, Kendall BE, Barter S, et al. Magnetic resonance imaging in central nervous system sarcoidosis. *Neurology* 1988; 38:378–383.

62. Sauter MK, Panitch HS, Kristt DA. Myelopathic neurosarcoidosis: Diagnostic value of enhanced MRI. *Neurology* 1991; 41:150–151.

63. Borucki SJ, Nguyen BV, Ladoulis CT, McKendall RR. Cerebrospinal fluid immunoglobulin abnormalities in neurosarcoidosis. *Arch Neurol* 1989; 46:270–273.

64. Constantinescu CS, Goodman DBP, Grossman RI, Mannon LJ, Cohen JA. Serum angiotensin-converting enzyme in multiple sclerosis. *Arch Neurol* 1997; 54:1012–1015.

65. Morrissey SP, Miller DH, Hermaszewski R, et al. Magnetic resonance imaging of the central nervous system in Behçet's disease. *Eur Neurol* 1993; 33:287–293.

66. Sharief MK, Hentges R, Thomas E. Significance of CSF immunoglobulins in monitoring neurologic disease activity in Behçet's disease. *Neurology* 1991; 41:1398–1410.

67. Devlin T, Gray L, Allen NB, et al. Neuro-Behçet's disease: Factors hampering proper diagnosis. *Neurology* 1995; 45:1754–1757.

68. Akman-Demir G, Baykan-Kurt B, Serdarglu P, Gurvit H, Yurdakul S, Yazici H, Bahar S, Aktin E. Seven-year follow-up of neurologic involvement in Behçet syndrome. *Arch Neurol* 1996; 53:691–694.

69. Layzer RB. Myeloneuropathy after prolonged exposure to nitrous oxide. *Lancet* 1978; 2:1227–1230.

70. Kinsella LJ, Green R. Anesthesia paresthetica: Nitrous oxide-induced cobalamin deficiency. *Neurology* 1995; 45:1608–1610.

71. Flippo TS, Holder WD. Neurologic degeneration associated with nitrous oxide anesthesia in patients with vitamin B12 deficiency. *Arch Surg* 1993; 128:1391–1395.

72. Schilling RF. Is nitrous oxide a dangerous anesthetic for vitamin B12-deficient subjects? *JAMA* 1986; 255:1605–1606.

73. Holloway KL, Alberico AM. Postoperative myeloneuropathy: a preventable complication in patients with B12 deficiency. *J Neurosurg* 1990; 72:732–736.

74. McMorrow AM, Adams RJ, Rubenstein MN. Combined system disease after nitrous oxide anesthesia: a case report. *Neurology* 1995; 45:1224–1225.

75. Lindenbaum J, Healton EB, Savage DG, et al. Neuropsychiatric disorders caused by cobalamin deficiency in the absence of anemia or macrocytosis. *N Engl J Med* 1988; 318:1720–1728.

76. Ransohoff RM, Jacobsen DW, Green R. Vitamin B12 deficiency and multiple sclerosis (letter). *Lancet* 1990; 335:1285–1286.

77. Chatterjee A, Yapundich R, Palmer CA, Marson DC, Mitchell GW. Leukoencephalopathy associated with cobalamin deficiency. *Neurology* 1996; 46:832–824.

78. Green R, Kinsella LJ. Current concepts in the diagnosis of cobalamin deficiency. *Neurology* 1995; 45:1435–1440.

79. Natowicz MR, Bejjani B. Genetic disorders that masquerade as multiple sclerosis. *Am J Med Genet* 1994; 49:149–169.

80. Hirose G, Bass NH. Metachromatic leukodystrophy in the adult. *Neurology* 1972; 22:312–320.

81. Hohenschutz C, Friedl W, Schlor KH, et al. Probable metachromatic leukodystrophy/pseudodeficiency compound heterozygote at the aryl-sulfatase A locus with neurological and psychiatric symptomatology. *Am J Med Genet* 1988; 31:169–175.

82. Klemm E, Conzelmann E. Adult-onset metachromatic leukodystrophy presenting without psychiatric symptoms. *J Neurol* 1989; 236:427–429.

83. Kolodny EH, Raghavan SS, Lott IT, Sergay SM. Low sulfatidase and demyelinating disease. *Neurology* 1981; 31:86.

84. Crome L, Hanefield F, Patrick D, Wilson J. Late-onset globoid cell leukodystrophy. *Brain* 1973; 96:841–848.

85. Kolodny EH, Raghavan S, Krivit W. Late-onset Krabbe disease (globoid cell leukodystrophy): Clinical and biochemical features of 15 cases. *Dev Neurosci* 1991; 13:232–239.

86. Verdru P, Lammens M, Dom R, Van Elsen A, Carton H. Globoid cell leukodystrophy: A family with both late-infantile and adult type. *Neurology* 1991; 41:1382–1384.

87. Thomas PK, Halpern JP, King RHM, Patrick D. Galactosylceramide lipidosis: Novel presentation as a slowly progressive spinocerebellar degeneration. *Ann Neurol* 1984; 16:618–620.

88. Zwesloot CP, Padberg GW, van Seters AP, Maaswinkel-Mooy PD, Onkenhout W. Adult adrenoleukodystrophy: The clinical spectrum in a large Dutch family. *J Neurol* 1992; 239:107–111.

89. Farrell DF, Hamilton SR, Knauss TA, Sanocki E, Deeb SS. X-linked adrenoleukodystrophy: Adult cerebral variant. *Neurology* 1993; 43:1518–1522.

90. Dooley JM, Wright BA. Adrenoleukodystrophy mimicking multiple sclerosis. *Can J Neurol Sci* 1985; 12:73–74.

91. DiMauro S, Moraes CT. Mitochondrial encephalomyopathies. *Arch Neurol* 1993; 50:1197–1208.

92. Barkovich AJ, Good WV, Koch TK, Berg BO. Mitochondrial disorders: Analysis of their clinical and imaging characteristics. *AJNR* 1993; 14:1119–1137.

93. Harding AE, Sweeney MG, Miller DH, et al. Occurrence of a multiple sclerosis-like illness in women who have a Leber's hereditary optic neuropathy mitochondrial DNA mutation. *Brain* 1992; 115:979–989.

94. Huang C-C, Wai Y-Y, Chu N-S, et al. Mitochondrial encephalomyopathies: CT and MRI findings and correlations with clinical features. *Eur Neurol* 1995; 35:199–205.

95. de Weerdt CJ, West LN. Neurological studies in families with Leber's optic atrophy. *Acta Neurol Scand* 1971; 47:541-554.

96. Franks WA, Sanders MD. Leber's hereditary optic neuropathy in women. *Eye* 1990; 4:482–485.

97. Lees F, MacDonald A-ME, Turner JWA. Leber's disease with symptoms resembling disseminated sclerosis. *J Neurol Neurosurg Psychiatry* 1964; 27:415–421.

98. Hunter SB, Ballinger WE, Rubin JJ. Multiple sclerosis mimicking primary brain tumor. *Arch Pathol Lab Med* 1987; 111:464–468.

99. Kalyan-Raman UP, Garwacki DJ, Elwood PW. Demyelinating disease of corpus callosum presenting as glioma on magnetic resonance scan: A case documented with pathological findings. *Neurosurgery* 1987; 21:247–250.

100. Kepes JJ. Large focal tumor-like demyelinating lesions of the brain: Intermediate entity between multiple sclerosis and acute disseminated encephalomyelitis? A study of 31 patients. *Ann Neurol* 1993; 33:18–27.

101. O'Neill BP, Illig JJ. Primary central nervous system lymphoma. *Mayo Clin Proc* 1989; 64:1005–1020.

102. Patchell RA. Primary central nervous system lymphoma in the transplant patient. *Neurol Clin North Am* 1988; 6:297–303.

103. Hurst RW, Kenyon LC, Lavi E, Raps EC, Marcotte P. Spinal dural arteriovenous fistula: The pathology of venous hypertensive myelopathy. *Neurology* 1995; 45:1309–1313.

104. Tobin WD, Layton DD. The diagnosis and natural history of spinal cord ateriovenous malformations. *Mayo Clin Proc* 1976; 51:637–646.

105. Aminoff MJ, Logue V. The prognosis of patients with spinal vascular malformations. *Brain* 1974; 97:211–218.

106. Aminoff MJ, Logue V. Clinical features of spinal vascular malformations. *Brain* 1974; 97:197–210.

107. Dhopesh VP, Weinstein JD. Spinal aterio-venous malformations simulating multiple sclerosis: Importance of early diagnosis. *Dis Nerv System* 1977; 38:848–851.

108. Deen HG, Nelson KD, Gonzales GR. Spinal dural arteriovenous fistula causing progressive myelopathy: Clinical and imaging considerations. *Mayo Clin Proc* 1994; 69:83–84.

IV

TREATMENT

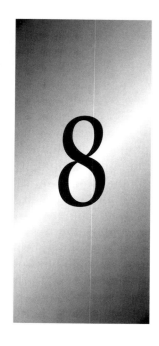

8 Immunology and Etiologic Concepts

Roland Martin, M.D., and Suhayl Dhib-Jalbut, M.D.

Although the etiology of multiple sclerosis (MS) is still not known, it currently is widely believed that a T cell–mediated autoimmune process is responsible for crucial aspects of its pathogenesis. This is supported by several lines of evidence, including a disease-associated genetic background, the pathohistologic findings, the response to immunomodulatory treatment, and similarities with an animal model, experimental allergic encephalomyelitis (EAE). Recently progress has been made in understanding of basic aspects of T cell recognition of myelin antigens, new findings in white matter pathology, advances in diagnostic magnetic resonance imaging (MRI) studies, and, for the first time, the development of effective immunotherapies. In this chapter we outline our current understanding of the immunology of MS and how this knowledge may be employed to design new treatment approaches.

Demyelination of central axons is considered the hallmark of MS and is characterized by damage to the myelin sheath and/or oligodendrocytes. Conduction block or conduction impairment results from the damage of the multilamellar myelin sheath, which is composed of myelin proteins and lipids, and, depending on the severity of the inflammatory process or as yet poorly understood mechanisms, axonal damage also may result (1–3). Multiple sclerosis may affect almost any part of

the central nervous system (CNS) white matter and cause a broad spectrum of clinical signs and symptoms. The course of MS most often starts as relapsing-remitting (RR), then changes to secondary progressive (SP) with incomplete recovery or steady progression. Some patients have only a primary progressive (PP) disease, which is characterized by an insidious onset, steady worsening, and an overall poorer prognosis. Because of the lack of specific laboratory tests, the diagnosis of MS is still largely clinical. A diagnosis of clinically definite MS requires a demyelinating disorder of the CNS, often occurring at young age and affecting at least two distinct sites in the CNS, with at least two temporally separate exacerbations and without an alternative explanation. Cerebrospinal fluid (CSF) analysis, MRI of the brain and spinal cord, and electrophysiologic findings may support the diagnosis. Its cause remains an enigma.

Most evidence points to an immunopathologic disease mechanism that is shaped both by an immunogenetic background and by exogenous factors. The pathologic findings of perivascular infiltrates of lymphocytes and monocytes and the local activation of resident microglia and astrocytes support an underlying immunologic mechanism, but the paucity of inflammation at later stages and the loss of axons and oligodendrocytes indicate that other factors may contribute to the chronic aspects of the disease. The course of MS and its clinical phenotypes are highly variable, and the lack of specific diagnostic or immunologic markers have made the investigation of the processes in humans difficult. Therefore, the immunologic aspects of MS have been studied extensively in a well-defined animal model, EAE, in which many questions related to the etiology, pathogenesis, and treatment of MS could be experimentally considered. Although these studies may improve understanding of many facets of the potential immunologic mechanism of MS, one must keep in mind that EAE is an "artificial" model elicited in inbred animal strains. Any observation in this model should therefore only be extrapolated to the human disease with caution.

This chapter outlines studies of immunogenetics, histopathology, cellular and humoral immune responses in MS, the most relevant observations from EAE experiments, and finally the examination of different treatment modalities, which together led to our current understanding of the immunology of MS.

POTENTIAL CAUSES OF MULTIPLE SCLEROSIS

Multiple sclerosis may be caused by exogenous agents such as viruses or bacteria, and epidemiologic data as well as similarities to infectious demyelinating diseases provide circumstantial evidence that favors an infectious etiology (4). Relapses often occur in close temporal relation to viral infections but not to other exogenous events (5). The prevalence of MS increases with latitude on both hemispheres and is particularly high (60 to 100 per 100,000 population) in Northern Europe and Northern America (6). These geographic variations could be due to genetic or environmental factors, such as nutrition, hygiene standards, or exposure to different pathogens. Studies of MS "epidemics," such as that in the Faroe Islands (6), where MS was first observed during World War II, suggested that an unknown pathogen, possibly a virus, was brought to the islands by British troops.

Further support for a viral etiology stems from parallels with infectious demyelinating diseases such as progressive multifocal leukoencephalopathy (PML), a disease that is mediated by the papovavirus JC (4,7). However, PML is characterized by large confluent areas of white matter damage in immunocompromised individuals (7). Another infectious demyelinating disease, HTLV-1–associated myelopathy/tropical spastic paraparesis/ (HAM/TSP) (8,9), is caused by the human T lymphotrophic virus type 1 (HTLV-1), a retrovirus that is closely related to HIV-1, which also causes adult T-cell leukemia (ATL). HAM/TSP was originally observed in circumscribed geographic areas (Southern Japan, Jamaica, and the Caribbean) (9), where it affects between 1 percent and 5 percent of HTLV-1–infected individuals.

Human lymphocyte antigen (HLA)–background, time of infection, and other as yet poorly understood factors may contribute to susceptibility. HAM/TSP may clinically mimic primary progressive MS, but differs from it by high titers of HTLV-1–specific antibodies in blood and CSF and the presence of proviral genome in cells of affected individuals (8). Demyelination in HAM/TSP is less marked than in MS and is accompanied by axonal loss. Recent studies suggest that HTLV-1–restricted cytotoxic T-lymphocytes (CTL) specific for regulatory or structural viral proteins found at high frequencies in blood, CSF, and at low numbers in the spinal cord could be effectors in producing CNS disease (10,11). The microglia is a likely target for HTLV-1, as demonstrated in cultures of adult human microglial cells (12). Infected microglia may produce proinflammatory cytokines that contribute to inflammation and demyelination. HTLV-2, a related retrovirus, may also cause CNS damage (13), but little is known about the pathogenesis and clinical aspects of this disease. Studies of HAM/TSP clearly demonstrate that a T-cell response against an infectious agent such as HTLV-1 can produce a demyelinating disease of the CNS.

In distinction to the aforementioned chronic entities, an acute monophasic demyelination termed *postinfectious encephalomyelitis* (PIE) may occur 10 to 40 days after infection with measles, varicella, or vaccinia virus (4,14). The pathology presents with demyelinating plaques of the same rather than different stages, and it is currently believed that demyelination is caused by a virus-induced immune response against myelin, such as after measles (14). Epidemiologic studies have shown that viral infections often precede relapses of MS (15), and a number of specific viruses, including measles, HTLV-1, herpesviruses, retroviruses, and others, have been implicated (4). However, although initial reports linking a specific virus and MS have not held up over time, it could be shown that myelin basic protein (MBP)–specific T cells can be found during postmeasles encephalomyelitis (14) and in the CSF during rubella panencephalitis (16) and Lyme radiculomyelitis (17). Although humanherpes virus 6 has recently been implicated in MS (18,19), it is more likely that infectious agents induce an immune response against self-antigens (5) or that infection of oligodendrocytes makes them more vulnerable to inflammation-mediated damage rather than implicating a single virus in the etiology of MS. Autoreactive T cells are part of the "normal" T cell repertoire, and strong stimuli such as virus infection may activate such cells, increase cytokine secretion, and concomitantly upregulate adhesion molecules and major histocompatibility complex (MHC) molecules, thus creating the necessary environment for autoimmune disease. Bacteria and viruses may induce autoreactivity or tissue damage by several mechanisms, including superantigens, i.e., proteins that are able to cause a potent activation of T cells expressing a specific T-cell receptor (TCR) variable chain (20) or through molecular mimicry (21). The latter involves crossreactivity of T cells or B cells with stretches of amino acids or conformational determinants that are shared between a virus and a myelin antigen (21). Understanding T cell recognition at the molecular level has allowed us to study molecular mimicry in more detail, and it appears that in some instances it is involved in induction of autoimmunity (22).

Naturally occurring demyelinating diseases of animals as well as experimental models for such diseases also mimic characteristics of MS. Theiler's murine encephalomyelitis virus (TMEV) may be induced in susceptible mouse strains by intracerebral inoculation (23,24). Inflammatory foci consist of infiltrates with macrophages, lymphocytes, and reactive astroglia (24), whereas later stages of inflammatory lesions typically show extensive demyelination, and lipid-containing macrophages, but sparing of axons and vessels. Demyelination in Theiler's encephalomyelitis is induced by a DTH response by MHC-class II–restricted, CD4+, TMEV-specific TH1 cells (23,25,26), and lymphokine-activated macrophages (25). The observations that demyelination also occurs in TMEV-inoculated nude mice and that virus-specific antibodies may react with myelin indicate that both humoral and cellular immune responses induced by TMEV contribute to the demyelinating process.

Demyelinating diseases induced by rat-adapted measles virus or neurotrophic mouse hepatitis virus (JHM) (27,28) are other examples. The latter is characterized by direct infection of oligodendrocytes. Myelin-reactive T cells develop in acutely infected animals, and an EAE-like disease can be transferred by MBP-sensitized T lymphocytes from these animals (27). T-cell reactivity to myelin components could result from the release of myelin from damaged oligodendrocytes or by induction of T cells that recognize determinants shared by virus and myelin proteins.

Finally, visna, a spontaneous lentivirus-induced leukoencephalomyelitis of sheep, is remarkably similar to MS (29,30), with its slowly progressive paralytic course due to inflammation and demyelination throughout brain and spinal cord. Although infectious virus could not be recovered from the CNS, viral nucleic acid has been demonstrated in a substantial number of cells (29,30). Immunosuppressive treatment temporarily delays progression, which suggests the involvement of immunologic mechanisms.

IMMUNOPATHOLOGIC FEATURES OF THE MULTIPLE SCLEROSIS LESION

Depending on the stage of the lesion, cell numbers, and phenotypes, the expression of immunologically relevant surface receptors, chemokines, and lymphokines may vary (31–39). Acute lesions are characterized by T lymphocytes, plasma cells, macrophages, and bare, demyelinated, or transected axons (32). The expression of endothelial cell activation markers and adhesion molecules, including vascular cell adhesion molecule-1 (VCAM-1), endothelial cell leukocyte adhesion molecule-1 (E-selectin/ELAM-1), MHC-class II antigens, intracellular adhesion molecule-1 (ICAM-1), and urokinase-activator receptor, is greatly enhanced on CNS endothelial cells in early lesions compared with the periplaque tissue (36). Each of these molecules may participate in cell adhesion and migration into the parenchyma. The presence of albumin, complement, and immunoglobulins in the tissue indicates disruption of the blood–brain barrier (BBB) and local production of immunoglobulins (37). The composition of T-cell phenotypes varies. Some studies documented a predominance of CD8+ over CD4+ cells, others higher numbers of CD4+ cells at the plaque edge and in the surrounding tissue (34,38,39). Active inflammation is shown by T cells positive for interleukin-2 (IL-2) receptors and MHC-class II antigens, as well as the local production of T-cell derived lymphokines such as interferon gamma (IFN-γ), tumor necrosis factor (TNF-α/β), and IL-2 (35,40–42). These lymphokines and chemokines contribute to the recruitment of cells from the bloodstream and at the same time induce the upregulation of surface markers, not only on these invading cells but also on cells of the CNS.

With respect to the effector mechanisms leading to myelin damage, IL-1, nitric oxide, and oxygen radicals are produced by activated macrophages and are believed to contribute to the overall inflammation as well as to tissue damage (43). Several factors, including complement, proteolytic enzymes, reactive nitrogen (NO), and oxygen species (O_2-), are probably involved in the direct destruction of myelin (55,56) and enhance immunoglobulin-mediated mechanisms (43,44). The expression of heat shock proteins (HSP), a group of phylogenetically conserved proteins that serve protective roles in cellular stress of various kinds including heat, irradiation, lymphokine exposure (particularly IFN-γ), HSP-65 (45) and HSP-90 (46) on oligodendrocytes in close neighborhood of T cells expressing the g/d TCR was observed in chronically active lesions, whereas a/b TCR T cells are more abundant in early active lesions (45–47). Subsequently, the expression of HSP in the CNS during inflammatory stress could lead to destruction of HSP-expressing resident cells by T cells specific for a bacterial HSP with shared peptide sequence (45–48).

LOCAL ANTIGEN PRESENTATION IN THE CENTRAL NERVOUS SYSTEM

In both EAE and MS, inflammatory demyelination is believed to be mediated by activated CD4+ T cells of the

Th1 phenotype that have the capacity to cross the blood–brain barrier (BBB) (49). Specialized endothelial cells (EC) joined by tight junctions form the BBB that normally excludes inflammatory cells and macromolecules from passive access to the CNS (50,51). The mechanism of T-cell migration across the BBB is thought to first involve adhesion due to cytokine-mediated upregulation of adhesion molecules on T-cells and their ligands on EC (51), followed by diapedesis across the endothelium. Another potential mechanism for T-cell invasion of the BBB could involve T-cell recognition of antigen presented by EC and subsequent CTL-mediated BBB damage (52–54). In the CNS compartment, T-cell reactivity is amplified through recognition of "relevant" antigen(s) presented by resident antigen-presenting cells (APCs) and in response to cytokines secreted by these cells. Antigen presentation in the CNS requires the induction of MHC/HLA class II molecules normally not expressed on glial cells, as well as the upregulation of adhesion and co-stimulatory molecules. IFN-γ and TNF-α secreted by migrating T-cells can induce these molecules on astrocytes and microglia and consequently render these cells competent APCs (55).

Although there is substantial evidence to support an immunologic function for both astrocytes (56–68) and microglia (59,61–63,68) in CNS inflammation, the specific role of each cell type in the pathogenesis of the MS lesion remains a subject of debate and controversy. This controversy centers on three main issues:

1. Is the microglia or the astrocyte the major APC in the CNS?
2. Can these cells initiate or simply perpetuate immune reactivity in the CNS?
3. Can these cells have a dual function in activating as well as downregulating immune reactivity in the CNS?

In MS, the microglia rather than the astrocyte is believed to be the major APC, based on the cellular distribution of HLA class II expression in the lesion (69), as well as the in vitro demonstration that astrocytes can only activate T cells after priming by microglia (70,71) or co-culture with microglia or IL-1 (66). In addition, the observation that human microglia but not astrocytes express the co-stimulatory molecule B-7 (65) favors the microglia as the the predominant APC in MS. Tantalizing in vitro animal studies suggest that perivascular microglia may have a role different from that of parenchymal microglia in regulating the immune response, in that the former is the dominant APC (70,72).

There is emerging evidence that astrocytes and microglia can also downregulate the cellular immune response in the CNS in the course of inflammation. Four

potential negative feedback mechanisms have been suggested; they are not mutually exclusive:

1. Astrocytes and microglia can secrete antiinflammatory cytokines such as transforming growth factor-β (TGF-β) and IL-10, which inhibit Th1 responses (73).
2. Overexpression of class II molecules on parenchymal microglia could lead to T-cell apoptosis (74).
3. If indeed astrocytes lack the B7 costimulatory molecule, these cells could downregulate the immune response in the CNS by anergizing T-cells.
4. Encephalitogenic CD4+ T cells can have cytotoxic function and lyse glial cells (57,60,75), thus downregulating their immune function (55).

The ability of CNS cells to present antigen is cytokine dependent. HLA Class II molecules and a host of other molecules involved in APC/T-cell interaction including adhesion and costimulatory molecules are not expressed under physiologic conditions but can be induced by IFN-γ. A number of mediators, including cytokines (76) and neurotransmitters (77,78), modulate the expression of IFN-γ–induced class-II expression, and this modulation appears to be cell type specific (79). Examples include the ability of type I IFNs (reviewed in Ref. 80), IL-10 (81), TGF-b (82), IL-4 (83), and GM-CSF (84) to inhibit class II expression on glial cells. The modulatory effect of IFN-β on glial cells class II expression is probably responsible in part for the therapeutic effect of IFN-β in MS (80). Similar inhibitory effects of IL-10 and TGF-β on class II expression underlie part of the rationale for the current use of these cytokines in MS clinical trials.

GENETIC FACTORS ASSOCIATED WITH MULTIPLE SCLEROSIS

The finding of different prevalence rates of MS (6) in different geographic areas has been considered to reflect environmental and genetic factors in the pathogenesis of this disease (85). However, it will be difficult to sort out what their relative roles are as long as individual factors are not identified. Evidence for a role of genetic factors in MS has been derived from family and twin studies (85–89). Most of the candidate genes, i.e., those of the HLA, TCR complex, GM allotypes 124, alpha-1 antitrypsin or the 5'-flanking region of the MBP gene (126), to name only a few, are linked either to the immune system or to myelin. Because disease association with HLA genes is by far the strongest, and because the role of other genes is often controversial, we focus on genes of the HLA complex. For more detail on genetic factors, the reader is referred to recent excellent reviews (90,91).

Major histocompatibility complex (HLA in humans) molecules play a crucial role in cellular immune responses to foreign and self-antigens, because T cells recognize antigen only in the context of self-HLA molecules (92). This is referred to as MHC/HLA-restricted antigen recognition and may provide an explanation for how disease susceptibility and HLA background may be related (93). In Caucasian MS populations, the strongest associations have been observed with HLA-DR2 Dw2 (this allele is now termed DR15 at the level of serologic typing and HLA-DRB1*1501 and -DRB5*0101 by oligonucleotide typing), whereas HLA-DR4 and -DR6 have been observed in Sardinian and Jordanian Arab MS patients, and DR4 in Mexican MS patients, respectively. The latter groups have considerably lower prevalence rates, and the distribution of HLA-DR molecules varies with respect to the frequency of single alleles (reviewed in Ref. 90).

HLA-class II genes are clustered in close proximity on chromosome 6, and therefore HLA-DR- and -DQ genes are inherited together within one haplotype, i.e., they are in linkage dysequilibrium. Due to their tight linkage, it is therefore still not clear whether HLA-DR and -DQ confer risk together or independently. Studies on frequencies of restriction fragment length polymorphisms (RFLP) and DQ genotypes have identified associations of certain segments with MS alleles 135–139. Several studies that are not covered here showed that 97 percent of 61 MS patients carried HLA-DR types (DR15Dw2, DR4, or DR6), which had been associated with disease in different ethnic groups (94), whereas another larger study found HLA-DR2 associated with disease and, as the second strongest association, HLA-DR3 (95). Multiple sclerosis–associated DQ molecules share polymorphic amino acid stretches of the membrane distal domain that is involved in antigen binding and contacting the TCR (94). Based on these results, it was speculated that a unique autoantigen or foreign antigen may be presented in the context of these DQ molecules, but even now the role of DQ as a restriction element is only poorly understood (94). Further studies on this subject documented a joint or independent contribution of DQb and DQa, whereas the role of HLA-DP is controversial at the present time.

Underscored by genetic findings, it is currently considered likely that at least the major two disease courses, relapsing-remitting (RR) and primary chronic progressive (PCP), represent two different entities. In RR MS, the HLA-class I molecules HLA-A3 and -B7 and the class II molecule HLA-DR2 are found more often, whereas HLA-A3, -B7, and -DR3 are more frequent in PCP MS (95). Another study demonstrated that HLA-DR15 Dw2 and DQw6 haplotypes were strongly associated with both forms of MS, but additional risk in RR MS was conferred by a different DQb pattern in patients with PCP MS (96). Attempts to link certain sequence motifs of the DQA1 or DQB1 molecules to disease (97) have so far not led to a clear understanding of which segments of disease-associated DR- or DQ molecules are associated with disease and how their presence translates into an abnormal immune response against myelin antigens. So far none of the DQ polymorphisms fully explain the disease association and, in summary, there is a weak association with certain HLA-class I genes and a stronger association with the class II alleles HLA-DR15 and -DQB1*0602 and DQA1*0102. No differences have been detected in the genomic DNA of DRb, DQa, and DQb genes derived from MS patients as compared with those from healthy individuals (98). Based on our current understanding of the cellular immune system, several possibilities exist as to how specific HLA-class II heterodimers may influence disease susceptibility. Unique autoantigens may be processed and presented preferentially in the context of certain HLA-DR- or -DQ molecules, but the presence of certain HLA-DQ antigens may also play a regulatory role (99).

Besides direct influences of HLA molecules, other genes that are inherited with the same complex haplotypes and are located near or between the HLA genes on chromosome 6 may also be associated with disease. These include TNF alleles, peptide transporters, HSPs, complement genes, or MOG, among others. Their role needs further investigation (100), but they certainly are interesting candidates that could contribute to disease susceptibility.

Another group of genes that have attracted attention during recent years are those that contribute to the TCR. Based on EAE experiments in which it was shown that certain TCRs are preferentially used by encephalitogenic T cells, it was believed that the TCR a- and b chains, which form the mature TCR heterodimer, represent good candidates for MS susceptibility genes. Although these studies initially documented an overrepresentation of certain TCR RFLP of either a- or b chain variable (V) or constant (C) regions (reviewed in Ref. 91) in MS patients of different geographic areas or in family members of MS, other studies using the same experimental strategies have failed to obtain similar results (101,102). One reason for this controversy is the genetic heterogeneity in the examined MS populations. At present, it is not clear how the presence of certain TCR germline would lead to autoimmune disease. However, it has been shown in experimental systems by germline alteration of TCR genes that this manipulation can induce autoreactive T cells and autoimmune disease (103).

Whole genome searches, which have recently been performed in several laboratories (104–106), as well as analyses of complex genetic disease such as SLE in mouse models (107), indicate that multiple genes are weakly associated with disease and form a quantitative trait. Future studies will have to identify these associated genes and their contributions to the pathogenesis of MS.

LESSONS FROM EXPERIMENTAL ALLERGIC ENCEPHALOMYELITIS

Experimental allergic encephalomyelitis (EAE) is an acute or chronic relapsing demyelinating disease induced in various susceptible animal strains (e.g., Lewis rats or SJL mice) by the injection of myelin or myelin components in appropriate adjuvants and is mediated by encephalitogenic T cells (108,109). During the last decades, various EAE models that differ with respect to the inducing myelin component, "clinical" phenotype, course, pathology, and immunologic hallmarks (i.e., involvement of humoral versus cellular immune mechanisms) have been studied extensively by a number of laboratories (110).

Pathology of the Demyelinating Lesion in EAE

The pathology of EAE varies considerably among different species and is dependent on the mode of induction and encephalitogen used. As examples, EAE in the SJL mouse is characterized by perivascular lymphomonocytic infiltrates, demyelination, and some remyelination in lesions of different ages, depending on whether the acute phase or later stages are analyzed (111). In Lewis rats, EAE shows an acute inflammatory process with limited demyelination. Such differences in pathology are also seen in EAE in outbred primates with a hyperacute and often fatal disease that is caused by a hemorrhagic encephalomyelitis in macaques, whereas in marmosets EAE produces perivascular inflammation and demyelination. It is currently not clear what causes these differences in EAE pathology, but the highly variable degrees of inflammation and demyelination, affected areas of the CNS, and clinical courses indicate that different mechanisms may be involved (112).

EAE Susceptibility in Different Animal Strains

Susceptibility differs between inbred rodent strains (110). Backcrossing experiments between resistant and susceptible strains and the generation of congenic animal strains indicated that genes of the major histocompatibility complex (MHC) are the most important susceptibility factor, but that other background genes also contribute to susceptibility. Some of the most thoroughly studied MHC genes are IAu and IAs in PL- and SJL mice, respectively, as well as RTIb in Lewis rats (reviewed in Refs. 110,112). How MHC genes and other immunologically relevant background genes influence disease susceptibility and why one strain shows a more acute inflammatory course and the other a more chronic and demyelinating course are not yet understood.

Encephalitogenic Myelin Components

Central nervous system myelin is produced by oligodendroglial cells. It consists of approximately 75 percent to 80 percent lipids and 20 percent to 25 percent proteins, including proteolipidprotein (PLP), myelin basic protein (MBP 1), the enzyme 2'3'-cyclic nucleotide 3' phosphodiesterase (CNPase), myelin-associated glycoprotein (MAG) myelin oligodendroglia glycoprotein (MOG), and others such as brain-specific creatine-kinase and tubulin (113,114). Proteolipidprotein and MBP are most abundant, representing 50 percent and 30 percent of myelin protein, respectively. Interactions between the hydrophobic PLP, the basic MBP, and myelin lipids are thought to account for the highly organized lamellar structure of mature myelin (113). Differential RNA splicing and posttranslational modifications result in size isoforms and charge isomers of most myelin antigens, and the relative composition of myelin with respect to the myelin proteins varies during ontogeny, during inflammatory states, and after remyelination (113).

Myelin Basic Protein

Myelin basic protein is located in the cytosol and exists in several isoforms because of differential splicing from seven exons of a single gene (115). The most prevalent form in mature myelin is the 18.5 kDa isoform. Although highly conserved, amino acid (AA) substitutions in the MBPs isolated from different species affect its encephalitogenic activity (116). Furthermore, size isoforms or posttranslational modifications, which may be expressed at higher levels during myelination or remyelination, can be relevant for the induction and perpetuation of demyelinating diseases (117–119). Myelin damage during the course of MS results in the release of MBP, which can then be detected in CSF and urine and may serve as a marker for myelin breakdown during active disease (120,121).

The MHC background of a given inbred mouse or rat strain influences the region of MBP that is encephalitogenic in that animal, e.g., the N-terminal region Ac1-11 induces EAE in PL/J and B10.PL mice, whereas a region in the middle of the molecule AA 89-100 is encephalitogenic in SJL/J mice. In the rat, the major encephalitogenic region is AA 69-86, and in rhesus monkeys AA 153-165. (For more detail, see reviews 116,122.)

Proteolipidprotein

Proteolipidprotein (PLP) is a 30 kDa highly hydrophobic transmembrane protein that interacts with myelin lipids and stabilizes opposing layers of the myelin membrane (123). Because of its physicochemical characteristics, PLP is harder to isolate and to work with in immunologic studies. Therefore, short synthetic peptides from the hydrophilic regions of PLP are often used for immunologic studies. Both PLP and its size isoform DM20 (25 kDa), which lacks AA 116-150 (124), are encephalitogenic in mice, guinea pigs, rats, and rabbits (reviewed in Ref. 112). Because of its exquisite expression in the CNS as opposed to MBP, which is found in both PNS and CNS, and because more pronounced demyelination is observed in PLP-induced disease, e.g., in SJL mice, it was speculated that PLP may be more important as an encephalitogen than MBP. The finding that tolerization with PLP, but not MBP, protects EAE induction with whole spinal cord homogenate further supported this notion (125). However, it is not clear whether this can be generalized to different strains.

Encephalitogenicity of Myelin Components Other Than MBP and PLP

Relatively less is known about less abundant myelin components such as CNPase, MAG, and MOG. Myelin oligodendroglia glycoprotein in particular has recently gained considerable attention because of findings in both EAE (125–127) and MS patients (128). Passive transfer by MOG (44-53)-specific T cells into naive Lewis rats leads to an intense perivascular inflammatory response, blood–brain barrier breakdown, but less parenchymal inflammation (129), and various MOG peptides have now been shown to be encephalitogenic in different species, including mice, rats, and marmosets. Experimental allergic encephalomyelitis could not so far be induced with MAG or CNPase. Experimental allergic encephalomyelitis induced with MOG, which is accessible on the outside of the myelin sheath, generates a humoral response manifested by MOG-specific antibodies that appear to play an important role in determining the extent of demyelination. Similar to MOG, humoral immune reactivity against lipids also occurs (130) and may increase the extent of demyelination. However, attempts to induce EAE with lipids alone generally have failed. These observations support the theory that antibody-mediated mechanisms (complement-mediated lysis, opsonization, enhanced antigen presentation by macrophages) may contribute to the severity of T cell–mediated autoimmune disease or may modify their clinical phenotype.

EAE Is a T Cell–Mediated Autoimmune Disease

Experimental allergic encephalomyelitis can be transferred from affected to naive animals by transferring immune cells, but not humoral factors, documenting the fact that EAE is a T cell–mediated autoimmune disease (108,109,131–133). This adoptive transfer or passive model of EAE (AT-EAE) has been used to study many immunologic questions, and it is now well accepted that EAE is mediated by CD4+ T cells that are specific for the portion of MBP or PLP that is encephalitogenic in the respective animal strain (116,122,134,135).

With respect to antigen recognition, T cells are not able to interact with conformational determinants, but only with short peptides that are derived from foreign or self-proteins and embedded into the antigen-binding cleft of MHC-class I or MHC-class II molecules, i.e., MHC- or HLA-restricted antigen recognition (92,136). Antigenic peptides may stem either from endogenously synthesized proteins (e.g., viral proteins, which are recognized in the context of MHC-class I molecules by CD8+ T cells) (137) or from exogenous proteins that are processed by proteolytic cleavage before they are presented on MHC-class II molecules to CD4+ T cells (137). The third component of this complex is the T-cell antigen receptor (TCR), a heterodimeric surface molecule consisting of an alpha chain and a beta chain (138). The TCR is formed from a limited number of germlines segments, i.e., the variable (V), junctional (J), and, only for the beta chain, segments for the diversity (D) regions with the nonpolymorphic constant (C) region. These are rearranged to form the TCR alpha-chain and beta-chain molecules (138). T-cell antigen receptor diversity results from the combination of VDJ segments with either C gene (beta chain) or from VJC (alpha chain). Over 50 variable (V) alpha-chain and beta-chain genes are known, and, together with N-nucleotide additions in the junctional regions, result in a further increase in TCR diversity, thus creating a T cell repertoire that is able to interact with virtually any self-MHC/peptide combination. Structural comparisons with antibody molecules and mutation analyses of antigen-specific TCR molecules have revealed that parts of the complementarity determinant region (CDR) CDR3 primarily interact with the antigenic peptide, whereas CDR1 and CDR2 are probably contacting peptide/MHC complex or MHC molecule alone (139). Understanding these three components, i.e., TCR, MHC, and peptide, the so-called trimolecular complex in EAE has provided important insights into the pathogenesis of EAE. Furthermore, these data have helped to design highly specific therapies for EAE. A number of excellent reviews dealing with the role of T cells in EAE have been published elsewhere (122,140,141).

Relationship of the MHC Background to the T-Cell Response in EAE

The encephalitogenic epitopes of MBP and PLP differ in various mouse and rat strains depending on their MHC-class II background (116). In PL/J mice and B10.PL mice, the encephalitogenic MBP peptide is recognized in the context of IAu, in SJL/J mice with IAs, and in B10RIII mice with IAr (142). In Lewis rats, MBP (69-86) is encephalitogenic in the context of (RT-1)a, MBP (110-129), and with (RT-1)w in Lou/M rats (143). The main encephalitogenic PLP peptide in SJL/J mice (restricted by IAs) is located in AA (139-151) (144), in SWR mice (IAq) in AA (103-116), and in Biozzi AB/H and NOD mice in AA (56-70) (145). Additional minor encephalitogenic regions exist for most of the susceptible strains and are sometimes recognized in the context of IE molecules rather than IA. Minor encephalitogenic determinants (146) often are not the target in the initial phase of MBP-specific or PLP-specific T cells but may become important at later stages or during chronic courses as a result of a process referred to as epitope spreading (147). Thus, the disease-associated MHC class II molecule determines which myelin peptides may preferentially bind and, as a consequence, are recognized by T cells, i.e., are immunodominant.

T-Cell Receptor Usage of Encephalitogenic T Cells

Because the TCR is the only unique structure within the trimolecular complex, attention quickly focused on this molecule and on attempts to delineate which TCRs are expressed by encephalitogenic T cells (147). It was both exciting and surprising when it was found that encephalitogenic T cells from Lewis rats and B10.PL and PL/J mice express a nearly identical, highly restricted TCR repertoire (Vb8.2 and Va4.3, respectively, in TCC recognizing MBP Ac1-11), although they are derived from different species (148,149). Sequencing of the junctional regions showed a limited usage of Db and Jb but to a lesser extent with four out of eight clones using Jb2.7, two Jb2.3, and two Jb2.5 (150). Each of the clones expressed the alpha chain Va4.3 (150). Similar results were obtained from studies with T-cell hybridomas established from B10.PL mice in response to the same MBP peptide (151). It was even more striking that encephalitogenic cells from Lewis rats, even though from a different species and specific for a different MBP epitope, expressed the same TCR Vb-chain, Vb8.2, which is identical to that expressed in B10.PL and PL/J mice (148,149,152) and also with very similar CDR3 regions.

Different from these results, the highly EAE-susceptible SJL mice, which have deleted a portion of their TCR germline including Vb8, show less restricted TCR usage in their encephalitogenic T cells, with Vb17 being the most prominent TCR chain (140). That a more heterogeneous TCR repertoire with TCR other than Vb8.2 may also be observed in Lewis rats was recently demonstrated and argues against the idea that a specific variable region is the most important factor for the development of certain autoimmune diseases (153). However, the

description of a restricted TCR usage has raised great interest in highly specific immunotherapies against the TCR (see subsequent section).

The EAE Lesion—Relevance of Immune Cells and Brain Resident Cells

Although EAE is considered a T cell–mediated disease, several lines of evidence indicate that additional factors are involved in disease production, phenotype, and course (154). This notion became obvious from both genetic studies but also experiments with transgenic mouse lines expressing the TCR derived from encephalitogenic B10 T cells in the germline of C57/B6 mice (154). The development of spontaneous EAE in these animals depends on the housing conditions. Although over 90 percent of peripheral T cells in this model express the transgenic TCR, only a few animals become sick under germ-free conditions, whereas mice in non–germ-free environments had a much higher rate of EAE (154). This supports the idea that nonspecific factors, possibly infections, contribute to T-cell activation and disease induction. This finding suggests that nonspecific factors associated with infections, possibly nonspecific activation of T cells, may contribute to disease production.

Once encephalitogenic cells have entered the CNS (see previous section for migration and local antigen presentation), they may amplify and/or mediate the local inflammatory response and demyelination in a number of ways: IFN-γ enhances the expression of MHC-class I and MHC-class II molecules on endothelial cells, astrocytes, and microglia; activates macrophages; stimulates the differentiation of cytotoxic T cells; and activates NK-cells. TNF-α/β (the latter is also termed LT-a; the first is secreted by many cells, including lymphocytes and monocytes, whereas the latter stems from T cells) show a large degree of homology and bind to the same surface receptor (155). Tumor necrosis factor, in particular TNF-b/LT-a, is considered an important factor in the pathogenesis of demyelinating lesions (156,157), damaging both endothelial cells, which leads to blood–brain barrier leakage, and oligodendroglial cells, which results in demyelination (158,159).

Although TNF secretion has previously been considered a major factor responsible for myelin damage, other potential mechanisms include toxic radicals (i.e., oxygen and nitrogen derivatives), antibody (see amplification by MOG-specific antibodies) and complement-mediated damage, killing of oligodendrocytes via Fas and Fas-ligand or homotypic CD56 interactions (see subsequent section). The relative importance of these effector pathways and whether encephalitogenic cells mediate damage directly or indirectly is not clear at present, either in EAE or in MS. However, LT-a has been identified as a crucial factor in EAE by blocking studies (156,157) and by knock-out mice (160), whereas similar studies in TNF-a knock-out mice or mice in which both cytokine genes had been deleted were less clear (161).

Humoral Immune Responses in MS Patients

One of the earliest known immunologic abnormalities in MS is the persistent secretion of oligoclonal immunoglobulins in the cerebrospinal fluid (162), now referred to as oligoclonal bands (OCB). Oligoclonal bands are one of the most sensitive, although nonspecific, markers for disease (up to 95 percent of patients are positive) (163). This limited diversity of persistently secreted antibodies is still puzzling, and although reactivity has been demonstrated against a number of common viruses such as measles, rubella, mumps, or herpes (163–165), even sophisticated techniques such as the use of phage display libraries have not identified a single pathogen that is recognized by CSF-Igs of many patients (166). Very recent observations suggest that an Alu-repeat with unknown function may be the target of the humoral response in some patients (167) and that a large percentage of MS patients are positive for antibodies against an immunodominant MBP peptide (85-99) (168–170). It is interesting that the same area is preferentially recognized by MBP-specific T cells derived from DR2+ MS patients (170,171), suggesting that the sustained antibody response may be driven by myelin-reactive T cells.

The OCB in MS may either be specific for an as yet unidentified pathogen or be the result of a dysregulation in immune responsiveness. The latter notion finds support by a lack of suppressor function (172,173) as well as increased Ig synthesis (173) in mitogen-driven assay systems, indicating that there may be an as yet ill-defined suppressive activity. Whether this is due to disturbances in CD8+ T cell function or lack of a subset of CD4+ helper T cells, termed *suppressor-inducer cells* (174), is not yet clear. However, defective CD4+ T cell function was also found in an antigen-specific system, i.e., the reduction of measles-specific cytolytic activity (175).

Multiple sclerosis patients certainly do not suffer from a general immunodeficiency; rather, they tend to react with a biased Th1 response, and, along these lines, they rarely suffer from severe allergies (176), which are associated with a Th2 biased response. Data obtained in EAE and in MS underscores that it will be important to follow these questions in more detail and try to correlate the data with clinical characteristics and MRI findings longitudinally.

Cellular Immune Responses to Myelin Antigens in Multiple Sclerosis

The elegant studies in EAE have helped to identify several encephalitogenic components of myelin, characterized the

T-cell response against these in great detail, and led to novel immunotherapeutic strategies (122,140), and they have also stimulated similar studies in MS (177). We outline next the current status of the most important studies and discuss their potential implications for the pathogenesis and therapy of MS. As already mentioned, evidence in MS is gathered by trying to correlate immunologic observations with clinical disease status or MRI parameters. Because this comparison is often not possible in a systematic way, many of the observations are in part controversial.

Frequency of Myelin-Specific T cells

Different EAE in which the potential pathogenicity of a T-cell population can be assessed directly by transfer into a healthy animal, one means to address this issue in MS was to compare the frequencies of myelin-reactive T cells in MS patients and controls. It was at first expected that myelin-specific T cells would only be found in patients, and therefore the observation that MBP-specific T cells can easily be isolated from controls was quite surprising (178); it has now been confirmed by many studies (179–187). Myelin-specific T cells are thus not a unique characteristic of MS but can be isolated from virtually every healthy individual, an observation that has shed new light on thymic selection of T cells. Autoreactive T cells are a constant component of our T-cell repertoire, and MS research therefore tried to underscore their role by comparing frequencies in MS patients with controls. Because MBP and PLP are by far the best examined myelin components, we focus mostly on them but also mention others that have recently received attention.

A number of different techniques have been employed to determine the frequencies of MBP-specific or PLP-specific T cells, i.e., ELISPOT assays, which measure individual cytokine-secreting cells, but also split-well cloning with and without precultivation in IL-2, and finally more sophisticated techniques, which followed individual T cells via their TCR. The results of these studies have not been completely conclusive (181,184,188–192). The absolute numbers of MBP-specific or PLP-specific T cells varied between approximately 1/1000 or more (specific TCR), $1/10^4$–$1/10^5$ (ELISPOT) to $1/10^6$–$1/10^7$ (split-well cloning), but, depending on the technique, there was a tendency toward elevated numbers in MS patients versus controls. Compared with the peripheral blood, the frequencies in the CSF were approximately 1–2 orders of magnitude higher (ELISPOT) (188). It is not yet clear how these largely different numbers can be explained, but most likely they depend on the very different techniques, which read out either too high or too low numbers. Another important factor relates to the origin of the expanded cells, i.e., whether they are derived from the naive or memory population. Although the former would be thought to mirror primarily the existing T-cell repertoire, one would assume that the latter may be more disease-relevant because they should have been expanded in vivo. Therefore, Zhang and coworkers precultivated the PBL in IL-2 before assessing their antigen-specificity in order to enrich for in vivo activated T cells (189). Their results show an increased number of in vivo activated MBP-specific and PLP-specific T cells in MS patients (189), which is in line with other reports documenting that hprt-mutant T MBP-specific (193) or PLP-specific (194) T cells, i.e., T cells that must have been activated and mutated in vivo, are found only in MS. A recent study that carefully compared the specificity, cytokine profiles, and other parameters of MBP-specific T cells from either naive (CD45RA) or memory (CD45RO) populations found similar frequencies, but otherwise striking differences, in clones from the two subgroups, shedding new light on the role of autoreactive T cells (Muraro PA, et al., manuscript in preparation). Finally, the comparison of frequencies of MBP-specific T cells in affected and unaffected family members (190–192) or even in discordant versus concordant identical twins (190) documented similar numbers of MBP-specific T cells within one set regardless of disease. In identical twins, differences in frequencies were observed between different sets, but within one set the numbers were very similar even if that pair was discordant (190). These findings may be interpreted as a sign that MBP-specific T cells can be expanded during myelin breakdown, but they could also indicate that the relative magnitude of the response primarily shows a predisposing "trait" for myelin reactivity. Exogenous factors may then determine whether myelin-reactive T cells are activated and expanded or not. The sometimes very high numbers in controls also document that their presence is certainly not sufficient to induce disease.

Fine-Specificity of MBP-Specific T-cells

The link between disease-associated MHC alleles and encephalitogenic epitopes in EAE provided interesting clues as to how the presence of a specific MHC molecule may determine the preferential recognition of a myelin peptide by pathogenic T cells. It was therefore no surprise that this question was also looked at in human myelin-specific T cells, particularly in the response to MBP. There are now extensive data about this topic from long-term T-cell lines (TCL) and T-cell clones (TCC) (171,179–187,195,196). Without addressing every detail of these studies, the following major observations have been made: The comparison of T cells from MS patients and controls did not show major differences with respect to fine-specificity. Data from large numbers of TCLs that had been generated by whole 18.5 kDa MBP in several studies documented a few immunodominant regions in the middle (residues 83-99)

(171,181–187,195–197). Whether there is also an immunodominant region in the N-terminal region is not clear at present (181,183,185,187,189). The potential disease relevance of the middle immunodominant region was further underlined by recognition in the context of several MS-associated HLA-DR molecules (DR15 Dw2, DR4 Dw4, DR4 Dw14, DR13 Dw19) (195), but also others that are not MS-related. Slightly different peptides [peptide 80-99 (197) and peptide 84-102 (184)] were recognized in the context of one of the two b-chains isotypically expressed in the HLA-DR15 Dw2 haplotype [DR2b encoded by DRB1*1501, and DR2a encoded by DRB5*0101 (198,199) and of HLA-DQw6 (184)]. Further mapping of the fine-specificity of (87-106)-specific TCL by truncated and Ala-substituted peptides revealed both nested epitopes in this region and a high degree of diversity with respect to fine-specificity (200). The demonstration of similar specificities in both patients and normals was initially disappointing, but the fact that the middle MBP epitope is immunodominant in DR+ MS patients and controls and encephalitogenic in two other species (SJL mice and Lewis rats) indicated that common features of these MHC molecules in different species are associated with demyelinating diseases. This notion is true not only for the middle region but also for the C-terminus, which is encephalitogenic in rhesus monkeys (201), and for MBP (peptide 111-129), which induces a chronic EAE in strain 13 guinea pigs (116). It currently is not clear whether these similarities in the recognition of certain MBP peptides are explained by similarities of proteolytic cleavage during processing of MBP or are due to other factors is currently not clear. Furthermore, a limited number of T-cell specificities might be present early during disease, and in some individuals a limited number of specificities might be present over longer periods of time (187,202).

Most of the aforementioned studies focused entirely on the most abundant MBP isoform (18.5 kDa). However, MBP exists in a variety of posttranslational modifications (leading, for example, to charge isomers due to citrullination of various numbers of arginines in the molecule) and size-isoforms (203). During recent years, it was demonstrated that such rather rare isoforms of MBP, such as amino acids encoded by exon 2 (118,204), citrullinated forms of MBP (i.e., C8), or Goli-MBP, may not only be encephalitogenic (205) but are also recognized by substantial numbers of T cells from MS patients (119).There is, for example, a stronger response to C8 in MS patients (Tranquill, Whitaker et al., unpublished results). It is interesting to note that C8, an MBP isoform with 6 citrulline modifications, is more neutral and usually occurs both early during myelin development and during remyelination (203). C8 is also accumulated in MS lesions during the course of the disease, and it has been speculated that, because of its neutral pH, C8 may destabilize the myelin bilayers because it is not able to form as tight interactions with acidic lipids. As a result, C8 may result in an increased vulnerability of myelin, providing an explanation of how immature myelin may not only serve as a target for the autoimmune T-cell response but also lead to easier breakdown of myelin and thus perpetuate disease (119).

Experiments that searched for molecular mimics of MBP demonstrated that T cell recognition by autoreactive CD4+ T cells is highly degenerate and that the MBP peptide is usually a suboptimal ligand (206). Using combinatorial peptide libraries or peptides with single and multiple aa substitutions led to the identification of molecular mimics with much higher, i.e., several orders of magnitude, stimulatory potency than the MBP peptide (206–208).

HLA-Restriction of MBP-Specific T Cells

Besides the fine specificity, it is clear from the results in EAE that the MHC/HLA background plays an important role in determining disease susceptibility. Therefore, it appeared to be of considerable interest to examine whether certain MBP peptides would be recognized preferentially in the context of the MS-associated HLA-DR- or HLA-DQ alleles. HLA-restriction of MBP-specific TCL was studied by blocking proliferation with monoclonal anti-DR-, -DP, or -DQ antibodies (181–184, 207) or by matching and mismatching effector and target cells in cytotoxicity assays with respect to their HLA-class II types. Each of the studies demonstrated preferential restriction of MBP-specific T cells by HLA-DR molecules (181–184,195,197,209), whereas only a few proliferative TCL recognized MBP in the context of HLA-DQ or HLA-DP (181,187). Each of the MS-associated HLA-DR alleles, DR2, -DR4 and -DR6, could present between five and nine different MBP peptides in cytotoxicity (183) or proliferation experiments (181,182). When studying individual peptides, a similar permissiveness was observed, e.g., the 87-106 and 152-170 peptides could both be presented by several HLA-DR molecules or even HLA-DQw6 (peptide 84-102) (195,196,210).

These data raised the question which factors are involved in determining the immunodominance of a certain myelin peptide. One explanation came from systematic in vitro peptide binding studies, which documented that MBP (peptide 83-99) binds with high affinity to the two MS-associated DR2 alleles, DR2a and DR2b but also to other alleles such as DR4 or DR13. This high binding affinity is related to the presence of ideal HLA-binding motifs that are overlapping each other in the MBP (peptide 83-99) molecule (196,198,199). However, high affinity binding cannot be the sole explanation for immunodominance. This is documented by MBP (peptide

111-129), which is highly immunodominant in the DR4 Dw4 (DRB1*0401) haplotype and nevertheless binds very poorly to this allele. In this instance, properties of the MBP-specific TCL, such as high affinity TCR and their relative overrepresentation in the TCR repertoire, seem to be the determining factor for immunodominance (see subsequent section) (211). "Promiscuous" binding (i.e., binding to several HLA-DR alleles) is not unique to the middle MBP peptide but had been reported previously for an important malaria circumsporozoite and for a tetanus toxin antigen (212,213). Myelin basic protein (peptide 83-99) is also preferentially recognized in the context of mouse (IAs, see above) and rat (RT-1) MHC molecules, supporting its potential relevance in DR2+ individuals. In summary of the aforementioned studies and experiments performed with T cells established from discordant and concordant identical twins (214), there is a tendency for MS-associated HLA-DR molecules in various populations (DR15 > DR4 > DR6 > others) to serve most often as restriction elements for T cells.

Considering the various HLA-DR haplotypes, each HLA-DR heterodimer consists of a monomorphic DR-a chain, which pairs with DR-b chains either encoded by a DRB1 or by a DRB3, -4, or -5 gene. Therefore, two DR heterodimers are encoded by each haplotype, and a total of four different DR chains may be coexpressed on the surface of cells in heterozygous individuals. It is important to keep in mind (and this is ignored by many studies of the restriction of MBP-specific T cells) that two DR-b chains are isotypically expressed on DR15 positive cells (encoded by DRB1*1501 and DRB5*0101). The two molecules are also called DR2a (DRB5*0101) and DR2b (DRB1*1501) and their relative role to serve as a restriction element for MBP-specific T cells in MS has been investigated in a few studies (197,215). At present, the relative importance of the two alleles cannot yet be assessed with certainty. From our own data and a few other reports, the following conclusions can be drawn: The preferential recognition of certain MBP peptides in the context of either DR2a or DR2b correlates with their peptide binding affinities (171,196), i.e., MBP (83-99) is immunodominant with both DR2a and DR2b and is the only peptide binding well to DR2b. In the context of DR2a, there are at least two more epitopes in the C-terminus (approximately 131-149 and 141-159) (171,196). None of the studies has so far examined sufficient numbers of TCL to conclude that DR2a is more important than DR2b in MS (171,196,197,199).

Taken together, there are so far no significant differences with respect to HLA-restriction between MBP-specific T cells from MS patients and controls. However, MS-associated HLA-DR molecules serve more often as restriction element and are highly permissive with respect to restricting several peptides. Immunodominance of a

MBP peptide in the context of a particular HLA-DR molecule relates to the presence of appropriate HLA-binding motifs and consequently high affinity binding but, in other instances, to the composition of the T-cell repertoire.

T-Cell Receptor Usage by MBP-Specific T Cells

The observation of a restricted TCR usage by encephalitogenic T cells was one of the most exciting findings during the last decade (187,191,200,214,216–222). It was hoped that, even if MBP-specific TCL show different specificities and restriction, such cells might share TCR chains that could then be employed for specific immunotherapies. TCR expression was examined either by V-region-specific antibodies or by PCR amplification with V-region family-specific primers. The initial observations that demonstrated a restricted usage of Vb17 and Vb12 in MBP (84-102)-specific T cells looked very promising, but it was not clear whether the set of clones, which was mostly derived from one patient, was sufficiently representative (218). Another study on this topic documented restricted Vb usage within individual patients but not interindividually (216). It is difficult to compare the two reports because the former focused on well-defined TCC specific for the immunodominant MBP peptide, whereas the latter contained limited information about specificity, and none of the TCC was specific for MBP (peptide 84-102). Again, a different study found a strikingly restricted usage of Vb5.2 and Vb6.1 in approximately 75 percent of MBP-specific TCL with different fine specificities and derived from DR2+ MS patients (219). These findings contrast with the first study, in which less than 10 percent expressed Vb5.2 or 6.1. Later investigations, which examined both fine specificity and TCR usage in large panels of MBP-specific TCL, found no overexpression of Vb5.2 beyond that which would be expected from the distribution in normal peripheral blood. The general consensus from most studies is that TCR usage in MBP-specific cells in general (200,217), or in TCL derived from selected patients or families (191), or in TCC specific for individual peptides, is heterogeneous (187). A recent report shed new light on the interaction between TCR usage, HLA restriction, and peptide specificity. Muraro and coworkers demonstrated that MBP peptide (111-129) is strongly immunodominant in the context of HLA-DRB1*0401 (previous designation, DR4 Dw4) (211). Different from MBP peptide (83-99), which is immunodominant in the context of DR2a and DR2b and binds with high affinity to these HLA-DR alleles (see previous), MBP peptide (111-129) binds very poorly to DR4 Dw4 molecules but is nevertheless immunodominant (211). In addition, MBP (111-129)-specific TCC show a restricted TCR usage, whereas MBP peptide (83-99)-specific TCC express very heterogeneous TCR

(200). In searching for an explanation of this discrepancy, it became clear that there are already parallels in EAE. In PL/J mice, IAu -restricted and MBP (Ac1-11)-specific TCC also express restricted numbers of TCR, and MBP (Ac1-11) binds very poorly to IAu. In contrast, in SJL mice, MBP peptide (89-101)-specific and encephalitogenic, IAs-restricted T cells are heterogeneous with respect to fine specificity and TCR usage, and the MBP peptide (89-101) binds very strongly to the IAs molecule. These differences are currently explained by the following hypothesis. The IAs-MBP (89-101) MHC/peptide [SJL mice; DR2-MBP(83-99) in humans] complex is held together tightly, and therefore the affinity requirements for TCR recognizing this complex are less stringent, i.e., it may be heterogeneous with respect to the combinations of Va/Vb chains and TCR CDR3 regions that meet this criteria. The opposite is the case with the IAu-MBP (Ac1-11) MHC/peptide complex [PL/J mice; DR4 - MBP (111-129) in humans], i.e., the MHC/peptide complex is rather unstable, and consequently only well-fitting or higher affinity TCR will be able to productively interact with these complexes. It is therefore not surprising that TCR usage is restricted in the latter situation. It must be stressed, however, that this reasoning is speculative. It is clear that a number of factors, such as MHC/peptide interactions and thus the availability of such complexes as well as selection of the T cell repertoire, both in the thymus and later during development, play important roles for immunodominance and CR usage.

Recent research has also compared the sequences of the junctional (CDR3) regions of specific clones in order to identify unique TCR sequences in MS patients. Despite overall heterogeneity, the comparison of CDR3 regions from in vivo–activated MBP-specific hypoxanthine-phosphoribosyl-transferase (hprt) negative T cells with those from TCR expressed in MS brains, TCR expressed by encephalitogenic T cells in EAE, and a human MBP-specific cytotoxic TCL from an MS patient showed strikingly similar amino acid stretches (223). Another study documented that the sequences of CDR3 regions from Va8-expressing T cells derived from bulk TCL that had been expanded by either MBP or tetanus toxoid (TT), show a limited degree of heterogeneity, but became more diverse with duration of disease, suggesting recruitment of new populations of T cells (224). Careful longitudinal studies of single TCRs, even though they could so far not link individual TCRs to fluctuations of disease activity, have found remarkable stability of T cell clones over years (225).

Combined, the aforementioned studies have documented how difficult it is to obtain conclusive information in the outbred human population of MS patients. So far, most if not all of the studies have suffered from the limited numbers of patients and controls, often small number of TCC, and the lack of stratification of patients with respect to disease duration, phenotype, and immunogenetic background. Therefore, despite increasing sophistication of immunologic techniques, there are still many unanswered questions. The influence of genetic background, most importantly differences in HLA expression, was eliminated in one report by comparing the expressed TCR a-chain repertoire of identical twins discordant or concordant for MS (214). Although the authors found similar TCR a-chain distributions in unstimulated PBL for each set of twin regardless of disease state, a remarkable skewing in the TCR a-chain repertoire was observed following stimulation with self-antigens (MBP) or foreign antigens (tetanus toxoid). Concordant twins had selected the same TCR Va-chains, whereas discordant twins used different ones (214). Whether the differences in TCR repertoires had developed before onset of disease and thus were predisposing, or whether they developed during the chronic disease, could not be addressed. The demonstration of different TCR repertoires in response to specific antigenic stimuli in individuals with identical immunogenetic backgrounds at least supported the idea that T cells and the TCR repertoire may be important for disease pathogenesis.

TCR Usage in the Brain

The aforementioned studies dealt with TCR expression of peripheral blood lymphocytes. Whether this reflects the disease-relevant cell population is not clear, and therefore other researchers examined the TCR a-chain and b-chain usage in the lesions of brain autopsy tissue derived from MS patients (33,46,220,221). One of these reports documented a limited Va-chain usage (Va10 in all three brains, Va8 and Va12 in two brains each, and two to four rearranged Va-chains in three MS brains) (220). Another study found a limited expression of Va and Vb chains in chronic but not in acute plaques (33). When the TCR expression in brain lesions was correlated with molecular HLA types, a limited degree of heterogeneity in Va and Vb chain expression was found (221). Seven of seven individuals with the HLA haplotype HLA-DR1*1501, DQA1*0102, DQB1*0602 expressed Vb5.2, and six of seven expressed Vb6.1 in lesion-derived T cells (221). Furthermore, the brain-derived TCR sequences shared important junctional amino acid stretches with a Vb5.2-expressing MBP-specific TCL from a DR15 positive MS patient (195), indicating that MBP-specific T cells with a specific junctional region may be specific for the immunodominant MBP peptide, restricted by DR15 and possibly involved in the pathogenesis of MS.

In summary, although we have learned a lot about the TCR usage in MS patients and made some important observations, i.e., shared sequences between rodents and humans, the demonstration of skewing of the TCR repertoire in discordant monozygotic twins, the increasing diversity of TCR with ongoing disease, the relationship between MHC/peptide binding and TCR diversity, as well as the shared TCR sequences in lesions and MBP (83-99)-specific T cells, we are far from understanding these interactions to the point that we can claim that a certain T-cell population is relevant for disease or could use TCRs for therapeutic purposes.

Phenotype and Function of MBP-Specific T Cells

CD4+ Th1 cells mediate the inflammatory process in EAE and virus-induced demyelinating diseases, but the extent of demyelination may be modified by myelin-specific antibodies, which suggests that Th2-mechanisms also play a role. This is underlined by the worsening of MS by IFN-γ (226). The role of other proinflammatory cytokines, i.e., TNF-α/β, on the demyelinating process, has been summarized before and is supported by the finding of increased TNF-α levels in the CSF during clinical exacerbations of MS (41,227) and by increased TNF-α secretion by DR2-restricted TCL from MS patients (228). Another sign of increased T-cell activation in MS is that IL-2 levels in the peripheral blood are also elevated (40,42).

The following characteristics were found for human MBP-specific T cells: Similar to encephalitogenic T cells, they belong almost exclusively to the CD4+ T lymphocyte phenotype (181,183–186,229). With respect to their function, most of the studies of human MBP-specific T cells focused on antigen-specific proliferation, but it was also documented that a large percentage are cytotoxic (183,189,209) and secrete significant amounts of IFN-γ and TNF-α/β (229,230). Whether myelin-specific cytotoxicity is involved in disease pathogenesis is not clear in EAE. It is interesting that human MBP-specific cytotoxicity can involve three different lysis mechanisms, i.e., Fas-Fas-ligand–mediated, apoptotic killing, perforin-mediated lysis and a novel type of target cell lysis that involves homotypic CD56/NCAM interactions (231,232). The latter is particularly attractive because the CD56-mediated lysis does not require the presence of autologous HLA-DR molecules. Oligodendrocytes do not express HLA-class II molecules but do express NCAM, a homologue of CD56, and it was recently shown that oligodendrocyte may in fact be lysed by CD56-expressing CD4+ T/NK cells (233). Although MBP-specific, cytotoxic Th1-like T cells are found in both patients and contro ls, the similarities with EAE-mediating T cells nevertheless suggest that such cells could play a role in the pathogenesis of MS. The involvement of activated T cells in the pathogenesis of MS is supported by increasing IL-2- and IFN-γ–secreting cells (186) and soluble IL-2 receptors (42) as well as increases in adhesion molecules expression (VLA3-6, LFA1 and LFA3, CD2, CD26 and CD44) on CSF T cell (234).

A small fraction of MBP-specific T cells are CD4/CD8 double positive and may not yet be fully differentiated (Martin R, Flerlage M, McFarland HF, unpublished results). Their role is not clear, and neither is that of CD8⁺ T cells, which may also be found in demyelinating lesions. This mostly cytolytic T cell population could lyse oligodendrocytes directly via a MHC-/HLA-class I–restricted cytolytic mechanism (235), but lysis may also be mediated through g/d T cells (236), a mechanism called *bystander lysis* or via CD56/NCAM, as discussed previously. CD8⁺, HLA-class I–restricted cytotoxic T cells with specificity for MPB, MAG, MOG, and PLP from patients and controls have successfully been established by using the knowledge of HLA-class I peptide-binding motifs (237). These cells secrete TNF-α, are capable of lysing oligodendrocytes (235), and may thus also be involved in tissue damage in MS white matter. Furthermore, as demonstrated by T-cell vaccination studies in EAE and also in MS, the CD8⁺ T-cell population could also contain regulatory T cells (238,239), which may exert their function in a number of ways: (a) direct recognition of myelin-specific T cells and interference by direct lysis of autoreactive T cells, or (b) indirectly via the release of modulatory cytokines such as IL-4, IL-10, and TGF-β. Cells that secrete IL-4 and TGF-β are elevated in the CSF of patients with optic neuritis or MS patients (240), although it is still difficult to interpret these observations. Our own data document that CD4⁺ MBP-specific T cells express a wide variety of cytokine phenotypes, with many intermediates from full Th1 to full Th2 cells (241). Different from the mouse system, where IL-10 was clearly categorized as a Th2 cytokine, the situation is less clear in human TCC, in which most clones secrete IL-10. The cytokine patterns are stable over long periods of time, suggesting that the in vivo commitment is kept during in vitro culture (241). Although there is a slight overrepresentation of Th1-like cells, the difference between cells from MS patients and controls is not drastic. However, according to results with PLP-specific T cells, Th1-cells are more abundant during clinical exacerbations, whereas Th0- and Th2-like cells are easier to expand in periods of remissions (242,243). The reduced requirements for co-stimulatory signals, such as B7.1-CD28 interactions, indicates a generally different activation state of MS T cells, which may mean that quantitatively or qualitatively less stimulus may be sufficient to drive the activation of myelin-specific T cells in MS (244,245).

The role of the activation requirements, functional phenotypes, involvement of oligodendrocyte cytolysis, and regulation of T-cell growth, e.g., by apoptosis or regulatory cytokines, are so far incompletely understood in EAE and even more so in MS. Recent studies indicate that there may be an imbalance in the Fas-Fas-ligand–mediated apoptotic pathway in MS (246). Further studies will hopefully allow us to determine which cells mediate disease, not only to develop a pathogenetic scenario but also to follow them along the disease course (i.e., as surrogate marker) and eventually to develop more specific therapies.

T-Cell Responses to Other Myelin Antigens

During recent years, antigens other than MBP or modified forms of MBP have received increasing attention because of improvements in isolation or recombinant expression and peptide synthesis, and also because the studies with human MBP-specific T cells were conclusive only to a limited degree. The antigens of interest included major myelin antigens such as PLP (247-250), and isoforms of MBP (29,30), but also minor antigens such as MOG (128,251,252), myelin-associated glycoprotein (MAG) (128,248,252,253), 2'3'-cyclic nuleotide 3' phosphodiesterase (CNPase) (254), transaldolase-H (Tal-H), a protein encoded by an HTLV-derived endogenous retroviral sequence (255), a-B crystallin, and a small heat shock protein expressed in myelin (256).

PLP is a highly conserved and extremely hydrophobic protein. Because of its high hydrophobicity, it is almost impossible to keep PLP in solution, and therefore most laboratories have switched either to the extramembraneous or cytosolic loops or to synthetic overlapping peptides spanning these extracellular domains (257). PLP-specific T cells could be established by various techniques both from peripheral blood and from CSF (194,248,249,258). Several areas of PLP, including PLP peptide (40-60) (248), PLP peptide (89-106) (249), and PLP peptide (184-209) (258), were recognized by a substantial number of TCL. In terms of phenotype and function, PLP-specific TCL are comparable to MBP-specific TCL, i.e., most of them are restricted by HLA-DR molecules, and many show cytotoxic activity (194,248,249,258). Also, when PLP-specific clones from MS patients in relapse or remission were established, the former tended to be preferentially Th1-like and the latter Th0-like, arguing for a role in disease (242). It is still controversial whether T-cell reactivity to PLP is increased in MS patients compared with controls because both increased reactivity in patients (189,250) and similar responses (184,248) have been reported.

The information about myelin-associated glycoprotein (MAG) is more limited. Only a few studies have addressed the question of whether MAG-specific T cells can be established from MS patients and controls (128,247,252,253). The data have been inconsistent and ranged from low-level reactivity only in patients with active disease (252) to elevated frequencies of MAG-specific T cells in both PBL and CSF of MS patients (259). This limited knowledge is probably due to difficulties isolating this large protein, which constitutes only a small fraction of total myelin proteins.

Following the interesting observations in EAE that antibodies against myelin oligodendroglia glycoprotein (MOG) enhance demyelination, a lot of attention has been focused on this protein (128,251,252). Although MOG is only found in minor quantities in CNS tissue, an enhanced MOG-specific T-cell response has been documented in MS patients even when primary proliferation was used as a readout (128). Information about the immunodominant areas of MOG in MS patients and controls is just beginning to emerge, and so far one of the encephalitogenic regions [MOG (35-55)] elicited strong responses, but an N-terminal region and more C-terminal also appear to be immunodominant (260).

Other groups employed different approaches, such as testing the T-cell response in MS patients against HPLC-separated fractions of MS-myelin (261). Surprisingly, the "classic" myelin components played a minor role within this material, and the T-cell response was preferentially directed against a small heat shock protein, a B-crystallin (256). Whether this protein is able to induce a demyelinating disease in animals is currently being examined.

The list of potential candidate autoantigens expanded further during the last few years. Reactivity of CSF antibodies against transaldolase-H (Tal-H), an oligodendrocyte enzyme that is encoded by an HTLV-I–derived gene, was found in a majority of tested MS patients and, although still preliminary, the same investigators also documented a Tal-H-specific T cell response (255).

The third most abundant myelin protein, CNPase, has also attracted interest, but so far very little is known both about the physiologic role of this enzyme or its potential involvement in demyelinating disease. CNPase-specific $CD4^+$ T cells can be generated by stimulation with whole native CNPase, CNPase peptides, or recombinant CNPase (254) (Kalbus M, Muraro P, et al., manuscripts in preparation). However, it was so far not possible to induce EAE with this protein in some of the EAE-susceptible strains (Sommer N, Sappler G, et al., unpublished results). Nor is there information about whether the CNPase-specific T-cell response is enhanced in MS patients.

Research in this area is complicated not only by the fact that many of these proteins are extremely difficult to isolate but also because all of them may occur in multiple posttranslationally modifications or size isoforms (119). As examples, amino acids encoded by exon 2 of the MBP gene, which are found in the 21.0 kDa MBP isoform, are not only encephalitogenic but also are a target for human T cells derived from MS patients (262). The same is true for two other MBP "derivatives," golli-MBP, an MBP protein with an N-terminal extension that is expressed in the thymus (263), and citrullinated C8-MBP (119). Each of these modified MBP forms is encephalitogenic. It is interesting that C8 appears not only earlier during myelin development than the mature and basic form of MBP but also during remyelination. It was found that the myelin of MS patients builds up more and more of the neutral C8 protein with increasing demyelination (see above). C8-specific TCL can be established from MS patients and controls (119), and recent data indicate an elevated response to C8 in patients (Whitaker JN, et al., manuscript in preparation).

What can we learn from the preceding data? It is obvious by now that T cells can be raised against almost any of the myelin components. Some of the studies indicate that the response to individual proteins or peptides are elevated in patients, but the numbers of individuals often were too small to allow definitive conclusions. Furthermore, only a few reports took into account whether T cells had been preactivated in vivo, or whether they were derived from memory versus naive cells or from CSF versus peripheral blood. Beyond these technical concerns, it is becoming increasingly clear that different disease phenotypes can be induced in different animal strains by different antigens (110). For example, MBP-induced disease in Lewis rats is a monophasic and inflammatory disease, whereas a chronic-relapsing course with marked demyelination is observed in MBP-induced or PLP-induced disease in SJL mice. If an astroglia constituent, S-100, is used to immunize Lewis rats, they will only suffer from inflammation without any clinical signs (264). Disease induction with MOG in BN rats is characterized by a severe and fulminant course of disease similar to that observed in the Marburg type of MS (Linington et al., personal communication), and in general the antigen specificity of encephalitogenic T lymphocytes appeared to determine at least in part the distribution of lesions in the CNS (265). If we wanted to extrapolate this information to MS, it is not too far-fetched to expect a wide variety of courses and phenotypes in the outbred human population, depending on an individual's immunogenetic background and the target autoantigen. In the future, we will therefore have to stratify the MS patients for similar studies according to their mostly involved CNS areas, HLA-type, course of disease, and so forth. Additionally, the question of specificity in autoimmune diseases may need to be revisited entirely based on our recent observations that autoantigens are unlikely to be the natural ligand for the T cells that we establish with MBP or other myelin compnents (206,208). Our recent data obtained with combinatorial peptide libraries show that T cells are highly degenerate in their recognition and that peptide ligands can be defined that are orders of magnitude more potent in triggering such cells than the autoantigenic peptide itself (206). This suggests that autoreactivity is probably a common and frequently occurring phenomenon, but that additional factors such as the upregulation of MHC density, adhesion molecules, and costimulatory molecules, both on the T cells and in the target tissue, are required to start the autoimmune damage of a certain target tissue.

LESSONS FROM MS TREATMENT

The concept that MS is an immune-mediated disease finds support in the response to immunosuppressive or immunomodulatory treatment (266,267). Corticosteroids that exert strong short-term antiinflammatory and immunosuppressive actions (269) are known to shorten the severity and duration of relapses, most likely by closing the blood–brain barrier, reducing edema in the lesions, and suppressing multiple immunologic functions. However, steroids do not alter the long-term course of MS. Immunosuppressants, including azathioprine and cyclophosphamide, may have some beneficial effects in terms of reducing exacerbation rate and clinical progression, although general agreement on the effectiveness of these drugs is lacking (266,270). During the past few years, two new treatments have been introduced and approved for MS, interferon-β (IFN-β) (267,268) and glatiramer acetate (271–273). IFN-b reduces the exacerbation rate and slows the clinical progression of disease, but the overall effect is moderate. Although type I interferons have been known for almost three decades, there is at present only an incomplete understanding of how IFN-β modulates disease activity in MS. Its action is thought to be mediated by antagonizing one of the major proinflammatory cytokines, i.e., IFN-γ, and through the induction of IL-10 (275), but this does not seem to account for its entire mechanism of action (96). Glatiramer acetate is probably as effective as IFN-β, but it has a milder side-effect profile. According to EAE experiments, glatiramer acetate primarily acts through interference with antigen presentation to autoreactive T cells, but in part also by inducing suppressive T cell populations. These treatments are considered important advances and have given us drugs of proven efficacy. However, they are still far from ideal in stopping disease activity completely, or even in reversing some of the clinical signs. Therefore, many new treatments are being developed or are already in clinical testing. These include vaccination with specific TCR variable chain-derived peptides or whole inactivated myelin-specific T cells (270), administration of growth factors (IGF-1), (275), immunomodulatory cytokines such as TGF-b (276) and IL-10 (277), and blockade of adhesion molecules with antibodies against CD4+, VCAM, and ICAM, oral tolerization with MBP (278), retinoic acid (279), MHC-peptide complexes, unspecific and family-specific phosphodiesterase inhibitors (280,281), and others. This list is not complete, but it provides the reader with an impression of the spectrum of different approaches. In the future, it is hoped that we will learn more about the disease pathogenesis of MS, in part through highly specific therapeutic strategies, but, more importantly, our therapeutic arsenal should improve and allow us to offer specifically tailored medication for the various stages and courses of disease. Using MRI and other sophisticated neuroimaging techniques, we will not only be able to diagnose MS earlier, but also employ this technique to monitor the efficacy of novel therapies (282–284).

DIRECTION OF FUTURE RESEARCH

In recent years, multiple sclerosis research has made significant progress in many areas, including the potential triggers of disease, its immunopathogenesis and diagnostic monitoring, and therapy. From what has proceeded, it is obvious that we need to learn more. Compared with animal experiments, many factors remain uncertain because conclusions with respect to the preceding topics are often based on indirect data and extrapolations from parallels with EAE. Myelin-specific T cells are thought to be involved in the disease process but are certainly not sufficient by themselves. Additional genetic factors, the so-called immunogenetic background, as well as exogenous triggers, are necessary for disease. However, so far we have no specific diagnostic markers, and it is not clear whether MS represents a single disease entity or a group of diseases that share a similar pathogenesis but have different triggers. Both clinical and genetic evidence indicate that the two major forms of MS, i.e., relapsing-remitting and primary chronic progressive, may be different. The many similarities between MS and EAE with respect to shared immunodominant epitopes, Th1-bias, and clinical phenotypes argue for common pathomechanisms, but many questions remain unanswered at present.

During the next years, it will be crucial to carefully assess which genes contribute to susceptibility, which MRI parameters best reflect the various stages of tissue damage, how we can address the lesion pathology by careful histopathologic evaluation, which immunologic markers may be useful to follow inflammatory activity, and how we may best treat early stages of MS without inflicting much harm. New therapeutic approaches will be important not only as a treatment but also as a means to understand the immunologic mechanisms involved in the pathogenesis of MS.

References

1. Martin R, McFarland HF, McFarlin DE. Immunological aspects of demyelinating diseases. *Annu Rev Immunol* 1992; 10:153–187.
2. Prineas JW. The neuropathology of multiple sclerosis. In: Vinken PJ, Bruyn GW, Klawans HL, Koetsier JC (eds.). *Handbook of clinical neurology, Demyelinating diseases.*

3rd ed. Amsterdam/New York: Elsevier Science, 1985:213–257.

3. Trapp BD, Peterson J, Ransohoff RM, et al. Axonal transection in the lesions of multiple sclerosis. *N Engl J Med* 1998; 338:278–285.

4. Johnson RT, Griffin DE. Virus-induced autoimmune demyelinating disease of the central nervous system. In: Notkins AL, Oldstone MBA (eds.). *Concepts in viral pathogenesis.* 2nd ed. New York: Springer, 1986:203–209.

5. Sibley WA, Bamford CR, Clark K. Clinical viral infections and multiple sclerosis. *Lancet* 1985; 1:1313–1315.

6. Kurtzke JF. Epidemiology of multiple sclerosis. In: Vinken PJ, Bruyn GW, Klawans HL, Koetsier JC (eds.). *Handbook of clinical neurology.* 3rd ed. Amsterdam/New York: Elsevier Science, 1985:259–287.

7. Levy RM, Bredeson DE, Rosenblum ML. Opportunistic central nervous system pathology in patients with AIDS. *Ann Neurol* 1988; 23(Suppl):7–12.

8. Jacobson S, Gupta A, Mattson DH, Mingioli ES, McFarlin DE. Immunological studies in tropical spastic paraparesis. *Ann Neurol* 1990; 27.

9. Osame M, Matsumoto M, Usuku K. Chronic-progressive myelopathy associated with elevated antibodies to human T-lymphotrophic virus type I and adult T-cell leukemia-like cells. *Ann Neurol* 1987; 21:117–122.

10. Jacobson S, Shida H, McFarlin DE, Fauci AS, Koenig S. Circulating CD8+ cytotoxic T lymphocytes specific for HTLV-I pX in patients with HTLV-I associated neurological disease. *Nature* 1990; 348:245–248.

11. Levin MC, Lehky TJ, Flerlage AN, et al. Immunologic analysis of a spinal cord–biopsy specimen from a patient with human T-cell lymphotropic virus type I–associated neurologic disease. *New Engl J Med* 1997; 336:839–845.

12. Dhib-Jalbut S, Hoffman PM, Yamabe T, et al. Extracellular human T-lymphotropic virus type I tax protein induces cytokine production in adult human microglial cells. *Ann Neurol* 1994; 36:787–790.

13. Jacobson S, Lehky T, Nishimura M, et al. Isolation of HTLV-II from a patient with chronic, progressive neurological disease clinically indistinguishable from HTLV-I-associated myelopathy/tropical spastic paraparesis. *Ann Neurol* 1993; 33:392–396.

14. Johnson RT, Griffin DE, Hirsch JS, et al. Measles encephalomyelitis: Clinial and immunological studies. *New Engl J Med* 1984; 310:137–141.

15. Sibley WA, Bamford CR, CLark K, Smith MS, Laguna JF. A prospective study of physical trauma and multiple sclerosis. *J Neurol Neurosurg Psychiatry* 1991; 54:584–589.

16. Martin R, Marquardt P, O'Shea S, Borkenstein M, Kreth HW. Virus-specific and autoreactive T-cell lines isolated from cerebrospinal fluid of a patient with chronic rubella panencephalitis. *J Neuroimmunol* 1989; 23:1–10.

17. Martin R, Ortlauf J, Sticht-Groh V, et al. *Borrelia burgdorferi*-specific and autoreactive T-cell lines from cerebrospinal fluid in Lyme radiculomyelitis. *Ann Neurol* 1988; 24:509–516.

18. Challoner PB, Smith KT, Parker JD, et al. Plaque-associated expression of human herpesvirus 6 in multiple sclerosis. *Proc Natl Acad Sci USA* 1995; 92:7440–7444.

19. Soldan SS, Berti R, Salem N, et al. Association of human herpes virus 6 (HHV-6) with multiple sclerosis: increased IgM response to HHV-6 early antigen and detection of serum HHV-6 DNA. *Nature Med* 1997; 3:1394–1397.

20. Kappler J, Kotzin B, Herron L, et al. Vb-specific stimu-

lation of human T cells by staphylococcal toxins. *Science* 1989; 244:811–813.

21. Wucherpfennig KW, Strominger JL. Molecular mimicry in T cell-mediated autoimmunity: viral peptides activate human T cell clones specific for myelin basic protein. *Cell* 1995; 80.

22. Zhao ZS, Granucci F, Yeh L, Schaffer PH, Cantor H. Molecular mimicry by herpes simplex virus-type 1: autoimmune disease after viral infection. *Science* 1998; 279:1344–1347.

23. Clatch RJ, Lipton HL, Miller SD. Characterization of Theiler's murine encephalomyelitis virus (TMEV)-specific delayed-type hypersensitivity responses in TMEV-induced demyelinating diseases: Correlation with clinical signs. *J Immunol* 1986; 136:920–927.

24. Chamorro M, Aubert C, Brahic M. Demyelinating lesions due to Theiler's virus are associated with central nervous system infection. *J Virol* 1986; 57:992–997.

25. Lipton HL, Dal Canto MC. Theiler's virus induced demyelination—prevention by immunosuppression. *Science* 1976; 192:62–64.

26. Peterson JD, Karpus WJ, Clatch RJ, Miller SD. Split tolerance of Th1 and Th2 cells in tolerance to Theiler's murine encephalomyelitis virus. *Eur J Immunol* 1993; 23:46–55.

27. Watanabe R, Wege H, ter Meulen V. Adoptive transfer of EAE-like lesions from rats with coronavirus-induced demyelinating encephalomyelitis. *Nature* 1983; 305:150–152.

28. Liebert UG, Hashim GA, ter Meulen V. Characterization of measles virus-induced cellular autoimmune reactions against myelin basic protein in Lewis rats. *J Neuroimmunol* 1990; 29:139–147.

29. Haase AT. Pathogenesis of lentivirus infections. *Nature* 1986; 322:130–136.

30. Narayan O, Sheffler D, Clements JE. Restricted replication of lentiviruses. *J Exp Med* 1985; 162:1954–1969.

31. Brück W, Schmied M, Suchanek G, et al. Oligodendrocytes in the early course of multiple sclerosis. *Ann Neurol* 1994; 35:65–73.

32. Raine CS. Multiple sclerosis and chronic relapsing EAE: Comparative ultrastructural neuropathology. In: J.F. Hallpike JF, C.W. Adams CW, W.W. Tourtellotte WW (eds.). *Multiple sclerosis.* Baltimore: Williams & Wilkins. 1983:413–478.

33. Wucherpfennig KW, Newcombe J, Li H, et al. T cell receptor Va-Vb repertoire and cytokine gene expression in active multiple sclerosis lesions. *J Exp Med* 1992; 175:993–1002.

34. Traugott U, Scheinberg LC, Raine CS. On the presence of Ia-positive endothelial cells and astrocytes in multiple sclerosis lesions and its relevance to antigen presentation. *J Neuroimmunol* 1985; 8:1–14.

35. Hofman FM, von Hanwehr RI, Dinarello CA. Immunoregulatory molecules and IL-2 receptors identified in multiple sclerosis brain. *J Immunol* 1986; 136:3239–3245.

36. Washington R, Burton J, Todd RF, et al. Expression of immunologically relevant endothelial cell activation antigens on isolated central nervous system microvessels from patients with multiple sclerosis. *Ann Neurol* 1994; 35:89–97.

37. Raine CS. Biology of disease: The analysis of autoimmune demyelination: Its impact on multiple sclerosis. *Lab Invest* 1984; 50:608–635.

38. Hauser SL, Bhan AK, Gilles F. Immunohistochemical

analysis of the cellular infiltrate in multiple sclerosis lesion. *Ann Neurol* 1986; 19:578–587.

39. Booss J, Esiri MM, Tourtellotte WW. Immunohistochemical analysis of T-lymphocyte subsets in the central nervous system in chronic progressive multiple sclerosis. *J Neurol Sci* 1983; 62:19–32.

40. Hartung H-P, Hughes RAC, Taylor WA, et al. T cell activation in Guillain-Barré syndrome and in MS: Elevated serum levels of soluble IL-2 receptors. *Neurology* 1990; 40:215–218.

41. Sharief MK, Hentges R. Association between tumor necrosis factor-a and disease progression in chronic progressive multiple sclerosis. *New Engl J Med* 1991; 325:467–472.

42. Sharief MK, Thompson EJ. Correlation of interleukin-2 and soluble interleukin-2 receptor with clinical activity of multiple sclerosis. *J Neurol Neurosurg Psychiatry* 1993; 56:169–174.

43. Hartung H-P. Immune-mediated demyelination. *Ann Neurol* 1993; 33:563–567.

44. Sanders ME, Koski CL, Robbins D. Activated terminal complement in cerebrospinal fluid in Guillain-Barré syndrome and multiple sclerosis. *J Immunol* 1986; 136: 4456–4459.

45. Selmaj K, Brosnan CF, Raine CS. Expression of heat shock protein-65 by oligodendrocytes in vivo and in vitro: implications for multiple sclerosis. *Neurology* 1992; 42:795–800.

46. Wucherpfennig KW, Newcombe J, Li H, Keddy C. Gamma delta T cell receptor repertoire in acute multiple sclerosis lesions. *Proc Natl Acad Sci USA* 1992; 89:4588–4592.

47. Selmaj K, Brosnan CF, Raine CS. Colocalization of lymphocytes bearing gamma delta T-cell receptor and heat shock protein hsp65+ oligodendrocytes in multiple sclerosis. *Proc Natl Acad Sci USA* 1991; 88:6452–6456.

48. Hvas J, Oksenberg JR, Fernando R, Steinman L, Bernard CC. Gamma delta T cell receptor repertoire in brain lesions of patients with multiple sclerosis. *J Neuroimmunol* 1993; 46:225–234.

49. Wekerle H, Linington C, Lassmann H, Meyermann R. Cellular immune reactivity within the CNS. *Trends Neuro Sci* 1986; 9:271–277.

50. Nathanson JA, Chun LL. Immunological function of the blood-cerebrospinal fluid barrier. *Proc Natl Acad Sci USA* 1989; 86:1684–1688.

51. Cannella B, Raine CS. The adhesion molecule and cytokine profile of multiple sclerosis lesions. *Ann Neurol* 1995; 37:424–435.

52. Burger DR, Ford D, Vetto RM, et al. Endothelial cell presentation of antigen to human T cells. *Hum Immunol* 1981; 3:209–230.

53. McCarron RM, Kempski O, Spatz M, McFarlin DE. Presentation of myelin basic protein by murine cerebral vascular endothelial cells. *J Immunol* 1985; 134:3100–3103.

54. McCarron RM, Spatz M, Kempski O, et al. Interaction between myelin basic protein-sensitized T lymphocytes and murine cerebral vascular endothelial cells. *J Immunol* 1986; 137:3428–3435.

55. Shrikant P, Benveniste EN. The central nervous system as an immunocompetent organ: role of glial cells in antigen presentation. *J Immunol* 1996; 157:1819–1822.

56. Fontana A, Fierz W, Wekerle H. Astrocytes present myelin basic protein to encephalitogenic T-cell lines. *Nature* 1984; 307:273–276.

57. Sun D, Wekerle H. Ia-restricted encephalitogenic T lymphocytes mediating EAE lyse autoantigen-presenting astrocytes. *Nature* 1986; 320:70–72.

58. Massa PT, ter Meulen V, Fontana A. Hyperinducibility of Ia antigen on astrocytes correlates with strain-specific susceptibility to experimental autoimmune encephalomyelitis. *Proc Natl Acad Sci USA* 1987; 84:4219–4223.

59. Cash E, Zhang Y, Rott O. Microglia present myelin antigens to T cells after phagocytosis of oligodendrocytes. *Cell Immunol* 1993; 147:129–138.

60. Dhib-Jalbut S, Kufta CV, Flerlage M, Shimojo N, McFarland HF. Adult human glial cells can present target antigens to HLA-restricted cytotoxic T-cells. *J Neuroimmunol* 1990; 29:203–211.

61. Frei K, Siepl C, Groscurth P, et al. Antigen presentation and tumor cytotoxicity by interferon-gamma-treated microglial cells. *Eur J Immunol* 1987; 17:1271–1278.

62. Hickey WF, Kimura H. Perivascular microglia cells of the central nervous system are bone marrow derived and present antigen in vivo. *Science* 1988; 239:290–292.

63. Williams K, Bar-Or A, Ulvestad E, et al. Biology of adult human microglia in culture: comparisons with peripheral blood monocytes and astrocytes. *J Neuropathol Exp Neurol* 1992; 51:538–549.

64. Williams K, Ulvestad E, Cragg L, Blain M, Antel JP. Induction of primary T cell responses by human glial cells. *J Neurosci Res* 1993; 36:382–390.

65. Williams K, Ulvestad E, Antel JP. Detection of immunoregulatory B7-1 and IL-10 in human adult microglia. *J Neuroimmunol* 1994; 54:150.

66. Williams KC, Dooley NP, Ulvestaad E, et al. Antigen presentation by human fetal astrocytes with the cooperative effect of microglia or the microglial-derived cytokine IL-1. *J Neurosci* 1995; 15:1869–1878.

67. Dhib-Jalbut S, Gogate N, Jiang H, Eisenberg H, Bergey G. Human microglia activate lymphoproliferative responses to recall viral antigens. *J Neuroimmunol* 1995; 65:67–73.

68. Ford AL, Goodsall AL, Hickey WF, Sedgwick JD. Normal adult ramified microglia separated from other central nervous system macrophages by flow cytometric sorting. Phenotypic differences defined and direct ex vivo antigen presentation to myelin basic protein-reactive CD4+ T cells compared. *J Neuroimmunol* 1995; 154: 4309–4321.

69. Hayes GM, Woodroofe MN, Cuzner ML. Microglia are the major cell type expressing MHC class II in human white matter. *J Neurol Sci* 1987; 80:25–37.

70. Sedgwick JD, Schwender S, Imrich H, et al. Isolation and direct characterization of resident microglial cells from the normal and inflamed central nervous system. *Proc Natl Acad Sci USA* 1991; 88:7438–7442.

71. Ma C-G, Zhang G-X, Xiao G-G, et al. Suppression of experimental autoimmune myasthenia gravis by nasal administration of acetylcholine receptor. *J Neuroimmunol* 1995; 58:51–60.

72. Hickey WF, Kimura H. Perviascular microglial cells of the CNS are bone-marrow derived and present antigen in vivo. *Science* 1988; 239:290–293.

73. Frei K, Fontana A. Cytokines in the brain. Antigen presentation in the CNS. *Mol Psychiatry* 1997; 2:96–98.

74. Klyushnenkova EN, Vanguri P. Ia expression and antigen presentation by glia: strain and cell-type specific differences amont rat astrocytes and microglia. *J Neuroimmunol* 1997; 79:190–201.

75. Fallis RJ, McFarlin DE. Chronic relapsing experimental

allergic encephalomyelitis. Cytotoxicity effected by a class II restricted T cell line specific for an encephalitogenic epitope. *J Immunol* 1989; 143:2160–2165.

76. Dhib-Jalbut S, McFarlin DE. Macrophages, microglia and other antigen-presenting cells in neurological disorders. *Prog Neuroendocrin Immunol* 1989; 2:86–95.

77. Frohman EM, van den Noort S, Gupta S. Astrocytes and intracerebral immune responses. *J Clin Immunol* 1989; 9:1–9.

78. Lee SC, Collins M, Vanguri P, Shin ML. Glutamate differentially inhibits the expression of class II MHC antigens on astrocytes and microglia. *J Immunol* 1992; 148:3391–3397.

79. Smith ME, McFarlin DE, Dhib-Jalbut S. Differential effect of interleukin-1 beta on Ia expression in astrocytes and microglia. *J. Neuroimmunol.* 1993; 46:97–104.

80. Dhib-Jalbut S. Mechanisms of IFNb action in multiple sclerosis. *Multiple Sclerosis* 1997; 3:397–401.

81. Frei K, Lins H, Schwerdel C, Fontana A. Antigen presentation in the central nervous system. The inhibitory effect of IL-10 on MHC class II expression and production of cytokines depends on the inducing signals and the type of cell analyzed. *J Immunol* 1994; 152:2720–2728.

82. Panek RB, Benveniste EN. Class II MHC gene expression in microglia. Regulation by the cytokines IFN-gamma, TNF-alpha, and TGF-beta1. *J Immunol* 1995; 154:2846–2854.

83. Suzumura A, Sawada M, Itoh Y, Marunouchi T. Interleukin-4 induces proliferation and activation of microglia but suppresses their induction of class II major histocompatibility complex antigen expression. *J Neuroimmunol* 1994; 53:209–218.

84. Hayashi M, Dorf ME, Abromson-Leeman S. Granulocyte-macrophage colony stimulating factor inhibits class II major histocompatibility complex expression and antigen presentation by microglia. *J Neuroimmunol* 1993; 48:23–32.

85. Ebers GC. Genetic factors in multiple sclerosis. *Neurol Clin* 1983; 1:645–654.

86. Compston A, Sadovnick AD. Epidemiology and Genetics of Multiple Sclerosis. *Curr Opinion Neurol Neurosurgery* 1992; 5:175–181.

87. Sadovnick AD, Armstrong H, Rice GP, et al. A population-based study of multiple sclerosis in twins: update. *Ann Neurol* 1993; 33:281–285.

88. Lynch SG, Rose JW, Smoker W, Petajan JH. MRI in familial multiple sclerosis. *Neurology* 1991; 40:900–903.

89. McFarland HF. Twin studies and multiple sclerosis. *Ann Neurol* 1992; 32:722–723.

90. Ebers GC, Dessa Sadovnick A. The role of genetic factors in multiple sclerosis susceptibility. *J Neuroimmunol* 1994; 54:1–17.

91. Oksenberg JR, Steinman L. The role of the MHC and T-cell receptor in susceptibility to multiple sclerosis. *Curr Opinion Immunol* 1990; 2:619–621.

92. Zinkernagel RM, Doherty PC. Restriction of in vitro T cell-mediated cytotoxicity in lymphocytic choriomeningitis within a syngeneic or semiallogeneic system. *Nature* 1974; 248:701–702.

93. Nepom GG, Erlich H. MHC class-II molecules and autoimmunity. *Annu Rev Immunol* 1991; 9:493–526.

94. Vartdal F, Sollid LM, Vandvik B, Markussen G, Thorsby E. Patients with multiple sclerosis carry DQB1 genes which encode shared polymorphic aminoacid sequences. *Hum Immunol* 1989; 25:103–110.

95. Epplen C, Jäckel S, Santos EJM, et al. Genetic predispo-

sition to multiple sclerosis as revealed by immunoprinting. *Ann Neurol* 1997; 41:341–352.

96. Olerup O, Hillert J, Frederikson S, et al. Primarily chronic progressive and relapsing/remitting multiple sclerosis: Two immunogenetically distinct disease entities. *Proc Natl Acad Sci USA* 1989; 86:7113–7117.

97. Haegert DG, Michaud M, Schwab C, Francis GS. Multiple sclerosis and HLA class II susceptibility and resistance genes. *J Neurosci Res* 1990; 26:66–73.

98. Cowan EP, Pierce ML, McFarland HF, McFarlin DE. HLA-DR and -DQ allelic sequences in multiple sclerosis patients are identical to those found in the general population. *Hum Immunol* 1991; 32:203–210.

99. Hirayama K, Matsushita S, Kikuchi I, Iuchi M, Ohta N, Sasazuki T. HLA-DQ is epistatic to HLA-DR in controlling the immune response to schistosomal antigen in humans. *Nature* 1987; 327:426–430.

100. Liblau R, van Endert PM, Sandberg-Wollheim M, et al. Antigen processing gene polymorphisms in HLA-DR2 multiple sclerosis. *Neurology* 1993; 43:1192–1197.

101. Hillert J, Leng C, Olerup O. T cell receptor alpha chain germline gene polymorphisms in multiple sclerosis. *Neurology* 1992; 42:80–84.

102. Hashimoto LL, Mak TW, Ebers CC. T cell receptor alpha-chain polymorphisms in multiple sclerosis. *J Neuroimmunol* 1992; 40:41–48.

103. Sakaguchi S, Ermak TH, Toda M, et al. Induction of autoimmune disease in mice by germline alteration of the T cell receptor gene expression. *J Immunol* 1994; 152:1471–1484.

104. Ebers GC, Kukay K, Bulman DE, et al. A full genome search in multiple sclerosis. *Nat Genet* 1996; 13:472–476.

105. Haines JL, Ter-Minassian M, Bazyk A, et al. A complete genomic screen for multiple sclerosis underscores a role for the major histocompatibility complex. The Multiple Sclerosis Genetics Group. *Nat Genet* 1996; 13:469–471.

106. Sawcer S, H.B. J, Feakes R, et al. A genome screen in multiple sclerosis reveals susceptibility loci on chromosome 6p21 and 17q22. *Nat Genet* 1996; 13:464–468.

107. Vyse TJ, Kotzin BL. Genetic susceptibility to systemic lupus erythematosus. *Annu Rev Immunol* 1998; 16:261–292.

108. Paterson PY. Transfer of allergic encephalomyelitis in rats by means of lymph node cells. *J Exp Med* 1960; 111:119–133.

109. Pettinelli CB, McFarlin DE. Adoptive transfer of experimental allergic encephalomyelitis in SJL/J mice after in vivo activation of lymph node cells by myelin basic protein: requirement for Lyt-1+2- T lymphocytes. *J Immunol* 1981; 127:1420–1423.

110. Wekerle H, Kojima K, Lannes-Vieira J, Lassmann H, Linington C. Animal models. *Ann Neurol* 1994; 36:S47–53.

111. Ludwin SK. CNS demyelination and remyelination in the mouse. An ultrastructural study of cuprizone toxicity. *Lab Invest* 1978; 39:597–612.

112. Martin R, McFarland HF. Immunological aspects of experimental allergic encephalomyelitis and multiple sclerosis. *Critical Rev Clin Lab Sci* 1995; 32:121–182.

113. Williams KA, Deber CM. The structure and function of central nervous system myelin. *Critical Rev Clin Lab Sci* 1993; 30:29–64.

114. Quarles RH, Morell P, McFarlin DE. Diseases involving myelin. In: Siegel G, Agranoff B, Albers RW, Molinoff P (eds.). *Basic neurochemistry*. 4th ed. New York: Raven Press, 1989:697–713.

115. Kamholz J, Toffenetti J, Lazzarini RA. Organization and

expression of the human myelin basic protein gene. *J Neurosci Res* 1988; 21:62–70.

116. Fritz RB, McFarlin DE. Encephalitogenic epitopes of myelin basic protein. In: Sercarz EE (ed.). Antigenic determinants and immune response. Chem. Immunol. 46. Ed. Karger, Basel: 1989; 46:101–125.

117. Segal BM, Raine CS, McFarlin DE, Voskuhl RR, McFarland HF. Experimental allergic encephalomyelitis induced by the peptide encoded by exon 2 of the MBP gene—a peptide implicated in remyelination. *J Neuroimmunol* 1994; 51:7–19.

118. Voskuhl RR, McFarlin DE, Stone R, McFarland HF. T-lymphocyte recognition of a portion of myelin basic protein encoded by an exon expressed during myelination. *J Neuroimmunol* 1993; 42:187–192.

119. Martin R, Whitaker JN, Rhame L, Goodin RR, McFarland HF. Citrulline-containing myelin basic protein is recognized by T-cell lines derived from multiple sclerosis patients and healthy individuals. *Neurology* 1994; 44:123–129.

120. Whitaker JN. Myelin encephalitogenic protein fragments in cerebrospinal fluid of patients with multiple sclerosis. *Neurology* 1977; 27:911–920.

121. Whitaker JN. The presence of immunoreactive myelin basic protein peptide in urine of persons with multiple sclerosis. *Ann Neurol* 1987; 22:648–655.

122. Zamvil SS, Steinman L. The T lymphocyte in experimental allergic encephalomyelitis. *Annu Rev Immunol* 1990; 8:579–621.

123. Lees MB, Brostoff S. Proteins of myelin. In: Morell P (ed.). *Myelin.* 2nd ed. New York: Plenum Press, 1984:197–224.

124. Macklin WB, Campagnoni CW, Deininger PL, Gardinier MV. Structure and expression of the mouse myelin proteolipid protein gene. *J Neurosci Res* 1987; 18:383–394.

125. Kennedy MK, L.-J. T, Dal Canto MC, et al. Inhibition of murine relapsing experimental autoimmune encephalomyelitis by immune tolerance to proteolipid protein and its encephalitogenic peptides. *J Immunol* 1990; 144: 909–915.

126. Amor S, Groome N, Linington C, et al. Identification of epitopes of myelin oligodendrocyte glycoprotein for the induction of experimental allergic encephalomyelitis in SJL and Biozzi AB/H mice. *J Immunol* 1994; 153:4349–4356.

127. Johns TG, Kerlero de Rosbo N, et al. Myelin oligodendrocyte glycoprotein induces a demyelinating encephalomyelitis resembling multiple sclerosis. *J Immunol* 1995; 154:5536–5541.

128. Kerlero de Rosbo N, Mendel I, Ben-Nun A. Chronic relapsing experimental autoimmune encephalomyelitis with a delayed onset and an atypical clinical course, induced in PL/J mice by myelin oligodendrocyte glycoprotein (MOG)-derived peptide: preliminary analysis of MOG T cell epitopes. *Eur J Immunol* 1995; 25:985–993.

129. Linington C, Berger T, Perry L, et al. T cells specific for the myelin oligodendrocyte glycoprotein mediate an unusual autoimmune inflammatory response in the central nervous system. *Eur J Immunol* 1993; 23:1364–1372.

130. Moore GWR, Traugott U, Mokhtarian F, Norton WT, Raine CS. Experimental autoimmune encephalomyelitis. A generation of demyelination by different myelin lipids. *Lab Invest* 1984; 51:416–424.

131. Stone SH. Transfer of allergic encephalomyelitis by lymph node cells in inbred guinea pigs. *Science* 1961; 134:619–621.

132. Panitch HS, McFarlin DE. Experimental allergic encephalomyelitis: Enhancement of cell-mediated transfer by concanavalin A. *J Immunol* 1977; 119:1134–1137.

133. Richert JR, Driscoll BG, Kies MW, Alvord EC. Adoptive transfer of experimental allergic encephalomyelitis: Incubation of rat spleen cells with specific antigen. *J Immunol* 1979; 122:494–496.

134. Zamvil S, Nelson P, Mitchell D, et al. T cell clones specific for myelin basic protein induce chronic relapsing EAE and demyelination. *Nature* 1985; 317:355–358.

135. Wraith DC, Smilek DE, Mitchell DJ, Steinman L, McDevitt HO. Antigen recognition in autoimmune encephalomyelitis and the potential for peptide-mediated immunotherapy. *Cell* 1989; 59:247–255.

136. Brown JH, Jardetzky TS, Gorga JC, et al. Three-dimensional structure of the human class II histocompatibility antigen HLA-DR1. *Nature* 1993; 364:33–39.

137. Germain RN. MHC-dependent antigen processing and peptide presentation: Providing ligands for T lymphocyte activation. *Cell* 1994; 76:287–299.

138. Davis MM, Bjorkman PJ. T-cell antigen receptor genes and T-cell recognition. *Nature* 1988; 334:395–402.

139. Jorgensen JL, Esser U, Fazekas de St. Groth B, Reay PA, Davis MM. Mapping T-cell receptor-peptide contacts by variant peptide immunization of single-chain transgenics. *Nature* 1992; 355:224–230.

140. Acha-Orbea H, Steinman L, McDevitt HO. T cell receptors in murine autoimmune diseases. *Annu Rev Immunol* 1989; 7:371–406.

141. Kumar V, Kono DH, Urban JL, Hood L. T cell receptore repertoire and autoimmune diseases. *Annu Rev Immunol* 1989; 7:657–682.

142. Jansson L, Olsson T, Hojeberg B, Holmdahl R. Chronic experimental autoimmune encephalomyelitis induced by the 89–101 myelin basic protein peptide in B10RIII (H-2r) mice. *Eur J Immunol* 1991; 21:693–699.

143. Hashim G, Vandenbark AA, Gold DP, Diamanduros T, Offner H. T cell lines specific for an immunodominant epitope of human basic protein define an encephalitogenic determinant for experimental autoimmune encephalomyelitis-resistant Lou/M Rats. *J Immunol* 1991; 146: 515–520.

144. Tuohy VK, Sobel RA, Lees MB. Myelin proteolipid protein-induced experimental allergic encephalomyelitis. Variations of disease expression in different strains of mice. *J Immunol* 1988; 140:1868–1873.

145. Amor S, Baker D, Groome N, Turk JL. Identification of a major encephalitogenic epitope of proteolipid protein (residues 56–70) for the induction of experimental allergic encephalomyelitis in Biozzi AB/H and nonobese diabetic mice. *J Immunol* 1993; 150:5666–5672.

146. Sercarz EE, Lehmann PV, Ametani A, et al. Dominance and crypticity of T cell antigenic determinants. *Annu Rev Immunol* 1993; 11:729–766.

147. Lehmann PV, Sercarz EE, Forsthuber T, Dayan CM, Gammon G. Determinant spreading and the dynamics of the autoimmune T-cell repertoire. *Immunol Today* 1993; 14:203–208.

148. Burns FR, Li X, Shen N, et al. Both rat and mouse T cell receptors specific for the encephalitogenic determinant of myelin basic protein use similar Va and Vb chain genes even though the major histocompatibility complex and encephalitogenic determinants being recognized are different. *J Exp Med* 1989; 169:27–39.

149. Zamvil SS, Mitchell DJ, Lee NE, et al. Predominant

expression of a T cell receptor Vb gene subfamily in autoimmune encephalomyelitis. *J Exp Med* 1988; 167:1586–1596.

150. Acha-Orbea H, Mitchell L, Timmermann L, et al. Limited heterogeneity of T cell receptors from lymphocytes mediating autoimmune encephalomyelitis allows specific immune intervention. *Cell* 1988; 54:263–273.

151. Urban JL, Kumar V, Kono DH, et al. Restricted use of the T cells receptor V genes in murine autoimmune encephalomyelitis raises possibilities for antibody therapy. *Cell* 1988; 54:577–592.

152. Chluba J, Steeg C, Becker A, Wekerle H, Epplen JT. T cell receptor b chain usage in myelin basic protein-specific rat T lymphocytes. *Eur J Immunol* 1989; 19: 279–284.

153. Sun D, Gold DP, Smith L, Brostoff S, Coleclough C. Characterization of rat encephalitogenic T cells bearing non-V beta 8 T cell receptors. *Eur J Immunol* 1992; 22:591–594.

154. Goverman J, Woods A, Larson L, et al. Transgenic mice that express a myelin basic protein-specific T cell receptor develop spontaneous autoimmunity. *Cell* 1993; 72:551–560.

155. Vassalli P. The pathophysiology of tumor necrosis factors. *Annu Rev Immunol* 1992; 10:411–452.

156. Ruddle NH, Bergman CM, McGrath KM, et al. An antibody to lymphotoxin and tumor necrosis factor prevents transfer of experimental allergic encephalomyelitis. *J Exp Med* 1990; 172:1193–200.

157. Broome Powell M, Mitchell D, Lederman J, et al. Lymphotoxin and tumor necrosis factor-alpha production by myelin basic protein-specific T cell clones correlates with encephalitogenicity. *Int Immunol* 1990; 2:539–544.

158. Selmaj K, Raine CS. Tumor necrosis factor mediates myelin and oligodendrocyte damage in vitro. *Ann Neurol* 1988; 23:339–346.

159. Zajicek JP, Wing M, Scolding NJ, Compston DAS. Interactions between oligodendrocytes and microglia. A major role for complement and tumor necrosis factor in oligodendrocyte adherence and killing. *Brain* 1992; 115:1611–1631.

160. Suen WE, Bergman CM, Hjelmstrom P, Ruddle NH. A critical role for lymphotoxin in experimental allergic encephalomyelitis. *J Exp Med* 1997; 186:1233–1240.

161. Frei K, Eugster HP, Bopst M, et al. Tumor necrosis factor alpha and lymphotoxin alpha are not required for induction of acute experimental autoimmune encephalomyelitis. *J Exp Med* 1997; 185:2177–2182.

162. Kabat EA, Wolf A, Bezer AE. The rapid production of acute disseminated encephalomyelitis in rhesus monkeys by injection of brain tissue with adjuvants. *Science* 1946; 104:362–363.

163. Tourtellotte WW. The cerebrospinal fluid in multiple sclerosis. In: Vinken PJ, Bruyn GW, Klawans HL, Koetsier (eds.). *Handbook of clinical neurology, Demyelinating diseases*. Amsterdam/New York: Elsevier Sci. 1985:79–130.

164. Martin R, Martens U, Sticht-Groh V, Dörries R, Krüger H. Persistent intrathecal secretion of oligoclonal, *Borrelia burgdorferi*-specific IgG in chronic meningo-radiculo-myelitis. *J Neurol* 1988; 235:229–233.

165. ter Meulen V, Stephenson JR, Kreth HW. Subacute sclerosing panencephalitis. In: *Comprehensive virology*. Vol. 18. ed: H. Fraenkel-Conrat and R.R. Wagner. Plenum, New York. 1983.

166. Cortese I, Tafi R, Grimaldi LME, et al. Identification of peptides specific for cerebrospinal fluid antibodies in multiple sclerosis by using phage libraries. *Proc Natl Acad Sci USA* 1996; 93:11063–11067.

167. Archelos JJ, Trotter J, Previtali S, et al. Isolation and characterization of an oligodendrocyte precursor-derived B-cell epitope in multiple sclerosis. *Ann Neurol* 1998; 43:15–24.

168. Warren KG, Catz I. Synthetic peptide specificity of anti-myelin basic protein from multiple sclerosis cerebrospinal fluid. *J Neuroimmunol* 1992; 39:81–89.

169. Warren KG, Catz I. Relative frequency of autoantibodies to myelin basic protein and proteolipid protein in optic neuritis and multiple sclerosis cerebrospinal fluid. *J Neurol Sci* 1994; 121:66–73.

170. Wucherpfennig KW, Catz I, Hausmann S, et al. Recognition of the immunodominant myelin basic protein peptide by autoantibodies and HLA-DR2 restricted T cell clones from multiple sclerosis patients: identity of key contact residues in the B-cell and T-cell epitopes. *J Clin Invest* 1997; 100:1114–1122.

171. Vergelli M, Kalbus M, Rojo SC, et al. T cell response to myelin basic protein in the context of the multiple sclerosis associated HLA-DR15 haplotype: peptide binding, immunodominance and effector functions of T cells. *J Neuroimmunol*, 1997.

172. Antel JP, Arnason BGW. Suppressor cell function in multiple sclerosis —correlation with clinical disease activity. *Ann Neurol* 1979; 5:338–342.

173. Reder AT, Arnason BGW. Immunology of multiple sclerosis. In: Vinken PJ, Bruyn GW, Klawans HL, Koetsier (eds.). *Handbook of clinical neurology, Demyelinating diseases*. Amsterdam/New York: Elsevier Sci. 1985: 337–395.

174. Morimoto CM, Hafler DA, Weiner HL, et al. Selective loss of the suppressor-inducer T-cell subset in progressive multiple sclerosis. Analysis with the anti-2H4 monoclonal antibody. *New Engl J Med* 1987; 316:67–72.

175. Jacobson SJ, Flerlage ML, McFarland HF. Impaired measles virus-specific cytotoxic T-cell response in multiple sclerosis. *J Exp Med* 1985; 162:839–850.

176. Oro AS, Guarino TJ, Driver R, Steinman L, Umetsu DT. Regulation of disease susceptibility: Decreased prevalence of IgE-mediated allergic disease in patients with multiple sclerosis. *J Allergy Clin Immunol* 1996; 97:1402–1408.

177. Hohlfeld R. Biotechnological agents of the immunotherapy of multiple sclerosis. Principles, problems and perspectives. *Brain* 1997; 120:865–916.

178. Burns J, Rosenzweig A, Zweiman B, Lisak RP. Isolation of myelin basic protein-reactive T-cell lines from normal human blood. *Cell Immunol* 1983; 81:435–440.

179. Burns JB, Littlefield K. Human T lymphocytes reactive with whole myelin recognize predominantly myelin basic protein. *J Neuroimmunol* 1989; 22:67–74.

180. Baxevanis CN, Reclos GJ, Servis C, et al. Peptides of myelin basic protein stimulate T lymphocytes from patients with multiple sclerosis. *J Neuroimmunol* 1989; 22:23–30.

181. Chou YK, Vainiene M, Whitham R, et al. Response of human T lymphocyte lines to myelin basic protein: association of dominant epitopes with HLA-class II restriction molecules. *J Neurol Sci* 1989; 23:207–216.

182. Richert J, Robinson ED, Deibler GE, et al. Evidence for multiple human T cell recognition sites on myelin basic protein. *J Neuroimmunol* 1989; 23:55–66.

183. Martin R, Jaraquemada D, Flerlage M, et al. Fine specificity and HLA restriction of myelin basic protein-specific cytotoxic T cell lines from multiple sclerosis patients
and healthy individuals. *J Immunol* 1990; 145:540–548.

184. Ota K, Matsui M, Milford EL, Mackin GA, Weiner HL,
Hafler DA. T-cell recognition of an immunodominant
myelin basic protein epitope in multiple sclerosis. *Nature*
1990; 346:183–187.

185. Pette M, Fujita K, Kitze B, et al. Myelin basic protein-
specific T lymphocyte lines from MS patients and healthy
individuals. *Neurology* 1990; 40:1770–1776.

186. Olsson T, Wei Zhi W, Höjeberg B, et al. Autoreactive T
lymphocytes in multiple sclerosis determined by antigen-
induced secretion of interferon-g. *J Clin Invest* 1990;
86:981–985.

187. Meinl E, Weber F, Drexler K, et al. Myelin basic protein-specific T lymphocyte repertoire in multiple sclerosis. Complexity of the response and dominance of nested
epitopes due to recruitment of multiple T cell clones. *J
Clin Invest* 1993; 92:2633–2643.

188. Olsson T, Sun J, Hillert J, et al. Increased numbers of T
cells recognizing multiple myelin basic protein epitopes
in multiple sclerosis. *Eur J Immunol* 1992; 22:1083–1087.

189. Zhang J, Medaer R, Hashim GA, et al. Myelin basic protein-specific T lymphocytes in multiple sclerosis and controls: Precursor frequency, fine specificity, and cytotoxicity. *Ann Neurol* 1992; 32:330–338.

190. Martin R, Voskuhl R, Flerlage M, McFarlin DE, McFarland HF. Myelin basic protein-specific T-cell responses
in identical twins discordant or concordant for multiple
sclerosis. *Ann Neurol* 1993; 34:524–535.

191. Joshi N, Usuku K, Hauser SL. The T-cell response to
myelin basic protein in familial multiple sclerosis: Diversity of fine specificity, restricting elements, and T-cell
receptor usage. *Ann Neurol* 1993; 34:385–393.

192. Voskuhl RR, Martin R, McFarland HF. A functional
basis for the association of HLA class II genes and susceptibility to multiple sclerosis: Cellular immune
responses to myelin basic protein in a multiplex family.
J Neuroimmunol 1993; 42:199–208.

193. Allegretta M, Nicklas JA, Sriram S, Albertini RJ. T Cells
responsive to myelin basic protein in patients with multiple sclerosis. *Science* 1990; 247:718–721.

194. Trotter JL, Hickey WF, van der Veen RC, Sulze L. Peripheral blood mononuclear cells from multiple sclerosis
patients recognize myelin proteolipid protein and
selected peptides. *J Neuroimmunol* 1991; 33:55–62.

195. Martin R, Howell MD, Jaraquemada D, et al. A myelin
basic protein peptide is recognized by cytotoxic T cells
in the context of four HLA-DR types associated with
multiple sclerosis. *J Exp Med* 1991; 173:19–24.

196. Valli A, Sette A, Kappos L, et al. Binding of myelin basic
protein peptides to human histocompatibility leukocyte
antigen class II molecules and their recognition by T cells
from multiple sclerosis patients. *J Clin Invest* 1993;
91:616–628.

197. Pette M, Fujita K, Wilkinson D, et al. Myelin autoreactivity in multiple sclerosis: recognition of myelin basic
protein in the context of HLA-DR2 products by T lymphocytes of multiple sclerosis patients and healthy
donors. *Proc Natl Acad Sci USA* 1990; 87:7968–7972.

198. Vogt AB, Kropshofer H, Kalbacher H, et al. Ligand
motifs of HLA-DRB5*0101 and DRB1*1501 molecules
delineated from self-peptides. *J Immunol* 1994; 153:
1665–1673.

199. Wucherpfennig KW, Sette A, Southwood S, et al. Structural requirements for binding of an immunodominant
myelin basic protein peptide to DR2 isotypes and for its
recognition by human T cell clones. *J Exp Med* 1994;
179:279–290.

200. Martin R, Utz U, Coligan JE, et al. Diversity in fine specificity and T cell receptor usage of the human CD4+ cytotoxic T cell response specific for the immunodominant
myelin basic protein peptide 87–106. *J Immunol* 1992;
148:1359–1366.

201. Karkhanis YD, Carlo DJ, Brostoff SW, Eylar EH. Allergic encephalomyelitis: Isolation of an encephalitogenic
peptide active in the monkey. *J Biol Chem* 1975;
250:1718–1722.

202. Salvetti M, Ristori G, D'Amato M, et al. Predominant
and stable T cell responses to regions of myelin basic protein can be detected in individual patients with multiple
sclerosis. *Eur J Immunol* 1993; 23:1232–1239.

203. Moscarello MA, Wood DD, Ackerley C, Boulias C.
Myelin in multiple sclerosis is developmentally immature. *J Clin Invest* 1994; 94:146–154.

204. Fritz RB, Zhao M-L. Thymic expression of myelin basic
protein (MBP). Activation of MBP-specific T cells by
thymic cells in the absence of exogenous MBP. *J
Immunol* 1996; 157:5249–5253.

205. Zhou SR, Moscarello MA, Whitaker JN. The effects of
citrullination or variable amino-terminus acylation on
the encephalitogenicity of human myelin basic protein in
PL/J mice. *J Neuroimmunol* 1995; 62:147–152.

206. Hemmer B, Fleckenstein B, Vergelli M, et al. Identification of high potency microbial and self ligands for a
human autoreactive class II-restricted T cell clone. *J Exp
Med* 1997; 185:1651–1659.

207. Vergelli M, Hemmer B, Kalbus M, et al. Modifications
of peptide ligands enhancing T cell responsiveness imply
large numbers of stimulatory ligands for autoreactive T
cells. *J Immunol* 1997; 158:3746–3752.

208. Hemmer B, Vergelli M, Pinilla C, Houghten R, Martin
R. Probing degeneracy in T-cell recognition using combinatorial peptide libraries. *Immunol Today* 1998;
19:163–168.

209. Richert JR, Robinson ED, Deibler GE, et al. Human
cytotoxic T-cell recognition of a synthetic peptide of
myelin basic protein. *Ann Neurol* 1989; 26:342–346.

210. Ota K, Matsui M, Milford EL, et al. T-cell recognition
of an immunodominant myelin basic protein epitope in
multiple sclerosis. *Nature* 1990; 346:183–187.

211. Muraro PA, Vergelli M, Kalbus M, et al. Immunodominance of a low-affinity MHC binding myelin basic protein epitope (residues 111–129) in HLA-DR4 (B1*0401)
subjects is associated with a restricted T cell receptor
repertoire. *J Clin Invest*, 1997.

212. Sinigaglia F, Guttinger M, Kilgus J, et al. A malaria T-
cell epitope recognized in association with most mouse
and human MHC-class II molecules. *Nature* 1988;
336:778–770.

213. Hammer J, Valsasnini P, Tolba K, et al. Promiscuous and
allele-specific anchors in HLA-DR binding peptides. *Cell*
1993; 74:197–203.

214. Utz U, Biddison WE, McFarland HF, McFarlin DE, Flerlage M, Martin R. Skewed T cell receptor repertoire in
genetically identical twins with multiple sclerosis correlates with disease. *Nature* 1993; 364:243–247.

215. Jaraquemada D, Martin R, Rosen-Bronson S, et al.
HLA-DR2a is the dominant restriction molecule for the

cytotoxic T cell response to myelin basic protein in DR2Dw2 individuals. *J Immunol* 1990; 145:2880–2885.

216. Ben Nun A, Liblau RS, Cohen L, et al. Restricted T-cell receptor Vb gene usage by myelin basic protein-specific T-cell clones in multiple sclerosis: predominant genes vary in individuals. *Proc Natl Acad Sci USA* 1991; 88:2466–2470.

217. Giegerich G, Pette M, Meinl E, Epplen JT, Wekerle H, Hinkkanen A. Diversity of T cell receptor alpha and beta chain genes expressed by human T cells specific for similar myelin basic protein peptide/major histocompatibility complexes. *Eur J Immunol* 1992; 22:753–8.

218. Wucherpfennig KW, Ota K, Endo N, et al. Shared human T cell receptor V beta usage to immunodominant regions of myelin basic protein. *Science* 1990; 248:1016–1019.

219. Kotzin BL, Karuturi S, Chou YK, et al. Preferential T-cell receptor Vb-chain variable gene use in myelin basic protein-reactive T-cell clones from patients with multiple sclerosis. *Proc Natl Acad Sci USA* 1991; 88:9161–9165.

220. Oksenberg JR, Stuart S, Begovich AB, et al. Limited heterogeneity of rearranged T-cell receptor V alpha transcripts in brains of multiple sclerosis patients. *Nature* 1990; 345:344–346.

221. Oksenberg JR, Panzara MA, Begovich AB, et al. Selection for T-cell receptor Vb-Db-Jb gene rearrangements with specificity for a myelin basic protein peptide in brain lesions of multiple sclerosis. *Nature* 1993; 362:68–70.

222. Richert J, Robinson E, Martin R, et al. Human T cell receptor (TCR) a and b gene expression in the response to myelin basic protein. *FASEB J* 1991; 5:A1680.

223. Allegretta M, Albertini RJ, Howell MD, et al. Homologies between T cell receptor junctional sequences unique to multiple sclerosis and T cells mediating experimental allergic encephalomyelitis. *J Clin Invest* 1994; 94:105–109.

224. Utz U, Brooks JA, McFarland HF, Martin R, Biddison WE. Heterogeneity of T-cell receptor a-chain complementarity-determining region 3 in myelin basic protein-specific T cells increases with severity of multiple sclerosis. *Proc Natl Acad Sci USA* 1994; 91:5567–5571.

225. Wucherpfennig KW, Zhang J, Witek C, et al. Clonal expansion and persistence of human T cells specific for an immunodominant myelin basic protein peptide. *J Immunol* 1994; 152:5581–5592.

226. Panitch HS, Hirsch RL, Schindler J, Johnson KP. Treatment of multiple sclerosis with gamma interferon: Exacerbations associated with activation of the immune system. *Neurology* 1987; 37:1097–1102.

227. Chofflon M, Juillard C, Juillard P, Gauthier G, Grau GE. Tumor necrosis factor alpha production as a possible predictor of relapse in patients with multiple sclerosis. *Eur Cytokine Netw* 1992; 3:523–531.

228. Zipp F, Weber F, Huber S, et al. Genetic control of multiple sclerosis: increased production of lymphotoxin and tumor necrosis factor-a by HLA-DR2+ T cells. *Ann Neurol* 1995; 38:723–730.

229. Hemmer B, Vergelli M, Calabresi P, et al. Cytokine phenotype of human autoreactive T cell clones specific for the immunodominant myelin basic protein peptide (83–99). *J Neurosci Res* 1996; 45:852–862.

230. Voskuhl RR, Martin R, Bergman C, Dalal M, Ruddle NH, McFarland HF. T helper 1 (TH1) functional phenotype of human myelin basic protein-specific T lymphocytes. *Autoimmunity* 1993; 15:137–143.

231. Vergelli M, Le H, van Noort JM, et al. A novel population of CD4+ CD56+ myelin-reactive T cells lyses target cells expressing CD56/neural cell adhesion molecule. *J Immunol* 1996; 157:679–688.

232. Vergelli M, Hemmer B, Muraro P, et al. Human autoreactive CD4+ T cell clones use perforin- or Fas–Fas ligand-mediated pathways for target cell lysis. *J Immunol* 1997; 158:2756–2761.

233. Antel JP, McCrea E, Ladiwala U, Qin YF, Becher B. Non-MHC-restricted cell-mediated lysis of human oligodendrocytes in vitro: relation with CD56 expression. *J Immunol* 1998; 160:1606–1611.

234. Svenningsson A, Hansson GK, Andersen O, Andersson R, Patarroyo M, Stemme S. Adhesion molecule expression on cerebrospinal fluid T lymphocytes: Evidence for common recruitment mechanisms in multiple sclerosis, aseptic meningitis, and normal controls. *Ann Neurol* 1993; 34:155–161.

235. Ruijs TCG, Freedman MS, Grenier YG, Olivier A, Antel JP. Human oligodendrocytes are susceptible to cytolysis by major histocompatibility complex class I-restricted lymphocytes. *J Neuroimmunol* 1990; 27:89–97.

236. Freedman MS, Ruijs TCG, Selin L, Antel JP. Peripheral blood g-d T cells lyse fresh human brain-derived oligodendrocytes. *Ann Neurol* 1991; 30:794–800.

237. Tsuchida T, Parker KC, Turner RV, McFarland HF, Coligan JE, Biddison WE. Autoreactive CD8+ T-cell responses to human myelin protein-derived peptides. *Proc Natl Acad Sci USA* 1994; 91:10859–10863.

238. Offner H, Hashim GA, Vandenbark AA. T cell receptor peptide therapy triggers autoregulation of experimental encephalomyelitis. *Science* 1991; 251:430–432.

239. Zhang J, Medaer R, Stinissen P, Hafler DA, Raus J. MHC-restricted depletion of human myelin basic protein-reactive T cells by T cell vaccination. *Science* 1993; 261:1451–1454.

240. Link J, Söderström M, Kostulas V, et al. Optic neuritis is associated with myelin basic protein and proteolipid protein reactive cells producing interferon-g, interleukin-4 and transforming growth factor-b. *J Neuroimmunol* 1994; 49:9–18.

241. Hemmer B, Vergelli M, Calabresi PA, et al. Cytokine phenotype of human autoreactive T cell clones specific for the immunodominant myelin protein peptide. *J Neurol Sci* 1996; 45:852–862.

242. Correale J, Gilmore W, McMillan M, et al. Patterns of cytokine secretion by autoreactive proteolipid protein-specific T cell clones during the course of multiple sclerosis. *J Immunol* 1995; 154:2959–2968.

243. Correale J, McMillan M, McCarthy K, Le T, Weiner LP. Isolation and characterization of autoreactive proteolipid protein-peptide specific T-cell clones from multiple sclerosis patients. *Neurology* 1995; 45:1370–1378.

244. Scholz C, Patton KT, Anderson DE, Freedman GJ, Hafler DA. Expansion of autoreactive T cells in multiple sclerosis is independent of exogenous B7 costimulation. *J Immunol* 1998; 160:1532–1538.

245. Lovett-Racke AE, Trotter JL, Lauber J, et al. Decreased dependence of myelin basic protein-reactive T cells on CD28-mediated costimulation in multiple sclerosis patients. A marker for activated/memory T cells. *J Clin Invest* 1998; 101:725–730.

246. Zipp F, Weller M, Calabresi PA, et al. Increased serum levels of soluble CD95 (Apo-1/Fas) in relapsing remitting multiple sclerosis. *Ann Neurol* 1998; 43:116–120.

247. Sun J-B. Autoreactive T and B cells in nervous system disease. *Acta Neurol Scand* 1993; 87(Suppl):1–56.

248. Pelfrey CM, Trotter JL, Tranquill LR, McFarland HF. Identification of a novel T cell epitope of human proteolipid protein (residues 40–60) recognized by proliferative and cytolytic CD4+ T cells from multiple sclerosis. *J Neuroimmunol* 1993; 46:33–42.

249. Pelfrey CM, Trotter JL, Tranquill LR, McFarland HF. Identification of a second T cell epitope of human proteolipid protein (residues 89–106) recognized by proliferative and cytolytic CD4+ T cells from multiple patients. *J Neuroimmunol* 1994; 53:153–161.

250. Sun JB, Olsson T, Wang W-Z, et al. Autoreactive T and B cells responding to myelin proteolipid protein in multiple sclerosis and controls. *Eur J Immunol* 1991; 21:1461–1468.

251. Sun J, Link H, Olsson T, et al. T and B cell responses to myelin-oligodendrocyte glycoprotein in multiple sclerosis. *J Immunol* 1991; 146:1490–1495.

252. Johnson D, Hafler DA, Fallis RJ, et al. Cell-mediated immunity to myelin-associated glycoprotein, proteolipid protein, and myelin basic protein in multiple sclerosis. *J Neuroimmunol* 1986; 13:99–108.

253. Zhang YD, Burger D, Saruhan M, Jeannet M, Steck AJ. The T-lymphocyte response against myelin-associated glycoprotein and myelin basic protein in patients. *Neurology* 1993; 43:403–407.

254. Rösener M, Muraro PA, Riethmüller A, et al. 2',3'-cyclic nucleotide 3'-phosphodiesterase: a novel candidate autoantigen in demyelinating diseases. *J Neuroimmunol*, 1997.

255. Banki K, Colombo E, Sia F, et al. Oligodendrocyte-specific expression and autoantigenicity of transaldolase in multiple sclerosis. *J Exp Med* 1994; 180:1649–1663.

256. van Noort JM, van Sechel AC, Bajramovic JJ, et al. The small heat-shock protein aB-crystallin as candidate autoantigen in multiple sclerosis. *Nature* 1995; 375:798–801.

257. Hafler DA, Benjamin DS, Burks J, Weiner HL. Myelin basic protein and proteolipid protein reactivity of brain- and cerebrospinal fluid-derived T cell clones in multiple sclerosis and postinfectious encephalomyelitis. *J Immunol* 1987; 139:68–72.

258. Greer JM, Csurhes PA, Cameron KD, McCombe PA, Good MF, Pender MP. Increased immunoreactivity to two overlapping peptides of myelin proteolipid protein in multiple sclerosis. *Brain* 1997; 120:1447–1460.

259. Link H, Sun J-B, Wang Z, et al. Virus-specific and autoreactive T cells are accumulated in cerebrospinal fluid in multiple sclerosis. *J Neuroimmunol* 1992; 38:63–74.

260. Kerlero de Rosbo N, Hoffmann M, Mendel I, et al. Predominance of the autoimmune response to myelin oligodendrocyte glycoprotein (MOG) in multiple sclerosis: reactivity to the extracellular domain of MOG is directed against three main regions. *Eur J Immunol* 1997; 27:3059–3069.

261. van Noort JM, El Quagmiri M, Boon J, van Sechel AC. Fractionation of central nervous system myelin proteins by reversed-phase high-performance liquid chromatography. *J Chromat B* 1994; 653:155–161.

262. Voskuhl RR, Robinson ED, Segal BM, et al. HLA restriction and TCR usage of T lymphocytes specific for a novel candidate autoantigen, X2 MBP, in multiple sclerosis. *J Immunol* 1994; 153:4834–4844.

263. Tranquill LR, Skinner E, Campagnoni C, et al. Human T lymphocytes specific for the immunodominant 83–99 epitope of myelin basic protein: recognition of golli MBP HOG 7. *J Neurosci Res* 1996; 45:820–828.

264. Kojima K, Berger T, Lassmann H, et al. Experimental autoimmune panencephalitis and uveoretinitis transferred to the Lewis rat by T lymphocytes specific for the S100b molecule, a calcium binding protein of astroglia. *J Exp Med* 1994; 180:817–829.

265. Berger T, Weerth S, Kojima K, Linington C, Wekerle H, Lassmann H. Experimental autoimmune encephalomyelitis: The antigen specificity of T lymphocytes determines the topography of lesions in the central and peripheral nervous system. *Lab Invest* 1997; 76:355–364.

266. Mackin GA, Dawson DM, Hafler DA, Weiner HL. Treatment of multiple sclerosis with cyclophosphamide. In: Rudick RA, Goodkin DE (eds.). *Treatment of multiple sclerosis*. London: Springer, 1992:199–216.

267. The IFNB Multiple Sclerosis Study Group and the University of British Columbia MS/MRI Analysis G. Interferon beta-1b in the treatment of multiple sclerosis: Final outcome of the randomized controlled trial. *Neurology* 1995; 45:1277–1285.

268. Jacobs LD, Cookfair DL, Rudick RA, et al. Intramuscular interferon beta-1a for disease progression in relapsing multiple sclerosis. *Ann Neurol* 1996; 39:285–294.

269. Myers LW. Treatment of multiple sclerosis with ACTH and corticosteroids. In: Rudick RA, Goodkin DE (eds.). *Treatment of multiple sclerosis*. London: Springer, 1992:135–156.

270. Hughes RAC. Treatment of multiple sclerosis with azathioprine. In: Rudick RA, Godkin DE (eds.). *Treatment of multiple sclerosis*. London: Springer, 1992:157–172.

271. Johnson KP, Brooks BR, Cohen JA, et al. Copolymer 1 reduces relapse rate and improves disability in relapsing-remitting multiple sclerosis: Results of a phase III multicenter, double-blind, placebo-controlled trial. *Neurology* 1995; 45:1268–1276.

272. Comi G, Filippi M, for the Copaxone MRI Study Group. The effect of glatiramer acetate (Copaxone®) on disease activity as measured by cerebral MRI in patients with relapsing-remitting multiple sclerosis (RRMS): A multicenter, randomized, double-blind, placebo-controlled study extended by open-label treatment. *Neurology* 1999; 52(6)(Suppl 2):A289.

273. Mancardi GL, Sardanelli F, Parodi RC, et al. Effect of copolymer-1 on serial gadolinium-enhanced MRI in relapsing remitting multiple sclerosis. *Neurology* 1998; 50:1127-1133.

274. Rudick RA, Ransohoff RM, Peppler R, VanderBrug Medendorp S, Lehmann P, Alam J. Interferon beta induces interleukin-10 expression: relevance to multiple sclerosis. *Ann Neurol* 1996; 40:618–627.

275. Liu X, Linington C, Webster HD, et al. Insulin-like growth factor-I treatment reduces immune cell responses in acute non-demyelinative experimental autoimmune encephalomyelitis. *J Neurosci Res* 1997; 47:531–538.

276. Racke MK, Dhib-Jalbut SD, Cannella B, et al. Prevention and treatment of chronic relapsing experimental allergic encephalomyelitis by transforming growth factor-b-1. *J Immunol* 1991; 146:3012–3017.

277. Rott O, Fleischer B, Cash E. Interleukin-10 prevents experimental allergic encephalomyelitis in rats. *Eur J Immunol* 1994; 24:1434–1440.

278. Weiner HL, Mackin GA, Matsui M, et al. Double-blind pilot trial of oral tolerization with myelin antigens in multiple sclerosis. *Science* 1993; 259:1321–1324.

279. Massacesi L, Castigli E, Vergelli M, et al. Immunosuppressive activity of 13-cis-retinoic acid and prevention of experimental autoimmune Encephalomyelitis in Rats. *J Clin Invest* 1991; 88:1331–1337.

280. Sommer N, Löschmann PA, Northoff GH, et al. The antidepressant rolipram suppresses cytokine production and prevents autoimmune encephalomyelitis. *Nature Med* 1995; 1:244–248.

281. Genain CP, Roberts T, Davis RL, et al. Prevention of autoimmune demyelination in non-human primates by a cAMP-specific phosphodiesterase inhibitor. *Proc Natl Acad Sci USA* 1995; 92:3601–3605.

282. Paty DW, Li DKB, The UBC MS-MRI Study Group and the IFN-b MS Study Group. Interferon beta-1b is effective in relapsing and remitting multiple sclerosis 2: MRI analysis results of a multi-center, randomized, double-blind, placebo-controlled trial. *Neurology* 1993; 43: 662–667.

283. McFarland HF, Frank JA, Albert PS, et. al. Using gadolinium-enhanced magnetic resonance imaging lesions to monitor disease activity in multiple sclerosis. *Ann Neurol* 1992; 32:758–766.

284. Stone LA, Frank JA, Albert PS, et al. The effect of interferon-b on blood-brain-barrier disruptions demonstrated by contrast-enhanced magnetic resonance imaging in relapsing-remitting multiple sclerosis. *Ann Neurol* 1995; 37:611–619.

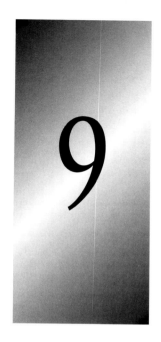

9 Therapy of Relapsing Forms

Kenneth P. Johnson, M.D.

The majority of multiple sclerosis (MS) patients begin their lifelong experience of the disease with an acute attack that most commonly involves the spinal cord or optic nerves (see Chapter 4). All MS attacks or relapses are serious, even those with only mild sensory symptoms, because each one reminds the patient of the disease and often brings on anxiety or depression. Many relapses are major neurologic events—unilateral blindness; significant hemiparesis; or a brainstem syndrome with incoordination, diplopia, nausea and vomiting, and so on—that require acute intervention and sometimes hospitalization.

Although all MS relapses are significant, the first and second relapses are particularly important because they announce and confirm the diagnosis and set patients on their chronic course. Because of their special significance, these relapses should be managed by the physician with special care. Proper, in-person discussion of the diagnosis, the phases and variability of the disease, and the available therapies, even if not required at once, is important to give the patient a sense of hope that he or she has some control over future events. The initial interview to discuss the diagnosis is best carried out with the patient and a support person—a spouse, a parent, or a friend. With the availability of relatively effective immunomodulatory therapies that alter the long-term course of MS, patients need to be aware of their place and usefulness at the onset of illness.

WHAT IS A RELAPSE?

According to the Poser (1) criteria, a relapse must include one or more neurologic symptoms, must last more than 24 hours, and must not be secondary to a metabolic change such as fever. Recent randomized trials of new therapies have required that symptoms last at least 48 hours and be accompanied by an objective change on neurologic examination (2), but this is perhaps too stringent a definition for routine practice. Most relapses evolve over one to seven days and most remit within one to three months, although occasionally improvement may be observed up to a year after onset. Because any area of the central nervous system (CNS) may be the site of a new plaque, the potential combination of symptoms is large but common relapses affect function conducted through restricted pathways, such as the spinal cord.

Minor elevations of body temperature or exposure to environmental heat or exertion may reproduce previously resolved MS symptoms (Uhthoff's phenomenon, see Chapter 4). Such experiences are not true relapses and disappear when the patient's temperature returns to normal. In such situations, it is important to consider associated symptoms, such as urinary or pulmonary complaints and so forth, which may point to a cryptic infection. It also is useful to explain the issue of heat intolerance to help patients control environmental exposure. Patients often describe brief focal symptoms that last minutes or a few hours with complete resolution. The source of these symptoms is poorly understood, but generally they are not treated and are not considered to be relapses.

TREATMENT OF ACUTE RELAPSES

Not all relapses require treatment. Mild focal sensory attacks, although they qualify as true relapses, usually are not treated unless they include unpleasant symptoms: pain, burning or boring numbness, and so forth. At times, relapses that start with sensory complaints expand to include other neurologic components, so it is best to maintain contact with a patient or warn him or her that additional symptoms that require appropriate therapy may develop.

Relapses are the clinical announcement that the disease is active. With MS disease activity, whether determined by new clinical symptoms or by enhancing lesions on the magnetic resonance imaging (MRI), patients usually experience increased fatigue. In fact, fatigue often precedes the onset of neurologic symptoms (see Chapter 2).

All significant relapses, i.e., those with visual, motor, pain, or incoordination components, require acute glucocorticosteroid (GCS) therapy. Although there is no evidence that steroid therapy alters the long-term course of MS (3), clinical experience shows that most relapses resolve more quickly and perhaps more completely with adequate GCS therapy.

Results from the acute optic neuritis trial published in 1993 (4) have helped standardize MS relapse therapy in the United States, where the following regimen is common.

- Methylprednisolone, 1000 mg by intravenous (IV) infusion daily for three to five days
- Prednisone oral taper, starting at 60 mg daily with decreasing doses over two to three weeks (optional).

There are numerous variations on this regimen. Some patients receive the IV methylprednisolone in two or four divided doses. Often no oral prednisone taper is included. Longer IV dosing (up to 7 days) or higher initial oral prednisone dose (80 mg daily) is occasionally prescribed.

Some controversy exists about the need to prescribe IV versus oral steroids. The Optic Neuritis Study Group has published five-year data that show significant benefit of IV versus oral GCS (5). However, a careful study comparing oral and IV methylprednisolone treatment of acute MS relapses showed no difference in clinical outcome between

groups of approximately 40 patients each followed for 24 weeks (6). In this double-blind comparative trial, patients received either three daily IV infusions of 1000 mg of methylprednisolone or 48 mg p.o. daily for seven days, 25 mg daily for seven days, then 12 mg daily for seven days. The investigators equated 48 mg of methylprednisolone with 60 mg of prednisone. The oral regimen obviously was easier for the patients and was less expensive.

Systemic GCS administration usually produces metabolic and immunologic change in many organ systems. A useful description of GCS pharmacology and mechanisms of action may be found in Chapter 10. It is worth emphasizing that the inhibiting effect of GCS on lymphocytes within the CNS compartment is significant, resulting in a reversible reduction in intrathecal immunoglobulin production (7) and a resultant reduction in cerebrospinal fluid (CSF) immunoglobulin. This may temporarily alter diagnostic tests such as the CSF immunoglobulin G (IgG) index and the presence of oligoclonal IgG bands.

High-dose systemic therapy with GCS commonly reduces serum potassium levels, so a potassium supplement is recommended, especially if an oral GCS taper is included. Potassium may be supplemented either with prescribed medications or with daily dietary additions, especially fruits or vegetables such as oranges, tomatoes, and bananas.

Current practice recommendations discourage the chronic use of GCS in the management of relapsing MS (see Chapter 10). Occasional patients appear to become quite steroid-dependent and may raise therapeutic dilemmas, primarily because of the toxic or adverse effects of long-term steroid use. These include lenticular cataracts, hypertension, gastrointestinal complaints, weight gain, acne, buffalo hump, personality change including psychosis, sleep disorders, and accelerated osteoporosis resulting in pathologic fractures, especially fractures of the femoral neck and vertebral collapse. Other long-term side effects include muscle weakness, myelopathy, diabetes, and increased susceptibility to infection.

Previously, corticotropin (ACTH) was widely used to treat acute MS relapses and probably was effective. The need to give an IV infusion for 10 days or more and the relative difficulty in obtaining ACTH have led to a major decline in its use, although some clinicians maintain the opinion that the acute adverse effects profile of ACTH is less than with high-dose GCS.

USE OF IMMUNOMODULATING AGENTS TO REDUCE RELAPSE FREQUENCY

A new era in MS management began in the spring of 1993 with the approval by the U.S. Food and Drug Administration (FDA) of interferon beta-1b (Betaseron) for relapsing-remitting MS. Since then, interferon beta-1a (Avonex) has been approved, and a second interferon beta-1a product (Rebif) has been successfully tested and may become available in the United States glatiramer acetate (Copaxone), which applies a different immunomodulatory approach, was approved in late 1996 and is available as an effective option. Understanding these medications, their proven indications, their long-term benefits where known, their adverse effects profile, and their limitations is essential for the comprehensive management of MS relapses.

Glatiramer Acetate

History

Glatiramer acetate (Copaxone) was first developed at the Weizmann Institute in Israel and was called copolymer I. It is a collection of random peptides of four amino acids, L-alanine, L-lysine, L-glutamic acid, and L-tyrosine, with a molecular weight of 4.7 to 11 kilodaltons. Although it was developed as a research tool to investigate immunologic mechanisms in experimental allergic encephalomyelitis (EAE), it soon became apparent that it prevented or modified EAE in several species (8). When it was shown to be effective in many EAE models, including subhuman primates, cautious studies were undertaken by Abramsky and co-workers (9) in patients with acute postinfectious encephalomyelitis and advanced MS. Bornstein and coworkers at the Albert Einstein College of Medicine in New York then began safety and dose-finding studies (10) with glatiramer acetate before completing an important pilot trial (11) in relapsing-remitting MS patients, in which the relapse rate was

significantly lowered, an affect on disability was shown, and patient tolerance was excellent. A subsequent two-center study of 108 patients with more advanced primary and secondary progressive disease showed a positive therapeutic trend (12).

In 1986, commercial development of glatiramer acetate was undertaken by Teva Pharmaceuticals Ltd. in Israel. After developing a well-standardized product that was acceptable to the FDA, a pivotal phase III double-blind, placebo-controlled, multicenter trial was initiated at 11 U.S. universities in October 1991. Results of this successful trial were first reported in 1995 (2). The trial, which was first planned for 24 months, was extended for approximately six additional months (13), after which all interested patients were switched to glatiramer acetate and continued to be followed in an organized study. The glatiramer acetate investigation continued into its seventh year as of 1998, providing continuing information on the long-term benefit of treatment on relapses, disability, tolerability, and safety.

Mechanisms of Action of Glatiramer Acetate

Glatiramer acetate blocks both acute and relapsing EAE as well as EAE produced by several encephalogens, including proteolipid protein, myelin-associated oligodendrocyte glycoprotein, and myelin basic protein, and their encephalogenic peptides (14). In human cells it is not human lymphocyte antigen (HLA) restricted (15). It appears to have a relatively disease-specific mode of action, with little effect on experimental thyroiditis or myasthenia gravis.

Glatiramer acetate has been shown to block the interaction of various encephalogenic peptides with HLA class II molecules on antigen-presenting cells (APC), bind-

TABLE 9-1
Long-Term Immunomodulating Agents for Multiple Sclerosis

| | Beta Interferon | | Glatiramer Acetate | |
	1B Betaseron	1A Avonex	1A Rebif*	Copaxone
Dose	8 MIU	6 MIU	6 MIU or 12 MIU	20 mg
Route	SC	IM	SC	SC
Frequency	QOD	weekly	3 x/week	daily

SC—subcutaneous
IM—intramuscular
QOD—every other day
* Not available in United States. Available in Canada and many European countries.

ing rapidly and avidly to the class II molecular cleft (16,17). More specifically, it binds promiscuously to HLA DR molecules (15,18), which have a strong association with MS (19). These actions appear to interfere with sensitization of pathogenic T lymphocyte populations. Glatiramer acetate also has been shown to induce Th2 (anti-inflammatory) lymphocytes in EAE (20). This mode of action is thought to occur within the CNS, resulting in so-called "bystander" suppression at the site of the MS lesion, and thereby reducing inflammation, demyelination, and axonal damage.

Glatiramer Acetate in Clinical Practice.

The original hypothesis in developing glatiramer acetate was that long-term, continuous dosing would reduce the occurrence of relapses and lower or delay the risk of fixed disability. Results of the multicenter, placebo-controlled trial (2) and its extension (13) showed that glatiramer acetate achieved these goals, which led to FDA approval in 1996 and the commercial availability of glatiramer acetate in the United States in April 1997.

After two years of daily glatiramer acetate treatment, the relapse rate was reduced 29 percent versus placebo, whereas at ± 30 months the difference was 32 percent (13). The effect on slowing of disability was evaluated by neurologic evaluation every three months. The data were analyzed by multiple statistical methods (13). All but one showed a significant difference favoring glatiramer acetate and were generally more robust than that shown for the interferons (IFNs).

All interested participants in the glatiramer acetate pivotal trial have been maintained in an organized open-label study, including those receiving placebo, who were switched to active drug. After six years of observation, the annual relapse rate has fallen to 0.16, i.e., the risk of a relapse every five to six years, whereas the affect on disability is substantially better than predicted from natural history studies of MS.

No MRI component was included in the original trials. An Italian study (21) showed that glatiramer acetate therapy significantly reduces the occurrence of gadolinium-enhanced lesions when patients were scanned monthly for 12+ months before therapy and then for 12+ months while receiving the drug. A large European-Canadian, double-blind, placebo-controlled MRI trial of glatiramer acetate was recently completed and reported in the Spring of 1999. After nine months during which patients were scanned monthly, there was a highly significant benefit for glatiramer acetate over placebo for both number and volume of enhancing lesions as well as the number of new T2 lesions and volume of T2 lesions. The clinical relapse rate was significantly reduced by 33 percent in the treated cohort (41).

Who Should Be Treated?

Opinion has crystallized among MS experts that early therapy, soon after diagnosis, be recommended. A reemerging awareness of the importance of axonal damage and brain atrophy as fundamental aspects of MS, using neuropathologic (22) and MRI techniques, has led to the conclusion that axonal loss, in addition to demyelination and inflammation, is closely related to progressive disability. To minimize or delay axonal damage and secondary CNS atrophy, immunomodulatory therapy should be initiated early in the course of MS.

The concept of benign MS is traditional and it is true that ± 10 percent of patients follow a benign course for years or even decades. Unfortunately, this is a retrospective finding and it is impossible to determine at the time of diagnosis which patients will follow a benign course. Therefore, the current recommendation is to start therapy early in most patients. Glatiramer acetate should be considered as a first-line agent (Table 9-1). It also is the only option for MS patients who fail IFN therapy because of disease activity or intolerable adverse effects. Glatiramer acetate probably is the best choice for childhood and adolescent MS because it is well tolerated and, unlike the IFNs, has no adverse effect on endocrine function and does not cause the menstrual irregularities that are known to complicate IFN therapy.

Initiation of Glatiramer Acetate Therapy

In-depth patient instruction regarding the purpose of glatiramer acetate therapy, a review of the available data on long-term benefit, and the potential for adverse effects is essential. Because the adverse effects profile is favorable for glatiramer acetate, initiation of therapy generally is easier, but continuing support during the early months is recommended. No laboratory abnormalities have been reported with glatiramer acetate therapy, so monitoring is not required.

Adverse Effects of Glatiramer Acetate Therapy

Even though it must be injected daily, the safety and patient tolerance profile of glatiramer acetate is excellent. Broad experience has defined two adverse effects: injection site reactions and an immediate postinjection reaction.

Injection site reactions are common but mild and transient, in most cases lasting from 12 to 24 hours. No skin necrosis has been noted, but rare lipoatrophy has occurred. Some patients have reported burning pain that lasts three to five minutes, which is possibly related to failure to warm the medication to room temperature before injection.

The immediate postinjection reaction is both rare and benign yet of concern because it is frightening when first experienced. Patients report that within seconds or a few minutes of injecting glatiramer acetate, they experience flushing, chest tightness or pain, along with dyspnea, palpitation, and anxiety, all of which last from a few seconds to 30 minutes. The reaction is benign but of unknown cause. Extensive studies have failed to link it to myocardial dysfunction or to an allergic reaction. It also is rare, having occurred from one to seven times during the 30-month phase III trial in only 15 percent of patients. It is recommended that patients be informed of the reaction when initiating glatiramer therapy. In most cases, the glatiramer acetate program may successfully be continued following such a reaction. Of greater concern is the possibility that a patient will develop chest pain of a serious nature hours after the daily injection and incorrectly assume that it is due to glatiramer acetate and fail to seek appropriate diagnosis and care.

Studies have determined that almost all patients who receive glatiramer acetate develop binding antibodies that may reach high titers but then often fall to zero or to low levels after several months of continued dosing. No evidence of neutralizing antibodies has been found (23).

Interferon Beta

History

Investigation of human IFNs as potential therapies for MS began in the late 1970s, when two approaches were explored—chronic systemic administration and phased intrathecal dosing, both based on the premise that a virus was involved in the pathogenesis of MS. In the 15 years from 1978 to 1993, numerous trials were performed using different IFNs, routes of administration, doses, and patient populations, as historically noted by Jacobs and Johnson (24). Over time, the intrathecal route proved to be unacceptable and perhaps toxic and was abandoned.

The IFNs are classified as type I (alpha [IFNα] and beta [IFNβ]) and type II (gamma [IFNγ]). The type I IFNs are genetically related and have similar biologic (antiviral, antiproliferative, and immunomodulating) activity and are distinct from type II IFN. All have been produced by recombinant technology, and all have been tested as therapies for MS (25). A trial of fundamental significance in the understanding of MS took place in the mid-1980s, when Panitch and coworkers (26) gave IFNγ intravenously to 18 patients, seven of whom developed new, fortunately mild, relapses within a month. This study convincingly identified IFNγ as a key inflammatory cytokine in the pathogenesis of MS and raised the concept that inhibition of IFN could be of therapeutic benefit in MS. The type I IFNs inhibit IFNγ (27).

Mechanisms of Action of IFNβ

The therapeutic effect of IFNβ lies primarily in its ability to antagonize many of the undesirable effects of IFNγ and to close the opening of the blood–brain barrier that is characteristic of the acute MS plaque. Although it still is possible that a virus will be discovered to be involved in the cause of MS and that IFN functions as an antiviral, it is more likely that the IFNs act by way of their antiproliferative and immunomodulatory effects (28). The antiproliferative actions of IFNβ are consistent with its ability to inhibit proliferating encephalogenic T cells (29), which are considered to play a central role in formation of the MS plaque. Immunologically, whereas IFNγ enhances HLA class II expression on APC, IFNβ blocks this effect (30) and downregulates class II expression on several CNS cell types (31). Interferon also may stimulate production of Th2 suppressor or antiinflammatory T lymphocytes (32). In addition, IFNβ may have an inhibitory effect on the blood–brain barrier opening, which probably explains its major impact on reducing MRI gadolinium enhancement in active MS (33). Finally, it has been shown that IFNβ inhibits matrix metalloproteinases, which facilitate migration of T cells into the CNS (34). The possible function of IFNβ within the CNS compartment remains unclear.

Beta Interferon in Clinical Practice

A clear understanding of the purpose of IFNβ therapy and the findings of the various controlled trials is essential by both the patient and the physician. The pretrial premise on which each of the IFNβ clinical studies was based was that long-term dosing would reduce the relapse rate and, hopefully, the risk of increasing disability. Although IFNβ is termed a *treatment*, it may more appropriately be thought of as a preventive therapy or partial "vaccine-like" agent. When IFNβ-1b was first available, patients began therapy expecting to improve in terms of fixed disability. Emphasis on the preventive nature of IFNβ therapy and the need for long-term (measured in years) therapy is critical to successful use of these agents.

Who Should Be Treated?

Patients with well-defined, clinically definite MS should be considered for therapy because of the requirement for long-term use, the potentially troublesome side effects, and the cost. In addition to a history of creditable relapses, preferably with well-defined objective neurologic change, MRI confirmation of multiple CNS plaques is important. The presence of inflammatory CSF (elevated IgG index and/or oligoclonal IgG bands) and a modest CSF pleocytosis is confirmatory and useful. As noted in the glatiramer acetate section, therapy should be considered early, soon after diagnosis.

The indications for IFN use will change as additional studies and information become available. Although the initial controlled trials of IFNβ-1b and IFNβ-1a enrolled only relapsing-remitting patients, newer European-Canadian studies have shown that IFNβ-1b also has a significant benefit in controlling disability for more advanced secondary progressive patients (see Chapter 10).

Which IFNβ to Choose?

The choice of which commercial product to prescribe should be made in conjunction with the patient, considering lifestyle issues and the most recent data available on each agent. Each product has proven efficacy; however, considering that the pivotal trials were carried out using dissimilar protocols and recruited different types of patients, it is difficult to make exact comparisons. The IFNβ-1b study (35) and the IFNβ-1a (Rebif) study recruited a broad range of relapsing MS patients, from neurologically normal to those with moderately severe disability, whereas the IFNβ-1a (Avonex) study (36) enrolled a narrow range of relapsing patients with mild disability. There also were differences in the pretrial relapse experience. One pilot and two phase III beta IFN trials have been conducted and results published, whereas another large

phase III trial has been completed and reported. In all but one trial, multiple doses were compared, and in each case the higher dose was more effective, supporting the concept that, within the limits of patient tolerance (see subsequent section), a higher dose is more effective (Table 9-2). During the five-year IFNβ-1b trial (37), the annual percent reduction between groups (high-dose IFN versus placebo) was: year one—33 percent, year two—28 percent, year three—28 percent, year four—24 percent, and year five—30 percent. In the IFNβ-1a study (Avonex), a comparable intent to treat analysis showed a decrease in relapses of 18 percent over two years. Table 9-1 indicates the available doses and recommended schedules for interferon treatment.

Consideration of lifestyle may be an issue. The every other day, subcutaneous injections required with IFNβ-1b may be more troublesome than the weekly intramuscular injection of IFNβ-1a, especially for patients who must travel often.

Although the reduction in the relapse rate is more pronounced with IFNβ-1b, the available information suggests that IFNβ-1a (36-38) has an effect in slowing disability. The more recent IFNβ-1a (Rebif) trial also showed a significant effect on disability, especially at the higher dose (data not published). The substantial differences in how the trials were conducted and the type of patients recruited make direct disability comparisons difficult. In

TABLE 9-2
Comparison of Placebo-Controlled Interferon Beta Studies

	IFNβ-1b	IFNβ-1a		
	BETASERON	**AVONEX**	**REBIF**	
			LOW DOSE**	**HIGH DOSE**+
Study Characteristics				
Size	373	301	560	
EDSS Range	0–5.5	1–3.5	0–5.0	
Doses Tested	2	1	2	
Study Results				
% Relapse Reduction	31*	18	29	32
% Progressing	NS			
Placebo		35	38	
IFNβ Treatment		22		
Low Dose			30	
High Dose				24

EDSS, Expanded Disability Status Scale
* High dose, 8 MIU
** Low dose, 6 MIU
+ High dose, 12 MIU
NS, Not significant

the IFNβ-1b study, the difference between groups regarding disability was insignificant (p = 0.096), whereas in the IFNβ-1a trial it was significant (p = 0.02).

In regard to MRI change, all available IFNs produce a profound, rapid, and significant decrease on gadolinium enhancements (39). High-dose IFNβ-1b was shown to inhibit expansion of the T2 area of brain tissue involvement (burden of disease) significantly for more than four years (37), whereas IFNβ-1a controlled T2 expansion significantly for only one year (36).

Initiation of IFNβ Therapy

The ability to maintain patients on IFNβ therapy has been disappointing, especially because only long-term compliance, measured in years, is likely to provide real benefit. Two factors appear to be responsible: inadequate instruction and support at onset of treatment, and poorly tolerated side effects. Intensive education of the purpose of therapy and proper injection technique, along with discussion of realistic expectations, provided by a knowledgeable and empathetic MS nurse who is able to provide ongoing support in the first months of therapy, is probably the key to long-term success. Prompt attention to serious adverse effects, such as skin necrosis with IFNβ-1b or persistent flulike symptoms, is essential.

Several measures help reduce adverse effects of IFNβ, especially during the difficult initiation period. Using one half the recommended dose for two to four weeks, injecting at bedtime, and taking ibuprofen during the 24 hours after injection are all useful. Wide rotation of injection sites when using IFNβ-1b is essential.

Adverse Effects of IFNβ Therapy

Most of the commonly experienced adverse effects of IFNβ therapy are noted in Table 9-3, which details a study carried out at the University of Maryland with IFNβ-1b. The dropout rate as a result of adverse effects was relatively low during the first year, which was attributed to careful patient selection and education. Persistence of intolerable flulike symptoms was most prevalent in this series, although skin reactions and necrosis following subcutaneous IFNβ-1b injections are frequently cited as the primary cause of discontinuation. An increase in spasticity is commonly noted with IFNβ therapy. The symptoms are similar with IFNβ-1b and IFNβ-1a but less frequent with IFNβ-1a because of once-a-week dosing. Patients must be observed for laboratory deviations at three-month intervals when injecting IFNβ-1b, and all patients should be monitored regularly for evidence of depression, even though the evidence that IFNβ causes depression is debatable. Women should be warned to stop medication before attempting to become

TABLE 9-3
Withdrawals from IFNβ-1b (Betaseron) Therapy Over One Year (N167)

REASON FOR WITHDRAWAL	NUMBER
Persistent flulike symptoms	8
Dyspnea	3
Pregnancy	3
Increased spasticity	2
Skin reactions	2
Persistent headaches	2
Gastrointestinal symptoms	1
Thrombocytopenia (recurrent)	1
Total	22

pregnant or when pregnancy is confirmed. Pregnancy, of course, is not a side effect of IFNβ therapy but is a mandatory reason for stopping IFNβ use. Patients with small body mass and younger patients have an increased incidence of adverse effects (37).

Remarkable variation in patient tolerance to IFN therapy is noted. Many patients report few problems within weeks of onset, whereas other dedicated patients cannot tolerate a full dose of IFNβ-1b after a year of treatment and are usually switched to glatiramer acetate.

Neutralizing Antibodies

The importance of neutralizing antibodies to Type I IFNs as a cause of treatment failure is unclear. In the IFNβ-1b (35) study 38 percent and in the IFNβ-1a (36) study 22 percent of patients developed neutralizing antibodies in the original trials. Within months to years some patients raise high titers of neutralizing antibodies, which then decline even though dosing continues. Studies of comparable situations in which type I IFN is used therapeutically for various types of cancer clearly shows that persistent neutralizing antibodies reduce or block the clinical effect. In the current MS situation, patients who are doing well should be maintained on the initially prescribed IFN. For those who continue to have relapses (two to three per year) or show clear evidence of progression, the physician can obtain an IFN antibody titer, preferably on two samples drawn two or three months apart, or an enhanced MRI to assess for enhancing lesions. If there is clinical, antibody, or MRI evidence of active disease, the alternative, glatiramer acetate, should be considered. Neutralizing antibodies to IFNβ-1b cross-react with IFNβ-1a (40), arguing that switching from one IFN product to another will probably not be successful.

Direct Comparisons

The first study comparing the clinical effects of IFNβ-1b (Betaseron), IFNβ-1a (Avonex), and glatiramer acetate (Copaxone) was reported in the Fall of 1999. Approximately 450 patients in well-balanced groups were selected for each treatment and observed for 1+ years. Both glatiramer acetate and IFNß-1b had a significant effect on relapses and disability (EDSS), which was most pronounced for glatiramer acetate in the second six months. IFNβ-1a failed to significantly affect either the relapse rate or disability (42).

CONCLUSION

Glucocorticosteroid therapy should be considered for all significant MS relapses that involve visual, motor, coordination, and pain symptoms. Both IV and oral GCS probably are effective.

Several independent studies reported since 1993 show convincingly that long-term use of glatiramer acetate or beta interferon significantly lowers the MS relapse rate, reduces the number of enhancing and T2 lesions on MRI, and partially inhibits progression of fixed disability. The various clinical trials were conducted with the smallest statistically acceptable number of subjects for the shortest reasonable time to gain significant evidence of clinical effect for regulatory (FDA) approval. It is not reasonable to limit the use of these agents to the strict confines of the clinical trials. The same reasoning applies to appropriate insurance coverage for the broad relapsing MS population. New evidence indicates that these agents have a beneficial effect in the more progressive stages of disease, as was shown in the extended and open-label glatiramer acetate and European-Canadian IFNβ-1b trials.

Substantial evidence of axonal damage and CNS atrophy beginning soon after diagnosis argues strongly that immunomodulating therapy should be initiated early in the course of clinically definite MS.

The purpose for immunomodulating therapy of relapsing MS must be clearly understood by both the patient (and his or her support persons) and the treating physician. Careful patient education by a knowledgeable nurse, combined with frequent follow-up support, provides the best program for long-term therapeutic success.

References

1. Poser CM, Paty DW, Scheinberg L, et al. New diagnostic criteria for multiple sclerosis: Guidelines for research protocols. *Ann Neurol* 1983; 13:227–31.
2. Johnson KP, Brooks BR, Cohen JA, et al. Copolymer 1 reduces relapse rate and improves disability in relapsing-remitting multiple sclerosis: Results of a phase III multicenter, double-blind, placebo-controlled trial. *Neurology* 1995; 45:1268–1276.
3. Goodkin DE, Kinkel RP, Weinstock-Guttman B, et al. Randomized, double-masked study of bi-monthly high vs low dose intravenous methylprednisolone in relapsing-progressive multiple sclerosis. *Neurology.* In press.
4. Beck RW, Cleary PA, Trobe JP, et al. The effect of corticosteroids for acute optic neuritis on the subsequent development of multiple sclerosis. The Optic Neuritis Study Group. *N Engl J Med* 1993; 329:1764–1769.
5. The Optic Neuritis Study Group. Visual function 5 years after optic neuritis. *Arch Ophthalmol* 1997; 115: 1545–1552.
6. Barnes D, Hughes RAC, Morris RW, et al. Randomized trial of oral and intravenous methylprednisolone in acute relapses of multiple sclerosis. *Lancet* 1997; 349:902–905.
7. Baumhefner RW, Tourtellotte WW, Syndulkok, et al. Multiple sclerosis intra-blood-brain-barrier IgG synthesis: Effect of pulse intravenous and intrathecal corticosteroids. *Ital J Neurol Sci* 1989; 10:19–32.
8. Teitelbaum D, Sela M, Arnon R. Copolymer 1 from the laboratory to the FDA. *Isr J Med Sci* 1997; 33:280–284.
9. Abramsky O, Teitelbaum D, Arnon R. Effect of a synthetic polypeptide (Cop 1) on patients with multiple sclerosis and acute disseminated encephalomyelitis: preliminary report. *J Neurol Sci* 1977; 31:433–8.
10. Bornstein MB, Miller AI, Teitelbaum D, et al. Multiple Sclerosis: Trial of a synthetic polypeptide. *Ann Neurol* 1982; 11:317–9.
11. Bornstein MB, Miller AI, Slagel S, et al. A pilot trial of Cop 1 in exacerbating-remitting multiple sclerosis. *N Engl J Med* 1987; 317:408–14.
12. Bornstein MB, Miller AI, Slagle S, et al. A placebo-controlled, double-blind, randomized, two-center, pilot trial of Cop 1 in chronic progressive multiple sclerosis. *Neurology* 1991; 41:533–539.
13. Johnson KP, Brooks, BR, Cohen JA, et al. Extended use of copolymer 1 maintains clinical effect on multiple sclerosis relapse rate and degree of disability. *Neurology* 1998; 50:701–708.
14. Arnon R. The development of Cop 1 (Copaxone), an innovative drug for the treatment of multiple sclerosis: Personal reflections. *Immunol Lett* 1996; 50:1–15.
15. Fridkis-Hareli M and Strominger JL. Promiscuous binding of synthetic copolymer 1 to purified HLA-D molecules. *J Immunol* 1998; 160:4386–4397.
16. Teitelbaum D, Milo R, Arnon R, et al. Synthetic copolymer 1 inhibits human T-cell lines specific for myelin basic protein. *Proc Natl Acad Sci USA* 1992; 89:137–141.
17. Racke MK, Martin R, McFarland HF, et al. Copolymer-1–induced inhibition of antigen-specific T cell activation: Interference with antigen presentation. *J Neuroimmunol* 1992; 37:75–84.
18. Fridkis-Hareli M, Teitelbaum D, Gurevich E, et al. Direct binding of myelin basic protein and synthetic copolymer 1 to class II major histocompatibility complex molecules on living antigen-presenting cells. *Proc Natl Acad Sci USA* 1994; 91:4872–4876.
19. Martin R, Jaraquemada D, Flerlage M, et al. Fine specificity and HLA restriction of myelin basic protein-specific cytotoxic T cell lines from multiple sclerosis patients and healthy individuals. *J Immunol* 1990; 145:540–548.
20. Aharoni R, Teitelbaum D, Sela M, et al. Copolymer 1 induces T cells of the T helper type 2 that cross react with myelin basic protein and suppress experimental autoim-

mune encephalomyelitis. *Proc Natl Acad Sci USA* 1997; 94:10821–10826.

21. Mancardi GL, Sardanelli F, Parodi R, et al. Effect of copolymer 1 on serial gadolinium-enhanced MRI in relapsing remitting multiple sclerosis. *Neurology* 1998; 50:1127–1133.

22. Trapp BD, Peterson J, Ransohoff RM, et al. Axonal transection in the lesions of multiple sclerosis. *N Engl J Med* 1998; 338:278–285.

23. Johnson KP, Teitelbaum D, Arnon R, Sela M. Antibodies to copolymer 1 do not interfere with its clinical effect. *Neurology* 1995; 38:973.

24. Jacobs L, Johnson KP. A brief history of the use of interferons as treatment for multiple sclerosis. *Arch Neurol* 1994; 51:1245–1252.

25. Johnson KP. The historical development of interferons as multiple sclerosis therapies. *J Mol Med* 1997; 75:89–94.

26. Panitch HS, Hirsch RL, Schindler J, Johnson KP. Treatment of multiple sclerosis with gamma interferon: Exacerbations associated with activation of the immune system. *Neurology* 1987; 37:1097–1102.

27. Dhib-Jalbut S. Mechanisms of IFN action on multiple sclerosis. *Multiple Sclerosis* 1997; 3:397–401.

28. Arnason BG, Reder AT. Interferons and multiple sclerosis. *Clin Neuropharmacol* 1994; 17:495–547.

29. Noronha A., Toscas A, Jensen MA. Interferon beta decreases T cell activation and interferon gamma production in multiple sclerosis. *J Neuroimmunol* 1993; 46:145–154.

30. Ransohoff RM, Devajyothi C, Estes ML, et al. Interferon beta specifically inhibits interferon gamma induced class II major histocompatibility complex gene transcription in a human astrocytoma cell line. *J Neuroimmunol* 1991; 33(2):103–112.

31. Jiang H, Milo R, Swoveland P, et al. Interferon beta 1b reduces interferon gamma induced antigen presenting capacity of human glial and B cells. *J Neuroimmunol* 1995; 61:17–25.

32. Miller SD, Karpus WJ. The immunopathogenesis and regulation of T-cell-mediated demyelinating diseases. *J Immunol Today* 1994; 15:356–361.

33. Calabresi PA, Tranguill LR, Dambrosia JM, et al. Increases in soluble VCAM-1 correlate with a decrease in MRI lesions in multiple sclerosis treated with interferon beta 1b. *Ann Neurol* 1997; 41:669–674.

34. Stuve O, Dooley NP, Uhm JH, et al. Interferon beta 1b decreases the migration of T lymphocytes in vitro: Effects on matrix metalloproteinase-9. *Ann Neurol* 1996; 40:853–863.

35. The IFN Multiple Sclerosis Study Group. Interferon beta 1b is effective in relapsing-remitting multiple sclerosis. I. Clinical results of a multicenter, randomized, double-blind, placebo-controlled trial. *Neurology* 1993; 43:655–661.

36. Jacobs LD, Cookfair DL, Rudick RA, et al. Intramuscular interferon beta 1a for disease progression in relapsing multiple sclerosis. *Ann Neurol* 1996; 39:285–294.

37. The IFN Multiple Sclerosis Study Group and the University of British Columbia MS/MRI Analysis Group. Interferon beta 1b in the treatment of multiple sclerosis: Final outcome of the randomized controlled trial. *Neurology* 1995; 45:1277–1285.

38. Rudick RA, Goodkin DE, Jacobs LD, et al. Impact of interferon beta 1 a on neurologic disability in relapsing multiple sclerosis. *Neurology* 1997; 49:354–363.

39. Stone LA, Frank JA, Albert PS, et al. The effect of interferon beta on blood brain barrier disruption demonstrated by contrast-enhanced magnetic resonance imaging in relapsing remitting multiple sclerosis. *Ann Neurol* 1995; 37:611–619.

40. Khan OA, Dhib-Jalbut SS. Neutralizing antibodies to interferon β-1a (IFNβ 1a; Avonex™) and interferon β-1b (IFNβ 1b; Betaseron®) are cross-reactive. *Neurology* 1998; 51:310–311.

41. Comi G, Filippi M, et al. The effect of glatiramer acetate (Copaxone®) on disease activity as measured by cerebral MRI in patients with relapsing-remitting multiple sclerosis (RRMS): A multi-center, randomized, double-blind, placebo-controlled study extended by open-label treatment. *Neurology* 1999; 52(Suppl 2):A289 (abstract).

42. Khan O, Tselis A, et al. A prospective, controlled, open-label trial comparing the effects of Avonex, Betaseron, and glatiramer acetate on the relapse rate in patients with relapsing-remitting multiple sclerosis. *Ann Neurol* 1999; 46:938 (abstract).

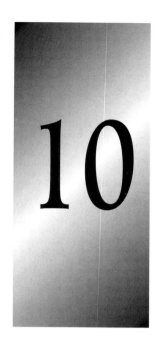

10 Treatment of Progressive Forms of Multiple Sclerosis

Donald E. Goodkin, M.D.

Multiple sclerosis (MS) is the most common cause of nontraumatic neurologic disability affecting young adults in the northern hemisphere. The socioeconomic consequences of progressive disability resulting from this disease are significant considering that between 1981 and 1992, 75 percent to 85 percent of MS patients in the United States, the United Kingdom, and Australia were unemployed and these individuals appear to be at particularly high risk for social isolation (1–3). Because acute and chronic active MS lesions are accompanied by largely irreversible axonal transection (4), early intervention is desirable. More effective treatments to stop or delay progression of disability resulting from MS are needed. In this chapter we review disease-modifying treatment options and emerging treatment options for patients with progressive forms of MS. The background and clinical experience with each therapy are presented. None of these treatments are curative and benefits from each are modest at best.

Progressive forms of MS include primary and secondary progressive MS and progressive-relapsing MS. We first review the clinical patterns of MS to illustrate an important consideration: the distinction between progressive and relapsing forms of MS is not always clear. Indeed, most clinical investigators agree that clinical trials that led to the approval of therapies for relapsing-remitting MS included many patients who met the current consensus definition for secondary progressive MS.

There is a notion that the treatments reviewed in this chapter may be most effective in patients with secondary progressive MS who experience gradual progression of disability accompanied by one or more exacerbations in the preceding two years. This is because a substantial number of patients enrolled in clinical trials for "chronic progressive" MS experienced gradual progression of disability and superimposed relapses. Whether treatments reviewed in this chapter are effective in patients with secondary progressive MS who have not experienced exacerbations for two or more years or in patients with primary or progressive-relapsing MS is not clear.

DEFINITIONS OF RELAPSING-REMITTING, SECONDARY PROGRESSIVE, PRIMARY PROGRESSIVE, AND PROGRESSIVE-RELAPSING MULTIPLE SCLEROSIS

The clinical course of MS follows a variable pattern but is generally characterized by acute episodes of worsening (exacerbations), gradual progression of disability, or combinations of both. After establishing international consensus for terminology, definitions for the most common clinical patterns of MS were proposed in 1996 (5).

First, patients with relapsing-remitting MS experience exacerbations with or without complete recovery (Figure 10-1, a, b). Approximately 85 percent of MS patients experience a relapse at disease onset. Relapsing-remitting patients are clinically stable between exacerbations. Second, patients with secondary progressive MS experience an initial relapse followed by gradual progression of disability with or without superimposed relapses (Figure 10-1, c, d). Approximately 50 percent of patients with relapsing-remitting MS convert to secondary progressive MS within 10 years of disease onset. Third, patients with primary progressive MS experience gradual progression of disability from disease onset without superimposed relapses (Figure 10-1 e, f). Approximately 10 percent of MS patients experience this clinical pattern. Fourth, patients with progressive-relapsing MS patients experience gradual progression of disability from disease onset that is later accompanied by one or more relapses. This clinical pattern affects approximately 5 percent of MS patients (Figure 10-1, g). The new definitions for clinical patterns of MS become confusing when reviewing clinical trials that were completed before 1996. For example, in trials for patients with "chronic progressive" MS, it generally is not clear how many study subjects experienced a secondary progressive, primary progressive, or progressive-relapsing clinical pattern. Similarly, it is not clear how many patients enrolled in earlier studies for relapsing-remitting MS would meet the current definition for secondary progressive MS.

Figure 10-1 illustrates the problem of distinguishing between relapsing-remitting MS with incomplete recovery (Figure 10-1,b) and secondary progressive MS accompanied by relapses (Figure 10-1, d). Patients generally are not reevaluated for months or years after an exacerbation has resolved. Thus on reevaluation it is not possible to determine whether progression of disability during the interval between exacerbations was gradual or a residual from the preceding exacerbation. The distinction between relapsing-remitting and secondary progressive MS with relapses is also difficult when reviewing monthly brain magnetic resonance imaging (MRI) scans. Both clinical forms show frequent gadolinium-enhancing lesions and greater T2-weighted lesion volumes than in patients with primary progressive MS (6). Thus it should not be surprising that the phase III clinical trials that led to the approval of interferon beta-1b, interferon beta-1a, and glatiramer acetate for relapsing-remitting (7,8) and relapsing forms (9) of MS probably included a substantial number of patients who would meet current consensus definition for secondary progressive MS. For these reasons, there are many clinicians who believe that therapeutic indications for interferon beta-1b, interferon beta-1a, and glatiramer acetate should be extended to patients with secondary progressive MS who during the preced-

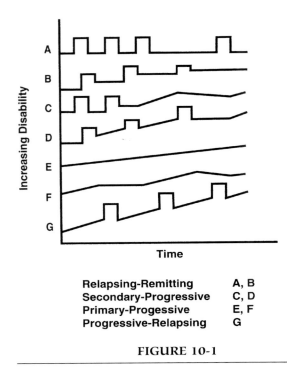

Relapsing-Remitting	A, B
Secondary-Progressive	C, D
Primary-Progessive	E, F
Progressive-Relapsing	G

FIGURE 10-1

Types and courses of multiple sclerosis.

ing two years experienced relapses superimposed upon gradual progression of disability.

TREATMENT OPTIONS FOR PATIENTS WITH PROGRESSIVE FORMS OF MULTIPLE SCLEROSIS

Interferon beta-1b, interferon beta-1a, and glatiramer acetate are reviewed in Chapter 11. Other treatment options for patients with progressive forms of MS reviewed in this section are listed alphabetically to facilitate location. The background and clinical experience with each treatment is provided. These treatments have in common various global immunosuppressant and specific immunomodulating actions. The use of treatments that globally suppress or selectively modulate the immune response of patients with MS is based on the hypothesis that the clinical manifestations of MS are attributable to self-directed immunity. Although unproven, this hypothesis is supported by the following empiric evidence derived from MS patients and animal models of the disease.

1. Clinical and histopathologic similarities between MS and animal models of chronic relapsing experimental allergic encephalomyelitis (EAE) (10);
2. Elevated intrathecal oligoclonal immunoglobulin production (11);
3. A characteristic distribution of cytokines and T-cell subsets within acute and chronic MS plaques (12);
4. Genetic linkage between disease susceptibility and specific HLA-DR haplotypes in several different ethnic groups and susceptibility loci associated with the T-cell receptor beta chain complex (13);
5. Diminished suppressor cell number and function and possible correlation of these abnormalities with disease activity (14);
6. Clinical worsening seen with the administration of interferon gamma (15); and
7. Transient benefit seen with immunosuppressive therapy (16).

Azathioprine

Background

Azathioprine is a purine analogue designed as a "pro drug" to permit the slow liberation of active metabolites 6-mercaptopurine and 6-thioinosinic acid into tissues. Because the maximal in vivo immunosuppressive effect requires three to six months of daily use, azathioprine is frequently combined with more rapidly acting corticosteroids. The precise mechanism of action is uncertain. Several studies have shown that azathioprine suppresses cell-mediated hypersensitivity reactions and produces alterations in antibody production (17). A preliminary report suggests that azathioprine reduces blood levels of tumor necrosis factor (TNF)-a and increases the suppressor-inducer T-cell subset in patients with MS (18).

Clinical Experience

In total, 21 clinical trials of azathioprine in MS have been published since the initial report in 1969 by Tucker and Kapphahn (19). Seven of these trials were controlled and involved either exacerbating or chronic progressive MS patients (20–26). It is not clear how many of the exacerbating or chronic progressive patients in those studies experienced gradual progression of disability with superimposed exacerbations (Figure 10-1, d). A meta-analysis of these seven studies demonstrates a small but significant benefit for azathioprine (27). The relative odds of remaining exacerbation-free for three years while taking azathioprine compared with placebo was 1.97 (27). This benefit compares favorably with the reduction in exacerbation rate reported with interferon beta and glatiramer acetate in relapsing-remitting MS (8,9). However, aza-

thioprine, like interferon beta 1-b, offers only a modest degree of protection against progression of disability. This modest benefit is of questionable significance and requires two to three years before becoming evident.

Toxicity with azathioprine is common but cessation of therapy is required in fewer than 10 percent of MS patients. Cessation of therapy is usually a result of drug-related fever, rash, or gastrointestinal intolerance. The incidence of malignancy associated with azathioprine therapy is not significantly greater than that observed in the general population (28–30).

The slight but consistent reduction in relapse rate, limited toxicity, drug availability, and cost helped to establish azathioprine as a commonly used immunosuppressant therapy in MS. Azathioprine is administered daily using oral doses of 1.5–2.5 mg per kg of body weight. In 1987 azathioprine was used as a standard disease-modifying treatment in some European MS treatment centers (31). The use of azathioprine appears to be less common since the emergence of oral methotrexate as a disease-modifying treatment option for patients with gradual progression of disability with superimposed exacerbations (see subsequent section, "Methotrexate").

2-Chlorodeoxyadenosine

Background

2-chlorodeoxyadenosine (cladribine) is an antilymphocyte agent that mimics the accumulation of deoxynucleotides in adenosine deaminase deficiency (32,33). This drug is reported to cause the death of lymphocytes by apoptosis and has relatively low toxicity toward other tissues. Unlike most other antilymphocyte drugs, it is equally effective against resting and dividing cells (32). The decision to explore the use of 2-chlorodeoxyadenosine in progressive forms of MS was based on the observation that the drug demonstrated prolonged lymphopenia and otherwise acceptable toxicity in the treatment of hairy cell leukemia, lymphomas, and autoimmune hemolytic anemia (34–36).

Clinical Experience

The results of a double-masked, phase II clinical trial comparing 2-chlorodeoxyadenosine and placebo were first reported in 1994 and updated in 1996 (37,38). Fifty-one patients with clinically definite or laboratory-supported definite (39) chronic progressive MS were randomized to receive either 0.1 mg of 2-chlorodeoxyadenosine per kilogram of body weight or placebo daily for one week each month for four months (37). Although this study was designed to include a two-year treatment phase, a preplanned interval analysis at one year demonstrated a therapeutic benefit in patients who were receiving active treatment. Thirty percent (7/23) of the placebo and 4 percent (1/24) of the actively treated patients experienced worsening as measured by a change of one or more points on the Kurtzke Expanded Disability Status Scale (EDSS) score (p < 0.02) (40). Significant benefits were observed at one year for active-treatment recipients as measured by mean paired difference (placebo minus 2-chlorodeoxyadenosine) in total T2-weighted lesion volumes and proportion of patients with gadolinium-enhancing volumes.

Although seven patients developed clinically significant thrombocytopenia, 2-chlorodeoxyadenosine was generally well tolerated. One 40-year-old woman died of fulminant hepatitis B eight days after her initial 2-chlorodeoxyadenosine infusion. It seems unlikely that this complication was treatment-induced because fulminant hepatitis has not been observed in more than 5,000 patients receiving cladribine for leukemia or lymphoma. A separate report suggested that 2-chlorodeoxyadenosine induced axonal peripheral polyneuropathy in six patients under treatment for refractory acute leukemia (41). These patients received 19–21 mg of 2-chlorodeoxyadenosine daily for five consecutive days, a total dose that is similar to that administered to patients with MS over four months.

The encouraging results of this preliminary study prompted a phase III study of patients with chronic progressive MS. In this study 159 patients were randomly assigned to receive placebo or one of two doses of cladribine (0.7 or 2.1 mg/kg). Patients were assessed monthly for 12 months, with evaluation of disability and six-monthly measures of gadolinium-enhanced MRI activity. In a preliminary report of the results from this study, treatments were well tolerated and produced dose-dependent thrombocytopenia (42). Mean disability as assessed by the EDSS and the Scripps Neurological Rating Scale (43), and the proportion of patients in whom treatment failed, was not different among the groups. However, subgroup analyses showed a trend toward greater stabilization of disease in females, patients with secondary progressive MS, and patients with a baseline EDSS score of between 3.5 and 5.0. A trend toward greater disease stability was observed in those with most pronounced lymphocyte nadir. Patients with primary progressive disease did not fare as well as patients with secondary progressive MS. The most dramatic effect was a greater than 90 percent suppression of gadolinium-enhancing lesions in the cladribine recipients. The final results of this study are awaited with considerable interest.

Cyclophosphamide

Background

Cyclophosphamide (CTX) is an alkylating agent that has both cytotoxic and immunosuppressive effects. Monthly intravenous (IV) cyclophosphamide administration in doses ranging from 1000 to 2000 mg per m^2 of body surface results in a pronounced reduction of the number of T helper or T inducer cells and a less striking decrease in suppressor or cytotoxic cells in patients with MS (44). Monthly pulses of IV cyclophosphamide for one year induced reductions in the numbers of suppressor or cytotoxic cells, natural killer cells, and antibody-dependent cellular cytotoxicity functions lasting from one to two months. In addition, reduced B cell numbers in these patients recovered in two to four months, whereas the recovery of helper cell subsets and total T cell numbers, helper/suppressor ratio, and proliferative responses to mitogens took more than four months (45). Others have found that the decrease in helper cell subset populations can still be demonstrated as long as 13.5 years after IV cyclophosphamide therapy (8 grams in 20 days) (46). Preliminary evidence indicates that cyclophosphamide normalizes increased interleukin-12 (IL-12) production in patients with chronic progressive MS and induces a Th2 cytokine switch (47).

Clinical Experience

In 1983 the results of a randomized, unblinded trial comparing (1) IV cyclophosphamide and corticotropin, (2) corticotropin alone, and (3) oral cyclophosphamide, corticotropin, and plasma exchange in 58 patients with chronic progressive MS were reported (48). A statistically significant reduction in the proportion of patients who experienced clinical progression was seen after 12 months in the patients receiving cyclophosphamide and corticotropin. Of the cyclophosphamide-corticotropin–treated group, 80 percent were stabilized or had improved EDSS scores at 12 months, compared with 20 percent of the group who received only corticotropin for 21 days. Although the benefits were no longer evident two years after therapy was initiated, this study appeared to offer a promising treatment option for patients with chronic progressive MS. Neurologists began to use this drug soon after this publication appeared.

Other investigators began to explore the possibility that booster injections of cyclophosphamide might prolong the clinical benefits reported with cyclophosphamide induction. In one study (49), patients with chronic progressive MS were randomly assigned to bimonthly cyclophosphamide booster injections (700 mg per m^2) or no further cyclophosphamide treatment following completion of the Hauser induction regimen (48). A trend that favored the patients treated with booster injections was observed, but this trend did not reach statistical significance. A subsequent report by the Northeast Cooperative Multiple Sclerosis Treatment Group suggested that bimonthly boosters were associated with prolonged clinical stability of chronic progressive MS patients (50). Of the patients initially treated with induction and subsequently treated with bimonthly cyclophosphamide boosters, 38 percent were stable or improved compared with 24 percent of the patients who received only induction therapy. These findings encouraged the use of cyclophosphamide induction and subsequent bimonthly cyclophosphamide boosters in clinical practice.

In a placebo-controlled, single-blind study of IV cyclophosphamide therapy, 22 patients with MS received IV cyclophosphamide without corticosteroids or corticotropin, and 20 control patients received IV folic acid (51). Twelve months after treatment, 64 percent of the cyclophosphamide-treated patients and 70 percent of the placebo-treated patients showed evidence of stable or improved functional status as measured by EDSS scores. The absence of any notable benefit found in this single-blind comparison of cyclophosphamide and folic acid, as well as the toxicity that occurred in similarly treated patients in clinical practice, began to dampen initial enthusiasm for the use of cyclophosphamide in patients with chronic progressive MS. Support for this therapy eroded further after the report of the Canadian Cooperative Multiple Sclerosis Study Group Trial of plasmapheresis and cyclophosphamide in MS (52). This multicenter, single-blind, randomized trial also failed to detect any important difference in treatment benefit in patients treated with IV cyclophosphamide and oral prednisone; daily oral cyclophosphamide, alternate-day prednisone, and weekly plasma exchange; and placebo medications and sham plasma exchange. The reasons for inconsistent results when using IV cyclophosphamide for patients with chronic progressive MS are not entirely clear but have been attributed to differences in drug doses, patient selection, and criteria used to define clinical deterioration (53,54). The final report from the Northeast Cooperative Multiple Sclerosis Treatment Group suggests that benefits observed with cyclophosphamide treatment may be restricted to patients younger than 40 years and those with a secondary progressive course as opposed to a primary progressive clinical course since disease onset (52). A study of pulse cyclophosphamide followed by treatment with interferon beta-1a in patients who are not responsive to beta interferons is now being organized by investigators in Boston and Cleveland.

In summary, clinical benefits observed with CTX therapy are generally marginal, and toxicity, including nausea, vomiting, alopecia, and potential sterility, are adverse effects. The benefits appear to be restricted to MS patients who are younger than 40 years and have secondary progressive disease. There is a general consensus that cyclophosphamide monotherapy has little benefit and significant toxicity in patients older than age 40 who have had a progressive course since disease onset.

Cyclosporine

Background

Cyclosporine is a cyclic undecapeptide that was initially isolated from two soil fungi and recognized as an antifungal metabolite. This drug has proven effective in preventing host versus graft and graft versus host responses when used alone or in combination with conventional agents, and it has been reported to be useful in treating a variety of putative autoimmune diseases in man (55). Interest in using this drug for human neurologic diseases, including MS, quickly followed these initial reports.

Much work has been done in the attempt to clarify cyclosporine's mechanism of action. Many of its in vitro effects can be explained by the observed inhibition of the production of a number of lymphokines, including interleukin-2 (IL-2), interleukin-3, migration inhibitory factor, and gamma interferon (56). Reduced levels of IL-2 messenger RNA (mRNA) inhibit IL-2 production (57), and the same mechanism appears to inhibit other lymphokines (58). However, cyclosporine appears to spare T lymphocytes that secrete a soluble factor that is critical for the expansion of nonspecific suppressor T cells. It appears possible that this T cell subpopulation belongs to the CD4+CD45R+ subset of T cells known as suppressor-inducer cells (59).

Clinical Experience

Three major studies have assessed the efficacy of cyclosporine in MS. The first (60) reported the results of a German multicenter, double-blind, controlled trial of 194 patients with clinically definite active relapsing MS: 98 patients were randomized to treatment with cyclosporine (5 mg/kg/day), and 96 patients underwent treatment with azathioprine (2.5 mg/kg/day). A review of the entry criteria for this study suggests that many of these patients had secondary progressive MS (5). Eighty-five patients in the cyclosporine group and 82 patients in the azathioprine group completed a treatment period of 24 to 32 months as stipulated by the study protocol. No significant changes were detected in EDSS, frequency of relapse, or overall treatment efficacy as assessed by patients and investigators at the end of the trial. Overall, only minor deterioration occurred in both groups during the trial. The incidence of side effects including hypertrichosis, gingival hyperplasia, paresthesias, elevated serum creatinine, and elevated blood pressure was more than two times more common in the cyclosporine group than in the azathioprine group. The authors concluded that cyclosporine as a single agent was not acceptable as the drug of final choice for the long-term immunosuppressive treatment of relapsing MS.

The second study was a double-blind, placebo-controlled trial with patients enrolled in centers in London (N = 44) and Amsterdam (N = 38) (61). Participants in this study had either relapsing or chronic progressive clinically definite MS. The patients were started on daily cyclosporine, 10 mg per kg of body weight for two months, which thereafter was adjusted to minimize toxicity for the final 22 months of observation. The mean daily maintenance dose differed at the two sites (London, 7.2 mg per kg, and Amsterdam, 5.0 mg per kg). A variety of outcome measures including the EDSS were used. Investigators in Amsterdam concluded that no beneficial effects were seen and that side effects from cyclosporine were a problem (62). However, the investigators at the London site reported a significant early benefit for the patients treated with cyclosporine. Patients in London had fewer relapses and a longer interval to first relapse on treatment over the two-year study and better overall functional assessments for the first six months of treatment (63).

The most recent study was a multicenter effort undertaken in the United States (64). In this study, clinically definite moderately disabled (EDSS 3.0 to 7.0) chronic progressive MS patients were randomized to receive cyclosporine (N = 273) or placebo (N = 274) for at least two years. The dosage was adjusted for toxicity, which resulted in trough whole-blood levels from 310 to 430 mg per mL. The mean worsening in EDSS score for cyclosporine-treated patients (0.39 ± 1.07 points) was significantly less (p = 0.002) than for placebo-treated patients (0.65 ± 1.08). Three primary efficacy criteria were used in this study: time to becoming wheelchair-bound, time to "sustained progression of disability," and a composite score of activities of daily living. Cyclosporine treatment delayed patients' ultimate confinement to wheelchair (p = 0.038), but statistically significant effects were not observed for the other criteria. It is difficult to directly compare this study with the German multicenter study because whole-blood trough levels and types of MS patients treated differed significantly.

Cyclosporine treatment did have a favorable effect on several secondary measures of disease outcome. A large and differential withdrawal rate (cyclosporine = 44 percent, placebo = 32 percent) complicated the analysis but did not appear to explain the observed effect of cyclosporine in delaying time to wheelchair confinement. Nephrotoxicity and hypertension were common side effects that accounted for most of the excess loss of patients in the cyclosporine arm of the study. The authors concluded that cyclosporine was associated with a modest benefit in the chronic progressive MS patients in the study, but these benefits were not evident until 18 to 24 months after initiation of therapy. Cyclosporine has never been widely used for the treatment of progressive forms of MS because of the delay in measurable benefit and the high incidence of drug-related adverse effects.

Methotrexate

Background

Low-dose (7.5 mg) weekly oral methotrexate (MTX) has been shown to be a relatively nontoxic, effective treatment for rheumatoid arthritis (RA) (65–70). Clinical investigators originally considered MTX to be a potential treatment for MS because of some similarities in the immune alterations and relapsing clinical courses seen in RA and MS patients. These similarities included reduced numbers of suppressor-inducer cells and increased ratio of helper-inducer to suppressor-inducer cells in the blood (71,72). Additionally, MTX was shown to inhibit the development of EAE (73).

The mechanisms responsible for the therapeutic efficacy of MTX in autoimmune disease are not known, but several known effects of MTX are potentially therapeutic when considered in the context of the present understanding of the immunopathogenesis of these diseases. These activities can be categorized as follows:

1. *Immunosuppressive activity.* An immunosuppressive effect of MTX is supported by the following observations: (1) significant decreases in immunoglobulin (Ig) M–rheumatoid factor levels have been observed in RA patients who improved clinically during MTX therapy (74); (2) serial assessments of T-cell subsets in RA patients treated with weekly, low-dose, oral MTX have demonstrated a significant increase in suppressor-effector (CD8+CD11+) cell numbers and a trend for increases in suppressor-inducer (CD4+2H4+) cells that paralleled clinical improvement (75); and (3) peripheral blood lymphocytes from RA patients receiving MTX that are grown in low-folate culture conditions show in vitro proliferation indices that are lower than those from normal individuals and from RA patients not being treated with MTX (76).

2. *Antiinflammatory activity.* An antiinflammatory effect of MTX has long been inferred by the observation that clinical manifestations of RA improve within a few weeks after initiating therapy and worsen just as quickly after the drug is discontinued (77). The following in vitro observations also support an antiinflammatory activity for MTX: (1) synthesis of the proinflammatory leukotriene B4 by peripheral blood neutrophils from MTX-treated RA patients is suppressed (78); and (2) the functional activity of IL-1 is decreased by MTX in vitro. This may be on the basis of binding of IL-1 to MTX by

virtue of a 60 percent sequence homology between IL-1b and dihydrofolate reductase (79), or inhibition of IL-1b binding to IL-1 receptors on target cells (80).

3. *Immunoregulation.* Methotrexate may also have significant immunoregulatory activities mediated by its antagonistic effect on histamine receptors located on cytotoxic T cells. It has been demonstrated that histamine binds to histamine-2 (H-2) receptors on cytotoxic T cells, thereby stimulating production of interferon gamma, which has been shown to upregulate major histocompatibility complex (MHC) class II expression on immunoactive cells (81). Histamine-2 receptor antagonists (H-2RA) have been used with some success in the treatment of psoriasis and pilot studies with H-2RA are already under way in MS.

Clinical Experience

There have been three published studies examining the toxicity and clinical efficacy of MTX in patients with MS. In the first pilot study, oral MTX (2.5 mg/day) and oral 6-mercaptopurine (75 mg/day) were administered to MS patients in alternating three-month cycles for 10 to 24 months (82). Although the study was randomized and blinded, the patient groups and outcome measures were poorly defined. Additionally, disease durations in the treatment groups were dissimilar. Thus, even though no therapeutic efficacy was evident, design limitations made the results of this study difficult to interpret. In the second pilot study, 45 patients with relapsing or chronic progressive MS were randomly assigned to receive one 2.5 mg tablet of methotrexate every 12 hours for three consecutive doses each week for one year (83). A marginally significant (p = 0.05) difference in the mean number of exacerbations favoring active treatment was seen in relapsing patients. However, no treatment group differences in progression of EDSS scores were noted in relapsing or chronic progressive patients.

In the third study, 60 patients with clinically definite chronic progressive MS, aged 21 to 60 years, with EDSS scores of 3.0 to 6.5, were randomly assigned to receive 7.5 mg of oral methotrexate or placebo one day each week for two years (84,85). The primary outcome measure for this phase II study was the rate of sustained "treatment failure" in the MTX and PLC arms of the study. As defined before study onset, patients could meet treatment failure requirements for the composite outcome variable in any of the following ways: (1) worsening of the entry EDSS (40) by ≥ 1.0 point for patients with an entry score of 3.0 to 5.0 or by ≥ 0.5 point for those patients with an entry EDSS score of 5.5 to 6.5; (2) worsening of the entry ambulation index (AI) (41) score of 2

to 6 by ≥ 1.0 point; or (3,4) worsening of ≥ 20 percent from baseline value on best performance of two successive Box and Block Test (BBT) or 9-Hole Peg Test (9HPT) (86) scores obtained with either hand. Thus the composite outcome measure was "disjunctive" (87) in that worsening of the designated amount on any of its components was taken to indicate treatment failure. Changes on any of the components of this composite outcome measure had to be sustained for two or more months to be designated as treatment failure.

A significant treatment effect was measured using the composite outcome. Sustained treatment failure was experienced by 51.6 percent of patients treated with MTX and 82.8 percent of patients treated with placebo (p = 0.011). Individually, EDSS, 9HPT, and BBT components of the composite outcome measure also favored MTX therapy. This effect was strongest for the 9HPT (p = 0.007) and was seen to a lesser extent by the BBT (p = 0.068) and the EDSS (p = 0.205). Sustained treatment failure as defined by change in AI did not differ between the groups. For the 19 patients who met criteria for treatment failure with the 9HPT, the median change in time from baseline 9HPT performance was 17.7 seconds and the median percent change from baseline was 45.7 percent. A significant treatment effect favoring methotrexate was also seen as measured by neuropsychological measures of information processing speed (p < 0.025), confrontational naming (p < 0.05), and prose recall (p < 0.05) (88). Adverse experiences were mild and no patient discontinued therapy as a direct result of therapy.

Thirty-five patients in this study were monitored with six-weekly brain MRI scans for six months. A treatment effect favoring MTX was observed measured by absolute change in T2-weighted total lesion area in this cohort. Change in T2-weighted total lesion area was significantly related to sustained progression of disability as measured by the 9HPT but not sustained progression measured by the EDSS (89).

Methotrexate appears to offer a relatively well tolerated treatment option for patients with chronic progressive MS. Its benefit appears to be most evident on tests of upper extremity function, and preliminary data suggest that patients with secondary progressive MS are more likely to experience treatment benefits than are patients with primary progressive MS.

Methylprednisolone

Background

Glucocorticosteroids (GCSs) are routinely used for the treatment of acute exacerbations of MS but their role as a disease-modifying therapy remains uncertain (90). Glucocorticosteroids have multiple and diverse effects on the cellular elements of the immune system, in general by inhibiting or increasing transcription of selected genes by acting through the GCS receptor. The following activities of GCSs are potentially relevant when considering GCSs as a disease-modifying treatment for MS.

1. ENDOTHELIUM, CAPILLARY PERMEABILITY, AND LEUKOCYTE CHEMOTAXIS

Leukocyte recruitment to sites of inflammation is dependent on the interaction of complementary surface adhesion molecules with those on endothelium. Histopathologic studies have shown upregulation of intercellular adhesion molecule-1 (ICAM-1) and vascular cell adhesion molecule-1 (VCAM-1) and leukocyte counter receptors leukocyte function-associated antigen-1 (LFA-1) and very late activation antigen-4 (VLA-4) in MS plaques (91). Glucocorticosteroids decrease E selectin and ICAM-1 expression in vitro, an effect that is reversed with RU 486, a steroid inhibitor (92). Leukocyte diapedesis in vivo is inhibited by dexamethasone, an effect mediated by lipocortin-1, which is induced by GCSs (93). Glucocorticosteroids inhibit inflammatory edema by reducing capillary permeability, the imaging correlate of which is a reduction of gadolinium enhancement on CT or MRI scans (94–96) This is seen as soon as eight hours after GCS administration, and edema reduction may be one of the most important steroid actions in the improvement of disability associated with acute MS attacks. Notably, this effect, which is dose dependent, is less effective with oral prednisone administered as 50 mg a day or 100 mg on alternate days than 60–120 mg every day (95). Despite dramatic reductions in gadolinium enhancement with GCSs, there is no consistent reduction in blood–brain permeability to albumin (97,98). The two molecules differ substantially in molecular weight (albumin 69,000 kilodaltons and gadolinium 300 kilodaltons), and only the latter is transported by the endothelial vesicular transport system. Thus, although the exact mechanism by which GCSs reduce capillary permeability is not known, it is likely to be at least in part due to reductions in transendothelial vesicular transport (97). It is also known that GCSs inhibit metalloproteases that are known to disrupt the blood–brain barrier and are elevated in the cerebrospinal fluid of MS patients (99).

2. MACROPHAGES AND MONOCYTES

Macrophages and monocytes are responsible for myelin phagocytosis, are capable of presenting antigenic fragments of myelin to T cells, are potently proinflammatory, and secrete myelinotoxic compounds. They have enhanced expression of MHC class II and chemotaxin receptors in MS plaques (100). Glucocorticosteroids induce a monocytopenia, with the peak effect at four to six hours and lasting 24 hours (101). In vitro GCSs inhibit chemo-taxis (102), enzyme release (103) and eicosanoid production (104), IgG- and CR3-mediated endocytosis (105), Fc receptor expression, phagocytosis, (106), proinflammatory cytokine release (107), and inducible nitric oxide synthase, which is known to promote EAE (108,109).

3. LYMPHOCYTES

A single intravenous dose of GCS decreases by redistribution of circulating CD4 (helper-inducer) T cells and B lymphocytes, but not CD8 (cytotoxic-suppressor) cell counts within four hours and levels return to normal in 24 hours (110,111). Glucocorticosteroids decrease lymphocyte proliferation to lectins and antigen, mixed lymphocyte responses, as well as cytokine release, including interferon gamma, which is known to increase MS exacerbations (112).

4. CYTOKINE PRODUCTION

Proinflammatory cytokines are the molecular mediators that determine the nature and kinetics of an immune response. There are three mechanisms by which GCSs inhibit proinflammatory cytokine expression. First, by repression of cytokine genes by binding to negative GRE. Glucocorticosteroids inhibit the transcription of interleukins 1,3–6,8, TNF (107,113,114), granulocyte-macrophage colony-stimulating factor (GM-CSF) (107), and interferon gamma (115) by the binding of the steroid receptor to negative GRE in these genes. Second, there is repression of gene expression by competitive binding to transcription factors as proinflammatory cytokines like TNF-a produce their cellular effects via activation of transcription factors AP-1 and NfkB. For example, there is potent steroid inhibition of AP-1 and NfkB binding to DNA by IL-1b and TNF-a (113) and the IL-2 gene and promoter has no negative GRE and steroids inhibit transcription by blocking AP-1 from DNA binding. Third, GCSs can inhibit proinflammatory cytokine expression by destabilizing cytokine mRNA, which will result in decreased translation. IL-1b mRNA stability is decreased, as shown by both steady-state measurements and pulse labeling (116). Examples of how such GCS activities may be of relevance in MS are that interferon gamma and TNF-a, which are inhibited by GCSs, appear to be important elements in the cascade of events culminating in demyelination. Administration of IFN-gamma increases MS exacerbations (112), elevated CSF TNF levels are associated with MS disease progression (117), and TNF administration augments whereas inhibition abrogates EAE (118,119).

Glucocorticosteroids induce TGFb-1 production from T cells in vitro (120), and administration of this cytokine is beneficial in EAE and is currently being evaluated in MS clinical trials. Glucocorticosteroids also downregulate IL-2 receptors modulating cytokine effects independent of repression or induction of their synthesis (121).

5. IMMUNOGLOBULIN PRODUCTION

Steroids decrease circulating B cell number and decrease serum immunoglobulin (Ig) levels within five days of treatment because of both decreased production and increased catabolism (122), and pulsed IV steroids induce a reversible reduction in intrathecal Ig synthesis (123,124).

Clinical Experience

Although corticotropin and GCSs hasten recovery from acute exacerbations of MS, their role in the long-term management of MS has not been rigorously investigated in a placebo-controlled clinical trial (125). Although it has been stated that chronic use of corticosteroids does not significantly slow progression of disability (125), there are only five studies that directly address this question. In 1961 the first study compared oral prednisone 10–15 mg with aspirin or placebo in 86 "moderately disabled" MS patients and demonstrated no difference in measures of disability, exacerbation rate, or patient self-assessment at 6 or 18 months (126). The methods of patient evaluation are not clear and the scoring system to determine progression of disability is not widely accepted or validated. The second study in 1965 reported the results of treatment of 76 patients with relapsing and progressive forms of MS with daily oral methylprednisolone, 8–12 mg or cyanocobalamin for 18 months (127). There were no differences in relapse rate, but there was less deterioration in the steroid recipients as measured by the pyramidal, cerebellar, and bladder functional systems scores of the EDSS (128). The third study of long-term management with corticotropin was reported in 1967 (129). In this study patients were treated with placebo or corticotropin, 15 to 25 units intramuscularly (IM) each day for 18 months. No treatment effect was observed. The fourth study was a randomized, double-masked trial of placebo or IV methylprednisolone, 500 mg administered intravenously for five days to 28 patients with chronic progressive MS. Improvement in pyramidal function was noted at one month. Unfortunately, it is difficult to interpret these results because the use of concomitant treatment for spasticity was not reported and the IV methylprednisolone recipients were more disabled than the placebo recipients at baseline (130).

Data from a recent phase II study suggest that higher doses of methylprednisolone may delay the time to onset of sustained progression of disability in patients with secondary progressive MS (131). In that study, 108 patients were randomly assigned to receive bimonthly pulses of 500 mg (high-dose) or 10 mg (low-dose) of methylprednisolone every eight weeks for two years. Each bimonthly pulse was administered intravenously once each day for three days, followed by a tapering course of methylpred-

nisolone administered orally starting on day 4 and concluding on day 14. High-dose recipients initiated their tapering dose of methylprednisolone at 64 mg and took the following doses on days 2–11: 64, 48, 48, 32, 32, 24, 24, 8, 8, 8 mg. Low-dose recipients initiated their tapering dose at 10 mg and took the following doses on days 2–11: 10, 8, 8, 6, 6, 4, 4, 2, 2, 2 mg. No treatment effect was evident with the primary outcome, the binomial comparison of the proportions of patients in each treatment group who after two years experienced sustained progression of disability (EDSS). However, a significant treatment effect was seen with the preplanned secondary outcome, a log rank comparison of the survival curves of the low-dose and high-dose recipients. Drug-related adverse events were observed more frequently in high-dose recipients, but serious drug-related adverse events were uncommon and cessation of study drug was only required in one patient (psychotic episode). Although the log rank comparison of survival curves favored the high-dose recipients, the design of this study does not enable us to know the optimal dose of methylprednisolone or whether low-dose recipients experience a treatment effect when compared with placebo recipients. A placebo-controlled phase III trial of methylprednisolone is necessary to answer these questions and clarify whether GCSs should become a disease-modifying treatment option for patients with secondary progressive MS.

Plasma Exchange

Background

Although it is generally accepted that MS is predominantly a cell-mediated inflammatory disorder, a role for autoantibodies or other proteinaceous substances in its pathogenesis has not been entirely excluded. This possibility, and the acknowledged effectiveness of plasma exchange in autoantibody- or immune-mediated disorders such as myasthenia gravis and Guillain-Barré syndrome, fostered an interest in plasma exchange as a possible therapy for patients with MS.

Clinical Experience

The first double-blind controlled trial of plasma exchange in patients with MS appeared in 1985 (132). Fifty-four patients with chronic progressive MS were randomized to receive active or sham plasma exchange. Patients who received active plasma exchange had 5 percent of their body weight exchanged per week for 20 weeks. All study participants received 1 mg of oral prednisone per kg of body weight every other day tapered after 15 weeks, and oral cyclophosphamide, 1.5 mg per kg daily during the 20-week treatment course. A significant difference in stabilization rates as measured by EDSS scores favoring the active plasma exchange was seen after 20 weeks. A second uncontrolled study of 200 patients with chronic progressive MS demonstrated an 83 percent stabilization or improvement rate as measured by change in EDSS scores (133). The clinical significance of this finding is difficult to interpret in the absence of a control group.

Initial enthusiasm for the use of plasma exchange as a potential therapy for chronic progressive MS was considerably reduced by the findings of the Canadian Cooperative Multiple Sclerosis Study Group (134). These investigators reported no notable difference in treatment failure rates in patients treated with either (1) oral prednisone plus 1 gram of IV cyclophosphamide every other day until the blood leukocyte count was less than 4500 per L, or a total dose of 9 grams was administered; (2) daily oral cyclophosphamide, 1.5–2.0 mg per kg, plus alternate-day oral prednisone and weekly plasma exchange; or (3) placebo tablets combined with sham plasma exchange. Nonetheless, a meta-analysis of the results from six prospective controlled clinical trials suggests that recipients of plasma exchange, when combined with an immunosuppressive drug, are less likely to experience a progression of disability than patients treated with immunosuppressive drugs alone (135). A phase III clinical trial is necessary to determine whether plasma exchange will have a role as a disease-modifying treatment option for patients with progressive forms of MS.

Total Lymphoid Irradiation

Background

Total lymphoid irradiation (TLI) was initially developed to treat Hodgkin's disease. Shortly thereafter it was used in the treatment of rheumatoid arthritis. The rationale for its use includes (1) its ability to induce a long-lasting suppression of T-cell immune responses in animals receiving skin grafts and bone marrow transplant (136); and (2) the absence of observed long-term sequelae, including hematologic malignancies (137). The beneficial effects seen with TLI in patients with rheumatoid arthritis (138) resulted in its application to patients with MS. In patients with MS, TLI and low-dose prednisone results in a marked reduction in the relative and absolute number of CD3+ T cells, CD4+ helper T cells, CD4+ CD45RA+ naive T cells, and CD19+ B cells for at least one year (139). It also is reported that a relatively greater susceptibility of CD4+ T cells combined with the generation of nonspecific suppressor cells appears to be partly responsible for the increased functional suppression observed in vitro after TLI (140). This restoration of functional suppression is hypothesized to downregulate the autoimmune response and lead to stabilization of disease activity in patients with MS (141).

Clinical Experience

Preliminary reports of the efficacy of TLI in stabilizing progressive MS were published shortly after its initial use in rheumatoid arthritis. The first controlled trial of TLI in the treatment of MS appeared in 1986 (142). Forty-five patients with chronic progressive MS were randomly assigned to receive TLI or placebo. A treatment effect favoring active therapy was seen in 24 patients up to 12 months after initiating treatment. This effect was most notable and sustained for up to 18 months in patients who had lymphocyte counts less than 850 per microliter three months after completing therapy (143). However, no patient characteristic predicted a sustained lymphopenia, and not all patients with sustained lymphopenia obtained a benefit from treatment.

Total lymphoid irradiation of patients with chronic progressive MS has been associated with at least five treatment-associated deaths (142). Three of the deaths were due to aspiration pneumonia in ambulatory patients with severe pretreatment bulbar dysfunction. One death was of unknown cause in a patient lost to follow-up but known to have severe MS before treatment (EDSS 8–9). The final death, which apparently was unrelated to therapy, was from a myocardial infarction that occurred 54 months after concluding treatment.

Modified TLI (i.e., without splenic irradiation) appears to provide similar clinical benefits without associated serious adverse events (144,145). In a double-blind controlled study, 46 chronic progressive MS patients were randomly assigned to receive; (1) modified TLI plus a tapered initial dose (30 mg) of oral prednisone, or (2) sham modified TLI and a tapered initial dose (30 mg) of oral prednisone. A significant treatment effect favoring active modified TLI plus oral prednisone was found as measured by a one-point improvement in the EDSS score sustained for six months. The treatment was not associated with severe toxicity. Modified TLI is currently considered an experimental treatment for patients with chronic progressive MS.

EMERGING TREATMENTS FOR PROGRESSIVE FORMS OF MULTIPLE SCLEROSIS

Interferon Beta

Background

Interferon beta-1b and interferon beta-1a are approved for use in patients with relapsing-remitting (7) and relapsing forms of MS (9). Earlier in this chapter we discussed the rationale for use of these treatments in patients with secondary progressive MS who experience gradual progression of disability and superimposed exacerbations. The role of these therapies for patients with gradual progression of disability without recent exacerbations remains unclear.

Clinical Experience

There are two ongoing phase III studies of the use of interferon beta in patients with secondary progressive MS. The first is a study of interferon beta-1b 8 MIU, administered subcutaneously every other day. This study, conducted by investigators in Europe and sponsored by Schering AG Berlin, Germany, includes 720 secondary progressive patients between 18 and 55 years with clinically definite MS for one or more years and EDSS scores 3.0 to 6.5. In the judgment of the investigators, patients must have experienced a relapsing-remitting course followed by progressive deterioration sustained for six or more months with or without superimposed relapses. The primary outcome is time to confirmed progression from baseline EDSS score (146). Secondary outcomes include a variety of clinical and MRI measures. Although this study was terminated after a preplanned interim analysis for reasons of "overwhelming efficacy," the results have not completed the peer review process or been presented in a scientific forum. It will be of particular interest to determine whether the response to treatment in patients who experience gradual progression of disability is different in those who do and do not experience superimposed relapses. The second is an ongoing study comparing placebo and two doses of interferon beta-1b, 8 MIU and 5 MIU/m2 body surface area up to a dose of 12 MIU administered subcutaneously every other day. This study includes more than 900 patients across 35 sites in North America. All patients with clinically definite MS for two or more years experienced a relapsing-remitting course followed by progressive deterioration sustained for at least six months. Patients may or may not have superimposed attacks; however, progression of disability cannot be solely attack related. At entry, EDSS scores range from 3.5 to 6.5 and patients may not have experienced an exacerbation in the preceding 60 days, taken immunosuppressive or cytotoxic therapy or other investigational drug for six months, received prior treatment with interferon, TLI, cladribine, or monoclonal antibodies. The treatment phase is three years and the primary outcome is time to progression of neurologic impairment defined by confirmed increase from the baseline EDSS score. Secondary outcomes include a variety of clinical and MRI measures. The final results from this study are not anticipated before the year 2000.

Mitoxantrone

Background

Mitoxantrone is an anthracenedione antineoplastic agent that intercalates with DNA and exerts a potent immunomodulating effect that suppresses humoral immunity, reduces T cell numbers, abrogates helper activity, and enhances suppressor function (147,148). It is highly effective in suppressing the development of acute EAE and prevents or delays relapse in a chronic relapsing model of EAE (149).

Clinical Experience

Mitoxantrone was administered in an open trial to 13 patients with chronic progressive MS (150). All patients received mitoxantrone 8 mg/m2 every three weeks for a total of seven infusions, with dosage adjustments depending on the hematologic profile at the nadir. The treatment was well tolerated, although four of seven women developed transient secondary amenorrhea. The postenrollment clinical course of these patients was more favorable than during the 18 months before enrollment. In a phase II study, 42 clinically active relapsing-remitting and secondary progressive were randomly assigned to mitoxantrone 20 mg IV and methylprednisolone 1 g IV each month (MxIVMP) or methylprednisolone 1 g IV alone (IVMP) each month for six months (151). Blinded analyses of MRI data showed significantly more MxIVMP than IVMP recipients without new enhancing lesions. Unblinded clinical assessments showed a significant improvement measured as change in EDSS score at months two to six in the MxIVMP recipients. The final mean improvement in EDSS score was greater than one point. There also was a significant reduction in the number of relapses and an increase in the number of patients free of exacerbation in the MxIVMP group. Additional studies of this promising therapy for patients with progressive forms of MS are needed.

References

1. Gulick EE, Yam M, Touw MM. Work performance by persons with multiple sclerosis: Conditions that impede or enable the performance of work. *Int J Nurs Stud* 1989; 26:301–311.
2. Maybery CP, Brown CR. Social relationships, knowledge and adjustment to multiple sclerosis. *J Neurol Neurosurg Psychiatry* 1984; 47:372–376.
3. Colville PL. Rehabilitation. In: Hallpike JF, Adams CWM, Tourtellotte WW (eds.). *Multiple sclerosis: Pathology, diagnosis, and management.* Baltimore: Williams & Wilkins, 1983:631–654.
4. Trapp BD, Peterson J, Ransohoff RM, et al. Axonal transection in the lesions of multiple sclerosis. *N Engl J Med* 1998; 338:278–285.

5. Lublin FD, Reingold SC. Defining the clinical course of multiple sclerosis: Results of an international survey. *Neurology* 1996; 46:907–911.

6. Losseff NA, Kingsley DPE, McDonald WI, Miller DH, Thompson AJ. Clinical and magnetic resonance imaging predictors of disability in primary and secondary progressive multiple sclerosis. *Multiple Sclerosis* 1966; 1:218–222.

7. IFNB Multiple Sclerosis Study Group. Interferon beta-1b is effective in relapsing-remitting multiple sclerosis: I. Clinical results of a multicenter, randomized, double-blind, placebo-controlled trial. *Neurology* 1993; 43:655–661.

8. Johnson KP, Brooks BR, Cohen JA, et al. Copolymer 1 reduces relapse rate and improves disability in relapsing-remitting multiple sclerosis: Results of a phase III multicenter, double-blind, placebo-controlled trial. *Neurology* 1995; 45:1268–1276.

9. Jacobs L, Cookfair D, Rudick R, et al. Intramuscular interferon beta-1a for disease progression in relapsing multiple sclerosis. *Ann Neurol* 1996; 39:285–294.

10. Lassman H. *Comparative neuropathology of chronic experimental allergic encephalomyelitis and multiple sclerosis.* Berlin: Springer-Verlag, 1983.

11. Walsh M, Tourtellotte W. The cerebrospinal fluid in multiple sclerosis. In: Hallpike J, Adams C, Tourtellotte W (eds.). *Multiple sclerosis: Pathology, diagnosis and management.* London: Chapman and Hall, 275–358.

12. Hofman FM, vonHanwehr RI, Dinarello CA, et al. Immunoregulatory molecules and IL2 receptors identified in multiple sclerosis brain. *J Immunol* 1986; 136:3239–3245.

13. Seboun E, Robinson M, Doolittle T, et al. A susceptibility locus for multiple sclerosis is linked to the T cell beta chain complex. *Cell* 1989; 57:1095–1100.

14. Morimoto C, Hafler DA, Weiner HL. Selective loss of suppressor inducer T cell subset in progressive multiple sclerosis: Analysis with anti-2H4 monoclonal antibody. *N Engl J Med* 1988; 316:67–72.

15. Panitch HS, Hirsch RL, Schindler J, Johnson KP. Treatment of multiple sclerosis with gamma interferon: Exacerbations associated with activation of the immune system. *Neurology* 1987; 37:1097–1102.

16. Rudick RA, Goodkin DE (eds.).*Treatment of multiple sclerosis: Trial design, results, and future perspectives.* New York: Springer Verlag, 1992.

17. Goodkin DE, Rudick RA, Ransohoff RM. Treatment of multiple sclerosis: Current status. Part 1. Clinical trials of experimental therapies. *Cleveland Clin J Med* 1992:59; 63–74.

18. Salmaggi A, Corsini E, La Mantia L, et al. Immunological monitoring of azathioprine treatment in multiple sclerosis patients. *J Neurol* 1977; 244:167–174.

19. Tucker WG, Kapphahn KH. A preliminary evaluation of azathioprine (Imuran) in the treatment of multiple sclerosis. *Henry Ford Hosp Med J* 1969; 17(2):89–91.

20. Swinburn WR, Liversedge LA. Long-term treatment of multiple sclerosis with azathioprine. *J Neurol Neurosurg Psychiatry* 1973; 36:124–126.

21. Ghezzi A, Di Falco M, Locatelli C, et al. Clinical controlled trial of azathioprine in multiple sclerosis. In: Gonsette DR, Delmotte P (eds.). *Recent advances in multiple sclerosis therapy.* Elsevier, Amsterdam, 1989.

22. Mertin J, Rudge P, Kremer M, et al. Double-blind controlled trial of immunosuppression in the treatment of multiple sclerosis: Final report. *Lancet* 1982; 2:351–354.

23. British and Dutch Multiple Sclerosis Azathioprine Trial Group. Double-masked trial of azathioprine in multiple sclerosis. *Lancet* 1988; 2:179–183.

24. Milanese C, La Mantia L, Salmaggi A, et al. Double blind controlled randomized study on azathioprine efficacy in multiple sclerosis: Preliminary results. *Ital J Neurol Sci* 1988; 9:53–57

25. Goodkin DE, Bailly RC, Teetzen ML, et al. The efficacy of azathioprine in relapsing-remitting multiple sclerosis. *Neurology* 1991; 41:20–25.

26. Ellison GW, Myers LW, Mickey MR, et al. A placebo-controlled, randomized, double-masked, variable dosage, clinical trial of azathioprine with and without methylprednisolone in multiple sclerosis. *Neurology* 1989; 39:1018–1026.

27. Yudkin PL, Ellison GW, Ghezzi A, et al. Overview of azathioprine treatment in multiple sclerosis. Lancet 1991; 338:1051–1055.

28. Hughes RAC. Treatment of multiple sclerosis with azathioprine. In: Rudick RA, Goodkin DE (eds.). *Treatment of multiple sclerosis: Trial design, results and future perspectives.* London: Springer-Verlag, 1992.

29. Kinlen LJ. Incidence of cancer in rheumatoid arthritis and other disorders after immunosuppressive treatment. *Am J Med* 1985; 78 (Suppl 1A):44–49.

30. Goodkin DE, Daughtry MM, VanderBrug-Medendorp S. The incidence of malignancy following cyclophosphamide (CTX) or azathioprine (AZA) treatment of multiple sclerosis (MS). *Ann Neurol* 1992; 32:257.

31. Lhermitte F, Marteau R, de Saxce H. Treatment of progressive and severe forms of multiple sclerosis using a combination of antilymphocyte serum, azathioprine and prednisone. Clinical and biological results. Comparison with a control group treated with azathioprine and prednisone only: 4-year follow-up. *Rev Neurol (Paris)* 1987; 143:98–107.

32. Carson DA, Wasson DB, Taetle R, Yu A. Specific toxicity of 2-chlorodeoxyadenosine toward resting and proliferating human lymphocytes. *Blood* 1983; 62:737–743.

33. Carson DA, Wasson DB, Beutler E. Antileukemic and immunosuppressive activity of 2-chloro-2'-deoxyadenosine. *Proc Natl Acad Sci USA* 1984; 81:2232–2236.

34. Piro LD. 2-Chlorodeoxyadenosine treatment of lymphoid malignancies. *Blood* 1992; 79:843–845.

35. Beutler E, Piro LD, Saven A, et al. 2-chlorodeoxyadenosine (2-CdA): A potent chemotherapeutic and immunosuppression nucleoside. *Leuk Lymphoma* 1991; 5:1–8.

36. Beutler E. Cladribine (2-chlorodeoxyadenosine). *Lancet* 1992; 340:952–956.

37. Sipe JC, Romine JS, Koziol JA, et al. Cladribine in treatment of chronic progressive multiple sclerosis. *Lancet* 1994; 344:9–13.

38. Sipe JC, Romine JS, Zyroff J, Koziol J, Beutler E. Treatment of multiple sclerosis with cladribine. In: Goodkin DE, Rudick RA (eds.). *Treatment of multiple sclerosis: Advances in trial design, results and future perspectives.* London: Springer-Verlag, 1996.

39. Poser CM, Paty DW, Scheinberg L, et al. New diagnostic criteria for multiple sclerosis: Guidelines for research protocols. *Ann Neurol* 1983; 13:227–231.

40. Kurtzke JF. Rating neurologic impairment in multiple sclerosis: An expanded disability scale (EDSS). *Neurology* 1983; 33:1444–1452.

41. Wong ET, Vahdat L, Tunkel RS, et al. Severe motor weakness from high-dose 2-chorodeoxyadenosine. *Ann Neurol* 1994; 36:293.

42. Rice G, the Cladribine Study Group. Cladribine and chronic progressive multiple sclerosis: The results of a multicenter trial. *Neurology* 1997; 48:1730 (abstract).

43. Sipe JC, Knobler RL, Braheny SL, et al. A neurologic rating scale (NRS) for use in multiple sclerosis. *Neurology* 1984; 34:1368–1372.

44. Moody DJ, Fahey JL, Grable E, et al. Administration of monthly pulses of cyclophosphamide in multiple sclerosis patients: Effects of long-term treatment on immunologic parameters. *J Neuroimmunol* 1987; 14:161–173.

45. Moody DJ, Fahey JL, Grable E, et al. Administration of monthly pulses of cyclophosphamide in multiple sclerosis patients: Delayed recovery of several immune parameters following discontinuation of long-term cyclophosphamide treatment. *J Neuroimmunol* 1987; 14:175–182.

46. Uitehaag, BMJ Nillesen WM, Hommes OR. Long-lasting effects of cyclophosphamide on lymphocytes in peripheral blood and spinal fluid. *Acta Neurol Scand* 1989; 79:12–17.

47. Comabella M, Balashov K, Smith D, Weiner HL, Khoury SJ. Cyclophosphamide treatment normalizes the increase IL-12 production in patients with chronic progressive MS and induces a Th2 cytokine switch. *Neurology* 1998; 50:A358.

48. Hauser SL, Dawson DM, Lehrich JR, et al. Intensive immunosuppression in progressive multiple sclerosis: A randomized, three-arm study of high-dose cyclophosphamide, plasma exchange, and ACTH. *N Engl J Med* 1983; 308:173–180.

49. Goodkin D, Plencner S, Palmer-Saxerud J, Teetzen M, Hertsgaard D. Cyclophosphamide in chronic progressive multiple sclerosis: Maintenance vs non-maintenance therapy. *Arch Neurol* 1987; 44(8):823–827.

50. Weiner HL, Mackin GA, Orav JA, et al. Intermittent cyclophosphamide pulse therapy in progressive multiple sclerosis: Final report of the Northeast Cooperative Multiple Sclerosis Treatment Group. *Neurology* 1993; 43:910–918.

51. Likosky WH, Fireman B, Elmore R, et al. Intense immunosuppression in chronic progressive multiple sclerosis: The Kaiser study. *J Neurol Neurosurg Psychiatry* 1991; 54:1055–1060.

52. The Canadian Cooperative Multiple Sclerosis Study Group. The Canadian cooperative trial of cyclophosphamide and plasma exchange in multiple sclerosis. *Lancet* 1991; 337:441–446.

53. Noseworthy JA, Vandervoort MK, Penman M, et al. Cyclophosphamide and plasma exchange in multiple sclerosis (letter). *Lancet* 1991; 337:1540–1541.

54. Weiner HL, Hauser SL, Dawson DM, et al. Cyclophosphamide and plasma exchange in multiple sclerosis (letter). *Lancet* 1991; 337:1033–1034.

55. Bach JF. Cyclosporine in autoimmune diseases. *Transplant Proc* 1989; 21:97–113.

56. Reem GH, Cook LA, Vilck J. Gamma interferon synthesis by human thymocytes and T lymphocytes by cyclosporine A. *Science* 1983; 221:63–65.

57. Elliott JF, Lin Y, Mitzel SB, et al. Induction of interleukin 2 messenger RNA inhibited by cyclosporin A. *Science* 1984; 226:1439–1441.

58. Colombani PM, Hess AD. T-lymphocyte inhibition by cyclosporine. Potential mechanisms. *Biochem Pharmacol* 1987; 36:3789–3793.

59. Rich S, Caprina MR, Arthelger C. Suppressor T cell growth and differentiation: Identification of a cofactor required from suppressor T cell function and distinct from interleukin 2. *J Exp Med* 1984; 159:1473–1490.

60. Kappos L, Patzold U, Poser S, et al. Cyclosporine versus azathioprine in the long-term treatment of multiple sclerosis—Results of the German Multicenter Study. *Ann Neurol* 1988; 23:56–63.

61. Rudge P, Koetsier JC, Mertin J, et al. Randomized double-blind controlled trial of cyclosporin in multiple sclerosis. *J Neurol Neurosurg Psychiatry* 1989; 52:559–565.

62. Beyer JOM. Second International Congress on Cyclosporine, Washington DC, USA, November 4–7, 1987 (Abstract). University of Texas Health Science Center. Organ Transplantation Center/The Division of Continuing Education, 1987.

63. Rudge P, Koetsier JC, Mertin J, et al. Randomized double-blind controlled trial of cyclosporin in multiple sclerosis. *J Neurol Neurosurg Psychiatry* 1989; 52:559–565.

64. The Multiple Sclerosis Study Group. Efficacy and toxicity of cyclosporine in chronic progressive multiple sclerosis: A randomized, double-blind, placebo-controlled clinical trial. *Ann Neurol* 1990; 27:591–605.

65. Weinblatt ME, Weissman BN, Holdsworth DE, et al. Long-term prospective study of methotrexate in the treatment of rheumatoid arthritis. 84-month update. *Arthritis Rheum* 1992; 35:129–137.

66. Kremer JM, Lee JK. A long term prospective study of the use of methotrexate in rheumatoid arthritis. Update after a mean of fifty-three months. *Arthritis Rheum* 1988; 31(5):577–584.

67. Furst DF, Kremer JM. Methotrexate in rheumatoid arthritis. *Arthritis Rheum* 1988; 31:305–314.

68. Rau R, Herborn G, Karger T, Werdier D. Retardation of radiologic progression in rheumatoid arthritis with methotrexate therapy. *Arthritis Rheum* 1991; 34:1236–1244.

69. Rustin GJS, Rustin F, Dent J, et al. No increase in second tumors after methotrexate chemotherapy for gestational trophoblastic tumors. *N Engl J Med* 1983; 308:473–476.

70. Zatarain E, Williams C, Fries JF. Comparison of adverse reactions of methotrexate and other disease modifying agents. *Arthritis Rheum* 1988; 31(Suppl):D84.

71. Reynolds WJ, Perra M, Yoon SJ, Klein NM. Evaluation of clinical and prognostic significance of T-cell regulatory subsets in rheumatoid arthritis. *J Rheumatol* 1985; 12:49–56.

72. Goto M, Miyamoto T, Nishioka K, Uchida S. T cytotoxic and helper cells are markedly increased and T suppressor and inducer cells are markedly decreased in rheumatoid synovial fluids. *Arthritis Rheum* 1987; 30:737–743.

73. Lisak RP, Heinz RG, Keis MW, Alvord EC. Dissociation of antibody production from disease suppression in the inhibition of allergic encephalomyelitis by myelin basic protein. *J Immunol* 1970; 104:1435–1446.

74. Alarcon GS, Schrohenloher RE, Bartolucci AA, et al. Suppression of rheumatoid factor production by methotrexate in patients with rheumatoid arthritis. Evidence for differential influences of therapy and clinical status on IgM and IgA rheumatoid factor expression. *Arthritis Rheum* 1990; 33:1156–1161.

75. Calabrese LH, Taylor JV, Wilke WS, Segal AM, Clough JD. Methotrexate (MTX) immunoregulatory T-cell subsets and rheumatoid arthritis: Is MTX an immunomodulator? *Arthritis Rheum* 1988; 31(Suppl 1):C20.

76. Hine RJ, Everson MP, Hardon JM, et al. Methotrexate therapy in rheumatoid arthritis patients diminishes lectin-induced mono-nuclear cell proliferation. *Rheumatol Int* 1990; 10:165–169.

77. Weinblatt ME, Coblyn JS, Fox DA, et al. Efficacy of low-dose methotrexate in rheumatoid arthritis. *N Engl J Med* 1985; 312:818–822.

78. Sperling RI, Benincaso AI, Anderson RJ, et al. Acute and chronic suppression of leukotriene B4 synthesis ex vivo in neutrophils from patients with rheumatoid arthritis beginning treatment with methotrexate. *Arthritis Rheum* 1992; 35:376–384.

79. Segal R, Yaron M, Tartakovsky B. Methotrexate: Mechanism of action in rheumatoid arthritis. *Semin Arthiris Rheum* 1990; 20:190–200.

80. Brody M, Bohm I, Bauer R. Mechanism of action of methotrexate: Experimental evidence that methotrexate blocks the binding of interleukin 1b to the interleukin 1 receptor on target cells. *Eur J Clin Chem Clin Biochem* 1993; 31:667–674.

81. Nielsen HJ, Hammer JH. Possible role of histamine in pathogenesis of autoimmune diseases: Implications for immunotherapy with histamine-2 receptor antagonists. *Medical Hypotheses* 1992; 39:349–355.

82. Neumann JW, Ziegler DK. Therapeutic trial of immunosuppressive agents in multiple sclerosis. *Neurology* 1972; 22(12):1268–1271.

83. Currier RD, Haerer AF, Maydrech EF. Low dose oral methotrexate treatment of multiple sclerosis: A pilot study. *J Neurol Neurosurg Psychiatry* 1993; 56(11):1217–1218.

84. Goodkin DE, Rudick RA, Vanderbrug-Medendorp S, et al. Low-dose (7.5 mg) oral methotrexate is effective in reducing the rate of progression of neurological impairment in patients with chronic progressive multiple sclerosis. *Ann Neurol* 1995; 37:30–40.

85. Low-dose, oral methotrexate for the treatment of chronic progressive multiple sclerosis. In: Goodkin DE, Rudick RA (eds.). *Treatment of multiple sclerosis: Advances in trial design, results and future perspectives.* London: Springer-Verlag, 1996.

86. Goodkin D, Hertsgaard D, Seminary J. Upper extremity function in multiple sclerosis: Improved assessment sensitivity with the use of the box & block and nine hole peg tests. *Arch Phys Med Rehabil* 1988; 69:850–854.

87. Goodkin DE, Rudick RA, Vanderbrug-Medendorp S, et al. Low-dose (7.5mg) oral methotrexate (MTX) for chronic progressive multiple sclerosis: Design of a randomized placebo-controlled trial with sample size benefits from composite outcome variable. Preliminary data on toxicity. *Online J Curr Clin Trials* (serial online) 1992 Sep 25; 1992(Doc No 19); 7723 words; 89 paragraphs.

88. Fischer JS, Goodkin DE, Rudick RA, et al. Low-dose (7.5 mg) oral methotrexate improves neuropsychological function in patients with chronic progressive multiple sclerosis. *Ann Neurol* 1994; 36:289.

89. Goodkin DE, Rudick RA, VanderBrug-Medendorp S, Daughtry MM, Van Dyke C. Low-dose oral methotrexate in chronic progressive multiple sclerosis: Analyses of serial MRIs. *Neurology* 1996; 47:1153–1157.

90. Andersson PB, Goodkin DE. Glucocorticosteroid therapy for multiple sclerosis: A critical review. *J Neurol Sci* (in press).

91. Cannella B, Raine CS. The adhesion molecule and cytokine profile of multiple sclerosis lesions. *Ann Neurol* 1995; 37:424–435.

92. Cronstein BN, Kimmel SC, Levin RI, Martiniuk F, Weissmann G. A mechanism for the antiinflammatory effects of corticosteroid: The glucocorticoid receptor regulates leukocyte adhesion to endothelial cells and expression of endothelial-leukocyte adhesion molecule 1 and intercellular adhesion molecule 1. *Proc Natl Acad Sci USA* 1992; 89:9991–9995.

93. Mancuso F, Flower RJ, Perrett M. Leukocyte transmigration, but not rolling or adhesion, is selectively inhibited by dexamethasone in the hamster post capillary venule. *J Immunol* 1995; 155:377–386.

94. Troiano R, Hafstein M, Ruderman M, Dowling P, Cook S. Effect of high dose intravenous steroid administration on contrast enhancing computed tomograpic scan lesions in multiple sclerosis. *Ann Neurol* 1984; 15:257–263.

95. Troiano RA, Hafstein MP, Zito G, et al. The effect of oral corticosteroid dosage on CT enhancing multiple sclerosis plaques. *J Neurol Sci* 1985; 70:67–72.

96. Barkhof R, Hommes OR, Scheltens P et al. Quantitative MRI changes in gadolinium-DTPA enhancement after high-dose intravenous methylprednisolone in multiple sclerosis. *Neurology* 1991; 41:1219–1222.

97. Burnham JA, Wright RR, Dreisbach J, Murray RS. The effect of high-dose steroids on MRI gadolinium enhancement in acute demyelinating lesions. *Neurology* 1991; 412:1349–1354.

98. Tourtellotte WW, Baumhefner RW, et al. Multiple sclerosis de novo CNS Ig G synthesis: Effect of ACTH and corticosteroids. *Neurology* 1980; 30:1155–1162.

99. Rosenberg, GA, Dencoff BS, Correa N, Reiners M, Ford CC. Effect of steroids on CSF matrix metalloproteinases in multiple sclerosis: Relation to blood-brain barrier injury. *Neurology* 1996; 46:1626–1632.

100. Muller-Ladner U, Jones JL, Wetsel RA, et al., Enhanced expression of chemotactic receptors in multiple sclerosis lesions. *J Neurol Sci* 1996; 144:135–141.

101. Fauci AS, Dale DC. The effect of in vivo hydrocortisone on subpopulation of human lymphocytes. *J Clin Invest* 1974; 53:240–246.

102. Rinehart JJ, Sagone AL, Balcerzak SP. Effects of corticosteroid therapy in human monocyte function. *N Engl J Med* 1975; 292:236–241.

103. Werb Z. Biochemical actions of glucocorticoids on macrophages in culture. Specific inhibition of elastase, collagenase and plasminogen activator secretion and effects on other metabolic functions. *J Exp Med* 1978; 147–169.

104. Flower RJ. Eleventh Gaddum memorial lecture. Lipocortin and the mechanism of action of the glucocorticoids. *Brit J Pharmacol* 1988; 94:987–1015.

105. Schreiber AD, Parson J, McDermott P, Cooper RA. Effect of corticosteroids on the human monocyte IgG and complement receptors. *J Clin Invest* 1975; 56:1189–1197.

106. Fries LF, Brickman CM, Frank MM. Monocyte receptors for the Fc portion of IgG increase in number in autoimmune hemolytic anemia and other hemolytic states and are decreased by glucocorticoid therapy. *J Immunol* 1983; 131:1240–1245.

107. Barnes PJ, Adcock I. Anti-inflammatory actions of steroids: Molecular mechanisms. *Trends Pharmacol Sci* 1993; 14:436–441.

108. Guyre PM, Girard MT, Morganelli PM, Manganiello PD. Glucocorticoid effects on the production and actions of immune cytokines. *J Steroid Biochem* 1988; 30(1–6): 89–93.

109. Brenner T, Brocke S, Szafer F, et al. Inhibition of nitric oxide synthase for treatment of experimental autoimmune encephalomyelitis. *J Immunol* 1997; 158(6):2940–2946.

110. Fauci AS. Mechanisms of corticosteroid action on lymphocyte subpopulations. II. Differential effects of in vitro hydrocortisone, prednisone and dexamethasone on in vitro expression of lymphocyte function. *Clin Exp Immunol* 1976; 24:54–62.

111. Fauci AS, Dale DC. The effect of in vivo hydrocortisone on subpopulation of human lymphocytes. *J Clin Invest* 1974; 53:240–246.

112. Panitch H, Bever C. Clinical trials of interferons in MS. What have we learned? *J Neuroimmunol* 1993; 46:155–164.

113. Adcock IM, Brown CR, Gelder CM, Shirasaki H, Peters MJ, Barnes PJ. Effects of glucocorticoids on transcription factor activation in human peripheral blood mononuclear cells. *Am J Physiol* 1995; 268(2 Pt 1):C331–338.

114. Almawi WY, Beyhum HW, Rahme AA, Rieder MJ. Regulation of cytokine and cytokine receptor expression by glucocorticoids. *J Leuk Biol* 1996; 60:563–572.

115. Boumpas DT, Paliogianni F, Anastassiou ED, Balow JE. Glucocorticosteroid action on the immune system: Molecular and cellular aspects. *Clin Exp Rheum* 1991; 9:4113–4123.

116. Amano Y, Lee SW, Allison AC. Inhibition by glucocorticoids of the formation of interleukin-1 alpha, interleukin-1 beta, and interleukin-6: Mediation by decreased mRNA stability. *Molec Pharmacol* 1993; 43(2):176–182.

117. Ruddle NH, Bergman CM, McGrath KM, et al. An antibody to lymphotoxin and tumor necrosis factor prevents transfer of experimental allergic encephalomyelitis. *J Exp Med* 1990; 172:1193–2000.

118. Kuroda Y, Shimamoto Y. Human tumor necrosis factor-alpha augments experimental allergic encephalomyelitis in rats. *J Neuroimmunol* 1991; 34:159–164.

119. Ayanlar-Batuman O, Ferrero AP, Diaz A, Jimenez SA. Regulation of TGF beta 1 gene expression by glucocorticoids in normal human T lymphocytes. *J Clin Invest* 1989; 88:1574–1580.

120. Stevens DB, Gould KE, Swanborg RH. Transforming growth factor-beta 1 inhibits tumor necrosis factor-alpha/lymphotoxin production and adoptive transfer of disease by effector cells of autoimmune encephalomyelitis. *J Neuroimmunol* 1994; 51(1):77–83.

121. Grabstein K, Dower S, Gillis S, Urdal, Larsen A. Expression of interleukin 2, interferon-gamma, and the IL 2 receptor by human peripheral blood lymphocytes. *J Immunol* 1986; 136:4503–4508.

122. Butler WT. Corticosteroids and immunoglobin synthesis. *Transplantation Proc* 1975; VII:49–53.

123. Durelli L, Cocito D, Riccio A, et al. High dose intravenous methylprednisolone in the treatment of multiple sclerosis: Clinical-immunologic correlations. *Neurology* 1986; 36:238–243.

124. Baumhefner RW, Tourtellotte WW, Syndulko K, Staugaitis A, Shapshak P. Multiple sclerosis intra-blood–brain-barrier IgG synthesis: Effect of pulse intravenous and intrathecal corticosteroids. *Ital J Neurol Sci* 1989; 10:19–32.

125. Myers LW. Treatment of multiple sclerosis with ACTH and Corticosteroids. In: Rudick R, Goodkin DE (eds.). *Treatment of multiple sclerosis: Trial design, results, and future perspectives.* New York: Springer Verlag, 1992:135–156.

126. Miller H, Newell DJ, Ridley A. Multiple sclerosis trials of maintenance treatment with prednisolone and soluble aspirin. *Lancet* 1961; 1:127–129.

127. Tourtellotte WW, Haerer AF. Use of an oral corticosteroid in the treatment of multiple sclerosis. *Arch Neurol* 1965; 12:536–545.

128. Kurtzke JF. On the evaluation of disability in multiple sclerosis. *Neurology* 1961; 2:686–694.

129. Millar JHD, Vas CJ, Noronha MJ, Leversedge LA, Rawson MD. Long term treatment of multiple sclerosis with corticotrophin. *Lancet* 1967; 2:429–431.

130. Milligan NM, Newcombe R, Compston DAS. A double-blind controlled trial of high dose methylprednisolone in patients with multiple sclerosis: 1. Clinical effects. *J Neurol Neurosurg Psychiatry* 1987; 50:511–516.

131. Goodkin DE, Kinkel RP, Weinstock-Guttman B, et al. Randomized, double-masked study of bi-monthly high vs low-dose intravenous methylprednisolone in relapsing-progressive multiple sclerosis. *Neurology* (in press).

132. Khatri BO, McQuillen MP, Harrington GJ, et al. Chronic progressive multiple sclerosis: Double blind controlled trial of plasmapheresis in patients taking immunosuppressive drugs. *Neurology* 1985; 35:312–319.

133. Khatri BO, McQuillen MP, Hoffman RG, et al. Plasmapheresis in chronic progressive MS: A long term study. *Neurology* 1991; 41:409–414.

134. The Canadian Cooperative Multiple Sclerosis Study Group. The Canadian cooperative trial of cyclophosphamide and plasma exchange in multiple sclerosis. *Lancet* 1991; 337:441–446.

135. Vamvakas EC, Pineda AA, Weinshenker BG. Meta-analysis of clinical studies of the efficacy of plasma exchange in the treatment of chronic progressive multiple sclerosis. *J Clinical Apheresis* 1995; 10:163–170.

136. Slavin SB, Reitz CP, Bieber HS, et al. Transplantation tolerance in adult rats using total lymphoid irradiation: Permanent survival of skin, heart and marrow allografts. *J Exp Med* 1978; 147:700–707.

137. Svaifler NJ. Fractionated total lymphoid irradiation; A promising new treatment for rheumatoid arthritis? Yes, no, maybe. *Arthritis Rheum* 1987; 30:109–114.

138. Field EDS, Strober RT, Hoppe A, et al. Sustained improvement of intractable rheumatoid arthritis after total lymphoid irradiation. *Arthritis Rheum* 1983; 26:937–946.

139. Rohowsky-Kochan C, Moinaro D, Devereux C, et al. The effect of total lymphoid irradiation and low-dose steroids on T lymphocyte populations in multiple sclerosis: Correlation with clinical and MRI status. *J Neurol Sci* 1997; 152:182–192.

140. Strober S, Kotzin B, Field E, et al. Treatment of autoimmune disease with total lymphoid irradiation: Cellular humoral mechanisms. *Ann NY Acad Sci* 1986; 475:285–295.

141. Weiner HL, Hafler DA. Immunotherapy of multiple sclerosis. *Ann Neurol* 1988; 23:211–222.

142. Cook SD, Troiano R, Zito G, et al. Effect of total lymphoid irradiation in chronic progressive multiple sclerosis. *Lancet* 1986; 1:1405–1411.

143. Cook SD, Devereux C, Troiano R. The treatment of patients with chronic progressive multiple sclerosis with total lymphoid irradiation. In: Cook SD (ed.). *Handbook of multiple sclerosis.* New York; Marcel Dekker, 1990:402–423.

144. Cook SD, Devereux C, Troiano R, et al. Combination total lymphoid irradiation and low dose corticosteroid therapy for progressive multiple sclerosis. *Acta Neurol Scand* 1995; 91(1):22–27.

145. Cook SD, Devereux C, Troiano R, et al. Modified total lymphoid irradiation and low dose corticosteroids in progressive multiple sclerosis. *J Neurol Sci* 1997; 152:172–181.

146. Polman CH, Dahlke F, Thompson AJ, et al. Interferon beta-1b in secondary progressive multiple sclerosis—outline of the clinical trial. *Multiple Sclerosis* 1995; 1:S51–S54.

147. Fidler JM, Dejoy SQ, Gibbons JJ. Selective immunomodulation by the antineoplastic agent mitoxantrone. I. Suppression of B lymphocyte function. *J Immunol* 1986; 137:727–732.

148. Fidler JM, Dejoy SQ, Gibbons JJ. Selective immunomodulation by the antineoplastic agent mitoxantrone. II. Non specific adherent suppressor cells derived from mitoxantrone-treated mice. *J Immunol* 1986; 136:2747–2754.

149. Lublin FD, Lavasa M, Viti C, Knobler RL. Suppression of acute and relapsing experimental allergic encephalomyelitis with mitoxantrone. *Clin Immunol Immunopathol* 1987; 45:122–128.

150. Noseworthy JH, Hopkins MB, Vandervoort MK, et al. An open-trial evaluation of mitoxantrone in the treatment of progressive MS. *Neurology* 1993; 43:1401–1406.

151. Edan G, Miller D, Clanet M, et al. Therapeutic effect of mitoxantrone combined with methylprednisolone in multiple sclerosis: A randomised multicentre study of active disease using MRI and clinical criteria. *J Neurol Neurosurg Psychiatry* 1997; 2:112–118.

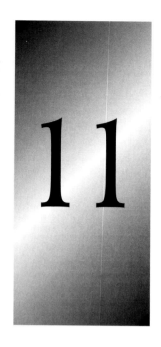

11 Emerging Therapies

Robert M. Elfont, M.D., Ph.D., R. Joan Oshinsky, M.D., Ph.D., and Fred D. Lublin, M.D.

Over the past decade multiple sclerosis (MS) has moved into the ranks of treatable conditions. However, current therapies are only partial, slowing disease progression and reducing relapse frequency and severity. It is clear that we need better approaches. The design of emerging and future therapies for MS should be directed toward more specific and less toxic treatments. This would lead us away from more broad-based immunosuppressive agents, with their attendant systemic toxicities.

Emerging therapies may be categorized into three main groups according to their degree of specificity for MS. In increasing order of specificity, these are therapies that induce immunosuppression, immunomodulatory therapies, and target-specific therapies. A fourth category, remyelination and growth factors, aims at promoting recovery.

THERAPIES THAT INDUCE IMMUNOSUPPRESSION

Chemotherapy

Many chemotherapeutic agents have been studied in MS, but none have provided compelling results. Cyclophos- phamide (1) and methotrexate (2,3) are presently used as therapies for select patients with rapidly progressing disease. The search for other cytotoxins with better therapeutic indices is ongoing.

Recently, mitoxantrone has been investigated in MS. In a study of 20 patients with relapsing-remitting MS who received either active drug or placebo, the mean exacerbation rate was reduced in the mitoxantrone-treated patients (4). In other studies mitoxantrone also reduced attack and progression rates in MS, with cardiotoxicity limiting the maximum cumulative dose (5). In a randomized, multicenter trial, in which 27 patients with relapsing-remitting MS received monthly intravenous (IV) infusions of mitoxantrone for one year and 24 patients received saline infusions, the mitoxantrone group showed a significant reduction in the mean number of exacerbations compared with the placebo group. There was no statistical benefit to treatment in terms of disease progression over two years as assessed by mean Expanded Disability Status Scale (EDSS) score, but the proportion of patients with a confirmed one-point or greater increase in their EDSS score was significantly reduced at two years in the mitoxantrone group (6). The number of gadolinium (gd)-enhancing lesions and the percentage of serial magnetic resonance imaging (MRI) scans showing no gd enhancement were greater in MS patients receiving mitoxantrone than expected based on historical controls (7). In patients with very active MS, monthly infusions of mitoxantrone in combination with methylprednisolone resulted in significantly more patients with no new enhancing lesions on MRI scan when compared with methylprednisolone treatment alone (6,8).

Immunosuppressant Drugs

A number of immunosuppressant drugs have been studied in MS. Several small studies conducted over the years have suggested that azathioprine, a purine synthesis inhibitor, may be minimally effective in treating MS, and the drug has gained a modicum of acceptance for the treatment of rapidly progressing disease. Recently, a dose of 2.5 mg per kg of body weight was assessed to have a marginal benefit on relapse frequency and disability without increasing the five-year risk of cancer. The drug mofetil (Mycofenloate) has a mechanism of action similar to that of azathioprine and may be of similar benefit in MS (9). Preliminary studies with tacrolimus, an immunosuppressant for the treatment of graft rejection, defined a concentration range that appeared to show efficacy and minimal toxicity in a small group of MS patients (10).

New immunosuppressant drugs are usually tested for an affect in experimental allergic encephalomyelitis (EAE), an animal model of MS. Two immunosuppressive malononitrilamides lessened the severity of attack in both acute and chronic relapsing EAE (11). Suramin, a polysulfonated napthylurea, also ameliorated EAE in mice (12). A new quinoline derivative reduced the percentage of myelin basic protrein (MBP)–reactive T cells generated in rats with EAE (13). Liposomes containing dichloromethylene diphosphonate suppressed clinical signs of EAE induced by adoptive transfer of encephalitogenic T cells in bone marrow chimera rats, eliminating more than 95 percent of marrow-derived macrophages and 68 percent of perivascular macrophages within spinal cord lesions (14). The usefulness of these drugs in the treatment of MS remains unknown.

Intravenous Immunoglobulin G

Intravenous immunoglobulin G (IV IgG) has proven useful in the treatment of a number of immune-mediated neurologic diseases, but its role in the treatment of MS remains uncertain. As reviewed by Dalakas, early case reports, open-label trials, and small controlled studies of IV IgG for the treatment of MS produced only variable, mild, or unsubstantiated benefit in some patients (15). A randomized, double-blind, multicenter trial did show that patients with relapsing-remitting MS benefited from monthly administration of IV IgG for two years, in terms of both their EDSS score and their relapse rate. Expanded Disability Status Scale scores were significantly decreased in the IV IgG–treated group and increased in the placebo groups, but the difference in scores between groups was less than half a point (16). In another double-blind, randomized study of 40 patients with relapsing-remitting MS who received IV IgG or placebo every two months for two years, there was a 38.6 percent reduction in the relapse rate in treated patients, with six patients in the IV IgG group but none in the placebo group remaining exacerbation-free throughout the study. Median time to first exacerbation was 233 days in the IV IgG group versus 82 days in the placebo group. Mean EDSS scores decreased by 0.3 in the IV IgG group and increased by 0.15 in the placebo group. Total MRI brain lesion score did not show a significant difference between groups (17). Another double-blind, randomized, placebo-controlled, phase III study is currently under way to evaluate safety and efficacy of IV IgG in the treatment of patients with primary or secondary progressive MS (18).

Anti–T-Cell Antibodies

Because regulatory CD4+ helper T cells play an integral role in autoimmunity, it has been postulated that reducing their numbers may be therapeutic in MS. In an open-label phase I trial of a humanized anti-CD4 antibody for treatment of MS, CD4+ cell counts decreased two hours after IV treatment and returned to baseline by three months. Six of 35 patients experienced stabilization of their disability after one year, but only two of 21 patients followed up for two years remained stable. After one year, nine of 17 patients were relapse-free. Serial MRI scans performed on a subgroup of patients showed stabilization of lesion burden for three months following treatment (19). In a phase II study, anti-CD4 monoclonal antibodies (MAbs) caused a substantial and long-lasting reduction in the number of circulating CD4+ T cells, but there was no significant effect on the number of gd-enhancing brain lesions on monthly MRI scans. Although there was a significant reduction in the number of clinical relapses, the finding may have been compromised by physician unblinding (20).

Treatment of both MS and EAE has been attempted by depleting a wider range of immune cells than only CD4+ T cells. A substantial reduction in disease activity as measured by gd-enhancing lesions on MRI was found in a pilot study of seven MS patients treated with CAMPATH-IH, an MAb that targets CD52 molecules on lymphocytes and monocytes (21). An anti-CD3 immunotoxin that transiently depletes T cells in blood and lymph nodes to 1 percent of their initial values administered, with or without cranial irradiation, to rhesus monkeys after they had developed an EAE-induced cerebrospinal fluid (CSF) pleocytosis. It either delayed or prevented the onset of paralysis. Histopathology in the treated animals revealed scant inflammatory plaques that contained very few T cells (22).

Bone Marrow Transplantation (BMT)

If the autoimmune theory of MS is correct, elimination of autoreactive lymphocytes, as accomplished by ablation of all leukocytes, should eradicate the disease. Bone marrow transplantation allows for reconstitution of the immune system following total myeloablation. Transplant of bone marrow from WAG rats, an EAE-resistant strain, to BUF rats, a strain susceptible to relapsing EAE, after ablating the BUF rats' endogenous marrow with irradiation or chemotherapy, induced remission of established EAE (23). A high degree of lymphoablation and complete replacement of host marrow by donor cells was necessary for successful treatment (24).

The outcome of BMT in EAE varies depending on the timing of the treatment during the course of the disease, and this may have implications for the use of BMT in MS. Myeloablation and syngeneic BMT, when performed at the peak of acute EAE, prevented glial scarring and reduced disease severity, but when performed late in the chronic phase did not significantly alter disease. In both circumstances the posttransplant immune system remained responsive to myelin epitopes (25).

Anecdotally, the clinical course of MS appeared to stabilize and MRI findings appeared to improve in a patient treated with allogeneic BMT for chronic mylogenous leukemia who had previously been diagnosed with MS (26). In a phase I/II study, 15 severely disabled patients with progressive MS underwent autologous blood stem cell transplant and treatment with antithymocyte globulin after receiving brain electrical activity monitoring (BEAM). One patient worsened neurologically at three months, and two patients had a relapse of their MS. Overall, improvement in disability was noted by EDSS. Allergy, infection, and neurotoxicity were significant complications of therapy (27). Bone marrow transplantation for MS is a highly complex therapy that carries substantial risk and should be attempted only at facilities with personnel experienced in both BMT and the evaluation of patients with MS. No standards for the type of MS patient to be considered for BMT have been established.

IMMUNOMODULATORY THERAPIES

Cytokines

The basic scientific data implicating cytokines in regulating the immune system coupled with the success of IFN-β as a treatment for MS have placed cytokine research at the center of the quest for new interventions in MS. In theory, any agent that provides or enhances the action of a Th-2 cytokine is potentially useful in combating MS, as is any agent that inhibits or opposes the action of Th-1 cytokines. The effects of many therapies for MS are believed to be, at least in part, mediated by changes in the relative concentrations of Th-1 and Th-2 cytokines.

Tumor Necrosis Factor (TNF)

Given the diverse and potent effects of TNF-α on immune function, appropriate manipulation of this Th-1 cytokine may hold great therapeutic promise. Surveys of serum cytokine concentrations in patients with MS have tended to associate elevation in TNF-α with worsening of disease (28,29). Increased expression of messenger RNA (mRNA) for TNF-α in peripheral blood monocyte cells (PBMC) similarly was found to correlate with worsening of MS (30,31). Conversely, expression of TNF-α mRNA was found to be reduced at the time of diagnosis of MS (32). Most, but not all, studies on in vitro TNF-α production by PBMCs isolated from patients with MS have supported the idea that TNF-α is involved in worsening of disease (33–37). TNF-α receptor expression on T cells and in soluble form also has been found to be increased in MS patients (38,39); not all studies have confirmed this (40,41).

TNF-α mRNA expression was increased in the central nervous system (CNS) of animals with EAE (42–45), predominantly in microglia and macrophages (42,46) but also in astrocytes (46). The findings from brains of patients with MS are in accord with the EAE studies (47,48). Analysis of TNF-α expression in cells from the CSF of patients with MS further implicates TNF-α in the disease (31,49,50). Studies that measure TNF-α levels in CSF are less clear-cut. Some showed elevated TNF-α concentrations in MS patients (51,52), whereas others did not (53,54). Higher levels of soluble TNF receptor were, however, found in the CSF of patients with MS compared with controls (55).

Interfering with endogenous TNF-α, whether with MAbs (56,57) or with a TNF-IgG fusion protein (58,59), has an almost uniformly salutary effect on EAE. Genetically augmenting the expression of TNF-α has the opposite affect on EAE (60,61).

Despite the evidence that TNF-α plays a deleterious role in EAE and MS, in an open-label phase I study of a humanized mouse monoclonal anti–TNF-α antibody the MAb caused gd-enhancing lesions of the brain, as well as increased CSF leucocyte counts and IgG indices, after each IV infusion (62). It should be noted that the action of MAbs need not always be inhibitory. Antibodies to a cell surface–signaling protein may inhibit the function of that protein but also may activate the protein by circumventing its ligand or by serving as an alternate ligand. Anti–TNF-α antibodies either enhanced, had no effect on, or inhibited EAE, depending on the antibody used (63). Nevertheless, the findings from the phase I clinical trial call into question whether the role of TNF-α in MS is an inciting one.

The action of a given cytokine may vary, depending on both the microenvironment into which the cytokine is released and the timing of its release. The precise role played by TNF-α in autoimmune demyelinating disease remains to be elucidated, but evidence from animal studies suggests that TNF-α is not strictly disease-promoting. For example, treatment of mice with a recombinant vaccinia virus system expressing a TNF-α construct inhibited EAE (63). Furthermore, mice with a homologous disruption of their gene encoding TNF-α, immunized with myelin oligodendrocyte glycoprotein (MOG) to induce EAE, developed severe neurologic impairment with high mortality and extensive inflammation and demyelination (64).

Phosphodiesterase Inhibitors

Phosphodiesterase inhibitors interfere with the production or processing of cytokines, most notably TNF-α, and therefore may be therapeutic in MS. Rolipram, a selective type IV phosphodiesterase inhibitor, reduced the clinical severity of EAE in rodents (65,66) and in a nonhuman primate (67). Although the production of TNF-α by macrophages was suppressed in vitro by the potent nonselective phosphodiesterase inhibitor propentofylline, the drug did not ameliorate EAE (66). Oral administration of pentoxifylline, another phosphodiesterase inhibitor, delayed the onset of clinical EAE and the infiltration of inflammatory cells into the CNS of mice, but without significantly altering the incidence or severity of disease (68). In eight patients with relapsing-remitting MS, oral pentoxifylline significantly reduced TNF-α and interleukin-12 (IL-12) mRNA expression and increased IL-4 and IL-10 expression (69). Clinical trials of pentoxifylline are ongoing.

Other Th-1 Cytokines

It is well established that the Th-1, proinflammatory cytokine, IFN-γ is integrally involved in EAE and MS. Although there are currently no drugs that specifically target IFN-γ, inhibiting IFN-γ secretion or antagonizing its action holds tremendous therapeutic potential. Disrupting the function of other Th-1 cytokines implicated in EAE and MS, namely IL-12, IL-6, IL-2, and IL-1, would theoretically be of similar benefit.

Exogenous IL-12 consistently exacerbated EAE in a number of different animal models (70-73), whereas inhibition of endogenous IL-12 had the opposite effect. A murine IL-12 antibody administered in vivo after lymph node cell transfer decreased the severity of EAE in mice (71).

Levels of IL-6 were elevated in the spinal cord and CSF of mice with EAE relative to controls, but anti–IL-6 had no significant effect on disease (63). In other experiments anti–IL-6 did, however, ameliorate EAE, even when given one day before the onset of neurologic signs. Paradoxically, the anti–IL-6 treatment was associated with increased levels of IL-6 activity in CSF and to a lesser extent in serum (74). In this regard, it is interesting that treating mice with a recombinant vaccinia virus to deliver an IL-6 gene construct also inhibited EAE (63).

Alpha Interferon

The Th-2 cytokine, IFN-α, shares many properties with the other major class I interferon, IFN-β, and may also be effective in treating MS. In a single-blind randomized trial, two of 12 patients with relapsing-remitting MS treated with recombinant interferon alpha-2a (r IF-α-2a) intramuscularly every other day for six months evidenced no clinical exacerbations or new or enlarging lesions on serial brain MRI scans versus seven of eight placebo-treated patients. Moreover, only one new MRI lesion was detected in the r IFN-α group as opposed to 27 new or enlarging lesions in the placebo group (75). Side effects were similar to those seen with IFN-β therapies (76,77). A randomized, placebo-controlled, double-blind trial of r IFN-α is under way in Norway (78).

Oral administration of IFN-α after recovery from the initial attack of chronic relapsing EAE in SJL/J mice suppressed relapses (79). The severity of clinical disease and the extent of inflammatory foci in the spinal cord were significantly decreased in Lewis rats with EAE fed IFN-α compared with mock-treated animals. The improvement seen in rats treated orally with IFN-α was greater than that seen in rats receiving the same dose subcutaneously (80). The optimally effective oral dose of murine IFN-α was superior in suppressing EAE than the optimally effective subcutaneous dose (81). Recombinant human IFN-α ingested at doses from 300 to100,000 U showed no toxicity in normal volunteers or in patients with relapsing-remitting MS. In the MS patients, serum levels of soluble intercellular adhesion molecule-1 (sICAM-1) and IL-2 decreased after ingesting 10,000 U of IFN-α. After ingesting 30,000 U the MS subjects showed decreased secretion of sICAM-1, IFN-γ, TGF-β, and IL-10 (82). Pilot studies looking at clinical outcome with oral IFN-a therapy are under way.

Other Th-2 Cytokines

The recently discovered IFN-τ, a type-I interferon originally identified as a pregnancy recognition hormone produced by trophoblast, prevented development of EAE as effectively as IFN-β but with less toxicity (83). Oral IFN-τ prevented paralysis in both acute and chronic-relapsing forms of murine EAE. Feeding of IFN-τ was as effective as intraperitoineal injection in preventing chronic-relapsing EAE (84). IFN-τ by either route induced CD4 T cells that secreted factors capable of inhibiting MBP-activation of T cells from mice with EAE, including IL-10 and TGF-β (85).

TGF-β 1 is an immunomodulatory peptide produced by monocytes and other immune cells. Among its many actions on immune cells are potent T cell–inhibiting activities (86). In vitro experiments suggest that TGF-β antagonizes many of the actions of IFN-γ (87). In contrast to reports that increased peripheral levels of TGF-β 1 inhibit EAE, transgenic mice that overexpress TGF-β 1 in the CNS were more susceptible to EAE, showing an earlier onset of symptoms, more severe clinical disease, and increased mononuclear cell infiltration in their spinal cords compared with nontransgenic littermates (88). In a phase I clinical trial TGF-β reduced the number of inflammatory cells in the CSF of patients with MS but also produced varying degrees of anemia, elevation of hepatocellular enzymes, and, most notably, nephrotoxicity without any discernible benefit in clinical or MRI parameters of disease progression (89).

Interleukin-10 has suppressive effects on autoantigen presentation and T cell–mediated immune reactions (90). Interleukin-10 either had no effect on EAE or worsened it (91) in some studies, but in other studies it delayed onset and reduced disease severity (92). Anti–IL-10 MAb, given just before the onset of signs, worsened EAE (91). When the migratory properties of memory T cells from lymph nodes of (SWRxSJL)F1 mice immunized with a PLP peptide were exploited to construct a site-specific vector for delivery of IL-10 cDNA into autoimmune inflammatory CNS lesions, the T-cell clones subsequently isolated demonstrated antigen-inducible expression of the IL-10 transgene and expressed cell surface markers consistent with the phenotype of normal memory T cells. Adoptive transfer of transfected T cells inhibited the onset of EAE and ameliorated neurologic and histologic signs in already established disease (93).

Experimental evidence indicates that IL-4 tends to have a beneficial immunomodulatory affect on EAE. In vivo administration of IL-4 protected animals from EAE and induced TGF-β–producing cells (94). Adoptive transfer of potentially encephalitogenic T cells, transduced with a retroviral gene construct to express IL-4, delayed the onset and reduced the severity of MBP-induced EAE in mice (95).

Chemokines

Like interferons and interleukins, chemokines constitute a subcategory of cytokine. Qualitatively increased levels of mRNAs encoding a variety of chemokines are widely expressed in the spinal cords of mice with EAE, variously localizing to microvascular endothelial cells, infiltrating immune cells, microglia, and/or astrocytes (96–99). Administration of antibodies to macrophage inflammatory protein-1α (MIP-1α) prevented the development of both acute and relapsing EAE and also ameliorated established clinical disease (97). Antibodies to monocyte chemoattractant protein-1 (MCP-1) significantly reduced the severity of relapsing EAE (100). The concentration of MIP-1α was significantly elevated in CSF from patients during MS exacerbation compared with patients who had noninflammatory neurologic diseases, and its concentrations in MS patients correlated with CSF leukocyte counts and protein content (101).

Adhesion Molecules

Cell-cell interactions, which are important in immune function, depend on the interplay of one or more pairs of cell adhesion molecules (CAMs). Altering the expression of CAMs is one way that cytokines exert influence over immune processes. Disrupting the interactions of complementary CAMs forms the basis for new treatment strategies in MS.

There are three categories of CAMs, the Ig supergene family, the selectin family, and the integrin family. A CAM from one category typically uses a CAM from another category as its ligand. Elevated serum and/or CSF levels of the selectins, E-selectin (102–104) and L-selectin (105,106), have been detected in patients with MS. So, too, have been elevated serum and/or CSF levels of the Ig supergene family members, ICAM-1 (102,107–110) and vascular cell adhesion molecule-1 (VCAM-1) (102,106,107,110–112). Circulating leukocytes from MS patients expressed higher levels of lymphocyte function-associated antigen-1 (LFA-1), an integrin that serves as the receptor for ICAM-I, than controls (113).

High levels of expression of ICAM-1 and LFA-1 as well as VCAM-1 and very late activation antigen-4 (VLA-4) were detected immunocytochemically in brains from patients with MS, particularly in chronic active lesions (47). Brain microvascular endothelial cells from MS patients also expressed higher levels of ICAM-1 than those from controls (113).

The integrins, which consist of α and β peptide chains, have provided ready targets for MAbs. Antibodies to CD11a and CD11b, members of the β2 integrin subfamily, have been useful in treating EAE. Antibodies to CD11a blocked induction of EAE, whereas anti-CD11b delayed onset and diminished clinical severity of EAE, even when injected after the first appearance of clinical signs (114). An MAb to a4 integrin also suppressed clinical and pathologic features of EAE (115). Monoclonal antibody to CD18, the common b-chain of a leuko-cyte integrin, administered at the onset of clinical disease, prolonged survival and reduced the extent of MRI-detected brain lesions in macaques with EAE (116). Coadministration in vivo of mAbs against LFA-1 and ICAM-1 suppressed EAE in Lewis rats (117). Clinical and MRI manifestations of EAE were only partially inhibited in rats treated with antibodies to ICAM-1 (118).

A humanized mouse mAb to the human a 4 integrin subunit of VLA-4 that blocked the interaction of leukocytes with VCAM-1 in vitro reversed active EAE in guinea pigs. This MAb currently is in phase II clinical trials for the treatment of acute MS exacerbations (119). A recently completed double-blind, placebo-controlled trial of a humanized anti-CD11/CD18 MAb failed to show a benefit in treating acute MS exacerbations.

B-7 Costimulatory Signal

T-cell activation requires both an antigen-specific signal, provided by the interaction of antigen, presented in the context of an appropriate major histocompatibility complex (MHC) class II molecule, with the T-cell receptor (TCR), and an antigen-independent costimulatory signal, provided by the interaction of either B7-1 (CD80) or B7-2 (CD86) on the APC with CD28 or CTLA-4 on the T-cell. Interfering with the costimulatory signal for T-cell activation may inhibit EAE. Systemic administration of CTLA-4Ig, an MAb that binds to both B7-1 and B7-2, suppressed clinical manifestations of EAE, even when given at a time when pathologic disease was already evident (120–122). However, costimulatory receptor blockade under some circumstances resulted in a seemingly paradoxical exacerbation of EAE (123–127). Whether blockade of CTLA-4 results in amelioration or exacerbation of EAE depends on whether it is the interaction of CTLA-4 with B7-1 (CD80) or B7-2 (CD86) that is principally disrupted. The majority of evidence indicates that interaction of CTLA-4 with the B7-1 molecule transduces a signal that is important for the activation of Th1-type T cells and that disruption of this signal improves EAE (124,128–131). That there was a higher percentage, and absolute number, of B7-1+ B lymphocytes in the CSF of patients with MS than in healthy individuals (132) raises the possibility that some form of anti-CTLA antibody may be therapeutic in MS.

Metalloproteinases

Metalloproteinases are enzymes that are involved in breaking down extracellular matrix and facilitating leukocyte migration. They also are responsible for the processing of cell surface cytokines, receptors, and other proteins involved in immune processes (133,134). Experimental

allergic encephalomyelitis in rodents is associated with expression of a number of metalloproteinases, principally in microglia, macrophages, and other immune cells within inflammatory lesions (135,136), and drugs that inhibit metalloproteinases have been effective in treating EAE (133). D-penicillamine, an inhibitor of gelatinase B, reduced mortality and morbidity in acute EAE and attenuated exacerbations in chronic relapsing EAE, even when administered after primary disease had developed (137). Injections of the hydroxamate matrix metalloproteinase inhibitor, Ro31-9790, similarly ameliorated EAE (138). BB-1101, a broad-spectrum inhibitor of metalloproteinase activity and TNF processing, also attenuated EAE (135).

Studies on brain tissue from patients with MS show changes in the distribution of the metalloproteinases in and about MS lesions, with different metalloproteinases being preferentially expressed in microvascular endothelial cells, blood vessel matrix, astrocytes, microglia, and infiltrating mononuclear cells at different stages of plaque development (139–141). Changes in metalloproteinase expression in the CNS of patients with MS are also reflected in their CSF concentrations (142–144). Interruption of metalloproteinase activity may have therapeutic potential in MS.

Final Common Pathways to Cell Death

Apoptosis

Apoptosis, or programmed cell death, is putatively involved in two important aspects of autoimmune demyelinating disease. Apoptosis may in part be responsible for oligodendrocyte and neuronal loss. It may also be necessary for deleting lymphocytes that have outlived their usefulness, including potentially self-injurious clones.

The best-characterized pathways for programmed cell death is the Fas system. Using immunohistochemistry, flow cytometry, and RT-PCR, immune cells expressing Fas and related molecules have been identified in the CNS of mice with EAE (145,146). Expression of Fas antigen on PBMCs (147) and soluble Fas in serum (148) is increased in patients with MS, but CSF levels of these molecules may not be (148,149). This has led to the idea that failure of apoptosis in the CNS may contribute to the pathogenesis of EAE and MS (149). Functional studies using genetic manipulation of apoptosis pathways have, however, indicated that disruption of apoptosis does not necessarily have a deleterious affect on EAE (150–153).

Bonetti and coworkers found that although Fas was constitutively present at low levels on oligodendrocytes and was upregulated in EAE, there was little evidence for active apoptosis, as assessed by chromosomal fragmentation (145). Nearly identical findings were obtained in their study of autopsy material in MS. However, other investigators studying markers of apoptosis in brains of patients with MS have concluded that there is significant apoptosis of oligodendrocytes. Vartanian and colleagues reported detecting apoptosis of oligodendrocytes at the advancing margins of chronic active MS plaques (155), whereas Dowling and coworkers found Fas ligand-bearing oligodendrocytes that showed DNA-labeling and morphologic changes in their nuclei characteristic of apoptosis in both acute and chronic MS lesions (156).

Nitric Oxide

Nitric oxide (NO), a free radical, can injure cells, as can the other reactive oxygen species (ROS) it generates. Nitric oxide, elaborated in inflammatory cells by the action of inducible NO synthase (iNOS), may contribute to the injury of oligodendrocytes and neurons in EAE or MS. A number of studies have demonstrated iNOS-expressing cells in the CNS of animals with EAE (157), mainly infiltrating cells (44,158), but also astrocytes and probably microglia (159). Increase of neuronal NOS in cerebral cortex and spinal cord has also been observed in EAE (160).

Because NO is transformed to peroxynitrite, and because peroxynitrite nitrates tyrosine residues, nitrotyrosine may be used as a marker for NO damage. Nitrotyrosine-positive cells were found in the brains and spinal cords of animals with EAE, both in perivascular infiltrates and in parenchymal cells (158,161,162).

Inasmuch as NO damages cultured astrocytes (163–166) and possibly cultured oligodendrocytes and neurons (167), one might predict that interfering with NO generation would reduce CNS tissue injury in EAE. Treatment with catalase, which scavenges the ROS H_2O_2, but not with superoxide dismutase, reduced the severity of EAE (168). The antioxidant butylated hydroxyanisole also decreased the incidence and severity of EAE (169), as did aminoguanidine, a selective inhibitor of iNOS (163,170). The inhibitor of iNOS induction, 2-phenyl-4,4,5,5-tetramethylimidazoline-1-oxyl-3-oxide, and the peroxynitrite scavenger, uric acid, both largely prevented clinical symptoms in EAE (171). Repeated injection of EUK-8, a synthetic catalytic scavenger of ROS, delayed onset and/or reduced severity of EAE (172). Intraventricularly administered antisense oligodeoxynucleotides complementary to iNOS also ameliorated EAE (173). However, not all compounds that inhibit NOS, interfere with ROS generation, or enhance free radical scavenging improved outcome in EAE (174–177).

Experimental allergic encephalomyelitis was induced more readily and resulted in more severe disease in mice containing a disrupted iNOS gene than in wild-type mice, implying that iNOS may play a protective role in autoimmune demyelinating disease (178). That dying cells, mainly inflammatory cells, were found in close proximity to iNOS-positive cells, or were themselves iNOS-positive, supports the view that NO may play an important role in eliminating inflammatory cells from the CNS (158).

As in EAE, CNS tissue pathology in MS tissue suggests involvement of NO pathways. Inducible NOS expression was demonstrated by polymerase chain reaction (PCR) or immunohistochemical techniques in monocyte-derived cells within MS plaques (171,179,180). Nitration of tyrosine residues in brain also was detected (171,179). Furthermore, NO metabolites were found to be raised in the serum of patients with MS as compared with controls (181), and in vitro NO production was higher in PBMCs isolated from patients with active MS lesions than from controls (182).

Neuronal Injury

Recently there has been renewed appreciation that neuronal loss and/or axonal transection plays a role in MS (183). Antibodies to an axolemma-enriched fraction antigen were detected in the CSF and serum of patients with MS in higher concentrations than in controls, indicating axonal injury (184). Moreover, axonal damage has been demonstrated immunocytochemically in both acute and chronic MS lesions (185,186). Magnetization transfer and proton MR spectroscopy also have provided evidence of neuronal or axonal injury in MS, showing that white matter of patients with MS, although appearing normal on conventional MRI sequences, often is not normal (187–192).

Neurons may be injured either directly or as bystanders in the immune attack of oligodendrocytes. The loss of trophic signals from oligodendrocytes also may be injurious to neurons. Still other mechanisms of neuronal injury may be operative in MS. Because excitotoxicity is a final common path to neuronal injury from a variety of insults, it is possible that it also plays a role in neuronal injury in EAE and MS. Despite the presence of reactive astrocytic gliosis, expression of glutamine synthetase and glutamate dehydrogenase—the astrocyte enzymes responsible for degradation of glutamate—was markedly reduced in mice with EAE.

Because excesses of glutamate may cause neuronal excitotoxicity, a decreased capacity of astrocytes to metabolize glutamate could contribute to neuronal injury in inflammatory demyelinating disease (193). The excitatory neurotoxicity of glutamate depends on its interaction with one or more of its receptors, including the N-methyl-D-aspartate (NMDA) receptor. The NMDA receptor antagonist, MK-801, restricted lesion formation and clinical disease in EAE. Because NMDA receptors are present on a variety of cell types other than neurons, including cerebrovascular endothelial cells, the action of MK-801 in EAE could just as well have been at this or some other site besides the neuron (194).

The evidence for excitotoxicity in MS presently is scant and contradictory. Cerebrospoinal fluid levels of the excitatory transmitters glutamate and/or aspartate have been reported to be increased (195), unchanged (196), or decreased (197) in MS, relative to appropriate controls. Putative neuroprotective agents under investigation in other neurologic diseases may one day be valuable adjuncts in the treatment of MS.

TARGET-SPECIFIC IMMUNOTHERAPIES

Native Myelin Peptides

Depending on the method of exposure to an antigen, a state of tolerance, rather than a state of immune activation, may be induced to the antigen in experimental animals or humans. However, the mechanism by which tolerance is induced remains elusive. Some experiments support the concept that high doses of IV MBP, which inhibit EAE, cause deletion of encephalitogenic, CD4+, MBP-specific, T cells via antigen-induced apoptosis (198,199). Other experiments support a mechanism that involves elaboration of immunomodulatory Th-2 cells (200). Still other work suggests that the ability of MBP to inhibit EAE depends on neither apoptosis nor the generation of Th-2 lymphocytes (201). An alternate mechanism by which MBP peptides could inhibit EAE is by acting on the antigen-presenting cells rather than the effector cells. High doses of these peptides or other peptides occupying MHC receptors could make the receptors inaccessible to autoantigens. That peptides irrelevant to myelin can block EAE if given in high enough concentrations, and that the inhibition may be overcome by the addition of naive APCs, supports this concept (202).

Genetically engineered viruses have been used as gene delivery systems to administer myelin-derived peptides for the induction of tolerance. Recombinant vaccinia viruses encoding MBP sequences protected mice from EAE (203) and delayed the onset of clinical EAE in marmosets (204). As with conventional modes of administering potential self-antigens, presentation by way of gene expression in a recombinant vaccinia virus may exacerbate autoimmunity instead of inducing tolerance in EAE (205).

Investigators have been studying inoculation with a synthetic MBP peptide by various routes as potential therapy in MS. In double-blind phase I trials, both intrathe-cal and IV injection of the peptide produced transient neutralization of free anti-MBP antibodies in CSF with no change in their bound levels. No adverse neurologic effects or systemic complications were encountered with administration of MBP synthetic peptides by either route (206). However, the transient neutralization of anti-MBP antibodies by the synthetic peptide did not prevent MS relapses (207).

Altered Peptide Ligands

Altered peptide ligands (APLs) may act as relatively inert competitors of autoimmunogenic native peptides at binding sites on lymphocytes and APCs, but they also may have more complex therapeutic modes of action. It is well established that native myelin peptides can be autoimmunogenic under one set of conditions and tolerogenic under other conditions. By using synthetic peptides whose amino acid sequences have been altered slightly from the naturally occurring myelin peptide, the risk of promoting autoimmunity might be reduced and tolerance-inducing properties may be enhanced. Just as repeated IV injections of an encephalitogenic epitope of MBP prevented MBP-induced EAE in mice, IV administration of substituted MBP peptide analogues also were effective in treating EAE, provided the peptide side chains presumed to interact with the TCR and MHC binding sites were preserved (208). L-alanine substitutions or conservative exchanges of the TCR contact residues of other MBP or PLP fragments also had protective effects on EAE (209,210).

Shift to a predominantly Th2 cytokine profile in treated animals after immunization with myelin-derived peptide may be a mechanism of action for APLs in EAE. An APL with a single amino acid substitution in an encephalitogenic PLP peptide inhibited induction of EAE with the native peptide. The T-cells generated in APL-protected animals still cross-reacted in vitro with potentially encephalitogenic antigens but produced decreased amounts of the Th1 cytokine, IFN-γ (211) and increased amounts of the Th2 cytokines, IL-4 and IL-10 (211,212), or TGF-β (213). Adoptive transfer of the T-cell lines generated from APL-treated animals also conferred protection from EAE (211,212). Looking at the effect of APLs on individual T-cell clones in vitro revealed that certain APLs could stimulate some Th-1 T-cell clones as well as some Th-2 T-cell clones (214,215). Given this, it is not surprising that certain APLs may enhance autoimmune responses (216).

As with native myelin peptides, APLs may have several mechanisms of action. Aside from competitive inhibition and exerting differential influences on Th1 and Th2 T-cell populations, APLs may also cause clonal deletion of autoreactive lymphocytes (217).

Treatment Based on Theory of Restricted T-Cell Receptor

Utilization

Many of the encephalitogenic T-cell clones elaborated within inbred strains of mice possessed the same amino acid or mRNA sequences in the β regions of the variable segments of their TCRs. This observation led to the theory that only T-cell clones using a restricted set of Vβ sequences had the potential to cause EAE or MS. Although the presence of restricted Vβ TCR utilization in outbred strains of animals has been called into question, the case for restricted Vβ utilization, even in humans, remains unsettled (218,219). For example, CSF cells from individuals with MS, expanded in vitro, expressed restricted numbers of Vβ genes, predominantly Vβ 2, whereas identically cultured PBMCs expressed a wide range of Vβ gene families (220). Similarly, when activated CD4+ T cells obtained from the CSF of patients with MS were selectively expanded in culture, an overrepresentation of several TCR Vβ gene families was noted, in this case predominantly members of the Vβ 6 family (221).

A study in which postnatal treatment of rats with an MAb specific for TCR Vβ 8.2 effectively eliminated Vβ 8.2-bearing cells and prevented EAE supported a role for immunotherapy directed toward a specific Vβ subset of TCRs. Furthermore, treatment with the Vβ 8.2-specific MAb as late as day 12 postimmunization suppressed clinical EAE (222). Treating mice with MAbs reactive against Vβ 8.2-specific regulatory CD4+ T cells increased the severity and duration of EAE and caused relapses in what, in this strain, is generally a self-limited disease (223). More equivocal results were obtained from other studies (224,225).

Immune Component Vaccination

In the course of an immune reaction anti-idiotype antibodies and T cells are formed that recognize unique elements on the proimmunogenic T-cells, i.e., the variable regions of the TCRs, which then serve to inhibit the initial immune response. This ability of the immune system to self-limit an immune reaction by responding to certain of its own elements constitutes the basis for attempting to treat autoimmune disease with various forms of autoantigen vaccination.

Vβ Elements

Because an immune response to the V region of the TCRs on the lymphocytes mediating autoimmune demyelinating disease may limit the disease process, it has been rea-

soned that vaccinating animals with the appropriate V region antigens would facilitate the immune system's endogenous downregulatory mechanisms. Injection of Vβ 8.2 peptides enhanced anti-idiotypic T cells and antibodies and reduced the severity of EAE in Lewis rats mediated by Vβ 8.2 effector cells (226). Although treatment of Lewis rats with a Vβ 8.2 peptide inhibited clinical EAE, Vβ 8.2+ T cells were still found in spinal cord infiltrates (227). The inhibitory immune reaction to an exogenous Vβ peptide thus does not seem to depend on complete deletion of T-cell clones bearing the homologous endogenous Vβ sequence. Instead, the salutary effect on EAE is probably brought about by boosting the reaction of anti-Vβ 8.2–specific regulatory T cells and is likely mediated as much, if not more, by soluble factors as by clonal deletion (228). Kumar and coworkers demonstrated that regulatory CD4+ T cells specific for a particular TCR peptide from the Vβ 8.2 chain become primed in mice spontaneously recovering from MBP-induced EAE. When clones of theses cells were injected into mice before inducing EAE they downregulated responses to the immunodominant epitope of MBP and protected against EAE (223). T-cell receptor peptide-specific regulatory T cells have also been shown to produce a soluble factor or factors that inhibit T-cell activation and protect against actively induced EAE (229).

If an immune response to a particular Vβ peptide is involved in downregulating the autoimmune attack in EAE, an inability of the immune system to respond to the relevant Vb element would be expected to worsen the disease. In Lewis rats tolerized as adults with Vβ 8.2 peptides (230), or as neonates to a comprehensive set of Vβ 8.2 epitopes (226), the severity of EAE increased. Moreover, injecting mice with a TCR peptide at one dose may promote self- regulatory T cells that respond to the deleterious TCR and protect from EAE, whereas at another dose the same peptide may induce tolerance to the self-injurious TCR and worsen disease (231).

As with the delivery of APL genes, Vβ TCR genes may be delivered to experimental animals by way of recombinant viral vectors. Immunization of mice with vaccinia virus recombinants expressing the Vβ 8.2 gene reduced clinical severity of EAE (232).

As noted previously, V gene biases among MBP-specific T-cell clones from some patients with MS have been reported. Injection of Vβ 5.2 and Vβ 6.1 peptides boosted the frequency of TCR peptide-specific T cells and reduced in vitro lymphocyte responses to MBP, in some cases with possible clinical benefit (228). On the basis of the findings of Wilson and coworkers that TCR Vβ 6 genes are overrepresented in CSF-derived T cells from MS patients (221), a phase I trial of two doses of a TCR Vβ 6 CDR2 region peptide vaccine was undertaken in 10 MS patients whose CSF T-cell populations were predominated by T cells with Vβ 6 mRNA. The patients treated with the higher dose showed a slight decrease in CSF cellularity, refractoriness of their CSF cells to proliferate in cytokine-supplemented expansion cultures, and a marked diminution in Vβ 6 mRNA levels from the CSF T-cells in these cultures. In the patients receiving the lower dose, CSF cellularity was the same as, or slightly increased over, prevaccination levels, CSF cells from one patient failed to grow in expansion cultures, and cultured CSF cells from two patients changed from an oligoclonal Vβ 6 pattern to a more polyclonal pattern (233).

Whole T-Cell Therapy in Humans

In a phase I clinical trial, five of eight patients with MS vaccinated with irradiated MBP-reactive T cells showed a decrease in the number of exacerbations in the two years after vaccination compared with the previous two years (a total of three versus 16). A similar decrease was not evidenced in matched control MS patients (a total of 10 versus 12). The mean increase in brain MRI lesion size in the vaccinated patients was 8 percent compared with 39.5 percent in the controls (234). The vaccinated patients also showed a moderate reduction in their disability scores relative to the control patients (235). T-cell vaccination induced predominantly CD8+ regulatory T cells capable of lysing the immunizing lymphocytes in a clonotype-specific manner and did not affect MBP-reactive clones not used for immunization (235). Vaccination resulted in a clonal depletion of circulating MBP-reactive T cells that persisted over a period of one to three years in the majority of recipients. In the three patients whose MS worsened after vaccination, circulating MBP-reactive T cells had reappeared. In those cases in which MBP-reactive T-cells were found, they differed in clonal origin from those of the immunizing clones, suggesting a shift in the T-cell repertoire to other MBP determinants (234,235).

REMYELINATION AND GROWTH FACTORS

Oligodendrocyte and Progenitors

Repair of damaged myelin in both rats and humans is believed to be mediated not only by surviving mature oligodendrocytes but also by newly generated oligodendrocytes from precursor cells (236). Only a portion of the oligodendrocyte progenitor cells in the adult rat spinal cord that are capable of differentiation are also capable of proliferation (237). Similarly, although chronic MS lesions contained significant numbers of oligodendrocyte precursor cells, they appeared relatively quiescent, not expressing the nuclear proliferation antigen recognized

by the Ki-67 antibody or forming remyelinating oligodendrocytes (238).

In rodents, transplanted neonatal glial progenitor cells remyelinated gliotoxin-induced CNS lesions (236). Transplantation of oligodendrocytes or their progenitors into the CNS of dogs with a mutation that causes focal demyelination resulted in significant repair of the lesions (239). Oligodendrocyte progenitor cells transplanted in the spinal cord of rats before induction of EAE showed greatly enhanced survival and migration compared with cells similarly transplanted in controls, suggesting that EAE-induced changes in the CNS microenvironment, possibly relating to the immune response, promote survival and migration of transplanted oligodendrocyte progenitors (240). In vitro, macrophage enrichment of aggregate brain cultures promoted myelination, further suggesting that macrophage-derived cytokines or growth factors may promote proliferation and differentiation of oligodendroglia or their progenitors (241).

Growth Factors

Growth factors, locally secreted peptides subserving a paracrine function, guide the development and differentiation of various cells and tissues. Insulin-like growth factor-I (IGF-I), platelet-derived growth factor (PDGF), fibroblast growth factor (FGF), and ciliary neurotrophic factor (CNTF) have all been detected in the CNS (242). These factors may exert influence over oligodendrocytes and may be useful in promoting remyelination.

Insulin-Like Growth Factor-I

Insulin-like growth factor-I improved clinical and pathologic outcomes in EAE (243,244). Axons in lesions of IGF-I–treated rats, but not of controls, were surrounded by regenerating myelin segments. The proportion of proliferating cells with oligodendroglia-like morphology and the relative mRNA levels for MBP and PLP also were higher in lesions of IGF-I–treated rats than controls. Furthermore, both the number of PLP mRNA-containing oligodendroglia and the relative PLP mRNA levels per oligodendrocyte were higher in lesions of IGF-I–treated rats (245). Insulin-like growth factor-I administered to Lewis rats after weakness from EAE had begun reduced clinical deficits, decreased lesion severity, and upregulated mRNA levels of MBP and PLP (246).

Whereas IGF-I may be of therapeutic benefit in EAE, the role of endogenous IGF-I in MS has yet to be established. For example, oligodendrocytes may respond to the trophic action of IGF in vitro, but patients with MS did not show significant changes in their levels of circulating IGF-I or IGF-binding proteins compared with healthy controls (247). Furthermore, the density of IGF-I receptors detected post mortem by binding of 125-I-IGF-I in the normal-appearing white matter or chronic plaques in brains from MS patients did not differ from their density in the white matter of control brains (248). Pilot studies to look at the effects of IGF-I in MS are under way.

Nerve Growth Factor

Micera and coworkers found that levels of NGF were enhanced in the thalamus and spinal cord of rats with EAE compared with control animals, and that the number of cells expressing mRNA for NGF in these two regions also was increased (249). Calza and colleagues also found that NGF content increased in the thalamus but decreased in the spinal cord and medulla, at times when cellular infiltration was most pronounced in the Lewis rat with EAE. Nerve growth factor receptors were also upregulated on the wall of blood vessels and some neurons in perivascular areas (160). Elevated levels of NGF protein, NGF mRNA, and low-affinity NGF-receptor mRNA were detected in several regions of the CNS of rats with EAE compared with untreated animals (250).

Levels of CSF NGF in patients with MS increased in the acute phase of the disease and decreased during remission (249,251).

Fibroblast Growth Factor

Exposure of postmitotic, terminally differentiating oligodendrocytes to FGF-2 resulted in downregulation of myelin-specific gene expression, increases in the length of cellular processes, reentrance into the cell cycle without accompanying mitosis, and altered expression of FGF receptors (252).

Ciliary Neurotrophic Factor

Ciliary neurotrophic factor significantly protected cultured oligodendrocytes from TNF-mediated and from serum deprivation-induced apoptosis but did not protect them from injury caused by activated CD4+ T-cells (253).

ANTIMICROBIAL THERAPY

It is outside the scope of this chapter to examine the role that latent or commensal infection may play in sustaining MS. Numerous candidate microorganisms have been investigated in this capacity. Most recently, *Chlamydia pneumoniae* (254) and humanherpes virus 6 have come under investigation (255–263). To the extent that a virus or atypical bacterial infection may be involved in MS, antibiotics and antiviral agents must be considered potential investigational therapies.

COMBINATION THERAPY

When combined in vitro, glatiramer acetate and IFN-β additively suppressed proliferation of MBP-specific T cells. Synthesis of the proinflammatory cytokines, IL-2 and IFN-γ, by MBP-specific lines was also additively inhibited (264). A phase I clinical trial to look at adding glatiramer acetate to established treatment with IFN beta-1a is currently under way. Neurologists have also begun, in select patients, combining either an IFN β or glatiramer acetate, with a nonspecific immunosuppressant or chemotherapeutic agent, but the practice is not supported by clinical data. Combining one immunomodulator with another, or with an immunosuppressant, could interfere with the beneficial action of either alone. Controlled clinical trials are under way to study some of these combinations.

References

1. Weiner HL, et al. Intermittent cyclophosphamide pulse therapy in progressive multiple sclerosis: Final report of the Northeast Cooperative Multiple Sclerosis Treatment Group. *Neurology* 1993; 43:910–918.
2. Goodkin DE, et al. Low-dose (7.5 mg) oral methotrexate reduces the rate of progression in chronic progressive multiple sclerosis. *Ann Neurol* 1995; 37:30–40.
3. Goodkin DE, et al. Low-dose oral methotrexate in chronic progressive multiple sclerosis: Analyses of serial MRIs. *Neurology* 1996; 47:1153–1157.
4. De Castro S, et al. Noninvasive assessment of mitoxantrone cardiotoxicity in relapsing remitting multiple sclerosis. *J Clin Pharmacol* 1995; 35:627–632.
5. Gonsette RE. Mitoxantrone immunotherapy in multiple sclerosis. *Multiple Sclerosis* 1996; 1:329–332.
6. Millefiorini E, et al. Randomized placebo-controlled trial of mitoxantrone in relapsing-remitting multiple sclerosis: 24-month clinical and MRI outcome. *J Neurol* 1997; 244:153–159.
7. Krapf H, et al. Serial gadolinium-enhanced magnetic resonance imaging in patients with multiple sclerosis treated with mitoxantrone. *Neuroradiology* 1995; 37:113–119.
8. Edan G, et al. Therapeutic effect of mitoxantrone combined with methylprednisolone in multiple sclerosis: A randomised multicentre study of active disease using MRI and clinical criteria. *J Neurol Neurosurg Psychiatry* 1997; 62:112–118.
9. Confavreux C, Moreau T. Emerging treatments in multiple sclerosis: Azathioprine and mofetil. *Multiple Sclerosis* 1996; 1:379–384.
10. McMichael J, et al. Computer-guided randomized concentration-controlled trials of tacrolimus in autoimmunity: Multiple sclerosis and primary biliary cirrhosis. *Ther Drug Monitor* 1996; 18:435–437.
11. Schorlemmer HU, Bartlett RR. Malononitrilamides (MNA 279 and MNA 715) have therapeutic activity in acute and chronic relapsing experimental allergic encephalomyelitis (EAE). *Inflammation Research* 1997; 46(Suppl 2):S163–S164.
12. Novales-Li P. Suramin exerts in vivo cytokine modulatory properties on splenocytes experimental allergic encephalomyelitis-induced SJL mice: Implications for

autoimmune disease therapy. *Immunopharmacology* 1996; 35:155–162.

13. Ohta Y, Fukuda S, Makino H. Reduction of disease causative T-cells in experimental autoimmune disease models by a new antirheumatic drug, TAK-603. *Immunopharmacology* 1997; 37:167–174.

14. Bauer J, et al. The role of macrophages, perivascular cells, and microglial cells in the pathogenesis of experimental autoimmune encephalomyelitis. *Glia* 1995; 15:437–446.

15. Dalakas, M.C. Intravenous immune globulin therapy for neurologic diseases. *Ann Intern Med* 1997; 126:721–730.

16. Fazekas F, et al. Treatment effects of monthly intravenous immunoglobulin on patients with relapsing-remitting multiple sclerosis: Further analyses of the Austrian Immunoglobulin in MS study. *Multiple Sclerosis* 1997; 3:137–141.

17. Achiron A, et al. Intravenous immunoglobulin treatment in multiple sclerosis. Effect on relapses. *Neurology* 1998; 50:398–402.

18. Poehlau D, et al. Intravenous immunoglobulin (IVIG) treatment for patients with primary or secondary progressive multiple sclerosis—Outline of a double-blind randomized, placebo-controlled trial. *Multiple Sclerosis* 1997; 3:149–152.

19. Rumbach L, et al. Biological assessment and MRI monitoring of the therapeutic efficacy of monoclonal anti-T CD4 antibody in multiple sclerosis patients. *Multiple Sclerosis* 1996; 1:207–212.

20. van Oosten BW, et al. Treatment of multiple sclerosis with the monoclonal anti-CD4 antibody cM-T412: Results of a randomized, double-blind, placebo-controlled, MR-monitored phase II trial. *Neurology* 1997; 49:351–357.

21. Moreau T, et al. CAMPATH-IH in multiple sclerosis. *Multiple Sclerosis* 1996; 1:357–365.

22. Hu H, et al. Depletion of T lymphocytes with immunotoxin retards the progress of experimental allergic encephalomyelitis in rhesus monkeys. *Cell Immunol* 1997; 177:26–34.

23. van Gelder M, van BD. Treatment of relapsing experimental autoimmune encephalomyelitis in rats with allogeneic bone marrow transplantation from a resistant strain. *Bone Marrow Transplant* 1995; 16:343–351.

24. van Gelder M, van Bekkum DW. Effective treatment of relapsing experimental autoimmune encephalomyelitis with pseudoautologous bone marrow transplantation. *Bone Marrow Transplant* 1996; 18:1029–1034.

25. Burt RK, et al. Effect of disease stage on clinical outcome after syngeneic bone marrow transplantation for relapsing experimental autoimmune encephalomyelitis. *Blood* 1998; 91:2609–2616.

26. McAllister LD, Beatty PG, Rose J. Allogeneic bone marrow transplant for chronic myelogenous leukemia in a patient with multiple sclerosis. *Bone Marrow Transplant* 1997; 19:395–397.

27. Fassas A, et al. Peripheral blood stem cell transplantation in the treatment of progressive multiple sclerosis: First results of a pilot study. *Bone Marrow Transplant* 1997; 20:631–638.

28. Hautecoeur P, et al. Variations of IL2, IL6, TNF alpha plasmatic levels in relapsing remitting multiple sclerosis. *Acta Neurol Belg* 1997; 97:240–243.

29. Pitzalis C, et al. Comparison of the effects of oral versus intravenous methylprednisolone regimens on peripheral blood T lymphocyte adhesion molecule expression, T cell

30. Rieckmann P, et al. Tumor necrosis factor-alpha messenger RNA expression in patients with relapsing-remitting multiple sclerosis is associated with disease activity. *Ann Neurol* 1995; 37:82–88.

31. Navikas V, et al. Augmented expression of tumour necrosis factor-alpha and lymphotoxin in mononuclear cells in multiple sclerosis and optic neuritis. *Brain* 1996; 119:213–223.

32. Musette P, et al. The pattern of production of cytokine mRNAs is markedly altered at the onset of multiple sclerosis. *Research Immunol* 1996; 147:435–441.

33. Correale J, et al. Patterns of cytokine secretion by autoreactive proteolipid protein-specific T cell clones during the course of multiple sclerosis. *J Immunol* 1995; 154: 2959–2968.

34. Glabinski A, Mirecka M, Pokoca L. Tumor necrosis factor alpha but not lymphotoxin is overproduced by blood mononuclear cells in multiple sclerosis. *Acta Neurol Scand* 1995; 91:276–279.

35. Philippe J, et al. In vitro TNF-alpha, IL-2 and IFN-gamma production as markers of relapses in multiple sclerosis. *Clin Neurol Neurosurg* 1996; 98:286–290.

36. Hermans G, et al. Cytokine profile of myelin basic protein-reactive T cells in multiple sclerosis and healthy individuals. *Ann Neurol* 1997; 42:18–27.

37. Wandinger KP, et al. Diminished production of type-I interferons and interleukin-2 in patients with multiple sclerosis. *J Neurol Sci* 1997; 149:87–93.

38. Martino G, et al. Tumor necrosis factor alpha and its receptors in relapsing-remitting multiple sclerosis. *J Neurol Sci* 1997; 152:51–61.

39. Bongioanni P, Meucci G. T-cell tumor necrosis factor-alpha receptor binding in patients with multiple sclerosis. *Neurology* 1997; 48:826–831.

40. D'Elios MM, et al. In vivo CD30 expression in human diseases with predominant activation of Th2-like T cells. *J Leukocyte Biol* 1997; 61:539–544.

41. Navikas V, et al. Soluble CD30 levels in plasma and cerebrospinal fluid in multiple sclerosis, HIV infection and other nervous system diseases. *Acta Neurol Scand* 1997; 95:99–102.

42. Renno T, et al. TNF-alpha expression by resident microglia and infiltrating leukocytes in the central nervous system of mice with experimental allergic encephalomyelitis. Regulation by Th1 cytokines. *J Immunol* 1995; 154:944–953.

43. Issazadeh S, et al. Cytokine production in the central nervous system of Lewis rats with experimental autoimmune encephalomyelitis: Dynamics of mRNA expression for interleukin-10, interleukin-12, cytolysin, tumor necrosis factor alpha and tumor necrosis factor beta. *J Neuroimmunol* 1995; 61:205–212.

44. Okuda Y, et al. Expression of the inducible isoform of nitric oxide synthase in the central nervous system of mice correlates with the severity of actively induced experimental allergic encephalomyelitis. *J Neuroimmunol* 1995; 62:103–112.

45. Sun D, et al. Production of tumor necrosis factor-alpha as a result of glia-T-cell interaction correlates with the pathogenic activity of myelin basic protein-reactive T cells in experimental autoimmune encephalomyelitis. *J Neurosci Res* 1996; 45:400–409.

46. Villarroya H, et al. Myelin-induced experimental allergic encephalomyelitis in Lewis rats: Tumor necrosis factor

alpha levels in serum and cerebrospinal fluid immunohistochemical expression in glial cells and macrophages of optic nerve and spinal cord. *J Neuroimmunol* 1996; 64:55–6461.

47. Cannella B, Raine CS. The adhesion molecule and cytokine profile of multiple sclerosis lesions. *Ann Neurol* 1995; 37:424–435.

48. McGuinness MC, et al. Human leukocyte antigens and cytokine expression in cerebral inflammatory demyelinative lesions of X-linked adrenoleukodystrophy and multiple sclerosis. *J Neuroimmunol* 1997; 75:174–182.

49. Rieckmann P, et al. Semi-quantitative analysis of cytokine gene expression in blood and cerebrospinal fluid cells by reverse transcriptase polymerase chain reaction. *Res Exp Med* 1995; 195:17–29.

50. Monteyne P, et al. Cytokine mRNA expression in CSF and peripheral blood mononuclear cells in multiple sclerosis: Detection by RT-PCR without in vitro stimulation. *J Neuroimmunol* 1997; 80:137–142.

51. Rentzos M, et al. Tumour necrosis factor alpha is elevated in serum and cerebrospinal fluid in multiple sclerosis and inflammatory neuropathies. *J Neurol* 1996; 243:165–170.

52. Drulovic J, et al. Interleukin-12 and tumor necrosis factor-alpha levels in cerebrospinal fluid of multiple sclerosis patients. *J Neurol Sci* 1997; 147:145–150.

53. Shaw MK, et al. Induction of myelin basic protein-specific experimental autoimmune encephalomyelitis in C57BL/6 mice: Mapping of T cell epitopes and T cell receptor V beta gene segment usage. *J Neurosci Res* 1996; 45:690–699.

54. Rovaris M, et al. Patterns of disease activity in multiple sclerosis patients: A study with quantitative gadolinium-enhanced brain MRI and cytokine measurement in different clinical subgroups. *J Neurol* 1996; 243:536–542.

55. Puccioni-Sohler M, et al. A soluble form of tumour necrosis factor receptor in cerebrospinal fluid and serum of HTLV-I-associated myelopathy and other neurological diseases. *J Neurol* 1995; 242:239–242.

56. Martin D, et al. Inhibition of tumor necrosis factor is protective against neurologic dysfunction after active immunization of Lewis rats with myelin basic protein. *Exp Neurol* 1995; 131:221–228.

57. Wiemann B, et al. Combined treatment of acute EAE in Lewis rats with TNF-binding protein and interleukin-1 receptor antagonist. *Exp Neurol* 1998; 149:455–463.

58. Korner H, et al. Tumor necrosis factor blockade in actively induced experimental autoimmune encephalomyelitis prevents clinical disease despite activated T cell infiltration to the central nervous system. *Eur J Immunol* 1997; 27:1973–1981.

59. Klinkert WE, et al. TNF-alpha receptor fusion protein prevents experimental auto-immune encephalomyelitis and demyelination in Lewis rats: An overview. *J Neuroimmunol* 1997; 72:163–168.

60. Probert L, et al. Spontaneous inflammatory demyelinating disease in transgenic mice showing central nervous system-specific expression of tumor necrosis factor alpha. *Proc Natl Acad Sci USA* 1995; 92:11294–11298.

61. Taupin V, et al. Increased severity of experimental autoimmune encephalomyelitis, chronic macrophage/microglial reactivity, and demyelination in transgenic mice producing tumor necrosis factor-alpha in the central nervous system. *Eur J Immunol* 1997; 27:905–913.

62. van Oosten BW, et al. Increased MRI activity and immune activation in two multiple sclerosis patients treated with the monoclonal anti-tumor necrosis factor antibody cA2. *Neurology* 1996; 47:1531–1534.

63. Willenborg DO, et al. Cytokines and murine autoimmune encephalomyelitis: Inhibition or enhancement of disease with antibodies to select cytokines, or by delivery of exogenous cytokines using a recombinant vaccinia virus system. *Scand J Immunol* 1995; 41:31–41.

64. Liu J, et al. TNF is a potent anti-inflammatory cytokine in autoimmune-mediated demyelination. *Nature Medicine* 1998; 4:78–83.

65. Sommer N, et al. The antidepressant rolipram suppresses cytokine production and prevents autoimmune encephalomyelitis [see comments]. *Nature Medicine* 1995; 1:244–248.

66. Jung S, et al. Preventive but not therapeutic application of Rolipram ameliorates experimental autoimmune encephalomyelitis in Lewis rats. *J Neuroimmunol* 1996; 68:1–11.

67. Genain CP, et al. Prevention of autoimmune demyelination in non-human primates by a cAMP-specific phosphodiesterase inhibitor. *Proc Natl Acad Sci USA* 1995; 92:3601–3605.

68. Okuda Y, et al. Pentoxifylline delays the onset of experimental allergic encephalomyelitis in mice by modulating cytokine production in peripheral blood mononuclear cells. *Immunopharmacology* 1996; 35:141–148.

69. Rieckmann, P, et al. Pentoxifylline, a phosphodiesterase inhibitor, induces immune deviation in patients with multiple sclerosis. *J Neuroimmunol* 1996; 64:193–200.

70. Segal BM, Shevach EM. IL-12 unmasks latent autoimmune disease in resistant mice. *J Exp Med* 1996; 184:771–775.

71. Leonard JP, et al. Regulation of the inflammatory response in animal models of multiple sclerosis by interleukin-12. *Crit Rev Immunol* 1997; 17:545–553.

72. Smith T, et al. Interleukin-12 induces relapse in experimental allergic encephalomyelitis in the Lewis rat. *Am J Pathol* 1997; 150:1909–1917.

73. Bright JJ, et al. Expression of IL-12 in CNS and lymphoid organs of mice with experimental allergic encephalitis. *J Neuroimmunol* 1998; 82:22–30.

74. Gijbels K, et al. Administration of neutralizing antibodies to interleukin-6 (IL-6) reduces experimental autoimmune encephalomyelitis and is associated with elevated levels of IL-6 bioactivity in central nervous system and circulation. *Molecular Med* 1995; 1:795–805.

75. Durelli L, et al. Interferon alpha treatment of relapsing-remitting multiple sclerosis: Long-term study of the correlations between clinical and magnetic resonance imaging results and effects on the immune function. *Multiple Sclerosis* 1995; 1(Suppl):S32–S37.

76. Durelli L, et al. Long term recombinant interferon alpha treatment in MS with special emphasis to side effects. *Multiple Sclerosis* 1996; 1:366–371.

77. Bongioanni MR, et al. Systemic high-dose recombinant-alpha-2a-interferon therapy modulates lymphokine production in multiple sclerosis. *J Neurol Sci* 1996; 143:91–99.

78. Nyland H, et al. Treatment of relapsing-remittent multiple sclerosis with recombinant human interferon-alfa-2a: Design of a randomised, placebo-controlled, double blind trial in Norway. *Multiple Sclerosis* 1996; 1:372–375.

79. Brod SA, et al. Oral administration of human or murine interferon alpha suppresses relapses and modifies adoptive transfer in experimental autoimmune encephalomyelitis. *J Neuroimmunol* 1995; 58:61–69.

80. Brod SA, et al. Modification of acute experimental autoimmune encephalomyelitis in the Lewis rat by oral administration of type 1 interferons. *J Interferon Cytokine Res* 1995; 15:115–122.

81. Brod SA, Khan M. Oral administration of IFN-alpha is superior to subcutaneous administration of IFN-alpha in the suppression of chronic relapsing experimental autoimmune encephalomyelitis. *J Autoimmunity* 1996; 9:11–20.

82. Brod SA, et al. Ingested IFN-alpha has biological effects in humans with relapsing-remitting multiple sclerosis. *Multiple Sclerosis* 1997; 3:1–7.

83. Soos JM, et al. The IFN pregnancy recognition hormone IFN-tau blocks both development and superantigen reactivation of experimental allergic encephalomyelitis without associated toxicity. *J Immunol* 1995; 155:2747–2753.

84. Soos JM, et al. Oral feeding of interferon tau can prevent the acute and chronic relapsing forms of experimental allergic encephalomyelitis. *J Neuroimmunol* 1997; 75:43–50.

85. Mujtaba MG, Soos JM, Johnson HM. CD4 T suppressor cells mediate interferon tau protection against experimental allergic encephalomyelitis. *J Neuroimmunol* 1997; 75:35–42.

86. Rollnik JD, et al. Biologically active TGF-beta 1 is increased in cerebrospinal fluid while it is reduced in serum in multiple sclerosis patients. *Acta Neurol Scand* 1997; 96:101–105.

87. Issazadeh S, et al. Interferon gamma, interleukin 4 and transforming growth factor beta in experimental autoimmune encephalomyelitis in Lewis rats: Dynamics of cellular mRNA expression in the central nervous system and lymphoid cells. *J Neurosci Res* 1995; 40:579–590.

88. Wyss-Coray T, et al. Astroglial overproduction of TGF-beta 1 enhances inflammatory central nervous system disease in transgenic mice. *J Neuroimmunol* 1997; 77:45–50.

89. Calabresi PA, et al. Phase 1 trial of transforming growth factor beta 2 in chronic progressive MS. *Neurology* 1998; 51:289–292.

90. Porrini AM, Gambi D, Reder AT. Interferon effects on interleukin-10 secretion. Mononuclear cell response to interleukin-10 is normal in multiple sclerosis patients. *J Neuroimmunol* 1995; 61:27–34.

91. Cannella B, et al. IL-10 fails to abrogate experimental autoimmune encephalomyelitis. *J Neurosci Res* 1996; 45:735–746.

92. Nagelkerken L, Blauw B, Tielemans M. IL-4 abrogates the inhibitory effect of IL-10 on the development of experimental allergic encephalomyelitis in SJL mice. *Internat Immunol* 1997; 9:1243–1251.

93. Mathisen PM, et al. Treatment of experimental autoimmune encephalomyelitis with genetically modified memory T cells. *J Exp Med* 1997; 186:159–164.

94. Inobe JI, Chen Y, Weiner HL. In vivo administration of IL-4 induces TGF-beta-producing cells and protects animals from experimental autoimmune encephalomyelitis. *Ann NY Acad Sci* 1996; 778:390–392.

95. Shaw MK, et al. Local delivery of interleukin 4 by retrovirus-transduced T lymphocytes ameliorates experimental autoimmune encephalomyelitis. *J Exp Med* 1997; 185:1711–1714.

96. Glabinski AR, et al. Central nervous system chemokine mRNA accumulation follows initial leukocyte entry at the onset of acute murine experimental autoimmune encephalomyelitis. *Brain Behav Immunity* 1995; 9:315–30.

97. Karpus WJ, et al. An important role for the chemokine macrophage inflammatory protein-1 alpha in the pathogenesis of the T cell-mediated autoimmune disease, experimental autoimmune encephalomyelitis. *J Immunol* 1995; 155:5003–5010.

98. Berman JW, et al. Localization of monocyte chemoattractant peptide-1 expression in the central nervous system in experimental autoimmune encephalomyelitis and trauma in the rat. *J Immunol* 1996; 156:3017–3023.

99. Miyagishi R, et al. Identification of cell types producing RANTES, MIP-1 alpha and MIP-1 beta in rat experimental autoimmune encephalomyelitis by in situ hybridization. *J Neuroimmunol* 1997; 77:17–26.

100. Karpus WJ, Kennedy KJ. MIP-1alpha and MCP-1 differentially regulate acute and relapsing autoimmune encephalomyelitis as well as Th1/Th2 lymphocyte differentiation. *J Leukocyte Biol* 1997; 62:681–687.

101. Miyagishi R, et al. Macrophage inflammatory protein-1 alpha in the cerebrospinal fluid of patients with multiple sclerosis and other inflammatory neurological diseases. *J Neurol Sci* 1995; 129:223–227.

102. Dore-Duffy P, et al. Circulating, soluble adhesion proteins in cerebrospinal fluid and serum of patients with multiple sclerosis: Correlation with clinical activity. *Ann Neurol* 1995; 37:55–62.

103. Tsukada N, et al. Soluble E-selectin in the serum and cerebrospinal fluid of patients with multiple sclerosis and human T-lymphotropic virus type 1-associated myelopathy. *Neurology* 1995; 45:1914–1918.

104. Giovannoni G, et al. Soluble E-selectin in multiple sclerosis: Raised concentrations in patients with primary progressive disease. *J Neurol Neurosurg Psychiatry* 1996; 60:20–26.

105. Mossner R, et al. Circulating L-selectin in multiple sclerosis patients with active, gadolinium-enhancing brain plaques. *J Neuroimmunol* 1996; 65:61–65.

106. Hartung HP, et al. Circulating adhesion molecules and tumor necrosis factor receptor in multiple sclerosis: Correlation with magnetic resonance imaging. *Ann Neurol* 1995; 38:186–193.

107. Droogan AG, et al. Serum and cerebrospinal fluid levels of soluble adhesion molecules in multiple sclerosis: Predominant intrathecal release of vascular cell adhesion molecule-1. *J Neuroimmunol* 1996; 64:185–191.

108. Rovaris M, et al. A comparison of conventional and fast spin-echo sequences for the measurement of lesion load in multiple sclerosis using a semi-automated contour technique. *Neuroradiology* 1997; 39:161–165.

109. Trojano M, et al. Soluble intercellular adhesion molecule-1 in serum and cerebrospinal fluid of clinically active relapsing-remitting multiple sclerosis: Correlation with Gd-DTPA magnetic resonance imaging-enhancement and cerebrospinal fluid findings. *Neurology* 1996; 47:1535–1541.

110. Rieckmann P, et al. Soluble adhesion molecules (sVCAM-1 and sICAM-1) in cerebrospinal fluid and serum correlate with MRI activity in multiple sclerosis. *Ann Neurol* 1997; 41:326–333.

111. Matsuda M, et al. Increased levels of soluble vascular cell adhesion molecule-1 (VCAM-1) in the cerebrospinal fluid and sera of patients with multiple sclerosis and human T lymphotropic virus type-1-associated myelopathy. *J Neuroimmunol* 1995; 59:35–40.

112. Calabresi PA, et al. Increases in soluble VCAM-1 correlate with a decrease in MRI lesions in multiple sclerosis

treated with interferon beta-1b. *Ann Neurol* 1997; 41:669–674.

113. Lou J, et al. Brain microvascular endothelial cells and leukocytes derived from patients with multiple sclerosis exhibit increased adhesion capacity. *Neuroreport* 1997; 8:629-633.

114. Gordon EJ, et al. Both anti-CD11a (LFA-1) and anti-CD11b (MAC-1) therapy delay the onset and diminish the severity of experimental autoimmune encephalomyelitis. *J Neuroimmunol* 1995; 62:153–160.

115. Kent SJ, et al. A monoclonal antibody to alpha 4 integrin suppresses and reverses active experimental allergic encephalomyelitis. *J Neuroimmunol* 1995; 58:1–10.

116. Rose LM, et al. Resolution of CNS lesions following treatment of experimental allergic encephalomyelitis in macaques with monoclonal antibody to the CD18 leukocyte integrin. *Multiple Sclerosis* 1997; 2:259–266.

117. Kobayashi Y, et al. Antibodies against leukocyte function-associated antigen-1 and against intercellular adhesion molecule-1 together suppress the progression of experimental allergic encephalomyelitis. *Cell Immunol* 1995; 164:295–305.

118. Morrissey SP, et al. Partial inhibition of AT-EAE by an antibody to ICAM-1: Clinico-histological and MRI studies. *J Neuroimmunol* 1996; 69:85–93.

119. Leger OJ, et al. Humanization of a mouse antibody against human alpha-4 integrin: A potential therapeutic for the treatment of multiple sclerosis. *Human Antibodies* 1997; 8:3–16.

120. Khoury SJ, et al. CD28-B7 costimulatory blockade by CTLA4Ig prevents actively induced experimental autoimmune encephalomyelitis and inhibits Th1 but spares Th2 cytokines in the central nervous system. *J Immunol* 1995; 155:4521–4524.

121. Perrin PJ, et al. Role of B7:CD28/CTLA-4 in the induction of chronic relapsing experimental allergic encephalomyelitis. *J Immunol* 1995; 154:1481–1490.

122. Arima T, et al. Inhibition by CTLA4Ig of experimental allergic encephalomyelitis. *J Immunol* 1996; 156:4916–4924.

123. Perrin PJ, et al. B7–mediated costimulation can either provoke or prevent clinical manifestations of experimental allergic encephalomyelitis. *Immunol Res* 1995; 14:189–199.

124. Racke MK, et al. Distinct roles for B7-1 (CD-80) and B7-2 (CD-86) in the initiation of experimental allergic encephalomyelitis. *J Clin Invest* 1995; 96:2195–2203.

125. Perrin PJ, et al. CTLA-4 blockade enhances clinical disease and cytokine production during experimental allergic encephalomyelitis. *J Immunol* 1996; 157:1333–1336.

126. Karandikar NJ, et al. CTLA-4: A negative regulator of autoimmune disease. *J Exp Med* 1996; 184:783–788.

127. Hurwitz AA, et al. Specific blockade of CTLA-4/B7 interactions results in exacerbated clinical and histologic disease in an actively-induced model of experimental allergic encephalomyelitis. *J Neuroimmunol* 1997; 73:57–62.

128. Miller SD, et al. Blockade of CD28/B7-1 interaction prevents epitope spreading and clinical relapses of murine EAE. *Immunity* 1995; 3:739–745.

129. Kuchroo VK, et al. B7-1 and B7-2 costimulatory molecules activate differentially the Th1/Th2 developmental pathways: Application to autoimmune disease therapy. *Cell* 1995; 80:707–718.

130. Perrin PJ, et al. Opposing effects of CTLA4-Ig and anti-CD80 (B7-1) plus anti-CD86 (B7-2) on experimental allergic encephalomyelitis. *J Neuroimmunol* 1996; 65:31–39.

131. Khoury SJ, et al. Ex vivo treatment of antigen-presenting cells with CTLA4Ig and encephalitogenic peptide prevents experimental autoimmune encephalomyelitis in the Lewis rat. *J Immunol* 1996; 157:3700–3705.

132. Svenningsson A, et al. Increased expression of B7-1 costimulatory molecule on cerebrospinal fluid cells of patients with multiple sclerosis and infectious central nervous system disease. *J Neuroimmunol* 1997; 75:59–68.

133. Chandler S, et al. Matrix metalloproteinases, tumor necrosis factor and multiple sclerosis: An overview. [Review] [95 refs]. *J Neuroimmunol* 1997; 72:155–161.

134. Moss ML, et al. Structural features and biochemical properties of TNF-alpha converting enzyme (TACE). *J Neuroimmunol* 1997; 72:127–129.

135. Clements JM, et al. Matrix metalloproteinase expression during experimental autoimmune encephalomyelitis and effects of a combined matrix metalloproteinase and tumour necrosis factor-alpha inhibitor. *J Neuroimmunol* 1997; 74:85–94.

136. Pagenstecher A, et al. Differential expression of matrix metalloproteinase and tissue inhibitor of matrix metalloproteinase genes in the mouse central nervous system in normal and inflammatory states. *Am J Pathol* 1998; 152:729–741.

137. Norga K., et al. Prevention of acute autoimmune encephalomyelitis and abrogation of relapses in murine models of multiple sclerosis by the protease inhibitor D-penicillamine. *Inflammation Research* 1995; 44:529–534.

138. Hewson AK, et al. Suppression of experimental allergic encephalomyelitis in the Lewis rat by the matrix metalloproteinase inhibitor Ro31-9790. *Inflammation Research* 1995; 44:345–349.

139. Maeda A, RA Sobel RA. Matrix metalloproteinases in the normal human central nervous system, microglial nodules, and multiple sclerosis lesions. *J Neuropathol Exp Neurol* 1996; 55:300–309.

140. Cuzner ML, Norton WT. Biochemistry of demyelination. *Brain Pathol* 1996; 6:231–242.

141. Anthony DC, et al. Differential matrix metalloproteinase expression in cases of multiple sclerosis and stroke. *Neuropathol Appl Neurobiol* 1997; 23:406–415.

142. Rosenberg GA, et al. Effect of steroids on CSF matrix metalloproteinases in multiple sclerosis: Relation to blood-brain barrier injury. *Neurology* 1996; 46:1626–1632.

143. Akenami FO, et al. Cerebrospinal fluid activity of tissue plasminogen activator in patients with neurological diseases. *J Clin Pathol* 1996; 49:577–580.

144. Akenami FO, et al. Cerebrospinal fluid plasminogen activator inhibitor-1 in patients with neurological disease. *J Clin Pathol* 1997; 50:157–160.

145. Bonetti B, et al. Cell death during demyelination: Effector but not target cells are eliminated by apoptosis. *J Immunol* 1997; 159:5733–5741.

146. White CA, McCombe PA, Pender MP. The roles of Fas, Fas ligand and Bcl-2 in T cell apoptosis in the central nervous system in experimental autoimmune encephalomyelitis. *J Neuroimmunol* 1998; 82:47–55.

147. Ichikawa H, Ota K, Iwata M. Increased Fas antigen on T cells in multiple sclerosis. *J Neuroimmunol* 1996; 71:125–129.

148. Inoue A, et al. Detection of the soluble form of the Fas molecule in patients with multiple sclerosis and human

T-lymphotropic virus type I-associated myelopathy. *J Neuroimmunol* 1997; 75:141–146.

149. Ciusani E, et al. Soluble Fas (Apo-1) levels in cerebrospinal fluid of multiple sclerosis patients. *J Neuroimmunol* 1998; 82:5–12.

150. Clark RB, Grunnet M, Lingenheld EG. Adoptively transferred EAE in mice bearing the lpr mutation. *Clin Immunol Immunopathol* 1997; 85:315–319.

151. Waldner H, et al. Fas- and FasL-deficient mice are resistant to induction of autoimmune encephalomyelitis. *J Immunol* 1997; 159:3100–3103.

152. Sabelko KA, et al. Fas and Fas ligand enhance the pathogenesis of experimental allergic encephalomyelitis, but are not essential for immune privilege in the central nervous system. *J Immunol* 1997; 159:3096–3099.

153. Malipiero U, et al. Myelin oligodendrocyte glycoprotein-induced autoimmune encephalomyelitis is chronic/relapsing in perforin knockout mice, but monophasic in Fas- and Fas ligand-deficient lpr and gld mice. *Eur J Immunol* 1997; 27:3151–60.

154. Bonetti B, Raine CS. Multiple sclerosis: Oligodendrocytes display cell death-related molecules in situ but do not undergo apoptosis. *Ann Neurol* 1997; 42:74–84.

155. Vartanian T, et al. Interferon-gamma-induced oligodendrocyte cell death: Implications for the pathogenesis of multiple sclerosis. *Molecular Med* 1995; 1:732–743.

156. Dowling P, et al. Involvement of the CD95 (APO-1/Fas) receptor/ligand system in multiple sclerosis brain. *J Exp Med* 1996; 184:1513–1518.

157. Cross AH, et al. Inducible nitric oxide synthase gene expression and enzyme activity correlate with disease activity in murine experimental autoimmune encephalomyelitis. *J Neuroimmunol* 1996; 71:145–153.

158. Okuda Y, et al. Nitric oxide via an inducible isoform of nitric oxide synthase is a possible factor to eliminate inflammatory cells from the central nervous system of mice with experimental allergic encephalomyelitis. *J Neuroimmunol* 1997; 73:107–116.

159. Tran EH, et al. Astrocytes and microglia express inducible nitric oxide synthase in mice with experimental allergic encephalomyelitis. *J Neuroimmunol* 1997; 74:121–129.

160. Calza L, et al. Time-course changes of nerve growth factor, corticotropin-releasing hormone, and nitric oxide synthase isoforms and their possible role in the development of inflammatory response in experimental allergic encephalomyelitis. *Proc Natl Acad Sci USA* 1997; 94:3368–3373.

161. Cross AH, et al. Evidence for the production of peroxynitrite in inflammatory CNS demyelination. *J Neuroimmunol* 1997; 80:121–130.

162. van der Veen RC, et al. Extensive peroxynitrite activity during progressive stages of central nervous system inflammation. *J Neuroimmunol* 1997; 77:1–7.

163. Brenner T, et al. Inhibition of nitric oxide synthase for treatment of experimental autoimmune encephalomyelitis. *J Immunol* 1997; 158:2940–2946.

164. Stewart VC, et al. Pretreatment of astrocytes with interferon-alpha/beta impairs interferon-gamma induction of nitric oxide synthase. *J Neurochem* 1997; 68:2547–2551.

165. Hua LL, et al. Selective inhibition of human glial inducible nitric oxide synthase by interferon-beta: Implications for multiple sclerosis. *Ann Neurol* 1998; 43:384–387.

166. Stewart VC, et al. Pretreatment of astrocytes with interferon-alpha/beta prevents neuronal mitochondrial respiratory chain damage. *J Neurochem* 1998; 70:432–434.

167. Xiao BG, et al. The cerebrospinal fluid from patients with multiple sclerosis promotes neuronal and oligodendrocyte damage by delayed production of nitric oxide in vitro. *J Neurol Sci* 1996; 142:114–120.

168. Ruuls SR, et al. Reactive oxygen species are involved in the pathogenesis of experimental allergic encephalomyelitis in Lewis rats. *J Neuroimmunol* 1995; 56:207–217.

169. Hansen LA, Willenborg DO, Cowden WB. Suppression of hyperacute and passively transferred experimental autoimmune encephalomyelitis by the anti-oxidant, butylated hydroxyanisole. *J Neuroimmunol* 1995; 62:69–77.

170. Okuda Y, et al. Aminoguanidine, a selective inhibitor of the inducible nitric oxide synthase, has different effects on experimental allergic encephalomyelitis in the induction and progression phase. *J Neuroimmunol* 1998; 81:201–210.

171. Hooper DC, et al. Prevention of experimental allergic encephalomyelitis by targeting nitric oxide and peroxynitrite: Implications for the treatment of multiple sclerosis. *Proc Natl Acad Sci USA* 1997; 94:2528–2533.

172. Malfroy B, et al. Prevention and suppression of autoimmune encephalomyelitis by EUK-8, a synthetic catalytic scavenger of oxygen-reactive metabolites. *Cell Immunol* 1997; 177:62–68.

173. Ding M, et al. Antisense knockdown of inducible nitric oxide synthase inhibits induction of experimental autoimmune encephalomyelitis in SJL/J mice. *J Immunol* 1998; 160:2560–2564.

174. Zielasek J, et al. Administration of nitric oxide synthase inhibitors in experimental autoimmune neuritis and experimental autoimmune encephalomyelitis. *J Neuroimmunol* 1995; 58:81–88.

175. Milford CM, et al. Testing lazaroids U-74389G and U-83836E for therapeutic value in experimental allergic encephalomyelitis in the Lewis rat. *Res Communications Molecular Pathol Pharmacol* 1995; 87:353–358.

176. Scott GS, Williams KI, Bolton C. A pharmacological study on the role of nitric oxide in the pathogenesis of experimental allergic encephalomyelitis. *Inflamm Res* 1996; 45:524–529.

177. Gold DP, et al. Nitric oxide and the immunomodulation of experimental allergic encephalomyelitis. *Eur J Immunol* 1997; 27:2863–2869.

178. Fenyk-Melody JE, et al. Experimental autoimmune encephalomyelitis is exacerbated in mice lacking the NOS2 gene. *J Immunol* 1998; 160:2940–2946.

179. Bagasra O, et al. Activation of the inducible form of nitric oxide synthase in the brains of patients with multiple sclerosis. *Proc Natl Acad Sci USA* 1995; 92:12041–12045.

180. De Groot CJ, et al. Immunocytochemical characterization of the expression of inducible and constitutive isoforms of nitric oxide synthase in demyelinating multiple sclerosis lesions. *J Neuropathol Exp Neurol* 1997; 56:10–20.

181. Giovannoni G, et al. Raised serum nitrate and nitrite levels in patients with multiple sclerosis. *J Neurol Sci* 1997; 145:77–81.

182. Sarchielli P, et al. Cytokine secretion and nitric oxide production by mononuclear cells of patients with multiple sclerosis. *J Neuroimmunol* 1997; 80:76–86.

183. Waxman SG. Demyelinating diseases—new pathological insights, new therapeutic targets [editorial; comment]. *New Engl J Med* 1998; 338:323–325.

184. Rawes JA, et al. Antibodies to the axolemma-enriched fraction in the cerebrospinal fluid and serum of patients with multiple sclerosis and other neurological diseases. *Multiple Sclerosis* 1997; 3:363–369.

185. Ferguson B, et al. Axonal damage in acute multiple sclerosis lesions. *Brain* 1997.

186. Trapp BD, et al. Axonal transection in the lesions of multiple sclerosis. *New Engl J Med* 1998; 338:278–285.

187. Loevner LA, et al. Microscopic disease in normal-appearing white matter on conventional MR images in patients with multiple sclerosis: Assessment with magnetization-transfer measurements. *Radiology* 1995; 196:511–515.

188. Filippi M, et al. A magnetization transfer imaging study of normal-appearing white matter in multiple sclerosis. *Neurology* 1995; 45:478–482.

189. Roser W, et al. Proton MRS of gadolinium-enhancing MS plaques and metabolic changes in normal-appearing white matter. *MR Med* 1995; 33:811–817.

190. Davies SE, et al. High resolution proton NMR spectroscopy of multiple sclerosis lesions. *J Neurochem* 1995; 64:742–748.

191. Narayanan S, et al. Imaging of axonal damage in multiple sclerosis: Spatial distribution of magnetic resonance imaging lesions. *Ann Neurol* 1997; 41:385–391.

192. De Stefano N, Federico A, Arnold DL. Proton magnetic resonance spectroscopy in brain white matter disorders. *Ital J Neurol Sci* 1997; 18:331–339.

193. Hardin-Pouzet H, et al. Glutamate metabolism is down-regulated in astrocytes during experimental allergic encephalomyelitis. *Glia* 1997; 20:79–85.

194. Bolton C, Paul C. MK-801 limits neurovascular dysfunction during experimental allergic encephalomyelitis. *J Pharmacol Exp Therapeut* 1997; 282:397–402.

195. Stover JF, et al. Neurotransmitters in cerebrospinal fluid reflect pathological activity. *Eur J Clin Invest* 1997; 27:1038–1043.

196. Klivenyi P, et al. Amino acid concentrations in cerebrospinal fluid of patients with multiple sclerosis. *Acta Neurol Scand* 1997; 95:96–98.

197. Aasly J, et al. Cerebrospinal fluid lactate and glutamine are reduced in multiple sclerosis. *Acta Neurol Scand* 1997; 95:9–12.

198. McFarland HI, et al. Amelioration of autoimmune reactions by antigen-induced apoptosis of T cells. *Adv Exp Med Biol* 1995; 383:157–166.

199. Racke MK, et al. Intravenous antigen administration as a therapy for autoimmune demyelinating disease. *Ann Neurol* 1996; 39:46–56.

200. Saoudi A, et al. Prevention of experimental allergic encephalomyelitis in rats by targeting autoantigen to B cells: Evidence that the protective mechanism depends on changes in the cytokine response and migratory properties of the autoantigen-specific T cells [see comments]. *J Exp Med* 1995; 182:335–344.

201. Tonegawa S. Tolerance induction and autoimmune encephalomyelitis amelioration after administration of myelin basic protein-derived peptide. *J Exp Med* 1997; 186:507–515.

202. Gautam AM. Self and non-self peptides treat autoimmune encephalomyelitis: T cell anergy or competition for major histocompatibility complex class II binding? *Eur J Immunol* 1995; 25:2059–2063.

203. Barnett LA, et al. Virus encoding an encephalitogenic peptide protects mice from experimental allergic encephalomyelitis. *J Neuroimmunol* 1996; 64:163–173.

204. Genain CP, et al. Inhibition of allergic encephalomyelitis in marmosets by vaccination with recombinant vaccinia virus encoding for myelin basic protein. *J Neuroimmunol* 1997; 79:119–128.

205. Wang LY, Fujinami RS. Enhancement of EAE and induction of autoantibodies to T-cell epitopes in mice infected with a recombinant vaccinia virus encoding myelin proteolipid protein. *J Neuroimmunol* 1997; 75:75–83.

206. Warren KG, Catz I. Administration of myelin basic protein synthetic peptides to multiple sclerosis patients. *J Neurol Sci* 1995; 133:85–94.

207. Warren KG, Catz I. The effect of intrathecal MBP synthetic peptides containing epitope P85 VVHF-FKNIVTP96 on free anti-MBP levels in acute relapsing multiple sclerosis. *J Neurol Sci* 1997; 148:67–78.

208. Samson MF, Smilek DE. Reversal of acute experimental autoimmune encephalomyelitis and prevention of relapses by treatment with a myelin basic protein peptide analogue modified to form long-lived peptide-MHC complexes. *J Immunol* 1995; 155:2737–2746.

209. Zhou SR, Whitaker JN. Active immunization with complementary peptide PBM 9-1: Preliminary evidence that it modulates experimental allergic encephalomyelitis in PL/J mice and Lewis rats. *J Neurosci Res* 1996; 45:439–446.

210. Stepaniak JA, Gould KE, Swanborg RH. Encephalitogenic T cells are present in Lewis rats protected from autoimmune encephalomyelitis by coimmunization with MBP73-84 and its analog. *J Neurosci Res* 1996; 45:447–454.

211. Nicholson LB, et al. An altered peptide ligand mediates immune deviation and prevents autoimmune encephalomyelitis. *Immunity* 1995; 3:397–405.

212. Nicholson LB, et al. A T cell receptor antagonist peptide induces T cells that mediate bystander suppression and prevent autoimmune encephalomyelitis induced with multiple myelin antigens. *Proc Natl Acad Sci USA* 1997; 94:9279–9284.

213. Santambrogio L, Lees MB, Sobel RA. Altered peptide ligand modulation of experimental allergic encephalomyelitis: Immune responses within the CNS. *J Neuroimmunol* 1998; 81:1–13.

214. Ausubel LJ, Krieger JI, Hafler DA. Changes in cytokine secretion induced by altered peptide ligands of myelin basic protein peptide 85-99. *J Immunol* 1997; 159:2502–2512.

215. Das MP, et al. Autopathogenic T helper cell type 1 (Th1) and protective Th2 clones differ in their recognition of the autoantigenic peptide of myelin proteolipid protein. *J Exp Med* 1997; 186:867–876.

216. Dressel A, et al. Autoantigen recognition by human CD8 T cell clones: Enhanced agonist response induced by altered peptide ligands. *J Immunol* 1997; 159:4943–4951.

217. Gaur A, et al. Amelioration of relapsing experimental autoimmune encephalomyelitis with altered myelin basic protein peptides involves different cellular mechanisms. *J Neuroimmunol* 1997; 74:149–158.

218. Pearson CI, et al. Induction of a heterogeneous TCR repertoire in (PL/JXSJL/J)F1 mice by myelin basic protein peptide Ac1-11 and its analog Ac1-11[4A]. *Molecular Immunol* 1997; 34:781–792.

219. Hemmer B, et al. Human T-cell response to myelin basic protein peptide (83-99): Extensive heterogeneity in antigen recognition, function, and phenotype. *Neurology* 1997; 49:1116–1126.

220. Usuku K, et al. Biased expression of T cell receptor genes characterizes activated T cells in multiple sclerosis cerebrospinal fluid. *J Neurosci Res* 1996; 45:829–837.

221. Wilson DB, et al. Results of a phase I clinical trial of a T-cell receptor peptide vaccine in patients with multiple sclerosis. I. Analysis of T-cell receptor utilization in CSF cell populations. *J Neuroimmunol* 1997; 76:15–28.

222. Imrich H, et al. Prevention and treatment of Lewis rat experimental allergic encephalomyelitis with a monoclonal antibody to the T cell receptor V beta 8.2 segment. *Eur J Immunol* 1995; 25:1960–1964.

223. Kumar V, Stellrecht K, Sercarz E. Inactivation of T cell receptor peptide-specific CD4 regulatory T cells induces chronic experimental autoimmune encephalomyelitis (EAE). *J Exp Med* 1996; 184:1609–17.

224. Whitham RH, et al. Treatment of relapsing autoimmune encephalomyelitis with T cell receptor V beta-specific antibodies when proteolipid protein is the autoantigen. *J Neurosci Res* 1996; 45:104–116.

225. Das MR, et al. Prior exposure to superantigen can inhibit or exacerbate autoimmune encephalomyelitis: T-cell repertoire engaged by the autoantigen determines clinical outcome. *J Neuroimmunol* 1996; 71:3–10.

226. Vainiene M, et al. Neonatal injection of Lewis rats with recombinant V beta 8.2 induces T cell but not B cell tolerance and increased severity of experimental autoimmune encephalomyelitis. *J Neurosci Res* 1996; 45: 475–486.

227. Buenafe AC, et al. Analysis of V beta 8.2 CDR3 sequences from spinal cord T cells of Lewis rats vaccinated or treated with TCR V beta 8.2-39-59 peptide. *J Immunol* 1995; 155:1556–1564.

228. Vandenbark AA, Hashim GA, Offner H. T cell receptor peptides in treatment of autoimmune disease: Rationale and potential. *J Neurosci Res* 1996; 43:391–402.

229. Kozovska MF, Yamamura T, Tabira T. T-T cellular interaction between CD4-CD8- regulatory T cells and T cell clones presenting TCR peptide. Its implication for TCR vaccination against experimental autoimmune encephalomyelitis. *J Immunol* 1996; 157:1781–1790.

230. Offner H, et al. Increased severity of experimental autoimmune encephalomyelitis in rats tolerized as adults but not neonatally to a protective TCR V beta 8 CDR2 idiotope. *J Immunol* 1995; 154:928–935.

231. Kumar V, et al. Recombinant T cell receptor molecules can prevent and reverse experimental autoimmune encephalomyelitis: Dose effects and involvement of both CD4 and CD8 T cells. *J Immunol* 1997; 159:5150–5156.

232. Chunduru SK, et al. Exploitation of the Vbeta8.2 T cell receptor in protection against experimental autoimmune encephalomyelitis using a live vaccinia virus vector. *J Immunol* 1996; 156:4940–4945.

233. Gold DP, et al. Results of a phase I clinical trial of a T-cell receptor vaccine in patients with multiple sclerosis. II. Comparative analysis of TCR utilization in CSF T-cell populations before and after vaccination with a TCR V beta 6 CDR2 peptide. *J Neuroimmunol* 1997; 76:29–38.

234. Medaer R, et al. Depletion of myelin-basic-protein autoreactive T cells by T-cell vaccination: Pilot trial in multiple sclerosis. *Lancet* 1995; 346:807–808.

235. Zhang I, J. Raus J. T cell vaccination in multiple sclerosis. *Multiple Sclerosis* 1996; 1:353–356.

236. Scolding NJ, et al. A proliferative adult human oligodendrocyte progenitor. *Neuroreport* 1995; 6:441–445.

237. Keirstead HS, Levine JM, Blakemore WF. Response of the oligodendrocyte progenitor cell population (defined by NG2 labeling) to demyelination of the adult spinal cord. *Glia* 1998; 22:161–170.

238. Wolswijk G. Chronic stage multiple sclerosis lesions contain a relatively quiescent population of oligodendrocyte precursor cells. *J Neurosci* 1998; 18:601–609.

239. Archer DR, et al. Myelination of the canine central nervous system by glial cell transplantation: A model for repair of human myelin disease. *Nature Medicine* 1997; 3:54–59.

240. Tourbah A, et al. Inflammation promotes survival and migration of the CG4 oligodendrocyte progenitors transplanted in the spinal cord of both inflammatory and demyelinated EAE rats. *J Neurosci Res* 1997; 50: 853–861.

241. Diemel LT, Copelman CA, Cuzner ML. Macrophages in CNS remyelination: Friend or foe? *Neurochem Res* 1998; 23:341–347.

242. Webster HD. Growth factors and myelin regeneration in multiple sclerosis. *Multiple Sclerosis* 1997; 3:113–120.

243. Liu X, Yao DL, Webster H. Insulin-like growth factor I treatment reduces clinical deficits and lesion severity in acute demyelinating experimental autoimmune encephalomyelitis. *Multiple Sclerosis* 1995; 1:2–9.

244. Liu X, et al. Insulin-like growth factor-I treatment reduces immune cell responses in acute non-demyelinative experimental autoimmune encephalomyelitis. *J Neurosce Res* 1997; 47:531–538.

245. Yao DL, et al. Insulin-like growth factor I treatment reduces demyelination and up-regulates gene expression of myelin-related proteins in experimental autoimmune encephalomyelitis. *Proc Natl Acad Sci USA* 1995; 92: 6190–6194.

246. Yao DL, et al. Insulin-like growth factor-I given subcutaneously reduces clinical deficits, decreases lesion severity and upregulates synthesis of myelin proteins in experimental autoimmune encephalomyelitis. *Life Sciences* 1996; 58:1301–1306.

247. Torres-Aleman I, Barrios V, Berciano J. The peripheral insulin-like growth factor system in amyotrophic lateral sclerosis and in multiple sclerosis. *Neurology* 1998; 50:772–776.

248. Wilczak N, De KJ. Insulin-like growth factor-I receptors in normal appearing white matter and chronic plaques in multiple sclerosis. *Brain Res* 1997; 772:243–246.

249. Micera A, De SR, Aloe L. Elevated levels of nerve growth factor in the thalamus and spinal cord of rats affected by experimental allergic encephalomyelitis. *Archives Italiennes de Biologie* 1995; 133:131–142.

250. De Simone R, et al. mRNA for NGF and p75 in the central nervous system of rats affected by experimental allergic encephalomyelitis. *Neuropathol Appl Neurobiol* 1996; 22:54–59.

251. Suzaki I, et al. Nerve growth factor levels in cerebrospinal fluid from patients neurologic disorders. *J Child Neurol* 1997; 12:205–207.

252. Bansal R, Pfeiffer SE. FGF-2 converts mature oligodendrocytes to a novel phenotype. [Review] [80 refs]. *J Neurosci Res* 1997; 50:215–228.

253. D'Souza SD, Alinauskas KA, Antel JP. Ciliary neurotrophic factor selectively protects human oligodendrocytes from tumor necrosis factor-mediated injury. *J Neurosci Res* 1996; 43:289–298.

254. Sriram S, Mitchell W, Stratton C. Multiple sclerosis associated with Chlamydia pneumoniae infection of the CNS. *Neurology* 1998; 50:571–572.

255. Challoner PB, et al. Plaque-associated expression of human herpesvirus 6 in multiple sclerosis. *Proc Natl Acad Sci USA* 1995; 92:7440–7444.

256. Carrigan DR, Harrington D, Knox KK. Subacute leukoencephalitis caused by CNS infection with human herpesvirus-6 manifesting as acute multiple sclerosis. *Neurology* 1996; 47:145–148.

257. Lycke J, et al. Acyclovir treatment of relapsing-remitting multiple sclerosis. A randomized, placebo-controlled, double-blind study. *J Neurol* 1996; 243:214–224.

258. Nielsen L, et al. Human herpesvirus-6 immunoglobulin G antibodies in patients with multiple sclerosis. *Acta Neurol Scand* 1997; 169 (Suppl):76–78.

259. Soldan SS, et al. Association of human herpes virus 6 (HHV-6) with multiple sclerosis: Increased IgM response to HHV-6 early antigen and detection of serum HHV-6 DNA. *Nature Medicine* 1997; 3:1394–1397.

260. Merelli E, et al. Human herpes virus 6 and human herpes virus 8 DNA sequences in brains of multiple sclerosis patients, normal adults and children. *J Neurol* 1997; 244:450–454.

261. Novoa LJ, et al. Fulminant demyelinating encephalomyelitis associated with productive HHV-6 infection in an immunocompetent adult. *J Med Virol* 1997; 52:301–308.

262. Braun DK, Dominguez G, Pellett PE. Human herpesvirus 6. *Clin Microbiol Rev* 1997; 10:521–567.

263. Martin C, et al. Absence of seven human herpesviruses, including HHV-6, by polymerase chain reaction in CSF and blood from patients with multiple sclerosis and optic neuritis. *Acta Neurol Scand* 1997; 95:280–283.

264. Milo R, Panitch H. Additive effects of copolymer-1 and interferon beta-1b on the immune response to myelin basic protein. *J Neuroimmunol* 1995; 61:185–193.

VI

SYMPTOM MANAGEMENT AND REHABILITATION

12 Introduction to Symptom and Rehabilitative Management: Disease Management Model

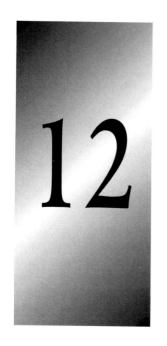

Catherine W. Britell, M.D., Jack S. Burks, M.D., and Randall T. Schapiro, M.D.

Multiple sclerosis (MS) affects multiple organ systems in the course of the disease, and thus it affects many facets of an individual's existence in different ways during the course of a lifetime.

The management of MS begins with the understanding that one cannot at this time "cure" the disease. Agents that alter the natural course of the disease have been developed, but they do not completely stop the disease. Fortunately, the quality of life of people with MS can be influenced by working to resolve the various problems that occur on a regular basis. This is the backbone of symptom management in MS (1).

Some symptoms appear because of demyelination within the brain and spinal cord; these are called primary symptoms. Among them are weakness; clumsiness; numbness; tingling; bladder, bowel, and sexual dysfunction; and visual problems. People with MS may also have complications of those primary symptoms. These are called secondary symptoms and include contractures, urinary tract infection, osteoporosis, muscle atrophy, and skin breakdown. Tertiary symptoms are the social, psychological, marital, and vocational problems associated with all chronic diseases.

Many and varied techniques and treatments are used to manage the numerous symptoms. The management of MS symptoms is complicated by the fact that the

disease is unpredictable. More often than is recognized, MS appears to be benign with a relapsing course but is followed by progression of the disease after several years. Symptoms may be prominent even in the early relapsing form.

Some symptoms are predictive of a more aggressive disease course. These symptoms include weakness, tremor, cognitive problems, and significant spasticity. Other symptoms tend to correspond to a milder course of the disease. Such symptoms often are sensory in origin and include numbness, tingling, visual blurring, and dizziness. Some symptoms, including bladder and bowel dysfunction and fatigue, are less predictable.

Many symptoms of MS resemble symptoms of other neurologic diseases, such as stroke or tumor, but some symptoms are relatively unique to MS. These include the electrical sensation coursing down the spine with the head flexed—Lhermitte's sign. Trigeminal neuralgia in a young person may be a sign of MS. Tonic spasms of the arm and leg are relatively unique to MS, as is an apractic hand called the "useless hand of Oppenheim."

Although attempts to localize and predict findings from magnetic resonance imaging localization are fraught with inaccuracy, anatomic localization may have prognostic significance. For example, the cerebral localization associated with cognitive problems is associated with a poor prognosis. Tremor associated with cerebellar outflow lesions also is an indicator of a poor clinical outcome. The paraparesis of spinal cord lesions may be an indicator of late-onset progressive spinal cord MS. Brainstem indicators of dysarthria, dysphasia, and internuclear ophthalmoplegia are associated with more active disease. Despite the localizable findings, many MS findings do not follow anatomic divisions. In fact, sensory abnormalities in MS are unlikely to fit anatomic mapping.

This multisystem involvement and these multifaceted functional needs may seem overwhelming to the patient, his or her family, and the health care provider with limited time and resources. However, quality of life for an individual with MS is highly dependent on how well his or her symptoms are managed and whether functional issues are addressed. It is important to develop a system of periodic comprehensive assessments and interventions that not only monitor and treat the effects of the disease on the various organ systems but also address the effects of the disease on the individual's physical, psychological, social, and vocational functioning. The best and easiest way to deliver comprehensive, holistic care is a productive stepwise plan with an interdisciplinary team of professionals working closely with the primary or principle care provider focused on the needs of the patient and the family.

THE HEALTH CARE TEAM

The concepts of interdisciplinary teamwork, team communication, and patient-centered multifaceted care have been mainstays of rehabilitative management for many years. However, these ideas and practices, as well as coordination of MS care, may be relatively new to some health care providers. A stable health care team consists of individuals with interest and expertise in MS care who share easy referral patterns, clear communication, and common goals and priorities for minimizing symptoms and maximizing function. Team members often can significantly enhance one another's effectiveness by prioritizing goals together and planning programs to optimally coordinate care. Although frequent team meetings may not be feasible in a primary health care setting, a common database often is possible, and good communication can make individual treatment programs maximally effective and efficient.

Primary care providers may be family medicine physicians, internists, neurologists, physiatrists, or non-physician health care providers, such as nurse practitioners, rehabilitation nurses, or physician assistants, who manage day-to-day health issues, address immediate complaints, oversee and interpret general health maintenance, and coordinate MS care and referral to other team members, health care providers, and/or community resources.

The health care team may include the following members, as patient needs dictate.

- The *neurologist,* when not the primary care physician, consults on neurologic care and symptom management, including immunotherapy, fatigue, behavioral disorders, spasticity, dysesthesia, and other neurologic and functional issues.
- The *physiatrist,* when not the primary care physician, consults on symptom management and functional issues, including spasticity, dysesthesia, fatigue, bladder and bowel management, musculoskeletal problems, weakness, incoordination, skin management, rehabilitation aids, and other functional issues.
- The *ophthalmologist* addresses problems associated (and not associated) with MS to maximize visual activity and coordination of vision.
- The *physical therapist* evaluates neuromuscular and musculoskeletal function and mobility issues and develops treatment programs for problems including range of motion, strength, coordination, spasticity, gait, and mobility.
- The *occupational therapist* evaluates issues of self-care, attendant management, and activities of daily living (ADLs), which may have neuromuscular, musculoskeletal, or cognitive aspects. He or she works with patients and families to modify the home, obtain equipment, and learn compensatory skills to overcome or adapt to functional impairment, and may be involved in workplace modification to maintain employment.
- The *rehabilitation nurse* addresses practical aspects of bowel and bladder management to maintain regular elimination, continence, and dignity. He or she deals with skin issues and pressure sore prevention, as well as many aspects of ADLs and home care.
- The *dietitian* assists patients and families to develop a healthy, nutritious diet and to prevent or treat obesity.
- The *psychologist* evaluates cognitive and emotional aspects of the patient's condition, diagnoses cognitive deficits, recommends compensatory measures, and counsels patients and families on the emotional sequelae of MS.
- The *social worker* assists patients and families in identifying community resources, sustaining income if possible, funding health and rehabilitative care, identifying and securing caregivers, and dealing with the many family issues that arise in the presence of a chronic illness.
- The *speech pathologist* diagnoses and treats communication and swallowing difficulties, and assists with daily planning and organizing for individuals

with cognitive dysfunction. Some speech pathologists also provide diagnostic testing for cognition.

- The *chaplain* or *minister* helps patients and families with their perspective of MS in their religious/spiritual belief system, while providing support around grief, loss, hope, and interpersonal and social issues.
- The *vocational rehabilitation counselor* tests and/or evaluates individuals to determine vocational strengths and weaknesses. He or she may work with employers and/or patient and family to recommend job accommodations to keep the patient working or to reemploy a patient who has become unable to perform his or her original job.
- The *therapeutic recreation specialist* works with patients and families to develop rewarding avocation/fitness pursuits appropriate to the patient's neuromuscular and psychological function. He or she may also be involved in respite and day care programs.
- The *driver education specialist* evaluates the patient's ability to drive, prescribes driving and/or vehicle modifications to make driving easier and safer, and recommends appropriate devices for vehicle ingress/egress and/or wheelchair or scooter transport.

FUNCTIONAL SYSTEMS MANAGEMENT

In the real health care world, it is not possible to address every problem of every patient on every visit. However, at least once a year, or more often if new symptoms or functional issues are developing, the principle care provider should systematically evaluate all the patient's health care and functional issues.

Neurologic Symptom Management

Every 6 to 12 months, or more often as symptoms change, the person with MS should have a neurologic examination to document the status of neurologic function. The examination should include complete manual muscle testing and sensory testing, testing of reflexes and muscle tone, gait evaluation, coordination testing, and visual acuity testing, as well as any laboratory or imaging studies indicated by clinical findings. Pain, fatigue, spasticity, weakness, tremor, incoordination, and sensory issues should be addressed. Immunotherapy or other treatments that may mitigate the course of the disease should be specifically addressed and discussed with the patient, at least on an annual basis. If the primary care provider is not skilled in dealing with the aforementioned issues, the patient should be referred to a specialist. Finally, it is essential to discuss plans for acute medical care in the event of an exacerbation or medical problems.

Musculoskeletal Function

When muscles are weak or the muscles across a joint become imbalanced as a result of MS, pain and damage to the joints and tendons may occur, particularly in the hips, knees, ankles, and shoulders. Limitation of joint motion often occurs when spasticity is present. If spasticity is untreated, the patient may develop contractures, which can severely limit gait, transfers, ADLs, and ease of attendant care. The physician or physical therapist should evaluate the range of motion of joints at least annually. Any tightness or contracture that has developed must be vigorously addressed by physical therapy and a home exercise program. Painful muscles, tendons, or joints should also be treated.

Nutrition

Proper nutrition helps to maintain health, and a formal dietary assessment should be done if problems are detected. Excessive weight gain must be avoided, as this will limit mobility, compromise skin integrity, and significantly affect self-esteem. A medically supervised weight reduction program should be initiated for overweight individuals. Ataxia or tremor sometimes make it difficult for the patient to eat independently, with resulting malnutrition. Swallowing disorders may make the patient afraid to eat. Frequent choking or aspiration can decrease nutritional intake. Unintentional weight loss should also be evaluated for causes related to other medical conditions, such as hyperthyroidism, cancer, or depression. Crash or "pop" diets can lead to electrolyte imbalance and physical deterioration.

General Health Screening

An appropriate general physical examination with routine cancer screening and attention to cardiovascular risk management should also be done every year. Multiple sclerosis is not a fatal disease, and other health problems are just as common in individuals with MS as in the general population. Good preventive health care is vital to maintaining functional status in the person with MS. The attribution of all a patient's symptoms to MS is fraught with hazards. It is important to evaluate each medical complaint for a non–MS-related cause.

Urinary Function

Urinary urgency, frequent nocturia, frequent infection, urinary incontinence, and/or urinary retention are all common in MS and must be addressed. It is possible to maintain dignified and healthy bladder emptying, freedom from infection, and a comfortable and reasonable "elimination lifestyle" with appropriate urinary management. People with MS should not tolerate incontinence, diapering, poor sleep, repeated infection, or skin problems related to bladder dysfunction. An evaluation by a urologist is indicated if these problems are significant and ongoing. A rehabilitation nurse who is trained in MS care can usually be of assistance with practical management suggestions.

Bowel Function

Although bowel problems are extremely common in MS, patients often have difficulty discussing the problem with a caregiver, so the caregiver sometimes needs to broach the subject. Even severe constipation or incontinence can be managed with the establishment of a bowel program. People with MS need not tolerate fecal incontinence or constipation. They need not take laxatives on a regular basis. The establishment of a bowel program is best undertaken with the help of a nurse who is trained in MS care.

Sexual Function

Because the person with MS faces so many other problems, sexual problems often are pushed to the background. Birth control, impotence, and female sexual problems all need to be addressed by the principal health care provider or the patient should be referred to a specialist who has expertise in this area. Sexual function and health in MS may be a multifaceted issue, involving much more than simply erectile function. The treatment of erectile dysfunction alone often is not sufficient to help couples deal with problems in their sexual relationship.

Mobility

The patient should be mobile in his or her home, neighborhood, and community with ease and safety. If mobility problems are present, orthoses (braces), aids (crutches, canes, walkers), or a wheeled mobility device (wheelchair or scooter) may be helpful. A good rule of thumb is that if the person with MS cannot perform work, community, social, church, or daily living activities because of mobility problems, some type of intervention is indicated. A rehabilitation therapist can best determine how to proceed with mobility issues. Loss of ability to drive safely is a difficult issue that must be addressed. Adaptive devices for the car may keep the patient driving safely much longer. If a mobility device is prescribed, the car may need to be modified. A skilled driver educator for the disabled often will be able to help address these issues. If the patient has lost vision and coordination to the point where even adapted driving cannot be done safely, he or she may benefit from training in the use of accessible public transportation. An occupational therapist often is helpful.

Activities of Daily Living

If there are problems with eating, dressing, bathing, toileting, maintenance of clothing and environment, shopping, cooking, or other necessary daily functions, an occupational therapy consultation may be helpful to the patient. The occupational therapist may also be helpful in modifying the work environment to make it accessible in order to keep the patient working.

Skin Integrity

If the patient loses sensation over the sitting area or other weight-bearing areas such as heels, elbows, or trochanters, he or she should be taught how skin sores occur and what preventive steps must be taken. If the patient spends a significant amount of time in a wheelchair, an optimal wheelchair cushion and appropriate fitting and positioning are essential. If any of these issues are of concern, a referral to a physical therapist or rehabilitation nurse specialist is indicated.

Cognitive Function and Psychological Issues

Cognitive issues are a common source of worry and upset to patients and their families. People with MS commonly experience difficulty with concentration, short-term memory, and attention. Other cognitive problems seen in MS include perceptual problems, executive functions, information processing, working memory, and communication. Depression or stress may also exacerbate the symptoms of cognitive dysfunction. If so, an evaluation by a psychologist who is skilled in working with people with MS is necessary. A treatment program is formulated to help maintain the patient's effectiveness at work, in the family, and in social settings. Depression often is a significant issue in MS and should be thoroughly evaluated and treated. Sleep disturbances may be related to depression, but many MS patients with sleep problems are not depressed. Other mechanisms such as medication side effects or sleep apnea need to be evaluated in such situations.

Speech, Communication, and Swallowing

If communicative ability is deteriorating because of dysarthria or word-finding problems, or if frequent choking or swallowing difficulties are occurring, a referral to a speech pathologist is indicated. Communication problems and dysphagia often are not discussed by the patients. Direct questioning is necessary to appreciate the problems. Some patients who aspirate and experience recurrent pneumonia do not perceive that they have a swallowing problem.

Social and Family Functioning

How a person with MS feels, functions, and lives depends to a great extent on his or her family and social support. A social worker often can help sort out finances, communication, parenting issues, caregiver and attendant issues, identification of community resources, and other things that are important to the family.

Vocational Functioning

For most people, a job is a significant part of his or her identity. Once a person loses a job or stops working because of a disability, it becomes twice as difficult to become reemployed. The health care system needs to be involved in this issue by dealing with functional issues such as mobility, bladder and bowel issues, cognitive issues, and job accommodation needs. A vocational counselor and/or occupational therapist can be helpful with job accommodations to keep the individual with MS comfortable and maximally effective in the workplace.

Recreation and Fitness

Fitness is exceedingly important in combating fatigue and maintaining maximal function. A medically prescribed and directed fitness program is helpful for weakness and incoordination. People with MS often are unable to take part in favorite personal or family recreational activities because of the fatigue or mobility issues associated with the disease. This will increase stress on the family. A recreational therapist can be extremely helpful in working with the patient and the family to develop rewarding recreation.

Spiritual Issues

A spiritual crisis often occurs when something bad happens to a person. Long-held beliefs and ideas about one's relationship to the universe may come into question, with resulting vulnerability to spiritual alienation and/or charlatanism. The practitioner often can help put the disease into a clearer perspective by helping the patient thoroughly understand the biology of MS and the unpredictability of the disease course. Intervention by a minister or chaplain with expertise in chronic disease and disability may help patients and families reground their spiritual lives.

PROACTIVE APPROACH

Although a comprehensive functional evaluation and management plan may seem impossibly complex, it can be implemented quickly and efficiently if one does it in an organized way, uses good survey tools, and works effectively with a health care team. By being aware of and periodically addressing all the patient's medical and functional problems, time is saved in the long run because problems are proactively addressed, complications are prevented, and crisis management is avoided. Identifying reasonable treatment goals and allowing the patient to prioritize them and meet them on his or her own schedule is ideal. This has the important effect of putting the patient in control. This approach takes the patient out of the "sick" role and promotes quality of life by allowing the person with MS to feel better and function better in the home, the community, and the workplace. A more rewarding relationship between the patient and his or her family, health care professional, and community is quite feasible.

THE DISEASE MANAGEMENT APPROACH TO MULTIPLE SCLEROSIS

The multifaceted problems encountered in MS can be overwhelming for the individual practitioner and patient. A new concept of treatment focuses on more than the individual symptoms (2,3). A comprehensive disease management approach has been adopted by some of the major comprehensive MS centers in the United States. However, disease management need not be confined to comprehensive centers.

The process of continually managing a disease from the time of diagnosis until death is feasible in any setting. Although the current managed care environment dictates the primary care physician as the gatekeeper; a disease management approach encompasses the concept of principal care. Under principal care, the MS specialist is responsible for the ongoing care of a person with a chronic illness. The principal care physician need not perform all the medical management but must make certain that medical management is provided.

Another disease management approach involves the comanagement of patients, by both the primary care physician and the specialist working in concert. In this situation, a nurse care coordinator is often the point person for the patient's care. That care coordinator is responsible for continual care through the appropriate health care professional. The care coordinator uses clinical practice guidelines or care pathways either to provide care directly or to triage care. The care coordinator also aids in the integration of the patient into the work and community environments.

The disease management process includes prevention, diagnosis, acute treatment, long-term treatment, community integration, and end-of-life management. The disease management model provides continuity with coordinated and comprehensive care in a cost-effective manner. It provides health care professionals with the "best practices" approach and is driven by practice guidelines and outcomes. The prevention part of disease management in MS focuses on secondary and tertiary prevention, including the prevention of medical complications and the reduction of disabilities and handicaps in spite of worsening neurologic impairment. Maintaining health, in addition to good medical care, can be carried out in any location of any size. The team members described in this chapter collaborate to promote the overall health care of the patient. Community integration such as vocation, advocation, social services, family services, and legal and/or advocacy services are integrated with the medical issues faced by the patients.

CONCLUSION

The various symptoms of MS are discussed by expert clinicians in the following chapters. The individual expertise reflected in these chapters, combined with the coordinated, comprehensive, collaborative approach, can result in optimal care. The approach can reduce the caregiver's burden and provide an educational model for the patient that allows him or her to have more control over the consequences of the disease. The overall goal of disease management is to achieve a whole that is greater than the sum of the treatment parts. The individual expertise in a system of care reduces long-term complications and results in healthier and happier patients.

References

1. Schapiro RT. *Symptom management in multiple sclerosis.* 3rd ed. New York: Demos, 1998.
2. Burks JS. Multiple sclerosis care: An integrated disease management model. *J Spinal Cord Med* 1998; 21(2): 113–116.
3. Burks JS. Is case management the solution to the managed care conundrum? *MS Quarterly Report* 1998; 17(2):4–7.

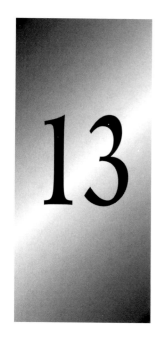

13 Clinical and Rehabilitation Outcome Measures

Linda Coulthard-Morris, M.A., L.P.C.

CURRENT STATUS OF OUTCOME MEASURES

There are no ideal outcome assessment measures in multiple sclerosis (MS). It is generally believed that the current MS impairment and disability measures are inadequate and lack the sensitivity to detect the types of changes experienced by people with MS. The development of precise and universally accepted assessment measures has been difficult, in part because of the very nature of the disease (1). The clinical course of MS is unpredictable and varies among patients and within patients over time.

Until recently the treatment options available for slowing the progression of MS were minimal, and as such the need to assess treatment outcomes was not paramount. With the recent development of numerous therapies such as Betaseron, Avonex, glatiramer acetate, intravenous immunoglobulin, or mitoxantrone, the demand for standardized assessment instruments has increased.

In response to this predicament, the National Multiple Sclerosis Society (NMSS) sponsored an international workshop in 1994 and organized the MS Clinical Outcomes Assessment Task Force to develop recommendations regarding the selection and development of appropriate clinical assessment measures for MS clinical trials

(2). The following list represents their most pertinent conclusions and recommendations for future MS clinical trials outcome measures:

1. The MS clinical outcome measure should reflect the extent of the disease process.
2. The MS clinical outcome measure should be multidimensional to reflect the principal ways MS affects an individual. The outcome measure should include components that assess gait and lower extremity function, arm function, visual function, and neuropsychological function. The MS clinical outcome measure should avoid redundant measures.
3. Individual components of the multidimensional MS clinical outcome measure should have high reliability, practicality, acceptability to patients, and cost-effectiveness. Measures that provide interval data are preferred over measures that provide categorical or ordinal data.
4. The MS clinical outcome measure should change over time as the severity of the disease worsens or improves.
5. The MS clinical outcome measure should be capable of demonstrating treatment effects.
6. Changes in the MS clinical outcome measure should be predictive of clinically meaningful change (p. 380)

LEVELS OF MEASUREMENT

There are four levels of measurement: nominal, ordinal, interval, and ratio. A *nominal* measure uses numbers to label different categories, for example, race, gender, or medical diagnosis. The most commonly used approach to scaling is the *ordinal* measure, which uses numbers to represent increasing order of the phenomenon being appraised, such as mild, moderate, and severe impairment. The numeric distance between each category is not equivalent. A change from mild to moderate is not necessarily equal to a change from moderate to severe. An *interval* measure is one in which the numbers assigned to the response categories are presumed to be equal. For example, the difference between 25 and 30 is the same as the difference between 50 and 55. A *ratio* measure also has equal intervals but includes a zero point. This makes it possible to conclude, for example, that one score is twice as much as another score.

SELECTION AND EVALUATION OF AN INSTRUMENT

When selecting an instrument, two properties must be considered: clinical usefulness and psychometric soundness (3). *Clinical usefulness* refers to how appropriate the selected instrument is in meeting the user's needs. Hobart and associates (3) outline the criteria for determining the usefulness of an instrument:

1. Time to administer
2. Ease of use
3. User-friendliness
4. Respondent burden
5. User manual or guidelines
6. Training requirements for users
7. Mode of rating (individual or team)
8. MS-specific vs. generic measure
9. Domain of use (in-patient/out-patient)

Psychometric Soundness refers to the psychometric properties of an instrument—reliability, validity, and sensitivity.

RELIABILITY

Reliability refers to the consistency, stability, or reproducibility of an instrument over time (3). It is the extent to which the same results are obtained when readministered to the same unchanged sample or phenomenon (4). The degree of consistency or agreement between two test scores is expressed in terms of a correlation coefficient *(r)*.

Perfect or ideal reliability would be expressed by a correlation coefficient or *r* value of 1.00. A correlation coefficient of 0.70 or higher is considered acceptable for both clinical and research purposes. In evaluating an instrument, there are several types of reliability to consider: *test-retest, interrater, intrarater, internal consistency, split-half,* and *alternative forms.*

Test-retest reliability (coefficient of stability) refers to the consistency or stability of test scores obtained by the same person on two different occasions under the same conditions. One difficulty in testing someone with MS is that test scores may fluctuate because the disease has changed, not because the measure is unreliable. When establishing the test-retest reliability of a new MS measure, testing should be conducted two weeks apart or less to minimize the changes of the patient's disease changing over that time period.

Interrater reliability refers to the consistency of test scores obtained between different observers or administrators of an instrument on the same patient at the same time. Cohen's kappa coefficient is considered the best measure for assessing interrater reliability.

Intrarater reliability is the consistency between scores obtained by the same observer on the same patient.

Internal consistency reliability examines the degree of homogeneity among the items or the degree to which the items correlate with each other. Internal consistency is only relevant when one domain or construct is being assessed. A multidimensional measure would not be expected to have high internal consistency because it is assessing many constructs or domains that may be relatively unrelated (4). Often internal consistency reliability is measured by Cronbach's alpha, which is based on the average correlation among items.

Split-half reliability is a method of assessing internal consistency in which the two halves (even and odd items) of the same test are compared using the Spearman-Brown formula.

Alternate-form reliability is the correlation between two forms or versions of the same test administered to the same person on two different occasions. Alternate forms of a test are used to avoid the difficulties encountered in test-retest reliability and are most appropriate for performance type tests in which learning can influence the results on the second administration of the test.

Intraclass correlation coefficient (ICC), a reliability coefficient assessing the stability of responses, can be used to measure intra- and interrater reliability. The use of ICC has several advantages over the traditional methods of correlation used in reliability studies. Granger and colleagues note that the ICC can be used to examine reliability among two or more raters or time points, can applied to ordinal level data without distortion when intervals between scores are assumed to be equal, and has been shown to be equivalent to nominal measures of agreement when scores are dichotomy (5).

VALIDITY

Validity refers to the extent to which an instrument measures what it purports or intends to measure and is the ultimate criterion for selecting an instrument (6). There are three basic type of validity: *content validity, criterion validity,* and *construct validity.*

Content validity examines the extent to which the content or items of the instrument measure the domain it is intended to evaluate. For example, if the domain being measured is fatigue, the items should all relate to fatigue.

Criterion validity refers to the extent to which the instrument measures its intended domain as compared with a criterion or "gold standard" instrument. There are two types of criterion validity: *concurrent validity* and *predictive validity. Concurrent validity* examines the relationship between an instrument and the criterion instrument when they are administered at the same time. *Predictive validity* occurs when the instrument being measured is compared with the criterion or gold standard instrument at a future time. Predictive validity also assesses the degree to which an instrument can accurately predict a future outcome or event. For example, certain exacerbations may be predictive of Expanded Disability Status Scale (EDSS) change.

Construct validity. Constructs are concepts with multiple attributes that often are theory driven and not directly measurable (i.e., quality of life) (6). There often is no gold standard or ideal instrument against which to validate a new instrument. In determining the construct validity of a new instrument, the new instrument goes through a series of studies that examine the relationship between the new instrument and similar *(convergent validity)* and different *(divergent validity)* instruments. *Convergent validity* is the degree to which an instrument correlates with other instruments measuring the same or a similar construct. *Divergent validity* or *discriminant validity* is the degree to which an instrument does not correlate with another instrument measuring a differing construct.

SENSITIVITY

Sensitivity or responsiveness is the degree to which an instrument is able to detect small but clinically significant changes. It may be considered a form of validity, and in this chapter it is included in the validity sections. Hobart and associates (3) outline three ways to determine sensitivity:

1. Serial administration of the instrument over time (pre- and post-treatment or several administrations of instrument (i.e., 3-, 6-, 9-, 12-month intervals)
2. Comparing the instrument against other criteria of change (i.e., staff and patient perception of change)
3. Comparing the instrument with other instruments of the same entity to assess relative responsiveness

For additional information regarding the psychometric evaluation of instruments, the reader is referred to references 6, 133, and 134.

WORLD HEALTH ORGANIZATION AND THE MINIMUM RECORD OF DISABILITY

There are numerous disability- and health-related measures available for assessing rehabilitation and clinical outcomes of people with MS. Most of these measures are "generic" to all patients with a chronic disease, whereas others have been specifically designed to assess the type of symptoms and problems experienced by people with MS. The most famous and widely used MS-specific outcome measure is the Minimum Record of Disability (MRD) published by the National Multiple Sclerosis Society (7). The MRD was designed to the follow classification of dysfunction developed by the World Health Organization (WHO). As the WHO applies to MS, the three types of dysfunction are: (1) *impairment*—clinical signs and symptoms produced by damage to the nervous system; (2) *disability*—the personal limitations imposed on the activities of daily living (ADLs) by the neurologic impairment; and (3) *handicap*—the social and environmental effects of the disability or impairment (8). The three measures included in the MDR are: (1) Expanded Disability Status Scale (impairment); (2) Incapacity Status Scale (disability); and Environmental Status Scale (handicap). The measures reviewed in this chapter, including the MDR scales, are outlined in Table 13-1.

IMPAIRMENT MEASURES

Impairments are the direct neurophysiologic consequences of the underlying pathology and refer to "... loss or abnormality of psychological, physiological, or anatomical structure or function" (9) It is important to note that not all pathology causes impairment.

Compared with disability measures, impairment measures tend to be less sensitive to change (10), tend to be disease-specific, and are most appropriate for diagnostic and assessment purposes. Despite its imperfections, the Expanded Disability Status Scale (EDSS) is the most widely used MS outcome measure (11). Several MS

TABLE 13-1
Index of the measures reviewed

IMPAIRMENT MEASURES

Kurtzke's Expanded Disability Status Scale/Functional
  System
Self-Administered Kurtzke and French Version
Scripps Neurological Rating Scale
Quantitative Examination of Neurological Function
Ambulation Index
Troiano Functional Scale

FUNCTIONAL MEASURES

Timed 25-Foot walk
9-Hole Peg Test
Paced Auditory Serial Addition Test-3

DISABILITY MEASURES

Barthel Index
Incapacity Status Scale
Functional Independence Measure

HANDICAP MEASURES

Environmental Status Scale
London Handicap Scale

HEALTH STATUS/QUALITY OF LIFE MEASURES

Sickness Impact Profile
Medical Rehabilitation Follow Along
Short Form (SF-36)
Short Form (SF-12)
Multiple Sclerosis Quality of Life-54
Multiple Sclerosis Quality of Life Inventory

---

impairment measures are available and are used in combination with the EDSS but none has been universally accepted. Other MS impairment measures include the Scripps Neurological Rating Scale, Quantitative Examination of Neurological Function, Troiano Functional Scale, and Ambulation Index. Unfortunately, none of these measures is significantly superior to the EDSS, and all have their own strengths and limitations.

Kurtzke Impairment System: Expanded Disability Status Scale (EDSS) and Functional Systems (FS)

In 1955 Kurtzke introduced the Disability Status Scale (DSS), an impairment and disability measure based largely on dysfunction in mobility that rated disease severity from 0 (normal) to 10 (death due to MS). In response to criticisms that the DSS lacked the necessary sensitivity to detect change, particularly in its middle range, an expanded version, the EDSS, was developed (12). The EDSS was formed by dividing each of the DSS steps into two (0, 1, 1.5, 2, 2.5, etc.).

Description

Kurtzke's system for assessing the neurologic impact of MS includes two scales: the Functional Systems (FS) and the Expanded Disability Status Scale (EDSS) (Table 13-2). The FS consists of eight single-item scales, with each scale rating the function of the eight major systems of the central nervous system (CNS)—the pyramidal, cerebellar, brainstem, mental, spasticity, sensory, visual, and bowel and bladder (13). The EDSS is a single-item scale that primarily measures ambulation impairment.

Reliability

In a multicenter cyclosporine clinical trial study, the EDSS demonstrated high test-retest reliability ($r = 0.93$) (14). Several studies have examined the interrater reliability of the EDSS with varying results (11). Results differ, in part because reliability is defined differently. For example, when reliability was defined as difference of ≤ 1.5 EDSS points, high interrater agreement was obtained (15). In their study, interrater agreement was high, with ICC ranging from 0.88 to 0.96 when assessing patients with an EDSS score between 1.0 and 3.5. Sipe and colleagues also report high interrater reliability, with a weighted kappa coefficient of agreement of 0.98 when agreement was defined as ≤ 1.0 EDSS point (two steps on the EDSS scale) (16).

Other studies have reported either varied or low interrater agreement. For example, Francis and colleagues reported varied interrater agreement ranging from $r = 0.32$ to 0.76 using Cohen's kappa coefficient on the EDSS (17). These results indicate that EDSS scores varied between 0 and 4.0 points among the three examiners. Pia Amato and associates reported a low interrater agreement (30 percent to 50 percent agreement) as expressed by the kappa index (18). Several studies report considerable interrater variability particularly within the middle range (4 to 5.5) (18).

Interrater reliability on Kurtzke's functional system (FS) is also low, with observer error accounting for 12 percent to 55 percent of the variation seen between individual FS scores (17). Low interrater agreement among neurologists on the FS has also been reported in other studies (19,20).

Validity

As expected, the EDSS is highly correlated with the DSS ($r = 0.99$) (21). The EDSS is also significantly correlated with other impairment measures such as the Scripps

TABLE 13-2A
Kurtzke's Functional System

A. PYRAMIDAL FUNCTIONS

0 = Normal
1 = Abnormal signs without disability
2 = Minimal disability
3 = Mild or moderate paraparesis or hemiparesis, severe monoparesis
4 = Marked paraparesis orhemiparesis, moderate quadraparesis, or monoplegia
5 = Paraplegia, hemiplegia, or marked quadriparesis
6 = Quadriplegia
V = Unknown

B. CEREBELLAR FUNCTIONS

0 = Normal
1 = Abnormal signs without disability
2 = Mild ataxia
3 = Moderate truncal or limb ataxia
4 = Severe ataxia, all limbs
5 = Unable to perform coordinated movements due to ataxia
V = Unknown
X = Used throughout after each number when weakness (grade or more on pyramidal) interferes with testing

C. BRAINSTEM FUNCTIONS

0 = Normal
1 = Signs only
2 = Moderate nystagmus or other mild disability
3 = Severe nystagmus, marked extraocular weakness or moderate disability of other cranial nerves
4 = Marked dysarthria or other marked disability
5 = Inability to swallow or speak
V = Unknown

D. SENSORY FUNCTIONS (1982 REVISION)

0 = Normal
1 = Vibration or figure-writing decrease only, in one or two limbs
2 = Mild decrease in touch or pain or position sense, and/or moderate decrease in vibration in one or two limbs; or vibratory (c/s figure-writing) decrease alone in three or four limbs
3 = Moderate decrease in touch or pain or position sense, and/or essentially lost vibration in one or two limbs; or mild decrease in touch or pain and/or moderate decrease in all proprioceptive tests in three or four limbs
4 = Marked decrease in touch or pain or loss of proprioception, alone or combined, in one or two limbs; or moderate decreased in touch or pain and/or severe proprioceptive decrease in more than two limbs
5 = Loss (essentially) of sensation in one or two limbs; or moderate decrease in touch or pain and/or loss of proprioception for most of body below the head
6 = Sensation essentially lost below the head
V = Unknown

E. BOWEL AND BLADDER FUNCTION (1982 REVISION)

0 = Normal
1 = Mild urinary hesitancy, urgency, or retention
2 = Moderate hesitancy, urgency, retention of bowel or bladder, or rare urinary incontinence
3 = Frequent urinary incontinence
4 = In need of almost constant catheterization
5 = Loss of bladder function
6 = Loss of bowel and bladder function
V = Unknown

TABLE 13-2A
continued

F. Visual (or optic) functions

0 = Normal
1 = Scotoma with visual acuity (corrected better than 20/30)
2 = Worse eye with scotoma with maximal visual acuity (corrected) of 20/30 to 20/59
3 = Worse eye with large scotoma, or moderate decrease in fields, but with maximal visual acuity (corrected) of 20/60
   to 20/99
4 = Worse eye with marked decrease of fields and maximal visual acuity (corrected) of 20/100 to 20/200; grade 3 plus
   maximal acuity of better eye of 20/60 or less
5 = Worse eye with maximal visual acuity (corrected) less than 20/200; grade 4 plus maximal acuity of better eye of
   20/60 or less
6 = Grade 5 plus maximal visual acuity of better eye of 20/60 or less
V = Unknown
X = Added to grades 0–6 for presence of temporal pallor

G. CEREBRAL (OR MENTAL) FUNCTIONS

0 = Normal
1 = Mood alteration only (does not affect DSS score)
2 = Mild decrease in mentation
3 = Moderate decrease in mentation
4 = Marked decrease in mentation (chronic brain syndrome moderate)
5 = Dementia or chronic brain syndrome-severe or incompetent
V = Unknown

OTHER FUNCTIONS

0 = None
1 = Any other neurologic finding attributed to MS (specify)
V = Unknown

Neurological Rating Scale (SNRS) ($r = 0.78$) (22), and with the lower extremity composite of the Quantitative Examination of Neurological Function (QENF) ($r = -0.69$) (23). Significant correlates were also reported between the EDSS and two quality of life measures, the SF-36 physical functioning subscale ($r = -0.79$) and the SIP physical total ($r = 0.81$) (24).

Changes on the EDSS and the Ambulation Index (AI) were significantly correlated (25). Furthermore, changes on EDSS were also positively correlated with the change in number of lesions on magnetic resonance imaging (MRI) (26).

Administration/Scoring

The EDSS can be administered by a neurologist or by a trained health care professional who has experience performing the examination. The amount of time necessary to complete the EDSS is 10 to 20 minutes. Functional Systems scores are designed to quantify the results of the neurologic examination. Each functional system is rated on a scale from 0 (normal function) to 5 or 6 (unable to per-

form the function). Findings on the FS are used to guide the scoring of the EDSS.

The EDSS is a 20-point scale, with scores ranging from 0 (no impairment) to 10 (death due to MS) in 0.5 increments. Scores between 0 and 3.5 are largely dependent on the history and findings of the neurologic examination in the appropriate grades of the functional systems. Scores between 0 and 4.5 indicate patients who are fully ambulatory, whereas scores of 5 or above primarily assess ambulation impairment. In scoring the EDSS and the FS it has been recommended that at least a two-step change (one point on the EDSS and two points on the FS) is necessary before concluding that MS status has changed (19,20).

Advantages

The content of Kurtzke's system is good in that it covers all the major neurologic areas affected by MS. Some of the Functional Systems (pyramidal, cerebellar, visual, mental) have been listed as promising scales by the NMSS Clinical Task Force. The wide use of the EDSS makes it

TABLE 13-2B
Kurtzke's Expanded Disability Status Scale (EDSS)

0	Normal neurologic exam (all grade 0 in functional systems [FS]; Cerebral grade 1 acceptable).
1.0	No disability, minimal signs in one FS (i.e., grade 1 excluding Cerebral grade 1).
1.5	No disability, minimal signs in more than one FS (more than one grade 1 excluding Cerebral grade 1).
2.0	Minimal disability in one FS (one FS grade 2, others 0 or 1).
2.5	Minimal disability in two FS (two FS grade 2, others 0 or 1).
3.0	Moderate disability in one FS (one FS 3, others 0 or 1), or mild disability in three or four FS (three/four FS grade 2, others 0 or 1) though fully ambulatory.
3.5	Fully ambulatory but with moderate disability in one FS (one grade 3) and one or two FS grade 2; or two FS grade 3; or five FS grade 2 (others 0 or 1).
4.0	Fully ambulatory without aid, self-sufficient, up and about some 12 hours a day despite relatively severe disability consisting of one FS grade 4 (others 0 or 1), or combinations of lesser grade exceeding limits of previous steps. Able to walk without aid or rest some 500 m.
4.5	Fully ambulatory without aid, up and about much of the day, able to work a full day, may otherwise have some limitation of full activity or require minimal assistance; characterized by relatively severe disability, usually consisting of one FS grade 4 (others 0 or 1) or combinations of lesser grades exceeding limits of previous steps. Able to walk without aid or rest for some 300 m.
5.0	Ambulatory without aid or rest for about 200 m; disability severe enough to impair full daily activities (for example, to work a full day without special provisions). (Usual FS equivalents are one grade 5 alone, others 0 or 1; or combinations of lesser grades usually exceeding specifications for step 4.0.)
5.5	Ambulatory without aid or rest for about 100 m; disability severe enough to preclude full daily activities. (Usual FS equivalents are one grade 5 alone, others 0 or 1; or combinations of lesser grades usually exceeding specifications for step 4.0.)
6.0	Intermittent or unilateral constant assistance (cane, crutch, or brace) required to walk about 100 m with or without resting. (Usual FS equivalents are combinations with more than two FS grade 3+.)
6.5	Constant bilateral assistance (canes, crutches, or braces) required to walk about 20 m without resting. (Usual FS equivalents are combinations with more than two FS grade 3+.)
7.0	Unable to walk beyond about 5 m even with aid, essentially restricted to wheelchair; wheels self in standard wheelchair and transfers alone; up and about in wheelchair some 12 hours a day. (Usual FS equivalents are combinations with more than one FS grade 4+; very rarely Pyramidal grade 5 alone.)
7.5	Unable to take more than a few steps; restricted to wheelchair; may need aid in transfer; wheels self but cannot carry on in a standard wheelchair for a full day; may require a motorized wheelchair. (Usual FS equivalents are combinations with more than one FS grade 4+.)
8.0	Essentially restricted to bed or chair or perambulated in wheelchair but may be out of bed itself for much of the day; retains many self-care functions; generally has effective use of arms. (Usual FS equivalents are combinations, generally grade 4+ in several systems.)
8.5	Essentially restricted to bed much of the day; has some effective use of arm(s); retains some self-care functions. (Usual FS equivalents are combinations, generally 4+ in several systems.)
9.0	Helpless bed patient; can communicate and eat (Usual FS equivalents are combinations, mostly grade 4+.)
9.5	Totally helpless bed patient; unable to communicate effectively or eat/swallow. (Usual FS equivalents are combinations, almost all grade 4+.
10	Death due to MS.

Source: Kurtzke JF. Rating neurologic impairment in multiple sclerosis: An expanded disability status scale (EDSS). *Neurology* 1983; 33:1444–1452.

a familiar, easy, and quantifiable method of communication among MS neurologists and other health care professionals. Whitaker and associates note that the EDSS allows simple comparison between patients or within a single patient over time (27). Although these comparisons may be simple, the low interrater reliability and low sensitivity of the EDSS to detect small changes make this problematic.

When comparing the EDSS with other standardized measures of physical function and impairment that focus on ambulation, the EDSS holds up well. The EDSS has demonstrated high convergent validity with the AI, SNRS, QENF (lower extremity composite), SF-36 (physical functioning subscale), and the SIP (physical total). In a longitudinal study, changes on the EDSS were found to be significantly correlated with changes in number of lesions on the MRI. However MRI changes are not always reflected by changes in EDSS, especially when the change is not related to mobility.

Disadvantages

The most common complaint about the EDSS is that it lacks the necessary sensitivity to detect the types of changes experienced by people with MS within a short period of time (1,11,22). Clinical trials need to be at least two to three years in length and require a large sample size in order to detect change (1).

Research indicates that two raters may rate a patient one standard deviation from his or her true score on the EDSS. Unfortunately, MS clinical trial researchers are defining clinically significant changes on the EDSS at a one grade change. With this amount of interrater variability, it is difficult to determine whether a changed EDSS score is due to a treatment effect or to error variance. For this reason, some researchers have recommended that at least a two-step change (one point on the EDSS and two points on the FS) be used to reliably conclude change in disease activity (19,20). Other investigators require sustained change—changes in the EDSS that persist for three to six months or more.

The EDSS was found to be less reliable at the lower ranges (28), meaning that it is not a reliable measure of impairment for MS patients who are mildly impaired and are not experiencing mobility problems. The distribution of scores of the EDSS was found to be bimodal, clustering at levels 3–4 and 6–7 (8,27) and relatively sparse in the middle range (4–5.5) (22,27,29). The incremental steps on the EDSS are inherently unequal. A change from EDSS score of 1 to 2 is not equal in disability to a change from a score of 5 to 6 (8,27) This particular problem, however, is not unique to the EDSS.

Comments

The EDSS continues to be the most widely used MS impairment measure despite its imperfections. The major complaints are that it lacks sensitivity in detecting disease status changes, has low interrater reliability, and does not accurately assess patient within the 4–5.5 point range. It predominantly measures ambulation and does not adequately assess many other impairment/disability domains (i.e., cognitive function, upper extremity function, and fatigue).

The Self-Administered Kurtzke

The self-administered Kurtzke, also referred to as the self-assessed EDSS, was specifically intended for MS patients to evaluate their own level of impairment (30). It was developed because the standard Kurtzke scale requires a neurologist to perform a physical examination in order to rate the functional systems. More recently, and independent of the original self-administered Kurtzke, the French also developed a self-assessment questionnaire (31). In this chapter, this measure is referred to as the French version of the self-administered Kurtzke. A possible third version may also be available. In a multicenter study, Italian MS neurologists devised a self-administered version of the MRD to be sent to patients who were not available for direct examination (32).

Description

Like the standard physician-administered Kurtzke, the self-administered Kurtzke is divided into two areas: functional systems (FS) and mobility (EDSS) (Table 13-3). The functional systems consists of eight items on a 4-point Likert scale (none, mild, moderate, and severe impairment). Mobility consists of 18 items that are divided into three groups: Able to walk (0 to 3.5), Able to walk only a limited distance (4.0 to 5.5), and Aids required or unable to walk (6.0 to 9.0).

The French version of the self-administered Kurtzke is also divided into the same two areas: functional systems (FS) and mobility (EDSS) (Table 13-4). The functional systems consists of 25 items: five pyramidal, three cerebellar, two brainstem; five bladder and bowel, five sensorial, three mental, and two visual. Functional systems are rated on a 4-point Likert scale (none, mild, moderate, and severe impairment). Mobility consists of 12 items ranging from no mobility impairment to restricted to bed.

Reliability

Interrater reliability or agreement between the self-administered and the standard physician-administered EDSS is high (Pearson $r = 0.90$) (30,31). As expected, interrater reliability decreases when low and high EDSS scores are analyzed separately. Scores between 0 and 3.5 had an average discrepancy of 1.6 on the EDSS, whereas higher scores (4.0 to 9.5) had a discrepancy of only 0.26 on the EDSS (30). Interrater agreement is best in the moderate to severe impairment range.

Consistent with results on the standard Kurtzke, interrater reliability on the FS generally is lower. Discrepancy on the FS between patient and physician rating range from an ICC $r = 0.26$ in the sensory to an ICC $r = 0.69$ in the pyramidal function (32). Similarly, Verdier-Taillefer and associates reported correlations ranging from lows of $r = 0.13$ (brainstem) and $r = 0.16$ (mental) to a high of $r = 0.66$ (pyramidal) (31).

Validity

No validity studies regarding the self-administered Kurtzke have been reported.

TABLE 13-3
Self-Administered Kurtzke

Instructions: Individuals with MS may experience difficulty in a number of different areas. For each of the 8 neurologic categories below, please indicate the degree of difficulty (none, minimal, moderate, or severe) that you are experiencing at the present time.

	NONE	MINIMAL DIFFICULTY, INTERFERES ONLY SLIGHTLY WITH FUNCTION	MODERATE DIFFICULTY, INTERFERES SIGNIFICANTLY WITH FUNCTION	SEVERE DIFFICULTY LITTLE OR NO FUNCTION IS POSSIBLE
1. Weakness in arm(s) and/or leg(s)	0	1	2	3
2. Tremor, clumsiness, or loss of balance	0	1	2	3
3. Double vision or slurred speech, or difficulty swallowing	0	1	2	3
4. Numbness or difficulty in feeling heat, pain or vibration in any part of the body	0	1	2	3
5. Frequency or urgent urination, awakening to urinate, not emptying the bladder completely, loss of bladder or bowel control, or constipation	0	1	2	3
6. Blurred vision in one or both eyes (even with glasses)	0	1	2	3
7. Difficulty with memory, calculation or reasoning	0	1	2	3
8. Stiffness or jerking of the muscles	0	1	2	3

OVERALL FUNCTION

On the following two pages are a number of statements that might be used to describe the overall function of MS patients. These statements are arranged in order from least severe (0) to most severe (9.0).

Instructions:

1. First locate the item that best describes your ability to walk.
   - If you are able to walk without limitations, please choose a statement under the section called "Able to Walk."
   - If you are able to walk only a limited distance, please choose a statement under the section called "Able to Walk Only a Limited Distance."
   - If you require aid(s) or assistance to walk or are unable to walk, please choose a statement under the section called "Aid(s) Required or Unable to Walk."
2. Circle the number of the one statement which best describes your overall condition at the present time.
3. In selecting your answer, refer back to your rating of the 8 neurologic categories listed.

Remember: Choose on *one* of the statements (0–9.0) which follow.

ABLE TO WALK

0.0 Essentially normal
1.0 Abnormality in *one* of the neurological categories but with no difficulty in function
1.5 Abnormality in *more than* one of the neurological categories but with no difficulty in function
2.0 Minimal difficulty in one of the neurological categories
2.5 Minimal difficulty in two of the neurological categories
3.0 Moderate difficulty in one of the neurological categories, able to walk
3.5 Moderate difficulty in one of the neurological categories and minimal difficulty in *one or more* of the neurological categories, able to walk

TABLE 13-3
continued

ABLE TO WALK ONLY A LIMITED DISTANCE

4.0   Able to walk without aid or rest at least 7 city blocks (500 meters or 1,625 feet)
       Self-sufficient, up and about some 12 hours a day (Relatively severe difficulty in one neurological category or moderate difficulty in several of the neurological categories)

4.5   Able to walk without aid or rest at least 4 city blocks (300 meters or 975 feet)
       May need minimal assistance, able to work a full day but may have some limitation of full activity (Relatively severe difficulty in one neurological category or moderate difficulty in several of the neurological categories)

5.0   Able to walk without aid or rest at least 2½ city blocks (200 meters or 650 feet)
       Disability is severe enough to limit full daily activities—for example: to work a full day without job modifications (Very severe difficulty in one of the neurological categories)

5.5   Able to walk without aid or rest at least 1 city block (100 meters or 325 feet)
       Disability is severe enough to *prevent* full daily activities (Very severe difficulty in one of the neurological categories or moderate difficulty in several of the neurological categories)

AID(S) REQUIRED OR UNABLE TO WALK

6.0   Assistance on *one* side (cane, crutch, brace) is required to walk approximately 1 city block (approximately 100 meters or 325 feet), with or without resting
       (Moderate difficulty in more than two neurological categories)

6.5   Constant assistance on both sides (canes, crutches, braces, walker) is required to walk about 20 meters (65 feet)
       (Moderate difficulty in more than two neurological categories)

7.0   Unable to walk more than about 5 meters (16 feet) even with aid
       Essentially restricted to wheelchair
       Can wheel self in standard wheelchair and can transfer alone
       Up and about in wheelchair some 12 hours a day
       (Severe difficulty in more than one neurological category or severe weakness only)

7.5   Unable to take more than a few steps, restricted to wheelchair
       Can wheel self in standard wheelchair and may need aid to transfer
       Cannot remain in wheelchair for a full day
       May require motorized wheelchair
       (Severe difficulty in more than one neurological category)

8.0   Essentially restricted to bed or chair
       Propelled by others in wheelchair
       May be out of bed part of the day
       Can use arms and able to care for self
       (Severe difficulty in several neurological categories)

8.5   Essentially restricted to bed much of the day
       Has limited use of arms
       Retains some self-care functions
       (Severe difficulty in several neurological categories)

9.0   Restricted to bed
       Cannot use arms
       Can speak, can eat if fed by others
       (Severe difficulty in several neurological categories)

Source: Scheinberg LC. Medical Rehabilitation Research and Training Center for MS, Department of Neurology, Albert Einstein College of Medical, Bronx, New York.

TABLE 13-4
Self-Administered Kurtzke (French Version)

Symptoms	None	Mild	Moderate	Severe
1. Weakness of right arm	0	1	2	3
2. Weakness of left arm	0	1	2	3
3. Weakness of right leg	0	1	2	3
4. Weakness of left leg	0	1	2	3
5. Leg stiffness or deficit at walk	0	1	2	3
6. Tremor	0	1	2	3
7. Clumsiness of arms	0	1	2	3
8. Lose of balance	0	1	2	3
9. Double vision	0	1	2	3
10. Difficulty in speaking and/or swallowing	0	1	2	3
11. Uncontrolled urinary urgency	0	1	2	3
12. Difficulty in urination, incomplete micturition or bladder emptying	0	1	2	3
13. Constipation	0	1	2	3
14. Loss of control of bladder	0	1	2	3
15. Loss of control of bowel	0	1	2	3
16. Difficulty in feeling a contact	0	1	2	3
17. Difficulty in feeling heat	0	1	2	3
18. Difficulty inh feeling pain	0	1	2	3
19. Pain or burning sensation in any part of the body	0	1	2	3
20. Bizarre feeling (pins and needles, constriction) in any part of the body	0	1	2	3
21. Difficulty with memory	0	1	2	3
22. Difficulty with calculation	0	1	2	3
23. Difficulty with reasoning or thinking	0	1	2	3
Level of vision (with glasses)	>7/10 (reading possible)	6/10–4/10 (recognition possible)	3/10 or 2/10 (distinction of forms)	<1/10 (loss of vision)
24. Right eye	0	1	2	3
25. Left eye	0	1	2	3

Source: Verdier-Taillefer MH, Roullet E, Cesaro P, Alperovitch A. Validation of self-reported neurological disability in multiple sclerosis. *International Journal of Epidemiology* 1994; 23:148–154.

Administration/Scoring

This questionnaire can be self-administered, administered by a health care professional, or administered by telephone. Direct observation may be used but it is not required. One generally allows 10 to 15 minutes for completion.

Separate scores are obtained for the FS and the EDSS (ambulation). On the French version of the self-administered Kurtzke, all items relating to a specific FS area are summed. For example, to score pyramidal function, sum responses to items 1 to 5. Total pyramidal function scores range from 0 to 15 points. On the self-administered Kurtzke, the different FS are represented by only one item, so no summing is required. On the self-administered Kurtzke, EDSS scores range from 0 to 9 points, and on the French version, EDSS scores range from 0 to 11 points.

Advantages

The self-administered Kurtzke is written in simple, non-technical language, making it easy for patients to understand and complete the test. With the development of this instrument, a patient's perception of neurologic functioning can be compared with the physician's rating of impairment. This comparison is useful in double-blind therapeutic trials and in cost-benefit studies of health care (33). It is also a useful impairment measure when conducting research by telephone interview or by mail.

The self-administered Kurtzke is a reliable measure of ambulation and is most appropriate for patients with moderate to severe ambulation difficulties. Some research indicates that patients can quite accurately assess their own neurologic symptoms. Patients reliably report symptoms such as weakness, stiffness, tremor, clumsiness, poor balance, visual difficulties, and bladder and bowel dysfunction (31).

Disadvantages

The self-administered Kurtzke has some of the same disadvantages as the physician-administered Kurtzke. On the EDSS, agreement between patients and physicians is best in the moderate to severe mobility range. Interrater reliability is lower with low EDSS scores. As with the standard physician-administered Kurtzke, discrepancies of FS scores on the self-administered Kurtzke are generally lower and varied.

Comments

This instrument is a useful measure for large-scale studies conducted by telephone or mail. It is most appropriate for moderate to severely impaired MS patients and is not suitable for MS patients who grossly distort their own impairment level (i.e., severe cognitive impairment or psychological denial).

Scripps Neurological Rating Scale

Scripps Neurological Rating Scale (SNRS), also referred to as the Neurological Rating Scale (NRS), was developed for clinical assessment of MS patients and has been used in several MS clinical trials (34).

Description

The SNRS is primarily based on a standard neurologic examination and assesses the following systems: mentation and mood, cranial nerves, lower cranial nerves, motor, DTRS, Babinski, sensory, cerebellar, and gait. It also includes a separate category for bowel, bladder, and sexual dysfunction.

Reliability

Test-retest reliability has not been reported on the SNRS. Interrater reliability was high, with a weighted kappa coefficient of 0.83 (34). Sharrack and Hughes noted that the degree of agreement was defined as a difference of no more than 10 points, which is a significant variation on a 100-point scale (11).

Validity

The correlation between the EDSS and SNRS was $r = 0.78$ (22). In comparing the EDSS and the SNRS, the EDSS shows more sudden changes compared with the SNRS, which showed more gradual changes. The EDSS usually remained unchanged for longer periods of time in contrast to the SNRS (22).

Administration/Scoring

The SNRS should be administered by a neurologist or a highly trained health care professional who understands how to complete a neurologic examination. It requires approximately 30 minutes to complete the SNRS.

The assignment of points on the SNRS is based on the neurologist's clinical assessment of each component in the neurologic examination. Scores on the SNRS are specially weighted for common fluctuating neurologic abnormalities, such as visual, motor, sensory, and cerebellar signs. On the SNRS, a neurologically normal person would receive a full score of 100 points. The maximum points possible for each system examined are mentation and mood (10 points), visual cranial nerves (21 points), other cranial nerves (5 points), strength for limbs (20 points), deep tendon relexes (8 points), Babinski sign

(4 points), sensory function for limbs (12 points), cerebellar function for limbs (10 points), and gait and balance (10 points). Bladder, bowel, and sexual dysfunctions are determined by subtracting the degree of impairment from the total SNRS score (maximum points subtracted is 10). Table 13-5 shows the SNRS scoring worksheet.

Advantages

Compared with the EDSS, the SNRS scores motor, sensory, and cerebellar functions separately and places more emphasis on upper limb function. There is evidence to suggest that the SNRS is a differentially sensitive measure of MS impairment compared with the EDSS (16,22). Changes in the clinical disease course tend to be more abrupt on the EDSS and more gradual on the SNRS.

Disadvantages

The SNRS lacks precision in defining degree of impairment, and the scoring options are vague (8,35). Guidelines for scoring the cranial nerves subscale (visual acuity,

TABLE 13-5
SNRS Scoring Worksheet*

SYSTEM EXAMINED	MAXIMUM POINTS	NORMAL	DEGREE OF IMPAIRMENT		
			MILD	MODERATE	SEVERE
Mentation and mood	10	10	7	4	0
Cranial Nerves:					
Visual Acuity	21	5	3	1	0
Fields, Discs, Pupils		6	4	2	0
Eye Movements		5	3	1	0
Nystagmus		5	3	1	0
Lower Cranial Nerves	5	5	3	1	0
Motor:					
RU	20	5	3	1	0
LU		5	3	1	0
RL		5	3	1	0
LL		5	3	1	0
DTRS:					
UE	8	4	3	1	0
LE		4	3	1	0
Babinski: R; L (2 ea)	4	4	—	—	0
Sensory:					
RU	12	3	2	1	0
LU		3	2	1	0
RL		3	2	1	0
LL		3	2	1	0
Cerebellar:					
UE	10	5	3	1	0
LE		5	3	1	0
Gait; Trunk and Balance	10	10	7	4	0
Special Category:					
Bladder/Bowels/Sexual Dysfunction	0	0	−3	−7	−10
Totals	100				

*Points assigned for each component of the neurologic examination are subtotaled, and points for autonomic dysfunction are subtracted, leaving the final SNRS score.
Source: Sipe JC, Knobler RL, Braheny SL, et al. A neurologic rating scale (NRS) for use in multiple sclerosis. *Neurology* 1984; 34:1368–1372.

fields, discs, pupils, eye movements, nystagmus) on the SNRS are also vague. Providing brief examples of mild, moderate, and severe impairment for each neurologic area would help guide the examiner. The SNRS does not designate symptom deficits, as on the Kurtzke FS, or adequately reflect cognitive dysfunction (27). The reverse scoring procedure (increasing score means decreasing impairment) makes comparing the SNRS with other impairment measures somewhat more difficult.

Comments

Like the Kurtzke system, the SNRS assesses impairment based on the neurologic examination, which makes it user-friendly to the neurologist. The scoring system is vague. Again, providing brief examples of mild, moderate, and severe impairment for each neurologic area would help guide the examiner and may help minimize interrater variation. Independent psychometric testing is needed before its usefulness can be completely determined.

Quantitative Examination of Neurological Function

The Quantitative Examination of Neurological Function (QENF), which was developed more than 25 years ago, was designed to objectively quantify neurologic status and function. The abbreviated form of the QENF test battery is called Neuroperformance Testing (NP). The QENF is a highly sensitive and comprehensive measure. It is appropriate for evaluating a wide range of abnormal and normal neurologic functions while also being responsive enough to detect small disease changes. In multiple sclerosis, the NP is used primarily to evaluate clinical trial outcomes.

Description

The QENF is a battery of timed performance tests that measure neurologic function. The QENF contains three predominant subscales: vision, upper extremity function, and lower extremity function. Examples of upper extremity tests are Purdue pegboard, finger tapping, cutting, dialing, and writing. Examples of tests for lower extremity functioning are foot tapping, tandem gait, and standing balance (23). The areas assessed by the QENF include cognition, strength, steadiness, reactions, speed, coordination, sensations, fatigue, gait, station, and selected ADL skills (36). The QENF consists of 57 different tests, 54 of which are administered to both the dominant and the nondominant body sides, producing a total of 111 measures for one complete examination (36). (Complete descriptions of the QENF tests can be found in references 36–38. The data sheets and instructions for administer-

ing the QENF are found in reference 38, Appendix A, B.) The NP as used in MS research includes the minimal set of tests considered most sensitive to change in MS (Table 13-6).

Reliability

The QENF has demonstrated high test-retest reliability with normal subjects and many patient groups, including MS patients. The NP test-retest reliability was found to be statistically significant, with Pearson correlation coefficient ranging from $r = 0.83$ for "Putting on a Shirt" to $r = 0.95$ for "Hand Tapping." The mean Pearson correlation coefficient for upper extremity tests was $r = 0.96$, for lower extremity tests $r = 0.93$, and the NP global composite was $r = 0.96$ (14). These test-retest reliability coefficients are higher than reported in an earlier NP study (23) Additional reliability information is also available (39).

Validity

The QENF has documented moderately high convergent validity with two other measures of ambulation. The lower extremity composite of the QENF correlated significantly with the EDSS and the Ambulation Index ($r = -0.69$ and -0.70, respectively) and was the most sensitive measure of treatment effect (23). There is also evidence to suggest that the bimanual upper extremity tasks on the NP are significantly correlated with cerebellar dysfunction in MS (40).

Administration/Scoring

The QENF can be administered by a neurologist, physical therapist, or other trained health care professional and should be administered in the morning, when fatigue is generally less of a factor. The length of time necessary to administer the QENF depends on the numbers of tests selected. To administer all 57 QENF tests would require considerable time, especially if fatigue is a factor. The NP version for MS requires 30 to 45 minutes (23).

Most NP tests allow two trials. The trials are timed in number of seconds (sec) necessary to complete the test. Each NP test score (e.g., hand tapping) is converted to a standard score based on the mean and standard deviation for that NP measure at baseline for all MS participants. Each NP composite is calculated as the average z-score value at a given time point (examination) over a set of comparable measures (14).

Advantages

The QENF is currently the most comprehensive assessment of neurologic function available (27). There is evi-

TABLE 13-6
The NP Tests for Multiple Sclerosis

Tests	Scoring
Symbol Digit Modalities Test	# correct in 90 sec
Upper Extremity Composit Tests	
Purdue pegboard—(avg R&L)	# correct in 30 sec
Finger tapping—(avg R&L)	avg # taps in three 10-sec trials
Shirt (avg 2 trials)	100/# of sec
Button (avg 2 trials)	100/# of sec
Zip (avg 2 trials)	100/# of sec
Bow (avg 2 trials	100/# of sec
Cutting (avg 2 trials)	100/# of sec
Dialing (avg 2 trials)	100/# of sec
Writing (v 2 trials)	100/# of sec
Lower Extremity Composit Tests	
Foot tapping—(avg R&L)	avg # taps in three 10-sec trials
Tandem gait (avg 2 trials)	steps/sec for 6–7 steps
Standing balance	# of sec up to 30 sec max
2 legs (avg eyes open/closed)	# of sec up to 30 sec max
1 leg eyes open (avg R&L)	# of sec up to 30 sec max
1 leg eyes closed (avg R&L)	# of sec up to 30 sec max
Rise (avg 2 trials)	100/# of sec

Source: Syndulko K, Tourtellotte WW, Baumhefner RW, et al. Neuroperformance evaluation of multiple sclerosis disease progresssion in a clinical trial: Implications for neurological outcomes. *Journal of Neurologic Rehabilitation* 1993; 7:153–176.

dence to suggest that it also is more sensitive than the EDSS and the AI in detecting disease progression and treatment effect (23). Furthermore, these changes in disease status were detected within the first year of the study. The content areas and many of the tests on the QENF are very similar or the same as those endorsed by the NMSS Clinical Outcomes Assessment Task Force.

Upper and lower extremity function can be assessed and scored separately. Not every test on the QENF must be used. A selective set of tests from the QENF may be employed based on the user's needs. For example, if the researcher is assessing the effectiveness of a new medication for intention tremors, select a few tests from the upper extremity subscale (i.e., Purdue pegboard, cutting, zip, and writing).

Disadvantages

The major disadvantages of the QENF are that it is time-consuming, complex, and costly (11,27). Selecting a subset of tests may make comparisons across studies difficult to interpret. For these reasons, the QENF has not been widely used. In response to these criticisms, a simplified version of the QENF was developed (41).

Comments

As recommended by the NMSS Task Force, more MS clinical trial studies are using quantitative tests like the QENF, and this has stimulated the use of performance-based measures in MS research.

Ambulation Index

The Ambulation Index (AI), also referred to as Hauser's Ambulation Index, was developed by Hauser and colleagues to quantify precise changes in gait (42). It has been used in several clinical trials outcome studies and is often used in conjunction with the EDSS to increase detection of ambulation changes, with the commonly observed range of EDSS scores between 4.0 and 6.0 (35).

Description

The AI is a lower extremity mobility test (Table 13-7). It is primarily a performance measure based on speed and the degree of assistance needed for walking 25 feet. It is a one-item test that grades mobility from 0 (asymptomatic and fully active) to 9 (restricted to wheelchair or unable to transfer self independently).

TABLE 13-7
Ambulation Index

Instructions: Time the patient's walk of 25 feet, after telling the patient to walk as quickly as he/she safely can.

0 **Asymptomatic**; fully active.

1 **Walks normally but reports fatigue** that interferes with athletic or other demanding activities.

2 **Abnormal gait** or episodic imbalance; gait disorder is noticeable to family and friends. Able to walk 25 feet in **10 seconds or less**.

3 **Walks** independently; able to walk 25 feet in **between 11–20 seconds**.

4 **Requires** unilateral support (cane, single crutch) to walk; uses support more than 80% of the time. Walks 25 feet in **20 seconds or less**.

5 **Requires** unilateral support but walks 25 feet in **greater than 20 seconds** or requires **bilateral support** (canes, crutches, walker) and walks 25 feet in **20 seconds or less**.

6 **Requires** bilateral support and walks 25 feet in **greater than 20 seconds**. (May use wheelchair on occasion*).

7 Walking limited to **several steps with bilateral support**; unable to walk 25 feet. (May use wheelchair most of the time).

8 Restricted to wheelchair; **able to transfer independently**.

9 Restricted to wheelchair; **unable to transfer independently**.

10 Bedridden.

---

* The use of a wheelchair may be determined by a patient's lifestyle and motivation. It is expected that patients in grade 7 will use a wheelchair more frequently than those in grades 5 or 6. Assignment of a grade in the range of 5–7, however, is determined by the patient's ability to walk a given distance and not by the extent to which a patient uses a wheelchair.
Source: Hauser SL, Dawson DM, Lehrich JR, et al. Intensive immunosuppression in progressive multiple sclerosis. *New England Journal of Medicine* 1983; 308:173–180.

Reliability

The AI has demonstrated high test-retest reliability ($r = 0.91$) (14) and interrater reliability ($r = 0.98$) (43). In another study, Cohen's kappa coefficient ranged from moderate to substantial (0.5 to 0.7) (17). The interrater error was notably lower on the AI (3.9 percent) as compared with the EDSS (17 percent).

Validity

The AI also was strongly associated with the SF-36 Physical Functioning scale ($r = -0.74$) and with the following SIP scales: Ambulation, Physical and Body Care, and Movement (all $r > 0.70$) (24). The AI is significantly correlated with a new impairment measure, the Multiple Sclerosis Impairment Scale (MSIS) ($r = 0.85$), and compared with the MSIS and the EDSS, the AI was found to be the most sensitive measure of clinical change (43). Changes on the AI significantly correlated with changes on the EDSS (25) and with change in number of lesions on MRI (26).

Administration/Scoring

The AI can be administered by any health care professional or trained assistant. The patient is timed walking 25 feet after being instructed to walk as quickly and safely as possible.

Advantages

The AI is a sensitive, reliable measure of lower extremity function based largely on direct observation. It is a widely used test of lower extremity function in MS clinical trial studies.

Disadvantages

Although the patient is timed walking 25 feet, the exact performance times are not used. The AI is an ordinal scale, in which the steps in the measure are not equivalent and the data are focused in the response category that best represents the patient's performance.

Comment

Although the AI is only a one-item scale, the response intervals are small and precise enough to detect the types of ambulation changes experienced by MS patients. The AI has demonstrated high reliability and validity. It is a widely used measure that is rapidly becoming a standard test of lower extremity function in MS clinical trial studies.

Troiano Functional Scale (TFS)

The Troiano Functional Scale (TFS) was developed for use in a therapeutic trial involving chronic progressive MS patients (44).

Description

The TFS is a mixed instrument, assessing both impairment and disability (Table 13-8). It consists of three components or items: gait, transfers, and ADLs. The gait item is rated on a 6-point Likert scale from normal to inability to stand or take a step. Activities of daily living item is rated on a 5-point Likert scale according to the type and amount of assistance required. The transfer item is rated on a 4-point Likert scale according to the amount of assistance required.

Reliability

No reliability data have been published.

Validity

No validity data have been published.

Administration/Scoring

The TFS can be self-administered or administered by a health care professional within a few minutes. Scores on the TFS range from 0 (independent) to 12 points (dependence).

Advantages

The TFS is a short, simple measure. It is a rapid assessment of disease progression for patients in the later stages of the disease (27).

Disadvantages

The reliability and validity of this measure are not known. There are only three items, one for each subscale. The scale intervals are too large, which makes it a less sensitive measure for patients with mild to moderate MS. It is heavily weighted on ambulation, does not adequately assess ADL function, and fails to address other symptoms such as bowel and/or bladder function.

Comment

The psychometric properties of this measure are not known. For this reason, the TFS should not used as a clinical trials outcome measure or as a clinical monitor of disease progression. The TFS does provide preliminary functional status information that can help guide the direction of further assessment.

FUNCTIONAL OUTCOME MEASURES

More MS clinical trial studies are including performance measures that tend to be more psychometrically sound, more sensitive to change than the EDSS, and easier to ana-

---

TABLE 13-8
Troiano Functional Scale

GAIT: _____

0   Normal

1   Abnormal, independent

2   Uses unilateral assistance device

3   Uses bilateral assistance device; may use wheelchair for longer mobility; walking is sufficient to serve various routine daily activities

4   Depends mainly on wheelchair for mobility; may stand and take some steps with bilateral assistance; walking not very useful for practical purposes, done largely for short transfers and exercise activity, preferably with supervision

5   No standing or step excluding active human support or rigid support such as Kim stander

ACTIVITIES OF DAILY LIVING: _____

0   Normal

1   Independent with minimum dysfunction; may choose to use assistance or device for speed and efficiency

2   Routinely uses partial human assistance for some dexterity functions (writing, managing utensils, button, etc.) and dressing and bathing of lower body

3   Uses substantial human assistance for most activities, including bathing and dressing lower and upper body; actively participates

4   Dependent for all activities; passive with no effective participation

TRANSFERS: _____

0   Slight or no difficulty

1   Uses arms to shift weight, sitting to standing, or sitting to sitting, from a straight chair or wheelchair; transfers are independent

2   Routinely uses assistance for most transfers; actively participates

3   Dependent for all transfers; passive with no effective participation

TOTAL _____

Source: Cook SD, Devereux C, Troiano R, Hafsten MP, et al. Effect of total lymphoid irradiation in chronic progressive multiple sclerosis. *Lancet* 1986; 1:1405–409.

lyze. On the other hand, performance type tests are also subject to variations in human judgment and tend to be more expensive and time-consuming to administer, possibly requiring equipment and a test administrator. The measures also tend to be multidimensional, covering lower extremity function, upper extremity function, visual function, and neuropsychological function. After analyzing all available measures, the NMSS Clinical Outcomes Assessment Task Force has found several promising measures (2) (Table 13-9).

The Multiple Sclerosis Functional Composite Measure

Based on further examination of the measures outlined in Table 13-9, the NMSS Task Force generated quantitative functional composites that showed high reliability, significant relationship with disease duration, changed over time and exhibited both concurrent and predictive validity based on the EDSS (45). The MS functional composite measures that have been strongly recommended and are being used in several MS clinical trials are:

1. Timed 25-Foot Walk
2. Nine-Hole Peg Test (average of right and left arms)
3. Paced Auditory Serial Addition Test—3" version

These three tests can constitute a single composite score by combining the individual standardized components (z-score) into an overall score (2).

Timed 25-Foot Walk Test

The Timed 25-Foot Walk test is a gait speed test. The AI and the Timed 25-Foot Walk test are basically the same test, but the scoring procedures differ. The Timed 25-Foot test uses the actual amount of time taken to complete the task and the AI, which is an ordinal measure, selects the response category that best represents the patient's performance.

Description

The Timed 25-Foot Walk test is a mobility and leg function performance test in which the patient is timed walking 25 feet. Patients who need assistance and patients who use a wheelchair and are unable to complete the test are noted as such.

Reliability

In examining test-retest reliability between the 5-meter and the 10-meter walk and between the walks completed on the first and second occasion, high correlations were found (Pearson $r = 0.95-0.99$) (46). In a similar MS

TABLE 13-9
Promising Clinical Outcome Assessment Measures

AMBULATION AND LEG FUNCTION

1. Ambulation Index
2. Timed 25-Foot Walk
3. Timed tandem gait
4. Pyramidal functional system score (FSS)
5. SNRS—lower extremity measure
6. QENF Lower limb composite

ARM FUNCTION

1. Cerebellar FSS
2. Nine-Hole Peg Test
3. Box and Block Test
4. Purdue Pegboard
5. QENF Upper limb composite

VISUAL FUNCTION

1. Visual FSS
2. Visual acuity
3. Cranial nerve subscore from the SNRS

NEUROPSYCHOLOGICAL FUNCTION

1. Mental FSS
2. Paced Auditory Serial Addition Test (2-second version)
3. Paced Auditory Serial Addition Test (3-second version)
4. Controlled Oral Word Association Test (CO-WAT)
5. Symbol Digit Modality Test (SDMT)

---

study, high interrater and test-retest reliability were reported (47). Individual test-retest variability can range from 0 percent to 40 percent, but most patients (95 percent) only varied their speed on each walk by less than 25 percent of the slowest time (46).

Validity

Concurrent validity, as assessed by Spearman rank-order correlation coefficients, was demonstrated by the significant relationship between walking speed and the Gait Abnormality Rating Scale ($r = -0.68$). Specific validity information on the Timed 25-Foot Walk test is still needed.

Administration/Scoring

The Timed 25-Foot Walk test is simple to use and can be administered by any trained person. The patient could administer the test himself/herself if given proper instructions (46). The test requires one to five minutes to complete, depending on ambulatory ability. The score is the actual amount of time it takes to complete the task.

Advantages

The test is a simple, objective, and observable mobility test that can reliably assess all levels of impairment. Because it is a performance test, ceiling and floor effect problems are minimized and statistical analysis of ambulation change is straightforward.

Disadvantages

A common complaint associated with any performance type test is "practice effects." This problem is minimized on the Timed 25-Foot Walk test by having the patient take practice trials until the time to complete the task stabilizes.

Comments

Gait speed has been shown to be a useful and reliable functional measure of a person's walking ability.

Nine-Hole Peg Test

The Nine-Hole Peg Test (9-HPT) was developed by Mathiowetz and associates to test fine manual dexterity (48). It is considered the best test of dexterity disability (49) and has been strongly recommended by the NMSS Clinical Outcomes Assessment Task Force a composite key clinical trials outcome measure. It is rapidly becoming a gold standard test of upper extremity function in many MS studies (25,50,51).

Description

The 9-HPT is an upper extremity function test that requires the following equipment (52):

1. Nine wooden dowels; 9 mm diameter, 32 mm long
2. Wood base with nine holes (10 mm diam, 15 mm deep) spaced 15 mm apart in three rows of three holes
3. Lid to base, with tray 100 mm square and 100 mm deep to hold pegs

Reliability

The 9-HPT has demonstrated high interrater reliability (left $r = 0.99$, right $r = 0.97$) and moderate to moderately high test-retest reliability (left $r = 0.43$, right $r = 0.69$) using the Pearson correlation coefficient (53). Significant practice effects between the two trials were noted for the right hand ($p < 0.001$) and the left hand ($p < 0.05$). Heller and associates have also reported high reliability values on the 9-HPT; however, individual interpretation of the 9-HPT results is difficult because the 9-HPT data were combined with the other upper extremity test and assessed by observer (54).

Validity

Concurrent validity of the 9-HPT has been demonstrated by its moderate association with the Purdue Pegboard using a Pearson correlation coefficient (right hand $r = -0.61$ and left hand $r = 0.53$) (53). Timed test of hand function, including the 9-HPT, correlated well with handicap (rank correlation $= 0.73$) (55). With neurologically impaired patients, the 9-HPT is sensitive enough to detect minor hand function impairments (55) and helped improve the low sensitivity of the EDSS for detecting functional changes in MS patients in the 3.0 to 6.5 EDSS point range (51).

Administration/Scoring

The 9-HPT can be administered quickly by a trained volunteer or health care professional. Most normal people can complete this test in 18 to 20 seconds (52). The patient is instructed to place the pegs in the holes as quickly as possible, while the test administer notes how long it takes to complete the task. Two variations have been used: timing the patient while placing the pegs into the holes and timing the patient while first placing and then removing the pegs (49). Scores can be obtained for either hand or both hands. Scores are calculated in two different ways: the length of time taken to place nine pegs, and the number of pegs placed in 50 seconds (49). Goodkin and colleagues have suggested a change of more than 20 percent in 9-HPT score as a basis for concluding that the functional ability of the patient has changed (50).

Advantages

The 9-HPT is a short, standardized measure of upper extremity function that is easy to administer. It is suitable for use with most MS patients except those whose arm mobility and function are severely limited (i.e., those who have spasticity or intention tremors). It is significantly more sensitive than the EDSS in detecting upper extremity change (50) and was found to be the most sensitive measure of upper extremity tests compared with the Frenchay Arm Test and finger tapping rate (54).

Disadvantages

The 9-HPT is not appropriate for assessing MS patients whose upper extremity mobility and function are severely impaired. A test of gross manual dexterity such as the Box and Block Test would be more suitable for such patients.

Comments

The 9-HPT is a simple, inexpensive, and portable measure of fine manual dexterity. It is reliable, valid, and probably the most sensitive measure of upper extremity manual dexterity available.

Paced Auditory Serial Addition Test (PASAT)

Developed by Gronwall, the PASAT is a multiple computational task that is designed to measure attention and information processing speed (56). Specifically, the PASAT measures how rapidly a person can perform numeric operations on digits held in short-term memory (57) and provides an estimation of the amount of information a person can handle at one time.

Description

The PASAT is a test in which a random series of numbers from one to nine is presented verbally to the patient via an audiotape. The patient is instructed to add pairs of numbers such that each number is added to the one immediately preceding it. For example, the second number is added to the first, the third number to the second, and so on. The patient much give the answer before the next number is presented. Some MS studies use the original version of the PASAT in which 50 single digits are presented in different sequences for each of four trials and presentation rates for the four trials are: 2.4-, 2.0-, 1.6-, and 1.2-second intervals (57,58). In other studies, patients listen to 61 single digits for one or two trials that are two seconds (hard condition) and/or three seconds (easy condition) in length (59,60) The NMSS Clinical Outcomes Assessment Task Force recommends using the three-second interval version of the PASAT (PASAT-3") to maximize participation. Other neuropsychologists may add a two-second interval version (PASAT-2") to obtain further information.

Administration/Scoring

The PASAT can be administered by a neuropsychologist, speech/language pathologist, or trained health care professional. The PASAT requires 10 to 15 minutes to complete the practice trials and the two test trials. A practice trial of 10 numbers is presented to ensure that the patient understands the task. Again, the patient is instructed to add every consecutive two digits in a row and give the answer verbally to the test administrator. The patient must give the answer before the next number is presented. Three different scores can be obtained: number of correct

responses, number of incorrect responses, and missing or no responses.

Reliability

Test-retest reliability is generally not used on the PASAT because readministered performance scores are significantly influenced by practice effects. For this reason, split-half reliability, a measure of internal consistency, is applied. The PASAT has demonstrated high split-half reliability ($r = 0.96$) (61).

Validity

The convergent validity of the PASAT has been demonstrated by its significant association with other measures of attention and memory such as the Stroop Test (60), the Paired Associate subtest of the Wechsler Memory Scale, Wechsler Memory Scale Memory Quotient, and the Rey Auditory-Verbal Learning Test (57). The PASAT has also demonstrated divergent validity. Compared with normal controls, MS patients scored significantly lower on the PASAT across all trial speeds (62). Compared with MS patients who were cognitively preserved, mildly cognitively impaired MS patients preformed worse on the PASAT, making fewer correct responses and having more missing answers (60).

The PASAT is a sensitive test of mild to severe MS cognitive slowness (58,60). It is significantly correlated with change in total lesion volume at one year ($r = -0.58$, $p < 0.001$) (59) and with retrieval of information from long-term memory (57).

Advantages

The PASAT is sensitive enough to detect slight changes in speed of information processing and attention and is significantly correlated with MRI changes. Compared with other similar measures, the PASAT is probably the most likely to detect mild cognitive impairments because of the multiple computations and the greater memory load differentiation the task requires (57). These features make the PASAT a valuable and practical measure of cognitive function changes in MS patients.

Disadvantages

The PASAT has clear ceiling and floor effects that may impact its usefulness in early- or late-stage MS. It is a difficult and frustrating test that is significantly influenced by practice effects. On the PASAT, this concern is handled in two ways—practice trials and the use of a different version on the second administration. Practice trials ensure that the patient understands the task and can be administered until performance stabilizes. Other factors known to affect test results include intelligence, age, and education (63). Performance on the PASAT shows much greater variability in lower IQ ranges, and results are generally poorer as age increases and educational level decreases. Patients who experience anxiety may require more practice trials than are normally provided before administrating this test.

Comments

The PASAT is a sensitive measure of impairments in information processing efficiency and attention/concentration even when the deficits are mild. It is appropriate for assessing most levels of cognitive impairment from mild to moderately severe. This test, which is frustrating and demanding for cognitively intact people, would not be appropriate for severely cognitively impaired patients.

DISABILITY MEASURES

Disability refers to ". . . any restriction or lack of ability to perform an activity within the range considered normal for a human being" (9). Rehabilitation makes its strongest impact in terms of influencing disability as evidenced by the hundreds of disability instruments available. Unlike impairment measures, disability measures tend to be generic and universally applied to every patient population. Most disability measures assess either ADLs or instrumental activities of daily living (IADLs). ADL instruments measure personal care activities such as dressing, eating, bathing, grooming, toileting, and mobility. IADL instruments also assess the patient's ability to adapt to the environment and include such domains as home management, money management, shopping, work, transportation, and social interactions. Determining ability to perform these activities is part of assessing overall functional status.

Barthel Index

The Barthel Index (BI) was developed by Mahoney and Barthel in 1965 to assess the functional status and mobility skills of neuromuscular and musculoskeletal patients (64). The Barthel Index is used primarily to determine functional status before and after treatment, to document treatment progress, and to indicate the amount of nursing care needed (65). It also has been used to identify patients who might be appropriate for rehabilitation.

Description

The BI is designed to assess the degree of independence a patient has in performing various self-care and mobility tasks. Each item measures a discrete ADL task function: bowels, bladder, grooming, toilet use, feeding, transfer, mobility, dressing, stairs, and bathing.

Reliability

The Barthel Index has demonstrated high test-retest reliability ($r = 0.89$) with severely disabled adults, interrater reliability ($r > 0.95$) (66), and Cronbach alpha internal consistency ($r = 0.98$) (67).

Validity

The BI has documented predictive and convergent validity. Predictive validity was demonstrated by successfully predicting mortality among stroke patients (66). Among patients who survived, intake scores predicted length of stay and rate of rehabilitation progress. Patients with a discharge BI score greater than 60 points were more likely be discharged to home (68); they were easier to manage and required less time and effort (66) than those who scored lower than 60 points (Granger's version).

Convergent validity was demonstrated by its significant correlation with another prominent disability measure, the PULSES Profile ($r = -0.74$ to 0.90) (66) (Note that the negative sign results because the two scales were inversely scored.) The BI also has documented the ability to discriminate between people with and without ADL disability and to predict level of disability (69).

In MS patients, the BI was found to be sensitive enough to detect change in the functional status of MS patients receiving inpatient rehabilitation (70). In this study the greatest functional changes occurred in MS patients with moderate and severe disability. The BI may be insensitive to improvements or gains made by mildly impaired MS patients.

Administration/Scoring

The BI can be self-administered, administered by health care professionals, or administered by telephone. It can be given to the patient, spouse, family member, or nurse, depending on who provides the most reliable information. Direct observation may be used but it is not required. Whether the ADL and mobility information is obtained from the patient or from another reliable source, the critical factor is to record what the patient does, not what the patient could do. It is realistic to allow 5–10 minutes to complete this measure.

Two versions of the original BI are now commonly used. Wade and Collin's version contains 10 ADL items and provides a total score that ranges from 0 (total dependence) to 20 (total independence) in 1-point increments (Table 13-10). Granger's version includes 15 ADL items

TABLE 13-10
The Barthel Index (Wade and Collin's Version)

BOWELS

0 = incontinent (or needs to be given enemata)
1 = occasional accident (once/week)
2 = continent

BLADDER

0 = incontinent, or catheterized and unable to manage
1 = occasional accident (max once per 24 hours)
2 = continent (for over 7 days)

GROOMING

0 = needs help with personal care
1 = independent face/hair/teeth/shaving (implements provided)

TOILET USE

0 = dependent
1 = needs some help, but can do something alone
2 = independent (on and off, dressing, wiping)

FEEDING

0 = unable
1 = needs help cutting, spreading butter, etc.
2 = independent (food provided in reach)

TRANSFER

0 = unable—no sitting balance
1 = major help (one or two people, physical), can sit
2 = minor help (verbal or physical)
3 = independent

MOBILITY

0 = immobile
1 = wheelchair independent including corners etc.
2 = walks with help of one person (verbal or physical)
3 = independent (but may use any aid, e.g., stick)

DRESSING

0 = dependent
1 = heeds help, but can do about half unaided
2 = independent (including buttons, zips, laces, etc.)

STAIRS

0 = unable
1 = needs help (verbal, physical, carrying aid)
2 = independent up and down

BATHING

0 = dependent
1 = independent (or in shower)

TOTAL (0–20)

Source: Collin C, Wade DT, Davies S, Horne V. The Barthel ADL Index: A reliability study. *International Disability Studies* 1988; 10:61–63.

and provides a total score that ranges from 0 (total dependence) to 100 (total independence) in 5-point increments (Table 13-11). The BI uses ordinal data and the weighting varies by item.

Granger and associates report that a score of 60 points is the cutoff point between independence and some dependence (66). They further state that a score between 40 and 20 points indicates severe dependence, whereas a score of 20 or below indicates total mobility and self-care dependence.

Advantages

The BI is a reliable and valid instrument of ADLs and mobility. It is simple to administer and easy to score because of its metric-like rating system (71,72). The BI includes bowel and bladder functioning items, which some other ADL measures have overlooked.

Disadvantages

The BI is not an ordered scale and the weights attributed to each item are somewhat arbitrary. Changes by a given number of points do not reflect equivalent changes in ADL function across different activities (65).

The BI has also been criticized for its definite ceiling effect (66). Changes at higher levels of functioning are not detected or measured by the BI (65). It is, however, sensitive enough to detect when a patient first needs personal assistance, which makes it a very useful clinical measure (72).

Although the number of ADL domains accessed appears to be adequate, specific subscale behaviors are not included. For example, dressing is one domain that is appraised in the original version. In Granger's version, upper and lower extremity dressing were evaluated separately, thus providing the assessor with additional information. Similarly, some of the items (transfers, feeding, toileting, and dressing) may be interpreted differently by different raters (73). Again, in referring to the dressing item, dressing is difficult because "half" could be interpreted as meaning that upper or lower half of the body is unaided, or half the effort and needs help with both halves. Most of the major disadvantages of this instrument are overcome by following the Barthel ADL Index Guidelines (Table 13-12).

Comments

The BI is one of the best known, highly recommended, and commonly used ADL instruments. It is best suited for assessing and monitoring various disabled populations, including MS patients. It is sensitive enough to detect when a patient first needs personal assistance and is best suited

TABLE 13-11
Barthel Index (Granger'sVersion)

INDEPENDENT		DEPENDENT		
INTACT	LIMITED	HELPER	NULL	ACTIVITY
10	5	1	1	Drink from cup/feed from dish
5	5	3	0	Dress upper body
5	5	2	0	Dress lower body
0	0	−2	0	Don brace or prosthesis
5	5	0	0	Grooming
4	4	0	0	Wash or bathe
10	10	5	0	Bladder continence
10	10	5	0	Bowel continence
4	4	2	0	Care perineum/cloth at toilet
15	15	7	0	Transfer, chair
6	5	3		Transfer, toilet
1	1	0	0	Transer, tub or shower
15	15	10	0	Walk on level 50 yards or more
10	10	5	0	Up and down stairs, 1 flight
15	5	0	0	Wheelchair/50 yds—if not walking
				Barthel Total Score

Source: Granger CV. Health accounting—functional assessment of the long-term patient. In: Kottke FJ, Stillwell GK, Lehmann JF (eds.). *Krusen's handbook of physical medicine and rehabilitation.* Philadelphia: WBSaunders, 1982.

for MS patients with moderate to severe disability. It is intended to provide only a brief assessment of the primary ADLs and mobility functions. It has been criticized for being too narrow in focus (65,74) and for not assessing such areas as general health status, communication skills, or psychosocial status (66). However, it is important to remember that it measures what it is designed and intended to measure. If more health status information is needed, comprehensive measures such as the Sickness Impact Profile and the Short Form-36 are available.

Incapacity Status Scale

The Incapacity Status Scale (ISS) was developed by Kurtzke (75) and Granger (76) to assess the physical limitations caused by MS that effect one's ability to perform ADLs. The ISS was derived from the PULSES Profile and the Barthel Index.

Description

This 16-item questionnaire assesses the functional status of MS patients on a 4-point Likert scale (0 = normal to 4 = loss of function) (Table 13-13). The 16 functional disability areas are stair climbing, ambulation, transfers, bowel function, bladder function, bathing, dressing, grooming, feeding, vision, speech and hearing, medical problems, mood and thought disturbances, mentation, fatigability, and sexual function. The first nine items assess the level of assistance needed to perform ADLs. The total ISS score primarily represents mobility status and level of independence in performing ADLs.

Reliability

The ISS has documented high internal consistency reliability ranging from a Cronbach's alpha of 0.86 (77) to a Cronbach's alpha of 0.93 (21). High ICC of 0.94 (21), and ICC values above 0.70 for most of the ISS items (78) also have been reported.

Validity

The construct validity of the ISS has been demonstrated by its high correlation with other standardized measures of disability and impairment. For example, the correlation between the ISS and the Disability Status Scale was $r = 0.81$ (7). The correlation between the ISS and the Long-Range Evaluation System was $r = 0.87$ (75). Support for the predictive validity of the ISS comes from the moderate correlation between the ISS and the number of hours of home assistance needed ($r = 0.74$) (79).

TABLE 13-12
The Barthel ADL Index Guidelines

1. The Index should be used as a record of what a patient does, NOT as a record of what a patient could do.
2. The main aim is to establish degree of independence from any help, physical or verbal, however minor and for whatever reason.
3. The need for supervision renders the patient NOT independent.
4. A patient's performance should be established using the best available evidence. Asking the patient, friends/relatives and nurses will be the usual source, but direct observation and common sense are also important. However, direct testing is not needed.
5. Usually the performance over the preceding 24–48* hours is important, but occasionally longer periods will be relevant.
6. Unconscious patients should score "0" throughout, even if not yet incontinent.
7. Middle categories imply that patient supplies over 50% of the effort.
8. Use of aids to be independent is allowed.

Bowels (preceding week)
If needs enema from nurse, then "incontinent."* Occasional = once a week.

Bladder (preceding 24–48 hours)
Occasional = less than once a day.
A catheterized patient who can completely manage the catheter alone is registered as "continent."

Grooming (preceding 24–48 hours)
Refers to personal hygiene: brushing teeth, fitting false teeth, doing hair, shaving, washing face.
Implements* can be provided by helper.

Toilet use
Should be able to reach toilet/commode, undress sufficiently, clean self, dress, and leave.
With help = can wipe self and do some other of above.*

Feeding
Able to eat any normal food (not only soft food). Food cooked and served by others. But not cut up.
Help = food cut up, patient feeds self.*

Transfer
From bed to chair and back. Dependent = No sitting balance (unable to sit); two people to lift.
Major help = one strong/skilled or two normal people. Can sit up. Minor help = one person easily OR needs any supervision for safety.

Mobility
Refers to mobility about house or ward, indoors. May use aid. If in wheelchair, must negotiate corners/doors unaided.
Help = by one, untrained person, including supervision/moral support.

Dressing
Should be able to select and put on all clothes, which may be adapted. Half = help with buttons, zips, etc., but can put on some garments alone.*

Stairs
Must carry any walking aid used to be independent.

Bathing
Usually the most difficult activity. Must get in and out unsupervised and wash self. Independent in shower = "independent" if unsupervised/unaided.*

* = items added or modified after study; asterisk at end, whole item added; asterisk in middle, phrase added or clarified.
Source: Collin C, Wade DT, Davies S, Horne V. The Barthel ADL Index: A reliability study. *International Disability Studies* 1988; 10:61–63.

TABLE 13-13
Incapacity Status Scale

1. **Stair Climbing** (Ability to ascend a flight of stairs of about 12 steps)

    0—Normal
    1—Some difficulty but performed
    2—Need for canes, braces, prostheses, or dependent upon banister to perform
    3—Need human assistance to perform
    4—Unable to perform; includes mechanical lifts

2. **Ambulation** (Ability to walk on level ground or indoors some 50 meters without rest)

    0—Normal
    1—Some difficulty but performed without aid
    2—Need for canes, braces, prostheses to perform
    3—Need for human assistance or use of manual wheelchair, which patient enters, leaves, and maneuvers without aid
    4—Unable to perform; includes perambulation in a wheelchair and motorized wheelchair

3. **Toilet/Chair/Bed Transfer** (Ability to enter and leave regular toilet and/or chair and/or bed; includes wheelchair transfer as indicated. The worst transfer function determines the grade)

    0—Normal
    1—Some difficulty but performed without aid
    2—Need for adaptive or assistive devices such as trapeze, sling, bars, lift, sliding board to perform
    3—Requires human aid to perform
    4—Must be lifted or moved about completely by another person

4. **Bowel Function**

    0—Normal
    1—Bowel retention not requiring more than high fibre diets, laxatives, occasional enemas or suppositories, self-administered
    2—Bowel retention requiring regular laxatives, enemas or suppositories, self-administered in order to induce evacuation; cleanses and disimpacts self
    3—Bowel retention requiring enemas or suppositories administered by another; disimpacted by another; needs assistance in cleansing; occasional incontinence; presence of colostomy tended by self
    4—Frequent soiling due either to incontinence or a poorly maintained ostomy device, which patient cannot maintain without assistance

5. **Bathing**

    0—Normal
    1—Some difficulty with washing and drying self though performed without aid whether in tub or shower or by sponge-bathing, whichever is usual for the patient
    2—Need for assistive devices (trapeze, sling, lift, shower or tub bar) in order to bathe self; need to bathe self outside of tub or shower if that is the usual method
    3—Need for human assistance in bathing parts of the body or in entry/exit/positioning in tub or shower
    4—Bathing performed by others (aside from face and hands)

6. **Dressing**

    0—Normal
    1—Some difficulty clothing self completely in standard garments, but accomplished by self
    2—Specially adapted clothing (special closures, elastic-laced shoes, front closing garments) or devices (long shoe horns, zipper extenders) required to dress self
    3—Need for human aid to accomplish; performs considerable portion him/herself
    4—Need for almost complete assistance, unable to dress self

TABLE 13-13
continued

7. **Grooming** (Care of teeth or dentures and hair, shaving, or application of cosmetics)

0—Normal
1—Some difficulty but all tasks performed without aid
2—Need for adaptive devices (electric razors or toothbrushes, special combs or brushes, arm rests or slings) but performed without aid
3—Need for human aid to perform some of the tasks
4—Almost all tasks performed by another person

8. **Feeding** (Ingestion, mastication, swallowing of solids and liquids, and manipulation of the appropriate utensils)

0—Normal
1—Some difficulty but performed without aid
2—Need for adaptive devices (special feeding)
3—Need for human aid in the delivery of food; dysphagia preventing solid diet; esophagostomy or gastrostomy maintained and utilized by self; tube-feeding performed by self
4—Unable to feed self or to manage ostomies

9. **Vision** (Rate of the basis of the worse of either visual acuity or double vision)

0—Normal vision. Can read print finer than standard newsprint with corrective lenses
1—Cannot read print finer than standard newsprint with corrective lenses or complains of double vision
2—Magnifying lenses or large print necessary for reading or double vision interferes with function
3—Can only read very large print such as major newspaper headlines
4—Legal blindness

10. **Speech and Hearing** (Verbal output and input for interpersonal communication purposes)

0—Normal; no subjective hearing loss; articulation and language appropriate to the culture
1—Impaired hearing or articulation not interfering with communication
2—Deafness sufficient to require hearing aid and/or dysarthria interfering with communication. Needs communication aids such as special keyboards, etc.
3—Severe deafness compensated for by sign language or lip reading facility and/or severe dysarthria compensated for by sign language or self-written communication
4—Severe deafness and/or dysarthria without effective compensation

11. **Medical Problems** (Presence of general medical and/or neurological and/or orthopedic disorders; this includes MS and related problems such as decubiti, contractures, and urinary tract infections)

0—No significant disorder present
1—Disorder(s) not requiring active care; may be on maintenance medication; monitoring not required more often than every three months
2—Disorder(s) requiring occasional monitoring by physician or nurse, more often than every three months but less often than weekly
3—Disorder(s) requiring regular attention (at least weekly) by physician or nurse
4—Disorder(s) requiring essentially daily attention by physician of nurse, usually in hospital

12. **Mood and Thought Disturbances** (This includes anxiety, depression, mood swings, euphoria, delusions, hallucinations, and thought disorder. The rating should reflect current behavior even if the patient is maintained on medication)

0—No observable problem
1—Disturbance is present at times, but does not interfere with day-to-day functioning
2—Disturbance does interfere with day-to-day functioning, but the person can manage without professional assistance except for occasional visits to maintain medication
3—Disturbance interferes with day-to-day functioning and consistently requires professional intervention beyond that required to maintain medication; e.g., requires psychotherapy or hospitalization
4—Despite medication and/or other intervention, disturbance is severe enough to preclude day-to-day functioning

TABLE 13-13
continued

14. Mentation (Disturbance in memory, reasoning, calculation, judgment, or orientation)

0—No observable problem

1—Disturbance is present but does not interfere with performance of everyday activities

2—Disturbance interferes with performance of everyday activities; the person may need to use lists or other prompting devices, but manages without the help of other people; the person is likely to be a poor historian

3—Disturbance is severe enough to require prompting or assistance from others for performance of everyday activities

4—Disturbance precludes the performance of most everyday activities; may include severe confusion, disorientation, or memory loss

15. Fatigability (This is a sense of overwhelming weakness or lassitude, which dramatically alters baseline motor and coordination (occasionally visual or sensory) functions. It may be transient or persistent for hours or even days, and occurs at varying frequency; a very common complaint in MS)

0—No fatigability

1—Fatigability present but does not notably interfere with baseline physical function

2—Fatigability causing intermittent and generally transient impairment of baseline physical function

3—Fatigability causing intermittent transient loss or frequent moderate impairment of baseline physical function

4—Fatigability that generally prevents prolonged or sustained physical function

16. Sexual Function

0—Sexually active as before and/or not experiencing some sexual problems. (No changes in patient's usual pattern of sexual activity; for example, no change in frequency and type of sex activities; and no changes in previous genital sensations, erections, and ejaculation in men, and vaginal lubrication and orgasm in women. This includes persons without previous sexual experience or who are voluntarily celibate.

Source: International Federation of Multiple Sclerosis Societies. *M.R.D. Minimal record of disability of multiple sclerosis*. New York: National Multiple Sclerosis Society, 1985.

Administration/Scoring

The ISS can be administered in 20 to 30 minutes by a trained health care professional or volunteer (7) and is appropriate for both inpatient and outpatient use. The ISS has been successfully administered by telephone (80) and has been self-administered when the patient is not severely cognitively impaired (78).

To score the ISS, the 16 item scores are totaled and will range from 0 to 64, with a low score indicating normal function and a high score indicating impairment or loss of function. It is worth noting that some researchers have analyzed ISS items separately, have eliminated items, and have divided ISS items into subscales based on factor analysis. When lower reliability items have been removed, the ISS is basically the same test as the Barthel Index with one additional item—speech/hearing (14). When analyzing ISS subscales separately, factors 1 and 2 (mobility and ADLs) have enough items to represent those constructs. Depending on the study, the third factor has either been bowel/bladder (14) or fatigue, psychic function, and physical problems (21).

Advantages

The ISS is a short, standardized measure of mobility and self-care. Compared with the BI, the ISS is generally more descriptive and provides additional information about fatigue, vision, speech/hearing, sexual functioning, mood, social interaction, and cognitive status.

Disadvantages

The ISS has been criticized for its emphasis on mobility and self-care (11,21). Examination of the item-total correlations suggests that mobility and self-care form a single dimension, which accounts for a good deal of the variance in total scores. The items whose content are unrelated to mobility and self-care have lower item-total correlations and may actually be part of a different dimension not adequately assessed by this instrument (i.e., fatigue, psychic function, and physical problems items).

The ISS has been criticized by Sharrack and Hughes (11) because the individual items were not sensitive enough to detect minor changes in clinical status. However, individual items should not be analyzed separately because they generally are less reliable and less sensitive to change. The high Cronbach's alpha (0.93) indicates that one homogeneous dimension underlies the items in a summed score and thus supports the use of summed total score on this scale.

Comments

When used and analyzed correctly, the ISS is a reliable and valid measure of mobility and self-care. It is an adequate test when used as a whole, but the third dimension of the test (fatigue, psychic function, and physical problems items) is weak and not sufficiently represented. The best attributes of the ISS, the mobility and self-care items, are essentially the same as the BI. Thus this author recommends using the BI instead of the ISS.

Functional Independence Measure

The Functional Independence Measure (FIM™) was developed by the American Academy of Physical Medicine and Rehabilitation and the American Congress of Rehabilitation Medicine (81). Originally derived from the Barthel Index, it is currently the most widely used and accepted measure of disability (82). It was specifically designed only for inpatient use. It is appropriate for screening, formal assessment, case management monitoring, and program evaluation of all types of rehabilitation inpatients (83).

Description

The FIM assesses the amount of assistance required to perform a variety of ADLs (Table 13-14). In measuring disability in this way, the FIM reflects the burden of care and the cost of disability (83). The FIM contains two subscales—motor function and cognitive function. The first 13 items on the FIM represent the motor function subscale and assess the following domains: self-care, sphincter control, transfers, and locomotion. The last five items represent the cognitive function subscale and relate to communication and social cognition. The FIM contains 18 items on a 7-point Likert scale (7 = completely independent to 1 = total assistance).

Reliability

Several studies have examined the reliability of the FIM and were summarized in a 1996 FIM review article (82). Reliability values were calculated across 11 studies and results revealed a median interrater reliability for the total FIM of 0.95 and a median test-retest reliability value of

0.95. The median reliability values for the six FIM subscales ranged from 0.95 for Self-Care to 0.78 for Social Cognition. These results are based on a large sample (1,568 patients) with a wide variety of disability levels and medical conditions.

Validity

In a recent MS study, the FIM was found to be highly correlated with other measures of disability (Barthel Index), and impairment (Environmental Status Scale) (84). Separate regressions of the measures resulted in R^2 values that were both above 0.81 ($p < 0.01$). All measures were found to be predictive of the burden of care as measured in minutes of assistance provided per day with an $R^2 = 0.78$ for the FIM ($p < 0.001$) In another MS study, the FIM was found to be sensitive or responsive enough to detect changes in people with progressive MS receiving inpatient rehabilitation (85).

Administration/Scoring

The FIM is designed to be administered by any trained clinician, regardless of discipline. Uniform Data System for Medical Rehabilitation offers a variety of training programs and conducts a two-stage credentialing process to ensure that facilities using the FIM are collecting data properly. The FIM generally requires less than 40 minutes to administer by either conference, observation, or telephone interview. The administrator must respond to each item and select the response that best describes the patient's current level of function. The item responses range from a high score of 7 (complete independence) to a low of 1 (total assistance). The highest total score is 126 and the lowest total score is 18. The guide for use of the Uniform Data Set, including the FIM, is also available (Dr. Carl Granger, UDSMR, SUNY at Buffalo, 232 Parker Hall, 3435 Main Street, Buffalo, NY 14214-3007). More information about the FIM is obtainable at: http://www.udsmr.org/products.htm.

Advantages

In summarizing the global merits of the FIM, Granger and Brownscheidle state, "The FIM helps quantify disability to discriminate between classes of subjects living in the community rather than in a nursing home or predict the cost of managing a person with disability if there is not further improvement. Furthermore, the FIM is evaluative, permitting one to detect clinically important change when it occurs" (83, p. 265).

Compared with the ISS, the FIM distinguishes between bladder and bowel function, separates bathing and transferring items, and includes perineal hygiene.

TABLE 13-14
Functional Independence Measure (FIM)

FIM™ instrument

Functional Independence Measure

LEVELS		
	7 Complete Independence (Timely, Safely) 6 Modified Independence (Device)	**NO HELPER**
	Modified Dependence 5 Supervision (Subject = 100%+) 4 Minimal Assist (Subject = 75%+) 3 Moderate Assist (Subject = 50%+) **Complete Dependence** 2 Maximal Assist (Subject =25%+) 1 Total Assist (Subject = less than 25%)	**HELPER**

	ADMISSION	DISCHARGE	FOLLOW-UP
Self-Care A. Eating B. Grooming C. Bathing D. Dressing - Upper Body E. Dressing - Lower Body F. Toileting	☐☐☐☐☐☐	☐☐☐☐☐☐	☐☐☐☐☐☐
Sphincter Control G. Bladder Management H. Bowel Management	☐☐	☐☐	☐☐
Transfers I. Bed, Chair, Wheelchair J. Toilet K. Tub, Shower	☐☐☐	☐☐☐	☐☐☐
Locomotion L. Walk/Wheelchair M. Stairs	☐☐ W Walk / C Wheelchair / B Both	☐☐ W Walk / C Wheelchair / B Both	☐☐ W Walk / C Wheelchair / B Both
Motor Subtotal Score	☐	☐	☐
Communication N. Comprehension O. Expression	☐☐ A Auditory / V Visual / B Both / V Vocal / N Nonvocal / B Both	☐☐ A Auditory / V Visual / B Both / V Vocal / N Nonvocal / B Both	☐☐ A Auditory / V Visual / B Both / V Vocal / N Nonvocal / B Both
Social Cognition P. Social Interaction Q. Problem Solving R. Memory	☐☐☐	☐☐☐	☐☐☐
Cognitive Subtotal Score	☐	☐	☐
TOTAL FIM Score	☐	☐	☐

NOTE: Leave no blanks; enter 1 if patient not testable due to risk

Source: Granger CV. UDSMR, SUNY at Buffalo, 232 Parker Hall, 3435 Main Street, Buffalo, NY 14214-3007.

These distinctions make the FIM more precise and more sensitive (84).

With MS patients, the FIM was found to be the best measure for assessing physical care needs as measured in minutes of assistance provided per day by another person in the home (84). The comparison measures used in this study were the Incapacity Status Scale, the Environmental Status Scale, and the Barthel Index.

Disadvantages

The ordinal nature of FIM data and the generic nature of the questions make this questionnaire particularly prone to ceiling and floor effects. The FIM was specifically designed for moderate to severely disabled inpatients, so it does not adequately assess less impaired patient populations. The FIM has been criticized for its lack of MS specificity—it does not include common MS symptoms such as fatigue, vision, and sexual dysfunction (86)—and for its lack of MS sensitivity. Although there is some evidence to suggest that the FIM is a sensitive measure (85), the sensitivity of this measure for MS patients is still being questioned, and further investigation is needed to resolve this argument.

Comment

The FIM is the gold standard disability measure and currently is the best comprehensive evaluation and outcomes monitor for all patient populations receiving inpatient rehabilitation. It is one of the best measures for assessing the physical and functional care needs of MS patients with moderate to severe disabilities.

HANDICAP MEASURES

The WHO defines handicap as ". . . a disadvantage for a given individual that limits or prevents the fulfillment of a role that is normal for that individual" (9) and is determined by comparing the expectations of the specific individual to the reference group's expectations within the same cultural, social, economic, and physical environment. The handicap domains assessed by the WHO include orientation, mobility, physical dependence, economic self-sufficiency, occupation, and social integration. It is important to realize that environmental factors, such as social expectations, prejudices, the legal system, family support, the physical environment, and financial matters, play a major role in determining handicap (52,87). This point becomes especially critical when assessing handicap measures. For example, some handicap measures may rate the patient as more handicapped if the physical environment has been changed to include adaptive equipment such as grab bars or hand controls. However, if the adaptive equipment allows the person to continue performing his or her normal family role, the person should be given a lower handicap rating.

In evaluating handicap measures, one should keep in mind Stewart's definition of a good handicap measure: "Any scale attempting to be a valid measure of handicap in neurorehabilitation must incorporate in its design an allowance for consideration of an individual patient's circumstances, including previous lifestyle and roles. It should be clear in its distinction between disability and handicap, cover those areas of handicap targeted for change in the rehabilitation process, and must be sensitive to any changes which may occur" (87, p. 314).

Environmental Status Scale (ESS)

The Environmental Status Scale (ESS) was based on the Socio-Economic Scale developed by Mellerup and associates (88).

Description

The ESS consists of seven items on a 0 (no handicap) to 5 (significant handicap) Likert scale (Table 13-15). The handicap dimensions assessed on this scale are work status, financial/economic status, personal residence or home, personal assistance, transportation, community assistance, and social activity.

Reliability

The ESS has documented high internal consistency reliability (Cronbach's alpha = 0.83) (7). Two studies have examined the interrater reliability of the ESS using ICC. Physician-patient agreement was above 0.70 for most of the ESS items (78). Interrater reliability made independently by two neurologists was $r = 0.97$ for the ESS (7).

Validity

To accurately assess the concurrence of the ESS, it should be compared with another handicap measure, not with impairment and disability measures. The ESS was found to be significantly correlated with the Disability Status Scale, an impairment measure, ($r = 0.76$) (12,13); with the FIM and Barthel Index (disability measures); and predictive of physical care needs (84). The ESS was also found to be sensitive enough to detect change in handicap status in 44 percent of MS patients receiving inpatient rehabilitation (70). Although researchers criticize the ESS for its "lack of sensitivity," they also admit that handicap changes may be influenced by short rehabilitation stay and not having enough time to change the home environment before discharge.

TABLE 13-15
Environmental Status Scale (ESS)

1. Actual work status

0—normal or retired (e.g., full-time worker, homemaker, student)
1—works full time but in a less demanding position
2—works more than half time at job, housework, or school
3—works between one-quarter and one-half time at job, housework, or school
4—works less than one-quarter time at job, housework, or school
5—unemployed, not able to do housework or to attend school

2. Financial/economic status

0—no MS-related financial problems
1—family maintains usual financial standard without external support; some financial disadvantages resulting from MS
2—family maintains usual financial standard with aid of some external financial support
3—family maintains usual financial standard by receiving basic disability pension as defined in location of residence
4—family maintains usual financial standard only because receiving all available financial assistance
5—family unable to maintain usual financial standard despite receipt of all available financial assistance

3. Personal residence/home

0—no change necessary
1—minor modification necessary
2—moderate modification necessary
3—major structural alteration or addition necessary
4—must move to satisfactory personal home
5—must live in a facility for dependent care because unable to continue any personal home (institutionalized)

4. Personal assistance required

0—none
1—minor help: relatives involved but personal independence is maintained
2—requires assistance for activities of daily living up to 1 hour per day from relative or others in the home
3—requires assistance for activities of daily living up to 3 hours per day from relatives or others in the home
4—requires more than 3 hours of personal assistance per day, but is able to live at home and does not need a constant attendant
5—requires a constant attendant or care in an institution, i.e., cannot be left alone for more than short periods such as 2–3 hours

5. Transportation

0—uses public transport with no problems, or drives
1—uses all forms of transport available despite minor difficulties, or drives with minor difficulty, e.g., needs handicap parking
2—uses some public transport despite difficulties, or needs hand controls to drive
3—cannot use public transport but can use private transport, cannot drive but may be driven by others
4—requires community (public or private agency) transport in a wheelchair
5—requires ambulance

6. Community services

0—none required
1—requires service only once per month or less frequently
2—requires not more than 1 hour per week
3—requires not more than average of 1 hour per day
4—requires 1–4 hours per day
5—requires more than 4 hours per day or institutionalized

TABLE 13-15
continued

7. Social activity

   0—socially active as before with no changes in the usual pattern of social activity, and no difficulty maintaining this pattern
   1—maintains usual pattern of social activity despite some difficulties
   2—some restrictions on social activity such as change in type or frequency of some activities or increased dependence on others
   3—significant restrictions on social activity; largely dependent on actions of others but still able to initiate some activity
   4—socially inactive except for the initiative of others
   5—no social activity; does not see friends or family; social contact is limited to that provided by community service providers, e.g., visiting nurse

Source: Stewart G, Kidd D, Thompson AJ. The assessment of handicap: An evaluation of the Environmental Status Scale. *Disability and Rehabilitation* 1995; 17:312–316.

Administration/Scoring

The original version of the ESS, which was developed by The International Federation of Multiple Sclerosis Societies, was based on a structured interview and reflected the worst level of handicap over time rather than the present situation. For rehabilitation outcome purposes, it is more appropriate to assess the patient's current handicap functioning, thus determining whether the intervention alters handicap. The ESS has been self-administered (78) and administered in an unstructured interview setting (87).

The structured interview and the instructions for scoring the ESS are included in the International Federation of Multiple Sclerosis Societies' *Minimal Record of Disability Handbook* (7). It requires 5–10 minutes to complete (87). A total handicap score is obtained by summing each item, which is scored from 0 to 5. Total scores range from 0 (no social handicap) to 35 (maximal handicap).

Advantages

The ESS is a reliable and valid measure and is the first MS-specific handicap instrument. It is short, simple to administer, and easy to score; it can be administered by a trained professional or volunteer.

Disadvantages

In a critical review of the ESS, Stewart and colleagues point out that because the ESS was developed from a socioeconomic measure, it represents a measure of current socioeconomic status rather than handicap (87). For example, the transportation item assesses type of transportation versus a person's ability to reach a desired destination. On the ESS, handicap is rated high when a person uses financial support, personal assistance, community services, or adap-

tative equipment. If the use of adaptative equipment allows a person to function or complete a desired social role, handicap should be rated low. Thus the use of services, assistance, and adaptative equipment may actually help decrease handicap rather than representing increased handicap as it does on the ESS.

Comment

The ESS was the first MS-specific handicap scale that primarily measured current socioeconomic status rather than handicap. It has not been widely accepted as a rehabilitation or clinical trials outcome measure in MS and will probably be replaced by the London Handicap Scale.

London Handicap Scale

The London Handicap Scale (LHS), developed by Harwood and associates, is a new handicap measure for chronic diseases (89).

Description

The LHS assesses the six handicap dimensions outlined by the WHO model—mobility, physical independence, occupation, social integration, orientation, and economic self-sufficiency (Table 13-16). It focuses on how the patient's health affects everyday life. It consists of only six items, with each item representing a handicap domain.

Reliability

The original reliability and validity study was conducted with 361 stroke inpatients (89). Longitudinal data on the 170 survivors were obtained 12 months after hospital dis-

TABLE 13-16
The London Handicap Scale

This questionnaire asks six questions about your everyday life. Please answer each question. Tick the box next to the sentence that describes you best. Think about things you have done over the last week. Compare what you can do with what someone like you who is in good health can do.

Getting around (mobility)
Think about how you get from one place to another, using any help, aids or means of transport that you normally have available.

Does your health stop you from getting around:
1. Not at all: You go everywhere you want to, no matter how far away.
2. Very slightly: You go most places you want to, but not all.
3. Quite a lot: You get out of the house, but not far away from it.
4. Very much: You don't go outside, but you can move around from room to room indoors.
5. Almost completely: You are confined to a single room, but can move around in it.
6. Completely: You are confined to a bed or a chair. You can not move around at all. There is no one to move you.

Looking after yourself (physical independence)
Think about things like housework, shopping, looking after money, cooking, laundry, getting dressed, washing, shaving and using the toilet.

Does your health stop you looking after yourself?
1. Not at all: You can doe everything yourself.
2. Very slightly: Now and again you need to little help.
3. Quite a lot: You need help with some tasks (such as heavy housework or shopping), but no more than once a day.
4. Very much: You can do some things but you need help more than once a day. You can be left alone safely for a few hours.
5. Almost completely: You need help to be available all the time. You can not be left alone safely.
6. Completely: You need help with everything. You need constant attention, day and night.

Work and Leisure (occupation)
Think about things like work (paid or not), housework, gardening, sports, hobbies, going out with friends, traveling, reading, looking after children, watching television and going on holiday.

Does your health limit your work or leisure activities?
1. Not at all: You can do everything you want to do.
2. Very slightly: You can do almost all the things you want to do.
3. Quite a lot: You find something to do almost all the time, but can not do some things for as long as you would like.
4. Very much: You are unable to do a lot of things, but can find something to do most of the time.
5. Almost completely: You are unable to do most things, but can find something to do some of the time.
6. Completely: You sit all day doing nothing. You can not keep yourself busy or take part in any activities.

Getting on with people (social integration)
Think about family, friends, and people you might meet during a normal day.

Does your health stop you getting on with people?
1. Not at all: You get on well with people, see everyone you want to see, and meet new people.
2. Very slightly: You get on well with people, but your social life is slightly limited.
3. Quite a lot: You are fine with people you know well, but feel uncomfortable with strangers.
4. Very much: You are fine with people you know well, but you have few friends and little contact with neighbors. Dealing with strangers is very hard.
5. Almost completely: Apart from the person who looks after you, you see no one. You have no friends and no visitors.
6. Completely: You don't get on with anyone, not even people who look after you.

TABLE 13-16
continued

Awareness of your surrounds (orientation)
Think about taking in and understanding the world around you, and finding your way around in it.

Does your health stop you understanding the world around you?
1. Not at all: You fully understand the world around you. You see, hear, speak, and think clearly, and your memory is good.
2. Very slightly: You have problems with hearing, speaking, seeing or your memory, but these do not stop you doing most things.
3. Quite a lot: You have problems with hearing, speaking, seeing, or your memory, which make life difficult a lot of the time. But, you understand what is going on.
4. Very much: You have great difficulty understanding what is going on.
5. Almost completely: You are unable to tell where you are or what day it is. You can not look after yourself at all.
6. Completely: You are unconscious, completely unaware of anything going on around you.

Affording the things you need (economic self-sufficiency)
Think about whether health problems have led to any extra expenses, or have caused you to earn less than you would if you were healthy.

Are you able to afford the things you need?
1. Yes, easily: You can afford everything you need. You have easily enough money to buy modern labor-saving devices, and anything you may need because of ill-health.
2. Fairly easily: You have just about enough money. It is fairly easy to copy with expenses caused by ill-health.
3. Just about: You are less well-off than other people like you; however, with sacrifices you can get by without help.
4. Not really: You only have enough money to meet your basic needs. You are dependent on state benefits for any extra expenses you have because of ill-health.
5. No: You are dependent on state benefits, or money from other people or charities. You can not afford things you need.
6. Absolutely not: You have no money at all and no state benefits. You are totally dependent on charity for your most basic needs.

Source: Harwood RH, Gompertz SE, Ebrahim S. Handicap one year after a stroke: Validity of a new scale. *Journal of Neurology, Neurosurgery, and Psychiatry* 1994; 57:825–829. (Copied with permission from the Medical Outcomes Trust.)

charge. The LHS has documented high test-retest reliability (Pearson r = 0.91) (89).

Validity

Construct validity was assessed by comparing the LHS with the Nottingham Health Profile (NHP) and the BI (89). The LHS was moderately correlated with the NHP (r = 0.69) and Barthel Index (r = 0.56) respectively. In an MS study, the LHS was sensitive enough to detect handicap changes following inpatient rehabilitation of progressive MS patients compared with MS controls who did not receive rehabilitation (85).

Administration/Scoring

This short and simple measure can be completed by the patient within a few minutes. The item responses are on a 6-point Likert scale ranging from 1 (no handicap) to 6 (extreme handicap). However, the overall score ranges from 1 (no handicap) to 0 (maximum handicap) because the matrix of scale weights enables the severity of disadvantages in each dimension to be combined. Harwood and coworkers (90) present the model for calculating the severity of handicap as:

$$\text{Handicap} = 0.456 + u_m + u_{pi} + u_{oc} + u_{si} + u_{or} + u_{ess}$$

The constant, 0.456, is added to the utility weights for each item and presented in Table 13-17. The scoring manual for the LHS is available from the Medical Outcomes Trust (91).

Advantages

The LHS is a simple, short measure that covers all the dimensions of handicap outlined in the WHO definition. It is a standardized measure that has been well received by the MS research community and will most likely replace the ESS.

TABLE 13-17
London Handicap Scale—Utility Weights

	PART UTILITY ASSOCIATED WITH LEVEL OF DISADVANTAGE*					
	1	2	3	4	5	6
Mobility ("getting around")	0.071	0.038	0.000	−0.036	−0.072	−0.108
Physical independence ("looking after yourself")	0.102	0.011	−0.021	−0.053	−0.057	−0.061
Occupation ("work and leisure")	0.099	−0.004	−0.014	−0.024	−0.035	−0.060
Social integration ("getting on with people")	0.063	−0.035	−0.007	−0.022	0.029	−0.041
Orientation ("awareness of your surroundings")	0.109	−0.008	−0.038	−0.051	−0.063	−0.075
Economic self-sufficiency ("affording the things you need")	0.100	0.067	0.033	−0.023	−0.067	−0.111

* 1 = no disadvantage, 6 = the most severe disadvantage
Source: RH, Rogers A, Dickinson E, Ebrahim S. Measuring handicap: The London handicap scale, a new outcome measure for chronic disease. *Quality in Health Care* 1994; 3:11–16.

Disadvantages

The LHS has been criticized for being a society-perceived rather than a patient-perceived handicap measure (92). In defense of this argument, Harwood was following the WHO definition of handicap, which is based on the social and environmental disadvantages that result from the underlying impairment and disability.

It is difficult to draw conclusions about the construct validity of the LHS when compared with a disability instrument (Barthel Index) and a quality of life measure (NHP). In assessing the convergent validity of the LHS, it should be compared with other measures of handicap. Research indicates that there is only a general or non-specific relationship between impairment, disability, and handicap (52,93). Reducing disability through rehabilitation may or may not impact impairment or handicap.

Comments

Although this is a fairly recent measure, whose first reliability and validity study results look promising, additional psychometric testing is needed. It does appear to be a very useful addition to the few measures of handicap that are already available.

HEALTH-RELATED QUALITY OF LIFE INSTRUMENTS

One of the most dramatic changes in the health care field in the last decade has been a shift from doctor-oriented to patient-oriented outcomes. Patients' perceptions of their own physical and psychosocial functioning has became a central theme in the development of the new multidimensional health-related quality of life (HRQOL) instruments. These comprehensive instruments generally incorporate physical, psychological, and social components into a single measure and try to assess the impact of an illness from the patient's perspective.

The Sickness Impact Profile

The Sickness Impact Profile (SIP) is a well-known, highly recommended, generic health status questionnaire. It was first developed in 1976 (94) and was revised in 1981 (95) as a measure of perceived health status. The SIP has been used to fulfill a variety of needs, including outcome measure, health survey, program planning, policy formulation, and monitoring patient progress. It was designed to be broadly applicable across types and severities of illness and across demographic and cultural subgroups (95).

Description

The SIP contains 136 behavioral items that describe changes in a person's behavior or performance because of an illness (Table 13-18). It measures two broad health status domains, physical and psychosocial functioning, and covers 12 content areas—work, recreation, emotion, affect, home life, sleep, rest, eating, ambulation, mobility, communication, and social interaction. The respondents mark items or statements that apply to them on a given day and are related to their health. The British version of the SIP, the Functional Limitations Profile (FLP), contains all the items of the SIP, but the wording of some the items have been changed (96).

TABLE 13-18
Sickness Impact Profile

Check *only* those statements that you are sure describe you today and are related to your state of health.

Sleep and Rest Subscale

_____ 1. I spend much of the day lying down in order to rest.
_____ 2. I sit during much of the day.
_____ 3. I am sleeping or dozing most of the time—day and night.
_____ 4. I lie down more often during the day in order to rest.
_____ 5. I sit around half asleep.
_____ 6. I sleep less at night, for example, wake up too early, don't fall asleep for a long time, awaken frequently.
_____ 7. I sleep or nap more during the day.

Emotion Subscale

_____ 1. I say how bad or useless I am, for example, that I am a burden to others.
_____ 2. I laugh or cry suddenly.
_____ 3. I often moan and groan in pain and discomfort.
_____ 4. I have attempted suicide.
_____ 5. I act nervous or restless.
_____ 6. I keep rubbing or holding areas of my body that hurt or are uncomfortable.
_____ 7. I act irritable and impatient with myself, for example, talk badly about myself, swear at myself, blame myself for things that happen.
_____ 8. I talk about the future in a hopeless way.
_____ 9. I get sudden frights.

Body Care and Movement Subscale

_____ 1. I make difficult moves with help, for example, getting into or out of cars or bathtubs.
_____ 2. I do not move into or out of bed or chairs by myself but am moved by a person or mechanical aid.
_____ 3. I stand only for short periods of time.
_____ 4. I do not maintain balance.
_____ 5. I move my hands or fingers with some limitation or difficulty.
_____ 6. I stand up only with someone's help.
_____ 7. I kneel, stoop, or bend down only by holding onto something.
_____ 8. I am in a restricted position all the time.
_____ 9. I am very clumsy in body movements.
_____10. I got in and out of bed or chairs by grasping something for support or using a cane or walker.
_____11. I stay lying down most of the time.
_____12. I change position frequently.
_____13. I hold onto something to move myself around in bed.
_____14. I do not bathe myself completely, for example, I require assistance with bathing.
_____15. I do not bathe myself at all but am bathed by someone else.
_____16. I use a bedpan with assistance.
_____17. I have trouble getting shoes, socks, or stockings up.
_____18. I do not have control of my bladder.
_____19. I do not fasten my clothing, for example, require assistance with buttons, zippers, shoelaces.
_____20. I spend most of the time partly undressed or in pajamas.
_____21. I do not have control of my bowels.
_____22. I dress myself but do so very slowly.
_____23. I got dressed only with someone's help.

Household Management Subscale

_____ 1. I do work around the house only for short periods of time or rest often.
_____ 2. I am doing lose of the regular daily work around the house than I would usually do.
_____ 3. I am not doing any of the regular daily work around the house than I would usually do.

TABLE 13-18
continued

_____ 4. I am not doing any of the maintenance or repair work that I would usually do in my home or yard.
_____ 5. I am not doing any of the shopping that I would usually do.
_____ 6. I am not doing any of the house cleaning that I would usually do.
_____ 7. I have difficulty doing handwork, for example, turning faucets, using kitchen gadgets, sewing, and carpentry.
_____ 8. I am not doing any of the clothes washing that I would usually do.
_____ 9. I am not doing heavy work around the house.
_____10. I have given up taking care of personal or household business affairs, for example, paying bills, banking, or working on the budget.

Mobility Subscale

_____ 1. I only got about within one building
_____ 2. I stay in one room.
_____ 3. I am staying in bed more.
_____ 4. I am staying in bed most of the time.
_____ 5. I am not now using public transportation.
_____ 6. I stay at home most of the time.
_____ 7. I am only going to places with rest rooms nearby.
_____ 8. I am not going into town.
_____ 9. I stay away from home only for brief periods of time.
_____10. I do not got around in the dark or in unlit places without someone's help.

Social Interaction Subscale

_____ 1. I am going out less to visit people.
_____ 2. I am not going out to visit people at all.
_____ 3. I show lose interest in other people's problems, for example, don't listen when they toll me about their problems, don't offer to help.
_____ 4. I often act irritable toward those around me, for example, snap at people, give sharp answers, criticize easily.
_____ 5. I show loss affection.
_____ 6. I am doing fewer social activities with groups of people.
_____ 7. I am cutting down the length of visits with friends.
_____ 8. I am avoiding social visits from others.
_____ 9. My sexual activity is decreased.
_____10. I often express concern over what might be happening to my health.
_____11. I talk less with those around me.
_____12. I make many demands, for example, insist that people do things for me, tell me how to do things.
_____13. I stay alone much of the time.
_____14. I act disagreeable to family members, for example, I act spiteful, I am stubborn.
_____15. I have frequent outbursts of anger at family members, for example, strike at them, scream, throw things at them.
_____16. I isolate myself an much as I can from the rest of the family.
_____17. I am paying less attention to the children.
_____18. I refuse contact with family members, for example, turn away from them.
_____19. I am not doing the things I usually do to take care of my children or family.
_____20. I am not joking with family members as I usually do.

Ambulation Subscale

_____ 1. I walk shorter distances or stop to rest often.
_____ 2. I do not walk up or down hills.
_____ 3. I use stairs only with mechanical support, for example, handrail, cane, crutches.
_____ 4. I walk up or down stairs only with assistance from someone else.
_____ 5. I get around in a wheelchair.
_____ 6. I do not walk at all.
_____ 7. I walk by myself but with some difficulty, for example, limp, wobble, stumble, have stiff legs.

TABLE 13-18
continued

_____ 8. I walk only with help from someone.
_____ 9. I go up and down stairs more slowly, for example, one step at a time, stop often.
_____ 10. I do not use stairs at all.
_____ 11. I got around only by using a walker, crutches, cane, walls, or furniture.
_____ 12. I walk more slowly.

Alertness Subscale

_____ 1. I am confused and start several actions at a time.
_____ 2. I have more minor accidents, for example, drop things, trip and fall, bump into things.
_____ 3. I react slowly to things that are said or done.
_____ 4. I do not finish things I start.
_____ 5. I have difficulty reasoning and starting problems, for example, making plans, making decisions, learning new things.
_____ 6. I sometimes behave as if I were confused or disoriented in place or time, for example, where I am, who is around, directions, what day it is.
_____ 7. I forget a lot, for example, things that happened recently, where I put things, appointments.
_____ 8. I do not keep my attention on any activity for long.
_____ 9. I make more mistakes than usual.
_____ 10. I have difficulty doing activities involving concentration and thinking.

Communication Subscale

_____ 1. I am having trouble writing or typing.
_____ 2. I communicate mostly by gestures, for example, moving my head, pointing, sign language.
_____ 3. My speech is understood only by a few people who know me well.
_____ 4. I often lose control of my voice when I talk, for example, my voice gets louder or softer, trembles, changes unexpectedly.
_____ 5. I don't write, except to sign my name.
_____ 6. I carry on a conversation only when very close to the other person or looking at him/her.
_____ 7. I have difficulty speaking, for example, get stuck, stutter, stammer, slur my words.
_____ 8. I am understood with difficulty.
_____ 9. I do not speak clearly when I am under stress.

Recreation and Pastime Subscale

_____ 1. I do my hobbies and recreation for shorter periods of time.
_____ 2. I am going out for entertainment less often.
_____ 3. I am cutting down on some of my usual inactive recreation and pastimes, for example, watching TV, playing cards, reading.
_____ 4. I am not doing any of my usual inactive recreation and pastimes, for example, watching TV, playing cards, reading.
_____ 5. I am doing more inactive pastimes in place of my other usual activities.
_____ 6. I am doing fewer community activities.
_____ 7. I am cutting down on some of my usual physical recreation or activities.
_____ 8. I am not doing any of my usual physical recreation or activities.

Eating Subscale

_____ 1. I am eating much loss than usual.
_____ 2. I feed myself but only by using specially prepared food or utensils.
_____ 3. I am eating special or different food, for example, soft food, bland diet, low-salt, low-fat, low-sugar.
_____ 4. I eat no food at all but am taking fluids.
_____ 5. I just pick or nibble at my food.
_____ 6. I am drinking less fluids.
_____ 7. I feed myself with help from someone else.

TABLE 13-18
continued

_____ 8. I do not feed myself at all but must be fed.

_____ 9. I am eating no food at all; nutrition is taken through tubes or intravenous fluids.

Work Subscale

1. Do you usually do work other than managing your home?　　　　　YES____NO____
   If you answered yes, go to question #5 on this subscale.
   If you answered no, answer questions #2 through #4 on this subscale.
2. Are you retired?　　　　　YES____NO____
3. If you are retired, was your retirement related to your health?　　　YES____ NO____
4. If you are not retired but are not working, is this related to your health?　　YES____ NO____

_____ 5. I am not working at all. (*If you checked this statement, skip all other questions.*)

_____ 6. I am doing part of my job at home.

_____ 7. I am not accomplishing as much as usual at work.

_____ 8. I often act irritable toward my work associates, for example, snap at them, give sharp answers, criticize easily.

_____ 9. I am working shorter hours.

_____10. I am doing only light work.

_____11. I work only for short periods of time or take frequent rents.

_____12. I am working at my usual job but with some changes, for example, using different tools or special aids, trading some tasks with others.

_____13. I do not do my job as carefully and accurately as usual.

Source: Skinner A. The Sickness Impact Profile Scoring Manual. Medical Outcomes Trust, 8 Park Plaza, #503, Boston, Massachusetts 02116, 1998. (Copied with permission from the Medical Outcomes Trust).

Reliability

The 136-item version of the SIP has demonstrated high test-retest reliability (0.88 to 0.92) (95). Cronbach's alpha coefficient for this version also was high ($r = 0.94$) (95).

Validity

Convergent and divergent validity was assessed by multitrait, multimethod technique. In comparing the SIP with other measures of functional status (Katz IADL and National Health Interviews Survey) and among different patient populations (hip replacement, arthritis, and hyperthyroidism), high correlations were obtained (95). The psychosocial dimension of the SIP is highly correlated with various psychological measures and appears to be strongly related to depression (97,98).

In MS research, the Physical Composite Total on the SIP was significantly correlated with the EDSS ($r = 0.81$), 9-HPT ($r = 0.45$), and AI ($r = 0.77$) (24). The Psychosocial Composite Total on the SIP was substantially correlated with the Modified Fatigue Impact Scale ($r = 0.62$) and the Mental Health Inventory ($r = -0.60$) (24). There is clear discrimination between the Physical and Psychosocial Composite scales. In comparing the sensitivity of the SIP with that of the EDSS, only the SIP scores changed significantly following exercise training (99). The exercise group improved on all components of the physical dimension of the SIP and showed improvements in social interaction, emotional behavior, home management, total SIP score, and recreation and pastime.

Administration/Scoring

The SIP can be self-administered or interviewer-administered and requires 20 to 30 minutes to complete. The SIP can be totaled by the 12 subscales, by broad domains (physical or psychosocial composite totals), or by item (74). The total score on the SIP ranges from 0 (better health) to 100 (poor health). To calculate the overall SIP score, one adds the scale values for each item checked across all subscales, divides by the maximum possible score for the SIP, and then multiplies the results by 100 to obtain the total SIP score (74). Bowling (74) notes that a normal population generally obtains a SIP score of 2 or 3, which increases to a score in the mid-30's for terminally ill cancer and stroke patients (74). Scoring and instructions for the SIP (100) and the FIP (96) are available.

Advantages

Because the SIP focuses on sickness-related behaviors, it can be applied to many patient populations for a number of different purposes, making cross-study comparisons possible. The comprehensive coverage of the SIP, its extensive development, and its emphasis on current performance makes it an excellent rehabilitation measure (101).

Disadvantages

The SIP has been criticized for two major reasons: its length and lack of sensitivity. According to Wilkin and associates, the SIP lacks a responsiveness to detect change over time in the same individuals (4). However, in at least one MS study, significant SIP score changes were reported following eight weeks of exercise therapy. More MS longitudinal studies using the SIP are needed before conclusions can be drawn regarding its sensitivity to detect change.

The SIP has been criticized by several researchers and practitioners who state that its length is an obstacle to routine use (4,101). In a 1993 study on stroke patients, early recovery patients complained that the SIP was too time-consuming and fatiguing (102). In response to this complaint, the short-form SIP-68 was developed (Table 13-19). The psychometric properties of the SIP-68 appear to be comparable to the longer version (103–105). The SIP-68 requires additional validation studies before the effectiveness and generalizability of this shorter version can be determined. A scoring manual for the SIP68 is available (105).

Although the Physical and Psychosocial Composite scales and many of the subscales are valid and applicable to MS, the lifestyle subscales are weak (i.e., Recreation and Pastimes), and the Communication Subscale and the Work Subscale need further validation (24). Ritvo and colleagues also note that interpretation of the Work Subscale varies dramatically, depending on whether the patient is currently employed, and thus may require separate analysis.

Comments

The SIP is a standardized, general-purpose health status questionnaire that is widely used as an outcome measure in the United States. It is useful in a wide variety of clinical and research settings, particularly those dealing with chronic illness. However, few MS studies have used the SIP< probably because it is long and time-consuming. With the development of the SIP-68, it is hoped more MS researchers and clinicians will use this valuable assessment and outcomes measure. Results indicate that, compared with the EDSS, the SIP is a sensitive and comprehensive measure that assesses the type of changes MS patient experience following rehabilitation therapy.

Medical Rehabilitation Follow Along/Lifeware

The Medical Rehabilitation Follow Along (MRFA) or Lifeware was developed by Granger and coworkers (5).

It was specifically designed for the early detection of the functional problems typically experienced and evaluated during outpatient rehabilitation therapy. Unlike the SIP and the SF-36, which were designed to assess the health status of the general population, the MRFA assesses the health status changes of various patient populations.

Description

The MRFA was developed using Rasch analysis to construct linear measures that function on an interval level. It combines the best attributes of several existing questionnaires into a single multidimensional health status questionnaire. There are three forms of the MRFA: the Musculoskeletal Form, the Neurological Form, and the Multiple Sclerosis Form. The number of items for each form varies. The Likert scale ranges also vary, depending on the health status domain being evaluated.

The Musculoskeletal Form of the MRFA consists of 31 patient report items, encompassing three domains:Physical Functioning, Pain Experience (pain scale), and Affective Well-Being. Components including body movement and control, effort, pain-free, a visual analog pain rating scale, placid, and life satisfaction assess these three domains. The components include items from other standardized instruments: the Functional Assessment Screening Questionnaire (FASQ), the Oswestry Scale, and the short-form McGill Pain Questionnaire.

The Neurological Form of the MRFA consists of 39 items. It examines four domains and "other"—Physical (neuromotor, effort); Pain Experience (pain scale); Affective Well-Being (placid, satisfaction); Cognition (neurocognitive); Other (driving, limitations).

The Multiple Sclerosis Form examines three domains and "other"—Physical (MS physical), fatigue, sphincter); Pain experience (pain scale); Affective Well-Being (placid, satisfaction); Other (vision, EDSS components).

Reliability

The initial validation study of the Musculoskeletal Form of the MRFA demonstrated overall high test-retest reliability. The ICC values, for the quality of daily living and physical functioning subscales range from $r = 0.74$ to $r = 0.97$, respectively. The ICC values for the items assessing pain and psychological well-being ranged from 0.36 to 0.93, respectively (5). The reliability data for the Neurological and Multiple Sclerosis Forms have not been published.

Validity

Validity studies for the Musculoskeletal Form of the MRFA have been completed using both raw scoring (106)

TABLE 13-19
The SIP-68

SOMATIC AUTONOMY

1. I get around in a wheelchair.
2. I get dressed only with someone's help.
3. I do not move into or out of bed by myself, but am moved by a person or mechanical aid.
4. I stand up only with someone's help.
5. I do not fasten my clothing, for example, require assistance with button, zippers, shoelaces.
6. I do not walk at all
7. I do not use stairs at all.*
8. I make difficult moves with help, for example, getting into or out of cars, bathtubs.
9. I do not bathe myself completely, for example, require assistance with bathing.
10. I do not bathe myself at all, but am bathed by someone else.
11. I do not have control of my bladder.
12. I am very clumsy in body movements.
13. I do not have control of my bowels.
14. I feed myself with help from someone else.
15. I do not maintain balance.
16. I use bedpan with assistance.
17. I am in a restricted position all the time.

MOBILITY CONTROL

1. I go up and down stairs more slowly, for example, one step at a time, stop often.*
2. I walk shorter distance or stop to rest often.*
3. I walk more slowly.*
4. I use stairs only with mechanical support, for example, handrail, cane, crutches.
5. I walk by myself but with some difficulty, for example, limp, wobble, stumble, have stiff leg.*
6. I kneel, stoop, or bend down only by holding on to something.*
7. I do not walk up or down hills.*
8. I get in and out of bed or chairs by grasping something for support or using a cane or walker.
9. I stand only for short periods of time.
10. I dress myself, but do so very slowly.
11. I have difficulty doing handwork, for example, turning faucets, using kitchen gadgets, sewing, carpentry.
12. I move my hands or fingers with some limitation or difficulty.

PSYCHIC AUTONOMY AND COMMUNICATION

1. I have difficulty reasoning and solving problems, for example, making plans, making decisions, learning new things.
2. I have difficulty doing activities involving concentration and thinking.
3. I react slowly to things that are said or done.
4. I make more mistakes than usual.
5. I do not keep my attention on any activity for long.
6. I forget a lot, for example, things that happened recently, where I put things, appointments.
7. I am confused and start several actions at a time.
8. I do not speak clearly when I am under stress.
9. I have difficulty speaking, for example, get stuck, stutter, stammer, slur my words.
10. I do not finish things I start.
11. I am having trouble writing or typing.

SOCIAL BEHAVIOR

1. My sexual activity is decreased.
2. I am cutting down the length of visits with friends.
3. I am drinking less fluids.

TABLE 13-19
continued

4. I am doing fewer community activities.
5. I am doing fewer social activities with groups of people.
6. I am going out for entertainments less often.
7. I stay away from home only for brief periods of time.
8. I am eating much less than usual.
9. I am not doing heavy work around the house.
10. I do my hobbies and recreation for shorter periods of time.
11. I am doing less of the regular daily work around the house than I would usually do.
12. I am cutting down on some of my usual inactive recreation and pastime, for example, watching TV, playing cards, reading.

EMOTIONAL STABILITY

1. I often act irritable toward those around me, for example, snap at people, give sharp answers, criticize easily.
2. I act disagreeably to family members, for example, I act spiteful, I am stubborn.
3. I have frequent outbursts of anger at family members, for example, strike at them, scream, throw things at them.
4. I act irritable and impatient with myself, for example, talk badly about myself, swear at myself for things that happen.
5. I am not joking with family members as I usually do.
6. I talk less with those around me.

MOBILITY RANGE

1. I am not doing any of the shopping that I would usually do.
2. I am not going into town.
3. I am not doing any of the house cleaning that I would usually do.
4. I am not doing any of the regular work around the house.
5. I stay at home most of the time.
6. I am not doing any of the clothes washing that I would usually do.
7. I am not going out to visit people at all.
8. I am getting around only within one building.
9. I have given up taking care of personal or household business affairs, for example, paying bills, banking, working on budget.
10. I do not get around in the dark or in unlit places without someone's help.

*Items assigned a positive score when "I do not walk at all" was scored positively.
Source: Post MWM, Bruni AF de, Witte LP de, Schrijvers A. The SIP-68: A measure of health-related functional status in rehabilitation medicine. *Archives of Physical Medicine and Rehabilitation* 1996; 77:440–445. (Copied with permission from the Medical Outcomes Trust).

and Rasch measures (107). The results provide support for the validity of inferences made from the raw score scales and Rasch measures of the MRFA for people with musculoskeletal problems. Convergent validity was determined by comparing the physical functioning and well-being/mental health scales from the MRFA with the corresponding scales on the SF-36. Significant correlations on physical functioning scales ($r = 0.83$) and on the well-being/mental health scales ($r = 0.57$) were obtained between the SF-36 and MRFA.

Administration/Scoring

The MRFA can be administered by interviewing the patient in person or over the telephone. Administration of the MRFA over the telephone can be difficult if the patient does not have the answer sheet to view. The Likert scale for each health domain or subscale varies, which may be confusing. Clinician-rated components of the Neurological Form can be completed with input from the patient or caregiver. The Mini-Mental State component requires questioning by the clinician. Completion of the Musculoskeletal Form of the MRFA requires 7–16 minutes.

Each domain or subscale on the MRFA Forms is scored separately. All scores are from 0 to 100, with the higher scores representing better functioning, less pain, less EDSS disability, less emotional distress, and so forth. Additional scoring information can be obtained by contacting Dr. C. V. Granger (UDSMR, SUNY at Buffalo, 232 Parker Hall 3435 Main Street, Buffalo, NY 14214-

3007) or on the internet: http://www.udsmr.org/products. htm or http://www.lifeware.org.

Advantages

The MRFA is the first health status instrument specifically designed to assess the types of problems experienced by outpatients receiving rehabilitation therapy. It is also the first outpatient rehabilitation instrument designed for early detection of functional problems in an effort to prevent secondary complications.

Disadvantages

The MRFA appears to be a good measure of physical functioning but it needs further refinement in other areas (i.e., the fear item, ICC = 0.36 and terror/panic item, ICC = 0.44). The original reliability study was completed on a relatively small sample of only 47 patients and included only the Musculoskeletal Form of the MRFA. Additional reliability and validity studies need to be completed on the Neurologic and Multiple Sclerosis Forms of the MRFA before definite conclusions can be made as to the usefulness of this instrument for MS. The sensitivity of the MRFA still needs to be established because the ability to detect change and demonstrate improvement with rehabilitation therapy is the primary purpose of this instrument.

Comments

The MRFA is the first outpatient rehabilitation measure to assess disability, handicap, and general health status, with an emphasis on prevention or early detection of secondary problems. It is important to remember that on the MRFA, the Multiple Sclerosis Form is only appropriate to use when assessing benign or mild MS patients. The wording of the MS Form assumes a higher level of physical functioning. The Neurological Form of the MRFA is best used when assessing all types of MS (benign, relapsing-remitting, and primary/secondary chronic progressive) or when both ambulatory and wheelchair-bound patients are being evaluated.

The 36-Item Short Form (SF-36)

The 36-item short form (SF-36) was designed to survey the health status of the general population in the Medical Outcomes Study (108,109). It has become a popular outcome instrument for a wide variety of patient groups, including MS patients. It is a multidimensional health questionnaire that captures most features of health that are important to all patients. The SF-36 has been used for health policy evaluations, general populations surveys, clinical research and practice, and other applications using various diverse populations (109).

Description

The SF-36 Health Survey measures two broad areas of health status, referred to as the physical composite summary (PCS) and the mental composite summary (MCS), and includes eight health subscales (Table 13-20). The subscales are (1) physical functioning, (2) social functioning, (3) role limitations because of physical health problems, (4) role limitations because of emotional problems, (5) mental health status (psychological distress and psychological well-being), (6) bodily pain, (7) vitality (energy/fatigue), and (8) general health perceptions. The SF-36 consists of 36 items, 35 of which comprise the eight subscales. One item pertains to perception of change in health over a one-year period and is scored separately (109).

Reliability

Several SF-36 reliability studies have been completed on a variety of groups, including working adults (110), the elderly (111), and a variety of patient populations (112–114). Internal consistency reliability coefficients determined by Cronbach's alpha range from $r = 0.78$ to a high of $r = 0.93$ across scales (114,115). Lower Cronbach alphas were reported on the social functioning subscale in two studies ($r \leqslant 0.76$) (110,113). Test-retest reliability range from $r = 0.60$ (social functioning) to $r = 0.81$ (physical functioning) (113). Based on the Medical Outcomes Study of 1,440 outpatients, reliabilities for the PCS and MCS (composite scores) were $r = 0.92$ and $r = 0.91$, respectively (116).

Validity

The SF-36 has demonstrated construct validity by correctly classifying various patients across the eight subscales (113,117,118). Convergent and discriminant validity have also been satisfactory. The SF-36 and Nottingham Health Profile were highly correlated on related subscales and less correlated on noncomparable dimensions (113). Compared with the Nottingham Health Profile, the SF-36 appears to be the more sensitive measure of lower levels of dysfunction and disability (110). The SF-36 also correctly classified or discriminated between groups with expected health differences (113).

In an MS research study, a significant correlation between the EDSS and the SF-36 physical subscale was reported ($r = -0.67$, p < 0.001) (119). No other SF-36 domains were significantly related to the EDSS. Compared with the general population (119,120) and with diabetes and epilepsy groups (121), MS patients tend to score significantly

TABLE 13-20
SF-36 Health Status Scale Information

Physical functioning	10	21	Limited a lot in performing all physical activities including bathing or dressing	Performs all types of physical activities including the most vigorous without limitations due to health
Role limitations due to physical problems	4	5	Problems with work or other daily activities as a result of physical health	No problems with work or other daily activities as a result of physical health, past 4 weeks
Social functioning	2	9	Extreme and frequent interference with normal social activities due to physical and emotional problems	Performs normal social activities without interference due to physical or emotional problems, past 4 weeks
Bodily pain	2	11	Very severe and extremely limiting pain	No pain or limitations due to pain, past 4 weeks
General mental health	5	26	Feelings of nervousness and depression all of the time	Feels peaceful, happy, and calm all of the time, past 4 weeks
Role limitations due to emotional problems	3	4	Problems with work or other daily activities as a result of emotional problems	No problems with work or other daily activities as a result of emotional problems, past 4 weeks
Vitality	4	21	Feels tired and worn out all of the time	Feels full of pep and energy all of the time, past 4 weeks
General health perceptions	5	21	Believes personal health is poor and likely to get worse	Believes personal health is excellent

Source: Wade JE, Sherbourne CD. The MOS 36-item short-form health survey (SF-36). *Medical Care* 1992;30:473-483. (Copied with permission from the Medical Outcomes Trust).

lower in the SF-36 domains of physical functioning, role limitations due to physical problems, and energy/vitality.

Administration/Scoring

The SF-36 can be reliably administered over the phone, face to face, or self-administered (122). It is a short questionnaire that generally requires less than 10 minutes to complete. For each subscale, items are coded, totaled, and transformed to a 0 to 100 scale, with 0 representing the poorest state of health and 100 indicating the best (110). The scoring information and instruction manuals are available from The Health Institute (115) or on the Internet at http://www.sf-36.com/.

Advantages

The SF-36 is currently the most widely used health status questionnaire, as documented by almost 600 publications. It is a comprehensive multidimensional measure that is useful in monitoring general and patient populations and is applicable across many social, demographic, and age groups. There are several uses for the SF-36, it being particularly helpful when comparing the relative burden of different diseases, differentiating the health benefits produced by different treatments, and evaluating individual patients. It also assesses many of the health concepts that are important to people with MS, such as fatigue, role limitations, physical function (120).

Disadvantages

The SF-36 has been criticized for its ceiling and floor effects (52). The range of health behavior responses is limited, resulting in large numbers of people obtaining the highest score possible (ceiling effect) or the lowest score possible (floor effect). Specifically, ceiling effects were reported for the role functioning and social functioning subscales (114).

Floor effects were found for the role limitation subscales (117) and the physical function subscale (123) and were highest among wheelchair-bound patients.

The utility and performance of the SF-36 varies depending on the population being assessed. Ziebland (124) found that the SF-36 adequately detected change in health status among homogenous treatment groups, but heterogenous group responses were too varied to determine correctly the impact of health interventions in the entire community. Compared with the SIP and the Nottingham Health Profile (NHP), the SF-36 appears to be less comprehensive and less suitable for the elderly (111). The SF-36 does not include a sleep disturbance subscale and provides only limited coverage of areas such as pain and emotional well-being. Items pertaining to work or vigorous activities were generally not applicable to the elderly or the severely disabled MS patients.

However, the SF-36 appears to be more sensitive when assessing more active, healthier populations. Compared with the SIP, only the SF-36 discriminated between patients with relatively good physical performance at the three-month follow-up in terms of their ability to work, play sports, and garden (125). These results indicate that the SF-36 appears to be a more sensitive mobility measure, whereas the SIP is a more comprehensive measure of health status.

Comments

The SF-36 is a well-established, standardized health status measure that has many applications (i.e., clinical trials, rehabilitation outcomes, and patient monitoring). Compared with the EDSS, the SF-36 provides significantly more information regarding the functional status and quality of life of MS patients. The inclusion of the energy/vitality subscale on the SF-36 makes it particularly relevant to people with MS. The major problem with the SF-36 is the considerable floor effects detected on the two role function subscales. This issue becomes a particular concern when assessing severely impaired MS patients. Therefore, Vickery and associates strongly recommend adding the MS ADL motor scale to reduce the floor effects on the physical function subscale (123).

Short-Form (SF-12)

SF-12 was developed as an alternative to the SF-36 for the purposes of monitoring large samples from general and patient populations (126) and in response to the need for shorter health survey measures (127).

Description

The SF-12 is a subset of items from the SF-36. Like the SF-36, the SF-12 measures two broad health status domains: physical well-being (the Physical Component Summary) and psychological well-being (the Mental Health Component Summary) (Table 13-21). The Physical Component Summary (PCS-12) domain evaluates physical functioning, physical role limitations, bodily pain, and general health. The Mental Health Component Summary (MCS-12) domain assesses vitality, social functioning, social role limitation, and mental health. The SF-12 consists of 12 items and assesses the same eight health domains as the SF-36.

Reliability

Many SF-12 reliability studies have been completed based on the general population (127), various patient populations (127,128), and with varying age groups (127). Test-retest reliability ranges from $r = 0.76$ (Mental Component Summary) to $r = 0.89$ (Physical Component Summary) (127).

Validity

To determine the validity of the SF-12, it was compared with the SF-36 across various physical and mental treatment groups over time (127,128). Correlations between the SF-12 and SF-36 for the PCS-12 and MCS-12 component summary scales were $r = 0.95$ and $r = 0.97$, respectively. The SF-12 produced the two summary scores (physical and mental) of the SF-36 with better than 90 percent accuracy (126,128). Mean scores on the SF-12 and SF-36 were almost identical and 95 percent confidence intervals (CIs) substantially overlap at both times across all treatment groups. Results from comparing the SF12 and the SF-36 were similar, indicating the same magnitude of ill health and degree of change over time.

Administration/Scoring

The SF-12 can be self-administered, administered over the phone, or administered face to face. It is a very short questionnaire that generally requires two minutes to complete (127). To assist examiners in scoring the SF-12, Kosinski (126) presented an sample scoring procedure for an individual patient (Table 13-22). In scoring the PCS-12 and the MSC-12, (1) summate the physical weights corresponding to the item response choice selected to score PCS-12 and summate the mental weights corresponding to the items response choices selected to score MCS-12; (2) standardize the PCS-12 score by adding the constant (56.57706) to the sum for the physical weights; and (3) standardize the MCS-12 score by adding the constant (60.75781) to the sum of the mental weights. This results in a final PCS-12 and MCS-12 score. Scores for each scale range from 0 to 100, with 0 representing the poorest state

---

TABLE 13-21
SF-12 Health Survey

---

1. In general would you say your health is:
   Excellent____   Very good____   Good Fair____   Poor____

The following items are about activities you might do during a typical day. Does **your health now limit you in these activities**? If so how much?

2. **Moderate activities**, such as moving a table, pushing a vacuum cleaner, bowling, or play golf

3. Climbing **several** flights of stairs

   Response categories: Yes, limited a lot; Yes, limited a little, No, not limited at all.

During the **past 4 weeks**, have you had any of the following problems with your work or other regular daily activities **as a result of your physical health**?

4. **Accomplished less** than you would like

5. Were limited in the **kind** of work or other activities

   Response categories: Yes; No

During the **past 4 weeks**, have you had any of the following problems with your work or other regular daily activities **as a result of any emotional problems** (such as feeling depressed or anxious)?

6. **Accomplished less** than you would like

7. Didn't do work or other activities as **carefully** as usual

   Response categories: Yes; No

8. During the **past 4 weeks**, how much did **pain** interfere with your normal work (including both work outside the home and housework)?

   Response categories: Not at all; a little bit; moderately; quite a bit; extremely

These questions are about how you feel and how things have been with you **during the past 4 weeks**. For each question, please give the one answer that comes closest to the way you have been feeling. How much of the time during the **past 4 weeks**.

9. Have you felt calm and peaceful?

10. Did you have a lot of energy?

11. Have you felt downhearted and blue?

    Response categories: All of the time; most of the time; a good bit of the time; some of the time; a little of the time; none of the time.

12. During the **past 4 weeks**, how much of the time has your **physical health or emotional problems** interfered with your social activities (like visiting with friends, relatives, etc.)?

    Response categories: All of the time; most of the time; some of the time; a little of the time; none of the time.

Source: Ware JE, Kosinski M, Keller SD. A 12-item short-form health survey: construction of scales and preliminary tests of reliability and validity. *Medical Care* 1996; 34:220-233.

---

of health and 100 indicating the best. Scoring information and instruction manuals are available from the Health Institute (129) or on the Internet at http://www.sf-36.com/.

Advantages

The SF-12 is a multidimensional measure of physical status and psychological well-being that is applicable across many patient groups. It is a standardized instrument that is short and easy to use. Its short length makes it realistic to administer on a large scale, such as in a national health status survey.

SF-12 summary scale scores (PCS and MSC) replicate those obtained on the SF-36 PCS and MSC with a high degree of accuracy. The fact that the SF-12 questionnaire is entirely a subset of the SF-36 makes comparison across studies useful. The SF-12 has received accreditation by the National Committee for Quality Assurance and has been translated into Spanish, French, German, Italian, and Japanese.

Disadvantages

Difficulties scoring the SF-12 appear to be the most frequent complaint. The SF-12 scoring protocol was

TABLE 13-22

SF-12 HEALTH SURVEY—SCORING SAMPLE

This questionnaire asks for your views about your health. This information will help keep track of how you feel and how well you are able to do your usual activities. Please answer every question by marking one box. If you are unsure about how to answer, please give the best answer you can.

1. In general, would you say your health is:

	Excellent	Very good	Good	Fair	Poor
(Physical)	0 ☐	−1.31872 ☐	−3.02396 ☑	−5.56461 ☐	−8.37399 ☐
(Mental)	0	−0.06064	0.03482	−0.16891	−1.71175

The following questions are about activities you might do during a typical day. Does your health now limit you in these activities? If so, how much?

2. Moderate activities, such as moving a table, pushing a vacuum cleaner, bowling, or playing golf

	Yes, Limited a Lot	Yes, Limited a Little	No, not limited at all
(Physical)	−7.23216 ☐	−3.45555 ☑	0 ☐
(Mental)	−3.93115	1.86840	0

3. Climbing several flights of stairs

(Physical)	−6.24397 ☐	2.68282 ☐	0 ☑
(Mental)	−2.73557	1.43103	0

During the past 4 weeks, have you had any of the following problems with your work or other regular daily activities as a result of your physical health?

4. Accomplished less than you would like

	Yes	No
(Physical)	−4.61617 ☑	0 ☐
(Mental)	1.44060	0

5. Were limited in the kind of work or other activities

(Physical)	−5.51747 ☐	0 ☑
(Mental)	1.66968	0

During the past 4 weeks, have you had any of the following problems with your work or other regular daily activities as a result of any emotional problems (such as feeling depressed or anxious)?

6. Accomplished less than you would like

	Yes	No
(Physical)	3.04365 ☐	0 ☑
(Mental)	−6.82672	0

7. Didn't do work or other activities as carefully as usual

(Physical)	2.32091 ☐	0 ☑
(Mental)	−5.69921	0

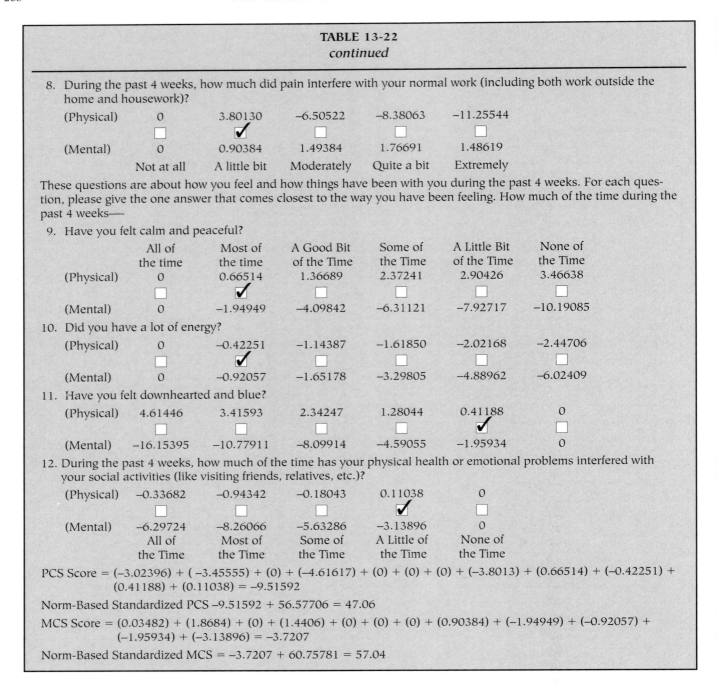

TABLE 13-22
continued

8. During the past 4 weeks, how much did pain interfere with your normal work (including both work outside the home and housework)?

	Not at all	A little bit	Moderately	Quite a bit	Extremely
(Physical)	0	3.80130 ✓	−6.50522	−8.38063	−11.25544
(Mental)	0	0.90384	1.49384	1.76691	1.48619

These questions are about how you feel and how things have been with you during the past 4 weeks. For each question, please give the one answer that comes closest to the way you have been feeling. How much of the time during the past 4 weeks—

9. Have you felt calm and peaceful?

	All of the time	Most of the time	A Good Bit of the Time	Some of the Time	A Little Bit of the Time	None of the Time
(Physical)	0	0.66514 ✓	1.36689	2.37241	2.90426	3.46638
(Mental)	0	−1.94949	−4.09842	−6.31121	−7.92717	−10.19085

10. Did you have a lot of energy?

(Physical)	0	−0.42251 ✓	−1.14387	−1.61850	−2.02168	−2.44706
(Mental)	0	−0.92057	−1.65178	−3.29805	−4.88962	−6.02409

11. Have you felt downhearted and blue?

(Physical)	4.61446	3.41593	2.34247	1.28044	0.41188 ✓	0
(Mental)	−16.15395	−10.77911	−8.09914	−4.59055	−1.95934	0

12. During the past 4 weeks, how much of the time has your physical health or emotional problems interfered with your social activities (like visiting friends, relatives, etc.)?

	All of the Time	Most of the Time	Some of the Time	A Little of the Time	None of the Time
(Physical)	−0.33682	−0.94342	−0.18043	0.11038 ✓	0
(Mental)	−6.29724	−8.26066	−5.63286	−3.13896	0

PCS Score = (−3.02396) + (−3.45555) + (0) + (−4.61617) + (0) + (0) + (0) + (−3.8013) + (0.66514) + (−0.42251) + (0.41188) + (0.11038) = −9.51592

Norm-Based Standardized PCS −9.51592 + 56.57706 = 47.06

MCS Score = (0.03482) + (1.8684) + (0) + (1.4406) + (0) + (0) + (0) + (0.90384) + (−1.94949) + (−0.92057) + (−1.95934) + (−3.13896) = −3.7207

Norm-Based Standardized MCS = −3.7207 + 60.75781 = 57.04

developed with the statistical software programmer in mind and, as such, it includes complicated algorithms (126). This problem was quickly rectified by publishing a simple visual scoring example (126).

Although the short length of this questionnaire is appealing, the tradeoff is loss of precise, detailed information. For example, vitality/energy was omitted on the SF-12. Unfortunately, fatigue is a major symptom and determinant of health status and quality of life for people with MS that needs to be assessed.

Most of the health status domains assessed on the SF-12 contain only one item. Consequently, the eight health status domains cannot be reliably analyzed separately as compared with the SF-36. On the SF-12, only the physical and mental composite summary scores can be analyzed (128).

Comments

The SF-12 is a brief, standardized health status questionnaire derived completely from the SF-36. The SF-12 is most appropriate when comparing MS patients with other populations (normal or patient) for general health status differences. Compared with other HRQOL measures, the SF-12 requires less time and money to administer. This may be an issue when resources are severely restricted and the decision is whether to asses health-related quality of life. For clinical trials, patient follow-up, or rehabilitation outcomes, other measures (SF-36, MSQLI, MRFA) provide more specific MS information.

The Multiple Sclerosis Quality of Life (MSQOL)-54

The MSQOL-54 is both a generic and an MS-specific measure of health-related quality of life (120). It was designed to evaluate the health-related quality of life (HRQOL) concerns common to all patient populations, while simultaneously assessing the most relevant concerns of people with MS. The generic core of the MSQOL-54 is the SF-36 measure, which allows comparisons with other patient populations. The MS-specific items were based on relevant quality of life issues derived from review of the literature. The original reliability and validity study included 179 adults with a definite diagnosis of MS and whose status ranged from newly diagnosed to severely impaired (120). Forty-one of the participants were ambulatory without assistance and had an average disease duration of nine years.

Description

The MSQOL-54 contains 54 items (SF-36 items and 18 MS-specific items), and 52 of the items are distributed into 12 subscale and two single items (Table 13-23). The 12 subscales on the MSQOL-54 are physical function, role limitations—physical, role limitations—emotional, pain, emotional well-being, energy, health perception, social function, cognitive function, health distress, overall quality of life, and sexual function. The two single items are change in health status and satisfaction with sexual function. The 18 MS-specific items provide additional information regarding cognitive function, sexual function, health distress, and overall quality of life. Two composite scores can be obtained on the MSQOL-54—physical health composite and mental health composite. The physical health composite includes the following subscales: physical function, health perceptions, energy/fatigue, role limitation—physical, pain, sexual function, social function, and health distress. The mental health composite includes health distress, overall quality of life, emotional well-being, role limitations—emotional, and cognitive function.

Reliability

Internal consistency reliability coefficients determined by Cronbach's alpha range from $r = 0.75$ (social function) to a high of $r = 0.96$ (physical function) across the 12 subscales (120). Lower Cronbach alphas were reported on the social functioning subscale in two studies ($r \leq 0.76$). Test-retest reliability for the 12 subscales, using ICC, range from $r = 0.67$ (role limitation—physical) to $r = 0.96$ (physical functioning) (120). Test-retest reliability for the physical health composite was $r = 0.87$ and for the mental health composite was $r = 0.87$.

Validity

The construct validity of the generic core of the MSQOL-54, the SF-36 has already been proven, but the MS-specific subscales or items on the MSQOL-54 have not. Convergent validity of this measure needs to be established by comparing it with other similar measures such as the Medical Rehabilitation Follow Along or the Multiple Sclerosis Quality of Life Inventory, which also contain MS-specific subscales.

Vickrey and colleagues base the construct validity of the MSQOL-54 on its moderate associations with symptom severity, ambulation status, role function, and mental health (120). Many of these significant relationships are based on their association with the generic core of the MSQOL-54, the SF-36. For example, MS symptom severity in the prior year and level of ambulation were significantly correlated with functional scales such as physical function, social function, and role limitations. Physical function was highly correlated with ambulation status. The pain subscale was associated with hospital admission in the prior year. Health distress and role limitations resulting from emotional difficulties were associated with depressive symptoms.

The question still remains whether the MSQOL-54 adds any significant contribution beyond the SF-36. In addressing this issue, Vickery and colleagues compared the SF-36 with the Quality of Life Questionnaire (QOLQ) for MS, the MS ADL Scale, and some MSQOL-54 items (cognitive function and sexual function) (123). In using a regression model to assess the best predictors of quality of life, the MSQOL-54 health distress subscale made a significant contribution to the model (p = 0.0004) and was entered second after the SF-36 physical function subscale.

Administration/Scoring

The MSQOL-54 can be self-administered or administered by a health care professional or volunteer. The amount of time needed to complete the MSQOL-54 ranges from 11

TABLE 13-23
Multiple Sclerosis Quality of Life (MSQOL)-54 Instrument

INSTRUCTIONS: The survey asks about your health and daily activities. Answer every question by circling the appropriate number (1, 2, 3,).

If you are unsure how to answer a question, please give the best answer you can and write a comment or explanation in the margin. Please feel free to ask someone to assist you if you need help reading or marking the form.

1. In general would you say your health is:

(circle one number)

Excellent 1
Very good 2
Good 3
Fair 4
Poor 5

2. **Compared to one year ago**, how would you rate your health in general **now**?

(circle one number)

Much better now than one year ago 1
Somewhat better now than one year ago 2
About the same 3
Somewhat worse now than one year ago 4
Much worse now than one year ago 5

3-12. The following questions are about activities you might do during a typical day. Does **your health** limit you in these activities? If so, how much? (Circle 1, 2, or 3 on each line)

	YES, LIMITED A LOT	YES, LIMITED A LITTLE	NO, NOT LIMITED AT ALL
3. Vigorous activities, such as running, lifting heavy objects, participating in strenuous sports	1	2	3
4. Moderate activities, such as moving a table, pushing a vacuum cleaner, bowling, or playing golf	1	2	3
5. Lifting or carrying groceries	1	2	3
6. Climbing several flights of stairs	1	2	3
7. Climbing one flight of stairs	1	2	3
8. Bending, kneeling, or stooping	1	2	3
9. Walking more than a mile	1	2	3
10. Walking several blocks	1	2	3
11. Walking one block	1	2	3
12. Bathing and dressing yourself	1	2	3

13-16. During the **past 4 weeks**, have you had any of the following problems with your work or other regular daily activities **as a result of your physical health**?
(Circle one number on each line)

	YES	NO
13. Cut down on the amount of time you could spend on work or other activities	1	2
14. Accomplished less than you would like	1	2
15. Were limited in the kind of work or other activities	1	2
16. Had difficulty performing the work or other activities	1	2

TABLE 13-23
continued

17-19. During the **past 4 weeks**, have you had any of the following problems with your work or other regular daily activities **as a result of any emotional problems** (such as feeling depressed or anxious) (Circle one number on each line)

	YES	No
17. Cut down on the amount of time you could spend on work or other activities	1	2
18. Accomplished less than you would like	1	2
19. Didn't do work or other activities as carefully as usual	1	2

20. During the **past 4 weeks**, to what extent has your physical health or emotional problems interfered with your normal social activities with family, friends, neighbors, or groups?

(circle one number)
Not at all 1
Slightly 2
Moderately 3
Quite a bit 4
Extremely 5

PAIN

21. How much **bodily** pain have you had during the **past 4 weeks**?

(circle one number)
None 1
Very mild 2
Mild 3
Moderate 4
Severe 5
Very severe 6

22. During the past 4 weeks, how much did pain interfere with your normal work (including both work outside the home and housework)?

(circle one number)
Not at all 1
A little bit 2
Moderately 3
Quite a bit 4
Extremely 5

23-32. These questions are about how you feel and how things have been with you **during the past 4 weeks**. For each question, please give the one answer that comes closest to the way you have been feeling.

How much of the time during the **past 4 weeks**...
(Circle one number on each line)

	ALL OF THE TIME	MOST OF THE TIME	A GOOD BIT OF THE TIME	SOME OF THE TIME	A LITTLE OF THE TIME	NONE OF THE TIME
23. Did you feel full of pep?	1	2	3	4	5	6
24. Have you been a very nervous person?	1	2	3	4	5	6
25. Have you felt so down in the dumps that nothing could cheer you up?	1	2	3	4	5	6
26. Have you felt calm and peaceful?	1	2	3	4	5	6
27. Did you have a lot of energy?	1	2	3	4	5	6

TABLE 13-23
continued

28. Have you felt downhearted and blue?	1	2	3	4	5	6
29. Did you feel worn out?	1	2	3	4	5	6
30. Have you been a happy person?	1	2	3	4	5	6
31. Did you feel tired?	1	2	3	4	5	6
32. Did you feel rested on waking in the morning?	1	2	3	4	5	6

33. During the **past 4 weeks**, how much of the time has your physical health or emotional problems interfered with your social activities (like visiting with friends, relatives, etc.)?

(circle one number)

Not at all 1
A little bit 2
Moderately 3
Quite a bit 4
Extremely 5

HEALTH IN GENERAL

34-37. How TRUE or FALSE is **each** of the following statements for you.
(Circle one number on each line).

	DEFINITELY TRUE	MOSTLY TRUE	NOT SURE	MOSTLY FALSE	DEFINITELY FALSE
34. I seem to get sick a little easier than other people	1	2	3	4	5
35. I am as healthy as anybody I know	1	2	3	4	5
36. I expect my health to get worse	1	2	3	4	5
37. My health is excellent	1	2	3	4	5

HEALTH DISTRESS

How much of the time during the **past 4 weeks**...
(Circle one number on each line)

	ALL OF THE TIME	MOST OF THE TIME	A GOOD BIT OF THE TIME	SOME OF THE TIME	A LITTLE OF THE TIME	NONE OF THE TIME
38. Were you discouraged by your health problems?	1	2	3	4	5	6
39. Were you frustrated about your health?	1	2	3	4	5	6
40. Was you health a worry in your life?	1	2	3	4	5	6
41. Did you feel weighed down by your health problems?	1	2	3	4	5	6

COGNITIVE FUNCTION

How much of the time during the **past 4 weeks**...
(Circle one number on each line)

	ALL OF THE TIME	MOST OF THE TIME	A GOOD BIT OF THE TIME	SOME OF THE TIME	A LITTLE OF THE TIME	NONE OF THE TIME
42. Have you had difficulty concentrating and thinking?	1	2	3	4	5	6
43. Did you have trouble keeping your attention on an activity for long?	1	2	3	4	5	6

TABLE 13-23
continued

44. Have you had trouble with your memory?	1	2	3	4	5	6
45. Have others, such as family members or friends, noticed that you have trouble with your memory or problems with your concentration?	1	2	3	4	5	6

SEXUAL FUNCTION

46-49. The next set of questions are about your sexual function and your satisfaction with your sexual function. Please answer as accurately as possible about your function **during the last 4 weeks only**. How much of a problem was each of the following for you **during the last 4 weeks only**. (Circle one number on each line)

MEN	NOT A PROBLEM	A LITTLE OF A PROBLEM	SOMEWHAT OF A PROBLEM	VERY MUCH A PROBLEM
46. Lack of sexual interest	1	2	3	4
47. Difficulty getting or keeping an erection	1	2	3	4
48. Difficulty having orgasm	1	2	3	4
49. Ability to satisfy sexual partner	1	2	3	4

(Circle one number on each line)

WOMEN	NOT A PROBLEM	A LITTLE OF A PROBLEM	SOMEWHAT OF A PROBLEM	VERY MUCH A PROBLEM
46. Lack of sexual interest	1	2	3	4
47. Inadequate lubrication	1	2	3	4
48. Difficulty having orgasm	1	2	3	4
49. Ability to satisfy sexual partner	1	2	3	4

50. Overall, how satisfied were you with your sexual function **during the past 4 weeks**?

(circle one number)

Very satisfied 1
Somewhat satisfied 2
Neither satisfied nor dissatisfied 3
Somewhat dissatisfied 4
Very dissatisfied 5

51. During the **past 4 weeks**, to what extent have problems with your bowel or bladder function interfered with your normal social activities with family, friends, neighbors, or groups?

(circle one number)

Not at all 1
Slightly 2
Moderately 3
Quite a bit 4
Extremely 5

52. During the past 4 weeks how much did pain interfere with your enjoyment of life?

(circle one number)

Not at all 1
Slightly 2
Moderately 3
Quite a bit 4
Extremely 5

TABLE 13-23
continued

QUALITY OF LIFE

53. Overall how would you rate your own quality of life? Circle one number on the scale below:

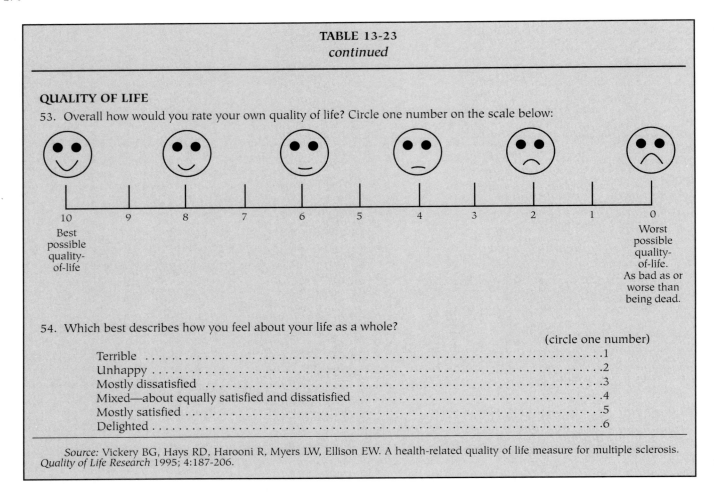

| 10 | 9 | 8 | 7 | 6 | 5 | 4 | 3 | 2 | 1 | 0 |

Best
possible
quality-
of-life

Worst
possible
quality-
of-life.
As bad as or
worse than
being dead.

54. Which best describes how you feel about your life as a whole?

(circle one number)

Terrible 1
Unhappy 2
Mostly dissatisfied 3
Mixed—about equally satisfied and dissatisfied 4
Mostly satisfied 5
Delighted 6

Source: Vickery BG, Hays RD, Harooni R, Myers LW, Ellison EW. A health-related quality of life measure for multiple sclerosis. *Quality of Life Research* 1995; 4:187-206.

to 18 minutes, but one should allow more time if the patient requires assistance (120). Subscale scores are obtained by transforming item scores to a 0 to 100 scale, with 0 representing the worst health and 100 indicating the best health state. Then average the transformed item scores to obtain a total subscale score. The physical and mental health composite score is created by the weighted linear combination of subscale scores. The scoring and composite weighing information is available in the MSQOL-54 manual (130).

Advantages

The MSQOL-54 is a comprehensive quality of life measure that specifically evaluates the types of problems experienced by people with MS. All of the multi-item subscales demonstrated adequate internal consistency reliability, and test-retest reliability met the 0.70 minimum standard for group comparison for all but one subscale (health perception) (120). The SF-36 generic core permits the MSQOL-54 to be compared with other chronic disease populations and with the general population. These features make the MSQOL-

54 a versatile measure that is appropriate for MS settings (clinical trials, rehabilitation, and clinical follow-up).

Disadvantages

Based on a review of the MS literature, the MSQOL-54 does include the most relevant MS symptoms. Unfortunately, the MSQOL-54 was constructed mainly by adding individual items to the SF-36, and some important MS symptoms were not adequately assessed (i.e., sexual and cognitive function). On the MSQOL-54, the sexual satisfaction includes only one item.

Problems with floor/ceiling effects were experienced on the two role limitation subscales (120). On the role limitation—physical subscale, nearly 50 percent of the MS patients scored the lowest possible score (floor effect). On the role limitation—emotional, 46 percent of MS patients scored the highest possible score (ceiling effect). The implications of the floor effect on the role limitation—physical subscale only becomes an issue when wheelchair-bound MS patients are being followed up longitudinally (120).

Comment

The MSQOL-54 is a standardized multidimensional health-related quality of life measure specifically for MS. It combines generic health-related problems (SF-36) with concerns most relevant to people with MS. Compared with the SF-36, MSQOL-54 provides additional information regarding health distress, which is the unique contribution of this measure. The MSQOL-54 does not adequately assess cognitive function or sexual function, so this measure needs further development. If the MSQOL-54 or the SF-36 is used when studying severely impaired or wheelchair-bound MS patients, floor effect can be limited by adding the MS ADL Scale—specifically, the motor subscale (131).

Multiple Sclerosis Quality of Life-Inventory

The Multiple Sclerosis Quality of Life Inventory (MSQLI), like the MSQOL-54, is both a generic and an MS-specific quality of life measure (24) . It was designed to measure the quality of life concerns common to all patient populations while concurrently addressing the most relevant concerns of people with MS. The generic core of the MSQLI is the SF-36 measure and as such allows comparisons with other patient populations. The MS-specific scales were based on relevant quality of life issues derived from extensive review of the quality of life literature. The MSQLI field testing was a multicenter study that included 300 MS patients whose status ranged from newly diagnosed to severely impaired (24).

Description

The MSQLI is a comprehensive quality of life measure that combines the best existing questionnaires or the best attributes of several existing questionnaires into a relatively brief assessment package. It consists of 138 items and 10 separate scales (Table 13-24). The scales assess the following quality of life domains: general health status, fatigue, pain, sexual satisfaction, bladder control, bowel control, vision, cognitive function, mental, and (10) social support. The MSQLI is comprised of the following 10 measures:

Health Status Questionnaire (SF-36)
Modified Fatigue Impact Scale (MFIS)
MOS Pain Effects Scale (PES)
Sexual Satisfaction Scale (SSS)
Bladder Control Scale (BLCS)
Bowel Control Scale (BWCS)
Impact of Visual Impairment Scale (IVIS)
Perceived Deficits Questionnaire (PDQ)
Mental Health Inventory (MHI)
Modified Social Support Survey (MSSS)

Note that the MSSS is a measure of perceived, not actual, support and refers to support from all sources.

Reliability

Most internal consistency reliability coefficients determined by Cronbach's alpha across all MSQLI measures were above 0.08 and ranged from $r = 0.67$ (SF-36—social functioning) to a high of $r = 0.97$ (MSSS total score). Individual alpha coefficients for all MSQLI scales and subscales are reported in Table 13-25.

Validity

The MSQLI has documented content, criterion-related, and construct validity (24). In demonstrating construct validity, the MSQLI was compared with a variety of other measures, including the EDSS/FS, SIP, Ambulation Index, 9-HPT, and UCLA Loneliness-Companionship Scale. For detailed information regarding correlations among all the measures, the reader is referred to the MSQLI manual (24).

Administration/Scoring

The MSQLI can be self-administered or administered by a trained health care professional in 45 minutes. If the abbreviated version is used, administration time is reduced to 30 minutes, but use of the full-length version is strongly recommend whenever possible (24). The MSQLI provides several scores, each assessing a different dimension of quality of life. Most measures are easily scored simply by adding raw scores for each scale or subscale to create a total score. These measures include the MFIS, PES, SSS, BLCS, BWCS, IVIS, and PDQ. Higher scores on these tests indicate greater problems. On the SF-36, MHI, and the MSSS, for each subscale, items are added, means are calculated, and scores are transformed to a 0 to 100 scale. Higher scores indicate better mental and physical health (SF-36, MHI) and high perceived support (MSSS). The scoring procedures for the MSQLI measures are also available (Dr. Nicholas G. LaRocca, NMSS, 733 Third Avenue, New York, NY, 10017).

Advantages

The MSQLI is a new comprehensive battery of measures that captures the richness and complexity inherent in a concept such as quality of life (24), while simultaneously assessing the most relevant concerns of people with MS. Based on cross-sectional data, reliability and validity have been demonstrated on both the generic and MS-specific measures included in the MSQLI. The MSQLI is a well-

TABLE 13-24
The MSQLI

Patient's Name: _____   Date: _____ /_____ /_____
                                                                     month   day   year

ID#: _____   Test#:   1   2   3   4

HEALTH STATUS QUESTIONNAIRE (SF-36)

INSTRUCTIONS:

This survey asks for your views about your health and daily activities. If you are marking your own answers, please circle the appropriate responses (0, 1, 2,...). If you need help in marking your responses, **tell the interviewer the number** of the best response (or what to fill in). **Please answer every question.** If you are not sure which answer to select, please choose the one answer that comes closest to describing you. The interviewer can explain any words or phrases that you do not understand.

1. In general, would you say your health is:

Excellent	Very Good	Good	Fair	Poor
1	2	3	4	5

2. For each statement please circle the one number that indicates how true or false that statement is for you.

	DEFINITELY TRUE	MOSTLY TRUE	NOT SURE	MOSTLY FALSE	DEFINITELY FALSE
a) I seem to get sick a little easier than other people.	1	2	3	4	5
b) I am as healthy as anybody I know.	1	2	3	4	5
c) I expect my health to get worse.	1	2	3	4	5
d) My health is excellent.	1	2	3	4	5

3. **Compared to one year ago**, how would you rate your health in general **now**?

Much Better	Somewhat Better	Same	Somewhat Worse	Much Worse
1	2	3	4	5

4. Now, think about the activities you might do on a typical day. Does **your health** limit you in the activities? If so, **how much?** Please circle 1, 2, or 3 for each item to indicate how much your health limits you.

	YES, LIMITED A LOT	YES, LIMITED A LITTLE	NO, NOT LIMITED AT ALL
a) **Vigorous activities**, such as running, lifting heavy objects, participating in strenuous sports	1	2	3
b) **Moderate activities**, such as moving a table, pushing a vacuum cleaner or bowling, or playing golf	1	2	3
c) Lifting or carrying groceries	1	2	3
d) Climbing **several** flights of stairs	1	2	3
e) Climbing **one** flight of stairs	1	2	3
f) Bending, kneeling, or stooping	1	2	3
g) Walking **more than a mile**	1	2	3
h) Walking **several blocks**	1	2	3
i) Walking **one block**	1	2	3
j) Bathing and dressing yourself	1	2	3

TABLE 13-24
continued

5. During the **past 4 weeks**, have you had any of the following problems with your work or other regular daily activities **as a result of your physical health**? Please circle "1" (Yes) or "2" (No) for each item.

		YES	NO
a)	Cut down on the **amount of time** you spent on work or other activities	1	2
b)	**Accomplished less** than you would like	1	2

During the **past 4 weeks**, have you had any of the following problems with your work or other regular daily activities **as a result of your physical health**? Please circle "1" (Yes) or "2" (No) for each item.

		YES	NO
c)	Were limited in the kind of work or other activities	1	2
d)	Had difficulty performing the work or other activities (for example, it took extra effort)	1	2

6. How much bodily pain have you had during the **past 4 weeks**?

None	Very mild	Mild	Moderate	Severe	Very severe
1	2	3	4	5	6

7. During the **past 4 weeks**, how much did pain interfere with your normal work (including work both outside the home and housework)?

Not at all	A little bit	Moderately	Quite a bit	Extremely
1	2	3	4	5

8. During the **past 4 weeks**, have you had the following problems with your work or other regular daily activities **as a result of any emotional problems** (such as feeling depressed or anxious)? Please circle "1" (Yes) or "2" (No) for each item.

		YES	NO
a)	Cut down on the **amount of time** you spent on work or other activities	1	2
b)	**Accomplished less** than you would like	1	2
c)	Did do work or other activities **less carefully** than usual	1	2

9. During the **past 4 weeks**, to what extent have your physical health or emotional problems interfered with your normal social activities with family, friends, neighbors, or groups?

Not al all	Slightly	Moderately	Quite a bit	Extremely
1	2	3	4	5

10. The next set of questions is about how you feel and how things have been with you during the **past 4 weeks**. For each question, please circle the one number for the answer that comes closest to the way you have been feeling.

How much of the time during the **past 4 weeks**...

		ALL OF THE TIME	MOST OF THE TIME	A GOOD BIT OF THE TIME	SOME OF THE TIME	A LITTLE OF THE TIME	NONE OF THE TIME
a)	did you feel full of pep?	1	2	3	4	5	6
b)	have you been a very nervous person?	1	2	3	4	5	6
c)	have you felt so down in the dumps nothing could cheer you up?	1	2	3	4	5	6
d)	have you felt calm and peaceful?	1	2	3	4	5	6
e)	did you have a lot of energy?	1	2	3	4	5	6
f)	have you felt downhearted and blue?	1	2	3	4	5	6
g)	did you feel worn out?	1	2	3	4	5	6
h)	have you been a happy person?	1	2	3	4	5	6
i)	did you feel tired?	1	2	3	4	5	6

TABLE 13-24
continued

11. Finally, during the past 4 weeks, how much of the time has your physical health or emotional problems interfered with your social activities (like visiting with friends, relatives, etc.)?

All of the time	Most of the time	Some of the time	A little of the time	None of the time
1	2	3	4	5

Patient's Name: _____   Date: _____/_____/_____
                                                                              month   day   year

ID#: _____   Test#:   1   2   3   4

MODIFIED FATIGUE IMPACT SCALE (MFIS)

Following is a list of statements that describe how fatigue may affect a person. Fatigue is a feeling of physical tiredness and lack of energy that many people experience from time to time. In medical conditions like MS, feelings of fatigue can occur more often and have a greater impact than usual. Please read each statement carefully, and then **circle the one number** that best indicates how often fatigue has affected you in this way during the **past 4 weeks**. (If you need help in marking your responses, **tell the interviewer the number** of the best response.) **Please answer every question.** If you are not sure which answer to select, please choose the one answer that comes closest to describing you. The interviewer can explain any words or phrases that you do not understand.

Because of my fatigue during the **past 4 weeks**…

	NEVER	RARELY	SOMETIMES	OFTEN	ALMOST ALWAYS
1. I have been less alert.	0	1	2	3	4
2. I have had difficulty paying attention for long periods of time.	0	1	2	3	4
3. I have been unable to think clearly.	0	1	2	3	4
4. I have been clumsy and uncoordinated.	0	1	2	3	4
5. I have been forgetful.	0	1	2	3	4
6. I have had to pace myself in my physical activities.	0	1	2	3	4
7. I have been less motivated to do anything that requires physical effort.	0	1	2	3	4
8. I have been less motivated to participate in social activities.	0	1	2	3	4
9. I have been limited in my ability to do things away from home.	0	1	2	3	4
10. I have had trouble maintaining physical effort for long periods.	0	1	2	3	4
11. I have had difficulty making decisions.	0	1	2	3	4
12. I have been less motivated to do anything that requires thinking.	0	1	2	3	4
13. my muscles have felt weak.	0	1	2	3	4
14. I have been physically uncomfortable.	0	1	2	3	4
15. I have had trouble finishing tasks that require thinking.	0	1	2	3	4
16. I have had difficulty organizing my thoughts when doing things at home or at work.	0	1	2	3	4
17. I have been less able to complete tasks that require physical effort.	0	1	2	3	4
18. my thinking has been slowed down.	0	1	2	3	4
19. I have had trouble concentrating.	0	1	2	3	4
20. I have limited my physical activities.	0	1	2	3	4
21. I have needed to rest more often or for longer periods.	0	1	2	3	4

TABLE 13-24
continued

Patient's Name: _____

ID#: _____

Date: _____ / _____ / _____
         month   day   year

Test#: 1 2 3 4

MODIFIED FATIGUE IMPACT SCALE—5-ITEM VERSION (MFIS-5)

Following is a list of statements that describe how fatigue may affect a person. Fatigue is a feeling of physical tiredness and lack of energy that many people experience from time to time. In medical conditions like MS, feelings of fatigue can occur more often and have a greater impact than usual. Please read each statement carefully, and then **circle the one number** that best indicates how often fatigue has affected you in this way during the **past 4 weeks**. (If you need help in marking your responses, **tell the interviewer the number** of the best response.) **Please answer every question**. If you are not sure which answer to select, please choose the one answer that comes closest to describing you. The interviewer can explain any words or phrases that you do not understand.

Because of my fatigue during the **past 4 weeks**...

	NEVER	RARELY	SOMETIMES	OFTEN	ALMOST ALWAYS
1. I have been less alert.	0	1	2	3	4
2. I have been limited in my ability to do things away from home.	0	1	2	3	4
3. I have had trouble maintaining physical effort for long periods.	0	1	2	3	4
4. I have been less able to complete tasks that require physical effort.	0	1	2	3	4
5. I have had trouble concentrating.	0	1	2	3	4

Patient's Name: _____

ID#: _____

Date: _____ / _____ / _____
         month   day   year

Test#: 1 2 3 4

MOS PAIN EFFECTS SCALE (PES)

INSTRUCTIONS

Individuals with MS can sometimes experience unpleasant sensory symptoms as a result of their MS (e.g., pain, tingling, burning). The next set of questions covers pain and other unpleasant sensations, and how they affect you. Please **circle the one number** (0, 1, 2,...) that best indicates the extent to which your sensory symptoms (including pain) interfered with that aspect of your life during the **past 4 weeks**. If you need help in marking your responses, **tell the interviewer the number** of the best response (or what to fill in). **Please answer every question**. If you are not sure which answer to select, please choose the one answer that comes closest to describing you. The interviewer can explain any words or phrases that you do not understand.

During the **past 4 weeks**, how much did these symptoms interfere with your...

	NOT AT ALL	A LITTLE	MODERATELY	QUITE A BIT	TO AN EXTREME DEGREE
1. mood	1	2	3	4	5
2. ability to walk or move around	1	2	3	4	5
3. sleep	1	2	3	4	5
4. normal work (both outside your home and at home)	1	2	3	4	5
5. recreational activities	1	2	3	4	5
6. enjoyment of life	1	2	3	4	5

TABLE 13-24
continued

Patient's Name: _____   Date: _____/_____/_____
                                                                month   day   year

ID#: _____   Test#:   1   2   3   4

SEXUAL SATISFACTION SCALE (SSS)

INSTRUCTIONS

The next series of questions concerns your intimate relationships and your satisfaction with your sex life. Many of these questions are very personal, but this is an important topic to cover. If you are marking your own answers, please **circle** the appropriate response (0, 1, 2,...). If you need help in marking your responses, tell the interviewer the number of the best response. **Please answer every question**. If you are not sure which answer to select, please choose the one answer that comes closest to describing you. The interviewer can explain any words or phrases that you do not understand.

1. Do you have a relationship with one primary partner?

    No [GO TO NEXT QUESTIONNAIRE] 0
    Yes 1

2. During the **past 4 weeks**, how satisfied have you been with the amount of affection expressed physically in your relationship?

Extremely Satisfied	Moderately Satisfied	Slightly Satisfied	Slightly Dissatisfied	Moderately Dissatisfied	Extremely Dissatisfied
1	2	3	4	5	6

3. During the **past 4 weeks**, how satisfied have you been with the variety of sexual activities you engage in with your partner?

Extremely Satisfied	Moderately Satisfied	Slightly Satisfied	Slightly Dissatisfied	Moderately Dissatisfied	Extremely Dissatisfied
1	2	3	4	5	6

4. During the **past 4 weeks**, how satisfied have you been with your sexual relationship in general?

Extremely Satisfied	Moderately Satisfied	Slightly Satisfied	Slightly Dissatisfied	Moderately Dissatisfied	Extremely Dissatisfied
1	2	3	4	5	6

5. How satisfied do you think your partner has been with your sexual relationship in general, during the **past 4 weeks**?

Extremely Satisfied	Moderately Satisfied	Slightly Satisfied	Slightly Dissatisfied	Moderately Dissatisfied	Extremely Dissatisfied
1	2	3	4	5	6

Patient's Name: _____   Date: _____/_____/_____
                                                                month   day   year

ID#: _____   Test#:   1   2   3   4

BLADDER CONTROL SCALE (BLCS)

INSTRUCTIONS

The next set of questions concerns bladder problems that can occur in MS. Many of these questions are very personal, but this is an important topic to cover. If you are marking your own answers, please **circle** the appropriate response (0, 1, 2,...) based on your bladder function during the **past 4 weeks**. If you need help in marking your responses, **tell the interviewer the number** of the best response. **Please answer every question**. If you are not sure which answer to select, please choose the one answer that comes closest to describing you. The interviewer can explain any words or phrases that you do not understand.

During the **past 4 weeks**, how often have you...

TABLE 13-24
continued

	NOT AT ALL	ONCE	TWO TO FOUR TIMES	MORE THAN WEEKLY BUT NOT DAILY	DAILY
1. lost control of your bladder or had an accident?	0	1	2	3	4
2. **almost** lost control of your bladder or had an accident?	0	1	2	3	4
3. altered your activities because of bladder problems?	0	1	2	3	4

4. During the **past 4 weeks**, how much have bladder problems restricted your overall lifestyle? (Please circle one number.)

Not at all
      0   1   2   3   4   5   6   7   8   9   Severely
                                            10

Patient's Name: _____ Date: _____ / _____ / _____

                                                       month   day   year

ID#: _____ Test#: 1 2 3 4

BOWEL CONTROL SCALE (BWCS)

INSTRUCTIONS

The next set of questions concerns bowel problems that can occur in MS. Many of these questions are very personal, but this is an important topic to cover. If you are marking your own answers, please **circle** the appropriate response (0, 1, 2,...) based on your bowel function during the **past 4 weeks**. If you need help in marking your responses, **tell the interviewer the number** of the best response. **Please answer every question**. If you are not sure which answer to select, please choose the one answer that comes closest to describing you. The interviewer can explain any words or phrases that you do not understand.

During the **past 4 weeks**, how often have you...

	NOT AT ALL	ONCE	TWO TO FOUR TIMES	MORE THAN WEEKLY BUT NOT DAILY	DAILY
1. been constipated?	0	1	2	3	4
2. lost control of your bowels or had an accident?	0	1	2	3	4
3. **almost** lost control of your bowels or almost had an accident?	0	1	2	3	4
4. altered your activities because of bowel control problems?	0	1	2	3	4

5. During the **past 4 weeks**, how much have bowel problems restricted your overall lifestyle? (Please circle **one** number.)

Not at all
      0   1   2   3   4   5   6   7   8   9   Severely
                                              10

TABLE 13-24
continued

Patient's Name: _____   Date: _____/_____/_____
                                                              month   day   year

ID#: _____   Test#:   1   2   3   4

IMPACT OF VISUAL IMPAIRMENT SCALE (IVIS)

INSTRUCTIONS

The following questions concern your vision and how any visual problems have affected your ability to do your daily activities. If you are marking your own answers, please **circle** the appropriate response (0, 1, 2,...) based on how your vision has been during the **past 4 weeks**. If you need help in marking your responses, **tell the interviewer the number** of the best response. **Please answer every question**. If you are not sure which answer to select, please choose the one answer that comes closest to describing you. The interviewer can explain any words or phrases that you do not understand.

During the **past 4 weeks**, how difficult did you find it to...

	NOT AT ALL DIFFICULT	SOMEWHAT DIFFICULT	EXTREMELY DIFFICULT	COULD NOT DO DUE TO VISUAL PROBLEMS
1. read or access personal letters or notes?	0	1	2	3
2. read or access printed materials, such as books, magazines, newspaper, etc.?	0	1	2	3
3. read or access dials, such as on stoves, thermostats, etc.?	0	1	2	3
4. watch television or identify faces from a distance?	0	1	2	3
5. identify house numbers, street signs, etc.?	0	1	2	3

Patient's Name: _____   Date: _____/_____/_____
                                                              month   day   year

ID#: _____   Test#:   1   2   3   4

PERCEIVED DEFICITS QUESTIONNAIRE (PDQ)

INSTRUCTIONS

Everyone at some point experiences problems with memory, attention, or concentration, but these problems may occur more frequently for individuals with neurologic diseases like MS. The following questions describe several situations in which a person may encounter problems with memory, attention or concentration. If you are marking your own answers, please **circle** the appropriate response (0, 1, 2,...) based on your cognitive function during the **past 4 weeks**. If you need help in marking your responses, **tell the interviewer the number** of the best response. **Please answer every question**. If you are not sure which answer to select, please choose the one answer that comes closest to describing you. The interviewer can explain any words or phrases that you do not understand.

During the **past 4 weeks**, how often did you...

	NEVER	RARELY	SOMETIMES	OFTEN	ALMOST ALWAYS
1. lose your train of thought when speaking?	0	1	2	3	4
2. have difficulty remembering the names of people, even ones you have met several times?	0	1	2	3	4
3. forget what you came into the room for?	0	1	2	3	4
4. have trouble getting things organized?	0	1	2	3	4

TABLE 13-24
continued

		NEVER	RARELY	SOMETIMES	OFTEN	ALMOST ALWAYS
5.	have trouble concentrating on what people are saying during a conversation?	0	1	2	3	4
6.	forget if you had already done something?	0	1	2	3	4
7.	miss appointments and meetings you had scheduled?	0	1	2	3	4
8.	have difficulty planning what to do in the day?	0	1	2	3	4
9.	have trouble concentrating on things like watching a television program or reading a book?	0	1	2	3	4
10.	forget what you did the night before?	0	1	2	3	4
11.	forget the date unless you looked it up?	0	1	2	3	4
12.	have trouble getting started, even if you had a lot of things to do?	0	1	2	3	4
13.	find your mind drifting?	0	1	2	3	4
14.	forget what you talked about after a telephone conversation?	0	1	2	3	4
15.	forget to do things like turn off the stove or turn on your alarm clock?	0	1	2	3	4
16.	feel like your mind went totally blank?	0	1	2	3	4
17.	have trouble holding phone numbers in your head, even for a few seconds?	0	1	2	3	4
18.	forget what you did last weekend?	0	1	2	3	4
19.	forget to take you medication?	0	1	2	3	4
20.	have trouble making decisions?	0	1	2	3	4

Patient's Name: _____

ID#: _____

Date: _____ / _____ / _____
month   day   year

Test#:   1   2   3   4

PERCEIVED DEFICITS QUESTIONNAIRE—5-ITEM VERSION (PDQ-5)

INSTRUCTIONS

Everyone at some point experiences problems with memory, attention, or concentration, but these problems may occur more frequently for individuals with neurologic diseases like MS. The following questions describe several situations in which a person may encounter problems with memory, attention, or concentration. If you are marking your own answers, please **circle** the appropriate response (0, 1, 2,...) based on your cognitive function during the **past 4 weeks**. If you need help in marking your responses, **tell the interviewer the number** of the best response. **Please answer every question**. If you are not sure which answer to select, please choose the one answer that comes closest to describing you. The interviewer can explain any words or phrases that you do not understand.

During the **past 4 weeks**, how often did you...

		NEVER	RARELY	SOMETIMES	OFTEN	ALMOST ALWAYS
1.	have trouble getting things organized?	0	1	2	3	4
2,	have trouble concentrating on things like watching a television program or reading a book?	0	1	2	3	4
3.	forget the date unless you looked it up?	0	1	2	3	4
4.	forget what you talked about after a telephone conversation?	0	1	2	3	4
5.	feel like your mind went totally blank?	0	1	2	3	4

TABLE 13-24
continued

Patient's Name: _____ Date: _____ / _____ / _____
                                                            month   day   year

ID#: _____ Test#:   1   2   3   4

MENTAL HEALTH INVENTORY (MHI)

The next set of questions are about how you feel, and how things have been for you during the **past 4 weeks**. If you are marking your own answers, please **circle** the appropriate response (0, 1, 2,…). If you need help in marking your responses, **tell the interviewer the number** of the best response. **Please answer every question**. If you are not sure which answer to select, please choose the one answer that comes closest to describing you. The interviewer can explain any words or phrases that you do not understand.

During the **past 4 weeks**, how much of the time…

	ALL OF THE TIME	MOST OF THE TIME	A GOOD BIT OF THE TIME	SOME OF THE TIME	A LITTLE BIT OF THE TIME	NONE OF THE TIME
1. has your daily life been full of things that were interesting to you?	1	2	3	4	5	6
2. did you feel depressed?	1	2	3	4	5	6
3. have you felt loved and wanted?	1	2	3	4	5	6
4. have you been a very nervous person?	1	2	3	4	5	6
5. have you been in firm control of your behavior, thoughts, emotions, feelings?	1	2	3	4	5	6
6. have you felt tense or high-strung?	1	2	3	4	5	6
7. have you felt calm and peaceful?	1	2	3	4	5	6
8. have you felt emotionally stable?	1	2	3	4	5	6
9. have you felt downhearted and blue?	1	2	3	4	5	6
10. were you able to relax without difficulty?	1	2	3	4	5	6
11. have you felt restless, fidgety, or impatient?	1	2	3	4	5	6
12. have you been moody, or brooded about things?	1	2	3	4	5	6
13. have you felt cheerful, lighthearted?	1	2	3	4	5	6
14. have you been in low or very low spirits?	1	2	3	4	5	6
15. were you a happy person?	1	2	3	4	5	6
16. did you feel you had nothing to look forward to?	1	2	3	4	5	6
17. have you felt so down in the dumps that nothing could cheer you up?	1	2	3	4	5	6
18. have you been anxious or worried?	1	2	3	4	5	6

Patient's Name: _____ Date: _____ / _____ / _____
                                                           month   day   year

ID#: _____ Test#:   1   2   3   4

MOS MODIFIED SOCIAL SUPPORT SURVEY (MSSS)

INSTRUCTIONS

People sometimes look to others for companionship, assistance, or other types of support. This questionnaire covers the types of support that would be available to you if you needed it. If you are marking your own answers, please **circle** the appropriate response (0, 1, 2,…) based on the support available to you during the **past 4 weeks**. If you need help in marking your responses, **tell the interviewer the number** of the best response (or what to fill in). **Please answer every question**. If you are not sure which answer to select, please choose the one answer that comes closest to describing you. The interviewer can explain any words or phrases that you do not understand.

TABLE 13-24
continued

How often is someone available…

	NONE OF THE TIME	A LITTLE OF THE TIME	SOME OF THE TIME	MOST OF THE TIME	ALL OF THE TIME
1. to help you if you are confined to bed?	1	2	3	4	5
2. to listen to you when you need to talk?	1	2	3	4	5
3. to give you good advice about a crisis?	1	2	3	4	5
4. to take you to the doctor if you need to go?	1	2	3	4	5
5. to show you love and affection?	1	2	3	4	5
6. to have a good time with?	1	2	3	4	5
7. to give you information to help you understand a situation?	1	2	3	4	5
8. to confide in or talk to about yourself or your problems?	1	2	3	4	5
9. to hug you?	1	2	3	4	5
10. to get together with for relaxation?	1	2	3	4	5
11. to prepare your meals if you are unable to do it yourself?	1	2	3	4	5
12. whose advice you really want?	1	2	3	4	5
13. to help with daily chores if you are sick?	1	2	3	4	5
14. to share your private worries and fears with?	1	2	3	4	5
15. to turn to for suggestions about how to deal with a personal problem?	1	2	3	4	5
16. to do something enjoyable with?	1	2	3	4	5
17. to understand your problems?	1	2	3	4	5
18. to love and make you feel wanted?	1	2	3	4	5

Patient's Name: _____

Date: _____ / _____ / _____
　　　　　　　　month　　　day　　　year

ID#: _____

Test#:　1　2　3　4

MOS MODIFIED SOCIAL SUPPORT SURVEY—5-ITEM VERSION (MSSS-5)

INSTRUCTIONS

People sometimes look to others for companionship, assistance, or other types of support. This questionnaire covers the types of support that would be available to you if you needed it. If you are marking your own answers, please **circle** the appropriate response (0, 1, 2,…) based on the support available to you during the **past 4 weeks**. If you need help in marking your responses, **tell the interviewer the number** of the best response (or what to fill in). **Please answer every question**. If you are not sure which answer to select, please choose the one answer that comes closest to describing you. The interviewer can explain any words or phrases that you do not understand.

How often is someone available…

	NONE OF THE TIME	A LITTLE OF THE TIME	SOME OF THE TIME	MOST OF THE TIME	ALL OF THE TIME
1. to take you to the doctor if you need to go?	1	2	3	4	5
2. to have a good time with?	1	2	3	4	5
3. to hug you?	1	2	3	4	5
4. to prepare your meals if you are unable to do it yourself?	1	2	3	4	5
5. to understand your problems?	1	2	3	4	5

TABLE 13-25
Informational on the MSQLI

	SCALES	SCORE RANGE	NUMBERS OF ITEMS	ALPHAS
SF-36	Physical Functioning	0–100	10	0.94
	Role-Physical	0–100	4	0.80
	Bodily Pain	0–100	2	0.91
	General Health	0–100	5	0.77
	Vitality	0–100	4	0.85
	Social Functioning	0–100	2	0.67
	Role-Emotional	0–100	3	0.75
	Mental Health	0–100	5	0.82
	Physical Component Summary Score	T-score	35	*
	Mental Component Summary Score	T-score	35	*
MFIS	Cognitive	0–40	10	0.95
	Physical	0–36	11	0.91
	Psychosocial	0–8	2	0.81
	Total	0–84	21	0.81
	Abbreviated Version	0–20	5	0.80
PES	Pain Effects Scale	6–30	6	0.86
SSS	Sexual Satisfaction Scale	4–24	4	0.91
BLCS	Bladder Control Scale	0–22	4	0.82
BWCS	Bowel Control Scale	0–26	5	0.78
IVIS	Vision-Reading	0–15	5	0.86
PDQ	Attention	0–20	5	0.82
	Retrospective Memory	0–20	5	0.86
	Prospective Memory	0–20	5	0.74
	Planning/Organization	0–20	5	0.85
	Total	0–80	20	0.93
	Abbreviated Version	0–20	5	0.84
MHI	Anxiety Scale	0–100	5	0.80
	Depression Scale	0–100	4	0.87
	Behav. & Emot. Control	0–100	4	0.78
	Positive Affect	0–100	4	0.83
	Total	0–100	18	0.93
	Abbreviated Version	0–100	5	0.82
MSSS	Tangible Support	0–100	4	0.87
	Emotional Support	0–100	8	0.95
	Affective Support	0–100	3	0.91
	Positive Support	0–100	3	0.92
	Total	0–100	18	0.97
	Abbreviated Version	0–100	5	0.88

constructed battery of validated tests that permits comparison of specific symptoms across studies and within a study. Most of the MS-specific measures included in the MSQLI are established scales.

Disadvantages

The length of the MSQLI may be an issue for some clinicians and researchers when time is an important factor. In response to this expected complaint, the developers have created abbreviated versions of some of the MSQLI measures. The psychometric properties of the abbreviated versions appear to be comparable to the longer versions. As with the MSQOL-54, the MSQLI has not yet been tested for sensitivity to MS changes in a longitudinal study.

Comments

The MSQLI is a promising new standardized multidimensional health-related quality of life measure that provides detailed information about the concerns most relevant to people with MS.

SUMMARY

There are numerous measures used in MS clinical trials and rehabilitation research—too many to be reviewed in this chapter. Here, the emphasis was on evaluating prevalent standardized instruments endorsed by the Medical Outcomes Trust and the NMSS Clinical Outcomes Assessment Task Force. Also reviewed were promising new measures and older measures commonly used but still in need of psychometric testing and development. The instruments in this chapter covered a broad array of MS outcome needs ranging from impairment, disability, handicap, to health-related quality of life. The depth and quality of the more recently constructed multidimensional health status measures are indicative of the progress the medical profession has made toward viewing medical and rehabilitation success from the patient's perspective.

For additional information regarding clinical and rehabilitation outcome measures, the reader is referred to the following references: 4,52,65,74, 132.

*A*cknowledgements

The author thanks Drs. Gary Cutter, Nicholas LaRocca, Harvey Retzloff, and Paul Retzlaff for their contributions.

*R*eferences

1. Rudick R, Antel J, Confavreux C, et al. Clinical outcomes assessment in multiple sclerosis. *Ann Neurol* 1996; 40:469–479.
2. Rudick R, Antel J, Confavreux C, et al. Recommendations from the national multiple sclerosis society clinical outcomes assessment task force. *Ann Neurol* 1997; 42:379–382.
3. Hobart JC, Freeman JA, Lamping DL. The evaluation of outcome measurement instruments. *MS Management* 1995; 2:6–12.
4. Wilkin D, Hallam L, Doggett MA. *Measures of need and outcome for primary health care.* New York: Oxford University Press, 1992.
5. Granger CV, Ottenbacher KJ, Baker JG, Sehgal A. Reliability of a brief outpatient functional outcome assessment measure. *Am J Phys Med Rehab* 1995; 74:469–75.
6. Johnston MV, Keith RA. Measurement standards for medical rehabilitation and clinical applications. In: Kraft GH (ed.). *Physical medicine and rehabilitation: Clinics of North America.* Philadelphia: WBSaunders, 1993; 4:425–49.
7. International Federation of Multiple Sclerosis Societies. *M.R.D. Minimal Record of Disability of multiple sclerosis.* New York: National Multiple Sclerosis Society, 1985.
8. Willoughby EW, Paty DW. Scales for rating impairment in multiple sclerosis: A critique. *Neurology* 1988; 38:1793–1798.
9. World Health Organization. *International classification of impairments, disabilities and handicaps.* Geneva: WHO, 1980.
10. Johnston MV, Wilerson DL, Maney M. Evaluation of the quality and outcomes of medical rehabilitation programs. In: DeLisa JB, Gans BM. *Rehabilitation medicine: Principles and practice,* 2nd ed. Philadelphia: JBLippincott, 1993:240–268.
11. Sharrack B, Hughes RAC. Clinical scales for MS. *J Neurol Sci* 1996; 135:1–9.
12. Kurtzke JF. Rating neurologic impairment in multiple sclerosis: An Expanded Disability Status Scale (EDSS). *Neurology* 1983; 33:1444–1452.
13. Kurtzke JF. One the evaluation of disability in multiple sclerosis. *Neurology* 1961; 11:686–694.
14. Syndulko K, Ke D, Ellison GW, et al. Comparative evaluations of neuroperformance and clinical outcome assessments in chronic progressive multiple sclerosis: 1. Reliability, validity and sensitivity of disease progression. *Multiple Sclerosis* 1996; 2:142–156.
15. Goodkin DE, Cookfair D, Wende K, et al. Inter- and intrarater scoring agreement using grades 1.0 to 3.5 or the Kurtzke expanded disability status scale (EDSS) *Neurology* 1992; 42:859–863.
16. Sipe JC, Romine JS, Koziol JA, et al. Cladribine in treatment of chronic progressive multiple sclerosis. *Lancet* 1994; 344:9–13.
17. Francis DA, Bain P, Swan AV, Hughes RAC. An assessment of disability rating scales used in multiple sclerosis. *Arch Neurol* 1991; 48:299–301.
18. Pia Amato M, Fratiglioni L, Groppi C, Siracusa G, Amaducci L. Inter-rater reliability in assessing functional systems and disability on the Kurtzke scale in multiple sclerosis. *Arch Neurol* 1988; 45:746–748.
19. Amato MP, Fratiglioni L, Groppi C, Siracusa G, Amaducci L. Interrater reliability in assessing function systems and disability basing on the Kurtzke scale in multiple sclerosis. *Arch Neurol* 1988; 45:746–748.
20. Noseworthy JH, Vandervoort MK, Wong CJ, Ebers GC. Inter-rater variability with the Expanded Disability Status Scale (EDSS) and Functional Systems (FS) in multiple sclerosis clinical trials. *Neurology* 1990; 40:971–975.
21. LaRocca N, Scheinberg L, Slater R. Field testing of a minimal record of disability in multiple sclerosis: The United States and Canada. *Acta Neurol Scand* 1984; 70 (Suppl 101):126–138.
22. Koziol JA, Frutos A, Sipe JC, Romine JS, Beutler E. A comparison of two neurologic scoring instruments for multiple sclerosis. *J Neurol* 1996; 243:209–213.
23. Syndulko K, Tourtellotte WW, Baumhefner RW, et al. Neuroperformance evaluation of multiple sclerosis disease progression in a clinical trial: implications for neurological outcomes. *J Neuro Rehab* 1993; 7:153–176.
24. Ritvo PG, Fischer JS, Miller DM, et al. *Multiple Sclerosis Quality of Life Inventory: A user's manual,* 1997. National Multiple Sclerosis Society, 733 Third Avenue, New York, NY 10017.

25. Rudick RA, Medendorp SV, Namey M, Boyle S, Fischer J. Multiple sclerosis progression in a natural history study: Predictive value of cerebrospinal fluid free kappa light chains. *Multiple Sclerosis* 1995; 1:150–155.

26. Khoury SJ, Guttmann CRG, Orav EJ, et al. Longitudinal MRI in multiple sclerosis. *Neurology* 1994; 44:2120–2124.

27. Whitaker JN, McFarland HF, Rudge P, Reingold SC. Outcomes assessment in multiple sclerosis clinical trials: A critical analysis. *Multiple Sclerosis* 1995; 1:37–47.

28. Weinshenker BG, Issa M, Baskerville J. Long-term and short-term outcome of multiple sclerosis. *Arch Neurol* 1996; 53:353–358.

29. Rodriguez M, Siva A, Ward J, et al. Impairment, disability, and handicap in multiple sclerosis: A population-based study in Olmsted County, Minnesota. *Neurology* 1994; 44:28–44.

30. Scheinberg LC, Feldman FM, Ratzker PK, et al. Self-assessment of neurological impairment in multiple sclerosis. Annual meeting of the American Academy of Neurology. *Neurology* 1986:36 (Suppl 1):284.

31. Verdier-Taillefer MH, Roullet E, Cesaro P, Alperovitch A. Validation of self-reported neurological disability in multiple sclerosis. *Intl J Epidemiol* 1994; 23:148–154.

32. Amato SA, Bergamaschi R, Logroscino G, et al. Accuracy of self-assessment of the minimal record of disability in patients with multiple sclerosis. *Acta Neurol Scand* 1993; 87:43–46.

33. Ratzker PK, Feldman FM, LaRocca NG. Self-assessment of neurological impairment in multiple sclerosis (unpublished manuscript).

34. Sipe JC, Knobler RL, Braheny SL, et al. A neurologic rating scale (NRS) for use in multiple sclerosis. *Neurology* 1984; 34:1368–1372.

35. Willoughby E. Impairment in multiple sclerosis. *MS Management* 1995; 2:13–16.

36. Potvin AR, Tourtellotte WW. The neurological examination: advancements in its quantification. *Arch Phys Med Rehabil* 1975; 56:425–437.

37. Davis R, Kondraske GV, Tourtellotte WW, Syndulko K. *Quantifying neurologic performance.* Philadelphia: Hanley & Belfus, 1989.

38. Potvin AR, Tourtellotte WW. *Quantitative examination of neurologic function* (Vol. I). Boca Raton: CRC Press, 1985a.

39. Potvin AR, Tourtellotte WW. *Quantitative examination of neurologic function* (Vol. II). Boca Raton: CRC Press, 1985b.

40. Baumhefner RW, Tourtellotte WW, Syndulko KW, et al, 1990.

41. Tourtellotte WW, Syndulko K. Two decades of experience using quantitative examination of neurologic functions. In: Davis R, Kondraske GV, Tourtellotte WW, Syndulko K (eds.). *Quantifying neurologic performance.* Philadelphia: Hanley & Belfus, 1989: 161–167.

42. Hauser SL, Dawson DM, Lehrich JR, et al. Intensive immunosuppression in progressive multiple sclerosis. *N Engl J Med* 1983; 308:173–180.

43. Ravnborg M, Gronbech-Jensen M, Jonsson A. The MS Impairment Scale: A pragmatic approach to the assessment of impairment in patients with multiple sclerosis. *Multiple Sclerosis* 1997; 3:31–42.

44. Cook SD, Devereux C, Troiano R, et al. Effect of total lymphoid irradiation in chronic progressive multiple sclerosis. *Lancet* 1986; 1:1405–409.

45. Fischer JS, Jak AJ, Kniker JE, Rudick RA, Cutter G. *Administration and scoring manual for the Multiple Sclerosis Functional Composite Measure (MSFC).* New York: Demos Medical Publishing, 1999.

46. Collen FM, Wade DT, Bradshaw CM. *Mobility after stroke: Reliability of measures of impairment and disability.*

47. Holden MK, Gill KM, Magliozzi MR, Nathan J, Piehl-Baker L. Clinical gait assessment in the neurologically impaired. Reliability and meaningfulness. *Phys Ther* 1984; 64:35–40.

48. Mathiowetz V, Weber K, Kashman N, Volland G. Adult norms for Nine Hole Peg Test of finger dexterity. *Occ Ther J Res* 1985; 5:24–38.

49. Wade DT. Measuring arm impairment and disability after stroke. *Intl Disability Studies* 1989; 11:89–92.

50. Goodkin DE, Hertsgaard D, Seminary J. Upper extremity function in multiple sclerosis: Improving assessment sensitivity with box-and-block and nine-hole peg tests. *Arch Phys Med Rehabil* 1988; 69:850–854.

51. Goodkin DE, Rudick RA, VanderBrug Medendorp S, et al. Low-dose (7.5 mg) oral methotrexate reduces the rate of progression in chronic progressive multiple sclerosis. *Ann Neurol* 1995; 37:30–40.

52. Wade DT. *Measurement in neurological rehabilitation.* New York: Oxford Medical Publications, 1992.

53. Mathiowetz V, Volland G, Kashman N, Weber K. Adults norms for box and block test of manual dexterity. *Am J Occ Ther* 1985; 39:386–391.

54. Heller A, Wade DT, Wood VA, et al. Arm function after stroke: Measurement and recovery over the first three months. *J Neurol Neurosurg Psychiatry* 1987; 50:714–719.

55. Grant R, Slattery J, Gregor A, Whittle IR. Recording neurological impairment in clinical trials of glioma. *J Neuro-Oncol* 1994; 19:37–49.

56. Gronwall DM. Paced auditory serial addition task: A measure of recovery from concussion. *Percept Motor Skills* 1977; 44:367–373.

57. Litvan I, Grafman J, Vendrell P, Martinez JM. Slowed information processing in multiple sclerosis. *Arch Neurol* 1988; 45:281–285.

58. Diamond BJ, DeLuca J, Kim H, Kelley SM. The question of disproportionate impairments in visual and auditory information processing in multiple sclerosis. *J Clin Exp Neuropsychol* 1997; 19:34–42.

59. Hohol MJ, Guttmann CRG, Orav J, et al. Serial neuropsychological assessment and magnetic resonance imaging analysis in multiple sclerosis. *Arch Neurol* 1997; 54:1018–1025.

60. Kujala P, Portin R, Revonsuo A, Ruutiainen J. Attention related performances in two cognitively different subgroups of patients with multiple sclerosis. *J Neurol Neurosurg Psychiatry* 1995; 59:77–82.

61. Egan V. PASAT: Observed correlations with IQ. *Personality and Individual Differences* 1988; 9:179–180.

62. DeLuca J, Johnson SK, Natelson BH. Information processing efficiency in chronic fatigue syndrome and multiple sclerosis. *Arch Neurol* 1993; 50:301–304.

63. Wiens, Fuller KH, Crossen JR. Paced auditory serial addition test: adult norms and moderator variables. *J Clin Exp Neuropsychol of* 1997; 19:473–483.

64. Mahoney FI, Barthel DW. Functional evaluation: The Barthel Index. *Maryland State Med J* 1965; 14:61–65.

65. McDowell I, Newell C. *Measuring health: A guide to rating scales and questionnaires.* New York: Oxford University Press, 1987.

66. Granger CV, Albrecht GL, Hamilton BE. Outcomes of comprehensive medical rehabilitation: Measurement of PULSES Profile and the Barthel Index. *Arch Phys Med Rehabil* 1979; 60:145–154.

67. Shiner D, Gross CR, Bronstein KS, et al. Reliability of the activities of daily living scale and its use in telephone interview. *Arch Phys Med Rehabil* 1987; 68:723–728.

68. Granger CV, Greer DS. Functional status measurement and medical rehabilitation outcomes. *Arch Phys Med Rehabil* 1976; 57:103–109.

69. Law M, Letts L. A critical review of scales of activities of daily living. *Am J Occ Ther* 1989; 43:522–528.

70. *Kidd D, Howard RS, Losseff NA, Thompson AJ. The benefit of inpatient neurorehabilitation in multiple sclerosis.* Clin Rehab 1995; 9:198–203.

71. Jacelon CA. The Barthel Index and other indices of functional ability. *Rehab Nurs* 1986; 11:9–11.

72. Wade DT, Collin C. The Barthel ADL Index: A standard measure of physical disability? *Intl Disability Studies* 1988; 10: 64–67.

73. Collin C, Wade DT, Davies S, Horne V. The Barthel ADL Index: A reliability study. *Intl Disability Studies* 1988; 10:61–63.

74. Bowling A. *Measuring health: A review of quality of life measurement scales.* Philadelphia: Open University Press, 1991.

75. Kurtzke JF. A proposal for a uniform minimal record of disability in multiple sclerosis. *Acta Neurol Scand* 1981; 64:110–129.

76. *Granger CV. Assessment of functional status: A model for multiple sclerosis.* Acta Neurol Scand 1981; 64:40–47.

77. Stuifbergen AK, Roberts GJ. Health promotion practices of women with multiple sclerosis. *Arch Phys Med Rehabil* 1997; 78:S3–S9.

78. Solari A, Amato MP, Bergamaschi R, et al. Accuracy of self-assessment of the minimal record of disability in patients with multiple sclerosis. *Acta Neurol Scand* 1993; 87:43–46.

79. LaRocca N. Analyzing outcomes in the care of persons with multiple sclerosis. In: Fuhrer MJ (ed.). *Rehabilitation outcomes: Analysis and measurement.* Baltimore: Brookes Publishing, 1987:151–162.

80. Francabandera FL, Holland NJ, Wiesel-Levison P, Scheinberg LC. Multiple sclerosis rehabilitation: Inpatient vs. outpatient. *Rehab Nurs* 1988; 12:251–253.

81. Hamilton BB, Granger CV, Sherwin FS, Zielezny M, Tashman JS. A uniform nation data system for medical rehabilitation. In: Fuhrer MJ (ed.). *Rehabilitation outcomes: Analysis and measurement.* Baltimore: Brookes Publishing, 1987:137–147.

82. Ottenbacher KJ, Yungwen H, Granger CV, Fiedler RC. The reliability of the Functional Independence Measure: A quantitative review. *Arch Phys Med Rehabil* 1996; 77:1226–1232.

83. Granger CV, Brownscheidle CM. Outcome measurement in medical rehabilitation. *Intl J Technol Assess Health Care* 1995; 11:262–268.

84. Granger CV, Cotter AC, Hamilton BE, Fiedler RC, Hens MM. Functional assessment scales: A study of persons with multiple sclerosis. *Arch Phys Med Rehabil* 1990; 71:870–875.

85. Freeman JA, Langdon DW, Hobart JC, Thompson AJ. The impact of inpatient rehabilitation on progressive multiple sclerosis. *Ann Neurol* 1997; 42:236–244.

86. Ketelaer P. Disability assessment in multiple sclerosis. *MS Mgmt* 1995; 2:17–20.

87. Stewart G, Kidd D, Thompson AJ. The assessment of handicap: An evaluation of the Environmental Status Scale. *Disability Rehab* 1995; 17:312–316.

88. Mellerup E, Fog T, Raun N, et al. The Socio-Economic Scale. *Acta Neurol Scand* 1981; 64(Suppl 87):130–138.

89. Harwood RH, Gompertz P, Ebrahim S. Handicap one year after a stroke: Validity of a new scale. *J Neurol Neurosurg Psychiatry* 1994a; 57:825–829.

90. Harwood RH, Rogers A, Dickinson E, Ebrahim S. Measuring handicap: The London Handicap Scale, a new outcome measure for chronic disease. *Quality in Health Care* 1994b; 3:11–16.

91. Harwood RH, Gompertz SE. *The London Handicap Scale scoring manual*, 1996. Medical Outcomes Trust, 8 Park Plaza, #503, Boston, MA 02116.

92. Carr AJ, Thompson PW. Personal viewpoint. Towards a measure of patient-perceived handicap in rheumatoid arthritis. *Br J Rheumatol* 1994; 33:378-82.

93. Whyte J. Toward a methodology for rehabilitation research. *Am J Phys Med Rehab* 1994; 73:428–435.

94. Bergner M, Bobbitt RA, Kressel S, et al. The Sickness Impact Profile: Conceptual formulation and methodology for the development of a health status measure. *Intl J Health Services* 1976; 6:393–415.

95. Bergner M, Bobbitt RA, Carter WB, Gilson BS. The Sickness Impact Profile: Development and final revision of a health status measure. *Med Care* 1981; 19:787–805.

96. Patrick DL, Peach H. *Disablement in the community.* Oxford: Oxford University Press, 1989.

97. Brooks WB, Jordan JS, Divine GW, Smith KS, Neelon FA. The impact of psychologic factors on measurement of functional status: Assessment of the Sickness Impact Profile. *Med Care* 1990; 28:793–804.

98. Temkin NR, Dikmen S, Machamer J, McLean A. General versus disease-specific measures: Further work on the Sickness Impact Profile for head injury. *Med Care* 1989; 27:S44–S53.

99. Petajan JH, Gappmaier E, White AT, et al. Impact of aerobic training on fitness and quality of life in multiple sclerosis. *Ann Neurol* 1996; 39:422–423.

100. Skinner A. *The Sickness Impact Profile Scoring Manual*, 1996. Medical Outcomes Trust, 8 Park Plaza, # 503, Boston, MA 02116.

101. Keith RA. Functional status and health status. *Arch Phys Med Rehabil* 1994; 75:478–483.

102. Schuling J, Greidanus J, Meijboom-De Jong B. Measuring functional status of stroke patients with the Sickness Impact Profile. *Disability Rehab* 1993; 15:19–23.

103. Bruin AF de, Buys M, Witt LP de, Diederiks JPM. The Sickness Impact Profile: SIP-68, a short generic version. *J Clin Epidemiol* 1994; 47:863–871.

104. Bruin AF de, Diederiks JPM, Witte LP de, Stevens FCJ, Philipsen H. The development of a short generic version of the Sickness Impact Profile. *J Clin Epidemiol* 1994; 47:407–418.

105. Post MWM, Bruni AF de, Witte LP de, Schrijvers A. *The Sickness Impact Profile scoring manual—68 scoring manual*, 1996b. Medical Outcomes Trust, 8 Park Plaza, # 503, Boston, MA 02116.

106. Baker JG, Granger CV, Ottenbacher KJ. Validity of a brief outpatient functional assessment measure. *Am J Phys Med Rehab* 1996; 75:356–363.

107. Baker JG, Granger CV, Fiedler RC. A brief outpatient functional assessment measure: Validity using Rasch measures. *Am J Phys Med Rehab* 1997; 76:8–13.

108. Stewart AL, Ware JE. *Measuring functioning and well-being.* Durham: Duke University Press, 1992.

109. Ware JE, Sherbourne CD. The MOS 36-Item Short-Form Health Survey (SF-36) I. Conceptual framework and item selection. *Med Care* 1992; 30:473–483.

110. Jenkinson C, Coulter A, Wright L. Short-form 36 (SF-36) health survey questionnaire: Normative data for adults of working age. *Br Med J* 1993; 306:1437–1440.

111. Hayes V, Morris J, Wolfe C, Morgan M. The SF-36 health survey questionnaire: Is it suitable for use with older adults?

112. Garratt AM, Ruta DA, Abdalla MI, Buckingham JK, Russell IT. The SF 36 health survey questionnaire: An outcome measure suitable for routine use within the NHS? *Br Med J* 1993; 306:1440–1444.

113. Brazier JE, Harper R, Jones NMB, et al. Validating the SF-36 health survey questionnaire: New outcome measure in primary care. *Br Med J* 1992; 305:160–164.

114. McHorney CA, Ware JE, Lu. JF, Sherbourne CD. The MOS 36-Item Short-Form Health Survey (SF-36): III. Tests of data quality, scaling assumptions, and reliability across diverse patient groups. *Med Care* 1994; 32:40–66.

115. Ware JE, Snow KK, Kosinski M, Gandeck B. *SF-36 Health Survey manual and interpretation guide,* 1993.The Health Institute, New England Medical Center, NEMC #345, 750 Washington Street, Boston, MA 02111.

116. Ware JE, Kosinski M, Bayliss MS, et al. Comparison of methods for scoring and statistical analysis of SF-36 health profile and summary measures: summary of results from the Medical Outcomes Study. *Med Care* 1995; 33 (Suppl):AS264–AS279.

117. McHorney CA, Ware JE, Raczek AE. The MOS 36-Item Short-Form Health Survey (SF-36): II. Psychometric and clinical tests of validity in measuring physical and mental health constructs. *Med Care* 1993; 31:247–263.

118. McHorney CA, Ware JE, Rogers W, Raczek AE, Lu JFR. The validity of relative precision of MOS short- and long-form health status scales and Darmouth COOP charts: Results from the Medical Outcomes Study. *Med Care* 1992; 30(Suppl):MS253–MS265.

119. Brunet DG, Hopman WM, Singer MA, Edgar CM, MacKenzie TA. Measurement of health-related quality of life in multiple sclerosis patients. *Can J Neuro Sci* 1996; 23:99–103.

120. Vickery BG, Hays RD, Harooni R, Myers LW, Ellison EW. A health-related quality of life measure for multiple sclerosis. *QOL Res* 1995; 4:187–206.

121. Hermann BP, Vickrey B, Hays RD, et al. A comparison of health-related quality of life in patients with epilepsy, diabetes and multiple sclerosis. *Epilepsy Res* 1996; 25:113–118.

122. Weinberger M, Oddone EZ, Samsa GP, Landsman PB. Are health-related quality-of-life measures affected by the mode of administration? *J Clin Epidemiol* 1996; 49:135–140.

123. Vickery BG, Hays RD, Genovese BJ, Myers LW, Ellison GW. Comparison of a generic to disease-targeted health related quality-of-life measures for multiple sclerosis. *J Clin Epidemiol* 1997; 50:557–569.

124. Ziebland S. The short-form 36 health status questionnaire: Clues from the Oxford region's normative data about its usefulness in measuring health gain in population surveys. *J Epidemiol Comm Health* 1995; 49:102–105.

125. Stuck G, Liang MH, Phillips C, Katz JN. The short-form-36 is preferable to the SIP as a generic health status measure in patients undergoing elective total hip arthroplasty. *Arthritis Care Res* 1995; 8:174–181.

126. Kosinski M. Scoring the SF-12 physical and mental health summary measures. *Med Outcomes Trust Bull* 1997; 5:3–4.

127. Ware JE, Kosinski M, Keller SD. A 12-item short-form health survey: Construction of scales and preliminary tests of reliability and validity. *Med Care* 1996; 34:220–233.

128. Jenkinson C, Layte R, Jenkinson D, et al. A shorter form health survey: Can the SF-12 replicate results from the SF-36 in longitudinal studies? *J Public Health Med* 1997; 19:179–186.

129. Ware JE, Kosinski M, Keller SD. *SF-12: Instruction and scoring manual,* 1995. The Health Institute, NEMC #345, 750 Washington Street, Boston, MA 02111.

130. Vickery BG. *MSQOL-54: Instruction and scoring manual,* 1998. UCLA, Department of Neurology, C-128 RNRC, Box 951769, Los Angeles, CA 90095-1769.

131. Gulick EE. The self-administered ADL scale for persons with multiple sclerosis. In: Waltz CF, Stricklan OL (eds.). *Measurement of nursing outcomes, Vol. I: Measuring client outcomes.* New York: Springer, 1988:128–159.

132. Herndon RM. *Handbook of neurologic rating scales.* New York: Demos Vermande, 1997.

133. LaRocca N. Statistical and methodologic considerations in scale construction. In: Munsat TL (ed.). *Quantification of neurologic deficit.* Boston: Butterworth Heinemann, 1989:49–67.

134. Nunnally JC, Bernstein JR. *Psychometric theory,* 3rd ed. New York: McGraw-Hill, 1994.

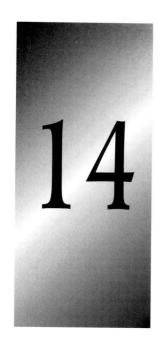

14 Fatigue

Lauren B. Krupp, M.D., and Leigh E. Elkins, Ph.D.

atigue is a frequent feature of multiple sclerosis (MS) and can be debilitating. Approximately two thirds of all individuals with MS report experiencing fatigue, and 14 percent to 28 percent report that it is their most disabling symptom (1–4). Unfortunately, despite its prevalence, it remains a perplexing clinical problem. This chapter reviews the clinical features, pathogenesis, and treatment of fatigue in MS.

CHARACTERISTICS OF FATIGUE

Many individuals report that fatigue is an initial manifestation of their MS, and relapses are often associated with increased fatigue. Fatigue is more common in individuals whose disease course is progressive (1). For example, in a large sample of 1,000 individuals with MS evaluated through the New York State MS Consortium (7), 33 percent of relapsing-remitting versus 55 percent of primary progressive or secondary progressive patients listed fatigue as moderate or severe. This pattern was also demonstrated in an earlier study of 47 individuals with MS undergoing neuropsychological testing (8) and in a more recent study of 100 individuals with MS and fatigue presenting to an outpatient clinic (4). However, there is only a weak association between fatigue and neurologic

impairment as measured by the Expanded Disability Status Scale (EDSS) (1–6), and fatigue is not significantly correlated with magnetic resonance imaging (MRI) measures of disease burden (9).

In general, MS fatigue worsens as the day progresses (10). A unique feature of MS fatigue is that it also is markedly affected by temperature. For more than 90 percent of individuals with MS, heat dramatically worsens their fatigue, whereas cool temperature brings relief (2,4). Fatigue in MS is exacerbated by a variety of other factors, including poor sleep, pain, psychological stressors, insufficient exercise, and side effects of medications.

Although fatigue in MS is independent of depression (2,5,6), psychological factors do influence fatigue perception. Vercoulen and coworkers demonstrated that focusing on both bodily sensations and a low sense of control contribute to fatigue in MS. In contrast, individuals who believe they can create an environment appropriate to their psychological and physical needs experience less fatigue and fatigue-related stress (11).

DEFINITION AND MEASUREMENT OF FATIGUE

Unfortunately, the variety of definitions and measurements have limited our understanding of MS fatigue.

Fatigue generally has been measured by either self-report, which requires an individual to describe and rate his or her fatigue; or performance, which requires an individual to attempt to sustain a level of physical or mental activity over time.

Self-Report Measures

Individuals with MS generally describe their subjective experience of fatigue as an overwhelming sense of tiredness, lack of energy, or feeling of exhaustion that has also been labeled "idiopathic lassitude" (12). This fatigue can be distinguished from symptoms of depression, which include lack of self-esteem, despair, or feelings of hopelessness. It is also distinct from limb weakness and sleepiness. Many patients have described their fatigue as similar to the feeling of exhaustion that often accompanies mild flulike illness.

A variety of instruments have been developed to assess self-reported fatigue in MS. Many of these measures focus on how the subjective feeling of fatigue compromises an individual's ability to function. For instance, the Fatigue Assessment Instrument (FAI) (13) is a 28-item questionnaire developed from studies of individuals with MS as well as other diseases. The FAI addresses overall severity of fatigue and allows for MS-specific features, such as exacerbation from heat, to be identified. The Fatigue Severity Scale (FSS) (5) is an abbreviated version of the FAI. Both the FSS total scores and the MS-specific features measured by the FAI were found to be sensitive for detecting improvements in studies of pharmacologic treatments for fatigue (9,14–18).

The Fatigue Impact Scale (FIS) (1) is another popular measure that assesses the impact of fatigue on daily functioning (3). The FIS has been incorporated into the MS-specific disability measure, the MSQOL-54, and has been demonstrated to be a strong predictor of mental and general health. Another commonly employed scale is the Multidimensional Assessment of Fatigue (MAF), which is a multidimensional rating of general fatigue originally developed with individuals who suffered fatigue as a result of rheumatoid arthritis (19). The MAF addresses fatigue severity, distress, timing, and interference across 14 typical activities of daily living.

Other scales address affective and cognitive features of fatigue. For example, the Functional Assessment of Multiple Sclerosis (FAMS) (20) is a measure that includes a "tiredness/thinking" subscale to address mental aspects of fatigue. The "tiredness/vigor" subscale of the Profile of Mood States (21) was sensitive to fatigue levels in an exercise study of people with MS (22).

Although all of these measures have been useful, the consistency of the subjective experience of fatigue among individuals is not clear. In turn, it has not been established whether subjective ratings accurately correspond to physiologic indications of fatigue. Another concern is that although some scales have been studied in large patient samples, none of the measures has been applied in longitudinal studies. The degree to which these instruments are sensitive to treatment effects or other interventions is also unclear (23).

Performance Measures

Fatigue may be physiologically defined as "the inability to maintain expected power output" (24,25). Fatigue can be objectively measured as an individual attempts to sustain a level of physical or mental performance. In physiologic studies of motor fatigue, the decrement in maximally generated force over time is evaluated during muscle contraction with an isometric gauge. For example, one study created a "fatigue index" by dividing the plot of force over time by the maximal force that is generated (14). Other studies of MS fatigue have examined changes in central motor drive and muscle metabolism during contraction of selected muscles of the upper or lower extremities (26,27).

People with MS also report that fatigue interferes with their ability to work efficiently on nonmotor tasks (e.g., reading, computing, or other cognitive functions). However, the fatigue of cognitive functioning is more complex to measure than motor or muscle fatigue. Caruso and colleagues (28) examined neuropsychological performance in a group of 18 MS participants before and after physical exercise and did not find any change in cognitive performances. However, cognitive fatigue may be an independent process. In this manner, cognitive fatigue may result from cognitive effort rather than physical effort.

In a more comprehensive study, Kujula and colleagues (29) compared the performance of MS participants with the performance of healthy controls on measures of attention before and after completion of a vigilance task. Relative to controls, MS subjects (including those with generally intact cognitive function) showed declines on the repeated measures of attention. These findings suggest that cognitive fatigue had developed in MS subjects but not in controls.

In a pilot study Elkins and coworkers (30) examined a range of cognitive functions before and after a cognitive demanding task in a group of MS subjects and healthy controls, matched according to age and education. Although at baseline there were no significant group differences on the neuropsychological measures, MS patients but not controls showed a clear decrement in performance over time on measures of memory and attention. This study suggests that both attention and memory are vulnerable to a fatigue effect in MS. Consistent with these findings was the observation by Sandroni and colleagues (31) that reaction time on memory tasks was slowed when MS patients were fatigued compared with when they were rested.

PATHOGENESIS

A variety of factors have been proposed to explain fatigue but none has been conclusively established as the cause. Motor fatigue is easily measured in MS and its pathogenesis has received the most focus. Although it is thought that involvement of premotor, limbic, or brain stem areas is a cause of decreased motivation or motor readiness, neuroimaging confirmation of this hypothesis is lacking. Electrophysiologic studies have proposed "twitch decline," a decline in central motor drive (32), as well as a drop in muscle torque during sustained contractions (33). Additional evidence for a central component to motor fatigue has been the observation of a reduction in motor evoked potentials in MS patients after walking without concomitant changes in measures of neuromuscular function (16). Abnormalities in peripheral motor function have also been observed in MS. Muscular fatigue has been associated with a decline in tetanic force, phosphocreatine, and intracellular pH in conjunction with intact neuromuscular transmission (27,34). Muscle biopsy in MS compared with controls indicates changes consistent with disuse and a greater reliance on anaerobic energy supply (35).

These studies of motor fatigue have contributed to our understanding of motor function in MS but do not explain the subjective or cognitive experiences of fatigue that most people describe. In most studies there is a lack of significant correlation between motor and subjective measures (32). For example, whereas in one study, 4-aminopyridine improved subjective fatigue as measured by the FSS, it did not alter most physiologic measures (18).

Immune factors have been linked to fatigue in MS. Medications such as interferon-alpha and interferon-beta produce prominent fatigue as an initial side effect (36,37). In animal studies, other cytokines including interleukin-1 and tumor necrosis factor have also been associated with either sleep induction or fatigue (38-41).

It has also been proposed that MS fatigue results from changes in neuroendocrine function or cerebral metabolism. Decreases in the brain supply of glucose could cause fatigue via either decreased blood glucose or impaired cerebral glucose metabolism. A positron emission tomography (PET) study of patients with MS identified a significant correlation between perceived fatigue as measured by the FSS and cerebral glucose availability (9). An increased concentration in the ratio of tryptophan to branched chain amino acids has been proposed to

mediate fatigue (42). Disruption in neurotransmitter systems including serotoninergic pathways interferes with attention and could also cause fatigue (43).

It appears likely that multiple contributing factors lead to the end result of an individual's experience of fatigue. Furthermore, as the different measurement approaches have indicated, what is labeled as fatigue in MS may actually represent separate and possibly independent processes.

EVALUATION

A proposed evaluation scheme is outlined in Figure 14-1. One of the first issues to be addressed in the MS patient with increased fatigue is whether there are signs of an impending relapse. New neurologic symptoms or signs accompanying fatigue could indicate increased disease activity. The possibility of infection or heat exposure as a cause of pseudoexacerbation should be considered. It is important to review medication history. Medications such as those used for spasticity, beta blockers, tricyclic antidepressants, benzodiazepines, and anticonvulsants may worsen fatigue.

It is critical to evaluate other symptoms that may contribute to fatigue. Potential cofactors that add to fatigue are pain, poor sleep, psychological stress, and deconditioning. Approximately 40 percent of MS patients experience severe pain (44). This pain may disrupt sleep, adding to stress and resulting in more fatigue. Therefore, fatigue that previously was manageable becomes intolerable. A review of systems that includes questions regarding headache, muscle pain, radicular pain, or back pain is an important part of the evaluation. Sleep problems such as sleep apnea, nocturnal myoclonus, or narcolepsy may occur in MS and contribute to fatigue (45–47). Assessment of sleep habits and observations by the patient's spouse or partner may help to identify previously undiagnosed sleep disorders.

Assessment of mood is critical to the evaluation of fatigue. Most people with MS have elevated depressive symptoms, although they may not meet the criteria for major depression. A simple office approach to the presence of mood disorders is to include self-report questionnaires such as the Beck Depression Inventory (BDI) (48) or the Center for Epidemiologic Studies Depression Scale (CES-D) (49) in the intake history. Obtaining a history for family psychiatric illness and examining the nature of the family unit and support systems are also components of a fatigue evaluation. For patients in whom overwhelming fatigue is associated with severe depression or in patients who are refractory to all forms of fatigue therapy, psychiatric referral may be of value.

At least at some point in their course, patients should be evaluated with a laboratory screen to exclude other

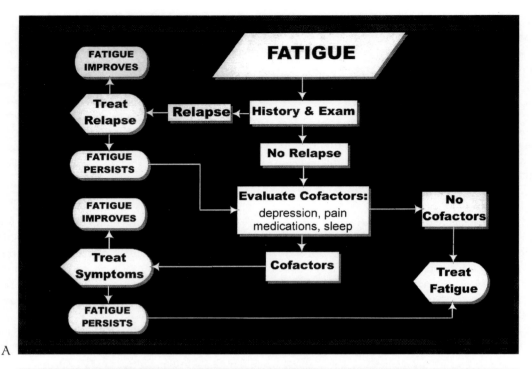

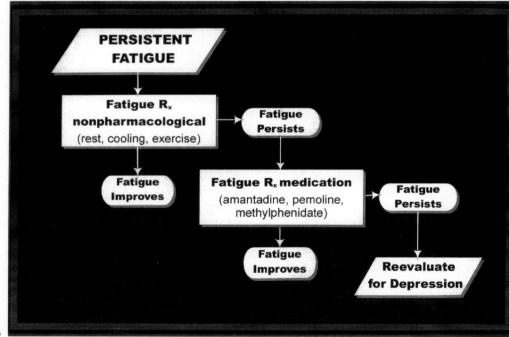

FIGURE 14-1

Initial (A) and subsequent (B) management of MS fatigue.

fatigue-producing conditions. Testing should include thyroid function tests, complete blood cell count, electrolytes, glucose, tests of liver function, antinuclear antibody, erythrocyte sedimentation rate, and urinalysis and culture.

Treatment

Fatigue treatment requires a multidisciplinary approach that should encompass the various factors that may contribute to fatigue severity. These include mood, level of physical activity, pain, medication, and sleep. Among the nonpharmacologic treatments, education and support are important. Patients are directly helped by recognizing fatigue as a genuine feature of MS.

Exercise is a powerful means to combat deconditioning and enhance self-esteem. The advantages of exercise on fatigue were demonstrated in a study of 54 patients randomly assigned to either 15 weeks of aerobic training or a nonexercise condition (22). Patients in the exercise condition experienced a significant reduction in fatigue as measured by the Profile of Mood States (POMS) at week 10 and had improvement in quality of life. However, improvement was not sustained at week 15. Self-reported physical state, social interaction, emotional behavior, and home management also improved. Whereas a graded exercise program is useful, overexertion may be detrimental. Carefully timed rest periods during the work day and avoidance of environmental factors that worsen fatigue (such as heat) may lessen fatigue and enhance productivity.

The use of rehabilitative services is associated with reduction in fatigue, as demonstrated in a study of 20 progressive MS patients who received an outpatient multidisciplinary rehabilitation program five hours a week for one year. Treated patients compared with a wait list control group had reduced fatigue and reduced MS-related symptoms at the one-year follow-up period (50).

Behavioral modification therapy is another effective means of combating fatigue. When behavioral techniques have been used to treat fatigue in individuals with chronic fatigue syndrome, there was a significant reduction in depression and fatigue components caused by mood disorder (51–53). Behavioral therapies on an individual or group basis can be easily applied in MS.

Often nonpharmacologic measures must be supplemented with medication. Treatments shown to be effective in randomized, double-blind, placebo-controlled trials are magnesium pemoline (pemoline), a central nervous system (CNS) stimulant, and amantadine hydrochloride (amantadine), an antiviral agent that also has antiparkinsonian effects (8,54–57)

In a Canadian multicenter MS fatigue treatment trial, amantadine significantly improved fatigue relative to placebo (56). In another study that comparing pemo-

line with placebo, no significant differences emerged but there was a trend in favor of pemoline (57) Forty-six percent of treated patients had excellent or good relief with pemoline compared with only 19.5 percent with placebo. Poorly tolerated side effects occurred in 25 percent of the pemoline group (56). In a placebo-controlled, randomized study comparing pemoline, amantadine, and placebo, amantadine but not pemoline was more effective than placebo (15). Side effects with either medication in this study were infrequent. Based on the relative benefit with amantadine and its low side effect–profile, this is the first-line medication to use for MS fatigue. If no benefit is seen, a second option is pemoline.

Other medications used on an anecdotal basis for fatigue include CNS stimulants such as methylphenidate (Ritalin) or dextroamphetamine. Central nervous system stimulants should be used with caution but have value in selected cases. They are contraindicated in patients with abuse potential. In a study examining the long-term efficacy and safety of 4-aminopyridine in MS, fatigue was a symptom frequently reported as improved with therapy (58). A pilot study in MS with 3,4-diaminopyridine reported subjective fatigue improvement in six of eight treated subjects but no change in physiologic fatigue measures (59). Future studies of 4-aminopyridine in the treatment of MS fatigue are under consideration.

Another pharmacologic strategy for fatigue is the use of antidepressant medication. This is clearly the treatment of choice for patients who have coexisting major depression, which is common in MS. Even patients who deny depressive symptoms may have definite responses to antidepressant medication. Agents with the least sedating properties are preferable, such as fluoxetine (Prozac), sertraline (Zoloft), nefazodone hydrochloride (Serzone), and desipramine (Norpramin).

In patients in whom fatigue is associated with sleep disorder, improved sleep hygiene is important. Exercise six hours before sleep may help, and patients should be cautioned not to look at the clock every few minutes. Medications for insomnia also may lessen fatigue. When fatigue is associated with anxiety, pharmacologic treatments that alleviate anxiety or panic attacks may provide benefit.

More direct treatments for MS fatigue are under investigation, including forms of 4-aminopyridine. At the time of this review, a multicenter clinical trial using interferon beta-1b (Betaseron) for secondary progressive MS is in progress, which includes assessment of fatigue among the outcome measures. It is hoped that this study will determine whether treatment with Betaseron lessens fatigue.

As we continue to understand the complex nature of fatigue in MS, improved therapies are likely to follow. Future studies that include separate analysis of motor, cognitive, and perceived components are likely to further advance management of this frequent and often disabling symptom.

References

1. Fisk JD, Pontefract A, Ritvo PG, Archibald CJ, Murray TJ. The impact of fatigue on patients with multiple sclerosis. *Can J Neurol Sci* 1994; 21(1):9–14.

2. Krupp LB, Alvarez La, LaRocca NG, Scheinberg L. Clinical characteristics of fatigue in multiple sclerosis. *Arch Neurol* 1988; 45:435–437.

3. Freal JE, Kraft GH, Coryell JK. Symptomatic fatigue in multiple sclerosis. *Arch Phys Med Rehabil* 1984; 65: 135–138.

4. Bergamaschi R, Romani V, Versino M Poli R, Cosi V. Clinical aspects of fatigue in multiple sclerosis. *Functional Neurol* 1997; 12:247–251.

5. Krupp LB, LaRocca NC, Muir-Nash J, Steinberg AD. The fatigue severity scale applied to patients with multiple sclerosis and systemic lupus erythematosus. *Arch Neurol* 1989; 46:1121–1123.

6. Vercoulen J, Hommes OR, Swanink C, et al. The measurement of fatigue in patients with multiple sclerosis: A multidimensional comparison with patients with chronic fatigue syndrome and healthy subjects. *Arch Neurol* 1996; 53:642–649.

7. New York State Consortium 1998. Unpublished data.

8. Grossman M, Armstrong C, Onishi K, et al. Patterns of cognitive impairment in relapsing-remitting and chronic progressive multiple sclerosis. *Neuropsychiatr Neuropsychol Behav Neurol* 1994; 7:194–210.

9. Roelcke U, Kappos L, Lechner-Scott J, et al. Reduced glucose metabolism in the frontal cortex and basal ganglia of multiple sclerosis patients with fatigue. A 18F-fluorodeoxyglucose positron emission tomographic study. *Neurology* 1997; 48:1566–1571

10. Van der Werf SP, Jongen PJH, Lycklama-Nijebolt GJ, Barkoff F, et al., *J Neurol Sci* 1998; 160:164–170.

11. Schwartz CE, Coulthard-Morris L, Zeng Q. Psychosocial correlates of fatigue in multiple sclerosis. *Arch Phys Med Rehabil* 1996; 77:165–170.

12. Shapiro RT. *Symptom management in multiple sclerosis.* 3rd ed. New York: Demos Medical Publishing, 1998.

13. Schwartz J, Jandorf L, Krupp LB. The measurement of fatigue: A new scale. *J Psychosom Res* 1993; 37:753–762.

14. Djaldetti R, Ziv I, Achiron A, Melamed E. Fatigue in multiple sclerosis compared with chronic fatigue syndrome: A quantitative assessment. *Neurology* 1996; 46:632–635.

15. Krupp LB, Coyle PK, Doscher C, et al. Fatigue therapy in multiple sclerosis: Results of a double-blind randomized parallel trial of amantadine, pemoline, and placebo. *Neurology* 1995; 45:1956–1961.

16. Schubert M, Wohlfarth KAI, Rollnick J, Dengler R. Walking and fatigue in multiple sclerosis: The role of the corticospinal system. *Muscle Nerve* 1998; 21:1068–1070.

17. Pepper C, Krupp LB, Friedberg F, Doscher C, Coyle PK. Comparison of psychiatric characteristics in chronic fatigue syndrome, multiple sclerosis, and depression. *J Neuropsych Clin Neurosci* 1993; 5:1–7.

18. Sheean G. Murray N, Rothwell J, Miller D., Thompsom A. An open labeled clinical and electrophysiological study of 3,4 diaminopyridine in the treatment of fatigue in multiple sclerosis. *Brain* 1998; 121:967–975.

19. Belza BL, Henke CJ, Yelin EH, Epstein WV, Gilliss CL. Correlates of fatigue in older women with rheumatoid arthritis. *Nurs Res* 1993; 42:93–99.

20. Cella DF, Dineen K, Arnason B, et al. Validation of the functional assessment of multiple sclerosis (FAMS) quality of life instrument. *Neurology* 1996; 47:129–139.

21. McNair DM, Lorr M, Droppleman LF. *Profile of mood states (POMS).* San Diego: Educational and Industrial Testing Service, 1992.

22. Petajan JH, Gappmaier E, White AT, et al. Impact of aerobic training on fitness and quality of life in multiple sclerosis. *Ann Neurol* 1996; 39:432–441.

23. Krupp LB, Soefer M, Pollina D, Smiroldo J, Coyle PK. Fatigue measures for clinical trials in multiple sclerosis. *Neurology* 1998; 50(Suppl):A126.

24. Dalakas MC, Mock V, Hawkins MJ. Fatigue: Definitions, mechanisms, and paradigms for study. *Semin Oncol* 1998 [Suppl 2]; 25(1):48–53.

25. Craig A, Cooper RE. Symptoms of acute and chronic fatigue. In: *Handbook of human performance.* New York: Academic Press 1992.

26. Rice CL, Vollmer TL, Bigland-Riticheie B. Neuromuscular responses of patients with multiple sclerosis. *Muscle Nerve* 1992:15:1123–1132

27. Sharma KR, Kent-Braun J, Mynhier MA, Weiner MW, Miller RG. Evidence of an abnormal intramuscular component of fatigue in multiple sclerosis. *Muscle Nerve* 1995; 18:1403–1411.

28. Caruso LS, LaRocca NG, Foley FW, et al. Exertional fatigue fails to affect cognitive function in multiple sclerosis. *J Clin Exp Neuropsychol* 1991; 13:74.

29. Kujala P, Portin R, Revonsuo A, Ruutiainen J. Attention related performance in two cognitively different subgroups of patients with multiple sclerosis. *J Neurol Neurosurg Psychiatry* 1995, 59:77–82.

30. Elkins LE, Pollina DA, Scheffer SR, Krupp LB. Effects of fatigue on cognitive functioning in multiple sclerosis. *Neurology* 1998; 50(Suppl):A126.

31. Sandroni P, Walker C, Starr A. "Fatigue" in patients with MS. *Arch Neurol* 1992; 49:517–524.

32. Sheehan, G L, Murray NMF, Rothwell, JC, Miller DH, Thompson AJ: An electrophysiological study of the mechanism of fatigue in multiple sclerosis. *Brain* 1997; 120:299–315.

33. Latash. M, Kalugina E, Orpett NJ, Stefoski D, Davis F. Myogenic and central neurogenic factors in fatigue in multiple sclerosis. *Multiple Sclerosis* 1996; 1:236–241.

34. Kent-Braun JA, Sharma KR, Miller RG, Weiner MW. Postexercise phosphocreatine resynthesis is slowed in multiple sclerosis. *Muscle Nerve* 1994; 17:835–841.

35. Kent-Braun JA, Ng AV, Castro M, et al. Strength, skeletal muscle composition, and enzyme activity in multiple sclerosis. *J Appl Physiol* 1997; 83:1998-2004.

36. Quesada. Clinical toxicity of interferons in cancer patients, a review. *J Clin Oncol* 1986; 4:234–243.

37. Neilly LK, Goodin DS, Goodkin DE, Hause SL. Side effect profile of interferon beta-1b in MS: Results of an open label trial. *Neurology* 1996; 46:552–554.

38. Moldofsky H, Lue FA, Eisen J, Keystone E, Gorczynski RM. The relationship of interleukin-1 and immune functions to sleep in humans. *Psychosom Med* 1986; 48:309–318.

39. Krueger JM, Walter J, Dinarello CA, Wolff SM, Chedid L. Sleep-promoting effects of endogenous pyrogen (interleukin-1). *Am J Physiol* 1984; 246:R994–R999.

40. Bertolone K, Coyle PK, Krupp LB, Doscher CA, Mehta PD. Cytokine correlates of fatigue in MS. *Neurology* 1993; 43:769S.

41. Chao CC, DeLa Hunt M, Hu S, et al. Immunologically mediated fatigue: A murine model. *Clin Immunopath* 1992; 64; 161–165.

42. Parry-Billings M, Blomstrand E, McAndrew N, Newsholme EA. A communicational link between skeletal muscle, brain, and cells of the immune system. *Intl J Sports Med* 1990; 11 (Suppl 2):122–128.

43. Heilman KM, Watson RT. Fatigue. *Neurology Network Commentary* 1997; 1:283–287.

44. Archibald CJ, McGrath P, Ritvo RG, et al. Pain in multiple sclerosis: Prevalence, severity, and impact on mental health. *Pain* 1994; 58:89–93

45. Caruso LS, LaRocca NC, Tyron W, et al. Activity monitoring of fatigued and non-fatigued persons with MS. *Sleep Res* 1991; 20:368.

46. Taphoorn MJ, van Someren E, Snoek FJ, et al. Fatigue, sleep disturbances, and circadian rhythm in multiple sclerosis. *J Neurology* 1993; 240:446–448.

47. Giancarlo T, Kapen S, Saad J, et al. Analysis of sleepiness and fatigue in multiple sclerosis. *Ann Neurol* 1987; 22:187.

48. Beck AT, Ward CH, Mendelson M. An inventory for measuring depression. *Arch Gen Psych* 1961; 4:561–571.

49. Radloff LS: CES-D scale: A self-report depression scale for research in the general population. *Appl Psychol Meas* 1977; 1:385–401.

50. Di Fabio RP, Soderberg, Choi T, Hansen CR, Schapiro RT. Extended outpatient rehabilitation: Its influence on symptom frequency, fatigue, and functional status for persons with progressive multiple sclerosis. *Arch Phys Med Rehabil* 1998; 79:141–146.

51. Deale AM, Chalder T, Marks I, Wessely S. Cognitive behavior therapy for chronic fatigue syndrome: A randomized controlled trial. *Am J Psychiatry* 1997; 408–414.

52. Friedberg F, Krupp LB. A comparison of cognitive behavioral treatment of chronic fatigue syndrome and primary depression. *Clin Infect Dis* 1994; 18:(Suppl 1):105–110.

53. Butler S, Chalder T, Ron M, Wessely S. Cognitive behaviour therapy in CFS. *J Neurol Neurosurg Psychiatry* 1991; 54:153–158.

54. Murray TJ. Amantadine therapy for fatigue in multiple sclerosis. *Can J Neurol Sci* 1985; 12(3):251–254.

55. Geisler MW, Sliwinski M, Coyle PK, et al. The effects of amantadine and pemoline on cognitive functioning in multiple sclerosis. *Arch Neurol* 1996; 53:185–188.

56. Canadian MS Research Group. A randomized controlled trial of amantadine in fatigue associated with multiple sclerosis. *Can J Neurol Sci* 1987; 14:273–278.

57. Weinshenker BG, Penman M, Bass B: A double-blind, randomized, crossover trial of pemoline in fatigue associated with multiple sclerosis. *Neurology* 1992; 42:1468–1471.

58. Polman CH, Bertelsmann FW, van Loenen AC, Koetsier JC. 4-Aminopyridine in the treatment of patients with multiple sclerosis. *Arch Neurol* 1994; 51:292.

59. Smits RCF, Emmen HH, Bertelsmann, et al. The effects of 4-aminopyridine on cognitive function in patients with multiple sclerosis: A pilot study. *Neurology* 1994; 44:1701–1705.

15 Spastic Paresis

Robert R. Young, M.D.

DEFINITIONS

Spastic paresis (1) refers to a syndrome with numerous physical signs such as exaggerated tendon reflexes (including clonus) and muscle hypertonia. Lance (2) defined spasticity, the simplest positive symptom within spastic paresis, as a velocity-dependent increased resistance of muscle to stretch due to activation of tonic stretch reflexes. In addition, there are other positive symptoms such as increased cutaneous (usually flexor) reflexes, autonomic hyperactivity, and pain in muscles or painful spasms. These signs of spasticity are almost always found together with a variable degree of paresis, a negative symptom that includes weakness, loss of dexterity, and fatigability. Together, these and other positive and negative symptoms characterize the clinical syndrome known as spastic paresis.

Although there are many different types of spastic paresis, *hemiplegic spasticity* with a flexed arm and extended leg (hemiplegic dystonia) without flexor spasms is obviously different from *spinal spasticity* seen following spinal cord injury (SCI), where legs (and arms if they are affected) are flexed and adducted (paraplegic dystonia), and heightened cutaneous reflexes with flexor spasms are the rule. Individuals with multiple sclerosis (MS) usually have the latter type of spastic paresis because many of their symptomatic lesions are within the spinal cord. The main difference, in terms of spasticity, between those with MS and those with SCI is that the former do not have autonomic dysreflexia, which is so common in the latter if the spinal level is at T6 or above. For the purposes of this chapter, those statements that concern individuals with SCI will also be taken to apply to individuals with MS. Obvious differences between MS and SCI outside the arena of spastic paresis (e.g., progression of symptoms, cognitive deficits, cerebellar ataxia, visual problems, and so forth) are not addressed here.

Spastic hyperreflexia has little relationship to a patient's disability; disability is largely due to paresis, for which there will be little effective therapy until methods are developed to facilitate regeneration and redirection of fibers within the CNS. In the meantime, pharmacologic and physical therapies are used to reduce the activity of stretch and cutaneous reflexes. All too often, clinicians do not consider the function of these reflexes during normal movements, nor do they ask whether exaggerated reflexes produce disorders of movement. Because, as described in a subsequent section, these reflexes can be reduced, they often are, whether that really helps the patient or not.

Clinically, it is obvious that no direct relationship exists between tendon jerks (phasic stretch reflexes) and muscle tone (tonic stretch reflexes). For example, following an acute stroke, tendon reflexes may be exaggerated early, whereas spastic muscle tone does not usually develop for several weeks, and in normal persons, no relationship has been demonstrated between reflex excitability and motor performance. Tendon jerks are hypoactive or absent in many fine athletes.

Central nervous system control of functional motor activity (for example, locomotion) involves complex interactions of spinal and supraspinal mechanisms. Rhythmic activation of leg muscles, which arises from activity in spinal interneuronal circuits, is modulated and adapted to the body's actual needs by means of many afferent inputs. Patterns of electromyography (EMG) activity in leg muscles, resulting from well-coordinated interactions between these different mechanisms, are translated into functionally modulated muscle tension by activation of the mechanical (contractile) properties of muscle fibers (3). Spinal programming of EMG activity, including reflex activities, is normally under supraspinal control. Disorders such as MS, which interfere with this supraspinal control, lead to characteristic abnormalities of gait, depending on exactly where and how large the causative lesion is; one can differentiate cerebellar gaits, extrapyramidal gaits, and hemiplegic gaits from gaits resulting from spastic paresis caused by MS (4). The point is that different pathophysiologies underlie different types of dysfunction in those with spastic paresis; it is unreasonable to act as if there is only one type of spastic paresis or one way to manage all those with spastic paresis.

NATURAL HISTORY

Little is known of the pathophysiology underlying the alterations in symptoms and signs that, following an acute CNS lesion, develop over months. Why, for example, is flaccid areflexic paresis ("spinal shock") present for weeks after a traumatic spinal cord injury? Following an acute stroke, tendon reflexes may be exaggerated within a few days, whereas spastic hypertonia develops over weeks and months.

What may underlie these neuronal reorganizations that occur following CNS lesions? Mendell (5) and Carr and coworkers (6) offered the following hypotheses: (1) development of new neural connections due to sprouting of new axon terminals, functional strengthening of preexisting synapses, or derepression of previously inactive connections; (2) alterations in the normal excitatory/inhibitory balance because of reductions in inhibition; and (3) denervation supersensitivity. Following a spinal cord lesion, sprouting of primary afferents as a possible cause of increased excitation and spasticity has not been demonstrated in cat (7) or in man (8). Reduction of presynaptic inhibition of immune response gene-associated antigen (Ia) afferent terminals has been demonstrated

(9,10) and seems to correlate with increased excitability of tendon reflexes. In addition to these neural changes, alterations in muscle mechanical properties occur in the leg extensors (11) and arm flexors (12), which may contribute to spastic hypertonia. Structural changes within spastic muscles and periarticular connective tissue occur soon after a CNS lesion (13) and are particularly prominent a year later (14,15).

THEORETIC MANAGEMENT CONCERNS

The first order of business when management decisions are to be made is to determine precisely what the patient's chief complaints really are and whether anything can be done about them. Paresis is responsible for a patient's major disability, and as yet nothing can be done to reverse lesion-induced disconnections within the motor system and thus alleviate paresis. Megadose steroids or N-methyl-D-aspartate (NMDA) receptor blockers are given acutely after a CNS injury to attempt to reduce some of the secondary damage to structures within the motor system, thus minimizing functional deficits. Functional electrical stimulation (FES) of paralyzed upper limb muscles, as well as bowel and bladder, in patients with spinal cord lesions is now commercially available, but FES is not yet in widespread use and is more difficult to employ in patients with MS or supraspinal lesions. Functional electrical stimulation to improve ambulation is still experimental. 4-Aminopyridine (4-AP), a potassium channel blocker, restores function in demyelinated CNS axons and has been shown to improve function in a few patients with spinal cord injury (16). None of these attempts to compensate for paresis is widely available yet, so attention turns to treatment of the positive symptoms.

Before doing so, one should remember that not all hyperreflexia needs to be treated; sometimes (such as with hyperactive tendon jerks) it is of little clinical significance and at other times it is actually useful (for example, the stiffly extended leg in hemiparesis that functions as a built-in crutch).

Treatment of spastic paresis by general physicians usually consists of giving pain pills or sleeping pills—neither of which address the primary problems causing discomfort or sleeplessness. Can we do better? Neurologists and physiatrists, in their efforts to help the paralyzed person, know they can reduce stretch reflex activity. If exaggerated reflexes are entirely responsible for increased muscle tone, their reduction might increase function in someone with spastic paresis; reducing stiffness in an antagonist muscle group might permit a weak agonist to be more effective. However, almost all studies of increased muscle tone and other spastic reflex activity have been done under passive conditions, with the patient relaxed, sitting, or lying (cf. 17,18), paying little attention to function. On the other hand, those investigations that were undertaken *during* functional movements of leg (19,20) and arm (12,21,22) did not demonstrate a cause-and-effect relationship between exaggerated reflexes and the disorders of function about which the patients were complaining. Although exaggerated stretch reflexes and other positive signs of spasticity are usually associated with deficits in functionally essential long-latency polysynaptic reflexes, the latter deficits are not caused by the former hyperreflexia. Force (i.e., tension) developed during functional movements appears not to depend, in those with spastic paresis, on exaggerated monosynaptic stretch reflexes (19). Total functional leg muscle activity is actually reduced in patients with spastic paresis of spinal or cerebral origin. Both electrophysiologic (15,21) and histologic (23,24) data document transformations of motor units that take place following MS or supraspinal lesions, suggesting that increased muscle tone in those circumstances is due, at least in part, to changes within muscle.

This default mode, in which a simpler spinal system regulates muscle tension following paresis due to a CNS lesion, is basically advantageous for a patient; stiff muscles provide support for the patient's body against gravity during gait and thus permit greater mobility. Rapid or highly coordinated movements are, however, no longer possible because of a lack of rapid and appropriate modulation of muscle activity to suit the environmentally imposed circumstances of the moment. Following a severe spinal or supraspinal lesion, these fail-safe mechanisms can overshoot the mark, with unwelcome sequelae such as painful spasms and spastic dystonia.

Optimal management of patients with spastic paresis must include classic rehabilitation techniques to train and develop residual motor function and to prevent secondary complications such as contractures. If antispastic drug therapy were shown to reduce muscle hypertonia and spasms only by weakening muscles (25), it would inevitably interfere with function. Such antispastic drug therapy, by reducing pain and facilitating their nursing care, would principally benefit only those patients who are already immobile. Fortunately, pharmacologic management of spasticity in MS is more useful and does more than simply weaken muscles.

PRACTICAL MANAGEMENT CONCERNS

Everyday management of patients with spastic paresis is largely empiric. Most well-controlled studies of antispastic drugs have focused on reflexes recorded under artificial conditions. The few studies that addressed the effects of antispastic drugs on functional movements failed to demonstrate significant benefits; they were not designed to document the considerable improvements that can follow antispastic therapy. For an overview of common methods for treating spasticity, see reviews by Glenn and Whyte (42) and Dietz (33).

Alleviating Causes of Increased Spasticity

Before beginning long-term medical therapy for spasticity (which should always precede surgical therapies), remember that painful flexor spasms and increased muscle tone can either be produced or exacerbated by nociceptive input from urinary tract infections, pressure sores, ingrown toenails, or broken bones, or by other drugs such as selective serotonin reuptake inhibitor (SSRI) antidepressants (26) and interferon beta-1b (27). Attention to such inciting factors may reduce the newly accentuated spasms or hypertonia without need for adding new antispastic medications.

Physical Therapy

Although very few well-controlled studies exist to prove it, physiotherapy may be helpful for those spastic patients who are either mobile or immobile. In those who retain some mobility, their residual motor functions should be strengthened and trained. In all patients, contractures of muscle and joints, which are difficult to treat once established, must be prevented, beginning at an early stage. Stretching paretic muscles, if done at least several times a day, can prevent painful contractures and even reduce spastic reflexes. Physiotherapy within a water-filled pool may be helpful; experiments have shown this to have profound effects on postural reflexes (28).

Different schools of physiotherapeutic practice exist, based on theoretic rationales, but none has been proven effective. Proprioceptive neuromuscular facilitation (PNF) and myofeedback techniques are said to activate spinal motoneurons by utilizing reflex mechanisms. In the techniques of Bobath and Vojta, which are primarily used to treat children with cerebral palsy, stereotyped movements are activated by such stimulation applied to dermatomes and joints. The Vojta method tries to activate complex movements that are believed to be programmed in the CNS. In contrast, the Bobath method tries to inhibit spasticity in flexor muscles of the arms and in extensors of the legs. Each school has its devotees, but there are no data to assist us in choosing one or the other method.

Physiotherapeutic techniques are intended to:

1. Avoid secondary complications such as pressure sores;
2. Prevent or try to treat contractures;
3. Reduce muscle hypertonia by stretching spastic muscles and by application of warm or cold packs;
4. Improve the patient's posture;

5. Develop and improve useful automatic movements and thus, perhaps, to induce voluntarily initiated and controlled complex movements;

6. Assist the patient in learning more coordinated movements by using tactile, auditory, vestibular, and visual cues; and

7. Supply supportive aids such as walkers, wheelchairs, crutches, orthoses, and special shoes.

Physiotherapy, to be maximally effective, should be part of a team approach that includes psychologists, social workers, and nurses, all of whom are focused on developing increased independence for the patient.

Special Locomotor Training

After complete spinal cord transection, cats can be trained to perform stepping movements on a treadmill with a pattern of leg muscle activation that resembles that observed in intact cats (29). This is taken as evidence for a central pattern generator, within the spinal cord, for gait. Clinical investigations (30) show that locomotor patterns can also be elicited and trained in patients with incomplete paraplegia or spastic hemiplegia. Special interactive locomotor training is performed on a treadmill with 20 percent to 30 percent of the subject's weight supported by a harness attached to the ceiling. As the subjects walk on the treadmill with reduced loading of their lower extremities, coordinated stepping movements and functional patterns of muscle activation can be facilitated with the help of therapists. Support of body weight is progressively reduced until subjects can walk, bearing their full weight, with a minimally abnormal gait. During this training, a progressively more normal locomotor pattern is developed, and patients profit functionally from such training, although it is expensive and demanding of the patient. Compared with normal locomotor patterns, patients continue to have greater variability in their EMG activity and, as in cats with spinal cord lesions, the EMG activity is less well modulated to suit the environment. Patients with complete spinal lesions also develop gait patterns using this type of locomotor training, but these patterns do not outlast the training session and are so far of no clinical benefit.

Systemic Medications

The aim of antispastic therapy is to reduce spasms and increased muscle tone without reducing the remaining voluntary power (31). Antispastic medications usually reduce the excess excitability of hyperactive spinal reflexes, although dantrolene weakens muscle directly. Different mechanisms of action attributed to these drugs include: (1) increased presynaptic inhibition of group I afferents, which leads to reduction of stretch reflex activity (baclofen, tizanidine, clonazepam, diazepam); (2) inhibition of excitatory interneurons within the spinal reflex pathways (tizanidine, glycine); and (3) reduced muscle contractility (dantrolene) (32,33).

If antispastic drugs were effective in achieving the aforementioned results, considering the importance of such reflexes for performance of useful movements, they might actually reduce functional movement. Clinical studies of tizanidine, diazepam, and baclofen have shown that reduction of hyperactive stretch or cutaneous reflexes usually is not associated with a significant improvement in motor function [tizanidine (34), diazepam (35), baclofen (36,37)]. Improvement in muscle spasms and clonus may even be associated with increased paresis [baclofen (36), baclofen versus tizanidine (25,38,39)].

Similar considerations also apply to dantrolene, which weakens all muscles by reducing release of calcium from sarcoplasmic reticulum, thus interfering with excitation/contraction coupling. To the extent that dantrolene reduces excess muscle tone, it produces weakness that usually makes physiotherapy less useful. In addition, dantrolene can be a hepatotoxin. It is not often used in the chronic therapy of patients with spastic paresis (40,41).

Weakness produced by the centrally acting antispastic drugs or by dantrolene obviously is more significant for mobile patients. In those who are leading a bed–chair existence, increased weakness may not be much of a problem, particularly if the medication reduces painful spasms and facilitates nursing care.

Although antispastic therapy is initiated with only one drug at a time, two or more drugs (e.g., baclofen and tizanidine) may eventually be needed simultaneously. Drug doses should be kept to the minimum needed for effective benefit, particularly in mobile patients, because most of these drugs can produce sedation or weakness if their blood levels are increased too rapidly or too far.

The most effective antispastic drugs are baclofen and tizanidine, with gabapentin and benzodiazepines, particularly clonazepam, being less widely used. They tend only to be effective in spasticity of spinal origin (i.e., MS, SCI, spinal tumors, spinal infarcts), having little effect on spasticity that follows cerebral lesions (42).

Baclofen is a gamma-amino butyric acid (GABA)-B agonist at the spinal level and supraspinally. Baclofen reduces stretch and especially cutaneous reflexes and also alleviates pain in patients with spasticity (43). Baclofen levels should be built up slowly to minimize drowsiness; withdrawing baclofen should also be done gradually to avoid rebound enhancement of spasms and to minimize the possibility of seizures or hallucinations. Baclofen can cause nausea, confusion, ataxia, and headache but has little cardio-hepato-renal toxicity.

Tizanidine is an imidazoline derivative that acts as an alpha-2-adrenergic agonist. Its clinical effects are similar to those of baclofen except that tizanidine may produce less weakness (35). Sedation can be minimized by starting with a low dose, which is slowly increased. Tizanidine often causes dry mouth and, because it is closely related to clonidine, should be used with care in patients who are taking medicine to lower blood pressure. Baclofen and tizanidine operate via different mechanisms and work well together.

Benzodiazepines, including clonazepam and diazepam, amplify the inhibitory action of GABA-A receptors, thereby increasing presynaptic inhibition, reducing the release of excitatory transmitters from afferent fibers, and reducing the gain of stretch and flexor reflexes. With these drugs, serious long-term side effects include development of tolerance, dependency, sleeplessness, and hallucinations. More acute side effects are weight gain, drowsiness, and potentiation of the effects with alcohol. Some of these adverse reactions are less pronounced with clonazepam (42,44).

Gabapentin has been shown to be effective in the treatment of spasticity in individuals with SCI (45) and MS (46,47). Although it is structurally related to the inhibitory neurotransmitter GABA, gabapentin does not activate or block GABA receptors, nor is it converted to GABA or a GABA agonist.

Memantine, which is not available in the United States, is an amantadine derivative that probably acts primarily as a noncompetitive NMDA-receptor antagonist (48); it is not effective in spasticity following cerebral lesions. It can produce agitation and dry mouth and should not be used in subjects who are pregnant or who have abnormal liver function studies.

Glycine, a naturally occurring inhibitory neurotransmitter, reduces experimentally induced hypertonia in animals, and several clinical investigations have shown that oral glycine alleviates symptoms of spasticity (49,50). A similar antispastic effect was described for its precursor, L-threonine (51), which is thought to modify spinal glycinergic transmission. Nevertheless, glycine has not yet been shown to be clinically useful.

Dantrolene diminishes activation of the intramuscular contractile apparatus but does not alter EMG activity; it may affect type I muscle fibers more than type II fibers. It is effective in all forms of spasticity because of its peripheral action, but it is not widely used because it is poorly tolerated by patients (41). In addition to weakness, dantrolene causes nausea, anorexia, and diarrhea. Liver necrosis has been reported, especially in women older than 35 who also take estrogens.

Intrathecal Baclofen

In patients with severe spasticity, even of spinal origin, oral antispastic drugs are generally not effective. Benefi-

cial effects are unsatisfactory and when drug levels are increased, adverse events such as drowsiness occur. However, chronic intrathecal baclofen, infused by an implanted programmable pump, almost always reduces spasticity, even of cerebral origin (31,52–56). The amount of intrathecal baclofen needed is tiny compared with oral doses. This small amount causes few cerebral side effects but is nevertheless very effective in alleviating spasms and increased muscle tone. Severe spasticity may be transformed into flaccid paresis, which, in the case of immobile patients, usually makes nursing care much easier. With follow-ups of almost 10 years, little tolerance has developed. For patients with severe spasticity, chronic intrathecal baclofen is a safe and effective adjunct to other forms of therapy, including physical therapy (57). Combined intrathecal baclofen and oral tizanidine is said to be more effective than either alone.

Before installing a pump, intrathecal baclofen should be tested acutely, using a lumbar puncture needle to inject a single 25–100 µg dose into lumbar cerebrospinal fluid, followed by monitoring of blood pressure and respiration for six hours. If a clear, useful effect is demonstrable, chronic therapy can be undertaken by the subcutaneous implantation of a programmable pump connected to a catheter. The intrathecal tip of the catheter should be placed in the thoracolumbar region. Adverse events related to pump or catheter failure may produce acute baclofen withdrawal, requiring emergency hospitalization. The pump/battery system must be replaced after four or five years. Other side effects include drowsiness and somnolence, occasionally associated with depression of respiration, as a result of a baclofen overdose from a bolus injection, pump malfunction, or misprogramming. Such patients should be admitted to an intensive care unit; no safe antidote is available. Although implantation of a baclofen pump is not difficult for a neurosurgeon, monitoring and reacting promptly to adverse events usually requires a well-trained team. Intrathecal baclofen is best managed in special centers.

Botulinum Toxin

Local injections of botulinum toxin (btx), which blocks release of acetylcholine from motor nerve endings, are effective in weakening any muscle for approximately three months (58). In patients with spastic paresis, focal muscle hypertonia can be satisfactorily treated by btx injections, using no more than 400 units of the American toxin (Botox) every three months. Widespread injections of many spastic muscles are not to be undertaken. Botulinum toxin injections into the external urethral sphincter also improves bladder function in patients with detrussor-sphincter dyssynergia.

Older Therapeutic Modalities

Neurosurgeons can alleviate spastic hyperreflexia by interrupting spinal reflex arcs. Selective dorsal rhizotomy, reducing afferent input, is effective in children with cerebral palsy (59–62). Dorsal longitudinal myelotomy is needed less often (63). Paresis and other abnormal movement patterns persist after spastic hyperreflexia is reduced (64). Infiltration of peripheral nerves or ventral roots with phenol or alcohol can transform a spastic paresis into a flaccid paresis (65). Ablative procedures are rarely undertaken today and phenol nerve blocks are less common because spasticity usually reappears after a number of months. Unwelcome sequelae, such as skin ulcerations as a result of sensory loss in the corresponding dermatomes, are also seen.

Beneficial effects on spasticity have been reported with functional electrical stimulation (FES) of the peroneal nerve during walking (66) and by transcutaneous electrical nerve stimulation (TENS) of several muscles (67,68). These effects, which are more obvious during phasic muscle activation, may be due to inhibition of EMG activity in the spastic extensor muscles. For most MS patients with moderate spasticity, this stimulation is unpleasant and too awkward to be used regularly.

Reduction in spastic stretch reflexes has been reported during chronic stimulation of the anterior cerebellum (69). Long-term spinal cord stimulation for control of spasticity in patients with SCI has recently been demonstrated to be neither efficacious nor cost-effective (70). In 18 of 20 patients with hemiplegic spasticity, TENS of the sural nerve produced a mild reduction in tone in tibialis anterior and triceps surae muscles outlasting the stimulation by 45 minutes (71).

Orthopedic surgeons lengthen shortened Achilles tendons in children with pes equinus deformities in an attempt to get the foot flat on the floor to improve gait (72). Such operations are now performed less often. Botulinum toxin is used repeatedly as the child grows to weaken the gastrocsoleus complex, get the foot flat on the floor, and improve balance and gait (73). After the child is grown, one Achilles-lengthening procedure may be needed.

SUMMARY

Optimal management of people with MS who are troubled by spastic paresis is a multidisciplinary endeavor. A physician, usually a neurologist or a physiatrist, with special interest in neurologic rehabilitation and management of MS should direct the team effort. Oral antispastic therapy is effective for symptoms and signs of mild to moderate spinal spasticity (flexor spasms and spastic dystonia of the flexor type in the legs) often seen in patients with MS. It only treats those positive symptoms and does little if anything for paresis, which is the major cause of disability. Therefore, before starting pharmacotherapy for spastic paresis, both the patient and the physician should be certain that their therapeutic goals are reasonable. Antispastic therapy does alleviate pain and spasms, which are seriously disabling symptoms, and facilitates hygiene and nursing care. These are admirable outcomes. In spite of the usefulness of antispastic therapy, it is underemployed. Nevertheless, it only rarely improves mobility or use of a paretic upper limb. For those with MS and severe spasticity, more invasive therapies (e.g., intrathecal baclofen) should more often be used than is now the case.

References

1. Young RR. Treatment of spastic paresis. *N Engl J Med* 1989; 320:1553–1555.
2. Lance JW. Symposium synopsis. In: Feldman RG, Young RR, Koella WP (eds.). *Spasticity: Disordered motor control.* Chicago: Year Book, 1980:485–495.
3. Gollhofer A, Schmidtbleicher D, Dietz V. Regulation of muscle stiffness in human locomotion. *Int J Sports Med* 1984; 5:19–22.
4. Dietz V. Human neuronal control of functional movements. Interaction between central programs and afferent input. *Physiol Rev* 1992; 72:33–69.
5. Mendell LM. Modifiability of spinal synapses. *Physiol Rev* 1984; 64:260–324.
6. Carr LJ, Harrison LM, Evans AL, Stephens JA. Patterns of central motor reorganization in hemiplegic cerebral palsy. *Brain* 1993; 116:1223–1247.
7. Nacimiento W, Mautes A, Toepper R, et al. B-50 (GAP-43) in the spinal cord caudal to hemisection: Indication for lack of intraspinal sprouting in dorsal root axons. *J Neurosci Res* 1993; 35:603–617.
8. Ashby P. Discussion I. In: Emre M, Benecke R (eds.). *Spasticity. The current status of research and treatment.* Carnforth: Parthenon, 1989:68–69.
9. Burke D, Ashby P. Are spinal "presynaptic" inhibitory mechanisms suppressed in spasticity? *J Neurol Sci* 1972; 15:321–326.
10. Delwaide PJ. Human monosynaptic reflexes and presynaptic inhibition. In: Desmedt JE (ed.). *New developments in electromyography and clinical neurophysiology.* Vol. 3. Basel: Karger, 1973:508–522.
11. Dietz V, Quintern J, Berger W. Electrophysiological studies of gait in spasticity and rigidity. Evidence that altered mechanical properties of muscle contribute to hypertonia. *Brain* 1981; 104:431–449.
12. Ibrahim IK, Berger W, Trippel M, Dietz V. Stretch-induced electromyographic activity and torque in spastic elbow muscles. *Brain* 1993; 116:971–989.
13. Malouin F, Bonneau C, Pichard L, Corriveau D. Non-reflex mediated changes in plantar flexion muscles early after stroke. *Scand J Rehab Med* 1997; 29:147–153.
14. Hufschmidt A, Mauritz KH. Chronic transformation of muscle in spasticity: A peripheral contribution to increased tone. *J Neurol Neurosurg Psychiatry* 1985; 48:676–685.
15. Sinkjaer T, Toft E, Larsen K, Andreassen S, Hansen H. Non-reflex and reflex mediated ankle joint stiffness in

multiple sclerosis patients with spasticity. *Muscle Nerve* 1993; 16:69–76.

16. Potter PJ, Hayes KC, Hsieh JT, et al. Sustained improvements in neurological function in spinal cord injured patients treated with oral 4-aminopyridine: Three cases. *Spinal Cord* 1998; 36:147–155.

17. Thilmann AF, Fellows SJ, Garms E. Pathological stretch reflexes on the 'good' side of hemiparetic patients. *J Neurol Neurosurg Psychiatry* 1990; 53:208–214.

18. Thilmann AF, Fellows SJ, Garms E. The mechanism of spastic muscle hypertonus: Variation in reflex gain over the time course of spasticity. *Brain* 1991; 114:233–244.

19. Berger W, Horstmann GA, Dietz V. Tension development and muscle activation in the leg during gait in spastic hemiparesis: The independence of muscle hypertonia and exaggerated stretch reflexes. *J Neurol Neurosurg Psychiatry* 1984; 47:1029–1033.

20. Dietz V, Berger W. Normal and impaired regulation of muscle stiffness in gait: A new hypothesis about muscle hypertonia. *Exp Neurol* 1983; 79:680–687.

21. Dietz V, Trippel M, Berger W. Reflex activity and muscle tone during elbow movements in patients with spastic paresis. *Ann Neurol* 1991; 30:767–779.

22. Powers RK, Campbell DL, Rymer WZ. Stretch reflex dynamics in spastic elbow flexor muscles. *Ann Neurol* 1989; 25:32–42.

23. Edstroem L. Selective changes in the size of red and white muscle fibres in upper motor lesions and Parkinsonism. *J Neurol Sci* 1970; 11:537–550.

24. Dietz V, Ketelsen UP, Berger W, Quintern J. Motor unit involvement in spastic paresis: Relationship between leg muscle activation and histochemistry. *J Neurol Sci* 1986; 75:89–103.

25. Hoogstraten MC, van der Ploeg RJ, van der Burg W, et al. Tizanidine versus baclofen in the treatment of spasticity in multiple sclerosis patients. *Acta Neurol Scand* 1988; 77:224–230.

26. Stolp-Smith KA, Wainberg M. Antidepressant exacerbation of spasticity. *J Am Paraplegia Soc* 1993; 16:140.

27. Bramanti B, Sessa E, Rifici C, et al. Enhanced spasticity in primary progressive MS patients treated with interferon beta-1b. *Neurology* 1998; 51:1720–1723.

28. Dietz V, Horstmann GA, Trippel M, Gollhofer A. Human postural reflexes and gravity. An underwater simulation. *Neurosci Lett* 1989; 106:350–355.

29. Barbeau H, Fung J. New experimental approaches in the treatment of spastic gait disorders. In: Forssberg H, Hirschfeld H (eds.). Movement disorders in children. *Med Sport Sci, Vol 36.* Basel: Karger, 1991:234–246.

30. Nesemeyanova TN. Physiological aspects in the restoration of motor function of spinal cord injury patients. In: Kao CC, Bunge RP, Reier PJ (eds.). *Spinal cord reconstruction.* New York: Raven, 1983:610–668.

31. Latash ML, Penn RD, Carcos DM, Gottlieb GL. Short-term effects of intrathecal baclofen in spasticity. *Exp Neurol* 1989; 103:165–172.

32. Young RR, Delwaide PJ. Drug therapy: Spasticity. *N Engl J Med* 1981; 304:28–33, 96–99.

33. Dietz V. Spasticity: exaggerated reflexes or movement disorder? In: Forssberg H, Hirschfeld H (eds.). Movement disorders in children. *Med Sport Sci, Vol. 36.* Basel: Karger, 1992:225–233.

34. Lapierre Y, Bouchard S, Tansey C, et al. Treatment of spasticity with tizanidine in multiple sclerosis. *Can J Neurol Sci* 1987; 14:513–517.

35. Bes A, Eyssette M, Pierrot-Deseilligny E, Rohmer F, Warter JM. A multi-centre, double-blind trial of tizanidine, a new antispastic agent, in spasticity associated with hemiplegia. *Curr Med Res Opin* 1988; 10:709–718.

36. Duncan GW, Shahani BT, Young RR. An evaluation of baclofen treatment for certain symptoms in patients with spinal cord lesions. *Neurology* (Minneap) 1976; 24:441–446.

37. Corston RN, Johnson F, Godwin-Austen RB. The assessment of drug treatment of spastic gait. *J Neurol Neurosurg Psychiatry* 1981; 44:1035–1039.

38. Bass B, Weinshenker B, Rice GP, et al. Tizanidine versus baclofen in the treatment of spasticity in patients with multiple sclerosis. *Can J Neurol Sci* 1988; 15:15–19.

39. Stien R, Nordal HJ, Oftedal SI, Slettebo M. The treatment of spasticity in multiple sclerosis: A double-blind clinical trial of a new antispastic drug tizanidine compared with baclofen. *Acta Neurol Scand* 1987; 75:190–194.

40. Meyler WJ, Bakker H, Kok JJ, Agoston S, Wesseling H. The effect of dantrolene sodium in relation to blood vessels in spastic patients after prolonged administration. *J Neurol Neurosurg Psychiatry* 1981; 44:334–339.

41. Anderson TP. (1982) Rehabilitation of patients with completed stroke. In: Kottke FJ, Stillwell GK, Lehmann JF (eds.). *Krusen's handbook of physical medicine and rehabilitation.* 3rd ed. Philadelphia: WB Saunders, 1982: 583–603.

42. Glenn MB, Whyte J . *The practical management of spasticity in children and adults.* Philadelphia: Lea & Febiger, 1990.

43. Hattab JR. Review of European clinical trials with baclofen. In: Feldman RG, Young RR, Koella WP (eds.). *Spasticity: Disordered motor control.* Chicago: Year Book, 1980:71–85.

44. Cendrowski W, Sobazyk W. Clonazepam, baclofen and placebo in the treatment of spasticity. *Europ Neurol* 1977; 16: 257–262.

45. Gruenthal M, Mueller M, Olson WL, et al. Gabapentin for the treatment of spasticity in patients with spinal cord injury. *Spinal Cord* 1997; 35:686–689.

46. Mueller ME, Gruenthal M, Olson WL, Olson WH. Gabapentin for relief of upper motor neuron symptoms in multiple sclerosis. *Arch Phys Med Rehabil* 1997; 78:521–524.

47. Dunevsky A, Perel AB. Gabapentin for relief of spasticity associated with multiple sclerosis. *Am J Phys Med Rehab* 1998; 77:451–454

48. Seif el Nasr M, Peruche B, Rossberg C, Mennel HD, Krieglstein J. Neuroprotective effect of memantine demonstrated in vivo and in vitro. *Europ J Pharmakol* 1990; 185:19–24.

49. Barbeau A. Preliminary study of glycine administration in patients with spasticity. *Neurology* (Minneap) 1974; 24:392.

50. Stern P, Bokonjic R. Glycine therapy in 7 cases of spasticity. A pilot study. *Pharmacology* 1974; 12:117–119.

51. Lee A, Patterson V. Double-blind study of L-threonine in patients with spinal spasticity. *Acta Neurol Scand* 1993; 88:334–338.

52. Mueller H, Zierski J, Dralle D, Boerner U, Hoffmann O. The effect of intrathecal baclofen on electrical muscle activity in spasticity. *J Neurol* 1987; 234:348–352.

53. Penn RD, Savoy SM, Corcos D, et al. Intrathecal baclofen for severe spinal spasticity. *N Engl J Med* 1989; 320: 1517–1521.

54. Ochs G, Struppler A, Meyerson BA, et al. Intrathecal baclofen for long-term treatment of spasticity: A multicentre study. *J Neurol Neurosurg Psychiatry* 1989; 52: 933–939.

55. Loubser PG, Narayan RK, Sandin KJ, Donovan WH, Russell KD. Continuous infusion of intrathecal baclofen: Long-term effects on spasticity in spinal cord injury. *Paraplegia* 1991; 29:48–64.

56. Coffey JR, Cahill D, Steers W, et al. Intrathecal baclofen for intractable spasticity of spinal origin: Results of a long-term multicenter study. *J Neurosurg* 1993; 78:226–232.

57. Stewart-Wynne EG, Silbert PL, Buffery S, Perlman D, Tan E. Intrathecal baclofen for severe spasticity: Five years experience. *Clin Exp Neurol* 1991; 28: 244–255.

58. Davis D, Jabbari B. Significant improvement of stiff-person syndrome after paraspinal injection of botulinum toxin A. *Mov Disord* 1993; 8: 371.

59. Laitinen LV, Nilsson S, Fugl-Meyer AR. Selective posterior rhizotomy for treatment of spasticity. *J Neurosurg* 1983; 1983; 58:895–899.

60. Peacock WJ, Staudt LA. Functional outcomes following selective posterior rhizotomy in children with cerebral palsy. *J Neurosurg* 1991; 74:380–385.

61. McLaughlin JF, Bjornson KF, Astley SJ, et al. Selective dorsal rhizotomy: Efficacy in an investigator-masked randomized clinical trial. *Dev Med Child Neurol* 1998; 40:220–232.

62. Wright FV, Sheil EM, Drake JM, Wedge JH, Neumann S. Evaluation of selective dorsal rhizotomy for the reduction of spasticity in cerebral palsy: A randomized controlled trial. *Dev Med Child Neurol* 1998; 40:239–247.

63. Putty TK, Shapiro SA. Efficacy of dorsal longitudinal myelotomy in treating spinal spasticity: A review of 20 cases. *J Neurosurg* 1991; 75: 397–401.

64. Giuliani CA. Dorsal rhizotomy for children with cerebral palsy: Support for concepts of motor control. *Phys Ther* 1991:248–259.

65. Scott BA, Weinstein Z, Chiteman R, Pulliam MW. Intrathecal phenol and glycerin in metrizamide for treatment of intractable spasms in paraplegia. *J Neurosurg* 1985; 63:125–127.

66. Stefanovska A, Gros N, Vodovnik L, Rebersek S, Acimovic-Janezic R. Chronic electrical stimulation for the modification of spasticity in hemiplegic patients. *Scand J Rehab Med* 1988; (Suppl)17:115–121.

67. Franek A, Turczynski B, Opara J. Treatment of spinal spasticity by electrical stimulation. *J Biomed Eng* 1988; 10:266–270.

68. Levin MF, Hui-Chan CW. Relief of hemiparetic spasticity by TENS is associated with improvement in reflex and voluntary motor functions. *Electroenceph clin Neurophysiol* 1992; 85:131–142.

69. Penn RD, Gottlieb GL, Agarwal GC. Cerebellar stimulation in man. Quantitative changes in spasticity. *J Neurosurg* 1978; 48:779–786.

70. Midha M, Schmitt JK. Epidural spinal cord stimulation for the control of spasticity in spinal cord injury patients lacks long-term efficacy and is not cost-effective. *Spinal Cord* 1998; 36:190–192.

71. Potisk KP, Gregoric M, Vodovnik L. Effects of trnascutaneous electrical nerve stimulation (TENS) on spasticity in patients with hemiplegia. *Scand J Rehab Med* 1995; 27:169–174.

72. Harryman SE. Lower-extremity surgery for children with cerebral palsy: Physical therapy management. *Phys Ther* 1991; 72:16–24.

73. Baumann JU. Behandlung kindlicher spastischer Fuss-Deformitäten. *Orthopäde* 1986; 15:191–198.

16 Weakness

Jack H. Petajan, M.D., Ph.D.

Weakness is an extremely important symptom in multiple sclerosis (MS), and it is the most feared symptom because it implies paralysis, loss of the ability to walk, and severe disability. Conservatively, it is experienced by at least half of the MS population, along with the phenomenon of motor fatigue, which is defined as a worsening of weakness as activity progresses. A person may begin walking without experiencing any symptoms whatsoever, subsequently develop a limp, and then, after walking just a short distance, develop such severe weakness in one lower extremity that walking becomes impossible.

A feeling of generalized weakness or lassitude in the absence of specific weakness of testable muscles may also be present. Patients may complain of being unable to perform daily activities because of a sense of generalized weakness, yet objective muscle testing may not disclose any muscle weakness whatsoever. Such patients may also have significant sensory deficits, heat intolerance, and a diurnal pattern of fatigue.

Weakness as a component of exacerbations is the least likely to completely recover. The extended disability status scale (EDSS) in its higher numbers depends crucially on an assessment of muscle strength and gait, so that weakness plays a significant role in determination of disability (1).

PHYSICAL ASSESSMENT OF MUSCLE STRENGTH

Benchmarks and Activities of Daily Living

When obtaining a history of the course of MS, it is essential to document performance of activities of daily living (ADLs). At what point did the patient experience difficulty walking on the level? When did climbing steps become so difficult that the patient required a railing? When did aids such as a cane become important, and was the cane used for strength or as a cue for better balance? If a wheelchair is used part-time for longer distances, this fact also needs to be recorded. It is also helpful to ask about specific activities such as rising from a squat, rising from a chair, climbing steps, and performing certain common daily activities such as working in the kitchen, dressing, combing the hair, and other self-maintenance activities. With this catalogue of activities in mind, a guided muscle test can be adapted to the individual patient. Follow-up of patients in the clinic can be facilitated by having them maintain a weekly log of selected activities.

Manual Muscle Testing Adapted to the Person with Multiple Sclerosis

It is helpful to use the Medical Research Council muscle grading system for evaluating muscle strength (2), but examination of patients with MS presents specific problems. For example, it is essential to evaluate hip flexion strength in the supine position because one may find that weakness is isolated to this function in patients with myelopathy. Additionally, the patient who has walked a considerable distance or who has been sitting in the waiting room for a period of time may manifest increased signs of spasticity and more muscle weakness than one who has previously been moving. It is preferred to test muscles with the patient in a specific posture. Most muscles can be tested in the ambulatory patient while he is standing. The patient should be observed both walking toward the examiner and walking away. Asymmetry of arm motion and gait rhythm should be noted. The patient is then asked to walk on heels and toes, and then to hop on each foot.

If any asymmetry of function is noted, the patient is asked to rise from a chair with his or her arms folded across the chest and, if this is accomplished well, to rise from a squatting position. A drift of the upper extremities can be determined with the patient extending the arms above shoulder level with the palms directed to the ceiling and the eyes closed. Pronation of the hand and slight drift of the upper extremity may indicate both weakness and corticospinal tract involvement. Shoulder abduction can be tested with the patient standing and the arms abducted. Biceps and triceps strength can be tested with the elbows flexed and the patient instructed to resist passive movement.

In a very strong patient in whom one suspects asymmetry of strength, it is essential to test muscles with the patient using the least mechanical advantage. For example, for the triceps, this is done with the elbow flexed; for the biceps, it is done with the elbow extended. Supraspinatus and infraspinatus can be tested with the patient standing with his arms at his side and the elbows flexed. Wrist extensors and flexors can be investigated with palms down; the intrinsic hand muscles innervated by the ulnar nerve are examined with the fingers spread. The thenar muscles can be tested with the palms supinated and the thumbs extended to the ceiling. Pronation and supination of the wrist are also examined. If there is concern for asymmetry of weakness of the ankle extensor muscles, the patient is told to balance on the examining table with one finger of each hand while he stands on the toes of one foot. A normal person can balance this way without tremor for at least one minute. Drift of the lower extremities can be determined with the patient prone and the knees flexed at 45 degrees. If weakness is more severe, drift can be assessed with the patient sitting and the knees extended.

Spasticity can be rated utilizing the Ashworth scale, which is dependent on the posture, state of rest, and effect of repeated stretches on the muscle (3). It is a scale of 1 to 5, with 1 being normal; 2, detectable resistance; 3, one "catch"; 4, more than one catch; and 5, unable to move the limb passively. Spasticity often is more apparent when the patient's posture resists gravity. The patient may have little resistance to passive movement while sitting, but will manifest the signs of a spastic paretic gait when attempting to walk. Resistance to passive movement decreases with repeated muscle stretches. Fewer than six stretches usually are required to achieve maximal relaxation, and only minutes of rest may restore stiffness to baselines (4)

When performing the neurologic examination, it is important to evaluate muscle strength first, before an assessment of coordination, in order to place the results of coordination tests in proper perspective. The patient who has spastic paresis of an upper extremity will have a slowness of rapid successive and fine movements of the fingers, which are proportionately related to the amount of weakness in the hand. This slowness and clumsiness is to be differentiated from ataxia, in which there is an irregularity of the movement, called *dyssynergia*, and failure to accurately reach a given target, or *dysmetria*. The path of the movement also is irregular, and the amount of irregularity is worsened by the amount of effort required to perform the movement.

Deep tendon reflexes are an important component of the neurologic examination and are directed at assessing weakness. Very brisk myotatic reflexes associated with spread of the muscle contraction to synergistic and sometimes antagonistic muscles as a consequence of the wave of vibration passing from the tendon to the muscle are often associated with weakness and inability to perform movements because of the marked increased sensitivity of the muscles to stretch. It is important to note that stretch reflexes can be obtained from virtually all muscles, particularly when they are overactive.

SYNDROMES OF WEAKNESS

Emulating "Stroke"

Because inflammatory demyelinative lesions may develop in many areas of the cerebral white matter, some of which may overlap the distribution of cerebral arteries, a motor syndrome similar to that of a patient with a cerebrovascular thrombosis may occur. An MS lesion may produce a syndrome typical of a capsular stroke, with hemiparesis or hemiplegia affecting most prominently the face and upper extremity, and to a lesser extent the lower extremity. The upper extremity is flexed in the decorticate posture. The lower extremity is extended, and the patient ambulates with a hemiparetic gait. Deep tendon reflexes are increased, and there is decorticate antigravity posture on the involved side. Plantar responses are extensor on the side of weakness. There may or may not be a hemisensory deficit or a visual field deficit, but a homonymous visual field deficit usually is not present. This may occur in a young person who has never had any symptoms of MS. If the dominant hemisphere is involved, the patient may even manifest aphasic disorder.

Paraparesis

Paraparesis is a common syndrome of MS. It usually is spastic in the early stages, and most commonly results from myelopathy, usually most severe in the cervical region. The patient often reports flexor spasms, usually worsened at night when he is falling asleep or with light stimulation of the skin. These spasms also may occur during the day or spontaneously. There may or may not be corresponding sensory deficits. It is important to inquire about urinary frequency and urgency, which may help corroborate the presence of involvement of the spinal cord. Weakness also may be flaccid if the involvement of the spinal cord is low or if one is examining a patient who has had paraparesis for many years. Under these circumstances, one may obtain adductor reflexes, spread of the knee jerks, but absent ankle jerks with extensor plantar responses bilaterally. There may be transsynaptic degeneration of motor neurons over time, with a dying back phenomenon responsible for flaccidity in the most distally innervated muscles.

Monoparesis

Monoparesis of an upper or lower extremity may occur and sometimes is associated with a sensory deficit highly suggestive of a typical dermatome and representing involvement of a spinal nerve. Indeed, electromyography may yield findings of denervation suggesting root compression (5). This syndrome, which emulates radiculopathy, results from an area of demyelination at the root entry zone in the spinal cord, probably with encroachment of the inflammation into the spinal gray matter.

Cranial Neuropathies

Cranial neuropathies may also occur. A very common pattern of weakness that may herald the onset of MS, is Bell's palsy, sometimes with hemifacial spasm and myokymia (6). A plaque or an area of inflammation in the pons that captures the facial nerve as it passes from the facial nucleus through the pons may produce a typical hemifacial palsy that subsequently resolves as the inflammation improves and remyelination occurs. Ectopic excitation of the nerve producing spasm and myokymia occur. Ptosis also may occur, sometimes with a variation suggestive of myasthenia gravis. Double vision

with partial involvement of the third nerve nucleus may produce unusual patterns of abnormal extraocular movements. Internuclear ophthalmoplegia resulting from involvement of the median longitudinal fasciculus may be seen by eliciting rapid saccades (7).

Sphincter Weakness

Sphincter weakness is a common complaint. It is necessary to document the severity of this problem by asking very direct questions: What is the frequency with which the urinary bladder is emptied during the day or night? Have there been any episodes of incontinence? Similarly, is there any bowel urgency, difficulty controlling the anal sphincter, or episodes of incontinence (8,9)?

Involuntary Movements

Accompanying weakness, a number of involuntary movements may occur. The most common of these are flexor and extensor spasms (10). These spasms usually involve the lower extremities with lesions caudal to the medullospinal junction that result in flexor spasms. Lesions above the level of the midbrain cause extensor spasms. Spasms may be so severe that the entire body is involved in the development of momentary postures of decorticate, decerebrate, or spinal rigidity. More rarely, dystonic syndromes may occur, with exaggerated associated movements and dystonic postures (11). This pattern of movement as a presenting symptom usually suggests the presence of gray matter disease rather than MS.

Myokymia and Fasciculations

Other involuntary movements include myokymia, usually of the mentalis muscles and sometimes associated with weakness of the facial muscles, and fasciculations that may occur in association with pseudoradiculopathy or neuropathic syndromes (12).

FACTORS THAT MODIFY WEAKNESS

Pain

Pain may have a number of causes (see Chapter 23). Contrary to popular belief, it also is a common complaint among MS patients (13). Painful paresthesias may affect movement and strength inasmuch as movements and pressure on the body may enhance the awareness of this symptom. It is what I call the "hot cup of coffee" syndrome in which muscle weakness develops as a consequence of spinal polysynaptic reflex activity that diminishes outflow from motor neurons as a protective avoidance response to pain. When this occurs in a lower extremity, it may severely impair gait or prevent walking altogether. In the immobilized patient who has developed muscle atrophy and joint contractures, pain arising from connective tissues may be elicited on muscle testing or efforts to move. Compression neuropathy may also be present in these patients, so that consideration must be given to an adequate diagnosis of the peripheral neuromuscular system in assessing muscle strength, especially in patients with disorders such as spastic paraparesis.

Body Temperature

An increase in body temperature of less than one half degree centigrade may greatly increase weakness and may be associated with the appearance of weakness when it was not otherwise present (14). Patients should be taught techniques of cooling and the importance of avoiding overheating. Adequate head covering in the sunlight is essential. Evaporative cooling may be enhanced by use of an atomizer to apply water to the body when heat exposure is unavoidable. Pre-exercise cooling in a tub of water that is first cooled from a tepid temperature to prevent abrupt exposure to very cold water can be tried. The human body has the capacity to develop regional heat sinks that serve to reduce body temperature after the cold stimulus has been removed. Preliminary studies of patients using this technique before aerobic exercise has indicated that an exercise period of at least one half hour can be accomplished following a half hour of cooling, with body temperatures just achieving baseline levels at the end of the exercise (15). Cooling can then be repeated using the same bath. Cold exposure, especially if sudden, can elicit a mass reflex, i.e., cold can increase spasticity. Some patients may attempt to take a cold bath but find themselves unable to do so because of the appearance of flexor and/or extensor spasms and the enhancement of such symptoms as paresthesias. As mentioned previously, it usually is advisable to use a tepid or neutral temperature bath that then is gradually cooled by the addition of cold water. Immersion of the lower half of the body in a gently agitated bath is the most effective way to accomplish the cooling of deep tissues. Because the heat capacity of water is very high, cooling may be accomplished more effectively than by evaporative loss or radiation. If the lower half of the body cannot be immersed, immersion of the legs alone may be adequate.

A variety of methods have been developed for body cooling and protection of the MS patient against the deleterious effects of elevated body temperature. Exercise should be performed in a cool environment. The application of a cooling vest, which circulates coolant around the chest wall, or wearing a cooling vest with frozen gel pads contained in it have been demonstrated to be effective ways of increasing heat loss and improving function. It also is possible to wear a cooling vest during exercise. Some investigators have shown both an acute or immediate effect of cooling on muscle strength and fatigue and a chronic effect, noting improvement over time (16). Acute effects have been demonstrated on such functions as the somatosensory evoked potential. It remains to be seen whether the effect of daily cooling on the immune system mediated by norepinephrine, cortisol, and other hormones may be helpful to the MS patient in the long term. In general, the effective use of cooling may enhance the performance of aerobic exercise, improving performance and ultimately fitness. Other functions such as vision, cognition, and sensation also improve.

Hydration

Many patients refrain from drinking water, especially during social occasions, because of poor bladder control. As a consequence, dehydration is a relatively common problem. Dehydration reduces circulating blood volume, which in turn enhances fatigue. Adequate hydration is absolutely essential, especially during exercise. When medications such as oxybutynin are prescribed, it is helpful to emphasize its use before social occasions so that the patient becomes accustomed to the effects of hydration without medication. If the patient must void more often than once every hour or so, this medication should be used during the day to help reduce the necessity of fluid restriction.

Psychological Factors

The presence of pain and anticipated injury during tests of motor performance and muscle testing may contribute significantly to modifying effort. When gait is being evaluated, the patient should be admonished not to hurry and to use a desultory gait. It is helpful to tell patients to imagine that they are going from the living room to the kitchen to obtain a glass of water.

It has been estimated that during the management of patients in a typical MS clinic, approximately 25 percent may have symptoms definable as conversion reactions, and more than half suffer from depression (17). Multiple sclerosis is an ideal condition for the suggestion of such syndromes in susceptible patients. Therefore, it is essential to make every effort to test motor performance in three different ways, by direct manual muscle testing and by the performance of two motor activities using the same neuromuscular system. Great discrepancy in performance should suggest to the examiner the possibility of functional weakness or the influence of nonneurologic factors. In such patients it often is difficult to obtain a history of previous episodes suggestive of conversion reaction. A history of physical, psychological, or sexual abuse may be obtained.

Fatigue and Its Assessment

Patients who have the syndrome of malaise or lassitude along with motor fatigue may perform abnormally during motor testing, making it extremely important to evaluate muscle strength under different circumstances. Motor examination may provide results that are very different from information about motor performance obtained during the history. For example, the patient may state that "I am rarely able to get out of bed, sleep one to two hours each afternoon, and have found myself unable to maintain a normal level of daily activities because of weakness," yet the motor examination may be mildly abnormal or normal. In such patients it is very important to establish a list of benchmarks for motor performance and compare these benchmarks with the results of objective testing of muscle strength to estimate the contribution of malaise to the fatigue syndrome.

PATHOPHYSIOLOGY OF WEAKNESS

Conduction Failure Within the Central Nervous System

As a consequence of demyelination and reduced current density at the nodes of Ranvier, the five- to sevenfold safety factor (the ratio of current available for saltatory conduction to that required for depolarization of the axon membrane) available at each node over which the resting membrane potential reverses may be inadequate (18). As a consequence, a block of conduction may occur. Furthermore, conduction failure may occur when interstimulus interval is less than 200 msec when weakness or spasticity is present (19). Increasing temperature makes conduction failure more likely because ionic conductance is increased and action potential duration is shortened (19). Furthermore, changes in the endoneurial environment, such as increased calcium concentration, may reduce the voltage sensitivity of sodium channels. Axonal loss occurring as a consequence of inflammatory demyelination may occur, which may "overload" remaining motor and sensory axons. It simply is not true that MS is only a demyelinating disease because there is evidence of neuroaxonal loss (20). Furthermore, as immobility leads to muscle atrophy, which may include the presence of abnormal innervation of skeletal muscles as a result of spastic posture associated with paresis, muscle metabolism is secondarily affected so that resting creatinine phosphate is reduced and the ability to generate creati-

nine phosphate after exercise is reduced (21). Gray matter involvement of the spinal cord not uncommonly produces radicular symptoms associated with findings of neurogenic atrophy. These changes contribute not only to paresis but also to metabolic changes that may occur within the muscle.

Central Fatigue

Central fatigue (reduced central drive) has been investigated in studies of the flexor pollicis brevis muscles fatigued by sustained voluntary contraction. Interpolated stimulation of the ulnar nerve and transcranial magnetic stimulation were used to estimate the contributions of central and peripheral factors to the development of fatigue. In MS patients without weakness, approximately 85 percent of the reduced force present at the end of 45 seconds of isometric contraction resulted from central fatigue. Only 20 percent of the fatigue was central in control subjects. No evidence of frequency-dependent conduction block (FDCB) was found in this study of MS subjects without weakness (22). However, FDCB may exist in patients with weakness because of the reduced number of central motor axons available for conduction of motor commands and more severe and extensive demyelination (23).

Using double magnetic stimulation at 120 percent of threshold, it has been demonstrated that a significant delay in conduction in response to the second pulse occurs at interpulse intervals of 75, 100, and 125 msec (24). These findings suggest an altered level of cortical excitability, possibly resulting from abnormal subcortical modulation, perhaps disinhibition, secondary to impaired input from the basal ganglia via the ventral lateral thalamus.

The Physiology of Immobility

The diagnosis and management of the muscle weakness that is often associated with abnormal muscle tone must be based on the understanding of the changes that occur in both the central and the peripheral neuromuscular systems as a consequence of demyelination and axonal loss in the central nervous system (CNS).

The presence of decorticate, decerebrate, and spinal postures is based on an interruption of motor pathways cephalad to the thalamus, the midbrain rostral to the red nucleus, and the bulbospinal junction, respectively. Activation of the descending reticular activating system, rubrospinal tract, and vestibulospinal systems varies depending on the state of arousal. Thus arousal plays an important role in the adjustment of muscle tone and the occurrence of flexor and extensor spasms. The gamma system that regulates muscle spindle bias represents the primary efferent pathway of the reticular system. An important action of baclofen is the augmentation of presynaptic inhibition through GABA-receptors that increase chloride conductance, leading to axonal membrane hyperpolarization. Abnormal postures are also mediated through direct facilitation of spinal motor neurons by descending influences on spinal interneurons.

Adaptation to pathologic change in the CNS occurs very rapidly. Animal studies have verified that changes in synaptic density and even the size of motor neurons and their axons occur in response to altered patterns of innervation. The amplitude of the myotatic reflex supporting the abnormal posture increases along with structural and neurochemical changes that support this increased activity.

Changes also can be found at all levels of the motor unit. Within days, nonused muscle fibers begin to atrophy, with more apparent reduction in minimum fiber diameters seen in type II or fast twitch fibers. However, both type I and type II fibers are affected, with oxidative capacity actually decreased more greatly in type I fibers. Muscle cells maintained in a shortened rest state lose sarcomeres. The elastic property of supporting connective tissue is reduced as elastin is replaced by collagen. It is absolutely essential to recognize the energy economy of the human body, which dispenses quickly with any nonused part. This downsizing includes blood volume, cardiac output, bone density, dermal thickness, and so forth, all of which serve the reduced metabolic and mechanical requirements of impaired function. It has been estimated that muscle mass (strength) decreases by 3 percent per day in the normal subject at bed rest (25–27).

Case Studies: Differential Diagnoses of Multiple Sclerosis and Weakness

Bell's Palsy

As mentioned previously, Bell's palsy may be a presenting symptom of MS and also may occur as a consequence of brainstem tumor, meningeal carcinomatosis, postinfectious neuropathy viral infection, sarcoid, and other causes.

A 25-year-old woman appeared with Bell's palsy, which had bothered her three years previously, although she made a complete recovery. She denied the presence of any other neurologic symptoms. An MRI performed at the time of the initial occurrence was normal. The only other point of interest in her history was a urinary frequency of 10 to 12 times per day with urgency. There were no other signs or symptoms suggestive of MS, but the patient's neurologic examination revealed brisk reflexes, an up-going toe opposite the site of the left Bell's palsy and significant impairment of vibration sense in both feet. Abdominal reflexes were absent. Subsequent MRI revealed the presence of pontine lesions, best seen

on the T2-weighted scan, and periventricular subcortical white matter lesions bilaterally. Cerebrospinal fluid revealed oligoclonal bands, increased immunoglobulin G (IgG) synthesis, and mild pleocytosis.

The diagnosis of MS in this patient emphasizes the importance of recurrent patterns of symptoms as a common feature of the illness and the presence of neurologic signs that are not symptomatic.

Radiculopathy

A 23-year-old woman appeared with clumsiness and numbness of the left upper extremity that had been present for two weeks. The thumb, the first and second fingers, as well as the palm, a band on the ventral forearm and upper arm extending into the shoulder, all were hypalgesic. Fine finger movements were reduced and there was mild weakness of both proximal and distal muscles of the upper extremity. Deep tendon reflexes revealed decreased or absent biceps and triceps jerks, normal brachioradialis jerks, and hyperactive reflexes elsewhere. Plantar responses were flexor. Vibration and position sense were significantly decreased in the thumb and first and second fingers and restored in the fifth finger. There was no neck pain or limitation of motion. Lhermitte's sign was absent.

A prior history was obtained of generalized paresthesias and fatigue with an intermittent pattern characteristic of "benign sensory MS." There also was increased urinary urgency and frequency. Cerebrospinal fluid evaluation on a previous occasion was reported as normal. Magnetic resonance imaging revealed a small number of subcortical white matter lesions. A repeat MRI of the cervical cord revealed a hemilateral white matter lesion extending from C6 to C7, corresponding to the patient's sensory involvement of the left upper extremity.

Neuropathy and "Pseudoneuropathy"

A 45-year-old male patient who was known to have MS of the chronic progressive type, but who was still ambulatory, was seen in the clinic with numbness of the left hand in a distribution "compatible with ulnar neuropathy." On examination of the hand, the second, third, and fourth fingers and the dorsal and ventral surface of the hand along its ulnar aspect were involved, and a short band of hypalgesia also was present, extending three inches proximal to the wrist crease. Although there was some clumsiness of finger motion of the left hand, no weakness could be detected in any of the intrinsic hand muscles innervated by the median or ulnar nerve. Electromyographic studies of the ulnar nerve and needle electrode examination of intrinsic hand and forearm muscles were entirely normal.

This patient has a pattern of sensory loss that is sometimes confused with peripheral neuropathy because the distribution of sensory loss strongly suggests peripheral nerve involvement. In most cases, careful examination of these patients will reveal that the sensory distribution does not conform precisely with the known patterns of peripheral sensory innervation. For example, in this patient the fourth finger was not split by sensory loss and the sensory loss also included the sensory distribution of the medial antebrachial cutaneous nerve.

Hemiparesis: Mimicry of the Capsular Stroke

Multiple sclerosis may present as a hemiparesis with a distribution of weakness similar to that of the patient who has had a capsular infarction. In these patients, there is hemisensory loss and, depending on cerebral dominance, there also may be dysphasia.

A 24-year-old woman was admitted emergently to the hospital when on awakening that morning she experienced right hemiplegia, sensory loss, and aphasia. A very large ring-enhancing lesion was found in the left subcortical white matter, with overlapping projections to both the sensory and motor cortex and encroaching on the thalamus. The differential diagnosis included acute cerebral infarction, brain tumor, and abscess. Only the history, which was strongly suggestive of optic neuritis that had occurred when the patient was in high school, suggested the diagnosis of MS, which was subsequently proven to be the cause of the patient's neurologic deficits. Motor neuron disease may also present as a hemiparesis with long-tract signs as well as scattered findings of lower motor neuron disease detectable only by electromyography. In these patients, sensory symptoms normally are absent and, if present, are attributable to peripheral nerve compression or injury.

Myasthenia Gravis

Multiple sclerosis and myasthenia gravis can be present concurrently. In most cases it is necessary to carry out electrodiagnostic studies and to evaluate acetylcholine receptor antibody in order to confirm the diagnosis. Weakness, easy fatigability, diplopia, ptosis, difficulty chewing and swallowing, with variation as a function of activity, may occur in both diseases. In these patients, it is sometimes difficult to determine which is contributing the most to the disability. In the patient with both diseases, there are no contraindications to treating the myasthenia gravis in the usual manner with thymectomy, prednisone, and pyridostigmine bromide, azathioprine, intravenous immunoglobulin, and apheresis, as well as other modes of therapy that are reserved for patients who do not respond.

Myopathic Disorders That Produce Proximal Weakness Such as Polymyositis

Limb girdle dystrophies and myotonic muscular dystrophy, which may present in adulthood, may also coexist with MS. One should not hesitate to perform electromyographic evaluation and even muscle biopsy to exclude these possibilities. In one large kindred studied in our clinic, both myotonic dystrophy and MS were present, often in the same individual. Because both illnesses may vary a great deal in severity, it became necessary to study each patient in detail with electromyography, genetic testing, cerebrospinal fluid examination, and MRI in order to assess the relative contribution of each disease.

Chronic Fatigue with Weakness

The complaints of patients with chronic fatigue syndrome overlap considerably with those of the fatigue associated with MS, which is estimated to affect approximately 85 percent of patients (28,29). There may be a history of possible viral infection or a period of worsening with viral infection. There may be nondescript neurologic symptoms such as numbness and tingling, transient blurring of vision, and even heat intolerance. The majority of patients will have an entirely normal neurologic examination. Magnetic resonance imaging with flare may indicate a small number of T2-weighted lesions in the subcortical white matter, but if the patient is over 50 years of age, such lesions may be present on the basis of small vessel disease. In the end it may be necessary to perform cerebrospinal fluid examination for IGG synthesis and oligoclonal bands. It is our practice to assess the spinal fluid for lactate in a search for possible mitochondrial disease of the brain, which may require magnetic resonance spectroscopy for detection. Follow-up of these patients over time may ultimately reveal the more typical signs and symptoms of MS.

Case History

A 28-year-old woman presented in 1995 with a history of severe fatigue following a flulike illness that had lasted for two months. When seen six months later, she was experiencing continued chronic fatigue and episodic numbness and tingling but had a perfectly normal neurologic examination. She remained in this condition until 1996, when she developed symptoms of radiculopathy affecting her left upper extremity, with a band of sensory loss suggesting a C5–6 dermatome but with extension into the upper arm and shoulder. Biceps and triceps reflexes were diminished. Biceps and triceps jerks were diminished to absent, with brisk reflexes everywhere else. Plantar responses were flexor. The remaining neurologic examination was normal. A previous MRI had been normal, but on this occasion the MRI of the cervical cord revealed a T2-weighted signal at the C6–7 level compatible with her pseudoradiculopathy. Spinal fluid examination and subsequent course were typical of MS.

TREATMENT OF MULTIPLE SCLEROSIS–RELATED WEAKNESS AS A COMPONENT OF EXACERBATION

Documentation of Changes in Motor Performance:

The documentation of increased weakness as a component of an exacerbation is very important and often difficult. It is not enough to simply receive a report from the patient that he feels weaker or less able to accomplish tasks of daily living. It may be helpful to document gait with a 25-foot walking time, counting steps, once a week (usually on a Saturday morning) with the patient providing the data during follow-up visits. The initial difficulty with gait is usually expressed as an increase in the number of steps that persists over a period of two to three weeks. The walking time increase usually follows the increase in the number of steps. The ability to rise from a squat or a chair or to climb steps may also be assessed. It is extremely important to document hip flexor weakness and its impact on gait. The time of day during which the examination is made and the patient's physical activity in the hour before the examination are also important. If the patient has been sitting in the examining room for a half hour or so, spastic stiffness may become worse and the patient may lose his ability to ambulate well. If the patient is seen in the afternoon, severe fatigue may be present, which may also affect the examination. Increased weakness is often accompanied by other symptoms and signs representing involvement of other areas of the nervous system. Visual loss, double vision, and changes in balance, coordination, and sensation may also help to define an exacerbation. The pattern of an exacerbation usually mimics other exacerbations that have been historically documented.

Chronic Weakness with Chronic Progressive Multiple Sclerosis

As stated previously, evaluating gait is extremely helpful in assessing the course of MS over time. In the chronic progressive patient, determination of gait at the same time of day once per month can be very useful, especially in definition of the patient who is developing secondary progressive disease. A list of benchmarks should also be obtained. Can the patient ambulate without assistance? What daily activities can he or she accomplish without assistance?

Modification of Environmental Aids

It is important to inquire about modification of the home environment to assist the patient with weakness to perform his or her daily activities. It is often surprising to find that no handholds are available, that the bath or shower are not accessible, or that there are areas in the house that may represent significant risk of injury, such as basement stairs. Placing important objects, clothing, dishes, and books within reach may not have been thought of. Many patients are reluctant to request aids for walking because they represent a benchmark of defeat. Explaining to the patient that walking aids simply provide a cue as to one's place in the environment so that gait can be improved may make them more acceptable. The patient with proprioceptive deficit who must focus on the horizon to maintain balance may find that a cane greatly facilitates awareness of the physical environment. A walker may be preferred when weakness supervenes so that more support by the upper extremities is required. Most patients should be trained in how to use a walker so that residual function of the lower extremities is maintained while the walker is being used. If there is a considerable difference between upper and lower extremity strength, some patients will use the walker as a way of substituting entirely for strength in the lower extremities. It should be emphasized that the walker is to be used to help maintain balance and to shift weight from one foot to the other while maintaining an erect posture with weight on both feet.

Maintaining Activities of Daily Living

As weakness progresses, it will be necessary to make significant modifications in the home environment to achieve the goals of living. Monitoring the decline in ability to perform ADLs is an essential component of the patient's history. The subtle changes that occur in habits of daily living will reflect the insidious progression of neurologic deficits. The slow progress toward immobility has consequences, the most significant of which is the loss of physical fitness. An occupational therapist can be helpful in facilitating the performance of daily activities and making life more acceptable. At the same time, it is important to introduce an exercise program and perhaps medication for treatment of fatigue.

THE ROLE OF EXERCISE

Aerobic Exercise

It has been shown that aerobic exercise for MS patients is possible and that it results in significant improvement in aerobic capacity and muscle strength. Most studies of the effects of exercise have been performed on individuals who are ambulatory or who have minor gait disability. After a 15-week aerobic training program using the Schwinn Aerdyne Cycle Ergometer, MS patients with an average disability score of EDSS 3.8 ± 0.3 improved aerobic fitness and muscle strength, and experienced less depression and anxiety than MS controls who received only social support (30). It is reasonable to assume that a person with MS who has the ability to exercise large muscle groups would improve aerobic capacity and strength. One issue that should be considered is the thermosensitive patient who may develop increased weakness with elevated body temperature, as discussed previously. Additional questions that have not been adequately addressed include whether coordination and balance and performance of ADLs can also be improved by aerobic exercise. It appears that the person with MS who has relatively little disability is still less mobile than the normal person, and may experience significant fatigue with a diurnal pattern (31). Improved aerobic fitness also decreases fatigue, but there has been little investigation of the carryover effects of improved fitness on other functions. For those who are capable of performing exercises such as t'ai chi, even to a limited extent, improved fitness and increased range of motion may result. Again, further investigation of this kind of exercise is needed. The other advantage of such exercises is that they are a "meditative ritual" that produces relaxation and reduces stress. The movements are very slow and extend into angles and postures not customarily assumed, which requires sustained attention.

Muscle Strengthening

Muscle strengthening should be a component of any exercise training program. An exercise prescription should be designed to increase strength in muscles that are important for aerobic exercise and performance of ADLs. Brief exercise "pulses" of 5 to 10 minutes are helpful and can be applied for general conditioning to weak muscle groups. A convenient estimate of the weights used is that the subject should be able to do approximately five repetitions over a complete range of motion without discomfort or fatigue. By the third set of repetitions, evidence of fatigue as inability to complete the cycle should be present. The patient who requires a wheelchair will predominantly use upper extremity exercise but may also be able to perform exercises that involve the lower extremities. A period of warm-up is essential to avoid the development of excessive flexor or extensor spasms. Passive range of motion exercises can be performed before active exercise to reduce rigidity and to ease the performance of active exercise. Even a few minutes of immobility can result in restoration of a degree of rigidity comparable to that which is present after sitting for many hours. As

few as six muscle stretches may be sufficient to reduce rigidity to plateau levels, at which point active exercise can begin. It is essential to be innovative in developing exercise programs for patients with severe disability. It is important to "keep wiggling" at all costs to avoid the serious consequences of immobility. This must be combined with an intelligent application of periods of rest ,which may occur two to three times per day. Even 10 minutes of rest in a horizontal position can be restorative.

Developing the Prescription for Muscle Strengthening

Assessment of the level of function. Patients may be classified into four functional categories: (1) no fatigue or thermal sensitivity; (2) normal but with fatigue (malaise and/or motor fatigue with or without thermal sensitivity; (3) mild to moderate motor disability usually affecting ambulation and requiring aids; ataxia may be present; (4) severe motor disability such that ADLs are not possible in many crucial areas such as walking, accomplishing transfers, dressing, and feeding. This assessment can usually be accomplished with a history and neurologic examination but knowledge of how disability affects performance in the home environment is often missing. A home visit by the therapist or physician is advantageous. The ecology of the home setting will determine whether exercises and accomplishable ADLs actually occur (32).

The unique distribution of weakness and the impact of fatigue on strength and ADLs must be considered. For convenience, physical activities and muscular fitness can be viewed in a graduated pyramidal manner (Figure 16-1) (32). At the base of the pyramid, the primary goal is maintenance of range of motion by slow passive stretch

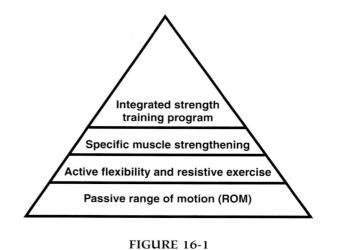

FIGURE 16-1

The muscular fitness pyramid.

for avoidance of contracture. Stretch needs to be performed daily, preferably in a background of small continuous passive activity such as rocking in a chair or using arm lifts.

The presence of muscle function accomplished only with gravity eliminated or against limb weight will require that the number of repetitions—usually less than 10 per cycle—be adjusted to the level of fatigue. Recovery of baseline muscle function without pain should occur within 24 hours. If baseline muscle function is not recovered, the exercise paradigm must be modified and reduced.

Patients with weakness who are unable to exercise against resistance will require selection of the appropriate weight and range of motion to maintain or increase strength. Therapists with experience in treating patients with neurologic disorders may be better able to cope with issues such as abnormal motor fatigue, involuntary movements, spasticity, and so forth. Data on muscle strengthening in patients with arthritis and the elderly are available, but there are few studies on patients with MS. However, several general principles are applicable (33,34). First, isokinetic exercise is preferred, with the maximal force applied at the end of the range of motion. Exercise devices available in rehabilitation settings can provide this condition but requirements are compromised in the home setting. Elastic bands can be used but the range of motion fatigues early, whereas training hardly occurs at the beginning of the movement. This can be partially minimized by setting a range of motion for training in which resistance is relatively constant. Short sets are performed over 90–60°, 60–30°, and 30–0°. Sandbags used over a defined range of motion can also be used to advantage. The intensity of exercise is selected based on measurement of a single maximal contraction (RM). In the MS patient this often requires additional time. The movement must be learned, sometimes in the presence of severe proprioceptive sensory deficit and poor attention. One session is usually devoted to learning the specific exercise. The RM is determined at the next session, at a time of the day when fatigue is minimal. Resistance is gradually increased so that "failure" occurs on the fourth to the sixth attempt, with about one minute of rest between. The procedure should be repeated two to three times in order to obtain the best estimate of RM. Resistance training paradigms currently consist of light to heavy sets of increasing resistance from 50–60 percent to 100 percent of the RM with up to 10 repetitions. They have been shown to result in significant improvement in strength in 90-year-old nursing home residents. Resistance and the number of repetitions may need to be reduced by up to 50 percent in the MS patient with motor fatigue. In addition, exercise capacity may change from week to week or even from day to day. The ability to accomplish a full range of motion against resistance will be limited by pain, contracture, motor fatigue, and fac-

tors that compromise motivation. It is more important to pursue and persist with a muscle strengthening program even if the number of repetitions originally planned cannot be accomplished. Periodic review of exercise capacity is essential.

For individuals with normal strength, with or without thermal sensitivity, a program of resistance exercises following the paradigm successful for the elderly would be most appropriate. The patient may be able to attend a rehabilitation facility or use resistance devices at home, providing isokinetic exercise with stable resistance through a full range of motion. Isometric exercise is of limited value beause it tends to minimize functional carry over and strength is not increased over a full range of motion.

Whenever possible, resistance exercises must be combined with an aerobic exercise program that is done three times per week. Preimposed exercise cooling is effective in promoting recovery from exercise.

Weakness and fatigue that prevent accomplishment of essential ADLs can rapidly lead to complete dependence on caregivers and severe consequences of immobility. A survey of daily activities will identify those that can be accomplished, albeit with some increased effort. The role of these activities in maintenance of fitness must be balanced with the efficiencies of everyday life. Can the patient grasp a glass of water and drink it with sufficient ease that he requires no assistance, or are minutes consumed to accomplish this simple task? It is essential that there be an emphasis on accomplishment because it is easy for the disabled person to experience life as a prison from which he is trying to escape.

For the ambulatory patient, functional independence must be encouraged whenever possible. Shopping, house maintenance activities, gardening, and play are all important venues for improved fitness.

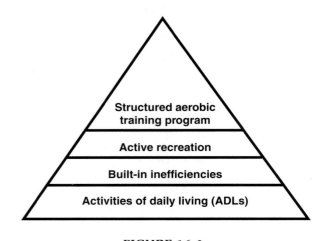

FIGURE 16-2

Role of physical activity or ADLs in monitoring fitness (32).

Studies of the behavioral consequences of improved fitness have shown that quality of life measures improve in proportion to the relative increase in fitness. Exercise is more likely to occur if it is experienced as recreation. As fitness improves, time spent participating in leisure activities also increases.

Exercise and Exacerbations

No significant increase in the rate or severity of MS exacerbations has been found in patients engaged in an exercise program (30). This corresponds well with prospective studies of the influence of stressors of all kinds on exacerbation rate, defined as the acquisition of new signs and symptoms (35). This observation is independent of the effect of emotional stress on such symptoms as spasticity, pain, and so forth, which may worsen under these conditions.

During an exacerbation, which may follow or be associated with a viral infection, the exercise regimen will usually be modified or discontinued for the period of recovery or treatment. Physical therapy should include modest exercise for maintenance of function, passive movement, and stretch. These activities will usually include walking, arm and leg lifts, and gentle water exercise followed by stretching. The duration of exercise will be determined by the level of fatigue, which is expected to be greater during the acute illness.

Because the patient in relapse may be experiencing significant alterations in neurologic status, a therapist with MS experience is preferred. Improvement in status may occur rapidly such that a set regimen of therapy may not be appropriate. For example, assistance with standing for increasing periods of time may graduate rapidly to the ability to walk, even without assistance. More research is necessary in the development of specific exercise protocols for people with various types of disabilities that may accompany weakness.

Motivation to Exercise

Participation in an exercise program requires the elusive factor of *motivation*. Separating exercise from socialization or a ritual component of daily living makes exercise burdensome and difficult to continue on a regular basis. It is best to emphasize the social and pleasure-giving aspects of exercise, which may include performing it with music and certainly, if at all possible, with other individuals. The person with MS generally will tell his or her physician that exercise can only be performed at a certain cost. It was initially believed that if people exercised on a regular basis, they would be able to do very little else because all of their "energy would be gone." In fact, the improvement in fitness results in less fatigue and improve-

ment in the quality of life because the individual is more able to participate successfully in more daily activities, especially recreation.

PASSIVE MOVEMENT AND STRETCH

Combining Stretch and Exercise

It is customary to combine stretch and exercise in the MS person without motor signs. Range of motion and stretch of major muscle groups should be performed following aerobic exercise. A planned regimen of stretch should include muscles of the shoulder and pelvic girdles as well as upper and lower extremities. As much "relaxed" time should be spent in stretching as in exercise. This is also an ideal time for socialization and meditation.

Stretch for the Patient with Long-Standing Motor Disability

The person with motor signs and symptoms who is experiencing weakness, and spastic decorticate, decerebrate, or spinal postures, presents an altogether different set of problems. A joint may be immobilized by contracture, and muscles may be atrophied in the patient with long-standing disease who has not received therapy. In the less involved patient, flexor or extensor spasms and some increased resistance to passive stretch may accompany normal strength and motor performance. Application of the exercise regimen followed by stretch must be appropriately adapted to the needs of each patient.

The immobilized patient with contracture: Following assessment of muscle strength and range of motion, heating or cooling of the muscle may reduce reflex response to passive stretch and holding of stretch against resistance. A daily range of motion regimen accompanied by volitional contraction with gravity eliminated can be applied. In most instances, a physical therapist is required to establish this routine. Such programs are not difficult to implement in the hospital but are often discontinued in the long-term care setting or at home. Home visits by a physical therapist are usually time limited. "Maintenance" therapy is not reimbursable and yet it is common knowledge that regression ocurs without continuing therapy. Therapy may be continued by a trained family member, or other methods of therapy can be used. Stiffness with reduced range of motion increases rapidly after cessation of passive stretch. This is easily demonstrated in the patient with spasticity. The increase in resistance develops in a matter of minutes. Methods for continuing passive stretch during the day include use of a rocking chair, moving against stabilized lower extremities, a mattress that inflates and deflates, and the use of pneumatic pillows that, when placed beneath the limb, can accomplish passive stretch with continuous movement. Passive movement and muscle stretch applied continuously to the paralyzed patient can maintain joint mobility, delay muscle atrophy, and reduce limb edema. In the hospital, most patients with lower limb paralysis are given pneumatic sequential compression devices to reduce edema and increase venous return, but they are not provided passive muscle stretch. However, such devices do reduce the incidence of pulmonary thrombo embolism arising from deep vein thrombosis in the legs. Unfortunately, such devices are not available to most homebound patients.

The spastic patient with varying degrees of muscle weakness: Range of motion and passive stretch can be applied following aerobic exercise. The strongest muscles will be those that support the spastic posture. For example, in the lower extremities, plantar flexion and knee extension will be most easily accomplished compared with lower extremity flexion. Volitional flexion may be assisted by the induction of reflex flexor spasm. This can usually be accomplished by manual stroking of the plantar or even the dorsal surface of the foot, or the lateral aspect of the leg. Gentle massage of the calf muscle may also facilitate flexion.

Standing is supported by extensor tone, most often present in patients with decorticate or decerebrate rigidity. In the MS patient, the tone may be periodically interrupted by flexor spasms that cause collapse of posture. Pain or touch stimuli can activate flexor spasms and lead to falls. Because of the variable nature of such spasms, it is not possible to use electrical stimulation of flexor reflex afferents to facilitate lower extremity function for purposes of improving gait. However, this may be possible in patients who have a more "fixed" deficit.

Hip flexion is essential for normal gait, and this movement is most severely affected in the MS patient with spasticity. Testing hip flexor strength with the patient supine provides a reasonable estimate of the ability to walk. Exercise to strengthen hip flexors should include a to-and-fro swinging exercise accomplished by pelvic movements that swing the unweighted extremity. In addition, hip joint contracture is common and appropriate stretch should be applied.

SPASMOLYTIC MEDICATION

Rigidity as well as flexor and extensor spasms may accompany weakness. These signs of spasticity may be modified by the use of baclofen (GABA-α agonist) and benzodiazepines. The primary indication for these medications is the presence of flexor and/or extensor spasms that interfere with sleep (36). Signs of spasticity or spastic rigidity can enhance weakness and may impair impor-

tant functions such as standing or walking. Therefore, it is important to adjust these medications carefully to achieve the desired end result. Tizanidine (Zanaflex), an alpha-2 agonist, reduces spasticity through another mechanism, i.e., presynaptic reduction in motoneuron excitability by reducing input to alpha motoneurons by the reticulospinal system located in the brainstem. Somnolence may be an adverse side effect of this medication. The dose must be increased gradually. A substantial benefit of this medication is that it is less likely than baclofen to produce weakness as it reduces spastic rigidity (37). Baclofen and tizanidine can be used together. For patients who require high doses of baclofen, or for those who are unresponsive or intolerant of other therapies, baclofen can be injected intrathecally by a programmable pump.

MEDICAL TREATMENT OF WEAKNESS AND FATIGUE

Many patients use a variety of stimulants, including caffeine, to enhance motor performance. Caffeine is used before anticipated ADLs that require physical activity. Adverse side effects of using stimulants later in the day include an increase in flexor and extensor spasms and impairment in the quality of sleep.

Amantadine has been demonstrated to be effective in the reduction of motor fatigue, most prominent in patients who have pyramidal signs (38). A dose of 100 mg twice a day is used. Muscle strength is increased, and the diurnal pattern of fatigue that impairs it is reduced. It appears to be more effective than pemoline (Cylert) in reducing motor fatigue.

A potassium channel blocking agent, 4-aminopyridine (4-AP), enhances a variety of neurologic functions, including strength, by improving conduction in the CNS (39). The pharmacologic effect is similar to that of cooling, which prolongs the duration of the nerve action potential and allows more current to be available for saltatory conduction. The medication has been found to be superior to 3-4-diaminopyridine in promoting conduction (40). Side effects include grand mal seizures, which occurred in two of 23 patients who were taking 4-AP on a long-term basis, from 6 to 43 months. A definite improvement in fatigue and vision was experienced. Hepatitis occurred in one patient (40)

NUTRITION AND VITAMINS

A peripheral component of weakness and fatigue has been identified in MS patients, especially those with weakness. Energy metabolism of the muscle is impaired as a function of neurologic motor deficit, with creatine phosphate recovery delayed following exercise (21). The ingestion of glucose before exercise may improve exercise tolerance and recovery. Such therapy needs to be verified by experiment. Serum carnitine, which facilitates the transport of fatty acids into mitochondria, is not abnormal in MS patients (41). In a manner similar to the general population, aging results in progressive reduction in the adequacy of mitochondrial function. Therefore, it is prudent to take vitamins that reduce the concentration of free radicals, such as vitamin E, and to ensure that such vitamins as thiamine, riboflavin, and pyridoxine (dose not to exceed toxic levels) are supplied to support mitochondrial function. Protein in the morning may help in delaying the development of fatigue in the afternoon. This aspect of diet requires further study because many people skip breakfast or do not ingest protein at that meal.

Added hydration must usually accompany or follow exercise. Sweat rates are more variable and less adequate in MS subjects. This abnormality can amplify the negative effects of heat stress.

PSYCHOLOGICAL FACTORS AND THEIR APPLICATION TO THE TREATMENT OF WEAKNESS

It is essential for people with MS to clearly define and experience their disability in as many ways as possible in order to "embrace it." This will require that they test themselves under a variety of circumstances to understand how their disability responds to various challenges. Only by extending themselves to the limits of disability is this definition possible. At the same time it is important to keep the goals of daily activities in mind so that assistance and aids are obtained when necessary.

Both patient and family must be educated with respect to the demands of the disability. There is no question that the patient with an energetic and capable support system does better in the long term. People with MS must become the cheerleaders for their support system. They must realize that when they ask for support, they are affirming the significance and importance of their caregivers. At the same time, it is important to acknowledge their support with signs of gratitude.

It is extremely difficult to be proactive in participating in exercise when both weakness and fatigue are present. Therefore, it is helpful when exercise is part of a social ritual and accomplishes something other than simply movement, which of itself is important. Exercise may be a component of meditation, socialization performed while listening or in rhythm with music, and a focal point of the day. Exercise should become an essential part of an "active" environment. Finally, humor applied in as many appropriate ways as possible is essential for survival in a world challenged by disability. The pleasure of daily interpersonal interaction is reduced when a sense of perspective is lost.

THE IMPORTANCE OF REST

So much emphasis has been placed on the importance of vigorous exercise and continuous activity during every waking moment in our society that the importance of rest has not been acknowledged. It is all right to be as quiet and immobile "as a stone." Being recumbent for even 10 minutes can do much to restore strength and vitality, especially in the thermosensitive patient who has been standing or sitting quietly for an hour or more. A period of rest of 10 or 15 minutes several times a day is restorative and can often substitute for more prolonged periods of rest that may include sleep. The influence of short periods of rest on neurologic function and the performance of daily activities needs to be assessed more thoroughly.

SUMMARY

Practical Management Guidelines

The survival of health clubs depends on the fact that many people are successful at initiating exercise programs but most cannot maintain them. This is an even greater problem for people with preexisting disability and fatigue. Socialization during exercise helps to enhance motivation. It has been demonstrated in repeated studies that setting modest goals for exercise results in more compliance with an exercise program than the "no pain—no gain" philosophy. The physician can help promote exercise by encouraging very modest programs of exercise, which may include using different exercise protocols from time to time and in different venues, especially recreation. It is also very helpful to follow up at a reasonable time, in three to four months, to evaluate how the exercise program is going.

Exercise with assessment of the VO_2 max is indicated for patients who are ambulatory and able to use either an exercise device, such as a treadmill or an exercycle, or are able to walk or run out of doors, with the usual concomitant assessment of cardiovascular status. Such patients should exercise at 60 perent to 65 percent of their maximum capacity for at least 20 minutes, three or more times per week. A five-minute warm-up period and a five-minute cool-down period should be applied. The exercise level may be increased every six weeks. This usually happens automatically as the individual becomes comfortable with the level of exercise. Various exercise venues can be used once the individual becomes familiar with the perceived level of effort that is necessary to achieve this level of training.

Modification of the exercise method will be necessary for individuals with more severe disability. The Schwinn Aerdyne Cycle Ergometer or other air-driven ergometers are helpful in this regard beause they are low-strain exercise devices that permit a subject to transfer force from weaker to stronger extremities. For individuals who use a wheelchair, it is possible for aerobic exercise to be performed using trunk and upper extremity muscles. The exercise system must be adapted to these patients. Rowing exercises and the use of light weights are helpful. For the patient who is unable to sustain exercise, the arms may be elevated above the head along with deep breathing, either actively or passively, in sessions of 10 to 20 repetitions two to three times per day. Anything that maintains movement of a part of the body that can be moved is extremely important. An adapted rocking chair and pneumatic pillows can facilitate passive movement. At the same time, the immobilized patient often is given an excessive amount of spasmolytic medication, which further enhances immobility. It is important to maintain appropriate amounts of these medications to diminish spasms while at the same time maintaining muscle tone.

References

1. Kurtzke JF. Rating neurological impairment in multiple sclerosis: Expanded Disability Status Scale (EDSS). *Neurology* 1983; 33:1444–1452.
2. Medical Research Council. *Aids to the examination of the peripheral nervous system.* London: Her Majesty's Stationary Office, 1976.
3. Ashworth B. Preliminary trial of corisprodol in multiple sclerosis. *Practitioner* 1964; 192:540–542.
4. Gappmeier E, Petajan JH. Effort of rest and passive stretch on quadriceps muscle stiffness in spastic paresis. Absract, American College of Sports Medicine, 1993.
5. Petajan JH. Electromyographic findings in multiple sclerosis: Remitting signs of denervation. *Muscle Nerve,* Special Lambert Symposium 1982:S157–S160.
6. Smith JK, McDonald WI. Spontaneous and evoked electrical discharge from a central demyelinating lesion. *J Neurol Sci* 1981; 55:39–47.
7. Ebers GC. Multiple sclerosis and other demyelinating diseases. In: Asbury AK, McKhann GM, McDonald WI (eds.). *Diseases of the nervous system.* Vol II. Philadelphia: WB Saunders, 1986, Chap. 102, pp. 1268–1281.
8. Betts CD, D'Mellow MT, Fowler CJ. Urinary symptoms and the neurological features of bladder dysfunction in multiple sclerosis. *J Neurol Neurosurg Psychiatry* 1993; 56:254–250.
9. Cobble ND, et al. In: Delisa JA, Gans B. *Rehabilitation medicine: Principles and practice.* 2nd ed. Philadelphia: JB Lippincott, 1993.
10. Andersson PB, Goodkin DE. Current pharmacologic treatment of multiple sclerosis symptoms. *West J Med* 1996; 165:313–317.
11. Treuchaut C, Bhatia KP, Marsden CD. Movement disorders in multiple sclerosis. *Movement Disord* 1995; 10:418–423.
12. Jacobs L, Kaba S, Pullicino P. The lesion causing continuous myokymia in multiple sclerosis. *Arch Neurol* 1994; 51:1115–1119.
13. Stenager E, Knudson L, Jensen K. Acute and chronic pain syndromes in multiple sclerosis. A five year follow-up study. *Ital J Neurol Sci* 1995; 16:629–632.
14. Guthrie TC. Visual and motor changes in patients with multiple sclerosis. *Arch Neurol Psychiatry* 1951; 65:437.
15. White AT, Wilson TE, Petajan JH. Effect of pre-exercise cooling on physical function and fatigue in multiple sclerosis patients. *Med Sci Sports Exercise* 1997; 29(5):S83.
16. Capello E, Gardella M, Leandre M, et al. Lowering body temperature with a cooling vest as symptomatic treatment for thermosensitive multiple sclerosis patients. *Ital J Neurosci* 1995; 16:533–539.
17. Johnson SK, Deluca J, Natelson BH. Depression in fatiguing illnesses: Comparing patients with chronic fatigue syndrome, multiple sclerosis, and depression. *J Affect Disord* 1996; 39:21–30.
18. Waxman SG. Membranes, myelin and the pathophysiology of multiple sclerosis. *N Engl J Med* 1982; 306:1529–1533.
19. Claus D, Weis M, Jahnke U, Plewe A, Brumholzl C. Corticospinal conduction studied with magnetic double stimulation in the intact human. *J Neurol Sci* 1992; 111:180–188.
20. Trapp BD, Peterson J, Ransoholl RM, et al. Axonal transection in the lesion of multiple sclerosis. *N Engl J Med* 1998; 338:278–285.
21. Sharma KR, Kent-Baun J, Mynhier MA, Weiner MW, Miller RG. Evidence of an abnormal intramuscular component of fatigue in multiple sclerosis. *Muscle Nerve* 1994; 17:1162–1169.
22. Sheean GL, Murray NM, Rothwell JC, Miller DH, Thompson AJ. An electrophysiologic study of the mechanism of fatigue in multiple sclerosis. *Brain* 1997; 120: 299–315.
23. Petajan JH, White AT, Tang PZ, Topaz S. Magnetic cortical stimulation (MCS) and fatigue in multiple sclerosis. Abstract, American Neurological Association, 1997.
24. Nielson JF. Frequency dependent conduction delay of motor evoked potentials in multiple sclerosis. *Muscle Nerve* 1997; 20:1264–1274.
25. Lamb LE, Stevens PM, Johnson RL. Hypokinesis secondary to chair rest from 4 to 10 days. *Aerospace Med* 1965; 35:755–763.
26. Katz R, Kumar VN. Effects of prolonged bed rest on cardiopulmonary conditioning. *Orthoped Rev* 1982; 11:89–93.
27. Kottke FJ. The effects of limitation of activity upon the human body. *JAMA* 1966; 196:825–830.
28. Krupp LB, Alvarez LA, LaRocca NG, Scheinberg L. Clinical characteristics of fatigue in multiple sclerosis. *Arch Neurol* 1988; 45:435–437.
29. Schwartz J, Jandorf L, Krupp LB. The measurement of fatigue: A new scale. *J Psychosom Res* 1993; 37:753–762.
30. Petajan JH, Gappmeier E, White AT, et al. Impact of aerobic training on fitness and quality of life in multiple sclerosis. *Ann Neurol* 1996; 39:432–441.
31. Ng AV, Kent-Braun J. Quantification of lower physical activity in persons with multiple sclerosis. *Med Science Sports Exercise* 1997; 29:517–523.
32. Petajan JH, White AT. Recommendations for physical activity in persons with multiple sclerosis. *Med Science Sports Exercise* 1998; in press.

33. Judge JO. Resistance training. *Topics Geriat Rehabil* 1993; 8(3):38–50.
34. Johnson JH, Searles LB, McNamara S. In-home geriatric rehabilitation, improving strength and function. *Topics Geriat Rehabil* 1993; 8(3):51–64.
35. Kurland LT. Trauma and multiple sclerosis. *Ann Neurol* 1994; 36(Suppl):533–537.
36. Davidoff RA. Pharmacology of spasticity. *Neurology* 1978; 28(Suppl):46–53.
37. Nance PW, Burgaresti J, Shellenberger K, et al. Efficacy and safety of tizanidine in the treatment of spasticity in patients with spinal cord injury. *Neurology* 1994; 44(Suppl 9):544–552.
38. Krupp LB, Coyle PK, Doscher C, et al. Fatigue therapy in multiple sclerosis: Results of a double-blind randomized, parallel trial of amantadine, pemoline, and placebo. *Neurology* 1995; 45:1956–1961.
39. Polman CH, Bertelsmann FW, van-Loenen AC, Koastles C. 4-aminopyridine in the treatment of patients with multiple sclerosis. *Arch Neurol* 1994; 51:292–296.
40. Polman CH, Bertelsmann FW, de-Waal R, et al. 4-aminopyridine is superior to 3,4-diaminopyridine in the treatment of patients with multiple sclerosis. *Arch Neurol* 1994; 51:1136–1139.
41. Fukuzawa T, Susaki H, Kikuchi S, Hamada T, Toshiro K. Serum carnitine and disabling fatigue in multiple sclerosis. *Psychiatry Clin Neurosci* 1996; 50:323–325.

17 Mobility

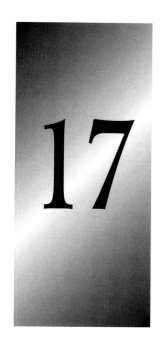

Jodie K. Haselkorn, M.D., M.P.H., Shayla E. Leer, M.P.T.,
Jacqueline A. Hall, M.S., O.T.R./L., and Debra J. Pate, M.S., C.T.R.S.

Limitations in activity and mobility are common problems among those who have multiple sclerosis (MS). Compared with most other chronic conditions, MS is not common. Nevertheless, it was the second most common condition linked with activity limitation in the three-year period from 1990 to 1992 (1). Of the 180,000 individuals with MS who participated in the National Health Interview Survey, 69.4 percent complained of limited activity. These statistics are comparable to those found in other surveys of people with MS (2). Fortunately, a number of causes for impaired mobility are remediable. This chapter introduces a framework for measuring and assessing the mobility problems that occur in MS, describes common assessment methods, and discusses techniques for management. It also distinguishes between medical professionals, who are referred to as physicians or clinicians, from trained attendants, referred to as caregivers.

FRAMING MOBILITY PROBLEMS IN MULTIPLE SCLEROSIS

The National Center for Medical Rehabilitation and Research (NCMRR) and the World Health Organization (WHO) have proposed useful frameworks to assist clin-

icians and researchers in assessing general problems encountered by people with disabilities. These frameworks assist the rehabilitation team in defining the problems, targeting interventions, and assessing outcomes at individual and global levels (3). The frameworks are dynamic and continue to evolve as we understand more about the consequences of this disease.

The National Center for Medical Rehabilitation and Research uses the terms *impairment, disability,* and *handicap* to describe the consequences of disease, disorder, or trauma. These terms are defined as follows: (1) *Impairment:* Any loss or abnormality of psychological, physiologic, or anatomic structure or function; (2) *Disability:* Any restriction or lack (resulting from an impairment) of ability to perform an activity in the manner or within the range considered normal for a human being; (3) *Handicap:* A disadvantage for a given individual, resulting from an impairment or a disability, that limits or prevents the fulfillment of a role that is normal (depending on age, gender, and social and cultural factors) for that individual. For example, in MS impairments such as fatigue, weakness, and spasticity can lead to a diminished ability to walk. If the person's employer does not have parking facilities near the worksite, this reduced ability to walk long distances may result in a handicap—unemployment.

These NCMRR terms parallel those put forth by the WHO's International Classification of Impairments, Disabilities, and Handicaps (ICIDH) (4). The ICIDH classification system describes the consequences of disease, disorder, or trauma at one of three levels: (1) *organ-level* changes in structure and function (impairment); (2) *person-level* changes in everyday activities (disability); and (3) *society-level* changes in social role (handicap) (ICIDH). These terms are linked in the ICIDH in a potential continuum beginning with *disease or disorder,* as follows:

Disease or disorder→Impairment→Disability→Handicap

The arrows mean "may lead to" and are not meant to indicate a necessary linear sequence across time. Little is known about how impairments (organ-level changes) influence disabilities (changes in a person's everyday activities), and how impairments and disabilities influence handicaps (society-level role functioning).

These two frameworks have relevance to the health care team addressing mobility problems in MS. One may identify spasticity, fatigue, weakness as *impairment* or *organ-level* changes and altered mobility as a *person-level* change or *disability*. A *societal problem* or *handicap* exists if alterations in mobility are associated with an individual's inability to perform household and occupational roles. To illustrate that these relationships are not linear, consider the professional golfer who developed a vascular disease that resulted in pain, which impaired ambulation. He was successful using adaptive equipment to golf and could perform his work. However, his impairment became a handicap when the golf tour did not at first recognize his accommodations as a legitimate means of pursuing his occupation.

ASSESSMENT TECHNIQUES

Although general frameworks can help clinicians conceptualize and classify the range of possible problems, specific instruments are useful in monitoring individual problems and, to some extent, in assessing the impacts of interventions on larger groups of individuals. Several of these instruments that have been used to classify problems in MS. Kurtzke's Functional System Scale (FSS) is an impairment-based instrument that evaluates eight domains of the central nervous system, scoring each domain from 0 to 6 (0 is normal and 6 is maximal impairment). The Expanded Disability Status Scale (EDSS) establishes severity with a score of 0 (normal) to 10 (death) (5). The lower range of the EDSS addresses impairments; scores 4 through 10 address disability, especially mobility (see Chapter 13). Other instruments used to assess impairments that may impact mobility in people with MS are the Ashworth spasticity scale, a variety of fatigue scales, and the Scripps Neurological Rating Scale.

The Functional Independence Measure (FIM), a task performance tool that measures individual disability, is used to assess individual and group outcomes after rehabilitation and to estimate caregiver burden (6). The FIM is a 13-item instrument that assesses disability in four domains: (1) self-care, (2) transfers, (3) locomotion, and (4) sphincter control. Each item is scored on a scale of 1 through 7 (1 is total assistance and 7 is independent). The Ambulation Index is another measure to assess disability.

The Craig Handicap Assessment and Reporting Technique (CHART) has been used to assess handicap (7). This instrument is based on dimensions of handicap identified and defined by the WHO (ICIDH) and assesses function along six handicap dimensions: (1) *orientation:* an individual's ability to orient to surrounding; (2) *physical independence:* an individual's ability to sustain a customary effective independent existence; (3) *mobility:* an individual's ability to move about effectively in his or her surroundings; (4) *occupation:* an individual's ability to spend time in the manner customary to that person's sex, age, and culture; (5) *social integration:* an individual's ability to participate in and maintain social relationships; and (6) *economic self-sufficiency:* an individual's ability to sustain customary socioeconomic activity and independence.

In recent years more attention has been focused not only on function but also on health-related quality of life (HRQL) (8). The relationship of function and quality of life is just beginning to be investigated (9). One of the best studied measures is the 36-Item Short-Form Health Survey (SF-36) (10,11). The SF-36 includes measures of physical function and HRQL. Some early work suggests that clinicians and individuals with MS agree regarding physical disability as measured by the physical functioning domain of the SF-36. However, they disagree regarding the overall health-related quality of life as assessed by the vitality, general health, and mental health aspects of the SF-36. On these later measures, people with MS rated themselves as functioning better than clinicians rated their function (12). Quality of life instruments have been developed for individuals with MS to address impairment, disability, handicap, and HRQL (13,14).

Breaking down issues facing the individual into either the NCMRR or the ICIDH classifications allows the clinician and individual with MS to target the most important areas to establish measurable goals for an intervention and to assess the outcome of an intervention.

ASSESSING AN INDIVIDUAL'S MOBILITY

A thorough history and comprehensive physical and functional examination are necessary to identify those impairments that cause decreased mobility in a person with MS.

The focus must be on determining which impairments cause the problem. Possible impairments that lead to mobility problems in people who have MS are illustrated in Table 17-1.

These problems may occur in isolation or in combination. A vicious cycle may be established when weakness (as a result of MS, fatigue, depression, and heat intolerance) leads to reduced exercise, which in turn leads to disuse atrophy, contracture, and deconditioning. Intervening in the cycle requires a thorough examination and an intervention plan that addresses both the primary and the secondary causes of reduced mobility.

An individualized assessment of mobility can identify problem areas and lead to a stepwise intervention program that builds on existing strengths, judicious use of pharmacologic interventions, and assistive technology when indicated. The assessment should cover all aspects of mobility, from joint range of motion and bed mobility to participation in the community and exercise for strength and endurance. For each aspect the assessment must consider whether the individual is independent or needs physical help or an assistive device.

MANAGEMENT OF MOBILITY PROBLEMS

Management of mobility problems must focus on the optimization of function. This section uses this functional perspective to discuss issues regarding range of motion, bed mobility, transfers, activities of daily living (ADLs), movement in the home and community with and without assistive technology, exercise for strength and endurance, and management of common symptoms that lead to impaired mobility.

TABLE 17-1
Impairments Associated with Decreased Mobility in Multiple Sclerosis

Primary
   Altered range of motion
   Weakness
   Deconditioning
   Balance
   Ataxia
Secondary
   Fatigue
   Depression
   Heat intolerance
   Pain
   Spasticity

Range of Motion

Maintenance of range of motion is key to preserving functional mobility. In the lower extremity the muscle groups most likely to be impacted by spasticity and to develop contractures are the iliopsoas, the hamstrings, and the gastrocnemius (Table 17-2). These muscle groups have a significant impact on everyday function, seating, and bed positioning. Individuals who have lower extremity spasticity or weakness in these groups should have a home exercise program that focuses on these muscle groups twice daily.

Contracture in the iliopsoas results in hip flexion contracture, which limits normal hip extension. Risk factors include positioning in bed with the hip flexed and pillows propped under the femur, use of an electric hospital bed, and prolonged sitting. Assessment for contracture can be made using the Thomas test (15). This screening test is done with the individual lying supine on a firm, flat surface and having or helping the person flex both hips to eliminate lumbar lordosis. The clinician has one hand under the lumbar spine to verify that it is flat and lowers the extremity to be tested with the other hand. Normal hip extension is between 0 degrees and −10 degrees. A normal test allows the hip and thigh to return to the bench or mat (or beyond) without increasing lumbar lordosis. An increased arched lumbar spine during the screen suggests a hip flexion contracture and lack of normal hip extension.

Contracture of the iliopsoas results in a functionally shorter limb on the affected side and poor push-off during the stance phase of ambulation. If an early contracture has developed, intervention is important because noninvasive intervention is effective only before the muscle has been replaced with nonpliable connective tissue. Contractures of 20 degrees to 30 degrees are associated with a marked inefficiency of gait. Maintaining range may be accomplished by lying prone on a hard surface. People who have good transfer skills can do this stretch on the floor while watching television or reading. Five minutes several times a day or one 20-minute period will help prevent shortening in this muscle group. A therapist can teach a caregiver techniques to stretch a contracted iliopsoas.

Contractures in the hamstrings result in a reduced ability to fully extend the knee. Risk factors for the development of this contracture include positioning with the hip and knee flexed, as is seen with prolonged bed rest, the use of electric beds, and prolonged wheelchair use. Screening for the presence of a contracture can be done using a straight leg raise. This contracture is often associated with a hip flexion contracture and results in an inefficient gait with hips and knees flexed. Isolated hamstring contractures greater than 20 degrees are associated with ambulation difficulties. Hamstring contractures may also lead to difficulties in transfers and in wheelchair posi-

	TABLE 17-2	
	Lower Extremity Range of Motion Deficits	
MUSCLE GROUP AT RISK	MUSCLE LENGTH SCREENING TESTS	RISK FACTORS
Iliopsoas	Thomas test	Prolonged sitting or bed rest with hips and knees in flexion
Hamstrings	Straight leg raise	Knees flexed during prolonged sitting or bolstering with pillows when in bed
Gastrocnemius	Dorsiflexion ROM at talocural joint with the knee extended	Prolonged bed rest, spastic plantarflexors with weak dorsiflexors

tioning if the knee is unable to extend far enough to appropriately place the lower leg.

In this case, range of motion can be maintained by a variety of active stretches done in a sitting or standing position. An individual can actively stretch the hamstring by placing one leg on a stool with a small towel rolled up under the ankle. He or she then leans forward, keeping the knee straight by applying slight pressure just above the kneecap with the hands. This position should be held for approximately 30 seconds and repeated five times. Passive stretch using a straight leg raise can also be done by a caregiver. A hamstring contracture may be stretched by prolonged static stretch with a low load applied over extended time or by using customized or off-the-shelf braces with adjustable knee joints that can slowly be increased into extension over time as the tissues lengthen.

Contractures in the gastrocnemius result in a plantarflexed foot and a functionally longer limb. This contracture is associated with poor foot clearance during the swing phase of gait, which increases the likelihood of a fall. During the stance phase, contracture changes the forces at the knee, which results in hyperextension of the knee and ineffective push-off. Assessment for contracture is done by dorsiflexing the foot with the knee initially flexed and slowly extending the knee. Normal range of motion will allow for at least 10 degrees of dorsiflexion with the knee fully extended. Range may be maintained by daily stretch done by active movement or by passive movement using caregiver assistance. It may be difficult to sort out the component that spasticity plays in reducing range of motion. Treatment of spasticity that limits mobility or a temporary tibial nerve block may be of assistance in conjunction with a program designed to treat contractures in the gastrocnemius.

Because the gastrocnemius is such a powerful muscle, treatment of contracture may require heat and a skilled therapist. One stretch can be done in the sitting position with the leg of the gastrocnemius that will be stretched positioned straight in front. The sole of the foot of the opposite leg should be positioned on the thigh of the straight leg. The individual can use a towel or a strap over the ball of the foot of the straight leg and pull back to stretch the calf. This stretch should be held for 30 seconds to one minute and repeated at least three times. If a contracture is organized and not able to be stretched, surgical release may be necessary. Preventive maintenance includes walking and standing if the individual is able to do so. Standing in a standing frame may be helpful if the individual has the bone density to support the weight. Caregivers can be trained to passively stretch the gastrocnemius and prevent contractures.

Management of lower extremity range of motion requires coordination among the providers who are responsible for the patient's overall care, spasticity management, mobility, and home care. It may take skilled therapy and modalities to initiate therapy. In chronic progressive conditions, therapy may need to be provided intermittently over time to maintain gains.

Unfortunately for individuals with MS, attention to range of motion is often placed at the bottom of the list of priorities that need attention. As medical interventions have progressed, we are able to prevent the previously most common causes of death—pneumonia and renal disease. Now we must ensure that people with MS do not develop range of motion problems that lead to lack of mobility, decubitus ulcers, sepsis, or even death.

Bed Mobility

Most people with MS are able to maintain bed mobility independently or with limited physical assistance. If maintaining bed mobility is a problem, a physical therapist can be instrumental in teaching techniques to optimize mobility and energy expenditure. Simple additions such as bed loops or handles along the sides of a regular mattress sometimes improve an individual's abilities in a standard bed. An occupational therapist or rehabilitation nurse can assist with these modifications. Hospital beds and trapeze equipment are sometimes necessary.

Individuals with very limited bed mobility and diminished sensation will likely need mattress overlays or specialty beds that keep skin pressure below capillary filling pressure to prevent decubitus ulcers. In addition, resting splints at the ankle, such as L'Nard or OSCARs, may help maintain dorsiflexion while minimizing pressure and skin breakdown over the calcaneus and the malleoli. The hand may also benefit from a resting or static splint to maintain range of motion and hygiene. A bladder and bowel program that optimizes skin integrity should also be considered. Consultation with an occupational therapist, a physical therapist, and a nurse specialized in skin management may be useful for those individuals with markedly reduced mobility.

Transfers

Most people with MS are able to transfer from a sitting position to a standing position or to a wheelchair. Adjustments such as high-seated chairs and raised toilet seats make these transfers easier for those with and without impairments, and they can usually be easily incorporated into a home. The most serious falls that generally occur are in the bathroom because of small spaces and numerous hard surfaces. Installing grab bars and adaptive equipment such as a shower seat and hand-held shower may be the key to preventing falls. For individuals who are unable to transfer independently, physical and occupational therapy consultants can provide the caregiver with transfer techniques that are safe for both the person with MS and the caregiver. In rare instances the caregiver may need a transfer lift system that could be either mechanical or power-driven and may use a sitting or standing technique.

The number of transfers per day may be excessively taxing for some people who live alone. Such individuals may benefit from a ceiling-mounted tracking system. This system is expensive but minimizes the number of transfers from bed to toilet, toilet to bath, and bath to wheelchair.

Activities of Daily Living

Usual activities of daily living(ADLs) can be taxing for a person with MS because of fatigue, weakness, spasticity, ataxia, and disuse weakness. Initial rehabilitation efforts should focus on management techniques that allow for efficient strategies to complete ADLs—bathing, dressing, toileting, eating, cooking, and so forth. People who cannot achieve control of their personal care cannot be expected to take on a strengthening and endurance program.

A person with MS who experiences fatigue during normal daily activities will greatly benefit from using energy conservation techniques and assistance to complete the necessary (but not particularly enjoyable) activities. People should set priorities and chose activities that optimize function and provide enjoyment. Activities should be balanced with rest periods, and a person may want to consider the use of assistive technology to participate in activities that might otherwise fatigue them. There are a variety of assistive devices that can help reduce energy expenditure during basic ADLs. A reacher and a sock aid, for example, can make dressing possible for someone who does not have full mobility.

Assistive Technology

The term *assistive technology* refers to any device that facilitates a person's independence. Assistive devices can be effective in helping to manage mobility problems. These devices should be prescribed in the setting of a thorough functional examination and should involve the rehabilitation team working closely with the person with MS to establish goals. Considerations of function, comfort, cosmesis, and cost are key to the acceptance of any assistive device. There is little role for off-the-shelf devices for those who are going to consistently use and benefit from a device for more than six to eight weeks. These devices should be customized to obtain the optimal benefit. The devices that are found tossed into a closet generally are those that have not been discussed with and "designed by" the person who needs the device.

Acceptance, adherence to use, and improved function are feasible when three conditions are met. First, the person who needs the device understands the purpose and relates to the improved function. Second, he or she has input into the design of a device that will become a part of her or his body image. Selection of color of materials, weight of components, and so forth all factor into adherence. Third, the person must be trained to use the device appropriately. For those who have a medical need for an assistive device, careful assessment, design, training, and education lead to enhanced function. It is ironic that people in medical need are deprived of similar benefit at a time when technology and personal wealth allow others to use these concepts to enhance sports performance.

Assistive devices that have had positive impacts on ambulation for individuals with MS are discussed in the following sections.

Ankle-Foot Orthoses

When foot drop resulting from an imbalance of strength in the dorsiflexors and plantar flexors exists, an ankle-foot orthosis (AFO) may improve the efficiency of gait. Plastic orthotics are lightweight and can be matched to skin color. Materials may include cutouts to minimize heat and moisture buildup.

The choice between an articulated and a nonarticulated AFO requires some consideration. An articulated AFO allows for easier transfer from a sitting to a standing position, makes driving a car easier, and provides stretch of the gastrocnemius. On the other hand, the motion and stretch of the gastrocnemius can trigger clonus at the ankle. Individual assessment will provide the best results. If an articulated ankle is selected, there are various hardware options to choose from to achieve desired mobility and stability at the ankle, as well as long-term wear. Whether an articulated ankle is selected, footplates that incorporate "neurodevelopmental" or "tone-inhibiting" features may minimize spasticity. These footplates usually extend the full length of the foot and provide foot stabilization through total contact proximal to the metatarsal heads, to the longitudinal arch, and at the navicula. A skilled therapist and orthotist working with the person with MS can develop a customized AFO that enhances safe mobility.

Indications for an AFO include weak dorsiflexors, an imbalance between weak dorsiflexors and spastic plantar-flexors, medial or lateral ankle instability, and some cases of quadriceps weakness. If a person is having a difficult time clearing the toes during the swing phase of the gait cycle, consideration of an AFO is in order. In some instances, quadriceps weakness can be controlled using an AFO with a dorsiflexion stop. Relative contraindications to a plastic AFO include peripheral vascular disease, diabetes (especially in the presence of peripheral vascular disease), poor or absent sensation, large alterations in volume because of fluctuating edema, uncontrolled spasticity, and poor eyesight. The clinician should avoid a scenario in which an ulcer is undetected or has a high risk of not healing. A lightweight double metal upright AFO installed into a leather shoe can be a suitable alternative when a plastic AFO is not feasible.

Many people do not want to accept a device that truly enhances his or her function based on the difficulties that accompany living with a chronic degenerative condition. Despite the many positive gains that these people make, the individual may focus on a decrease in physical function. An AFO or any other device may be perceived as "giving in" or as "the inevitable." The individual and her or his clinician must consult freely and explore all options to enhance function. It frequently is helpful to work with a specialist to help an individual accept disability and some of the necessary adjustments.

Ambulation Aids

Sixty-five percent of patients who survive 25 years after the diagnosis of MS are able to ambulate (16). However, many people with MS require an ambulation aid to improve balance and compensate for muscle weakness in order to walk safely.

A single-point cane can be useful to improve stability and balance, but the cane is limited because of the small base of support that it provides. A platform or four-point cane with pivoting options offers more support, especially on rough or uneven terrain. Forearm crutches, also referred to as Canadian or Lofstrand crutches, can be used when more support is needed. Axillary crutches are not appropriate for long-term mobility needs.

A walker provides the most stability and support for those who have weakness or balance deficits. There are a number of walkers on the market today, including some that have three or four wheels for easier maneuverability, pivoting wheels or crampons, and seats built in for rest when endurance is a problem. Walkers need to be prescribed by a qualified therapist or clinician who can consider the degree of hand function necessary to activate the breaks, the physical goals of the person, and the environment in which he or she will be ambulating.

Wheelchair Mobility and Prescription

Some people with MS, despite having adequate static strength, experience severe fatigue or heat intolerance. They can spend their daily energy allowance on the most basic mobility requirements. For such people, wheelchair mobility is medically justified even in the presence of a normal static clinical examination. Power mobility may also be medically justified in this group of people, even if the in-office examination suggests the ability to propel a manual wheelchair. Again, in order to obtain maximum independence, the full range of impairments and disabilities must be considered. Minor impairments in fatigue, vision, strength, sensation, coordination, and cognition are multiplicative and may trigger the need for power mobility.

When a wheelchair is prescribed, it must meet the goals of its user in the areas of comfort, appearance, and cost. Because MS is a long-term progressive disorder, custom prescription that is goal-directed generally will maximize benefits compared with off-the-shelf prescriptions. When ambulation initially becomes difficult, a manual wheelchair may be indicated only for long-distance mobility. At this stage, the clinician should consider a lightweight chair and cosmesis. The clinician must also keep in mind the predicted course of the person's MS and consider systems that allow for modification if the disease worsens.

There are two primary frames of manual chairs—rigid and folding. Rigid frames offer the greatest amount of seat adjustment, thereby optimizing posture and stability. The rigid frame offers the most energy-efficient push performance because energy is not lost in the crossbar system employed by the folding frame. The rigid frame chair is easily disassembled using quick-release axles to remove the tires and has a backrest that folds down. Rigid chairs tend to be lighter because there are fewer moving parts. On the other hand, a folding chair allows for quick stowage in an average automobile or an airplane. Many folding wheelchairs are taking advantage of advanced technology by using lighter materials, which results in less energy needed to push the chair.

Manual wheelchairs also come with a variety of modifications that make propulsion easier, such as plastic- or foam-coated hand-rims that provide a better grip for those who have motor or sensory impairments that affect hand function. For those who have decreased hand function, plastic- or foam-coated rims may help to provide a better grip utilizing friction to push forward. Spoke rims versus the "mag" type wheels can add more shock absorption and aid in reducing spasticity when operating on rough or uneven terrain. Brake extensions and grade aids can ease the use of wheel lock mechanisms and prevent the wheelchair user from rolling downhill on a grade. Until a person has had instruction in advanced wheelchair skills, the antitip or "wheelie" bars should be kept in a down position. A physical therapist who is trained in advanced wheelchair mobility can dramatically improve the function of qualified people who can potentially access the community.

Customized seating is essential for people with truncal weakness or sensory impairments. Seating issues for the person and the therapist to work out include adequate thoracolumbar support and trunk support. The seat cushion selected will depend on the need to optimize the stability of the pelvis and the amount of pressure the person can tolerate over the sacrum and ischial tuberosities.

There are numerous options for individually optimizing a person's mobility, even for a manual wheelchair. For a person to get optimal benefit and prevent potential problems, an assessment should be done by a qualified clinician who can recommend the system that best fits the person's needs.

For people who are unable to use a manual wheelchair because of fatigue, weakness, and lack of endurance, power mobility can be used to limit disability and handicap. The initial choices a clinician confronts are "power scooter" versus "power chair." People with MS often have strong preferences based on their experiences in the community.

Power scooters are available in many grocery stores and consequently may have greater community acceptance. They are good for shopping because they have a large storage capacity. They may also be easier to use at a table in a restaurant because the seat turns and the armrests can be adjusted. Scooters require trunk control and good upper body strength to operate the drive controls. On the other hand, a power wheelchair can be used even if the individual is quadriparetic. The higher quality of seating that can be achieved with a power wheelchair and the greater adaptability over time result in the majority

of power mobility prescriptions being written for power wheelchairs. Augmentative communication systems also tend to be more easily accommodated on power chair options. On the other hand, most power scooters can be broken down and stored in the trunk of a standard automobile, or a lift can be used to place them in the trunk or outside the automobile. Some power chairs are collapsible or can use a scooter lift, but the sturdier chairs require van transportation. Power chairs are more safely secured in a van and are easier for a caregiver to push if power is lost. The decision on which type of power mobility to start with requires a medical evaluation with thought to the person's short-term and long-term goals. This assessment should include a thorough physical and occupational therapy evaluation, recreational therapy evaluation for community mobility needs and leisure needs, speech therapy if indicated, and perhaps a social services consultation to optimize funding options.

Air Travel in a Wheelchair

Air carriers are obligated to make reasonable accommodations for people who use wheelchairs. However, individuals must work with the airline's "Special Needs Service Agent" well in advance of the trip to plan appropriate accommodations. When available, the person may want to work with a travel agent who specializes in the needs of wheelchair users.

If the person has a collapsible chair, he or she must inquire whether the chair can be placed inside the plane, which is desirable for most people. Collapsible wheelchairs that will not fit into a particular type of airplane or those that do not break down require storage as "luggage" in the cargo hold. In either case, a person will probably need to use the airline aisle chair for transport to his or her seat.

People with mobility problems are not permitted to sit near emergency exits and at times are not permitted to use aisle seats. Those who are dependent on another person for mobility are required to travel with an attendant who can assist in the event of an emergency. With or without assistance, a person with MS may not be able to access a bathroom in flight because of the architectural features of the bathroom or the unavailability of an "aisle chair" during flight. Proper personal hygiene safeguards are advised. These safeguards may include bladder and bowel programs before the flight; the use of a condom, indwelling catheter, or pad before departure; and a plan for as prompt as possible clean-up after the flight.

The decision to store a wheelchair in the cargo hold is not to be made lightly. Many of the custom power chairs cost as much as a good automobile and replacement may take months. If an individual's wheelchair must go into the cargo hold, proper storage, even crating, should be considered. The individual should consider purchasing insurance because the wheelchair will be valued as luggage—in fact, as one piece of the luggage allotment. Power mobility users must be aware of battery restrictions. Some types of batteries are either denied transport or must be packed as hazardous cargo, whereas other battery types have few or no restrictions.

Connecting flights also require considerable attention to detail. Given the relative lack of available wheelchairs at arrival or departure gates—even for those who reserve them—a connecting flight can be missed while the individual waits for a chair on the ground. Extra time to connect is the only safe approach at this time.

EXERCISE FOR INCREASED STRENGTH AND ENDURANCE

Once an individual, with or without an assistive device, is able to move around his or her home and community, it is appropriate to add exercise to the management plan for leisure, strength, and endurance.

Until relatively recently, it was believed that individuals with neuromuscular disease would not benefit from exercise above and beyond their usual ADLs and ambulation, and that in fact it could be detrimental. There especially was controversy regarding the role of strengthening in conditions that affect the upper motoneuron system, particularly in the presence of spasticity. Recent literature suggests that exercise programs do improve strength and endurance in individuals who have MS without neurologic compromise (17–21).

People with MS who are heat intolerant may find it difficult to adhere to an exercise program. Exercising in a cool environment or using a cool pool may enhance the person's ability to participate in an exercise program. However, research suggests that for cooling to be effective, core temperature needs to be reduced using a cooling device, for example, or by precooling in a cool pool or tub of water (22). Numerous cooling vests are available and the impacts of pre-exercise immersion is under study.

An exercise program should be balanced so that it not only optimizes the benefits of increased strength and endurance but also allows optimal participation in ADLs, leisure activities, and social domains.

SYMPTOM MANAGEMENT

A brief overview of the medical and rehabilitation management of a number of common symptoms that contribute to the mobility problems of people with MS is presented in the following sections.

Fatigue

Successful management of fatigue is essential to maintaining mobility for people with MS. Fatigue is discussed in detail in Chapter 14, and evidence-based management strategies have been recommended (23).

Spasticity

Spasticity is often defined clinically as the increase in rate-dependent reflexes. People with MS and clinicians should define what they consider "spasticity," and patients should define what they consider the undesirable effects of spasticity. For instance, individuals should define what the "problem" is. From a medical standpoint it is valid to treat pain, lack of sleep, decreasing range of motion, cosmesis, loss of skin integrity, and so forth.

A helpful approach to spasticity management may be found in the use of oral pharmacologic agents such as baclofen, tizanidine, diazepam, and dantrolene. The clinician should titrate these agents to minimize a specific impairment or to maximize particular functions. For example, the goal of a medication might be to reduce spasticity in the gastrocnemius and quadriceps, to optimize ambulation on flat surfaces within the home, to navigate five stairs to the sidewalk, and to walk 100 feet in the community without a rest. The clinician must also be careful to weigh the side effects and benefits of any of these agents. For example, a clinician can titrate a medication to reduce the stretch reflexes, but the individual with MS may find that transfers are more difficult because of a loss of functional knee extension or push-off that was previously associated with increased "tone" in the quadriceps or gastrocnemius. Treatment in this case would achieve reduced spasticity but at the cost of decreased mobility. Similarly, spasticity may be reduced, but the side effects of the agents may be associated with a perception of increased fatigue or weakness, also leading to a reduction in mobility.

Neurolytic or spasmolytic blocks with alcohol, phenol, or botulinum toxin may have a positive impact on mobility, especially if only a few muscles are involved. For instance, a person may have spasticity in the gastrocnemius and posterior tibialis, preventing them from effectively activating the antagonist tibialis anterior and peroneus longus and brevis, which results in poor quality ambulation as a result of planter flexion and inversion. In this case, selective use of blocks in the lower extremity of the gastrocnemius and posterior tibialis muscles may be effective. Selective blocks have the advantage of having few or no systemic side effects, but they are invasive and expensive. The blocks require readministration every six weeks to six months.

Intrathecal administration of baclofen or opioids has also been shown to have a positive effect on mobility. This treatment should be titrated to appropriately match the functional goals of the person with MS. For people who are severely impaired by MS, intrathecal administration may be the only alternative to preserve range of motion, minimize pain, preserve skin integrity, and enhance quality of life.

Spasticity management is also discussed in Chapter 15, and Clinical Practice Guidelines for the management of spasticity in MS are in process under the auspices of the Multiple Sclerosis Council of Clinical Practice Guidelines.

Ataxia

Of all of the impairments associated with MS, ataxia may be the most vexing to manage. Rehabilitation techniques that minimize the disability associated with ataxia are limited. Perhaps the most effective are those that use small weights applied to the distal extremity or use weighted assistive devices. Appropriate devices include weighted utensils, lightweight ankle weights, or weighted walkers, each of which has the effect of dampening the movement and enhancing function.

There are isolated reports in the literature and anecdotal reports suggesting that the use of isoniazid or clonazepam may be helpful. Careful consideration of the risks and benefits must be considered on a case-by-case basis. For example, sedating medication may reduce tremor, but also may increase the risk of falls and aspiration pneumonia and decrease cognitive function. Providers may want to videotape the patient's analysis before and after a course of treatment or use a gait laboratory to demonstrate improvement. The use of a blinded observer to measure the outcome, and even a pharmacist establishing a double-blind "n of one" study, may be warranted. Some centers have reported somewhat positive effects with stereotactic thalamotomy or thalamic stimulation (24).

CONCLUSIONS

Mobility impairments are common in people with MS, but they do not have to result in major disability and handicap. Numerous studies have demonstrated that rehabilitation techniques are useful in maintaining an individual's independence by limiting impairments, disability, and handicap (25–29).

Rehabilitation techniques range from individualized exercise programs to customized adaptive equipment, tailored pharmacologic therapy, and caregiver training. Appropriate rehabilitation approaches include "overrehabilitation" to optimize function for the future (30). Appropriate rehabilitation settings include inpatient, outpatient, and in-home treatment.

References

1. Vital and Health Statistics. Prevalence of Selected Chronic Conditions: United States, 1990–92, Table 22.
2. Aronson KJ. Quality of life among persons with multiple sclerosis and their caregivers. *Neurology* 1997; 48:74–80.
3. Whiteneck GG. The 44th annual John Stanley Coulter Lecture. Measuring what matters: Key rehabilitation outcomes. *Arch Phys Med Rehabil* 1994; 75:1073–1076.
4. World Health Organization. *International classification of impairments, disabilities and handicaps*. Geneva: WHO, 1980.
5. Kurtzke JF. Rating neurologic impairment in multiple sclerosis: An expanded disability status scale—EDSS. *Neurology* 1983; 33:1444–1452.
6. Granger CV, Cotter AC, Hamilton, BB, et al. Functional assessment scales: A study of persons with multiple sclerosis. *Arch Phys Med Rehabil* 1990; 71:870–875.
7. Whiteneck GG, Charlifue SW, Gerhart, KA, Overholser JD, Richardson GN. Quantifying handicap: A new measure of long-term rehabilitation outcomes. *Arch Phys Med Rehabil* 1992; 73:519–526.
8. Gill TM, Feinstein AR. A critical appraisal of the quality-of-life measurements. *JAMA* 1994; 272:619–626.
9. Keith RA. Functional status and health status. *Arch Phys Med Rehabil* 1994; 75:478–483.
10. Ware WE Jr, Sherbourne CD. The MOS 36-Item Short Form Health Survey (SF-36). I. Conceptual framework and item selection. *Med Care* 1992; 30:487–483.
11. McHorney CA, Ware WE Jr, Raczek AE. The MOS 36-Item Short Form Health Survey (SF-36).
12. Rothwell PM, McDowell Z, Wong CK, Dorman PJ. Doctors and patients don't agree: Cross sectional study of patients' and doctors' perceptions and assessments of disability in multiple sclerosis. 1997; 314:1580–1583.
13. Vicrey BG, Hays RD, Harooni R, Meyers LW, Ellison GW. A health-related quality of life measure for multiple sclerosis. *Quality of Life Research* 4:187–206.
14. Ritvo PG, Fischer JS, Miller DM, et al. *Multiple sclerosis quality of life inventory: A user's manual*. New York: National Multiple Sclerosis Society, 1997.
15. Kendall F, McCreary E, Provance P. *Muscle testing and function*. 4th ed. Williams & Wilkins, Baltimore, 1993.
16. Lechtenberg R. *MS fact book*. Philadelphia: FA Davis, 1988.
17. Ponicheter-Mulcare JA. Exercise and multiple sclerosis. *Med Sci Sports Exerc* 1993; 25:451–465.
18. Ponicheter JA, Rodgers MM, Glaser RM. Concentric and eccentric isokinetic lower extremity strength in multiple sclerosis and able-bodied. *J Orthop Sports Phys Ther* 1992; 16:114–122.
19. Petajan JK, Gappmaier E, White AT, et al. Impact of aerobic training on fitness and quality of life in multiple sclerosis. *Ann Neurol* 1996; 39:432–442.
20. Kraft, GH, Alquist AD, de Lateur BJ. Effect of resistive exercise on physical function in multiple sclerosis. *Arch Phys Med Rehabil* 1996; 33:328–329.
21. Tantucci C, Massucci M, Piperno R, Grassi V, Sobini CA. Energy cost of exercise in multiple sclerosis patients with low degree of disability. *Mult Scler* 1996; 2:161–167.
22. Kraft GH, Alquist AD. Effect of microclimate cooling on physical function in multiple sclerosis. *MS: Clin Lab Res* 1996; 2:114–115.

23. Fatigue and Multiple Sclerosis. Evidence based management strategies for fatigue in multiple sclerosis. Council of Clinical Practice Guidelines. October 1998. Paralyzed Veterans of America.

24. Geny C, Nguyen JP, Pollin B, et al. Improvement of severe postural cerebellar tremor in multiple sclerosis by chronic thalamic stimulation. *Mov Disord* 1996; 11:489–494.

25. Freeman JA, Langdon DW, Hobart JC, Thompson AJ. The impact of inpatient rehabilitation on progressive multiple sclerosis. *Ann Neurol* 1997; 42:236–244.

26. Erigenson JS. The cost-effectiveness of multiple sclerosis rehabilitation: A model. *Neurology* 1981; 31:1316–1322.

27. Crewe NM, Athelstan GT. Functional assessment in vocational rehabilitation: A systematic approach to diagnosis and goal setting. *Arch Phys Med Rehabil* 1981; 62:299–305.

28. Forer SK, Miller LS. Rehabilitation outcome: Comparative analysis of different patient types. *Arch Phys Med Rehabil* 1980; 61:359–365.

29. Jonsson A, Dock J, Ravnborg MH. Quality of life as a measure of rehabilitation outcome in patients with multiple sclerosis. *Acta Neurol Scand* 1996; 93:229–235.

30. Fabio RP, Choi T, Soderber J, Hansen CR. Health-related quality of life for patients with progressive multiple sclerosis: Influence of rehabilitation. *Phys Ther* 1997; 77: 1704–1716.

18 Vertigo, Imbalance, and Incoordination

Robert M. Herndon, M.D., and Fay Horak, Ph.D.

Vertigo, imbalance, and incoordination are frequent problems in multiple sclerosis (MS), and their management often is challenging. They put individuals at risk for falls and injury, which complicates management and increases disability. A fall with a fracture is a common event that moves a patient from being ambulatory with a cane or a walker to permanent wheelchair status. It may be as simple as a wrist fracture, but more commonly it is a compression fracture of a vertebra or a hip fracture. The risk of fracture is substantially increased by osteoporosis, which is common in MS because of decreased mobility, steroid use, and sometimes by lack of hormone replacement in postmenopausal women. If the patient with severe weakness and spasticity cannot walk for several days, he or she will decondition and may never walk again.

Additionally, imbalance necessitates the use of attention and cognitive efforts directed at balance and gait to compensate for normally automatic systems, which are not functioning. As a result, some MS patients literally cannot "walk and chew gum" or indeed walk and talk at the same time. Imagine what it would do to *your* ability to function if you had to think about each step you took. You could not mentally rehearse your day's schedule or your shopping list or the lecture you are preparing while you were walking. All your attention would need to be focused on walking. This problem affects a host of functions, including memory. If the person with MS does not pay attention to walking, he will lose his balance. Because of spasticity and impaired coordination, he no longer has the reflexes and speed to catch himself once he is off balance and cannot relax fast enough after starting to fall to minimize injury.

Because essentially every part of the brain is involved in balance in one way or another and there are extensive interactions between the systems involved in balance, it is not surprising that imbalance is a frequent problem in a disease that may cause damage in as many areas as MS. To understand imbalance one fundamental principle must be understood: *The brain is much better adapted to dealing with and compensating for missing information than it is for dealing with incorrect or misleading (distorted) information, and delayed information is false or misleading.*

The mechanism(s) responsible for balance disorders in MS may be dissected. The cause of imbalance may be an isolated lesion in a single system or pathway or, more commonly, may involve multiple lesions affecting two or more sensory and motor systems. If only one system is significantly affected, compensation may be reasonably effective. Compensation becomes increasingly complex when additional pathways are affected and compensatory mechanisms become increasingly less effective as involvement becomes more widespread and severe.

To treat balance disorders in individuals with MS, it is important to understand the physiologic mechanisms that underlie normal balance and coordination, the ways in which demyelinating lesions affect these functions, and the compensatory mechanisms and strategies used by patients to deal with the problem. This chapter reviews the nature of the dysfunction that leads to imbalance and/or incoordination, the types of testing available, and general management. Formal testing is only occasionally necessary, but an understanding of testing and how balance and coordination are perturbed in MS is important for management and prevention of injury.

Balance in stance and gait involves the integration of three sensory systems, the generation of appropriate motor activity, and the ability to adapt and modify sensorimotor behavior based on changing contexts, environments, and intentions (1,2). The sensory systems critical for balance are the proprioceptive (muscle, joint, and skin senses), visual, and vestibular (head position and movement) systems. These systems provide information that tells us where we are in relation to the support surface and how our bodies are moving through space. Motor outputs coordinate movements of the limbs, trunk, and head to control the body's center of mass in response to external perturbations and in anticipation of self-generated postural perturbations associated with voluntary movement.

Difficulty with balance and coordination occurs if any of these three major systems is malfunctioning or if the ability to integrate and coordinate the motor response is impaired. Control of balance is complex and involves essentially every part of the central nervous system. Therefore, damage to almost any part of the nervous system because of MS may affect balance.

The *proprioceptive system* extends from the peripheral nerves in the extremities through the full length of the dorsal columns of the spinal cord to the nucleus gracilis and cuneatus, then to the cerebellum, and by way of the medial lemniscus and thalamus to the parietal cortex. This system provides information on the location of our limbs and body, the amount of pressure or force being exerted, and in which direction and how fast the limbs and body are moving. Because of the extensive length of the pathways, the proprioceptive system is the most frequently involved sensory system in balance disorders in MS. Without this system, we would not know where our legs or arms are in space without looking at them and precise movement would be impossible.

Multiple sclerosis causes delayed neural conduction in a number of pathways, including the proprioceptive pathways (3). With delayed conduction, the brain still receives some information regarding limb position and movement, but it is delayed in time and degraded because of conduction failure in some axons as well as axonal destruction (4,5). The brain reacts as if it has reliable information when, in fact, because of the delay, the information is too old to act on properly. Thus the patient may feel he is swaying a little when he has already exceeded the limits of balance and is falling.

Delayed proprioception also delays the onset of automatic balance responses to external perturbations. The latency of balance responses are directly correlated with sensory conduction delays in the spinal cord. When the latencies of onset of some postural muscles are delayed more than others, a discoordinated and ineffective postural movement may result. Patients with MS who attempt to continue to rely on delayed, abnormal proprioceptive information may actually show improved balance when they are forced to use vestibular or visual senses instead of proprioception for balance, such as on unstable, compliant, or moving surfaces. Dorsal column stimulation may improve balance in MS because it removes proprioceptive misinformation by disrupting dorsal column function, thus forcing the person to depend on the vestibular and visual systems for balance. Delayed and distorted proprioception undoubtedly is the most common single cause of imbalance in MS

The *visual system* extends from the optic nerves through the optic tracts to the lateral geniculate body of the thalamus, then to the brainstem and to the optic radiations that extend through the parietal, temporal, and occipital white matter to the occipital cortex, and from there to many areas involved in analysis of visual information and control of eye movements. Visual information also goes from the lateral geniculate body by way of the superior colliculus to the brainstem, where there are extensive connections with the vestibular system. Vision is used not only to avoid obstacles in a predictive manner during gait, but also to differentiate self-motion from motion of the environment.

Visual motion in the form of looming or receding optic information in the central visual field or optic flow in the peripheral visual fields is used to determine the direction and velocity of our body motion in stance and gait. Visual information is especially important for reducing slow drift of the head and trunk in space.

Problems with vision alone normally do not cause imbalance. However, we depend on vision to compensate when the proprioceptive or vestibular system is malfunctioning. Although visual information is normally too slow, compared with proprioception, to be used to trigger equilibrium responses, it may become the primary system for balance when proprioception is extensively impaired. People with impaired proprioception often become excessively visually dependent for balance. They often have little difficulty indoors, where there are nearby walls and other large stationary visual reference points. However, spatial orientation may be impaired outdoors, away from close visual reference points, when visual motion of the environment may be interpreted as self-motion. These patients may lose their balance, not because of delayed or absent equilibrium responses, but because they make an inappropriate equilibrium response to environmental motion, which they incorrectly interpret as self-motion (6). If questioned carefully, patients with visual dependence for balance will report that standing out in the open in confusing visual environments such as shopping malls and heavy traffic areas gives them even more difficulty than walking in stationary visual environments.

The *vestibular system* signals the position of the head against gravity as well as changes in the angular and linear velocity of the head (7). It includes the vestibular apparatus in the inner ear, cranial nerve VIII, and the dorsolateral pons, extending through the brainstem to the inferior colliculus by way of the restiform body to the cerebellum and connecting rostrally to the temporal lobe. The vestibular nuclei in the brainstem receive convergent information from the vestibular, visual, and proprioceptive systems to control stability of the eyes, head, and trunk in space as well as to integrate the senses for perception of spatial orientation. Disorders of the vestibular system are associated with vertigo, unstable gaze during head movement, gait ataxia, and imbalance. Vertigo and poor gaze stability in themselves impair balance. Both vertigo and gaze stability problems resulting from vestibular deficits are usually worsened by head movements. These patients have much greater difficulty walking while turning the head than walking with the head aimed straight ahead.

Vestibular problems may also result in lost or distorted sensory information informing an individual about which way is "up" and whether he is moving or stationary. A vestibular loss type of balance deficit may not be apparent on normal clinical examination because patients with profound bilateral loss of vestibular function show no vertigo. They also may have normal balance in stance and in reaction to external perturbation if they are on a firm surface (allowing use of proprioceptive information) and looking at a stationary environment (using visual information).

When proprioceptive and visual information is not available, a loss of vestibular function results in "free falls," without any attempt at compensatory equilibrium responses. This occurs in such situations as standing or walking on a compliant surface (e.g., sand or foam), in the dark, or with the eyes closed. Distorted, rather than lost, vestibular function may allow a person to use vestibular information when necessary on compliant surfaces with the eyes closed but may result in excessive visual-dependence or surface-dependence for balance (8). Multiple sclerosis often produces central vestibular deficits that involve the brainstem, cerebellar pathways,

or cortical pathways. These deficits take much longer to compensate for than peripheral vestibular deficits involving the vestibular apparatus or cranial nerve VIII (9).

The *motor system* is extremely complex and may be responsible for several different problems with balance. Delays in conduction in the pyramidal tract, as determined using magnetically evoked motor responses, do not appear to correlate well with imbalance. Apparently, the brain is able to compensate for a delay in the motor response if it has good information about what the limb is doing. This is not surprising if one considers that the sensory system is designed to monitor motor responses continuously and to adjust the speed and force of the movement to the need. Patients with MS who have difficulty using online sensorimotor systems for balance tend to rely more on predictive systems, if they are available. The longer the delayed latencies of equilibrium response, the more important becomes the predictive control of posture.

Unlike pyramidal system involvement, cerebellar involvement *does* lead to imbalance. Cerebellar incoordination and tremor are among the most difficult MS symptoms to treat and often are incapacitating. Different balance problems will result, depending on what parts of the cerebellum are affected (10). Midline cerebellar involvement of the anterior lobe will result in hypermetric equilibrium responses, excessive anterior-posterior postural sway, an inability to use prediction to scale response magnitudes, and postural instability when standing on compliant surfaces (11–13).

In contrast, posterior lobe involvement results in tilting postural alignment, even with the eyes open (14). Spinocerebellar pathway involvement may result in excessive lateral or omnidirectional sway. Because many parts of the cerebellum may be involved simultaneously, often in combination with other sensory and motor involvement, the resulting balance deficits are complex and mixed (15). It is important to understand that much of what passes for cerebellar symptomatology, such as ataxia, incoordination, and imbalance, may in fact be due to delayed sensory feedback. Although it may be difficult to compensate for severe cerebellar deficits, some techniques may help with problems related to delayed proprioceptive feedback. For example, doing things under visual control will go a long way to compensate for imbalance and incoordination caused by delayed proprioception, although some training often is necessary to make optimal use of visual input.

HISTORY TAKING IN IMBALANCE

The first step in dissecting the cause(s) of imbalance is taking a careful history. When and under what circumstances does the patient have balance problems? Was there other evidence of an acute exacerbation of the disease when the imbalance occurred, such as cranial nerve involvement, that might provide a clue to the level of involvement? Was vertigo associated with the imbalance? If present, was the vertigo a sensation that the environment or the individual was spinning, or was it a sensation of tilt or movement of the ground? Was tinnitus or hearing loss associated with the imbalance? Is the problem constant or intermittent? Is standing or walking out in the open without any nearby visual reference points or supports a problem? If a large object nearby such as a bus moves, does it cause imbalance? Does visual blurring accompanying the imbalance?

If the history reveals that the imbalance is mainly a problem out in the open, away from nearby visual reference points, is it worse when standing than when walking? If there is no vertigo, the problem almost certainly is one of delayed proprioception, the most common cause of imbalance in MS. On the other hand, vestibular pathways are involved if there is a history of vertiginous episodes and the imbalance is accompanied by vertigo or a sensation that the world is tilted. If eye movement is disordered and depth perception is impaired, this in and of itself usually will not cause imbalance, but it will impair the ability to compensate for proprioceptive problems and aggravate the imbalance.

Neurologic examination in the patient with the new onset or worsening of imbalance should be performed with particular attention to evidence of brainstem lesions, visual system involvement, proprioceptive impairment, or a change in coordination. Brainstem lesions almost invariably involve several cranial nerves and affect eye movements in addition to any vestibular or proprioceptive involvement, and also may involve cerebellar pathways. Facial numbness, altered taste, dysarthria, and dysphagia are common in brainstem attacks. Hearing loss may occur less commonly, particularly if the zone of entry of cranial nerve VIII is involved. Disordered eye movement is common with nystagmus, which, depending on the location of the lesion, may be of the central or peripheral type. Rebound nystagmus and internuclear ophthalmoplegia are common and indicate some brainstem involvement.

Visual impairment alone generally does not result in imbalance. If new visual impairment causes imbalance, either other areas are involved in the current attack or the proprioceptive or vestibular system already was affected and the patient has become visually dependent. In that case, a prior history of imbalance will usually be present.

In some instances, more formal and detailed testing is needed to sort out the factors that contribute to imbalance. Formal testing may include testing on a balance platform (platform posturography), rotation chair testing for vestibular function, and sensory and motor evoked potentials.

PLATFORM POSTUROGRAPHY

Platform posturography is carried out on a special platform that measures both the motor responses to external support surface perturbations and the use of sensory information for spatial orientation (16). The latencies of muscle EMG and surface force response to support surface translations and rotations may provide information about the extent of proprioceptive conduction delays in the spinal cord and brainstem pathways that affect postural control.

Postural sway during stance under different sensory conditions is measured by estimating the center of body mass motion from forces at the surface. Sensory organization testing with posturography uses six different sensory conditions to isolate vestibular, visual, and proprioceptive components of balance. They consist of three visual conditions with a stable platform and the same three conditions with a "sway-referenced" platform. A sway-referenced platform provides an unstable base that rotates in proportion to the patient's forward and backward center of mass sway such that proprioception from the support surface cannot be used for spatial orientation, thus forcing the patient to depend on visual and/or vestibular cues. The visual surround may also be sway-referenced, making visual information unreliable as a reference for spatial orientation.

During sway-referencing, the visual surround moves in proportion to anterior-posterior body sway, providing incorrect visual cues so that the patient must actively ignore visual cues to retain balance. The three conditions are shown in Figure 18-1.

Using the platform, the amount of postural sway may be quantified in each of the six conditions.

- In condition 1, visual, vestibular, and proprioceptive cues are all available.
- In conditions 2 and 3, proprioceptive and vestibular cues are available, but visual cues are either absent (condition 2) or misleading (condition 3). Comparing sway in conditions 2 and 3 with condition 1 tells you whether the patient is visually dependent for balance. Patients who are extremely visually dependent may fall or sway excessively when eyes are closed (conditions 2 and 5) or the visual surround is sway-referenced (conditions 3 and 6). Some patients are only visually dependent when the visual surround is sway-referenced and show normal balance with the eyes closed.
- Conditions 4, 5, and 6 alter proprioceptive cues for postural orientation. Balance in condition 4 is dependent on vision and vestibular senses. Balance in conditions 5 and 6 is dependent on vestibular sense because proprioception is altered and visual cues are either absent (condition 5) or misleading

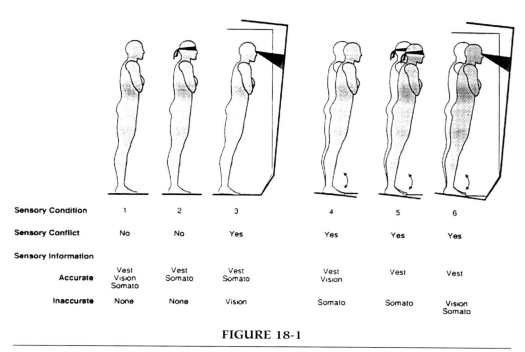

Sensory Condition	1	2	3	4	5	6
Sensory Conflict	No	No	Yes	Yes	Yes	Yes
Sensory Information						
Accurate	Vest Vision Somato	Vest Somato	Vest Somato	Vest Vision	Vest	Vest
Inaccurate	None	None	Vision	Somato	Somato	Vision Somato

FIGURE 18-1

(1) Eyes open with stable visual surround; (2) Eyes closed (Romberg test); (3) Eyes open with sway-referenced visual surround; (4) Eyes open with stable visual surround, sway-referenced platform; (5) Eyes closed, sway-referenced platform; and (6) Eyes open with sway-referenced visual surround, and sway-referenced platform.

(condition 6). A patient who falls or shows excessive sway in conditions 4 to 6 is surface-somatosensory–dependent for balance; he or she must have reliable surface information for postural orientation in order to balance (e.g., vision and vestibular information is insufficient or inadequate). Patients who fall or show excessive sway only in conditions 5 and 6 have a vestibular loss pattern of sensory organization. They can balance using either visual or surface proprioceptive information but cannot balance when both vision and proprioceptive information is altered and vestibular information must be relied on for balance.

By measuring balance in these motor and sensory conditions and correlating it with somatosensory evoked potentials, motor evoked responses, vestibular testing, and other data, it is possible to draw a number of conclusions regarding balance in the patient with MS and what may be done to improve it. It also is possible to specifically predict dangerous environments in which a particular patient is at high risk for a fall.

The patient should have no difficulty standing in the first three conditions, in which visual information alone is altered if proprioceptive sensation from the legs, particularly the ankles and feet, is normal and the vestibular

system is functioning normally. If proprioceptive information is delayed significantly by slowed conduction velocities, a marked increase in sway and perhaps falls will occur in conditions 2 and 3, but no further worsening or even a relative improvement in performance will be seen on conditions 4 to 6.

With a delay in dorsal column conduction, a marked increase in sway and perhaps falls will occur in conditions 2 and 3, but no further worsening or even a relative improvement in performance will be seen on conditions 4 to 6. Improvement in balance may occur on the sway-reference platform in patients with delayed proprioceptive conduction because they may switch from attempting to use incorrect and misleading support surface information to using the more reliable visual and vestibular information. By relying on delayed proprioceptive information, the nervous system perceives that the body has only moved a little when in fact it already may be moving beyond the limits of balance. Again, the brain has much greater difficulty compensating for misinformation than for absence of sensory information.

Vestibular system evaluation involves a careful history. It is unusual to have significant vestibular dysfunction in MS patients who have not experienced either true vertigo (spinning dizziness) or a sensation that either they or their environment is tilted. Tinnitus also is a frequent accompaniment of vestibular system dysfunction. Rarely, Meniere's syndrome (vestibular hydrops) complicates MS-related imbalance; it is marked by a feeling of fullness in the ears, tinnitus, hearing loss, and episodic acute attacks of vertigo so severe that the patient cannot stand or walk. In the absence of a history of vertigo, vestibular dysfunction rarely is a significant factor in imbalance in MS. If vestibular system involvement is suspected on the basis of the history, formal vestibular testing and/or platform posturography may be indicated.

ASSESSMENT AND TREATMENT OF BALANCE DISORDERS IN MULTIPLE SCLEROSIS

The assessment of imbalance in MS for treatment purposes involves first looking at the history and clinical findings and determining the cause of the imbalance. One can make a good estimate of the source(s) of imbalance by paying attention to the circumstances in which it occurs and looking at the neurologic examination in terms of evidence for proprioceptive delay, such as increased sway in the Romberg test and evidence of cerebellar involvement, being careful to distinguish "sensory ataxia" from cerebellar ataxia and looking for evidence of disordered vestibular function.

Several important items in the history may help to delineate the cause of imbalance in a particular patient. First, a history of vertigo or recurring tinnitus suggests significant vestibular involvement. The absence of such a history makes vestibular problems unlikely. A history of imbalance out in the open or on uneven ground, with much better balance indoors where there are visual objects near by at eye level, suggests proprioceptive impairment and the use of vision to compensate. These patients are dependent on vision to compensate for impaired proprioception. This may be confirmed by observing increased sway or loss of balance on Romberg testing.

Careful observation of the patient's balance standing and walking and walking in stressed conditions, such as tandem gait (field sobriety test), and general observations on strength, sensation, and coordination during the standard neurologic examination all contribute. Weakness, spasticity, and slowed motor conduction contribute surprisingly little to imbalance in MS—much less than one would expect *a priori*. On the other hand, a few MS patients have significant limb and truncal ataxia because of cerebellar pathway involvement. In such cases, the limb ataxia usually is pronounced and the cerebellar character is easily recognized.

The majority of patients with imbalance resulting from MS have markedly prolonged somatosensory evoked potentials with significant delays in the proprioceptive pathway from the legs. This is compensated for by using the vestibular and visual systems to maintain balance. If specifically asked, many of these patients will say that they have little trouble inside but have trouble both standing and walking out in the open where there are no close visual cues to tell them which way their body is moving.

Such patients will benefit significantly from the use of a cane in those situations in which visual cues are diminished, as in the dark or out in the open. In this case, the cane is not for support but is another point of contact with the ground, providing more immediate and amplified proprioceptive cues using a shorter neural pathway to improve balance. It is recommended that the patient obtain an attractive cane, a thorn stick, or a walking stick because a cane that sits at home in the closet is of little use. Alternatively, if leg weakness is a significant problem and the patient needs support, a forearm cane may be needed because simply compensating for the delayed proprioception will not relieve the problem.

If significant acute or intermittent vertiginous component is present, it may be treated with meclizine in a dose of 12.5 to 25 mg three or four times a day. Alternatively, anticholinergic medications such as a transdermal scopolamine skin patch may be helpful, but it should not be used for prolonged periods of time. During recovery from exacerbations accompanied by vertigo, short-term use of stimulants such as pemoline (Cylert) or methylphenidate (Ritalin) may be helpful. Unfortunately, there is little that will help if the problem is primarily cerebellar ataxia. Drug therapy has minimal benefit because medications such as clonazepam (Klonopin) reduce tremor in proportion to their sedation effects, i.e., the more the patient is sedated, the less the tremor is noticed. Balancing the beneficial medication effects on tremor with the side effects of sedation is difficult. A weighted walker so the patient does not fall backward may be useful. In some patients, wrist weights will slow the cerebellar tremor enough to allow a slight improvement in use of the hands.

Stereotactic surgery occasionally has been used to control cerebellar tremor, but results have been mixed and this procedure generally is considered as a last resort. When significant vestibular dysfunction is present, instruction in precautions to avoid falls and injury is indicated. Attempts at vestibular rehabilitation also may be helpful, although improvement takes longer and results tend to be less satisfactory with central vestibular disorders than with end-organ disease (17–20)

In summary, careful clinical assessment will allow dissection of the cause or causes of imbalance in MS and permit appropriate decision regarding management.

References

1. Horak FB, Macpherson JM. Postural orientation and equilibrium. In: Smith JL (ed.). *Handbook of physiology.*

"Section 12: Exercise: Regulation and integration of multiple systems." New York: Oxford University Press, 1996:255–292.

2. Horak FB. Adaptation of automatic postural responses. In: Bloedel J, Ebner TJ, Wise SP (eds.). *Acquisition of motor behavior in vertebrates.* Cambridge, MA: MIT Press, 1996:57–58.

3. Jones SJ. Clinical assessment of central nervous system axons: Evoked potentials. In: Waxman SG, Kocsis JD, Stys PK (eds.). *The axon: Structure, function and pathophysiology* New York: Oxford University Press, 1995: 629–647.

4. Waxman SG, Kocsis JD, Black JA. Pathophysiology of demyelinated axons. In: Waxman SG, Kocsis JD, Stys PK (eds.). *The axon: Structure, function and pathophysiology.* New York: Oxford University Press, 1995:438–461.

5. Trapp BD, Peterson J, Ransohoff RM, et al. Axonal transection in the lesions of multiple sclerosis. *N Engl J Med* 1998; 338:278–285.

6. Black FO, Wall C III, Nasher LM. Effect of visual and support surface references upon postural control in vestibular deficient subjects. *Acta Otolaryngol (Stockh)* 1983; 95:199–210.

7. Black FO, Shupert CL, Horak FB, Nashner LM. Abnormal postural control associated with peripheral vestibular disorders. In: Pompeiano O, Allum JHJ (eds.). *Progress in brain research,* Vol 76. Amsterdam: Elsevier Science Publishers, B.V., 1988:263–275.

8. Black FO, Nashner LM. Postural control in four classes of vestibular abnormalities. In: Igarshi M, Black FO (eds.). *Pathological disorders and postural control.* Basel: S. Karger, 1985:271–281.

9. Pfaltz CR. Central compensation of vestibular dysfunction. I. Peripheral lesions. *Adv Otorhinolaryngol* 1983; 30:335–348.

10. Diener HC, Dichgans J, Muller A, Thron A, Poremba M, Rapp H. Correlation of clinical sign with CT findings in patients with cerebellar disease. *J Neurol* 1986; 233:5–12.

11. Horak FB, Nashner LM. Central programming of postural movements: Adaptation to altered support surface configurations *J Neurophysiol* 1986; 55:1369–1381.

12. Horak FB, Nashner LM, Diener HC. Postural strategies associated with somatosensory and vestibular loss. *Exp Brain Res* 1990; 82:167–177.

13. Timmann D, Horak FB. Prediction and set-dependent scaling of early postural responses in cerebellar patients. *Brain* 1997; 120:327–337.

14. Dichgans J, Diener HC, Mauritz KH. What distinguishes the different kinds of postural ataxia in patients with cerebellar diseases. *Adv Otorhinolaryngol* 1983; 30:285–287.

15. Horak FB, Nashner LM, Diener HC. Abnormal scaling of postural responses in cerebellar patients. *Soc Neurosci Abstr* 1986; 12:1419.

16. Nashner LM, Black FO, Wall C III. Adaptation to altered support and visual conditions during stance: Patients with vestibular deficits. *J Neurosci* 1982; 2:536–544.

17. Herdman SJ. Physical therapy treatment for vestibular hypofunction. In: Herdman SJ, Borello-France DF, Whitney SL (eds.). *Vestibular rehabilitation.* Philadelphia: FA Davis, 1992.

18. Horak FB, Jones–Rycewicz C, Black FO, Shumway-Cook A. Effects of vestibular rehabilitation on dizziness and imbalance. *Otolaryngol Head Neck Surg* 1992; 106:175–180.

19. Shepard NT, Telian SA. Programmatic vestibular rehabilitation. *Otolaryngol Head Neck Surg* 1995; 112:173–182.

20. Shumway-Cook A, Horak FB. Rehabilitation strategies for patients with vestibular deficits. In: Arenberg IK (ed.). *Dizziness and balance disorders.* Amsterdam: Kugler Publications, 1993:677–691.

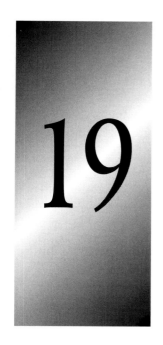

19 Neuro-Ophthalmic Signs and Symptoms

Elliot M. Frohman, M.D., Ph.D., Carol F. Zimmerman, M.D., and Teresa C. Frohman, B.A.

Multiple sclerosis (MS) is one of the most frequent neurologic conditions to produce neuro-ophthalmologic signs and symptoms. These manifestations can be divided into those that involve the visual sensory system and those that affect ocular motor function. The disease process can produce a broad diversity of abnormalities such that essentially any portion of the visual sensory system can be affected, including the retina, optic nerve, chiasm, postchiasmal pathways, and the visual sensory cortices and their connections. It has been estimated that up to 80 percent of MS patients will at some time have disease involvement of this system and that up to 50 percent will initially present with such abnormalities as a first manifestation of the disease (1,2). Furthermore, essentially all eye movement abnormalities known have been described in patients with MS. This provides a framework for the understanding of neuro-ophthalmic signs and symptoms in MS. Particular emphasis is placed on understanding currently proposed mechanisms that give rise to disorders of visual processing and ocular dysmotility.

VISUAL SENSORY ABNORMALITIES

Optic Neuritis

The term *optic neuritis* refers to inflammation of the optic nerve. In MS the demyelination is presumed to be due to inflammation and is one of the most common manifestations of MS. Optic neuritis occurs as the initial presenting symptom in 35 percent to 62 percent of patients (1,3) and in its isolated form it is probably a *forme fruste* of the disease.

Optic neuritis may be acute, chronic, or subclinical. Acute optic neuritis, the most common and easily diagnosed type, is characterized by sudden unilateral vision loss, which may progress over hours to days. Bilateral simultaneous presentation is rare, but sequential involvement of the fellow eye is common. The central visual disturbance may be mild or severe. Some patients are aware of peripheral visual field defects. Many patients notice color desaturation and difficulty seeing in dim illumination. Ninety percent of patients have concomitant pain in or around the eye, usually mild to moderate in severity and worse with eye movement (4,5). Some patients describe positive visual phenomena such as flashes of light (photopsias) that may be precipitated by eye movement (6) or, less commonly, by sound (7). These phenomena, like the Lhermitte's sign and other paroxysmal symptoms in MS, probably are due to ephaptic transmission.

Patients with optic neuritis occasionally describe a sense of disorientation, especially when in motion such as in moving traffic. This misperception may relate to the discrepancy in conduction velocity and latency between the two optic nerves and can be demonstrated by the Pulfrich effect (8,9). From the perspective of a patient with optic neuritis, a swinging pendulum moving in one plane will appear to travel in an elliptical pattern. This probably occurs because visual information derived from the affected optic nerve arrives at the cortex later than visual information from the unaffected nerve. Many patients complain of loss of depth perception, often out of proportion to that predicted by the level of central acuity.

Uhthoff's Symptom

In the early nineteenth century the German ophthalmologist Uhthoff (Figure 19-1) described transient desaturation of color vision during physical exercise in a patient with MS. Demyelinating plaque lesions were found within the optic nerve (10). Transient reversible neurologic dysfunction in response to exercise or exposure to heat is now referred to as Uhthoff's symptom. The high prevalence of Uhthoff's symptom in MS makes it a useful clue in the diagnostic assessment of patients with suspected demyelinating disease (11,12), but it is not pathognomonic for MS. Uhthoff's symptom has been described in optic neuropathy from Leber's hereditary optic neuropathy (LHON) (13), tumor (11), and vascular insufficiency syndromes, such as carotid artery disease and giant cell arteritis (14).

The Uhthoff's phenomenon can be produced by exposure to high ambient temperatures, with hot baths

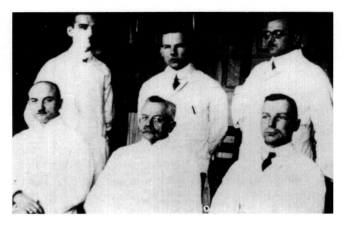

FIGURE 19-1

Wilhelm Uhthoff (seated in the center) with his assistants. (From Selhorst JB, Saul RF. Uhthoff and his symptom. *J Neuro-Ophthalmol* 1995; 15:63–69.)

or showers, and with the ingestion of hot food or liquid. The symptoms generally last for minutes but may persist for hours (15). In some patients, identical symptoms can occur with exposure to cold conditions, the "inverse Uhthoff's symptom" (16). Exercise, illness, and emotional stress can also precipitate symptoms. Although originally described in the optic nerve, temperature and exercise can also produce reversible fluctuations in many other neurologic functions, including alteration of focal sensory or motor function, ambulation disturbance, change in bowel, bladder or sexual function, and cognitive impairment.

Uhthoff's phenomenon is probably due to elevated temperature causing a decrement in axonal conduction in partially or completely demyelinated fibers (9,17,18). The mechanism for the Uhthoff's phenomenon may relate to the neuronal safety factor, which corresponds to the ratio of action potential current generated by the neuronal impulse to the minimum quantity of current necessary to maintain conduction. Temperature elevation increases the neuronal excitation threshold and decreases the action potential duration, which ultimately reduces the safety factor (19). Extremes of temperature are not necessarily crucial; temperature escalations in the axon as small as 0.5°C can produce reversible conduction block in demyelinated fibers (20,21). Reducing temperature can improve conduction (22). Davies (23) has shown that hyperventilation can reduce the visual evoked potential (VEP) latency and improve axonal conduction in response to respiratory alkalosis and changes in ionized calcium.

Despite the strong association of temperature elevation and the production of Uhthoff's symptom, investigators have shown that exercise in the absence of significant temperature elevation is sufficient to produce neurologic fluctuations, which suggests that a metabolic factor may play a role in some patients (24) (Figure 19-2).

Although there is no evidence that patients with frequent Uhthoff's symptoms have a worse prognosis over the course of their MS, caution must be exercised during conditions that precipitate the symptoms, as patients may be unable to move or function sufficiently to protect themselves. Reducing body temperature by taking cold showers, ingesting cold beverages, or using cooling devices has been beneficial in many patients. Ingestion of ice water has been shown to improve neuronal conduction in the optic nerve as measured by pattern shift visual evoked potentials (pVEPs) with corresponding improvement in visual acuity (22) (Figure 19-3). Pharmacologic intervention for heat sensitivity may be effective with agents that can prolong action potential duration, such as the potassium channel antagonists 4-aminopyridine (4-AP) and 3,4-diaminopyridine (3,4-DAP) (25).

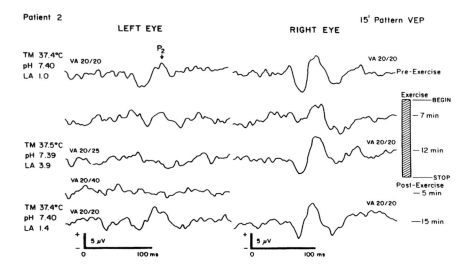

Patient 2

15' Pattern VEP

LEFT EYE   RIGHT EYE

FIGURE 19-2

The progressive decrease and ultimate loss of the P2 amplitude during exercise (stationary cycling) and independent of temperature. There was a corresponding decline in visual acuity from in the left eye from 20/20 to 20/40 with a decrease in venous pH and an increase in lactic acid. After cessation of exercise, conduction block was reversed and visual acuity was restored. (From Selhorst JB, Saul RF. Uhthoff and his symptom. *J Neuro-Ophthalmol* 1995; 15:63–69.)

CLINICAL ASSESSMENT

The diagnosis of optic neuritis is a clinical one. Examination should confirm optic nerve dysfunction in a patient with a history that is compatible with optic neuritis. Central acuity is usually reduced, but 10 percent of patients have preserved central vision of at least 20/20 (5). It is important to recognize that patients with optic neuritis who retain normal or near-normal acuity often have reduced color vision and contrast sensitivity that may seem out of proportion to central visual disturbance. Color vision can be easily tested using Hardy-Rand-Ritter or Ishihara pseudoisochromic tests or the Farnsworth-Munsell 100 hue test; the latter may be more sensitive in detecting demyelinating optic neuropathy (5,26). Although some visual abnormalities may be quite subtle, a careful clinical examination, including color testing, can be nearly as sensitive as neurophysiologic testing. In one study of MS patients, color vision, visual field, and red-free ophthalmoscopy were judged equally useful as VEP; only 8 percent of patients with abnormal pVEPs had a normal neuro-ophthalmic examination (27).

Virtually all patients with unilateral optic neuritis have a relative afferent pupillary defect (RAPD, or Marcus Gunn pupil) in the affected eye. An RAPD may be demonstrated objectively by the swinging flashlight test or subjectively by asking the patient to compare brightness of a light source in the affected eye with that in the unaffected eye. If an RAPD is not observed, one must consider the possibility of coexisting optic neuropathy in the fellow eye or question the diagnosis of optic neuropathy (including optic neuritis) in the affected eye.

Central visual field loss (central scotoma) has long been accepted as the hallmark of optic neuritis, accounting for more than 90 percent of visual field defects (28). It is now recognized that virtually any visual field defect can occur, including cecocentral, paracentral, arcuate, hemialtitudinal, hemianopic, peripheral constriction, and diffuse suppression (Figure 19-4). In patients entering the Optic Neuritis Treatment Trial (ONTT), localized defects were only slightly more common than diffuse defects (51.8 percent and 48.2 percent, respectively). Only 8 percent of affected eyes demonstrated central or cecocentral defects, whereas 20 percent showed nerve fiber layer defects (arcuate, altitudinal, or nasal step) (29). Confrontational visual field techniques may be used to screen patients but are probably insensitive compared with those performed using the Goldmann perimeter or automated threshold perimetry (Humphrey, Octopus, and others).

The optic disc in optic neuritis may appear normal (retrobulbar optic neuritis) or swollen (anterior optic neuritis or papillitis). Retrobulbar involvement occurs in two thirds of patients with acute optic neuritis (5). The normal appearance of the fundus in acute retrobulbar optic neuritis has inspired the adage that the patient sees nothing and the physician sees nothing. The optic disc becomes pale weeks to months after the initial episode, depending on the location of the lesion along the optic nerve. Hemorrhage at the disc margin is uncommon, occurring in less than 6 percent of patients with optic neuritis (5). Anterior optic neuritis associated with lipid exudates in the macula (macular star) suggests neuroretinitis and is not associated with MS. When acute anterior optic neuritis occurs in a patient with a previous history of optic neuritis in the fellow eye, fundus findings may mimic the Foster-Kennedy syndrome. Historically, this syndrome of disc swelling on one side and optic atrophy in the fellow eye was attributed to a sphenoid meningioma; although it has been described in MS (Figure 19-5), it is more commonly seen in sequential anterior ischemic optic neuropathy.

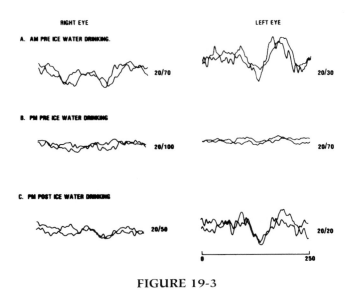

FIGURE 19-3

Ice water ingestion promotes improvement in optic nerve function. A 49-year-old man with MS demonstrated decline in visual acuity as the day progressed. He noted that the ingestion of ice water would significantly improve his visual acuity for approximately 30 minutes. *A,* VEPs were performed in the morning before ice water ingestion. There is a delay in the positive peak and visual acuities of 20/70 OD and 20/30 OS. *B,* By the afternoon there is severe conduction block without evidence of the evoked potential concomitant with a marked degradation in visual acuity; 20/100 OD and 20/70 OS. *C,* After the ingestion of ice water, there is a significant improvement in visual acuity in association with the reappearance of positive peaks; 20/50 OD and 20/20 OS. (From Scherokman BJ, Selhorst JB, Waybright EA, et al. Improved optic nerve conduction with ingestion of ice water. *Ann Neurol* 1985; 17:418–419.)

Visual Evoked Potentials

Visual evoked cortical potentials (VECPs or VEPs) record electrical activity of the occipital lobe in response to visual stimuli. Pattern reversal stimulus presentation (pVEP) yields more reproducible results than flash techniques (fVEPs) (30). However, flash VEP can be used to confirm visual pathway integrity when the P100 is not seen with pattern VEPs.

With pVEP testing, the patient sits one meter from a video monitor and observes a checkerboard pattern of black and white checks that reverses at a frequency of approximately 2 Hz. This produces a retinal signal that projects through the visual pathways. Surface electrodes over the occipital lobes record, amplify, and analyze the cortical evoked responses over multiple trials (generally 32 to 128). Each eye is stimulated individually, especially when the optic nerve is the primary interest; if a retrochi-

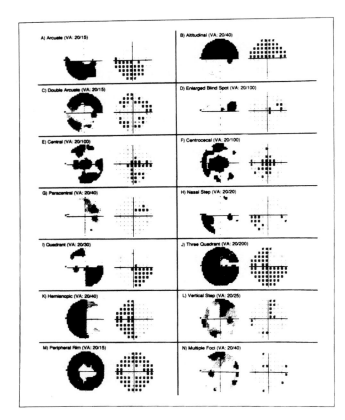

FIGURE 19-4

Monocular visual field defects associated with acute optic neuritis and defined by static Humphrey automated perimetry. (From Keltner JL, Johnson CA, Spurr JO, Beck RW, the Optic Neuritis Study Group. Baseline visual field profile of optic neuritis: The experience of the Optic Neuritis Treatment Trial. *Arch Ophthalmol* 1993; 111:231–234.)

asmal lesion is suspected, binocular hemifield stimulation is recommended but may be technically difficult.

The VEP reflects central visual activity because the central retinal fibers project to the surface of the occipital lobe (nearer to the recording electrodes), whereas more peripheral retinal fibers project deeper into the calcarine fissure. In addition, cortical representation of central (foveal) vision is larger than that for peripheral vision. The fovea is optimally stimulated by check size of 10 to 15 minutes, whereas parafoveal regions are stimulated by larger check sizes (50 minutes) (31). A range of check sizes is recommended for optimum stimulation. Generally, 15 to 30 minutes is sufficient, but larger patterns up to 50 to 70 minutes may be needed when central vision is severely reduced. The stimulus check size should be sufficiently large to optimize the amplitude of the evoked potential.

The first large positive peak (downward deflection by convention) occurs at approximately 100 milliseconds and is termed the P100. More peripheral visual field ter-

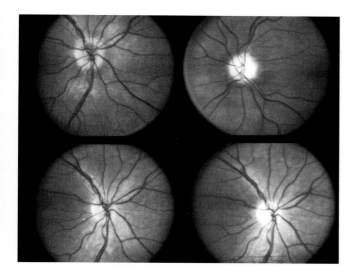

FIGURE 19-5

Anterior optic neuritis in a 39-year-old MS patient with the pseudo–Foster Kennedy syndrome. *Upper left,* the right optic disc shows mild edema and hyperemia, with blurring of the disc margin. There are no hemorrhages or exudates. *Upper right,* the left optic disc is pale, with loss of the nerve fiber layer. *Lower left,* after two weeks of steroid therapy the right optic disc is no longer edematous. Visual acuity is 20/200. *Lower right,* two months later visual acuity has improved to 20/40, color vision remains defective, and there is a small central scotoma. The optic disc has definite temporal pallor. (From Miller NR, Fine SL. *The ocular fundus in neuro-ophthalmologic diagnosis.* Saint Louis: C. V. Mosby Company, 1977:21.)

ritories evoke a later and smaller positive peak (P135), which can produce the so-called W-configuration. The first positive peak (P100) occurring after the first negative change (N75) should be defined carefully because confusion occasionally arises when the P135 is larger than a smaller abnormal P100. In such circumstances the P100 latency can be incorrectly read.

Optic neuritis characteristically causes prolongation of the P100 latency and decreased amplitude. A delay of greater than three standard deviations compared with control data is significant, but a difference in the interocular latencies (usually 8 to 10 milliseconds) is the most sensitive criterion for abnormal VEP in patients with MS (32,33). The VEP is abnormal in 47 percent to 85 percent of patients with MS, depending on patient selection, criteria for MS, and testing conditions (32,34). In one study, the VEP was abnormal in 85 percent of patients with clinically definite MS, 58 percent in those with probable MS, and 38 percent in those with possible MS (34). The VEP in the symptomatic eye adds little to the diagnosis in patients with a strong clinical suspicion of optic neuritis; however, the VEP may be

abnormal in up to 50 percent of patients with suspected MS and no history of optic neuritis (subclinical optic neuropathy) (27,35–37). Recovery from optic neuritis with improvement of visual acuity parallels improvement in the amplitude of the VEP, but latency usually remains delayed (30,38). However, 19 percent to 35 percent of patients with optic neuritis eventually normalize their VEP (39,40).

Abnormalities of the VEP indicate dysfunction at any point along the visual pathways from the retina to the striate cortex and are not pathognomonic for demyelinating optic neuropathy. Other disorders can cause VEP disturbance, including compressive lesions, congenital anomalies of the optic nerve, glaucoma, hereditary and toxic optic neuropathy, and papilledema. Optic neuritis is the most likely condition to cause prolonged latency, whereas other conditions tend to cause a greater reduction in VEP amplitude. Numerous factors affect VEP latency and/or amplitude, including pupillary diameter, age, refractive error, media opacity (cataract), and fixation (41). Visual evoked potential testing is most useful in establishing the presence of optic neuropathy in patients suspicious for MS, particularly in those with clinically silent lesions. The VEP may also help quantify response to experimental therapies. The potassium channel antagonists 4-AP and 3,4-DAP have been shown to improve VEP latency and amplitude, implying improved optic nerve conduction (25,42).

Magnetic Resonance Imaging and Optic Neuritis

Acute lesions in MS are associated with inflammation, which leads to a breakdown of the blood–brain barrier and is characterized by leakage of gadolinium on magnetic resonance imaging (MRI) (4,43). Lesions in the optic nerve may be difficult to detect with conventional MRI. The detection rate of intraorbital lesions has been greatly improved with newer techniques of fat suppression before and after intravenous (IV) gadolinium (4). Enhancing lesions show increased signal intensity, which may be obscured by the surrounding fat signal in nonsuppressed studies. Short T1 inversion recovery sequences (STIR) are also useful in the orbit; in contrast to enhanced studies, active lesions on STIR show decreased intensity, the so-called "negative enhancement" (44). Lesions in other areas of the brain are better seen on more T2-weighted sequences. Newer fluid attenuation inversion recovery (FLAIR) sequences are particularly sensitive in detecting demyelination lesions but are not specific. (Figure 19-6). Gadolinium enhancement on MRI is demonstrated in the optic nerves of the majority of patients with acute optic neuritis. Although there are no direct pathologic data for correlation, optic nerve enhancement on MRI probably signifies inflammation and conduction block and is associated with a reduction in VEP amplitude. In most patients,

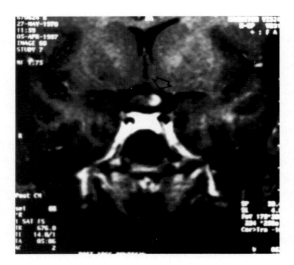

FIGURE 19-6

T1-weighted coronal MRI with fat suppression and gadolinium infusion. Note enhancement of the left intracranial optic nerve *(arrowhead)*.

enhancement is no longer observed one month after the onset of optic neuritis and correlates with recovery of visual acuity and improvement of VEP amplitudes (38,44).

Abnormalities on MRI in the periventricular and other white matter areas are seen in 30 percent to 70 percent of patients with isolated optic neuritis (5,46,47) and in 90 percent to 98 percent of patients with clinically definite MS (48). The presence of MRI lesions is a strong predictor of the risk of developing clinically definite multiple sclerosis (CDMS) (49), and the risk appears to be cumulative. Frederiksen (50) reported that 23 percent of patients with optic neuritis and MRI lesions progressed to CDMS over a 10-month follow-up period, whereas none with normal MRI developed CDMS. Morrisey (51) reported that 23 of 26 patients (82 percent) with abnormal MRI progressed compared with one of 16 with normal MRI within 5.5 years of the onset of optic neuritis. The ONTT data suggest that the risk is directly related to the number of MRI lesions; five years after acute optic neuritis, CDMS developed in 16 percent of patients with no MRI lesions, 37 percent in patients with 1 to 2 lesions, and 51 percent in patients with three or more lesions (52,53).

Most practitioners now perform MRI in patients who have had a singular event of optic neuritis and an otherwise normal neurologic examination. The diagnosis of optic neuritis is still a clinical one, and studies have shown that MRI adds little to the diagnosis in patients who have typical presenting symptoms. Of the 457 patients who met ONTT entry criteria for optic neuritis, only 2 patients (0.4 percent) had a compressive lesion mimicking optic neuritis (54). However, recent studies increasingly suggest that

prognosis and treatment options relate to the demonstration of demyelinating lesions on brain MRI. Patients with acute optic neuritis and abnormal MRI who were treated with IV methylprednisolone had a reduced risk of progression to CDMS during the first two years compared with those with normal MRI (*see* Treatment of Optic Neuritis). Magnetic resonance imaging is a valuable adjunct to paraclinical investigations (cerebrospinal fluid, evoked potentials, and so forth) to provide confirmatory evidence for the diagnosis of MS (laboratory-supported definite MS) (49,55). Until recently, early diagnosis was of limited benefit when no effective treatment was available. However, disease-modifying agents such as interferon and glatiramer acetate are now available, and early diagnosis and identification of those patients at risk may be crucial for timely therapeutic intervention that may control and limit the disease process and thereby reduce exacerbations, delay progression of disability, and limit neurologic deficits (56–58).

Magnetic resonance imaging is useful in establishing initial disease burden so that the activity of existing lesions and formation of new lesions can be monitored. New MRI lesions may reflect ongoing disease activity, even in the absence of clinically progressive symptoms. We believe that evidence of ongoing disease activity, derived from interval neurologic examination and serial MRI, is an indication for treatment with disease-specific agents or modification of existing therapy.

We recommend that all patients with optic neuritis undergo MRI to establish the diagnosis, facilitate counseling of the individual regarding his or her risk of MS, and guide decisions for treatment. Despite the strong correlation of MRI lesions with clinical MS, the exact predictive role of MRI in patients with isolated optic neuritis needs further study, particularly in the subset of patients with normal MRI.

Natural History of Acute Optic Neuritis

The natural course of acute optic neuritis is variable. Visual acuity typically worsens over the first days to two weeks after the onset of symptoms. Decline in color vision, visual field, and contrast sensitivity closely parallel the decline in acuity. Most patients then recover rapidly, achieving most of their improvement by five weeks. Some patients continue to recover for up to a year. The mean visual acuity 12 months after the onset of optic neuritis is 20/15. Fewer than 10 percent have visual acuity less than 20/40 at one year (29,59,60). Despite recovery of vision to 20/15 or to "near-normal," most patients are aware of differences in the quality of the vision compared with their premorbid vision or to the unaffected fellow eye. Persistent deficits in contrast sensitivity, color vision, and depth perception are common in these patients and in asymptomatic patients.

In patients whose presenting symptom is isolated optic neuritis, the risk of developing MS is approximately 30 percent after five to seven years. In long-term follow-up studies (up to 30 years), 75 percent of women and 34 percent of men developed CDMS (61–64). Factors associated with a higher rate of conversion to MS include recurrent neurologic events (fourfold increase), HLA antigens (fourfold increase in those with HLA-DR2), cerebrospinal fluid abnormalities, and brain MRI evidence of neuroanatomic dissemination (65).

Differential Diagnosis of Optic Neuritis

Numerous infectious or inflammatory disorders other than demyelinating disease may cause optic neuritis (Table 19-1A) (66). Ancillary studies (antinuclear antibody assay, syphilis serologies, chest radiograph, cerebrospinal fluid analysis) are of low yield in patients with typical isolated optic neuritis, and an exhaustive search for causative conditions is rarely indicated. Of course, patients with a suspicious history or atypical clinical findings should have more directed diagnostic evaluation. Patients with anterior optic neuritis and significant vitritis should be evaluated for syphilis, tuberculosis, sarcoidosis, and Lyme disease. Neuroretinitis, which is characterized by a macular star, is never associated with MS.

Acute optic neuritis can usually be distinguished from other causes of optic neuropathy and other ophthalmic conditions on clinical grounds (Table 19-1B) (66,67). History is usually suggestive in patients with compressive optic neuropathy from intracranial tumors, anterior ischemic optic neuropathy, sinus disease, and radiation-induced optic neuropathy. Patients whose presenting symptom is bilateral anterior optic neuritis should be evaluated for papilledema (optic disc edema caused by increased intracranial pressure). Leber's hereditary optic neuropathy (LHON), a mitochondrial disorder that usually causes bilateral central visual loss, may convincingly mimic optic neuritis, especially in young men in the acute stages before the fellow eye is involved. Hyperemia and telangiectasis of the disc in acute LHON may be difficult to distinguish from true disc swelling without fluorescein angiography. Drusen (hyaline bodies in the optic nerve) may mimic optic disc swelling (pseudopapilledema) and cause visual field loss, but acute visual loss from drusen is rare.

Subclinical Optic Neuropathy

Many patients with MS have asymptomatic (subclinical) optic neuropathy (68,69). According to the ONTT, 48 percent of patients with unilateral optic neuritis and no history of fellow eye involvement demonstrated visual field abnormalities in the asymptomatic eye. Abnormalities in color vision and contrast sensitivity were demonstrated in 21.7 percent and 15.4 percent of these patients, respectively, consistent with subclinical demyelination (68).

TABLE 19-1A
Causes of Optic Neuritis Other Than Demyelination

Viral and parainfectious
  Adenovirus
  Coxsackie
  Cytomegalovirus
  Human immunodeficiency virus
  Hepatitis A
  Herpes zoster
  Epstein-Barr virus
  Measles
  Mumps
  Rubella
  Varicella zoster
Postvaccination
Syphilis
Lyme disease
Tuberculosis
Mycobacterium pneumoniae
Sarcoidosis
Vasculitides (systemic lupus erythematosus, Wegener's)
Autoimmune
Sinus infection
Bee venom
Toxoplasmosis
Cat-scratch disease

TABLE 19-1B
Optic Neuropathies and Ophthalmic Conditions Mimicking Optic Neuritis

Neuroretinitis
Big blind spot syndrome
Leber's hereditary optic neuropathy
Diabetic papillitis
Ischemic optic neuropathy
Central retinal vein occlusion
Venous stasis retinopathy
Optic disc drusen
Central serous retinopathy
Carcinomatous meningitis
Infiltrating neoplasm (lymphoma)
Radiation-induced optic neuropathy
Paraneoplastic disorder

Chronic Optic Neuritis

Some patients with MS complain of visual disturbances yet have never experienced an identifiable episode of acute optic neuritis. Visual acuity often is 20/20, but careful testing of color vision, contrast sensitivity, quantitative threshold perimetry, and VEP often uncovers subtle optic nerve dysfunction in one or both eyes. Most clinicians have now discarded the diagnosis of chronic optic neuritis; with computerized tomography (CT) and MRI, it was determeined that many cases of "chronic optic neuritis" were in fact due to compressive lesions. However, chronic optic neuritis almost certainly occurs in MS patients and is probably underrecognized. Most patients already have established MS and complain of either a stable or a progressive visual disturbance (66). Optic atrophy, if not present initially, develops slowly over time. There is no current treatment, and it remains to be seen if disease-modifying agents for MS, such as interferon-β and glatiramer acetate, will affect the course of chronic demyelinating optic neuritis.

Optic Neuritis in Childhood

Optic neuritis in children differs from that in adults in several aspects. Childhood optic neuritis more often is anterior; 70 percent to 100 percent of children have swollen optic discs compared with 35 percent of adults (5,70–72). Bilateral and simultaneous involvement (60 percent to 100 percent) is far more common in children, and 56 percent to 83 percent follow a viral syndrome or other systemic illness (73–75). Riikonen reported that 33 percent occurred after a vaccination (74). Prognosis for recovery of vision is generally excellent, with most series reporting good or complete return of visual acuity or visual function in 75 percent to 100 percent of children. Pattern visual evoked potentials are more likely to normalize in children (55 percent versus 10 percent) (70).

Optic neuritis in children often is responsive to systemic steroids. Farris and Pickard treated six children with acute bilateral optic neuritis with IV methylprednisolone followed by a tapering course of oral prednisone. All patients demonstrated rapid improvement of vision during treatment (75). Steroid dependency is common, and some children may require a slower taper of the oral medication. We agree with Beck (69) and others that children with optic neuritis should undergo brain MRI and lumbar puncture, and most should be treated with IV methylprednisolone, followed by a slowly tapering dose of oral prednisone. The optimum dose of methylprednisolone is not well established; 10–20 mg/kg/day seems reasonable, although we have used divided doses as high as 45 mg/kg/day with no adverse side effects.

As in adults, optic neuritis is one of the most common manifestations of MS in children. In 17 children with definite MS, 77 percent had one or more episodes of optic neuritis, compared with 24 percent who had visual symptoms resulting from ocular motor disorders associated with brainstem lesions and 24 percent with cerebellar disease (76). Isolated optic neuritis in children seems to carry a lower risk of eventually developing MS (15 percent) (70).

Neuromyelitis Optica (Devic's Disease)

Bilateral optic neuritis in association with transverse myelitis is known as neuromyelitis optica or Devic's disease. This disorder is thought by many clinicians to represent an aggressive variant of MS, although there are distinct clinical and pathologic differences. Like MS, Devic's disease has a predilection for younger adults but has been described in all ages (77–79). Most cases of acute optic neuritis in MS are unilateral, whereas optic neuritis in Devic's disease is almost always bilateral and simultaneous; if the optic neuritis is unilateral, the fellow eye is usually affected within hours to days. Typically, the vision loss is severe, often to no light perception. The vision loss precedes the paraparesis in up to 76 percent of patients, but may occur at the same time or afterward. Primary progressive or relapsing paraparesis ultimately leads to paraplegia or quadriplegia in most patients. Despite the profound vision loss on presentation, most patients (but not all) do recover some vision (7).

All patients with Devic's disease have extensive involvement of the spinal cord, but the histopathology reported in the literature varies. Necrotizing cavitary degeneration with liquefactive changes, which is unusual in MS, is common in Devic's disease. Gliosis, a hallmark of MS, is less prominent in Devic's disease. Some patients, however, show chronic demyelinating lesions typical of those seen in MS, and others demonstrate perivenous infiltration of mononuclear cells in the white and gray matter with perivascular zones of demyelination, suggestive of postinfectious encephalomyelitis (80,81). The cerebrospinal fluid in patients with Devic's disease typically shows a mild pleocytosis, but oligoclonal bands and abnormal immunoglobulin G (IgG) synthesis rate and index are less common (82).

The major threat to life in Devic's disease is respiratory compromise as a result of lesions extending into the upper cervical spinal cord and lower brainstem. Advances in supportive care have improved the mortality rate in Devic's disease from as high as 50 percent to approximately 10 percent (78). Complete recovery is possible in some patients despite a period of complete paraplegia. Corticosteroids may hasten recovery in some patients with Devic's disease. For those with a progressive or relapsing clinical course, the choice immunomodulating therapy is still not certain. We have found that some patients clinically stabilize with azathioprine and intermittent pulse steroids.

Chiasmal and Postchiasmal Involvement of the Visual System

Demyelinating lesions in the optic chiasm may occur in isolation or may involve the adjacent optic nerve and/or optic tract. Patients with isolated lesions in the chiasm may have more subtle symptoms and findings. Central acuity and color vision may be normal and an afferent defect may be absent. Visual field defects typically demonstrate bitemporal features. Chiasmal enlargement and gadolinium enhancement may be demonstrated by MRI (83,84).

Patients with lesions of the chiasm and proximal optic nerve may present with features of acute optic neuritis on the side of the optic nerve lesion and temporal visual field suppression in the fellow eye *(junctional scotoma)*. Inferonasal retinal ganglion cells that subserve the superotemporal visual field cross in the chiasm and project slightly anteriorly in the contralateral optic nerve (Wilbrand's knee) before their posterior course in the optic tract. A lesion at the junction of the proximal optic nerve and adjacent chiasm may therefore cause a central or nerve fiber defect on the side of the affected optic nerve and a superotemporal defect in the fellow eye. A lesion of the optic tract causes a hemianopia opposite the side of the lesion. Because there are relatively more nasal retinal fibers (subserving temporal visual field), a tract lesion may cause an afferent pupillary defect on the side of the temporal field loss or contralateral to the tract lesion.

Unfortunately, lesions may not be isolated, and segments of optic nerve, chiasm, and tract may all be affected simultaneously. Virtually any visual field defect has been attributed to chiasm lesions. In the ONTT, 5.1 percent of patients with acute optic neuritis had bitemporal visual field defects and 8.9 percent had homonymous hemianopias (29).

Approximately two thirds of patients with optic neuritis and silent cerebral lesions seen on MRI have involvement of the optic radiations (47). In one postmortem study, 85 percent of MS patients had lesions of the optic radiations (85). Despite the frequent involvement of the postchiasmal visual sensory pathways, fewer than 10 percent of patients have homonymous field defects (29). Optic nerve lesions are more likely than retrochiasmal lesions to cause symptoms, probably because of the higher density of myelinated axons in the optic nerve, in contrast to the broader dispersal of fibers in the optic radiations. Nevertheless, complete or incomplete, congruous and incongruous, homonymous field defects have all been described secondary to lesions in the optic radiations (86). On rare occasions bilateral altitudinal hemianopia occurs secondary to damage to the superior or inferior portions of both occipital lobes (87).

Treatment of Optic Neuritis

Corticosteroids have long been the cornerstone of therapy for optic neuritis despite conflicting studies of effectiveness. The rationale for the use of these agents is based on their immunosuppressive and immunomodulatory effects. A number of immunologic perturbations are now recognized in MS, including a defect in suppressor cell function, the redistribution of lymphocytes into the CNS compartment, increased expression of cytokines and immune adhesion molecules, and the activation of CNS macrophages (microglial cells) (88). The principal effects of corticosteroids in the treatment of MS appear to be related to their antiinflammatory and antiedema effects.

No established guidelines existed for the treatment of optic neuritis until recently. The ONTT, a multiinstitutional study, was developed to evaluate the efficacy of corticosteroid treatment in acute optic neuritis and to explore the relationship between optic neuritis and MS (29). In this major trial, 457 patients between the ages of 18 and 45 presenting within eight days of onset of a first episode of unilateral optic neuritis were randomized to placebo, oral prednisone (1 mg/kg/day for 14 days), or IV methylprednisolone (250 mg every 6 hours for 72 hours followed by 11 days of oral prednisone 1 mg/kg/day).

The period of visual recovery was rapid irrespective of treatment; the majority of patients began to recover within two weeks, and almost all improved within the first month. The speed of recovery of visual acuity, visual field, and contrast sensitivity in the group treated with IV methylprednisolone was statistically more rapid compared with the oral prednisone–treated group and the placebo group (59,60). After six months 94 percent of patients had achieved a visual acuity of 20/40 or better and 75 percent had improved to 20/20 or better. Most patients showed little change in vision between six months and five years of follow-up. At five years 87 percent had 20/25 vision or better.

Within two years of the study onset, the rate of development of MS was only 7.5 percent in the IV methylprednisolone group compared with 14.7 percent in the prednisone group and 16.7 percent in the placebo group (89). After two years, however, the cumulative incidence of MS was comparable across all the groups (90). Brain MRI findings of demyelinating lesions in patients with optic neuritis were highly predictive of progression to definite MS. At three years MRI abnormalities remained strong predictors of MS; 43.1 percent of patients with three lesions on baseline MRI developed MS, whereas only 2.7 percent of patients with two lesions progressed to MS.

After five years the probability of a patient having a new episode of optic neuritis was 19 percent in the affected eye, 17 percent in the fellow eye, and 30 percent in either eye (52). One half of the patients who experienced recurrent optic neuritis did so within the first year, and two thirds did within the first two years. Treatment with oral prednisone alone was associated with a higher rate of recurrent optic neuritis. In the oral prednisone group, 30 percent of patients experienced recurrence compared with 16 percent in the placebo group and 14 percent in the IV methylprednisolone group (52).

It is not clear why treatment of optic neuritis with oral prednisone was associated with an increased rate of recurrence. One theory is that high doses of steroids may produce immunomodulating effects not seen with lower doses (91). In fact, low-dose prednisone therapy may preferentially diminish suppressor cell function. This immunologic defect (recognized in patients with MS) may promote escalation in the TH1 proinflammatory limb of the immune response network (92–95). In experimental allergic encephalomyelitis (EAE), an animal model of inflammatory demyelination, Reder has shown that corticosteroid dosing significantly influences clinical exacerbations (96).

Although treatment with corticosteroids may not appear to significantly alter the course of optic neuritis in the short run, some clinicians might argue that any acceleration in the course of recovery might justify the administration of a generally safe and well-tolerated agent. One might also look beyond the more focal episode of optic neuritis to the broader issue of the generalized demyelinating process. Corticosteroids may interfere with the elaboration of cytokines and expression of adhesion molecules, may influence lymphocyte trafficking, and may limit the process of epitope or determinant spreading, which in turn might limit clinical exacerbations. Furthermore, the early use of corticosteroids for clinical exacerbations may enhance the potential effectiveness of disease-modifying agents, such as interferon and copolymer-1. Future studies are needed to clarify the role of corticosteroids in the treatment of acute optic neuritis and other forms of exacerbation of MS.

Treatment is recommended for most patients who present with acute optic neuritis, provided there are no contraindications to the use of corticosteroids. In most patients 1,000 mg/day of methylprednisolone may be administered as a single daily IV infusion for three to five days, followed by a tapering dose of oral prednisone over two to six weeks. Intravenous methylprednisolone is well tolerated in healthy young adults (97) and often can be given in an outpatient setting. Oral prednisone, at least in the conventional dose of 1 mg/kg/day, is contraindicated as the sole treatment, although some practitioners are exploring the use of higher doses (2–5 mg/kg/day or more).

Ocular Inflammation in Multiple Sclerosis

Uveitis (inflammation of the iris, ciliary body, or choroid) is reported in 2 percent to 27 percent of MS patients, far more than in the general population (98–100). Anterior uveitis (iridocyclitis) involves the iris or ciliary body and is characterized by cells and flare in the anterior chamber (seen with slit-lamp biomicroscopy), keratic precipitates, posterior synechiae, lens opacities, and anterior vitreous cells. Pars planitis is inflammation of the peripheral retina and ciliary body characterized by cells and debris in the vitreous and "snowbank formation" along the pars plana of the ciliary body. It is thought to occur in 2 percent to 27 percent of MS patients (99–101). When pars planitis is seen in conjunction with perivenular phlebitis, the condition is referred to as intermediate uveitis. Uveitis, iridocyclitis, and pars planitis may occur together or in isolation. The symptoms may be mild to severe, and complications are directly proportional to the extent and severity of the inflammation. Complications of ocular inflammation include glaucoma, cataract, macular edema, retinal detachment, and vitreous hemorrhage (102).

Retinal venous sheathing occurs in 10 percent to 20 percent of patients with MS (98,100) (Figure 19-7) and represents active periphlebitis or sclerosis that is a direct sequela of inflammation (98). Histologically, there is a perivenular cellular infiltrate consisting largely of lymphocytes and plasma cells around small peripheral retinal veins

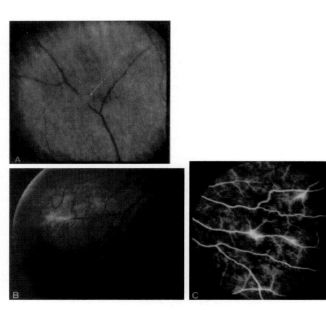

FIGURE 19-7

Retinal venous sheathing in MS. *A,* A focal area of perivenular phlebitis obscures a segment of the blood column in the superior temporal vein *(arrow). B,* Focal sheathing of retinal veins in another patient with MS. *C,* During the venous phase of fluorescein angiography multiple sites of leakage is observed along retinal veins. (From Miller NR. *Clinical Neuro-Ophthalmology.* Baltimore: Williams & Wilkins, 1995:4305.)

(98,103). Fluorescein angiography may show increased permeability of the vessels with leakage of dye around the veins. This may occur independent of inflammation elsewhere in the eye. The principal vascular abnormalities occur in the peripheral retina and can only be optimally seen with the indirect ophthalmoscope during dilated fundus examination. This peripheral distribution suggests that perivascular sheathing may be widely underrecognized.

Granulomatous periphlebitis has also been described (98) but is usually associated with uveitis. Granulomatous inflammation is often seen in the eye and is associated with infection (viral, protozoan, helminth, bacterial, fungal) or diseases of unknown etiology (e.g., sarcoidosis, Behçets disease, Vogt-Koyanagi-Harada syndrome, Eales' disease), but periphlebitis is common only in sarcoid. The periphlebitis in sarcoid is usually described as resembling "dripping candle wax" and is usually associated with vitritis or uveitis.

Focal granulomatous and nongranulomatous retinitis in the absence of retinal periphlebitis has been demonstrated pathologically in MS (98). Electroretinograms in patients with MS have shown reduction in some or all components of the response, which parallels the severity of the systemic disease and optic atrophy observed in these patients (104). Retinal dysfunction may occur in patients with MS in the absence of ophthalmoscopic lesions.

Perivenous retinal sheathing probably represents a hallmark of the pathophysiology of MS, perivenular inflammation, and may be an indicator for future development of MS when observed in patients with optic neuritis (105). The occurrence of retinal periphlebitis and retinitis in areas free of myelin and oligodendrocytes raises questions about the role of myelin as the primary target triggering the ocular inflammatory response in MS patients.

EYE MOVEMENT ABNORMALITIES IN MS

Some form of eye movement abnormality is observed in up to three fourths of patients with MS. Essentially all known eye movement disorders have been described in patients with MS, with the possible exception of ocular masticatory myorhythmia, which is seen exclusively in Whipple's disease. The neurophysiologic understanding of eye movement abnormalities and their recognition in the neurology clinic can facilitate the accurate localization of CNS lesions and thereby aid in the diagnosis of patients with suspected MS. It is imperative to appreciate that many ocular motor disturbances can be extremely subtle and easily overlooked on clinical examination. Furthermore, discrete ocular motor abnormalities may be subclinical and only elucidated with the use of neurophysiologic techniques such as oculography.

In MS patients, abnormalities in the ocular motor apparatus can produce disorders of rapid gaze shifting (saccades), pursuit eye movements, vestibular ocular reflexes, visual fixation, ocular alignment, and gaze holding. Whereas most of the lesions that are responsible for the occurrence of these abnormalities reside in the brainstem and cerebellum, demyelination in the cerebral hemispheres can also be responsible for disorders of ocular motility.

Involvement of ocular motor control pathways before the abducens nucleus for horizontal eye movements, and cranial nerve nuclei III and IV, and the interstitial nucleus of Cajal (INC) in the dorsal midbrain for vertical eye movements, produce supranuclear deficits that can be distinguished from nuclear insults by the integrity of vestibular ocular reflexes (VOR). Alternatively, nuclear insults produce abnormalities in the VOR because the final common pathway for horizontal and vertical vestibular-induced eye movements are controlled by neurons in the respective cranial nerve nuclei and in the INC.

The Ocular Motor Apparatus

Eye movements can be divided into those that produce gaze shifts and those that promote gaze stabilization. The objective of all distinct ocular motor mechanisms is to provide for the achievement of foveation across a variety of visual circumstances. The fovea is the portion of the retina with the highest visual acuity, so maintaining image focus on this structure promotes visual fixation and image processing.

Saccades represent the most rapid eye movements and produce shifts of gaze to a new fixation target. Smooth pursuit eye movements allow foveation while tracking a slowly moving target. While the head is steady, visual fixation is maintained by processes that inhibit gaze shifts and unwanted spontaneous activity originating from ocular motor burst neurons. During head movements, visual fixation on static objects is achieved by the recruitment of vestibular mechanisms (VORs) that correspondingly move the eyes in an equal and opposite direction to maintain foveation. With sustained head rotation or environmental movement, with the head steady, optokinetic nystagmus (OKN), which combines slow pursuit eye movements punctuated by saccadic refixations, promotes the reestablishment of image focus. Finally, vergence movements represent an evolutionary adaptation for frontal vision with binocularity. Vergence movements involve eye movements in opposite directions for simultaneous foveation.

All conjugate eye movements are associated with neural commands, which have been characterized by velocity and position information (106). For saccades, the velocity command, which is referred to as the pulse, generates the initial sequence for movement of the eyes. The velocity signals for conjugate eye movements are derived from the paramedian pontine reticular formation (PPRF) neurons for horizontal eye movements and from the rostral interstitial nucleus of the medial longitudinal fasciculus (riMLF) burst neurons in the rostral midbrain for vertical movements. The position element or step is derived from the velocity information by a process called neural integration (107). The step function essentially acts to overcome the elastic restoring forces of orbital tissue and thereby promotes gaze holding. The neural integrators for horizontal eye movements include the medial vestibular nucleus (MVN) and the nucleus prepositus hypoglossi (NPH). The INC is an important component of the vertical neural integrator.

Saccadic Eye Movements

The saccadic apparatus includes neurons in the frontal eye field (FEF), which project to a number of subcortical structures that serve to mediate rapid gaze shifts to remembered targets (Figure 19-8). This circuitry has a strong influence over saccadic initiation by direct connections with the superior colliculus (SC) and via connections with the caudate nucleus. The SC receives visual information from the retina and striate cortex concerning the contralateral hemifield. Information processing in the SC is important for the execution of accurate contralateral saccades with horizontal and vertical components. In addition to projections to the SC, the FEF has a primary excitatory influence on caudate neurons that project to the pars reticulata of the substantia nigra (SN). Neurons in the SN are inhibitory on the SC, so the FEF provides for feed forward inhibition that promotes saccadic initiation.

An alternative descending saccadic pathway involves a direct FEF projection, which runs through the anterior limb of the internal capsule to PPRF for horizontal saccades and to the riMLF for vertical saccades. Bilateral stimulation of the FEF is necessary for vertical saccades.

The PPRF contains excitatory burst neurons that produce the supranuclear horizontal saccadic eye velocity command sequence (the pulse). These neurons project to the adjacent VI nerve nucleus. The abducens nucleus consists of two types of neurons that mediate conjugate horizontal eye movements. Projection neurons innervate the ipsilateral lateral rectus muscle, whereas abducens interneurons decussate to the contralateral pons and via the medial longitudinal fasciculus (MLF) innervate the medial rectus subnucleus of cranial nerve III, which ultimately projects to the medial rectus muscle (Figure 19-9).

The parietal cortex also participates in the production of saccades and has a direct projection to the SC. In contrast to the FEF, the parietal cortex is more involved

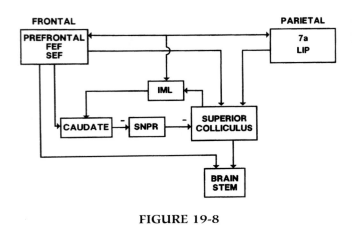

FIGURE 19-8

A block diagram of the major structures that participate in the control of saccades. FEF: frontal eye fields; SEF: supplementary eye fields; IML: intramedullary lamina of thalamus; LIP: lateral intraparietal area; SNPR: substantia nigra, pars reticulata. (From Leigh JR, Zee DS. *The neurology of eye movements,* 2nd ed. Philadelphia: FA Davis, 1991:103.)

in the production of saccades to novel visual stimuli than to remembered targets. The important dichotomy between the frontal and parietal lobes concerns internally generated voluntary saccades in the former and externally generated reflexive saccades in the latter. Essentially there are two parallel descending pathways for voluntary saccades that are parcellated functionally on the basis of target identity (Figure 19-8).

Cerebellar Pathways in Eye Movement Control

The dorsal vermis and fastigial nuclei are key cerebellar structures concerned with the control of saccadic accuracy and in the calibration of the size of the saccadic pulse. Lesions within these regions typically give rise to inaccurate saccades (dysmetria). Saccadic dysmetria is characterized by hypermetric or overshoot saccades and on occasion hypometric saccades. Macrosaccadic oscillations can be produced by lesions similar to those that lead to saccadic dysmetria.

Cerebellar control of saccades can be understood if one considers the neuroanatomic circuitry. Caudal to the excitatory burst neuron area of the PPRF is an area of the medullary reticular formation (MRF) containing inhibitory burst neurons (IBN) that project to the contralateral abducens nucleus. Firing of both excitatory burst neurons (EBN) and IBNs on the left side, for example, would provide an excitatory pulse to the left abducens nucleus for a leftward saccade and concurrent inhibition of the antagonist muscles; the right lateral rectus and the left medial rectus via interneurons in the MLF. Both the PPRF and the MRF receive excitatory projec-

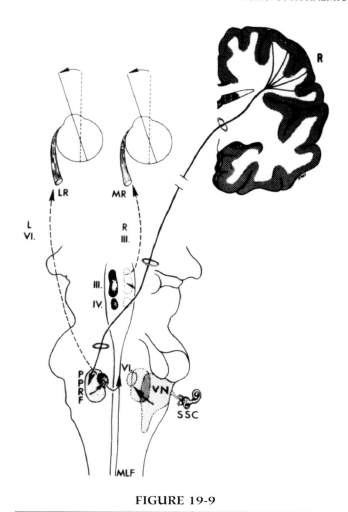

FIGURE 19-9

For conjugate horizontal gaze to the left, initial activity is generated in the right frontal cortex (frontal eye field 8 of Brodman). This pathway descends in the anterior limb of the internal capsule and subsequently decussates at the midbrain-pontine junction. These fibers then synapse in the paramedian pontine reticular formation (PPRF) on the left. Neurons in the PPRF directly project to the homolateral abducens nucleus (VI). There are two types of neurons in the abducens nucleus; projection neurons that innervate the ipsilateral (left) lateral rectus muscle and interneurons that innervate the contralateral *(right)* medial rectus subnucleus of cranial nerve III, via the medial longitudinal fasciculus (MLF). Neurons in the medial rectus subnucleus of III then proceed to innervate the medial rectus muscle. Also labeled, vestibular nucleus (VN) and semicircular canals (SSC). (From Glaser JS. *Neuro-Ophthalmology,* 2nd ed. Philadelphia: JB Lippincott, 1990:362.)

tions from the contralateral fastigial nucleus via the uncinate fasciculus (hook bundle of Russell). This pathway crosses the midline and bends around the superior cerebellar peduncle (SCP) en route to the brainstem. A demyelinating lesion in the right fastigial nucleus, or of the left deep cerebellar white matter in the region of the SCP, would result in decreased excitation of EBNs and IBNs on the left and could account for the hypometria of leftward saccades. Hence, with a left hook bundle lesion, one sees hypermetric saccades to the right, away from the side of the lesion (contrapulsion) (Figure 19-10) (108,109).

Fastigial cells have also been implicated in decelerating ipsilateral saccades. Cells in the right fastigial nucleus, which excite IBNs on the left, fire before the end of rightward saccades, inhibiting abducens motor neurons on the right side. Failure to generate this inhibition would result in a prolongation of the pulse applied to the right abducens motoneurons and consequently produce hypermetric saccades.

Fastigial neurons receive inhibitory projections from Purkinje cells (PCs) in the ipsilateral cerebellar vermis. These PCs receive climbing fiber input from the contralateral inferior olive via the inferior cerebellar peduncle (ICP) and mossy fiber input via the middle cerebellar peduncle. When a climbing fiber excites a PC, there is a refractory period, with diminished PC inhibitory acitivity on fatigial neurons. A lesion of the ICP thereby results in a net increase in PC inhibition of fastigial neurons. A lesion of the right ICP (as in the lateral medullary syndrome) causes increased right PC activity and right fastigial inhibition. This leads to ipsipulsion with hypermetric rightward saccades and hypometric saccades to the left (110) (Figure 19-10).

The flocculus is part of the vestibulocerebellum and is involved in the stabilization of visual images on the retina. This structure is important for gaze holding, smooth pursuit eye movements, and fixation suppression of the VOR during tracking of a visual target with the eyes and head. Lesions of the flocculus produce horizontal gaze-evoked nystagmus, primary position downbeat nystagmus, saccadic (low gain) pursuit, rebound nystagmus, postsaccadic drift (glissades), and a loss of VOR suppression, all of which are commonly seen in patients with MS. These abnormalities reflect the role played by the flocculus in the modulation of the brainstem neural integrator network for retinal stabilization. In addition to the role of the flocculus in neural integration, the NPH and MVN play central roles and are anatomically linked to the flocculus. Taken together, two principal components of saccadic innervation are controlled by the cerebellum; pulse size and pulse-step (velocity-position) match.

Fixation Instability (Saccadic Intrusions)

For steady gaze fixation, pause cells, which reside between the rootlets of the abducens nucleus, tonically inhibit burst neurons and thereby prevent the occurrence

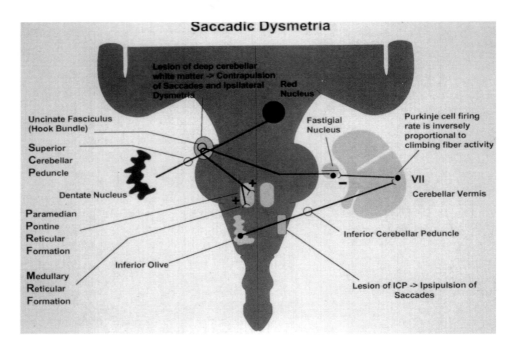

FIGURE 19-10

Diagram for saccadic ipsipulsion and contrapulsion. Increased Purkinje cell firing in the cerebellar vermis causes tonic inhibition of caudal fastigial nucleus cells. These neurons pass over the contralateral superior cerebellar peduncle in the uncinate fasciculus before making excitatory connections onto the paramedian pontine reticular formation (PPRF) and rostral medullary reticular formation (MRF). Horizontal saccades toward the side of the lesion are hypermetric (ipsipulsion), and saccades away from the lesion are hypometric because of lack of fastigial facilitation of the contralateral excitatory and inhibitory burst neurons in the PPRF and MRF, respectively. Interruption of the same circuit caused by a lesion in the deep cerebellar white matter in close proximity to the superior cerebellar peduncle causes saccadic contrapulsion because of uncinate fasciculus involvement and ipsilateral limb dysmetria due to dentatorubral pathway interruption. (From Frohman EM, Solomon D, Zee DS. Nuclear, supranuclear, and internuclear eye movement abnormalities in multiple sclerosis. *Intl MS J* 1996; 2:79–89.)

of unwanted saccadic pulses. Saccadic intrusions are spontaneously generated involuntary eye movements, which disrupt steady fixation. A variety of intrusions have been classified, all of which can be seen in patients with MS (Figure 19-11). Square-wave jerks are 1- to 5-degree eye movements away and back from the neutral position. Movements of 10 to 40 degrees in excursion are referred to as macrosquare wave jerks and large to-and-fro eccentric movements across the midline represent macrosaccadic oscillations.

Ocular flutter is a saccadic intrusion that is characterized by horizontal back-to-back saccades without an intersaccadic latency. Opsoclonus is similar but is characterized by both horizontal and vertical back-to-back saccades. Finally, microsaccadic flutter is a binocular condition with similar back-to-back saccades, but these movements are generally seen only on ophthalmoscopy or eye movement

recordings. Patients typically complain of shimmering, jiggling, or wavy vision. Dizziness and dysequilibrium are also described. It is important to point out that this condition must be distinguished from superior oblique myokymia, which is strictly monocular and characterized by a strong torsional component, and from ocular microtremor, opsoclonus, and voluntary nystagmus (111). Patients with MS occasionally experience steady fixation that is punctuated by paroxysmal episodes of diplopia. Such events typically recur multiple times per day and often resolve after treatment with carbamazepine (112,113).

Saccadic Abnormalities

Deficits in saccadic eye movements often may be demonstrated in MS patients on bedside examination. The three principal saccadic abnormalities seen in MS patients are

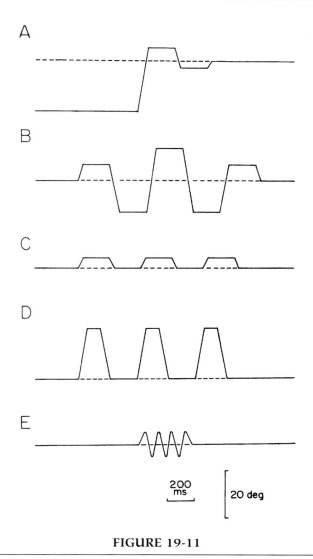

A

B

C

D

E

200 ms

20 deg

FIGURE 19-11

Saccadic oscillations. *A*, Dysmetria: inaccurate saccades. *B*, Macrosaccadic oscillations: hypermetric saccades about the position of the target. *C*, Square-wave jerks: small uncalled-for saccades away from and back to the position of the target. *D*, Macrosquare-wave jerks: large, uncalled-for saccades away from and back to the position of the target. *E*, Ocular flutter: to-and-fro, horizontal back-to-back saccades without an intersaccadic interval. Opsoclonus consists of horizontal and vertical back to back saccades without intersaccadic intervals (From Leigh JR, Zee DS. *The neurology of eye movements*, 2nd ed. Philadelphia: FA Davis, 1991:115.)

prolongation in the saccadic reaction time (SRT), decreased saccadic velocity (SV), and diminished saccadic accuracy (SA). These various parameters relate to distinct neurophysiologic processes. Saccadic reaction time or latency corresponds to the central neural conduction time and relates to conduction in the entire visual-oculomotor pathway. Saccadic velocity most likely correlates with

the function of burst neurons in the PPRF. Saccadic accuracy is expressed as a percentage ratio of the saccade amplitude to target amplitude and is probably determined by cerebellar or cerebellar pathway processing.

A number of oculographic investigations in MS patients have demonstrated discrete abnormalities in saccadic eye movements. Mastaglia showed abnormalities of SRT, SV, and SA in a significant number of patients with clinically definite and clinically probable MS (114). In one study, 19 of 20 patients with MS showed abnormally long saccadic initiation time (115). The most frequent saccadic abnormality identified in MS involves slowing of ocular adduction, consistent with internuclear ophthalmoplegia (INO). By objective measures, slowing is typically bilateral, even in many cases that are clinically determined to be unilateral.

Internuclear Ophthalmoplegia

Internuclear ophthalmoplegia is one of the neuro-ophthalmologic hallmarks of MS and is present in 17 percent to 41 percent of patients (116,117). This eye movement abnormality is produced by damage to the MLF in the brainstem tegmentum. The MLFs are a pair of white matter fiber tracts that extend through the pons and mesencephalon where they lie near the midline just under the fourth ventricle (Figure 19-12). The MLF both ascends and descends within the brainstem tegmentum and interacts with eye movement control structures that are

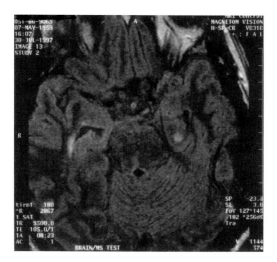

FIGURE 19-12

Proton density weighted MRI from an MS patients with a bilateral INO demonstrates a high signal abnormality in the rostral pontine tegmentum. The lesion extends from the subependymal zone of the fourth ventricle ventrally into the medial tegmentum, in the region of the MLF *(arrow)*.

involved in horizontal and vertical eye movements. The interruption of ascending axons that arise from the internuclear neurons in the abducens nucleus probably explains the adduction deficit in INO.

The cardinal clinical feature of INO is ocular disconjugacy during horizontal saccades secondary to slowing of adducting eye movements. Despite adduction weakness, convergence is intact in the majority of cases, consistent with normal integrity within the vergence pathways, including the fibers that derive from the medial rectus subnucleus of cranial nerve III.

The adduction abnormality in INO can take three principal forms: (1) complete adduction paresis, which is distinctly uncommon; (2) ocular limitation in association with decreased adduction velocity (Figure 19-13); and (3) diminished adduction velocity without ocular limitation (Figure 19-14).

Loss of both velocity and position coded information necessary for adduction during conjugate eye movements are involved when the lesion is complete. Patients with such lesions present with velocity slowing and diminished ability to adduct the eye beyond the midline. With partial lesions, attenuation of velocity and position coded information results in reduced adduction velocity without ocular limitation.

In its most subtle form, the range of adduction is normal, whereas only the velocity is reduced. This latter form of INO can often be overlooked on clinical exami-

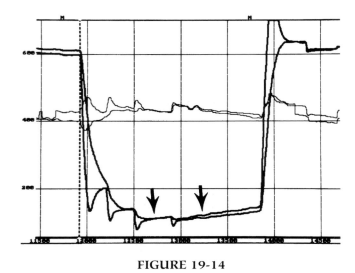

FIGURE 19-14

From a patient with bilateral INO. A leftward saccade shows evidence of adduction slowing and abduction nystagmus. However, both eyes approximate an LED target at 20 degrees to the left without limitation *(arrows)*.

nation and may only be evident on formal oculographic recording (116,118) (Figure 19-14). In one study, more than 80 percent of MS patients with INO had only slight or no restriction of adduction (116). The dissociation between saccade speed and range of motion may reflect the inability of demyelinated fibers to maintain high-frequency discharges, but with preservation of their ability to faithfully carry low-frequency discharges. Hence, the saccadic pulse of innervation is deficient, causing adduction to be slow, whereas the saccadic step is spared, allowing the range of adduction to be full (119).

It would be interesting to know whether there is a pathologic correlation between partial and complete lesions in INO. Could it be that in partial lesions, which are characterized by velocity slowing without limitation, demyelination occurs without axonal loss, whereas both occur in the latter? Such findings would have significant implications concerning strategies to promote neurologic recovery. If therapeutic agents that are able to facilitate remyelination can be identified, neurologic recovery would be expected only in those lesions with axonal preservation.

The main difference between the paresis of adduction with an ocular motor nerve palsy and that associated with an INO is that in the latter adduction induced by vergence is generally spared unless the MLF lesion is sufficiently rostral to involve the medial rectus subnucleus within the cranial nerve III nuclear complex (anterior INO of Cogan). It is the preservation of vergence tone that probably explains the lack of exotropia in most patients with INO (120). When bilateral MLF lesions

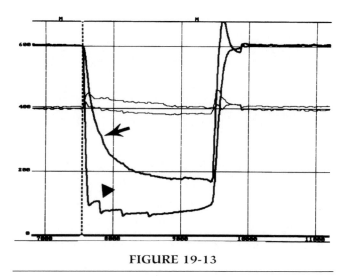

FIGURE 19-13

From a patient with bilateral INO (right to left). This eye movement tracing was derived from a high-speed (250 Hz), two-dimensional infrared oculography device (SMI, Germany). During a leftward saccade there is evidence of adduction slowing in the right eye *(arrow)* in addition to ocular limitation. The abducting left eye exhibits characteristic nystagmus *(arrowhead)*.

extend rostrally to involve the medial rectus subnuclei, patients become exotropic and manifest signs of adduction paresis, the so-called WEBINO (walleyed and bilateral INO) syndrome (121) (Figure 19-15).

Abduction Nystagmus in Internuclear Ophthalmoplegia

Horizontal dissociated nystagmus is another cardinal feature of INO and is most prominent in the abducting eye (Figures 9-13 and 9-14). Although there are many explanations for this observation, the most likely mechanism involves an adaptive response to overcome the weakness of the contralateral medial rectus (122,123). The pulse portion of the saccade is created primarily by the agonist muscle, and the step portion by more nearly equal contributions of the agonist and antagonistic muscles.

To overcome adduction weakness or slowing in INO, the increase in the pulse would have to be relatively greater than the increase in the step. Because of Herring's law of equal innervation, this change in innervation would have to go to both eyes. Thus, the conjugate adaptive response, while improving the accuracy and speed of the weak eye, would cause abnormalities of the pulse and step of innervation to the strong eye. An increase in size of the saccadic pulse and the change in the match between the sizes of the pulse and step produce saccadic overshoot (hypermetria) followed by a brief backward postsaccadic drift (Figures 9-13 and 9-14).

Abduction Slowing in Internuclear Ophthalmoplegia

Occasional patients with INO demonstrate abduction slowing on the side of the INO (119,124). In the context of adduction weakness, a small degree of abduction slowing might be expected because of the loss of the contribution of the off-pulse of innervation when the medial rectus is acting as an antagonist (125). Bronstein has demonstrated that the more prominent the INO and the larger the lesion as seen on MRI, the more likely there will be slowing of abduction in the same eye (posterior INO of Lutz) (124).

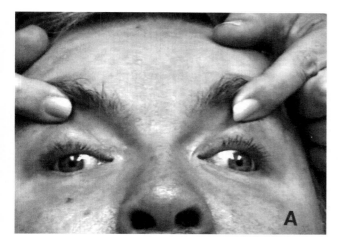

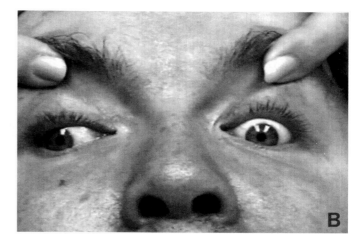

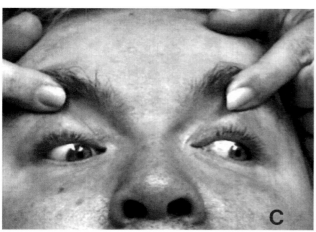

FIGURE 19-15

An MS patient with the WEBINO (walleyed, bilateral INO) syndrome. *A,* When looking straight ahead, the eyes are deviated outward (walleyed). *B,* With attempted gaze to the right, there is clear evidence of a left INO with ocular limitation. *C,* With attempted left gaze, there is a right INO, also with limitation. In this patient, convergence was absent, consistent with the anterior INO of Cogan. The walleyed appearance of such patients probably relates to the convergence dysfunction that occurs when MLF lesions are sufficiently rostral to involve the vergence pathways of horizontal gaze.

Vertical Eye Movements in Internuclear Ophthalmoplegia

Patients with bilateral INO often show characteristic patterns of vertical eye movement abnormalities. Disturbances of vertical gaze holding, inadequate vertical VORs, and abnormal optokinetic and pursuit responses are seen (126,127). Furthermore, bilateral lesions in the MLF abolish the vertical VOR in monkey (128). It is estimated that approximately half of the fibers contained within the MLF are related to vestibular-mediated eye movements (129). Approximately one third of patients with MS and INO demonstrate a vertical VOR disorder (116). These abnormalities probably reflect the interruption in MLF projection pathways between the vestibular nuclei (and the NPH), the trochlear and oculomotor nuclei, and the INC. It is important to note that vertical saccades and quick phases of vertical nystagmus are spared in INO because these eye movements are controlled at sites rostral to control pathways traveling in the MLF. Vertical pursuit defects can be seen in patients with INO, probably secondary to interruption in pursuit pathways that course through the MLF.

Diagnosis of Internuclear Ophthalmoplegia

The diagnosis of INO typically is based on clinical examination in which disconjugate horizontal saccades are seen. In Muri's study of 34 cases of INO in patients with MS, all had saccadic disconjugacy (116). The principal symptoms of INO are diplopia, blurred vision, and oscillopsia (the illusion of environmental movement), although many patients are asymptomatic. Vertigo also frequently occurs but probably reflects lesions that involve pathways outside the MLF. The cause of diplopia may involve adduction paralysis and/or skew deviation, which is not uncommonly associated with INO. Oscillopsia often relates to abduction nystagmus but may also be produced by a decrease in the gain of the VOR during either vertical or horizontal head movement. Some patients with INO have con-

comitant nystagmus, which may also contribute to oscillopsia. This occasionally presents with a dissociated pattern with downbeat nystagmus in one eye and torsional movements in the other (130).

The diagnosis of INO can be confirmed neurophysiologically by a number of eye movement tracking techniques. These techniques can identify a variety of abnormalities in patients with INO, including slowing of adduction saccades, abduction nystagmus, and diminished adduction saccadic amplitude. The ratio of saccade pairs (abducting eye/adducting eye) for individual saccadic parameters, the versional disconjugacy index (VDI), represents a sensitive measure of the disconjugacy seen in patients with INO (131). This type of analysis minimizes technique dependent intra- and interindividual variations seen with absolute saccade parameter values. The most elegant study to date is that of Flipse and coworkers (132), in which sharp distinctions between normals and patients with INO could be demonstrated by analysis of saccadic ratios (abducting eye/adducting eye) of peak acceleration and velocity.

Whereas bilateral INO is most commonly associated with demyelinating disease, unilateral INO typically is seen in patients with brainstem vascular occlusive disease. Nevertheless, unilateral INO does occur in patients with MS. However, a significant number of patients with clinically apparent unilateral INO have been found to have bilateral INO on formal neurophysiologic testing. Although MS is the most common cause of INO (120,133,134), the differential diagnosis is broad (135–137) (Table 19-2).

The One-and-a-Half Syndrome

The combination of a gaze palsy in one direction and INO on attempted gaze contralaterally is referred to as the one-and-a-half syndrome (138). This syndrome is produced by a lesion that damages either the PPRF or abducens nucleus together with the MLF on the same side. This combination gives rise to an ipsilateral gaze palsy in addition to

TABLE 19-2	
Causes of Internuclear Ophthalmoplegia (INO)	
Multiple sclerosis	Stroke
Infection	Neoplasms
Trauma	Mass effect
Drugs	Progressive supranuclear palsy
Wernicke's encephalopathy	Myasthenia gravis
Thyroid eye disease	Metabolic derangement
Chiari malformation	Syringobulbia
Miller-Fisher syndrome	

INO on attempted gaze to the side opposite the lesion (Figure 19-16). Patients with the one-and-a-half syndrome often present with the eye on the side opposite the lesion in exotropia. This is referred to as paralytic pontine exotropia and is the result of a tendency of the eyes to deviate contralaterally to the side of a gaze palsy. However, the eye on the affected side cannot move medially secondary to an INO, so only the contralateral eye deviates.

Because a gaze palsy can be the basis of a nuclear or supranuclear lesion, if VOR testing causes improvement in the abducting eye but not in the adducting eye, one can assume an INO secondary to a MLF lesion on one side and a PPRF lesion on the opposite side. Damage to the MLF on one side and to the VI fascicle on the other side can mimic a horizontal gaze palsy. An ipsilateral INO and VI fascicle lesion can produce paralysis of both adduction and abduction in one eye (monocular horizontal gaze paralysis).

An associated feature in some patients with INO is skew deviation. Skew deviation is a supranuclear vertical ocular misalignment, with the higher eye on the side of the lesion in midpontine and midbrain lesions and the lower eye on the side of the lesion in medullary lesions. The higher eye is observed to undergo incyclotorsion, whereas the lower eye undergoes excyclotorsion. Patients often exhibit a head tilt (typically away from the high eye) and may experience a perceptual deviation in the subjective visual vertical, in addition to vertical diplopia. Taken together, these features are referred to as the ocular tilt or torsion reaction (Figure 19-17).

In a study using infrared reflection oculography, the highest yield of saccadic abnormalities were observed when analyzing saccades and VOR suppression together, where deficits were seen in 29 of 31 clinically definite MS patients, 10 of 17 clinically probable MS patients, and 24 of 31 possible MS patients (117). Vestibular ocular reflex suppression refers to the ability to cancel the VOR during combined smooth eye–head tracking. This suppression may be derived from a smooth pursuit command or by some independent cancellation signal. The value of VOR suppression in the assessment of eye movement abnormalities has been further supported by Sharpe, who found impaired VOR suppression in 75 percent of 20 patients with MS and normal saccadic velocities (139). Taken together, these findings suggest that the combined analysis of saccades and VOR suppression is a sensitive detector of brainstem and cerebellar pathway disease in MS.

Vertical Saccadic Abnormalities

The riMLF in the midbrain tegmentum contains the burst neurons for vertical and torsional saccades and OKN quick phases. Each riMLF has burst neurons for upward and downward eye movements and neurons for torsional quick phases on that side. The riMLF projects to the ipsilateral third and fourth cranial nerve nuclei, which inner-

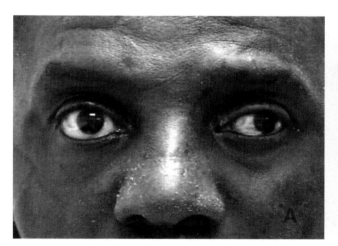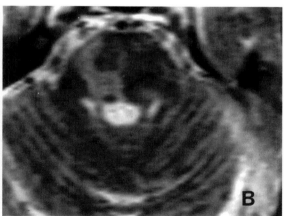

FIGURE 19-16

The one-and-a-half syndrome. *A,* This MS patient presented with an exotropia of the left eye when looking straight ahead (paralytic pontine exotropia). He had a complete inability to gaze to the right (right gaze palsy) and a right INO on attempted left gaze. The only preserved eye movement was left eye abduction. *B,* A T2-weighted MRI shows an extensive right pontine lesion *(arrow)* including involvement of the tegmentum region. In this syndrome, there is involvement of the abducens nucleus and adjacent MLF. If the gaze palsy normalizes with oculocephalic maneuvers, this may signify involvement of the PPRF (a supranuclear structure) with preservation of the abducens nucleus. The latter structure is used in the final pathway for vestibular induced horizontal eye movements.

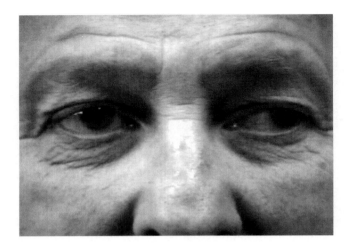

FIGURE 19-17

Combined INO and skew deviation. This MS patient demonstrates evidence of a right INO and a commitant right hyperdeviation. On attempted left gaze, there is right adduction slowing and limitation. The hyperdeviation was on the basis of a skew deviation.

vate the ipsilateral inferior rectus and inferior oblique and contralateral superior rectus and superior oblique. The two riMLFs are connected by the posterior and ventral commissures.

When demyelination occurs in the dorsal midbrain, Parinaud's syndrome may occur; it is characterized by diminished upward saccades, convergent retraction nys-

tagmus on attempted upward saccades, or when viewing a down-moving OKN tape, and near-light dissociation (Figure 19-18). Other features of Parinaud's syndrome may include skew deviation, fixation instability (square-wave jerks), convergence spasm or divergence paralysis, irregular pupils (correctopia), pseudoabducens palsy (a slower moving abducting eye during horizontal saccades, perhaps related to convergence excess), downward gaze preference (setting-sun sign), downbeating nystagmus, and abnormalities of vertical smooth pursuit and VOR eye movements. More isolated lesions may produce limited syndromes such as upgaze or downgaze palsies. These may occur with or without preservation of VOR-induced vertical eye movements, depending on the integrity of the INC, the midbrain center for vertical VORs.

Subclinical Eye Movement Abnormalities

Oculography in MS patients has demonstrated subclinical eye movement abnormalities. Solinger and Baloh described 13 of 16 MS patients without clinically apparent eye movement disorders, who on oculographic analysis demonstrated saccadic or pursuit abnormalities (118). In another study, 80 percent of clinically definite MS patients, 74 percent of clinically probable MS patients, and 60 percent of possible MS patients exhibited subclinical eye movement abnormalities (140). In 27 patients with disease isolated to the spinal cord, 14 patients had subclinical deficits. When SRT, SV, and SA were analyzed together, abnormalities were seen in 48 percent of patients

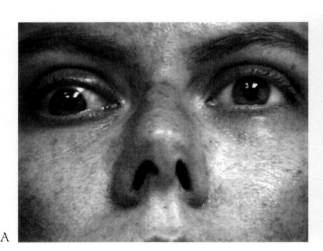

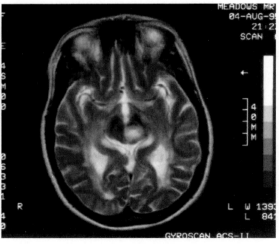

FIGURE 19-18

Parinaud's syndrome in MS. *A,* This MS patient presented with a left hyperdeiviation, anisocoria with left midriasis and near light dissociation, convergent retraction nystagmus, and vertical ophthalmoparesis. Other findings included right hypesthetic hemiparesis. *B,* A T2-weighted MRI demonstrates a large left midbrain plaque involving the tegmentum and cerebral peduncle.

with clinically normal eye movements (114). These studies suggest that an analysis of eye movements could be useful in patients who are under evaluation for the diagnosis of MS and do not meet the basic criterion of two events in space and time as established by Poser (49). The demonstration of a subclinical abnormality in ocular motor function may elucidate evidence for disease dissemination and provide additional confirmatory evidence for the diagnosis of MS.

Nuclear and Fascicular Lesions

Ocular motor palsies with consequent diplopia are uncommon in MS. Nevertheless, they have been observed and most frequently affect the sixth and third cranial nerves (141,142). Of the infranuclear lesions that occur in MS, sixth nerve paresis is the most common (143). Moster found that 12 percent of the 49 patients he evaluated with isolated lateral rectus palsies had demyelination (144). Hence, the presentation of an unexplained isolated ocular motor palsy in a young patient should raise suspicion about the possibility of MS.

The abducens nucleus, which is located in the pontine tegmentum, contains motor neurons that innervate the ipsilateral lateral rectus and interneurons that decussate in the MLF and innervate the contralateral medial rectus subnucleus. Abducens nucleus involvement can be distinguished from abducens nerve injury in that the former produces a gaze palsy to the side of the lesion, whereas the latter produces only an ipsilateral lateral rectus palsy. Bilateral horizontal gaze palsy secondary to a midline pontine lesion has been reported in MS (145).

Oculomotor (cranial nerve III) palsies occasionally occur (146) and partial fascicular (upper and lower division) and nuclear lesions have also been observed in MS patients (147). Trochlear nucleus and nerve lesions are even less common but have been reported (148). A unique ocular motor syndrome combines an INO with a contralateral hyperdeviation secondary to superior oblique weakness. Neuroanatomically, the lesion was localized to the caudal midbrain involving the MLF and trochlear nucleus (149) (Figure 19-19).

Ptosis on the basis of a brainstem lesion can present in a unilateral or bilateral form. When on the basis of oculomotor dysfunction, fascicular lesions give rise to unilateral ptosis, whereas nuclear lesions produce bilateral ptosis because of involvement of the central caudal nucleus. This nucleus is unpaired and contains cells that project to both levator palpebre superioris muscles. Horner's syndrome can also produce ptosis, albeit more mild than the degree of ptosis observed with cranial nerve III lesions.

Paroxysms of forced eye closure (blepharoclonus) have been described in MS. This disorder may be precip-

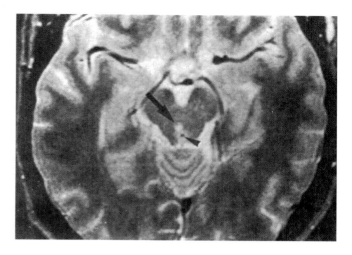

FIGURE 19-19

Combined right INO and left trochlear nerve paresis in a 41-year-old man with MS. A T2-weighted axial MR image demonstrates a punctate high signal intensity lesion *(arrow)* ventral to the cerebral aqueduct *(arrowhead)* at the level of the caudal midbrain. This lesion probably damaged the right MLF and the predecussation portion of the right trochlear nerve or the trochlear nucleus. (From Vanooteghem P, Dehaene I, Van Zandycke M, Casselman J. Combined trochlear nerve palsy and internuclear ophthalmoplegia. *Arch Neurol* 1992; 49:108–109.)

itated by eccentric eye movements or may occur abruptly while looking straight ahead (150) (Figure 19-20).

Pursuit Eye Movements

The neuroanatomic pathways for smooth pursuit involves cortical and subcortical structures and commences with the processing of visual information in the afferent visual apparatus (Figure 19-21). Retinal slip (the deviation of a target visual image away from the fovea) represents the error signal that is processed centrally and generates the command sequence for pursuit eye movements. Information from the lateral geniculate nucleus of the thalamus is projected onto the striate cortex, which then projects to the middle temporal (MT) visual area located in the superior temporal sulcus. This structure is important for the processing of motion stimuli. The medial superior temporal (MST) visual area is another striate target and is involved in the development of an ocular motor command signal based on expected target parameters such as target velocity and position (efference copy). Lesions here produce a deficit in ipsilateral pursuit. The MT and MST project to the FEF and dorsolateral pontine nucleus, both of which mediate ipsilateral pursuit. The dorsolateral pontine nucleus (DLPN) pro-

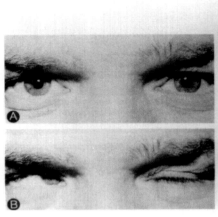
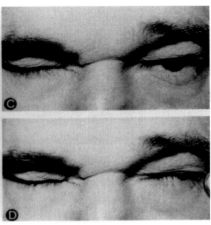

FIGURE 19-20

Gaze-evoked blepharoclonus. *A,* A 37-year-old man with MS. Ocular motor abnormalities included bilateral INO, skew deviation, and upgaze nystagmus. There was no defect when looking straight ahead. *B,* Bilateral blepharoclonus was observed with gaze to the left. The asymmetry of eye closure was probably secondary to a concomitant right facial palsy. *C,* A different MS patient with bilateral facial weakness. Asymmetric blepharoclonus occurred while looking straight ahead. *D,* Blepharoclonus was intensified with attempted left gaze. (From Keane JR. Gaze evoked blepharoclonus. *Ann Neurol* 1978; 3:243–245.)

jects to the flocculus and dorsal vermis. The flocculus projects to the vestibular nuclei (part of the neural integrator), which ultimately projects to the oculomotor nuclei. The pursuit pathways run in the posterior limb of the internal capsule.

Lesions within the descending pursuit pathway give rise to a variety of deficits, including low gain and high gain pursuit. In low gain pursuit, eye movements do not keep pace with the target object, so catch-up saccades must be incorporated to reestablish foveation (Figure 19-22). In patients with high gain pursuit, eye movements are excessive compared with the target object and back-up saccades must be used. In Mastaglia's study, 30 of 42 MS patients had abnormalties of pursuit eye movements (114). Although pursuit abnormalties are common in MS patients, these eye movements are dependent on patient cooperation and fatigue and are therefore not as reliable as saccadic deficits in differentiating between physiologic variation and true pathology.

Vestibular Dysfunction and Nystagmus

The vestibular system is involved in the control of compensatory eye movements in response to head movement with the goal of maintaining visual fixation. Vestibular mechanisms also influence postural tone and ambulation through the descending vestibulospinal tract. Information processing within the peripheral and central vestibular apparatus also contributes to our perception of head and body attitude with respect to the gravitational field.

Patients with MS are not infrequently affected by alterations in vestibular function that can give rise to oscillopsia, gait instability, and spatial disorientation. In addition to vestibular abnormalities, all forms of nystagmus have been seen in patients with MS. These repetitive eye movement abnormalities often degrade visual acuity, may produce oscillopsia and spatial disorientation, and ultimately exacerbate gait instability.

Basic Vestibular Physiology

The vestibular sense is mediated by two relatively simple reflexes. The VOR ensures best vision during head motion by stabilizing the line of sight, also called gaze. The vestibulospinal reflex (VSR) helps keep the head and body upright. Two phylogenetically old sensors within the labyrinth—the semicircular canals (SCCs) and the otolith organs—respond to acceleration and thereby transduce the motion and the position of the head into central biologic signals that produce these reflexes.

The SCCs sense angular acceleration to determine head rotation. Because of the mechanical properties of the labyrinth, the position of the cupula within the ampula, and hence the signals on primary vestibular afferents, encode head velocity. During angular head movement, endolymph within the SCC moves relative to the cupula, a membrane that spans the canal. When the cupula is deflected, processes of adjacent hair cells are displaced, producing either depolarization or hyperpolarization, depending on the direction of cupular movement. In the case of eye movements, the SCCs provide the input for the compensatory slow phases of the angular VOR in response to head rotation. These compensatory eye movements keep objects of visual interest on the fovea centralis, the retinal area of highest visual acuity.

The otolith organs (utricle and saccule) sense linear acceleration to detect both head translation and the position of the head relative to the pull of gravity (i.e., uprightness). Linear acceleration causes relative motion of the gelatinous matrix of the otolithic macula, in which are buried calcium carbonate crystals (otoconia). This causes the processes from otolith hair cells, which extend into the macula, to bend and so change their firing rate. In the case of eye movements, the otoliths provide the input for static ocular counteroll in response to head tilt and the input for the compensatory slow phases of the linear VOR in response to head translation. The SCCs and otoliths also provide

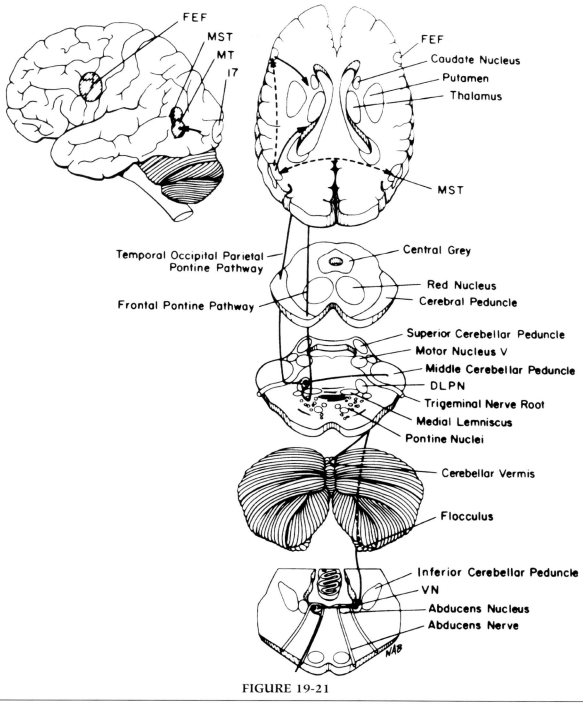

FIGURE 19-21

Hypothetical scheme for horizontal pursuit eye movements. Primary visual cortex *(area 17)* projects to the homologue of the middle temporal (MT) visual area, which in humans lies at the temporal-occipital-parietal junction. Middle temporal visual area projects to the homologue of the medial superior temporal (MST) visual area and also to the frontal eye fields (FEF). The medial superior temporal visual area also receives inputs from its contralateral counterpart. Medial superior temporal visual area projects through the retrolenticular portion of the internal capsule and posterior portion of the cerebral peduncle to the dorsolateral pontine nucleus (DLPN). The DLPN also receives inputs that are important for pursuit from the FEF, which descend in the medial portion of the cerebral peduncle. The DLPN projects, mainly contralaterally, to the flocculus, paraflocculus, and ventral uvula of the cerebellum; projections also pass to the dorsal vermis. The flocculus projects to the ipsilateral vestibular nuclei (VN), which in turn project to the contralateral abducens nucleus. (From Leigh JR, Zee DS. *The neurology of eye movements,* 2nd ed. Philadelphia: FA Davis:207.)

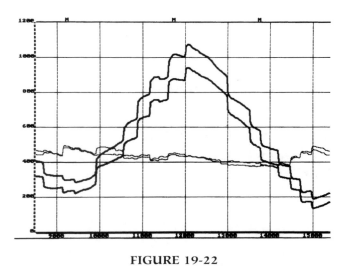

FIGURE 19-22

Low gain or saccadic pursuit. An infrared oculography tracing from an MS patient. Attempted smooth pursuit of a target moving in a triangular waveform demonstrated diminished velocity compared with the target and catch-up saccades to reachieve foveal refixation. Rightward pursuit is depicted by movement of the tracing upward, whereas leftward pursuit corresponds to downward movement of the tracing.

information for vestibulospinal reflexes that keep the head and body upright. The SCCs and the otoliths can detect motion in three dimensions (i.e., around any or all of the three axes of rotation: pitch (vertical), yaw (horizontal), and roll (torsion); and around any or all of the three axes of translation: fore and aft, side to side, and up and down.

The Velocity-Storage Mechanism

To improve the low-frequency response of the angular VOR, a central velocity-storage mechanism perseverates activity coming from the vestibular periphery by integrating the peripheral SCC signal. Velocity storage increases the time constant (the time for an exponential function to decay to 37 percent of its initial value) of the VOR from a value of approximately six seconds, based on activity in peripheral afferents, to a value of 15 to 20 seconds, based on the actual nystagmus response. The ability of the angular VOR to reliably transduce head velocity to low-frequency stimuli is improved in this way. Another equivalent measure of the time constant can be calculated during low-frequency sinusoidal rotations from the difference in timing (or shift in the phase relationship) between maximum head speed and maximum eye speed. The action of the velocity-storage mechanism is the basis for a common clinical neuro-otologic sign in patients with vestibular imbalance, head-shaking nystagmus, which is discussed subsequently.

Anatomic Projections

The SCCs and otolith organs are innervated by peripheral processes from bipolar neurons in the vestibular (Scarpa's) ganglion, which is located in the internal auditory canal. The superior division of the eighth cranial nerve innervates the anterior and horizontal SCC and the utricle; the inferior division innervates the posterior SCC and the saccule. The nerve from the ganglion to the brainstem is maintained by Schwann cell–derived myelin. However, the proximal few millimeters of the nerve, and the root entry zone within the pontomedullary junction, are covered by central myelin derived from oligodendrocytes and can therefore be a target of demyelination in MS.

Central projections from the SCCs are predominantly to the rostral portions of the vestibular nuclei complex (medial and superior vestibular nuclei); those from the otolith organs are predominantly to the caudal portions of the vestibular nuclei complex (lateral and inferior vestibular nuclei). There are also primary projections from the labyrinth to the vestibular portions of the cerebellum (nodulus and uvula). Second-order vestibular neurons project to the ocular motor nuclei, forming the substrate for the VOR. For horizontal head movement to the right (and leftward eye movements during straight ahead fixation), the right horizontal SCC is activated and projects to the right MVN, which in turn projects to the contralateral abducens nucleus.

With upward head movements during straight ahead fixation, afferents from each posterior SCC are excited, and the eyes move downward by primary projections to the contralateral inferior rectus and ipsilateral superior oblique muscles. Secondary projections and inhibitory projections to antagonist muscles are also important. Likewise, downward head rotation produces excitation in afferents from the anterior SCCs, which is relayed to the contralateral inferior oblique and ipsilateral superior rectus muscles, producing upward eye movement (Figure 19-23). The otolith organs give rise to the central projections that innervate the supranuclear structures that control vertical alignment of the eyes as well as torsional eye movements.

Other projections from the vestibular nuclei are to the cerebellum and more rostrally to the thalamus and cerebral cortex, including areas in the parietoinsular region and other vestibular association cortices. The vestibular contribution to sensations of head and body motion and position probably reach consciousness through these rostral projections.

Clinical Symptoms and Signs of Vestibulopathy

Because demyelination in MS so frequently occurs in brainstem and cerebellar pathways, it is not surprising that

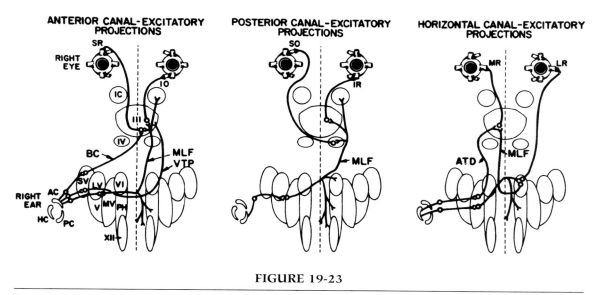

FIGURE 19-23

Summary of probable direct connections of the VOR based on findings from a number of species. III: oculomotor nuclear complex; IV: trochlear nucleus; VI: abducens nucleus; XII: hypoglossal nucleus; AC: anterior semicircular canal; ATD: ascending tract of Deiters; BC: brachium conjunctivum; HC: horizontal or lateral semicircular canal; IC: interstitial nucleus of Cajal; IO: inferior oblique muscle; IR: inferior rectus muscle; LR: lateral rectus muscle; LV: lateral vestibular nucleus; MLF: medial longitudinal fasciculus; MR: medial rectus muscle; MV: medial vestibular nucleus; PC: posterior semicircular canal; PH: prepositus nucleus; SV: superior vestibular nucleus; SO: superior oblique muscle; SR: superior rectus muscle; and V: inferior vestibular nucleus; VTP: ventral tegmental pathway. (From Leigh JR, Zee DS. *The neurology of eye movements*, 2nd ed. Philadelphia: FA Davis, 1991:35.)

abnormal vestibular sensations are a common feature of MS. These sensations include oscillopsia, spatial disorientation, and postural imbalance. Patients often describe difficulty with driving, walking in large open spaces, or moving about in crowded environments such as shopping malls and supermarkets. These sensory-rich environments provoke and intensify sensory conflicts, which may precipitate feelings of disorientation and vegetative symptoms such as nausea and vomiting. The majority of patients with MS experience balance difficulties at some point during the course of the disease. It has been estimated that approximately 20 percent of patients experience true vertigo, whereas the prevalence rate at any given time is probably less than 5 percent (151).

Vestibular dysfunction in patients with MS is not always clinically apparent. In one study, only four of 50 patients with MS and a normal otologic examination showed a normal pattern on electronystagmogram. The abnormalities seen consisted of positional or spontaneous nystagmus, directional preponderance, decreased caloric responses, or lack of fixation suppression of caloric induced nystagmus (152). These findings suggest that a detailed neuro-otologic examination can uncover evidence of brainstem disease in patients without findings on routine examination.

Vestibular signs and symptoms may reflect static (head still) and/or dynamic (head moving) disturbances. Static disturbances occur because in normal subjects there are balanced, tonic levels of discharge in the vestibular nerve and nuclei when the head is still. Unilateral lesions create such static disturbances and lead to a spontaneous nystagmus in the absence of any head motion. When the otoliths are affected unilaterally, diplopia and tilt of the head and body can occur.

Static vestibular imbalance also commonly leads to vegetative symptoms, including nausea, vomiting, diaphoresis, and occasionally hypotension and syncope. Dynamic disturbances occur in unilateral lesions because of a loss of the normal push-pull relationship—activity from one labyrinth increases as that from the other decreases—that produces compensatory responses to head motion. Bilateral lesions lead to dynamic disturbances because of an overall loss of function but rarely give rise to vertigo, nystagmus, or vegetative symptoms.

Static Imbalance

Spontaneous nystagmus (with the head still) is the hallmark of an imbalance in the tonic levels of activity mediating the angular VOR. When peripheral in origin, spontaneous nystagmus characteristically is damped by visual fixation and is increased or only becomes apparent when fixation is eliminated. Hence, for the VOR, one must do the equivalent of a Romberg test and look for spontaneous nystagmus with the patient wearing Frenzel goggles (magnifying lenses that prevent the patient from using visual fixation to suppress spontaneous nystagmus) or during ophthalmoscopy (with the opposite eye occluded to prevent fixation). The intensity of nystagmus is compared with that observed when the patient is fixating on a visual target.

The intensity of nystagmus usually depends on the position of the eye in the orbit. Nystagmus arising from a peripheral lesion—and most central lesions—is more intense (slow-phase velocity higher), or may only be evident, when gaze is pointed in the direction of the quick phase (Alexander's law), although the opposite sometimes occurs with central lesions.

Pure vertical or pure torsional nystagmus almost always has a central origin because of the improbability of selectively involving both anterior or both posterior SCCs (for a pure vertical nystagmus) or only the anterior and posterior SCCs in one labyrinth (for a pure torsional nystagmus). A mixed horizontal-torsional nystagmus usually indicates a peripheral lesion involving the entire vestibular nerve or all the SCC within one labyrinth.

Skew Deviation

Skew deviation is a vertical misalignment of the eyes that cannot be explained on the basis of an ocular muscle palsy. Skew is the hallmark of an imbalance in the tonic levels of activity underlying otolith-ocular reflexes. Skew deviation is a naturally occurring component of the righting reflex that occurs in lateral-eyed animals in response to lateral tilt of the body so that they can keep their eyes aligned with the horizontal meridian and their head and body upright. Presumably, in frontal-eyed animals this phylogenetically old pattern of eye deviation emerges when otolith inputs become unbalanced in a nonphysiologic way.

Patients with a skew deviation complain of vertical and sometimes torsional (one image tilted with respect to the other) diplopia. There also may be a cyclorotation (ocular counterroll) of both eyes associated with an illusion of tilt of the visual world. The head may also be tilted, usually toward the side of the lower eye. Together, skew deviation, ocular counterrolling, and head tilt constitute the ocular tilt reaction; the vestibulo-ocular and vestibulocollic components of the righting reaction in response to lateral tilt of the head and body.

Skew deviation is best detected using the tools and techniques of the ophthalmologist—objectively with cover testing or subjectively with a red glass or Maddox rod. With the alternate cover test, one looks for a vertical corrective movement, on switching the cover from one eye to the other, as an index of a vertical misalignment. Alternatively, one can use a red glass or a Maddox rod to dissociate the images seen by the two eyes, and then ask whether the patient sees one image above the other, indicating a vertical misalignment. The effect of the position of the eye in the orbit and of left and right head tilt on the skew should also be recorded, especially to exclude a fourth nerve palsy.

The hallmark of a fourth nerve palsy is a vertical misalignment that is greatest with the affected eye down and medial. The adducting eye is higher, and the misalignment is greater with the head tilted toward the side of the higher eye. Skew deviations tend to be relatively comitant, i.e., the degree of misalignment changes little with different directions of gaze, although this is not always the case. Ocular counterroll is difficult to detect clinically without photographic means, but if the amount of counterroll is large, it can be appreciated by the tilt of the imaginary line that connects the macula and the optic disk. Skew deviations may occur with cerebellar lesions; which eye is higher alternates, depending on whether gaze is directed to the left or to the right. The abducting eye usually is higher in cerebellar lesions.

The ocular tilt reaction can occur with lesions anywhere in the otolith-ocular pathway, peripheral labyrinth, vestibular nerve, vestibular nucleus in the medulla, medial longitudinal fasciculus in the pons or caudal midbrain, and the interstitial nucleus of Cajal, rostral to the oculomotor nucleus. With peripheral and vestibular nucleus lesions, the lower eye is on the side of the lesion. The otolith-ocular pathway crosses at the level of the vestibular nucleus such that with lesions above the decussation, the higher eye is on the side of the lesion. The head usually is tilted toward the side of the lower eye.

Dynamic Disturbances

Disturbances of vestibular function provoked by head motion or a change in head position reflect abnormalities in gain (amplitude), direction, and/or timing (phase) of the VOR and VSR, or occasionally mechanical disruptions in the labyrinth (e.g., benign paroxysmal positional vertigo and perilymphatic fistula). Dynamic disturbances occur with both unilateral and bilateral vestibular disturbances. The angular VOR can be tested at the bedside both by observing the effect of head rotation on visual acuity and by looking at the eye movements themselves in response to head rotation.

Dynamic visual acuity is a measure of the patient's best corrected visual acuity using a distance acuity chart with the head still, and then with the head passively rotated, first horizontally, then vertically, at a frequency of approximately 2 Hz, so as to prevent visual-following reflexes from helping to stabilize the eyes. Normal individuals may lose one line of acuity during head shaking, whereas patients with a complete loss of labyrinthine function usually lose approximately five lines. Partial vestibular dysfunction in which the VOR gain is diminished also results in degradation of visual acuity with head movement.

Examination of the induced slow phases of the VOR can be useful in assessing the integrity of VOR gain. The patient's head is oscillated back and forth in yaw (horizontal), in pitch (vertical), and in roll (torsion) with the subject instructed to fix on the examiner's nose. The observation of corrective saccades (usually catch-up) signifies an abnormal VOR gain. High-acceleration head thrusts are also used in the assessment of VOR gain, with the eyes beginning approximately 15 degrees away from primary position in the orbit and the amplitude of the head movement such that the eyes end near the primary position of gaze. Again, the presence of corrective saccades is a sign of an abnormal VOR gain.

Assessment of head-shaking nystagmus (HSN) is another way to look for an imbalance of dynamic vestibular function. First, with Frenzel goggles in place or by having the patient gaze ahead into white featureless paper (Ganzfeldt), the patient is instructed to shake the head vigorously but carefully approximately 30 times, side to side, with the chin pitched slightly down (to put the planes of the lateral semicircular canals in the plane of head rotation). The eyes are then carefully observed for evidence of nystagmus following the head shaking. Normal individuals have at most a beat or two of HSN. With a unilateral loss of labyrinthine function, there usually is a vigorous eye nystagmus with slow phases initially directed toward the lesioned side, which is followed by a reversal phase with slow phases directed toward the intact side.

The initial phase of HSN arises because there is an asymmetry of peripheral inputs during high-velocity head rotations; a larger amplitude response is transmitted centrally during rotation toward the intact side than toward the affected side. This asymmetry leads to an accumulation of activity during the head shaking within the vestibular nuclei in the velocity-storage mechanism. The nystagmus following head shaking in patients with a vestibular imbalance reflects the decay of activity within the velocity-storage mechanism.

Central lesions resulting from cerebellar dysfunction may also lead to head-shaking nystagmus, often with a vertical nystagmus appearing after horizontal head shaking (so-called cross-coupled nystagmus). Asymmetries in the central velocity-storage mechanism may also lead to a horizontal HSN, again making it necessary to measure rotational responses so that any HSN can be properly interpreted.

Central Lesions

The last few millimeters of the eighth cranial nerve, before entry to the brainstem at the pontomedullary junction, is covered by oligodendrocyte derived myelin. A lesion here can be indistinguishable from a process affecting the peripheral labyrinth. Furthermore, plaques of demyelination at the root entry zone or within the MVN can produce vestibular dysfunction that is difficult to differentiate from other peripheral vestibular syndromes.

In one study, 10 of 20 MS patients with features of peripheral vestibulopathy had canal paresis on caloric testing (153). Nevertheless, their nystagmus was not suppressed by fixation, which pointed to a central origin. Magnetic resonance imaging analysis using image matrix grids demonstrated that the primary lesion in these patients was within the MVN. It should be recalled that the MVN receives inputs from the cristae of the SCCs, the maculae of the otoliths, the visual (optokinetic) system, and proprioceptors in the neck. Hence, a demyelinating lesion in the root entry zone or in the MVN can produce a "central canal paresis" with features of a peripheral vestibular syndrome.

Oscillopsia in association with peripheral vestibular lesions often resolves quickly as compensatory mechanisms come into play, whereas such compensation generally does not occur as rapidly with brainstem disorders. Involvement of the central pathways required for compensation probably explains the persistent dysfunction seen in some patients with MS.

Vestibular Ocular Reflex Cancellation

When the head is tracking a moving target or when a fixation target is moving at the same velocity as the head (as in reading while moving in a vehicle), the VOR is normally suppressed or canceled in order to maintain a stable image. Vestibular ocular reflex cancellation can be assessed at the bedside by asking patients to fixate on their outstretched thumbs while rotating the head and arm together. Normally, there should be no movement of the eyes in the orbit during this maneuver. When VOR cancellation is deficient, vestibular nystagmus is observed, with quick phases in the direction of head rotation. Slow-phase eye movements move the eyes off the target in a direction opposite to the direction of head movement, and the rapid saccadic movements reestablish fixation on the target.

Poor VOR suppression is seen in patients with cerebellar disease, especially with lesions of the flocculus. A number of medications have been associated with this abnormality, including antiepileptic agents, hypnotic sedative drugs, and tricyclic antidepressants. Sharpe has shown not only that abnormalities of the VOR are common in asymptomatic patients with MS but also that 75 percent of 20 patients had impaired VOR suppression (154).

Increased VOR amplitude (gain) is commonly seen in patients with MS who have cerebellar lesions. It is characterized by slow phases that are too fast, which necessitates back-up corrective saccades during head motion (155,156). Patients with MS can also exhibit caloric hyperexcitability. Consistent with the central localization, there was impaired attenuation of caloric-induced nystagmus with visual fixation in most patients (157). A prolonged duration of vestibular nystagmus with increased amplitude and frequency has also been shown in 20 percent to 70 percent of patients with MS (158).

Paroxysmal Vestibular Disorders

Patients with MS occasionally present with paroxysms of vertigo, which are stereotyped and may represent one of a variety of paroxysmal attacks that occur in these patients (159). Such paroxysms are occasionally precipitated by hyperventilation, a phenomenon also seen in patients with perilymphatic fistula, petrous bone cholesteatoma, acoustic neuroma, and microvascular compression of cranial nerve VIII. In patients with MS, these paroxysms usually can be managed effectively with membrane-stabilizing agents such as carbamazepine or phenytoin or with acetazolamide. These attacks probably represent episodes of abnormal electrical excitability in demyelinated CNS vestibular pathways (160,161). Ephaptic or axonal cross-transmission has been offered as one mechanistic explanation. The differential diagnosis of these episodes includes the more common causes of vestibulopathy—transient ischemic attacks in vertebrobasilar insufficiency, benign paroxysmal positioning vertigo, vestibular neuritis, Meniere's syndrome, perilymphatic fistula, migraine, vascular compression syndrome, seizures, and drug toxicity. Distinguishing among these conditions is often difficult because vestibulopathy caused by MS can present with features of a peripheral or central disorder.

Nystagmus

Essentially every form of nystagmus has been described in patients with MS and occurs in as many as 40 percent to 60 percent of patients (162) (Table 19-3). Nystagmus is a repetitive to-and-fro movement of the eyes. When pathologic, it reflects abnormalities in the mechanisms that hold images on the retina. A disturbance of any of these mechanisms may cause drifts of the eyes—the slow phases of nystagmus during attempted steady fixation. Corrective quick phases or saccades then reset the eyes. The analysis of the waveform of the slow phases of nystagmus can often help localize the causative lesion. Con-

TABLE 19-3 *Types of Nystagmus in Multiple Sclerosis*	
Gaze-evoked	Periodic alternating
Multidirectional	Rebound
Upbeat	Dissociated (INO)
Downbeat	See-saw
Torsional	Pendular
Convergent-retraction	Mixed

stant velocity drifts of the eyes with corrective quick phases produce jerk nystagmus, which usually is caused by an imbalance of vestibular or possibly optokinetic or pursuit drives.

Lesions of the peripheral vestibular apparatus (labyrinth or cranial nerve VIII) usually cause a mixed horizontal-torsional nystagmus, with slow phases directed toward the side of the lesion. Peripheral vestibular nystagmus is suppressed during fixation because smooth pursuit is preserved. The physician may evaluate suppression of nystagmus at the bedside using the ophthalmoscope; when the fixating eye is transiently covered, drifts of the optic disk and retinal vessels may appear or increase in velocity if an underlying vestibular imbalance exists. Frenzel glasses also can be used to remove fixation and elicit nystagmus.

Nystagmus induced by a change in head position frequently results from degenerative changes in the labyrinth, which cause the posterior SCC to become sensitive to gravity. Positioning the patient in a head-hanging posture (below a plane parallel to the ground), with the head turned toward the involved side, may induce nystagmus and vertigo (the Hallpike-Dix maneuver). The nystagmus typically can take up to 30 seconds to commence and has predominant vertical and torsional components that move the eyes in a plane parallel to that of the posterior SCC being stimulated. Nystagmus usually abates after 10 to 15 seconds. When the patient sits up, the nystagmus may transiently reappear but with the slow phases directed to the opposite direction observed in the head-hanging position. Repeating the postural testing may induce further episodes, but they usually become progressively less severe with repetitive testing. When this typical clinical picture is present, the patient's nystagmus and vertigo probably are caused by benign labyrinthine disease. A single maneuver to dislodge the abnormal debris usually abolishes the vertigo. This vestibular disturbance is so common—and so treatable—that it should be specifically looked for, even in patients with MS. When posturally induced nystagmus does not have these features, disease of the CNS, especially the posterior fossa, must be considered.

Positional nystagmus of the "central type" can be an early sign of MS (163). This form of nystagmus can be distinguished from peripheral positioning nystagmus because it most often is purely horizontal, vertical, or torsional, conjugate, without latency, nonfatigable, lasts greater than 30 seconds, and is related to lesions within the brainstem or cerebellum.

Nystagmus caused by disease of the central vestibular connections may be purely torsional, purely vertical (downbeat or upbeat), or purely horizontal (without a torsional component), or it may have a pattern that mimics peripheral vestibular lesions. Smooth pursuit usually is affected as well, so the velocity of the slow-phase drift of central vestibular nystagmus does not diminish with fixation. Purely torsional nystagmus usually reflects intrinsic brainstem involvement. Downbeat nystagmus can be seen in MS patients with cerebellar or brainstem disease, probably in relation to disruption of the central projections from the posterior SCC. Upbeat nystagmus in primary position occurs with lesions at the pontomedullary or pontomesencephalic junction or within the fourth ventricle and probably reflects involvement of the central projections from the anterior canal system.

Periodic alternating nystagmus (PAN)—horizontal jerk nystagmus that changes direction approximately every two minutes—is a form of central vestibular nystagmus and usually is caused by lesions in the nodulus of the cerebellum. It can be treated successfully with baclofen, a gamma-aminobutyric acid (GABA)-β agonist.

Nystagmus on attempted eccentric gaze and with slow phases that show a declining exponential time course results from an unsustained eye position command. This gaze-evoked nystagmus commonly occurs as a side effect of certain medications, especially anticonvulsants, hypnotics, and tranquilizers, and with disease of the vestibulocerebellum or its brainstem connections in the MVN and NPH. Gaze-evoked nystagmus also may explain Alexander's law. With prolonged eccentric gaze, gaze-evoked nystagmus may dampen and actually change direction. It is then called centripetal nystagmus and is often followed by rebound nystagmus when the eyes return to the primary position (slow phases are directed toward the prior position of eccentric gaze). Rebound nystagmus usually coexists with other cerebellar eye signs, such as saccadic pursuit and diminished VOR cancellation.

Pendular nystagmus consists of a slow phase that is a sinusoidal oscillation rather than a unidirectional drift. Quick phases may be superimposed. Acquired pendular nystagmus may be a manifestation of MS, toluene intoxication, or a sequela of brainstem infarction. Pendular nystagmus is characterized by a sinusoidal oscillation, in the range of 2 to 6 Hz, rather than by a unidirectional drift and rapid quick phase. It may become more jerky on eccentric gaze. Pendular nystagmus may appear elliptical,

depending on the presence and relative phase of a sinusoidal vertical and horizontal component; oblique trajectories are rare, but torsional (sometimes incorrectly referred to as rotatory) components are not uncommon.

In patients with MS, pendular nystagmus is the form of nystagmus that produces the most distressing symptoms, including oscillopsia, poor visual acuity, nausea, disorientation, and instability (Figure 19-24). Acquired pendular nystagmus frequently is disconjugate and may even be horizontal in one eye and vertical in the other eye. In one study of acquired pendular nystagmus, 12 of 16 patients had MS. All 12 patients had a defect in convergence and six patients had bilateral INO (164). In patients with MS who have demyelination in the central tegmental tract within the Guillain-Mollaret triangle (consisting of the pathway between the cerebellar dentate nucleus and the contralateral red and inferior olivary nuclei), one observes pendular nystagmus and palatal tremor (oculopalatal myoclonus). This often is associated with subsequent inferior olivary hypertrophy that can be seen on MRI.

Patients with MS and pendular nystagmus often have tremor of the head and limbs as well as truncal titubation and ataxia (165). Primarily vertical pendular oscillations, predominant in one eye, may also be seen in patients with MS who have absent or markedly diminished visual acuity (often secondary to optic neuritis) in that eye, a condition referred to as the Heiman-Bielschowsky phenomenon (166) (Figure 19-25). Similarly, it has been proposed that binocular dissociation in pendular nystagmus may relate to asymmetries in optic neuropathy (167). Differential conduction times across the two optic nerves could affect

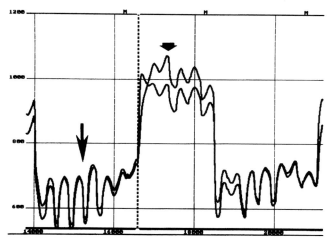

FIGURE 19-24

Acquired pendular nystagmus in MS. This infrared oculogram demonstrates horizontal pendular waveforms while the patients looks straight ahead (*arrow*) and with eccentric gaze to the right (*arrowhead*).

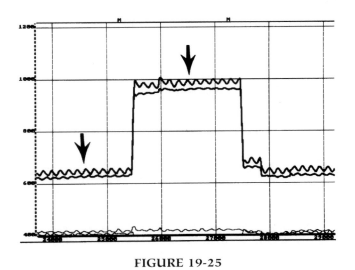

FIGURE 19-25

The Heiman-Bielschowsky phenomenon. This infrared oculo-gram was derived from an MS patient with a history of multiple episodes of optic neuritis. Visual acuity was 20/40 OD and 20/800 OS. Funduscopic examination shows severe optic disc pallor on the left with only mild temporal pallor on the right. The oculogram demonstrates striking asymmetric vertical pendular nystagmus. The more visually compromised left eye was associated with the larger amplitude nystagmus *(arrows)*.

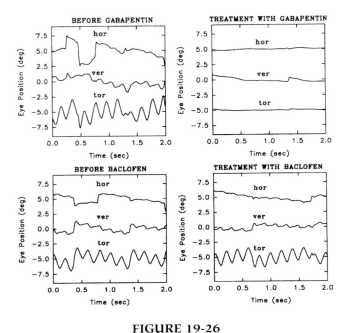

FIGURE 19-26

Effect of gabapentin and baclofen on acquired nystagmus in an MS patient. Gabapentin essentially abolished all components of the patient's nystagmus, whereas baclofen slightly reduced the vertical component. (From Averbuch-Heller L, et al. A double-blind controlled study of gabapentin and baclofen as treatment for acquired nystagmus. *Ann Neurol* 1997; 41:818–825).

visual feedback to the cerebellum, which is critical for the control of eye movements.

Other forms of nystagmus include convergence-retraction nystagmus, which occurs with midbrain lesions and usually coexists with upgaze paralysis (Parinaud's syndrome). In some cases convergence nystagmus may consist of asynchronous adducting saccades. It is not known whether adducting saccades alone can account for retraction or whether cocontraction of the extraocular muscles must occur as well.

Seesaw nystagmus, in which one eye elevates and intorts while the other eye depresses and extorts, also occurs with midbrain lesions and may be related to an imbalance in activity in structures (interstitial nucleus of Cajal) that receive projections from the labyrinthine otolith organs (163).

Dissociated nystagmus, which is greatest or present only in the abducting eye, most commonly occurs in INO. The mechanism of abducting nystagmus in INO is not known, although several hypotheses have been proposed (123). One hypothesis suggests that convergence is used to help adduct the weak eye, leading to abducting nystagmus in the other eye. Alternatively, an adaptive increase in saccadic innervation might help adduct the weak eye but, because of Hering's law of equal innervation, also would lead to abduction overshoot and nystagmus in the other eye. Other investigators have sug-

gested that the abducting nystagmus occurs because the lesion in the MLF interrupts either an ascending inhibitory pathway to the contralateral medial rectus muscle motoneurons or a descending excitatory pathway to contralateral abducens motoneurons. Finally, dissociated nystagmus in INO may reflect asymmetric gaze nystagmus because of involvement of structures outside but adjacent to the MLF. One or more of these mechanisms probably are responsible for the dissociated nystagmus in any patient with INO.

Treatment of Nystagmus

The treatment of nystagmus in MS is one of the most difficult challenges to the neurologist. Many pharmacologic agents have been used, most with only a modicum of effectiveness. Those agents that are successful in some patients may be ineffective in others. Such differences may relate to the variability of lesions between patients, involving different anatomic sites and affecting different neurotransmitter systems. Perhaps the best understood form of nystagmus is PAN, which occasionally occurs in patients with MS (169). Periodic alternating nystagmus is thought to result from dysfunction of the cerebellar nodulus, mani-

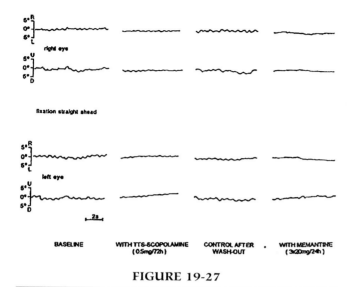

right eye

fixation straight ahead

left eye

| BASELINE | WITH TTS-SCOPOLAMINE (0.5mg/72h) | CONTROL AFTER WASH-OUT | WITH MEMANTINE (3x20mg/24h) |

FIGURE 19-27

Effect of scopolamine and memantine on acquired pendular nystagmus in a patient with MS. Scopolamine slightly diminished the amplitude of the nystagmus, whereas memantine induced almost complete cessation of nystagmus. Recordings are via DC-EOG with fixation straight ahead. R = right; L = left; U = up; D = down. (From Starck M, et al. Drug therapy for acquired pendular nystagmus in multiple sclerosis. *J Neurol* 1996; 627:1–8.)

festing as an instability in the velocity-storage mechanism. The projection from the nodulus to the vestibular nuclei uses GABA as the neurotranmitter. In this disorder, a GABA-β agonist, baclofen, restores deficient GABA activity in the vestibular nuclei and is effective in most patients who have this form of nystagmus (170,171).

In downbeat or upbeat nystagmus, clonazepam, a GABA-α agonist, has diminished the nystagmus and oscillopsia (172). Baclofen and scopolamine also have demonstrated some benefit.

In acquired pendular nystagmus, a variety of agents have been useful in selected patients. Averbuch-Heller and colleagues recently demonstrated that gabapentin, an anticonvulsive agent, significantly decreased pendular nystagmus (173) (Figure 19-26). Memantine, a glutamate antagonist, can dramatically abolish pendular nystagmus in patients with MS and may contribute to an improvement in visual acuity (174) (Figure 19-27).

References

1. Leibowitz U, Alter M. Optic nerve involvement and diplopia as initial manifestations of multiple sclerosis. *Acta Neurol Scand* 1968; 44:70–80.
2. Kuroiwa Y, Shibasaki H. Clinical studies of multiple sclerosis in Japan. I. A current appraisal of 83 cases. *Neurology* 1973; 23:609–617.
3. Wikström J, Poser S, Ritter G. Optic neuritis as an initial symptom in multiple sclerosis. *Acta Neurol Scand* 1980; 61:178–185.
4. Celesia GG, Kaufman DI, Brigell M, et al. Optic neuritis: A prospective study. *Neurology* 1990; 40:919–923.
5. Optic Neuritis Study Group. The clinical profile of optic neuritis: Experience of the optic neuritis treatment trial. *Arch Ophthalmol* 1991; 109:1673–1678.
6. Davis FA, Bergen D, Schauf C, McDonald WI, Deutsch W. Movement phosphenes in optic neuritis: A new clinical sign. *Neurology* 1976; 26:110–1104.
7. Lessell S, Cohen MM. Phosphenes induced by sound. *Neurology* 1979; 29:1524–1527.
8. Rushton D. Use of Pulfrich pendulum for detecting abnormal delay in the visual pathway in multiple sclerosis. *Brain* 1975; 98:283–296.
9. Regan D, Murray TJ, Silver R. Effect of body temperature on visual evoked potential delay and visual perception in multiple sclerosis. *J Neurol Neurosurg Psychiatry* 1977; 40:1083–1091.
10. Uhthoff W. Untersuchungen über die bei der multiplen Herdslerose Vorkommenden Augenstörungen. *Arch Psychiat Nervenkr* 1890; 21:55–116–303–410.
11. Nelson DA, Jeffreys WH, McDowell F. The effects of induced hyperthermia on some neurological diseases. *Arch Neurol Psychiat* 1958; 79:31–39.
12. Davis FA. The hot bath test in the diagnosis of multiple sclerosis. *J Mount Sinai Hosp NY* 1966; 33:280–282.
13. Smith JL, Hoyt WF, Susac JO. Ocular fundus in acute Leber's optic neuropathy. *Arch Ophthalmol* 1973; 90:349–354.
14. Raymond LA, Sacks JG, Choromokos E. Short posterior ciliary artery insufficiency with hyperthermia (Uhthoff's symptom). *Am J Ophthalmol* 1980; 90:619–623.
15. Goldstein JE, Cogan DG. Exercise and the optic neuropathy of multiple sclerosis. *Arch Ophthalmol* 1964; 72:168–176.
16. Honan WP, Heron JR, Foster DH, Snelgar RS. Paradoxical effects of temperature in multiple sclerosis. *J Neurol Neurosurg Psychiatry* 1987; 50:1160–1164.
17. Mathews WB, Read DJ, Pountney E. Effect of raising body temperature on visual and somatosensory evoked potentials in patients with multiple sclerosis. *J Neurol Neurosurg Psychiatry* 1979; 42:250–255.
18. Persson HE, Sachs C. Visual evoked potentials elicited by pattern reversal during provoked visual impairment in multiple sclerosis. *Brain* 1981; 104:369–382.
19. Bode DD. The Uhthoff phenomenon. *Am J Ophthalmol* 1978; 85:721–722.
20. Davis FA, Jacobson S. Altered thermal sensitivity in injured and demyelinated nerve: A possible model of temperature effects in multiple sclerosis. *J Neurol Neurosurg Psychiatry* 1971; 34:551–561.
21. Rasminsky M. The effects of temperature on conduction in demyelinated single nerve fibers. *Arch Neurol* 1973; 28:287–292.
22. Scherokman BJ, Selhorst JB, Waybright EA, et al. Improved optic nerve conduction with ingestion of ice water. *Ann Neurol* 1985; 17:418–419.
23. Davies HD, Carroll WM, Mastaglia FL. Effects of hyperventilation on patternreversal visual evoked potentials in patients with demyelination. *J Neurol Neurosurg Psychiatry* 1986; 49:1392–1396.
24. Selhorst JB, Saul RF, Waybright EA. Optic nerve conduction: Opposing effects of exercise and hyperventilation. *Trans Am Neurol Assoc* 1981; 106:101–105.

25. Bever CT, Young D, Anderson PA. The effects of 4-aminopyridine in multiple sclerosis patients: Results of a randomized, placebo-controlled, double-blind, concentration-controlled, crossover trial. *Neurology* 1994; 44:1054–1059.

26. Ménage MJ, Papakostopoulos D, Dean Hart JC, Papakostopoulos S, Gogolitsyn Y. The Farnsworth-Munsell 100 hue test in the first episode of demyelinating optic neuritis. *Brit J Ophthal* 1993; 77:68–74.

27. Nikoskelainen E, Falck B. Do visual evoked potentials give relevant information to the neuro-ophthalmological examination in optic nerve lesions? *Acta Neurol Scand* 1982; 66:42–57.

28. Miller NR. Optic neuritis. In: *Walsh and Hoyt's clinical neuroophthalmology,* 4th ed. Baltimore: Williams & Wilkins, 1982:227–248.

29. Keltner JL, Johnson CA, Spurr JO, Beck RW, Optic Neuritis Study Group. Baseline visual field profile of optic neuritis: The experience of the Optic Neuritis Treatment Trial. *Arch Ophthalmol* 1993; 111:231–234.

30. Halliday AM, McDonald WI, Mushin J. Visual evoked response in diagnosis of multiple sclerosis. *Br Med J* 1973; 4:661–664.

31. Bodes Wollner I, Ghialardi MF Mylin LH. The importance of stimulus selection in VEP preactice: The clinical relevance of visual physiology. In: Cracco RQ, Bodes-Wollner I (eds.). *Frontiers of clinical neuroscience: Evoked potentials.* New York: Alan R. Liss, 1986:15–27.

32. Warner J, Lessell S. Neuro-ophthalmology of multiple sclerosis. *Clin Neurosci* 1994; 2:180–188.

33. Drislane FW. Use of evoked potentials in the diagnosis and follow-up of multiple sclerosis. *Clinical Neuroscience* 1994; 2:196–201.

34. Chiappa KH. Pattern-shift evoked potentials: Interpretation. In: Chiappa KH (ed.). *Evoked potentials in clinical medicine,* 2nd ed. New York: Raven Press, 1990:111–154.

35. Wright CE, Drasdo N, Harding GFA. Pathology of the optic nerve and visual association areas: Information given by the flash and pattern evoked potential, and the temporal and spatial contrast sensitivity function. *Brain* 1987; 110:107–120.

36. Ashworth B, Aspinall PA, Mitchell JD. Visual function in multiple sclerosis. *Doc Ophthalmol* 1990; 73:209–224.

37. Pinckers A, Cruysberg JRM. Colour vision, visually evoked potentials and lightness discrimination in patients with multiple sclerosis. *Neuro-Ophthalmol* 1992; 12:251–256.

38. Halliday AM, McDonald WI, Mushin J. Delayed pattern-evoked responses in optic neuritis in relation to visual acuity. *Trans Ophthalmol Soc UK* 1973; 93:315–324.

39. Hely MA, McManis PG, Walsh JC, McLeod JG. Visual evoked responses and ophthalmological examination in optic neuritis. A follow-up study. *J Neurol Sci* 1986; 75:275–283.

40. Heinrichs IH, McLean DR. Evolution of visual evoked potentials in optic neuritis. *Can J Neurol Sci* 1988; 15:394–396.

41. Sokol S. The visually evoked cortical potential in optic nerve and visual pathway disorders. In: Fishman GA Sokol S (eds.). *Electrophysiologic testing in disorders of the retina, optic nerve, and visual pathway.* San Francisco: American Academy of Ophthalmology, 1990:105–141.

42. van Diemen HAM, Polman CH, van Dongen MMMM, et al. 4-aminopyridine induces functional improvement in multiple sclerosis patients: A neurophysiological study. *J Neurol Sci* 1993; 116:220–226.

43. Kermode AG, Thompson AJ, Tofts PS. Breakdown of the blood-brain barrier precedes symptoms and other MRI signs of new lesions in multiple sclerosis. *Brain* 1990; 113:1477–1489.

44. Youl BD, Turano G, Miller DH, et al. The pathophysiology of acute optic neuritis: The association of gadolinium leakage with clinical and electrophysiological deficits. *Brain* 1991; 114:2437–2450.

45. Kaufman DI, Pernicone JR. Advances in MRI and the impact on neuro-ophthalmology. *Sem Ophthalmol* 1992; 7:122.

46. Beck RW, Arrington J, Murtagh FR, Cleary PA, Kaufman DI, Optic Neuritis Study Group. Brain magnetic resonance imaging in acute optic neuritis: Experience of the Optic Neuritis Study Group. *Arch Neurol* 1993; 50:841–846.

47. Hornabrook RSL, Miller DH, Newton MR, et al. Frequent involvement of the optic radiation in patients with acute isolated optic neuritis. *Neurology* 1992; 42:77–79.

48. Miller DH, Newton MR, van der Poel JC, et al. Magnetic resonance imaging of the optic nerve in optic neuritis. *Neurology* 1988; 38:175–179.

49. Poser CM, Paty DW, Scheinberg L, et al. New diagnostic criteria for multiple sclerosis: Guidelines for research protocals. *Ann Neurol* 1983; 13:227–231.

50. Frederiksen JL, Larsson HBW, Henriksen O. Magnetic resonance imaging of the brain in patients with acute monosymptomatic optic neuritis. *Acta Neurol Scand* 1989; 80:512–517.

51. Morrissey SP, Miller DH, Kendall BE. The significance of brain magnetic resonance imaging abnormalities at presentation with clinically isolated syndromes suggestive of multiple sclerosis. *Brain* 1993; 116:135–146.

52. Optic Neuritis Study Group. Visual function 5 years after optic neuritis: Experience of the Optic Neuritis Study Group. *Arch Ophthalmol* 1997; 115:1545–1552.

53. Optic Neuritis Study Group. The five-year risk of multiple sclerosis after optic neuritis: Experience of the Optic Neuritis Treatment Trial. *Neurology* 1997; 49:1404–1413.

54. Beck RW, Cleary PA, Anderson MM, et al. A randomized, controlled trial of corticosteroids in the treatment of acute optic neuritis. *N Engl J Med* 1992; 326:581–588.

55. Paty DW, Li DKB, the UBC MS/MRI Study Group, the IFNB Multiple Sclerosis Study Group. Interferon beta-1b is effective in relapsing-remitting multiple sclerosis: II. MRI analysis results of a multicenter, randomized, double-blind, placebo-controlled trial. *Neurology* 1993; 43:662–667.

56. The IFNB Multiple Sclerosis Study Group. Interferon beta-1b is effective in relapsing-remitting multiple sclerosis: I. Clinical results of a multicenter, randomized, double-blind, placebo-controlled trial. *Neurology* 1993; 43:655–661.

57. Jacobs LD, Cookfair DL, Rudick RA. Intramuscular interferon beta-1a for disease progression in relapsing multiple sclerosis. *Ann Neurol* 1996; 39:285–294.

58. Johnson KP, Brooks BR, Cohen JA, et al. Copolymer 1 reduces relapse rate and improves disability in relapsing-remitting multiple sclerosis: Results of a phase III multicenter, double-blind, placebo-controlled trial. *Neurology* 1995; 45:1268–1276.

59. Beck RW, Cleary PA, Optic Neuritis Study Group. Optic Neuritis Treatment Trial: One-year follow-up results. *Arch Ophthalmol* 1993; 111:773–775.

60. Beck RW. The Optic Neuritis Treatment Trial: Implications for clinical practice. *Arch Ophthalmol* 1992; 110:331–332.

61. Cohen MM, Lessell S, Wolf PA. A prospective study of the risk of developing multiple sclerosis in uncomplicated optic neuritis. *Neurology* 1979; 208:213.

62. Francis DA, Compston DAS, Batchelor JR, McDonald WI. A reassessment of the risk of multiple sclerosis developing in patients with optic neuritis after extended follow-up. *J Neurol Neurosurg Psychiatry* 1987; 50:758–765.

63. Rizzo JF, Lessell S. Risk of developing multiple sclerosis after uncomplicated optic neuritis: A long-term prospective study. *Neurology* 1988; 38:185–190.

64. Sandberg-Wollheim M, Bynke H, Cronqvist S. A long-term prospective study of optic neuritis: Evaluation of risk factors. *Ann Neurol* 1990; 27:386–393.

65. Kesselring J. *Multiple sclerosis*. Cambridge, UK: Cambridge University Press, 1997;

66. Beck RW. Optic neuritis. In: Miller NR, Newman NJ (eds.). *Walsh and Hoyt's clinical neuroophthalmology*, 5th ed. Baltimore: Williams & Wilkins, 1998:599–647.

67. Sedwick LA. Optic neuritis. *Neurol Clin* 1991; 9: 97–114.

68. Beck RW, Kupersmith MJ, Cleary PA, Katz B, Optic Neuritis Study Group. Fellow eye abnormalities in acute unilateral optic neuritis: Experience of the Optic Neuritis Treatment Trial. *Ophthalmology* 1993; 100:691–697.

69. Patterson VH, Heron JR. Visual field abnormalities in multiple sclerosis. *J Neurol Neurosurg Psychiatry* 1980; 43:205–208.

70. Kriss A, Francis DA, Cuendet F, et al. Recovery after optic neuritis in childhood. *J Neurol Neurosurg Psychiatry* 1988; 51:1253–1258.

71. Kennedy C, Carroll FD. Optic neuritis in children. *Arch Ophthalmol* 1960; 63:747–755.

72. Meadows SP. Retrobulbar and optic neuritis in childhood and adolescence. *Trans Ophthalmol Soc UK* 1969; 89:603–638.

73. Koraszewska-Matuszewska B, Samochowiec-Donocik E, Rynkiewicz E. Optic neuritis in children and adolescents. *Klin Oczna* 1995; 97:207–210.

74. Riikonen R. The role of infection and vaccination in the genesis of optic neuritis and multiple sclerosis in children. *Acta Neurol Scand* 1989; 80:425–431.

75. Farris BF, Pickard DJ. Bilateral postinfectious optic neuritis and intravenous steroid therapy in children. *Ophthalmology* 1990; 97:339–345.

76. Steinlin MI, Blaser SI, MacGregor DL, Buncic JR. Eye problems in children with multiple sclerosis. *Pediatr Neurol* 1998; 12:207–212.

77. Jeffery AR, Buncic JR. Pediatric Devic's neuromyelitis optica. *J Pediatr Ophthalmol Strabismus* 1996; 33:223–229.

78. Whitham RH, Brey RL. Neuromyelitis optica: Two new cases and a review of the literature. *J Clin Neuroophthalmol* 1985; 5:263–269.

79. Filley CM, Sternberg PE, Norenberg MD. Neuromyelitis optica in the elderly. *Arch Neurol* 1984; 41:670–672.

80. Allen IV, Kirk J. Demyelinating diseases. In: Adams JH, Duchen LW (eds.). *Greenfield's neuropathology*, 5th ed. New York: Oxford University Press, 1992:447–520.

81. Mandler RN, Davis LE, Jeffery DR, Kornfeld M. Devic's neuromyelitis optica: A clinicopathological study of 8 patients. *Ann Neurol* 1993; 34:162–168.

82. Piccolo G, Franciotta DM, Camana C, et al. Devic's neuromyelitis optica: Long-term follow-up and serial CSF findings in two cases. *J Neurol* 1990; 237:262–264.

83. Kerty E, Eide N, Nakstad P, Nyberg-Hansen R. Chiasmal optic neuritis. *Acta Ophthalmol* 1991; 69:135–139.

84. Newman NJ, Lessell S, Winterkorn JMS. Optic chiasmal neuritis. *Neurology* 1991; 41:1203–1212.

85. Lehoczky T. Pathologic changes in the optic system in disseminated sclerosis. *Acta Morphol Acad Sci Hung* 1953; 4:395–408.

86. Plant GT, Kermode AG, Turano G, et al. Symptomatic retrochiasmal lesions in multiple sclerosis: Clinical features, visual evoked potentials, and magnetic resonance imaging. *Neurology* 1992; 42:68–76.

87. Vighetto A, Grochowicki M, Callieco R, et al. Altitudinal hemianopia in multiple sclerosis. *Neuro-Ophthalmol* 1991; 11:25–27.

88. Luccinetti CF, Rodriguez M. The controversy surrounding the pathogenesis of the multiple sclerosis lesion. *Mayo Clin Proc* 1997; 72:665–678.

89. Beck RW, Cleary PA, Trobe JD, et al. The effect of corticosteroids for acute optic neuritis on the subsequent development of multiple sclerosis. *N Engl J Med* 1993; 329:1764–1769.

90. Beck RW, Optic Neuritis Study Group. The Optic Neuritis Treatment Trial: Three-year follow-up results. *Arch Ophthalmol* 1995; 113:136.

91. Kupersmith MJ, Kaufman D, Paty DW, et al. Megadose corticosteroids in multiple sclerosis. *Neurology* 1994; 44:14.

92. Corbett JJ, Cruse JM. Corticosteroids and optic neuritis. *Neurology* 1993; 43:634.

93. Frey BM, Frey FJ, Holford NHG, Lozada F, Benet L. Prednisolone pharmacodynamics assessed by inhibition of the mixed lymphocyte reaction. *Transplantation* 1990; 33:578–584.

94. Haynes BF, Fauci AS. The differential effect of in vivo hydrocortisone on the kinetics of subpopulations of human peripheral blood thymus-derived lymphocytes. *J Clin Invest* 1978; 61:703–707.

95. Mix E, Olsson T, Correale J, Kostulas V, Link H. CD4+, CD8+, and CD4–, CD8– T-cells in CSF and blood of patients with multiple sclerosis and tension headache. *Scand J Immunol* 1990; 31:493–501.

96. Reder AT, Thapar M, Jensen MA. A reduction in serum glucocorticoids provokes experimental allergic encephalomyelitis: Implications for treatment of inflammatory brain disease. *Neurology* 1994; 44:2289–2294.

97. Chrousos GA, Kattah JC, Beck RW, Cleary PA, Optic Neuritis Study Group. Side effects of glucocorticoid treatment: Experience of the Optic Neuritis Treatment Trial. *JAMA* 1993; 269:2110–2112.

98. Arnold AC, Pepose JS, Hepler RS, Foos RY. Retinal periphlebitis and retinitis in multiple sclerosis: I. Pathological characteristics. *Ophthalmology* 1984; 91:255–261.

99. Breger BC, Leopold IH. The incidence of uveitis in multiple sclerosis. *Am J Ophthalmol* 1966; 62:540–545.

100. Bamford CR, Ganley JP, Sibley WA, Laguna JF. Uveitis, perivenous sheathing and multiple sclerosis. *Neurology* 1978; 28(2):119–124.

101. Zierhut M, Foster CS. Multiple sclerosis, sarcoidosis, and other systemic diseases in patients with pars planitis. *Dev Ophthalmol* 1992; 23:447.

102. Malinowski SM, Pulido JS, Folk JC. Long-term visual outcome and complications associated with pars planitis. *Ophthalmology* 1993; 100:818–825.

103. Toussaint D, Perier O, Verstappen A, Bervoets S. Clinicopathological study of the visual pathways, eyes, and cerebral hemispheres in 32 cases of disseminated sclerosis. *J Clin Neuroophthalmol* 1983; 3:211–220.

104. Gills JP Jr. Electroretinographic abnormalities and advanced multiple sclerosis. *Invest Ophthalmol* 1966; 5:555–559.

105. Lightman S, McDonald WI, Bird AC, et al. Retinal venous sheathing in optic neuritis: Its significance for the pathogenesis of multiple sclerosis. *Brain* 1987; 110:405–414.

106. Leigh J, Zee D. *The neurology of eye movements.* Philadelphia: FA Davis, 1991.

107. Skavenski AA, Robinson DA. Role of abducens neurons in the vestibular ocular reflex. *J Neurophysiol* 1973; 36:724–738.

108. Ranalli P, Sharpe JA. Contrapulsion of saccades and ipsilateral ataxia: A unilateral disorder of the rostral cerebellum. *Ann Neurol* 1986; 20:311–316.

109. Straube A, Buttner U. Pathophysiology of saccadic contrapulsion in unilateral rostral cerebellar lesions. *J Neuro-ophthalmol* 1994; 3:7.

110. Solomon D, Galetta SL, Liu GT. Possible mechanisms for horizontal gaze deviation and lateropulsion in the lateral medullary syndrome. *J Neuro-ophthalmol* 1995; 15:26–30.

111. Ashe J, Hain TC, Zee DS, et al. Microsaccadic flutter. *Brain* 1991; 114:461–472.

112. Todman DH. A paroxysmal ocular motility disorder in multiple sclerosis. *Aust NZ J Med* 1988; 18:785–787.

113. Twomey JA, Espir MLE. Paroxysmal symptoms as the first manifestations of multiple sclerosis. *J Neurol Neurosurg Psychiatry* 1980; 43:296–304.

114. Mastaglia FL, Black JL, Collins DWF. Quantitative studies of saccadic and pursuit eye movements in MS. *Brain* 1979; 102:817–834.

115. Ochs AL, Hoyt WF, Stark L, et al. Saccadic initiation time in multiple sclerosis. *Ann Neurol* 1978; 4:578–579.

116. Muri RM, Meienberg O. The clinical spectrum of internuclear ophthalmoplegia in multiple sclerosis. *Arch Neurol* 1985; 42:851–855.

117. Meienberg O, Muri R, Rabineau PA. Clinical and oculographic examinations of saccadic eye movements in the diagnosis of multiple sclerosis. *Arch Neurol* 1986; 43:438–443.

118. Solinger LD, Baloh RW, Myers L, et al. Subclinical eye movement disorders in patients with multiple sclerosis. *Neurology* 1977; 27:614–619.

119. Zee DS. Internuclear ophthalmoplegia: Pathophysiology and diagnosis. *Bailliere's Clin Neurol* 1992; 1:455–470.

120. Cogan, D.G. Internuclear ophthalmoplegia, typical and atypical. *Arch Ophthalmol* 1977; 84:583–589.

121. McGettrick P, Eustace P. The w.e.b.i.n.o. syndrome. *Neuro-ophthalmology* 1985; 5:109–115.

122. Baloh RW, Yee RD, Honrubia V. Internuclear ophthalmoplegia. I.Saccades and dissociated nystagmus. *Arch Neurol* 1978; 35:484–489.

123. Zee DS, HainTC, Carl JR. Abduction nystagmus in internuclear ophthalmoplegia. *Ann Neurol* 1987; 21:383–388.

124. Bronstein AM, Rudge P, Gresty MA, Du Boulay G, Morris J. Abnormalities of horizontal gaze: Clinical, oculographic, and magnetic resonance imaging findings. II. Gaze palsy and internuclear ophthalmoplegia. *J Neurol Neurosurg Psychiatry* 1990; 53:200–207.

125. Kommerell G, Olivier D, Theopold H. Adaptive programming of phasic and tonic components in saccadic eye movements. Investigations in patients with abducens palsy. *Invest Ophthalmol Vis Sci* 1976; 15:657–660.

126. Evinger LC, Fuchs AF, Baker R. Bilateral lesions of the medial longitudinal fasciculus in monkeys: Effects on the horizontal and vertical components of voluntary and vestibular induced eye movements. *Exp Brain Res* 1977; 28:1–20.

127. Ranalli PJ, Sharpe JA. Vertical vestibulo-ocular reflex, smooth pursuit and eye-head tracking dysfunction in internuclear ophthalmoplegia. *Brain* 1988; 111:1299–1317.

128. Jenkyn LR, Margolis G, Reeves AG. Reflex vertical gaze and the medial longitudinal fasciculus. *J Neurol Neurosurg Psychiatry* 1978; 41:1084–1091.

129. Pola J, Robinson DA. An explanation of eye movements seen in internuclear ophthalmoplegia. *Arch Neurol* 1976; 33:447–452.

130. Nozaki S, Mukuno K, Ishikawa S. Internuclear ophthalmoplegia associated with ipsilateral downbeat nystagmus and contralateral incyclorotary nystagmus. *Ophthalmology* 1983; 187:210–216.

131. Ventre J, Vighetto A, Bailly G, Prablanc C. Saccade metrics in multiple sclerosis: Versional velocity disconjugacy as the best clue? *J Neurol Sci* 1991; 102:144–149.

132. Flipse JP, Straahof CSM, Van der Steen J, et al. Binocular saccadic eye movements in multiple sclerosis. *J Neurol Sci* 1997; 148:53–65.

133. Smith JL, Cogan DG. Internuclear ophthalmoplegia: A review of 58 cases. *Arch Ophthalmol* 1959; 61:687–694.

134. Crane TB, Yee RD, Baloh RW, Hepler RS. Analysis of characteristic eye movement abnormalities in internuclear ophthalmoplegia. *Arch Ophthalmol* 1983; 101:206–210.

135. Atlas SW, Grossman RI, Savino PJ, et al. Internuclear ophthalmoplegia: MR-anatomic correlation. *Am J Neuro-radiol* 1986; 8:243–247.

136. Schmidt D. Signs in ocular myasthenia and pseudomyasthenia. Differential diagnostic criteria: A clinical review. *Neuro-Ophthalmology* 1995; 15:21–58.

137. Mauri L, et al. Evaluation of endocrine ophthalmopathy with saccadic eye movements. *J Neurol* 1984; 231: 182–187.

138. Wall M, Wray SH. The one-and-a-half syndrome—A unilateral disorder of the pontine tegmentum: A study of 20 cases and review of the literature. *Neurology* 1983; 33:971–980.

139. Sharpe JA, Goldberg J, Lo AW, et al. Visual-vestibular interaction in multiple sclerosis. *Neurology* 1981; 31:427–433.

140. Reulen JPH, Sanders EACM, Hogenhuis LAH. Eye movement disorders in multiple sclerosis and optic neuritis. *Brain* 1983; 106:121–140.

141. Ivers RR, Goldstein NP. Multiple sclerosis: A current appraisal of symptoms and signs. *Proc Mayo Clin* 1963; 38:457–466.

142. Rush JA, Younge BR. Paralysis of cranial nerves III, IV, and VI. *Arch Ophthalmol* 1981; 99:76–79.

143. Keane JR. Bilateral sixth nerve palsy: Analysis of 125 cases. *Arch Neurol* 1976; 33:681–683.

144. Moster ML, Savino PJ, Segott RC, et al. Isolated sixth nerve palsies in younger adults. *Arch Ophthalmol* 1984; 102:1328–1330.

145. Joseph R, Pullicino P, Goldberg CD, et al. Bilateral pontine gaze palsy: Nuclear magnetic resonance findings in presumed multiple sclerosis. *Arch Neurol* 1985; 42:93–94.

146. Miller N. Multiple sclerosis and related demyelinating diseases. In: Miller NR (ed.). *Clinical neuro-ophthalmology*. Baltimore: Williams & Wilkins, 1995:4324.

147. Ksiazek SM, Repka MX, Maguire A, et al. Divisional oculomotor nerve paresis caused by intrinsic brainstem disease. *Ann Neurol* 1989; 26:714–718.

148. Savitsky N, Rangell L. The ocular findings in multiple sclerosis. *Proc Assoc Res Nerv Dis* 1950; 28:403–413.

149. Vanooteghem P, Dehaene I, Van Zandycke M, Casselman J. Combined trochlear nerve palsy and internuclear ophthalmoplegia. *Arch Neurol* 1992; 49:108–109.

150. Keane JR. Gaze evoked blepharoclonus. *Ann Neurol* 1978; 3:243–245.

151. Herrera WG. Vestibular and other balance disorders in multiple sclerosis. *Neurol Clin* 1990; 2:407–420.

152. Aantaa E, et al. Electronystagmographic findings in multiple sclerosis. *Acta Otolaryngol* 1973; 75:1–5.

153. Francis DA, et al. The site of brainstem lesions causing semicircular canal paresis: An MRI study. *J Neurol Neurosurg Psychiatry* 1992; 55:446–449.

154. Sharpe JA, et al. Visual-vestibular interaction in multiple sclerosis. *Neurology* 1981; 31:427–433.

155. Baloh RW, et al. Vestibulo-ocular function in patients with cerebellar atrophy. *Neurology* 1975; 25:160–168.

156. Alpert JN. Failure of fixation suppression: A pathologic effect of vision on caloric nystagmus. *Neurology* 1974; 24:891–896.

157. Noffsinger D, et al. Auditory and vestibular aberrations in multiple sclerosis. *Acta Otolaryngol* 1972; 303(Suppl):192–198.

158. Huygen PLM. Vestibular hyperreactivity in patients with multiple sclerosis. *Adv Oto-Rhino-Laryngol* 1983; 30:141–149.

159. Twomey JA, Espir MLE. Paroxysmal symptoms as the first manifestations of multiple sclerosis. *J Neurol Neurosurg Psychiatry* 1980; 43:296–304.

160. Mathews WB, et al. (eds.). *McAlpine's multiple sclerosis*. New York: Churchill Livingstone, 1985.

161. Osterman PO, Westerberg CE. Paroxysmal attacks in multiple sclerosis. *Brain* 1975; 98:189–202.

162. Abb L, Schaltenbrand G. Statistische Untersuchungen zum Problem der multplen Sklerosen. II. Mitteilung. Das Drankheitsbild der multiple Sklerose. *Deutsch Z Nervenheilk* 1956; 174:199.

163. Katsarkas A. Positional nystagmus of the "central type" as an early sign of multiple sclerosis. *J Otolaryngol* 1982; 11:91–93.

164. Greasty MA, et al. Acquired pendular nystagmus: Its characteristics, localizing value and pathophysiology. *J Neurol Neurosurg Psychiatry* 1982; 45:431–439.

165. Aschoff JC, et al. Acquired pendular nystagmus with oscillopsia in multiple sclerosis: A sign of cerebellar nuclei disease. *J Neurol Neurosurg Psychiatry* 1974; 37:570–577.

166. Smith JL, et al. Monocular vertical oscillations of amblyopia: The Heimann-Bielschowsky phenomenon. *J Clin Neuro Ophthalmol* 1982; 2:85–91.

167. Barton JJS, Cox TA. Acquired pendular nystagmus in multiple sclerosis: Clinical observations and the role of optic neuropathy. *J Neurol Neurosurg Psychiatry* 1993; 56:262–267.

168. Samkoff LM, Smith CR. See-saw nystagmus in a patient with clinically definite multiple sclerosis. *Eur Neurol* 1994; 34:228–229.

169. Keane JR. PAN with downward beating nystagmus. *Arch Neurol* 1974; 30:399–402.

170. Halmagyi GM, et al. Treatment of periodic alternating nystagmus. *Ann Neurol* 1980; 8:609–611.

171. Furman JMR, et al. Vestibular function in periodic alternating nystagmus. *Brain* 1990; 113:1425–1439.

172. Currie JN, Matsuo V. The use of clonazepam in the treatment of nystagmus-induced oscillopsia. *Ophthalmology* 1986; 93:924–932.

173. Averbuch-Heller L, Tusa RJ, Fuhry L, et al. A double-blind controlled study of gabapentin and baclofen as treatment for acquired nystagmus. *Ann Neurol* 1997; 41:818–825.

174. Starck M, Albrecht H, Pollmann W, Straube A, Dieterich M. Drug therapy for acquired pendular nystagmus in multiple sclerosis. *J Neurol* 1996; 627:1–8.

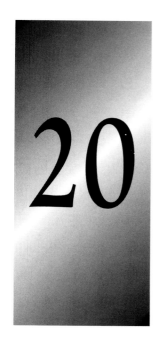

20 Paroxysmal Disorders

Aaron Miller, M.D.

Whereas typical relapses of multiple sclerosis (MS) consist of symptoms that persist for days to weeks or longer, an unusual feature of the disease is the occurrence of brief paroxysms of neurologic dysfunction. These phenomena tend to recur in stereotypical fashion over a period of time. When they do, most MS authorities consider the *cluster* of episodes to represent an exacerbation of MS. Although these paroxysmal symptoms differ remarkably in their clinical features, they nonetheless behave similarly in several respects, including their temporal profile and response to therapy.

Paroxysmal symptoms can occur at any time during the course of MS. Notably, several authors have documented the episodes as the initial manifestation of the disease (1–8). With the advent of prophylactic immunotherapy for MS, it has become particularly important to recognize that such phenomena may herald the disorder so that opportunity for early initiation of treatment is not lost.

PAROXYSMAL SYMPTOMS

Paroxysmal Pain

Trigeminal Neuralgia

Trigeminal neuralgia (TN) is probably the most fre-
quently occurring paroxysmal symptom in MS. This condition, like that of other forms of trigeminal neuralgia, is characterized by sudden, severe jabs of pain, occurring most often in the distribution of the second and third divisions of the nerve. These jolts, which are often described as *lancinating* or resembling an *electric shock*, may occur repetitively and often are triggered by sensory stimuli. The pain may be prompted by a light touch to the area, chewing, or as little as a gentle breeze.

Using a definition of trigeminal neuralgia as "brief, severe, paroxysmal pain within the distribution of the trigeminal nerve that could not be attributed to dental or other causes," but not requiring a trigger, Hooge and Redekop (9) reported 35 patients from a population of 1,882 individuals with MS, for an incidence of 1.9 percent. This prevalence was considerably higher than the 4.3 of 100,000 occurrence reported in the Rochester, Minnesota, population experience with trigeminal neuralgia (10). The pain began an average of 11.8 years after the first symptoms of MS. However, in five patients, trigeminal neuralgia was the initial manifestation of the disease, preceding the next symptoms by 1 to 11 years.

In this series, the age of onset of trigeminal neuralgia was younger than is typically seen in the idiopathic disorder only in those patients for whom it was the initial manifestation of the disease. In those individuals whose trigeminal pain was the first symptom, the syndrome began at a mean age of 38.2 years, significantly different from the 53.2 years of those whose disease began first. Gender distribution did not differ among those patients with idiopathic trigeminal neuralgia compared with the MS population.

Another significant difference between MS patients with TN and patients with idiopathic TN was the frequent coexistence of other signs of brainstem dysfunction. At the onset of the neuralgia, 3 of 23 MS patients had diminished facial sensation, whereas 10 of 23 patients had other brainstem signs. These authors found bilateral occurrence in 14 percent, considerably different from the 4 percent to 5 percent typically reported with the idiopathic disorder.

In an earlier report, Rushton and Olafson reported the Mayo Clinic experience between 1948 and 1962 (10). The authors reviewed all cases of MS and trigeminal neuralgia and found the disorders coexisting in 35 individuals. It is important to note, however, that this paper excluded patients with objective sensory or motor deficits involving the fifth cranial nerve. In their series, symptoms of MS preceded trigeminal neuralgia in 30 patients, by 1 to 29 years. In four instances, the trigeminal neuralgia occurred one month to three years before other evidence of MS.

In contrast to the more recent series cited previously, in this study the mean age of onset in the TN/MS patients—45.2 years—was statistically significantly younger than the 50.7 year mean age of onset for the general population of TN patients. Like the Vancouver experience, this study also found a greater incidence of bilaterality (11 percent) in the TN/MS patients compared with those without the demyelinating disease. Notably, 7 of 35 patients in this series reported the occurrence of painless paresthesias in the face preceding the onset of trigeminal neuralgia by 4 to 21 years.

Treatment options and responses do not appear to differ significantly for TN/MS compared with the idiopathic disorder. Patients often respond to anticonvulsants, particularly carbamazepine. In the Vancouver series, 27 patients were treated with carbamazepine. Ten patients experienced complete relief and another 10 reported partial response. Four patients had to discontinue the drug because of side effects, whereas two other patients experienced no improvement. Gabapentin has recently been reported to be effective (11). Interestingly, Reder and Arnason have observed a response to misoprostol, a long-acting prostaglandin E_1 analogue, in six of seven patients with TN/MS who had failed conventional pharmacotherapy (12).

A recent study reported the findings on magnetic resonance imaging (MRI) in seven consecutive patients with TN/MS (13). Of the five subjects with unilateral involvement, three patients had vascular compression of the fifth nerve at the root entry zone on the symptomatic side and one patient had an epidermoid tumor distorting the nerve. A demyelinating plaque was identified in only one patient, affecting the trigeminal nerve at the root entry zone in the pons.

In the two patients with bilateral pain, neurovascular compression was identified on both sides in one patient and on one side in the other patient. Microvascular decompression eliminated the pain in the two patients on whom the procedure was performed. Unfortunately, one of these—the patient with the demyelinating plaque—died of pulmonary infection five days after surgery. Another reported patient who underwent microvascular decompression experienced only partial relief.

Surgical therapy is a viable option for trigeminal neuralgia. Hooge and Redekop reported that of 14 patients undergoing radiofrequency rhizotomy, eight became pain-free and five others had partial relief (9). Two patients (one of whom also had radiofrequency rhizotomy) experienced complete relief and partial relief, respectively.

In another series, Brisman reported his consecutive experience with radiofrequency electrocoagulation (RFE) of the gasserian ganglion and the retrogasserian rootlets in patients with TN/MS and patients with isolated TN (14). Bilateral procedures were performed in 31 percent of the former, compared with 10.5 percent of the latter. The average age at first RFE in the idiopathic group was 63.5, significantly older than the age of 50 for the TN/MS group. In the TN/MS group, 13 of 16 patients had evidence of other brainstem involvement (four with internuclear ophthalmoplegia, eight with nystagmus, and one with abnormal brainstem auditory-evoked response). The procedural results did not show a statistically significantly different ipsilateral recurrence rate in the TN/MS group compared with that of the TN without MS group.

In another study, Kondziolko and coworkers reported good or excellent results of glycerol rhizotomy in 53 patients with TN/MS after a median follow-up period of 36 months [15]. The reoperation rate was 30 percent.

Other Pain

Paroxysmal pain can also occur elsewhere in the body. In their report of 14 of their own patients with paroxysmal symptoms, Twomey and Espir included six patients with pain, three of whom also experienced paresthesias (4). In a review of the literature by these authors, they encountered reports of nine other patients, seven of whom were male. The pain usually involved a single limb. Few authors have commented on the pain quality, but Osterman and Westenberg described one patient with an "ache" lasting 5 to 10 seconds and occurring approximately 12 times daily (16).

Patients with these pain syndromes have a response to pharmacologic therapy that is similar to the response of patients with trigeminal neuralgia. Twomey and Espir noted a response to carbamazepine in seven of the nine patients noted previously.

Tonic Spasms

A distinctive feature of MS is the occurrence of a paroxysmal dystonia, which has been variably referred to as *tonic spasms* or *tonic seizures*. It is preferable to avoid the latter term because these episodes are not epileptic.

Several authors (4,7,8,17–22), particularly Matthews (1), have provided detailed descriptions of these phenomena. The episodes are unilateral, almost always involving the arm, with or without the leg, and are "remarkably consistent in the extent of involvement of the spell from day to day." The episodes are brief, usually less than a minute. They occur frequently, often several or more times a day, and tend to occur in clusters. Pain, at times severe, is sometimes a feature. Episodes are at times precipitated by hyperventilation or movement.

Matthews reported 15 patients, in two of whom the tonic seizures, as he called them, were the initial manifestation of MS. All episodes were unilateral, involving the arm and, in nine cases, also the leg. The arm assumed variable positions, but the leg always showed extension at the hip and knee, with plantar flexion of the foot. Pain was present in seven patients. Movement or sensory stimulation precipitated the spasms in 13 patients, and three of seven patients (where queried) reported spasms triggered by hyperventilation. The longest observed episode was 90 seconds, and the longest was estimated by a patient at two minutes.

In 11 of Matthews's patients, the paroxysms appeared abruptly and persisted for two days to two months, resolving either spontaneously or with treatment, and not recurring when the medication was discontinued. The other four patients had a different temporal pattern, with infrequent episodes occurring over a period of one to four years. Five of the patients had other types of paroxysmal symptoms.

Matthews's detailed description of one of his patients, a 48-year-old woman with a 10-year history of MS, is illustrative of this clinical feature:

> . . . on putting her left foot to ground on getting out of bed one morning, she felt a "peculiar, horrid" sensation in the foot, rapidly spreading up the leg and then involving the left arm. The arm and leg became stiff and she had to sit down, but the attack passed off in about 30 seconds. During the next two weeks she experienced similar attacks with great frequency, often having three in 15 minutes and over 30 in a day. The attacks all began in the foot and followed a stereotyped pattern, the foot being inverted, and foot and toes plantar flexed, the upper limb semi-flexed at the elbow and fully flexed at the wrist and metacarpophalangeal joints, the fingers being extended at the interphalangeal joints. The limbs were held stiffly in this position and she experienced severe pain in the hand and foot. Voluntary movement was possible at the proximal joints of the limbs but not distally. No clonic movement ever occurred. On one occasion she was able to observe herself in the looking-glass during an attack and noticed that her face was drawn up to the left side. She was able to speak during the attacks, but would have to sit down until the spasm passed off in about a minute. Contact of the foot with the ground was apt to bring on an attack and at times she was reduced to hopping across the room on her right leg. The attacks would occur in bed and would waken her from sleep, particularly if she turned on to her left side. Consciousness was never lost or disturbed and the attacks were not followed by headache or by weakness of the affected limbs.

Twomey and Espir (4), in a review of the literature, collected 64 patients with "tonic seizures." All had abrupt attacks without warning, with 29 patients experiencing precipitating factors, most with tactile stimulation or trunk movements. Simultaneous bilateral involvement was noted in 10 patients, usually involving only the legs, but including all four limbs in three patients. Some patients have been reported to have transient premonitory or coexistent sensory symptoms.

Joynt and Green reported four patients in whom "tonic seizures" were the initial presentation of MS (17). One patient experienced an estimated 500 to 1000 attacks over a six-month period. Another patient had approximately 30 episodes daily, each lasting only 5 to 10 seconds, over a six-week period. These authors provided strong evidence against an epileptogenic basis for the spells by recording six normal electroencephalograms during the episodes and failing to observe any "postictal" weakness in at least two cases.

In another series of patients presenting with paroxysmal dystonia, Berger and coworkers noted that four of eight patients experienced pain, and another patient had an ipsilateral electrical sensation (7). The authors contributed the additional observation that "autonomic disturbances, such as piloerection, profuse perspiration, facial flushing, and hyperactive bowel sounds, may also accompany the paroxysmal dystonia."

The topographic distribution of the spasms may at times differ from the usual pattern described by Matthews (1). Patients have been described in whom the episodes have involved both arms, or one arm and both legs, or all four limbs.

In one unusual patient, clusters of spasms occurred on either side. "The initial cluster of 12 left-sided spasms in six months was followed by 10 similar clusters, with variable remission intervals, over five years. Within a cluster, spasms were unilateral and stereotyped, although the side and extent of the body involved varied from cluster to cluster" (7).

Most cases of tonic spasms have been presumed to be secondary to lesions in the spinal cord. However, Maimon and coworkers reported an apparent association between the episodes and a plaque in the contralateral internal capsule, as demonstrated by magnetic resonance imaging (MRI) (18). The tonic spasms occurred three weeks after a mild hemiparesis, at which time the only lesion on brain MRI was in the contralateral internal capsule. When the patient was reimaged 10 months later because of new symptoms, the capsular lesion had disappeared.

Most authors report successful therapy with carbamazepine, often in very low doses (4,7,23–26). Other anticonvulsants or baclofen may also be effective (1,22,25).

Paroxysmal Dysarthria and Ataxia

Although it has been reported somewhat less commonly than tonic spasms, paroxysmal dysarthria, with or without ataxia, has nonetheless been noted by many authors (3,4,16,26–34). In their review of the literature, Twomey and Espir collected 47 cases (4). They noted that "each episode starts with slurring of speech, which is usually accompanied by ataxia of gait and more rarely by incoordination of one or both upper limbs." The average duration of the attacks was 15 seconds. Ten of these cases were those reported earlier by Matthews, who noted that dysarthria was never the only component. Paroxysms of six patients began with sensory symptoms (burning, numbness, or tingling) in the face, always unilaterally; two of these patients also had sensory symptoms in a limb, which occurred either ipsilateral or contralateral to the facial sensation. Two patients said that during the attack they could not use the arm contralateral to the paresthesias. Two of Matthews's patients also experienced tonic spasms. Twomey and Espir further noted diplopia occurring during the attacks in three patients.

These authors observed that 21 of the 47 patients had precipitating factors for at least some of the attacks. Hyperventilation was most commonly noted, but sudden movement of a part of the body has also been a trigger. One woman reported episodes occurring after sexual intercourse, although most attacks of paroxysmal dysarthria occur spontaneously.

Paroxysmal Diplopia

Osterman and Westerberg reported three patients with paroxysmal diplopia (16). Episodes occurred up to 50 times daily, each lasting about 60 seconds. In one patient, relatives observed strabismus during an attack.

Paroxysmal Hemiataxia and Paresthesias

Two patients, also reported by Osterman and Westerberg, experienced episodes of hemiataxia and paresthesias (16). These individuals reported attacks beginning with unpleasant prickling and sometimes painful sensation on the side of the face and ipsilateral arm, followed immediately by ataxia of the contralateral arm and leg. The episodes lasted 10 to 30 seconds and recurred as often as five times an hour. One of these patients had accompanying dysarthria.

Other Paroxysmal Sensory Symptoms

Seven cases of paroxysmal paresthesias were noted by Twomey and Espir (4). The symptom usually was confined to one limb, lasted an average of 15 seconds, and occasionally was unpleasant.

Another unusual symptom in MS is paroxysmal itching, which has been described by several authors (5,6,35). Yamamoto and coworkers reported three Japanese women, in one of whom the episodes were the first manifestation of MS (5). The attacks occurred and ended abruptly in each woman, lasted from several seconds to several minutes, and recurred at least five to six times per day. The attacks often awakened patients from sleep. The distribution of the itching varied, involving the face, extremities, or trunk, often in a symmetric or segmental pattern.

Osterman and Westberg (16) and then Osterman (35) earlier reported similar cases. However, their patients experienced attacks as many as 80 times daily, with an average paroxysm of five minutes. The episodes typically were precipitated by sensory stimuli.

Episodes of paroxysmal itching are likely to respond to anticonvulsant agents such as carbamazepine or phenytoin. However, ibuprofen was effective in one patient who declined treatment with phenytoin (36).

Paroxysmal Akinesia

Whereas all the paroxysmal symptoms described previously may be considered "positive" phenomena, negative symptoms may also occur in the form of paroxysmal akinesia. Twomey and Espir identified 18 such cases in the literature (4). "Characteristically there is sudden loss of power of a limb or limbs described by the patients as 'knees locking,' 'legs collapsing,' 'legs don't go,' or 'unexpected falls' followed by rapid recovery." In all 12 cases of Zeldowicz, the symptom was reported to be the initial manifestation of MS (2). Attacks of paroxysmal akinesia have been described as occurring as frequently as four times an hour. Although the legs are usually involved, Castaigne described a patient whose right hand became weak for 10 to 20 seconds while playing the piano (22).

Lhermitte's Sign

Although eponymically named for Lhermitte, these electric shock–like sensations were originally described by Marie and Chatelin (37) in 1917, and the following year they were specifically noted by Beriel and Devic (38). Lhermitte and coworkers did not describe a patient until 1924 (39), but his name was apparently linked to the phenomenon—actually a symptom, rather than a sign—by McAlpine in his 1955 text (40).

Most typically considered to be a complaint of "electric shocks" down the spine when the neck is flexed, the distribution varies from patient to patient. Karchandani and coworkers reviewed the literature as well as their own series (41). These authors identified 38 patients with the symptom from their own population of 114 MS patients. Twelve of these subjects had never reported their symptoms to a physician before being specifically queried in this study; and in 16 percent of patients it was part of the initial attack.

Although most often described as an "electric shock" (30 patients), two patients described "pain"; two, "tingling, pins and needles"; two, "ripples or shivers"; one, "hair standing on end"; and one, "fizzing." In 11 patients, the sensation radiated down the spine only; in seven patients, to the spine and both legs; in four patients, to the spine, arms, and leg; in three patients, to the spine and arms only; in seven patients, up and down the spine; and in one patient, down an arm and a leg unilaterally. Five other patients described variable radiation. The symptoms were always brief, usually lasting less than two seconds.

Lhermitte's sign is strongly associated with MS in the minds of most neurologists. However, it occurs in a variety of myelopathic conditions, having been particularly noted in 25 percent of cases of subacute combined degeneration (42) and in radiation myelopathy (43).

Although the precise basis for Lhermitte's sign is not known, hints come from the experimental feline studies of Smith and McDonald (44), who found that sensory fibers traversing demyelinating lesions were most mechanically sensitive. These authors suggested that demyelination and axonal preservation were more important than the presence of severed axons. "The spread of sensation could indicate ephaptic activation of adjacent demyelinated axons in the posterior columns." Karchandani and colleagues further observed that the spinal cord is most mobile in the neck (41). During flexion, the cervical cord changes length by several centimeters and the denticulate ligaments tighten, resulting in much more

deformation of the cord than noted by Smith and McDonald in their experiments.

UHTHOFF'S SYMPTOM

In 1889 Uhthoff described transient visual blurring associated with exercise in patients with MS (45). Other types of transient symptoms may similarly occur with exertion. The phenomenon is generally believed to result from minor temperature elevation, as patients who experience symptoms during vigorous workouts generally improve rapidly as they cool down.

Scholl and coworkers studied the phenomenon in 81 patients with a first episode of isolated optic neuritis (46). In 40 patients (49.5 percent), the symptom occurred at some point during the attack, and within two weeks of onset in 16 percent of patients. The episodes continued for months to years in some patients. A typical attack consisted of blurring of vision in the affected eye, usually generalized, but sometimes more pronounced centrally, coming on after 5 to 20 minutes of the provoking factor. These authors did not restrict their use of the term to elicitation by exercise (which did occur in 52.5 percent of patients). Other provocateurs included hot bath or shower (27.5 percent); hot weather (27.5 percent); stress, anxiety, or anger (12.5 percent); tired, end of day (10 percent); hot food or drink (7.5 percent); cooking (5 percent); or other specific activity (7.5 percent). Sensitivity to a specific provocative factor was very stereotyped for a particular individual.

It is interesting that the occurrence of Uhthoff's symptoms was statistically significantly more often associated with an initial MRI typical of MS, by Paty's criteria (87 percent compared with 55 percent) (47). Furthermore, clinically definite MS, using the Poser criteria (48), developed significantly more often (57.5 percent) in patients with Uhthoff's symptom than in those without (29.3 percent) after a mean follow-up of 3.5 years.

Previous studies in optic neuritis had shown an incidence of Uhthoff's symptom of 29 percent in one retrospective study (49), but 15 of 29 of these patients could have the phenomenon provoked by heating. Another prospective study found that 33 percent of patients experienced the transient visual blurring (50).

Headache

Headache has been reported to occur as part of MS exacerbations. In one retrospective series, Freedman and Gray reported that in 44 of 1,113 patients, migraine-like headaches heralded one or more exacerbations (51). Their observation that half of the episodes beginning with headache were brainstem attacks is noteworthy.

More germane to the consideration of paroxysmal symptoms are the several reports of sudden severe headache. One man was awakened from sleep by the "worst headache" of his life two days before developing an oculomotor nerve paresis (52). Magnetic resonance imaging revealed more than 30 white matter lesions, but the only brainstem abnormality was in the cerebellar peduncle. Another patient was awakened from sleep by a severe nonthrobbing left hemicrania (53). The headache was replaced by facial numbness two hours later. Lesions in the lateral pons, along with multiple other areas of abnormal signal, were observed on MRI.

Perhaps the most striking case, reported by Haas and coworkers, was a 16-year-old girl who suddenly developed an intense headache, described as the worst in her life, followed 10 hours later by diplopia (54). The headache was bifrontal, with radiation to the occiput and temples, and was unaccompanied by nausea. Brain MRI showed the only abnormality to be an area of increased signal on T2 imaging, which enhanced with gadolinium, in the periaqueductal gray area of the midbrain. Raskin earlier had reported a series of patients (non-MS) who developed headache immediately or soon after electrodes were implanted in the periaqueductal gray region (55). The authors of this case report believe it "supports the contention of Raskin that perturbations within the periaqueductal gray can generate headache."

Seizures

Compared with the usual incidence of epilepsy of 0.5 percent in the general population (56), seizures clearly occur more frequently in patients with MS. Estimates of the frequency in MS vary from 1.8 percent to as much as 10.8 percent (56–62). Most estimates cluster in the range of 2 percent to 4 percent. In a recent study of 2,353 MS patients, Ghezzi and coworkers noted a prevalence of 1.7 percent in the overall series, but 2.3 percent when only patients with definite MS were considered (56). As Matthews notes, "Epilepsy undeniably occurs both as an initial symptom and in the course of the disease, but an uncritical assumption of a causal connexion can be misleading. Fits, occurring in close relationship to, or as an integral part of, a relapse are clearly acceptable. As might be expected, such fits frequently present focal features, and an occasional but rather characteristic patterns is the onset of very frequent focal motor seizures" (57).

The precise reason for the increased prevalence of seizures in the MS population is not clear. However, one explanation may be the high frequency of plaques adjacent to the cerebral cortex. In one pathologic series, 25 percent of plaques were found in this location. Such lesions may act as irritative foci and trigger the seizures. In the series of Ghezzi and coworkers (56), MRI scans showed such a location of lesions in three of 12 patients, although, somewhat surprisingly, they had generalized seizures.

The question of whether to provide long-term anticonvulsant therapy for patients experiencing seizures in the context of MS has not been well studied. In some circumstances, a seizure—usually partial in nature—may be related by localization to a gadolinium-enhancing lesion on MRI (63,64). In this situation, chronic treatment may not be warranted because such patients may be seizure-free after the acute inflammatory phase of the lesion has resolved (63). This tends to be approximately four weeks, on average, if one can draw this conclusion from the mean duration of gadolinium enhancement.

Miscellaneous Disorders

Although disorders of micturition are common in MS, Yoshimura and coworkers reported the very unusual occurrence of paroxysmal urinary incontinence (65). Episodes of epigastric pain were followed by urinary incontinence. The attacks lasted approximately 20 seconds, recurred within an interval of about five minutes, and occurred in clusters of one to two hours several times a day. The symptom was associated with a lesion in the right rostral pons, which was demonstrated on MRI. Paroxysms promptly ceased with treatment with carbamazepine, 200 mg daily.

Another unusual paroxysmal attack was the occurrence of convergence spasm (66). Episodes occurred 80 times per day for up to 20 seconds at a time and were provoked irregularly by hyperventilation. A dorsomedial lesion at the level of the quadrigeminal bodies, seen on MRI, may have been responsible. The episodes were terminated by treatment with bromocriptine after valproate and methylprednisolone failed to alleviate the symptoms and carbamazepine produced intolerable side effects. The attacks resumed when bromocriptine was temporarily discontinued. Presentation of MS with paroxysmal spasm of the superior rectus and levator palpebrae has also been reported (67).

Yet another peculiar phenomenon was the occurrence of visually induced paroxysmal nausea and vomiting (68). Any type of movement in the patient's field of vision would lead to intense nausea, followed by vomiting if the movement persisted. Closure of the eyes or the cessation of movement would abruptly terminate the symptoms, which would occur paroxysmally over three to four hours.

PATHOPHYSIOLOGY

The pathophysiology of paroxysmal symptoms is not certain and has been subject to considerable speculation. The most widely held view is that these phenomena, especially the more complex events such as tonic spasms, result from "ephaptic transmission" or the lateral spread of excitation from one axon to another. Ekbom and coworkers, in discussing "seizures" of spinal origin, initially postulated spread of abnormal excitation to contiguous neural structures (20). This view was expanded by Osterman and Westerberg, who suggested that the episodes resulted from transversely spreading activation of "damaged axons" in spinal cord tracts (16). The hypothesis finds support from the pathologic studies of Prineas and Connell, which showed that within MS plaques naked axons may be juxtaposed without intervening glial tissue, thus facilitating the possibility of laterally spreading excitation (69).

Other theories for the cause of paroxysmal symptoms have been suggested but find little evidence in support. These include effects of hypoxia on demyelinated axons (28) and the possibility that the state of abnormal axonal excitability bears some similarity to tetany (1). Hyperventilation has often been noted to trigger a variety of paroxysmal attacks, and it has been suggested that this may be related to a reduction in ionized calcium after overbreathing (1).

TREATMENT

Anticonvulsants have been the mainstay of therapy for a wide variety of paroxysmal symptoms. Phenobarbital, which was first tried because of the phenomenologic similarity of tonic seizures to focal epilepsy, was initially successful. Subsequently, carbamazepine has become the treatment of choice (23), with phenytoin a second choice. The former may be remarkably effective, often terminating paroxysms within hours of an initial small dose. In all probability, the benefits of these drugs result from a prominent effect on the axonal membrane. A newer anticonvulsant, gabapentin, has also proved useful (11). In prescribing these drugs, particularly carbamazepine, the clinician must be wary of the possibility that the patient may experience increased weakness, which could limit therapy.

Khan and Olek have reported the use of bromocriptine in the treatment of two patients with paroxysmal paresthesias (70). Both patients had failed therapy with other agents, including carbamazepine in one patient. Bromocriptine was also successfully used by Postert and coworkers in the treatment of a patient with paroxysmal convergence spasm (66). In addition, Khan has effected relief of paroxysmal symptoms with the use of ibuprofen (36).

References

1. Matthews WB. Tonic seizures in disseminated sclerosis. *Brain* 1958; 81:193–206.

2. Zeldowicz L. Paroxysmal motor episodes as early manifestations of multiple sclerosis. *Can Med Assn* 1996; 84: 937–941.

3. Perks WH, Lascelles RG. Paroxysmal brain stem dysfunction as presenting feature in multiple sclerosis. *Br Med J* 1976; 2:1175.

4. Twomey JA, Espir MLE. Paroxysmal symptoms as the first manifestations of multiple sclerosis. *J Neurol Neurosurg Psychiatry* 1980; 43:296–304.

5. Yamamoto M, Yabuki S, Hayabara T, Otsuki S. Paroxysmal itching in multiple sclerosis: A report of three cases. *J Neurol Neurosurg Psychiatry* 1981; 44:19–22.

6. Koeppel MC, Bramont C, Ceccaldi M, Habib MH, Sayag J. Paroxysmal pruritus and multiple sclerosis. *Br J Dermatol* 1993; 129:597–598.

7. Berger JR, Sheremata WA, Melamed E. Paroxysmal dystonia as the initial manifestation of multiple sclerosis. *Arch Neurol* 1984; 41:747–750.

8. Heath PD, Nightingale S. Clusters of tonic spasms as an initial manifestation of multiple sclerosis. *Ann Neurol* 1982; 12:494–495.

9. Hooge JP, Redekop WK. Trigeminal neuralgia in multiple sclerosis. *Neurology* 1995; 45:1294–1296.

10. Rushton JG, Olafson RA. Trigeminal neuralgia associated with multiple sclerosis. *Arch Neurol* 1965; 13:383–387.

11. Solaro C, Uccelli A, Inglese M, et al. Gabapentin is effective in treating paroxysmal symptoms in multiple sclerosis. *Neurology* 1998; 50(Suppl 4):A147.

12. Reder AT, Arnason BGW. Trigeminal neuralgia in multiple sclerosis relieved by a prostaglandin E analogue. *Neurology* 1995; 45:1097–1100.

13. Meaney JFM, Watt JWG, Eldridge PR, et al. Association betwen trigeminal neuralgia and multiple sclerosis: Role of magnetic resonance imaging. *J Neurol Neurosurg Psychiatry* 1995; 59:253–259.

14. Brisman R. Trigeminal neuralgia and multiple sclerosis. *Arch Neurol* 1987; 44:379–381.

15. Kondziolko D, Lunsford LD, Bissonette DJ. Long-term results after glycerol rhizotomy for multiple sclerosis-related trigeminal neuralgia. *Can J Neurol Sci* 1994; 21:137–140.

16. Osterman P, Westerberg CE. Paroxysmal attacks in multiple sclerosis. *Brain* 1975; 98:189–202.

17. Joynt RJ, Green D. Tonic seizures as a manifestation of multiple sclerosis. *Arch Neurol* 1962; 6:293–299.

18. Maimon D, Reder AT, Finocchiaro F, Recupero E. Internal capsule plaque and tonic spasms in multiple sclerosis. *Arch Neurol* 1991; 48:427–429.

19. Lance JW. Sporadic and familial varieties of tonic seizures. *J Neurol Neurosurg Psychiatry* 1963; 26:51–59.

20. Ekbom KA, Westerberg CE, Osterman PO. Focal sensory-motor seizures of spinal origin. *Lancet* 1968; 1:67.

21. Shibaski H, Kuroiwa Y. Painful tonic seizures in multiple sclerosis. *Arch Neurol* 1974; 30:47–51.

22. Castaigne P, Cambier J, Masson M, et al. Les manifestations motrices paroxystiques de la sclerose en plaques. *Presse med* 1970; 78:1921–1924.

23. Espir MLE, Millac P. Treatment of paroxysmal disorders in multiple sclerosis with carbamazepine (Tegretol). *J Neurol Neurosurg Psychiatry* 1970; 33:528–531.

24. Kuroiwa Y, Shibasaki H. Painful tonic seizures in multiple sclerosis. Treatment with diphenylhydantoin and carbamazepine. *Folia psychiat neurol jap* 1968; 22:107–119.

25. Voiculescu V, Pruskauer-Apostol B, Alecu C. Treatment with acetazolamide of brain stem and spinal paroxysmal disturbances in multiple sclerosis. *J Neurol Neurosurg Psychiatry* 1975; 38:191–193.

26. Andermann F, Cosgrove JBR, Lloyd-Smith D, Walters AM. Paroxysmal dysarthria and ataxia in multiple sclerosis. *Neurology* 1959; 9:211–215.

27. De Castro W, Cambell J. Periodic ataxia. *JAMA* 1967; 200:8923–8924.

28. Espir MLE, Watkins SM, Smith HV. Paroxysmal dysarthria and other transient neurological disturbances in disseminated sclerosis. *J Neurol Neurosurg Psychiatry* 1966; 29:323–330.

29. Espir MLE, Walker ME. Carbamazepine in multiple sclerosis. *Lancet* 1967; 1:280.

30. Harrison M, McGill JI. Transient neurological disturbances in disseminated sclerosis. A case report. *J Neurol Neurosurg Psychiatry* 1969; 32:230–232.

31. Matthews WB. Paroxysmal symptoms in multiple sclerosis. *J Neurol Neurosurg Psychiatry* 1975; 38:617–623.

32. Netsell R, Kent RD. Paroxysmal ataxic dysarthria. *J Speech Hearing Dis* 1976; 41:93–109.

33. Parker HL. Periodic ataxia. *Coll Pap Mayo Clin* 1946; 38:642–645.

34. Wolf P, Assmus H. Paroxysmale dysarthrie und ataxia. *J Neurol* 1974; 208:27–38.

35. Osterman PO. Paroxysmal itching in multiple sclerosis. *Br J Dermatol* 1976; 95:555–558.

36. Khan OA. Treatment of paroxysmal symptoms in multiple sclerosis with ibuprofen. *Neurology* 1994; 44:571–572.

37. Marie P, Chatelin C. Sur certains symptomes d'origine vraisemblablement radiculaire chez les blesse du crane. *Rev Neurol (Paris)* 1917:24:336.

38. Beriel T, Devic E. Sur un cas de douleurs a type de decharge dans la sclerose en plaques. *Lyon Med* 1918; 141:559.

39. Lhermitte J, Bollak NM. Les douleurs a type de decharge electrique consecutives a la flexion cephalique dans la sclerose en plaque. *Rev Neurol (Paris)* 1924; 2:36–52.

40. McAlpine D, Compston ND, Lumsden CE. *Multiple sclerosis*. Edinburgh: Livingstone, 1955:81–82.

41. Kanchandani R, Howe JG. Lhermitte's sign in multiple sclerosis: A clincal survey and review of the literature. *J Neurol Neurosurg Psychiatry* 1982; 45:308–312.

42. Gautier-Smith PC. Lhermitte's sign in subacute combined degeneration of the cord. *J Neurol Neurosurg Psychiatry* 1973; 36:861–863.

43. Boden G. Radiation myelitis of the cervical spinal cord. *Br J Radiol* 1948; 21:464–469.

44. Smith KJ, McDonald WI. Spontaneous and mechanically evoked activity due to central demyelinating lesion. *Nature* 1980; 286:154–155.

45. Uhthoff W. Untersuchungen uber die bei der multiplen Herdsklerose vorkommenden Augenstorungen. *Arch Psychiatr Nervenkr* 1889:21:303–410.

46. Scholl GB, Song HS, Wray SH. Uhthoff's symptoms in optic neuritis: Relationship to magnetic resonance imaging and development of multiple sclerosis. *Ann Neurol* 1991; 30:180–184.

47. Paty DW, Oger JJF, Kastrukoff LF, et al. MRI in the diagnosis of MS: A prospective study with comparison of clinical evaluation, evoked potentials, oligoclonal banding, and CT. *Neurology* 1988; 38:180–184.

48. Poser CM, Paty DW, Scheinberg L, et al. New diagnostic criteria for multiple sclerosis: Guidelines for research protocols. *Ann Neurol* 1983; 13:227–231.

49. Edmund J, Fog T. Visual and motor instability in multiple sclerosis. *Arch Neurol* 1955; 73:316–323.

50. Perkin GD, Rose FC. Prognosis for the development of multiple sclerosis. In: GD Perki, FC Rose (eds.). Optic neuritis and its differential diagnosis. Oxford: Oxford University Press. 1979:226–248.

51. Freedman MS, Gray TA. Vascular headache: A presenting symptom of multiple sclerosis. *Can J Neurol Sci* 1989; 16:63–66.

52. Galer BS, Lipton RB, Weinstein S, Bello L, Solomon S. Apoplectic headache and oculomotor nerve palsy: An unusual presentation of multiple sclerosis. *Neurology* 1990; 40:1465–1466.

53. Nager BJ, Lanska DJ, Daroff RB. Acute demyelination mimicking vascular hemicrania. *Headache* 1989; 29:423–424.

54. Haas DC, Kent PF, Friedman DI. Headache caused by a single lesion of multiple sclerosis in the periaqueductal gray area. *Headache* 1993; 33:452–455.

55. Raskin NH, Hosobuchi Y, Lamb Sl. Headache may arise from perturbation of brain. *Headache* 1987; 27:416–420.

56. Ghezzi A, Montanini R, Basso PF, Zaffaroni M, Massimo E, Cazzullo CL. Epilepsy in multiple sclerosis. *Eur Neurol* 1990; 30:218–223.

57. Matthews WB. Epilepsy and disseminated sclerosis. *Quart J Med* 1962; 31:141–155.

58. Boudouresques J, Khalil R, Ali Cherif A, et al. Epilepsie et sclerose en plaques (`a propos de 8 observations electrocliniques). *Revue neurol* 1975; 131:729–735.

59. Kinnunen E, Wikstrom J. Prevalence and prognosis of epilepsy in patients with multiple sclerosis. *Epilepsia* 1986; 27:729–733.

60. Conomy JP, Schiffer RB. Epilepsy in multiple sclerosis, an electroencephalographic and clinical study of 15 cases. *J Neurol* 1988; 235(Suppl):S65.

61. Fuglsang-Frederiksen V, Thygesen F. Seizures and psychopathology in multiple sclerosis: An encephalographic study. Discussion and pathogenesis *Acta Psychiat Neurol Scand* 1952; 27:17–41.

62. Cendrowski W, Majkowski J. Epilepsy in multiple sclerosis. *J Neurol Sci* 1972; 17:389–398.

63. Thompson AJ, Kermode AG, Moseley IF, Macmanus DG, McDonald WI. Seizures due to multiple sclerosis: Seven patients with MRI correlations. *J Neurol Neurosurg Psychiatry* 1993; 56:1317–1320.

64. Truyen L, Barkof F, Frequin STFM, et al. Magnetic resonance imaging of epilepsy in multiple sclerosis: A case control study. Implications for treatment trials with 4-aminopyridine. *Multiple Sclerosis* 1996; 1:213–217.

65. Yoshimura N, Nagahama Y, Ueda T, Yoshida O. Paroxysmal urinary incontinence associated with multiple sclerosis. *Urol Int* 1997; 59:197–199.

66. Postert TH, McMonagle U, Buttner Th, et al. Paroxysmal convergence spasm in multiple sclerosis. *Acta Neurol Scand* 1996; 94:35–37.

67. Ezra E, Plant GT. Paroxysml superior rectus and levator palpebrae spasms: A unique presentation of multiple sclerosis. *Br J Ophthalmol* 1996; 80:187–188.

68. Khan OA, Sandoz GM, Olek MJ, Kuta AJ. Visually induced paroxysmal nausea and vomiting as presenting manifestations of muliple sclerosis. *J Neurol Neurosurg Psychiatry* 1995; 59:342–343.

69. Prineas JW, Connell F. The fine structure of chronically active multiple sclerosis plaques. *Neurology* 1978; 28:68–75.

70. Khan OA, Olek MJ. Treatment of paroxysmal symptoms in multiple sclerosis with bromocriptine. *J Neurol Neurosurg Psychiatry* 1995; 58:253.

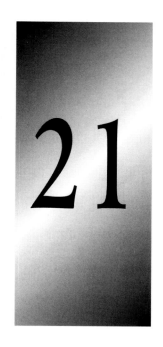

21 Dysarthria

Pamela Miller Sorensen, M.A., C.C.C.-S.L.P.

THE DIFFERENTIAL DIAGNOSIS AND PATHOPHYSIOLOGY OF DYSARTHRIA

Definitions of Dysarthria and Dysphonia

The term *dysarthria* describes motor speech disorders. Spasticity, weakness, slowness, and/or ataxic incoordination of the muscles in the lips, tongue, mandible, soft palate, vocal cords, and diaphragm may result from MS. Therefore, articulation, intelligibility, rate, and naturalness of speech may be compromised.

Dysphonia refers to voice disorders. Dysarthria in MS is usually accompanied by dysphonia because the muscle groups, structures, and neural pathways are shared for both speech and voice production. Therefore, voice quality, nasal resonance, pitch control, loudness, and emphasis may also be affected in MS.

The Processes of Normal Speech and Voice Production

It is important to understand the speed and complexity of normal speech and voice production to ensure quality evaluation and treatment of dysarthria and dysphonia in MS. These normal processes are overlapping and require that the following five systems work together rapidly and smoothly (Figure 21-1):

1. *Respiration*—using the diaphragm to quickly fill the lungs fully, followed by slow, controlled exhalation for speech
2. *Phonation*—using the vocal cords and air flow to produce voice of different pitch, loudness, and quality
3. *Resonance*—raising and lowering the soft palate to direct the voice to resonate in the oral and/or nasal cavities and further affect voice quality
4. *Articulation*—making quick, precise movements of the lips, tongue, mandible, and soft palate for clarity of speech
5. *Prosody*—combining all elements for a natural flow of speech with adequate speaking rate, appropriate pauses, and variations in loudness, emphasis, and melodic line to enhance meaning (2).

Prevalence of Dysarthria in Multiple Sclerosis

Speech impairment has long been considered a principal symptom of MS. In a lecture entitled "Disseminated Sclerosis: Its Symptomatology," which was published in 1877, Charcot presented the characteristic triad of signs

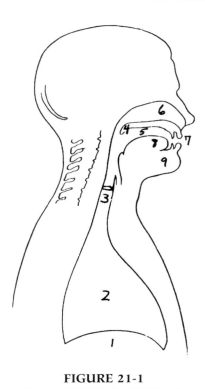

FIGURE 21-1

Aerodynamic model of speech production. *Respiration:* 1. Diaphragm; 2. Lungs. *Phonation:* 3. Vocal cords. *Resonance:* 4. Soft palate; 5. Oral cavity; 6. Nasopharynx. *Articulation:* 4. Soft palate; 7. Lips; 8. Tongue; 9. Mandible. [Adapted from Netsell (1)].

of what today is called MS: nystagmus, intention tremor, and scanning speech (3). Scanning speech has since been considered a hallmark of MS by many health care professionals. Even as recently as 1993, the results of a survey of speech-language pathologists revealed that dysarthria is believed to have a high prevalence in MS (4).

Although dysarthria is believed to be highly prevalent in MS, a review of the literature indicates otherwise. Results of three published studies demonstrate that 41 percent to 44 percent of the MS population experience speech or voice impairments, whereas only 23 percent perceive expressive communication disorders in themselves (5–7). Darley and coworkers (5) found that 41 percent of the 168 MS patients in their Mayo Clinic Study had specific speech deviations. In a community-based survey of 278 people with MS in Sweden, Hartelius and Svensson (6) reported that 44 percent of the 200 respondents perceived "impairment of speech and voice after the onset of their disease." In a cross-sectional survey of 656 individuals with MS, Beukelman and Kraft (7), reported that 23 percent of the 590 respondents perceived "speech and other communication disorders" in themselves.

The aforementioned findings indicate that dysarthria is not as universal a sign of MS as often believed. The majority (59 percent) of MS subjects were found to be essentially normal in terms of impact on the listener, and 56 percent to 73 percent perceived no significant speech, voice, or expressive communication disorders in themselves.

Underlying Pathophysiology of Dysarthria in Multiple Sclerosis

Multiple sclerosis can cause demyelinating lesions in many different areas of the brain and central nervous system (CNS). Areas of MS demyelination typically occur in the periventricular white matter of the brain, brainstem, cerebellum, and/or spinal cord. MS plaque, or scarring of brain tissue, can interrupt the transmission of the message between the brain and the muscles in the lips, tongue, soft palate, vocal cords, and diaphragm. Because these muscles control the quality of speech and voice, dysarthria and dysphonia may result. Dysarthria in MS is typically a resulting mixture of spastic and/or ataxic involvement.

Course of Symptoms of Dysarthria in Multiple Sclerosis

A variety of speech and voice problems can occur due to the nature of MS. The presence, type, severity, and different manifestations depend on the type of disease process, and the extent and location of MS plaque and demyelination. Because of the relapsing nature of some forms of MS, problems with speech and voice may come and go. They may temporarily worsen with exacerbations, paroxysmal episodes, and fatigue; or they may deteriorate over time if there is a progressive disease course with involvement of multiple neurologic systems.

Common Features of Dysarthria in Multiple Sclerosis

Darley and coworkers (5) published the most comprehensive scientific study to date that objectively identifies features of dysarthria in MS. In their 38-month study at the Mayo Clinic, 168 MS patients were formally evaluated by neurologists and assigned to one of eight groups. Assignment depended on which combination of neurologic involvement was seen: cerebrum, cerebellum, brainstem, and/or spinal cord. A formal diagnostic battery was administered by speech-language pathologists, and results were categorized into dimensions of deviant speech and voice. Computer analysis of 41 different factors was performed: 17 speech, 4 respiration, 13 neurologic, and 7 background history. Table 21-1 summarizes their findings

TABLE 21-1
Rank Order of Deviations in Speech and Voice in Multiple Sclerosis

PERCENT (N=168)	DEVIATION	DESCRIPTION
77%	Loudness control	(reduced, mono, excess, or variable)
72%	Harsh voice quality	(strained, excess tone in vocal cords)
46%	Imprecise articulation	(distorted, prolonged, irregular)
39%	Impaired emphasis	(phrasing, rate, stress, intonation)
37%	Impaired pitch control	(monopitch, pitch breaks, high, low)
35%	Decreased vital capacity	(reduced breath support and control)
24%	Hypernasality	(excessive nasal resonance)

of the seven most common characteristics of dysarthria and dysphonia in MS (5).

Misconceptions about Scanning Speech in Multiple Sclerosis

Scanning speech was once regarded as a hallmark of MS, but that notion has since been disputed. In a lecture in 1877, Charcot (3) described scanning speech as ". . . a slow, drawling manner, and sometimes almost unintelligible . . . the words are as if measured or scanned; there is a pause after every syllable, and the syllables themselves are pronounced slowly." However, in their 1962 neurology text, Grinker and Sahs (8) reported that "Charcot's triad of nystagmus, intention tremor and scanning speech, long considered pathognomonic of MS, is rarely seen in the early cases. . . . The slurring, monotony, irregular pauses and ebb of volume are identical to those encountered in other cerebellar diseases." Brain (9) also disagreed with Charcot: "Dysarthria in multiple sclerosis may be due either to spastic weakness, or ataxia of the muscles of articulation, or to a combination of these factors . . .

the 'scanning speech', sometimes regarded as typical, is exceptional." Darley and colleagues (5) also found that only 14 percent of the 168 MS patients in their study exhibited scanning speech (which they defined as excess and equal stress on spoken words).

Differential Diagnoses of Dysarthria in Multiple Sclerosis

There are three types of dysarthria associated with MS: *spastic, ataxic,* and *mixed dysarthria.* The differential diagnosis depends on the extent and location of demyelination and the specific speech, voice, and physical signs that result. Mixed dysarthria is most common in MS because of the typical involvement of multiple neurologic systems.

To facilitate differential diagnoses, Tables 21-2, 21-3, and 21-4 outline the speech and voice manifestations in each type of dysarthria and describe the associated neuromuscular and physical signs (10).

In MS, a mixed spastic-ataxic dysarthria is typical. Speech, voice, neuromuscular, and physical signs may be

TABLE 21-2
Spastic Dysarthria: Due to Bilateral Lesions of Corticobulbar Tracts

SPEECH AND VOICE SIGNS	NEUROMUSCULAR AND PHYSICAL SIGNS
Harsh, strained voice quality	Hypertonicity (excess muscle tone)
Pitch breaks	Bilateral spasticity
Imprecise articulation	Restricted range of motion (jaw)
Slow rate of speech	Reduced speed of movement
Reduced breath support and/or control	Bilateral hyperreflexia
Reduced or monoloudness	Sucking and jaw jerk reflexes
Short phrases, reduced stress	Cortical disinhibition
Hypernasality	Pseudobulbar crying or laughing

TABLE 21-3
Ataxic Dysarthria: Due to Bilateral or Generalized Lesions of the Cerebellum

SPEECH AND VOICE SIGNS	NEUROMUSCULAR AND PHYSICAL SIGNS
Vocal tremor	Intention tremor: head, trunk, arms, hands
Irregular articulation breakdown	Broad-based, ataxic gait
Dysrhythmic rapid alternating movements of the tongue, lips, and mandible	Nystagmus and irregular or jerky eye movements
Excess and equal stress: scanning speech	Balance or equilibrium problems
Excess and variable loudness	Hypotonicity
Prolonged phonemes and intervals	Overshooting, slow, voluntary movements

any combination of those listed in Tables 21-2 and 21-3. Identifying whether these specific signs have spastic and/or ataxic features can help determine the location of MS lesions and the appropriate plan of treatment.

Referral and Treatment Considerations

Accurate differential diagnosis of dysarthria guides treatment considerations. Referral to a speech-language pathologist or other specialist(s), as well as decisions about appropriate medications and rehabilitation management, can then be made.

THE PHARMACOLOGIC MANAGEMENT OF DYSARTHRIA IN MULTIPLE SCLEROSIS

Review of the Literature

To date, there are no published studies that report the efficacy of specific medication trials for the treatment of

dysarthria or dysphonia in MS. Reports of drug trials for the treatment of dysarthria in other related disorders follow and may serve as a model for future investigation in MS.

1. Biary and coworkers (11) reported the effective dosage of 0.25 to 0.5 mg of clonazepam for the treatment of parkinsonian dysarthria (N=11). Most improvement was noted in their short rushes of speech, variable rate, imprecise articulation, and inappropriate silences. Higher doses were less effective and commonly associated with drowsiness.
2. Critchley (12) and Nakano and colleagues (13) found that amantadine and anticholinergic drugs did not produce a noticeable improvement in the speech of people with Parkinson's disease.
3. Busenbark and coworkers (14) analyzed the effect of 168 mg/day of methazolamide on essential voice tremor (N=7) and found no significant difference in physician or patient scores of vocal tremor severity. Furthermore, adverse reactions, including drowsiness, paresthesias, dizziness, and confusion, were common.

TABLE 21-4
Mixed Dysarthria: Due to Bilateral, Generalized Lesions of Multiple Areas in the Cerebral White Matter, Brainstem, Cerebellum, and/or Spinal Cord

SPEECH AND VOICE SIGNS	NEUROMUSCULAR AND PHYSICAL SIGNS
Impaired loudness control (reduced, monoloudness, or excess and variable)	Any combination of spastic and ataxic features, as mentioned in Tables 21-2 and 21-3
Harsh or hypernasal voice quality	
Vocal tremor or intermittent aphonia	
Impaired articulation (imprecise, distorted, prolonged, or irregular breakdowns)	
Impaired emphasis (slow, prolonged intervals or sounds, reduced, or excess and equal stress)	
Impaired pitch control (monopitch or pitch breaks, too low or too high)	

4. The National Institutes of Health (NIH) published a Consensus Development Conference Statement in 1990 on the clinical use of botulinum toxin (botox) (15). Botox injections were reported to be a "safe and effective treatment of adductor spasmodic dysphonia . . . and a promising treatment for abductor spasmodic dysphonia and vocal tremors." However, they cited relative contraindications for "diseases of neuromuscular transmission" and "generalized neurologic disorders" (vs. focal dystonias). They warned that undesired regional effects, presumably due to diffusion, can cause short-lived but serious risks, such as airway obstruction and dysphagia. The NIH reported that the value of botox for treatment of spasticity caused by brain or spinal cord lesions is under investigation.

Pharmacologic Management of Symptoms

The rationale for neuropharmacologic intervention is to change the symptoms of dysarthria by affecting the neurochemical substrates underlying these pathways (11). Dysarthria in MS is typically a resulting mixture of spastic and/or ataxic involvement. Problems with speech and voice may also be complicated by MS fatigue. Therefore, evaluation of medication trials for spasticity, ataxia, tremor, and/or fatigue, in conjunction with therapy by a speech-language pathologist, is recommended.

Medications for Spasticity

Spasticity is increased muscle tone caused by lesions in the neural pathways of the brain and spinal cord that affect movement. Muscle tightness, spasms, clonus, and increased reflexes may result. Weakness is almost always present with spasticity (16). (See also Chapter 15.)

Some spasticity medications have a direct action on skeletal muscles and act presynaptically to suppress excitatory transmission. Other spasticity medications reduce the excitatory transmission in the spinal cord (17).

Because spasticity and weakness occur together, retaining some spasticity may be beneficial to counteract the weakness for better speech and voice production. Therefore, medications are started at low doses, with gradual adjustments based on patient response. A combination of baclofen and tizanidine may have a combined positive effect on reducing spasticity while minimizing the side effects. Adding small doses of diazepam (Valium) is another option (16). Intrathecal baclofen is often effective in patients with severe lower extremities spasticity who fail oral medications. Motor point blocks (phenol or botox injections) and surgical ablation procedures are rarely used because of the beneficial effects of the other treatments.

TABLE 21-5 *Oral Spasticity Medications*	
First-line treatments	Baclofen (Lioresal)
	Tizanidine (Zanaflex)
Second-line treatments	Dantrolene (Dantrium)
Other treatments	Diazepam (Valium)
	Clonazepam (Klonopin)
	Cyclobenzaprine (Flexeril)

Spasticity can effect speech and voice in many specific ways during respiration, phonation, articulation, and resonance. Too much muscle tone can restrict full range of motion of the diaphragm, thus reducing breath support, and causing inadequate loudness during speech. Excess tone in the vocal cords can result in a harsh, strained voice quality with pitch breaks. Increased tone can also restrict speed, strength, and range of motion of the jaw, lips, tongue, and soft palate, causing imprecise articulation, slow rate of speech, and occasional hypernasality. All of these characteristics are found in spastic dysarthria and dysphonia.

It is important to balance the goals of reducing excess tone while maintaining functional strength for respiratory, phonatory, and oral motor control. A speech-language pathologist can help monitor the effectiveness of various drug trials through periodic formal evaluation of specific dimensions of deviant speech and voice. Also, the efficacy of combining spasticity medications with traditional speech or voice therapy can be objectively studied.

Medications for Tremor and Ataxia

Tremor is a movement disorder with an involuntary, relatively rhythmic pattern. Although integration of many locations in the CNS are involved in the process, the cerebellum is primarily responsible for coordinating and fine-tuning complex movement. Several types of tremor may occur in MS as a result of demyelination in the cerebellum and its pathways. *Intention tremor*, observed as "increased oscillating movement when engaged in purposeful tasks," is common in MS (2). Either fine tremor or wide, jerking, shaking movements, also called *ataxia* or *cerebellar tremor*, may be seen in MS (16).

Tremor can be one of the most disabling symptoms of MS (2). It may affect any muscle group, including the arms, legs, trunk, head, vocal cords, jaw, lips, and tongue. Therefore, significant interference with the daily functions of walking, self-care, sitting balance, head control, writing, swallowing, speech, and voice may result. Tremor and ataxia increase energy consumption during purposeful movement, which may add to MS fatigue and reduce overall endurance for mobility, self-care, and communication (16).

Unfortunately, tremor is reported to be one of the most difficult symptoms to treat (2,16,17). No medication specifically for tremor control has been developed. However, some medications designed to treat other conditions have been found to have secondary antitremor properties(2). Muscle relaxants, antiseizure medications, and certain beta blockers have been tried on people with MS. Smith and Schapiro (2) listed the following possible drug trials, singly or in combination, in an effort to control tremor:

Inderal (Propranolol)
Klonopin (Clonazepam)
Mysoline (Primidone)
Laniazid or Isotamine (Isoniazid)
Glutethimide

They stated that although these medications are not usually effective for MS-related tremor, it is impossible to predict the response in individuals. Thompson (17) agreed that propranolol, clonazepam, and carbamazepine are rarely of value. Theriot (16) stated that medications tend to work best if tremor is fairly fine and does not involve more central parts of the body. Hallet and coworkers (18) documented some benefit with isoniazid in combination with pyridoxine to suppress tremor in a small portion of their MS subjects with severe postural cerebellar tremor. Rice and associates (19) reported a preliminary study of intravenous ondansetron in severe cerebellar tremor with encouraging results.

As mentioned earlier, botox injections have been shown to be "safe and effective with adductor spasmodic dysphonia . . . and a promising treatment for abductor spasmodic dysphonia and vocal tremor," according to a Consensus Development Conference Statement published in 1990 by the NIH. The NIH recommended an interdisciplinary team approach in botox therapy for speech and voice disorders, including otolaryngologist, speech-language pathologist, neurologist, and electromyographer. The standard procedure is injection of minute quantities of botulinum neurotoxin type A into specific muscles by highly specialized physicians. This provides "blocking at the neuromuscular junction, which can alleviate muscle spasm due to excessive neural activity of central origin, or can weaken a muscle for therapeutic purposes" (15).

There are no published reports of botox therapy for the vocal tremor in MS patients. The NIH cited relative contraindications for "diseases of neuromuscular transmission" and "generalized neurologic disorders" (which characterize MS). The temporary but serious risks of airway obstruction and dysphagia, although documented as rare, are other factors to consider in the decision.

When choosing a medication for trial, goal setting with the patient is very important, so that the sedating side effects of these drugs can be weighed against functional outcomes (16). Ataxic dysarthria resulting from MS has very specific dimensions of deviant speech and voice that are caused by generalized, demyelinating lesions in the cerebellum. A speech-language pathologist can provide objective measurement of the characteristic vocal tremor, diadochokinetic rate, irregularity of articulation breakdown, variability of loudness, excess and equal stress, and dysprosody. Use of electronic aids such as a tape recorder, specialized speech/voice laboratory computer software, and electromyographic biofeedback equipment can provide objective pre- and postdrug trial information and help with ongoing decision making.

Medications for Fatigue

Fatigue has long been considered one of the most common and disabling symptoms in MS (20). Published studies report somewhat promising results with amantadine (21–24) and pemoline (21,25) as pharmacologic interventions for fatigue in MS. Smith and Schapiro (2) described the action of the following medications used in MS fatigue management. Amantadine is an anti-influenza virus medication that is sometimes effective in relieving fatigue in MS through some unknown mechanism. Pemoline (Cylert), a mild CNS stimulant used primarily for attention deficit hyperactivity disorder and narcolepsy, is also used to treat fatigue. Fluoxetine (Prozac) has been prescribed with MS patients because of its positive dual effects on depression and fatigue. Thompson (17) stated that the use of the potassium channel blockers, 3-4 diaminopyridine and 4-aminopyridine, may also have a role in the management of MS fatigue. However, the last two drugs have not been studied adequately and are not yet approved by the U.S. Food and Drug Administration (FDA). (See also Chapter 14.)

Schapiro (26) classified four distinct types of fatigue in MS, each with its own recommended treatment strategies (Table 21-6).

It is important to differentially diagnose the type of fatigue so that the appropriate treatment decisions are made. There are a variety of fatigue scales that address the multidimensional aspects of fatigue in MS (see Chapter 14).

Symptoms of dysarthria and dysphonia may be complicated by fatigue in MS. Patients may complain of slurred speech or a weak voice during times of fatigue or after talking for long periods. This difficulty is understandable when considering the speed and complexity of finely coordinated oral, laryngeal, and respiratory movements that are required for normal speech and voice production. Lassitude and neural fatigue appear to be the two types that may temporarily worsen symptoms of dysarthria and dysphonia. Choosing the appropriate treatment strategies, and objectively monitoring the effect of specific medications on speech and voice, are ideally

TABLE 21-6
Treatment Strategies for Types of Fatigue in MS

Type of Fatigue	Features	Treatment Strategies
Normal	Less sleep Possible nocturia	Rest, possibly sleep medications Urodynamics, bladder medications
Neural	Short circuiting, exercise-induced muscle weakness	Temporarily cease activity Allow nerve conduction to resume
Depression	Feeling of lethargy, sadness, hopelessness	Refer for psychiatric diagnosis, psychotherapy, antidepressant trial
Lassitude	Overwhelming tiredness that seems unrelated to activity level or time of day	Relaxation, Energy conservation Symmetrel (Amantadine) Cylert (Pemoline) Prozac (Fluoxetine)

accomplished by a team approach with the physician and speech-language pathologist.

REHABILITATION MANAGEMENT OF DYSARTHRIA: AN INTERDISCIPLINARY APPROACH

People with MS are ideally seen by a team of health care professionals because demyelinating lesions of MS may impact many areas of function, including bladder, ambulation, self-care, vision, swallowing, cognition, communication, interpersonal relationships, and employment. An interdisciplinary approach requires that each team member become familiar with critical features of these functions so that timely and appropriate referrals across disciplines are made.

Referral Process and the Treatment Team

Preliminary identification of speech and voice problems may be accomplished by the patient, family, nurse, therapist, or physician during informal conversation. Features to observe are loudness, voice quality, nasality, clarity of articulation, intelligibility, and naturalness of conversational flow. Questions to ask, which guide appropriate referrals to a speech-language pathologist, are listed in Table 21-7. Formal evaluation and determination of candidacy for treatment can then follow.

The referral process may be initiated by the patient, family, or any health care professional (Figure 21-2). The physician then writes the order for "Speech/voice evaluation and treatment by a speech-language pathologist." Based on individual needs, other medical referrals may also be made to:

1. A *neurologist* for differential neurologic diagnosis and prescription of medications to manage the disease course and secondary symptoms.
2. A *physiatrist* for functional assessment of patients with multiple needs, for symptom management, and coordination of therapy by the rehabilitation team.
3. An *otolaryngologist* for consultation and direct observation of the vocal cords to determine laryngeal status and rule out serious pathologies.

TABLE 21-7
When to Refer to a Speech-Language Pathologist

Questions to ask:
1. Are problematic speech and voice characteristics detracting from the message that is being communicated?
2. Are speech and voice adequate for the patient's daily communication needs? Keep in mind that a person who is unemployed and living with a spouse of 20 years has communication needs that are different from those of a teacher or public speaker.
3. Are speech, voice, and communication problems interfering with the person's quality of life? (e.g., resulting in social isolation, public avoidance, or limitation in current job).
4. Are speech, voice, and communication problems perceived as troublesome by the patient or family?

Initiates → Request	Evaluates Medically → and Writes Referral(s)	Evaluates Dysarthria → Refers and Treats	Coordinates Therapy Goals with Team
			Patient and caregiver
Patient	Primary care physician		Physician and nurse
Family	Neurologist	Speech-language	Occupational therapist
Nurse	Physiatrist	pathologist	Physical therapist
Therapist	Otolaryngologist		Biofeedback therapist
			Psychotherapist
			Vocational rehabilitation counselor

FIGURE 21-2

Model of the Referral Process for Interdisciplinary Management of Dysarthria

After the *speech-language pathologist* formally evaluates respiration, oral motor function, speech, and voice, referrals are made to the appropriate disciplines based on individual needs. Coordination of goals and possible joint therapy sessions may be arranged. Specific overlapping roles of professional disciplines involved in optimizing speech, voice, and communication skills follow:

1. The *patient and caregiver* can provide direction in goal setting specific to their communication needs by furnishing information about the variability of speech and voice performance in different situations and the impact of these communication problems on relationships, community activities, and quality of life.

2. The *referring physician and nurse* are given feedback about the results of the speech/voice evaluation and the treatment plan. Additional referrals to medical specialists (neurologist, otolaryngologist, physiatrist) and the rehabilitation team (occupational therapist, physical therapist, biofeedback therapist, psychotherapist, and/or vocational rehabilitation counselor) can then be discussed. Medical procedures and medications trials (for spasticity, ataxia, tremor, and/or fatigue) may also be considered.

3. An *occupational therapist* can provide expertise in the areas of: (a) proper positioning for optimal speech and voice production; (b) adaptive equipment to improve sitting balance, head control, and respiratory support; (c) recommendations about the patient's best mode for operating augmentative communication devices based on available visual-motor skills; and (d) energy conservation techniques for fatigue management.

4. A *physical therapist* can provide additional information about neuromuscular and physical findings to aid in the differential diagnosis of dysarthria. Data about the location and degree of spasticity, weakness, tremor, ataxia, and/or motor planning problems affecting gait and mobility can be compared with deviations found in respiration, phonation, articulation, resonance, and prosody. The variability of speech and voice production during different physical activities can also be evaluated and later incorporated into the transfer phase of dysarthria therapy. The physical therapy principles of stretching, exercise, and/or stabilization can be followed by both disciplines, although for different muscle groups and purposes.

5. A *biofeedback therapist* can provide expertise, ideally during joint therapy sessions, in the use of computerized EMG/biofeedback equipment, with visual and auditory feedback, to (a) enhance the patient's self-monitoring/self-correction of optimal positioning and muscle control during speech and voice production; (b) learn relaxation techniques to reduce tremor and spasticity in specific muscle groups used for phonation and articulation; and (c) use diaphragmatic breathing to improve respiratory support for speech.

6. A *psychotherapist*, especially in moderate to severe cases of dysarthria, may (a) provide support to the patient and family around the frustrations of the communication difficulties; (b) help the patient deal with feelings of loss resulting from the possible impact on job, significant relationships, and self-image; and (c) work with the treatment team in addressing the issues of social isolation and public avoidance.

7. A *vocational rehabilitation counselor* may be involved to facilitate reemployment. A speech-language pathologist may advise the vocational rehabilitation counselor about the patient's cognitive-communication status and recommend job accommodations, communication equipment, and necessary support in the new job setting.

Motor Speech/Voice Evaluation

Evaluation of dysarthria and dysphonia include both formal and informal measures. Standard procedures include obtaining background information; examining the structure and function of the oral peripheral mechanism (lips, teeth, tongue, mandible, soft and hard palates); evaluating respiratory support by timing how long "ah" or "eee" can be sustained (normal = 20+ seconds); describing laryngeal function by analyzing the quality of the sustained phonation (smooth, irregular, tremulous, harsh, breathy); determining speed and coordination of the articulators, referred to as diadochokinetic rate, when repeating "puh-tuh-kuh" as rapidly and evenly as possible (normal = 10–12 in 5 seconds); and classifying deviations in respiration, phonation, articulation, resonance, and prosody perceived during spontaneous conversation. (See Appendix I.)

Formal published measures include:

1. Articulation tests that help determine general versus specific dysarticulation patterns; identify performance on specific phonemes; and analyze types, positions, and contexts of errors. Bernthal and Bankson (27) give a detailed review of various articulation tests available. However, because of the pattern of irregular articulatory breakdown in generalized neurologic disorders such as MS, formal articulation tests are rarely necessary.
2. Intelligibility ratings in words and sentences where tape-recorded responses are transcribed by unbiased judges who are unfamiliar with the material (*Assessment of Intelligibility of Dysarthric Speech*) (28).
3. Oral reading rate of phonetically balanced reading passages that yield an objective rating of words per minute (wpm), and subjective information about other elements of prosody, such as phrasing and naturalness of flow (Figure 21-3) (29).
4. Transcription analysis of a three-minute tape-recorded spontaneous speech sample (i.e., Job Task: a detailed description of the patient's job) that can yield information about speaking rate (wpm); breath support/control (number of spoken words per breath unit); articulation precision; intelligibility (number of words understood/total words spoken); and stress, intonation, and flow of conversational speech.

Screening hearing, vision, and cognitive status also has important implications for treatment planning. Speech therapy involves active listening and self-monitoring, which rely on good auditory acuity and discrimination skills. Mustillo (30) reported that although peripheral hearing loss through pure tone audiometry is of low prevalence in MS, central auditory deficits are frequently found through brainstem auditory evoked responses (62%–80%). This may affect discrimination of speech sounds in noisy backgrounds, binaural information processing, loudness function, and sound lateralization. Visual symptoms such as optic neuritis, nystagmus, double vision, visual scanning, and eye teaming difficulties are often found in MS. This may affect decisions about referrals, visual stimuli to use in therapy, and appropriateness of certain augmentative communication devices. Rao and coworkers (31) found a high prevalence of cognitive deficits in individuals with MS (40%–60%), although to a typically mild degree. Formal cognitive testing can rule out the problems that are characteristic of MS, such as difficulty with attention, speed and capacity of information processing, memory, and verbal fluency. Rao developed a 20–30 minute Neuropsychological Screening Battery for MS (32). which assesses these specific areas. Objective information about cognitive status can facilitate decision making about new learning and memory strategies to employ in dysarthria therapy and guide expected outcome.

> You wished to know all about my grandfather. Well, he is nearly ninety-three years old; he dresses himself in an ancient black frock coat, usually minus several buttons; yet he thinks as swiftly as ever. A long flowing beard clings to his chin, giving those who observe him a pronounced feeling of the utmost respect. When he speaks, his voice is just a bit cracked and quivers a trifle. Twice each day he plays skillfully and with zest upon our small organ. Except in the winter when the ooze or snow or ice prevents, he slowly takes a short walk in the open air each day. We have often urged him to walk more and smoke less, but he always answers, "Banana oil!" Grandfather likes to be modern in his language.

Rate = 133 words/_____ minute(s) or _____ wpm.

FIGURE 21-3

My Grandfather: A phonetically balanced oral reading passage.

Development of an Individualized Treatment Plan

Treatment decisions are based on the results of evaluation and tailored to the individual's needs. There are many clinical considerations involved in treatment planning, including the type and severity of dysarthria; the specific deviant features of respiration, phonation, articulation, resonance and/or prosody; the course and severity of the MS disease process; the timing of other medical interventions; and the number and severity of other symptoms (especially cognitive-behavioral and visual-motor involvement). A process-specific treatment approach, which identifies types of deficits and their underlying pathophysiology, is preferred for guiding therapy decisions. Other important clinical considerations include the present communication needs and environment, as well as future concerns (i.e., school, vocation, and what the disease process may bring) (33).

Principles of Treatment

Normal speech patterns may not be a realistic goal; therefore, training of specific compensatory skills through drill and neuromuscular facilitation become the emphasis in therapy (34). Improvement in adequacy, intelligibility, efficiency, and naturalness of communication, with reduction in the handicapping effects, are the measurable functional outcomes of dysarthria therapy. The general principles that underlie treatment for dysarthria include theories of motor learning (Figure 21-4), models of aerodynamic speech production (Figure 21-1), and the communication process (Figure 21-5), and the World Health Organization's (WHO) conceptual framework of impairment, disability, and handicap with chronic disorders (Table 21-8).

Dysarthria is a motor speech disorder, so theories of motor learning apply to its treatment. Weismer and Cariski (35) summarized that for acquisition of a new motor skill to be effective, massed practice with knowledge of results, or immediate, precise feedback, is required. Thus, retention, or the ability to reproduce this new skill the next day or week, can follow. The ultimate goal of dysarthria therapy is then met during the generalization phase, when consistent, independent transfer of the new skill in different speaking situations, at various locations, and with new communication partners is achieved. Johns (36) agreed that "drill" or the "systematic practice of specifically selected and hierarchically ordered exercises" with active self-monitoring and knowledge of results is essential for generalization of new compensatory skills for dysarthria. Schmidt (37) also recommended systematically altering practice, thus encouraging different information processing during the acquisition phase, so that retention and transfer of the new speech skill are enhanced. These theories of motor learning form the basis of procedures to follow in dysarthria therapy, when new motor speech skills are to be trained.

The aerodynamic model of speech production (Figure 21-1) provides the functional framework for analyzing anatomic and physiologic deviations that affect respiration, phonation, resonance, articulation, and prosody. Understanding the interdependence of these five processes guides the planning of where to begin in dysarthria ther-

apy. Treatment decisions about which specific skills to emphasize, and in what order, can then be determined.

The communication process model (Figure 21-5) provides the context within which treatment planning occurs. Dysarthria may cause a breakdown in the communication cycle. It is often recommended to incorporate the primary communication partner and other listeners in treatment sessions, especially with moderate to severe dysarthria. This provides an opportunity for the speaker to transfer new skills to different situations, and also for the listener to learn active communication skills, such as how to cue the patient, give feedback, and clarify the message heard.

Treatment often begins with individual sessions to acquire and retain the new speech skills, then moves toward practicing these specific dysarthria compensations in group therapy. Sullivan and coworkers (37) found significant improvement in maintaining new dysarthria compensations outside therapy, six months after discharge, by providing the videotapes of group sessions and written practice for home program follow-up. Antonius and colleagues (37) identified dimensions of situational difficulty to be considered in dysarthria treatment planning, such as familiarity of the communication partner, size of the audience, demand for speed and intelligibility, emotional load, and environmental adversity. They further described compensatory strategies to resolve communication breakdowns, such as instructing the partner in how to cue and clarify the message, improving precision in the second attempt, modifying the wording, eliminating environmental barriers, and avoiding difficult situations. They also suggested classification of the perceived reactions of communication partners as helpful, solicitous, or punishing. This information assesses the need for treatment strategies to improve the active listening skills and attitudes of people in the dysarthric speaker's environment.

Acquisition → Knowledge of Results →
Retention → Generalization

FIGURE 21-4

Theory of motor learning.

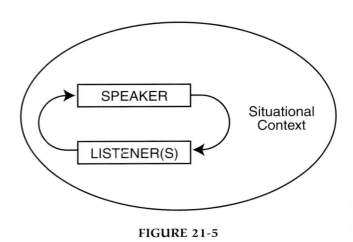

FIGURE 21-5

The communication process.

TABLE 21-8
Dysarthria as a Chronic Disorder

WORLD HEALTH ORGANIZATION CLASSIFICATIONS	DEFINITIONS AND CONSEQUENCES	APPLIED TO DYSARTHRIA	OUTCOME MEASURES
Impairment	Any loss or abnormality of psychological, physiological, or anatomical structure or function.	A neurogenic motor speech impairment that is characterized by slow, weak, imprecise and/or uncoordinated movements of the speech musculature.	Respiratory capacity and control. Phonatory function: target voice quality. Articulatory precision. Velopharyngeal function: reduced hypernasality.
Disability	Any restriction or lack of ability (resulting from an impairment) to perform an activity in a manner or within the range considered normal.	The disability (resulting from the motor speech impairment) is characterized by reduced intelligibility, rate and naturalness of speech.	Intelligibility in words, sentences and conversation. Speaking rate. Naturalness: breath units, phrasing, logical pauses, stress and intonation patterns.
Handicap	A disadvantage for a given individual (due to an impairment or disability) which limits or prevents the fulfillment of a role that is normal for that person (based on age, sex, educational, vocational, social, and cultural factors).	The handicap (resulting from the speech disability) may limit or prevent communication with others. It involves the negative self-perception and/or reaction of communication partners, which may then impact the social, educational, and vocational opportunities of the dysarthric speaker.	Speech and communication adequacy of speaker. Perceptions of speaker and listener. Cuing skills of the communication partner(s). Social, vocational, and community integration.

Adapted from Fey. (33)

The framework adopted by the WHO for differentially classifying chronic disorders in terms of impairment, disability, and handicap has been applied to dysarthria (33). Table 21-8 defines dysarthria from these three viewpoints and describes the appropriate outcome measures to use in each situation (38). Dysarthria therapy often begins with treating the impairments in respiration, phonation, resonance, and articulation, but must next shift to addressing the resulting functional limitation or disability that affects speech intelligibility, rate, and naturalness. Ultimately, dysarthria therapy should address the handicap or negative impact on social, educational, and vocational opportunities by emphasizing speaker adequacy and the skills and attitudes of the patient's communication partners. Yorkston and Bombardier (39) developed two questionnaires that begin to address the issues of disability and handicap in dysarthria; they are entitled *The Communication Profile for Speakers with Motor Speech Disorders* and *The Communication Profile for Spouses of Speakers with Motor Speech Disorders.*

Treatment Candidacy

Not all patients with dysarthria are potential treatment candidates merely because they have speech and voice problems (36). Prognosis for improvement relates to the severity and progression rate of the MS disease process, the response to medical intervention, the type and number of speech-related systems involved, as well as other cognitive-behavioral and visual-motor symptoms, the supportiveness of the communication partner and environment, and the motivation and stimulability for improvement noted in the patient. After formal evaluation by a speech-language pathologist and possible trial therapy, the potential for significant gains in longer term therapy can be judged.

Types of Treatment Approaches

There are a variety of treatment approaches to use in dysarthria therapy that depend on the specific problems identified and the expected outcome. Rehabilitation techniques may include proper positioning; stabilization; oral exercises; diaphragmatic breathing; voice and articulation drill; active self-monitoring; using behavioral compensations; prosthetic or electronic devices; eliminating behaviors that interfere with the message; enhancing communication skills between the dysarthric speaker and partner; transferring new skills in group therapy and the community; educating and training those at school, work, or in the family about the nature of the disorder and appropriate interaction strategies; and augmenting speech with alternative communication devices when indicated (33). The selection of appropriate treatment approaches and decisions about where to begin in therapy depend on which deviant speech dimension(s) are most disabling to speech intelligibility and naturalness.

The following tables list a variety of treatment approaches used for specific MS-related problems with *loudness control* (Table 21-9), *voice quality* (Table 21-10), *articulation* (Table 21-11), and *prosody* (Table 21-12). Traditional dysarthria therapy approaches in MS often address improvement of loudness, voice quality, and articulation, with the ultimate goal of adequate intelligibility. Refinement of prosodic features are often overlooked. However, enhancement of the dysarthric speaker's ability to identify and match the normal aspects of stress and intonation patterns, rate, and rhythm can result in more natural speech, which is perceived as ultimately less handicapping in the community.

After adequate intelligibility is achieved in therapy, adjustments in rate and naturalness ideally follow. The speech of MS patients with dysarthria may be perceived as bizarre because of the unusual patterns of monotony, pauses at illogical places, and inconsistent control of pitch, loudness, and duration. To treat reduced and monoloudness, monopitch, and excess and equal stress, the patient may learn improved stress patterning. This technique practices meaningful selective emphasis on key words in phrases and sentences by saying them louder, longer, and with higher pitch. For example, the following question-answer drill requires the dysarthric speaker to add stress to the pivotal word that focuses the meaning appropriately: "Who ate the sandwich?". . . "BOB ate the sandwich.". . . "What did Bob eat?". . . "Bob ate the SANDWICH." Normal variation of melodic line within a breath unit is also practiced to further enhance meaning and reduce monotony. Treatment approaches may include identifying and matching the typical "falling" pitch contour when making statements and the conventional "rising" melodic line when asking questions.

Techniques to control rate and use pauses in meaningful places play an important role in speech intelligibility and naturalness. They allow for more precise articulatory movements; better timing of the processes of respiration, phonation, articulation, and resonance;

TABLE 21-9 *Loudness Control*	
PROBLEMS	**TREATMENT APPROACHES**
Reduced loudness	Medication trial for spasticity and/or fatigue
	Proper sitting positioning, trunk and head support
	Breath support and control exercises
	Learn diaphragmatic breathing technique
	Use spirometer to monitor adequate inspiration for speech
	Use tape recorder, Voice lite, or speech lab computer software to monitor adequacy of loudness
	Practice phrasing (maximum # words/breath unit) when reading aloud, then while conversing
	Use portable voice amplifier (Figure 21-6)
Monoloudness	Tape-record reading passages with specific words underlined to meaningfully emphasize and say louder
	Transfer new skill from oral reading to conversation
Excess and variable	Medication trial for tremor and ataxia
	Sitting posture, trunk stabilization and head control
	Relaxation techniques and EMG/biofeedback for enhanced muscle during smooth respiration for speech and easy onset of voicing
	Tape recorder, Voice lite, or speech lab computer software to monitor loudness bursts
	Practice new skill during reading aloud and conversation

improved respiratory patterning for speech; and more time for the listener to "fill in the gaps" and enhance understanding. Normal speakers naturally vary the length of breath units and insert pauses where it makes syntactic and semantic sense. Dysarthric speakers' breath units are often shorter and more regular because of reduced breath support and control. Therapy may emphasize increasing the number of words per breath and varying

TABLE 21-10
Voice Quality

PROBLEMS	TREATMENT APPROACHES
Harsh, strained voice quality	Medication trial for spasticity
	Exercises to enhance respiration for speech
	Relaxation techniques and EMG/biofeedback to monitor laryngeal muscle control and easy onset of voicing
	Open mouth and "yawn-sigh" approaches during speech drill
	Tape recorder and computer software, such as Visipitch, for identifying and matching target voice quality
	Practice new skill in words, sentences, and conversational groups
Hypernasality	Soft palate exercises to improve velopharyngeal competence (VPC)
	Increase breath support for speech
	Articulation drill with plosives and their contrasting nasal glides (i.e., using /b, m/ and /d, n/ word pair lists)
	Open mouth approach to direct more oral than nasal air flow
	Slow rate of speech to allow extra time for velar movements
	Tape recorder for identifying and matching target voice quality
	Practice new skill in words, sentences, and conversational groups
	Possible palatal lift prosthesis to allow velopharyngeal closure (VPC) (Figure 21-7)
Vocal tremor	Medication trial for tremor and ataxia
	Evaluate candidacy for botox injection
	Sitting posture, trunk stabilization, and head control
	Relaxation techniques and EMG/biofeedback to control tremor and aim for smooth phonation
	Tape recorder and speech lab computer software for monitoring phonation breaks and identifying target voice quality
	Practice new skill during reading aloud and conversation

TABLE 21-11
Articulation

PROBLEMS	TREATMENT APPROACHES
Imprecise articulaton or Irregular articulatory breakdowns	Medication trial for spasticity, tremor, ataxia, and/or fatigue
	Proper sitting positioning, trunk and head support
	Oral exercises of the lips, tongue, soft palate and mandible to improve range of motion, strength, speed, and coordination
	Enhancement of breath support and respiratory control for speech
	Relaxation techniques and EMG/biofeedback to monitor and control the tone and movement of specific articulators and the timing of respiration, phonation, and articulation
	Identification of error patterns and specific articulation drill
	Practice such behavioral compensations as slow rate, overarticulation, phrasing, and strategic pauses during reading aloud and conversational groups
	Use a pacing board (Figure 21-8) or delayed auditory feedback (DAF) unit (Figure 21-9) to slow the rate of speech and allow active self-monitoring and self-correction
	Use a tape recorder or speech lab computer software to monitor articulation precision
	Practice new skill during reading aloud and conversational groups, with an emphasis on articulation clarity, intelligibility, and naturalness of speech
	Train the dysarthric speakers to attend to the listener, solicit feedback, and inform communication partner(s) of how best to cue them
	Use alternative communication devices when severe to profound deficits indicate, ranging from simple alphabet or word boards with headlight pointers, to more sophisticated electronic and portable speech output computer systems

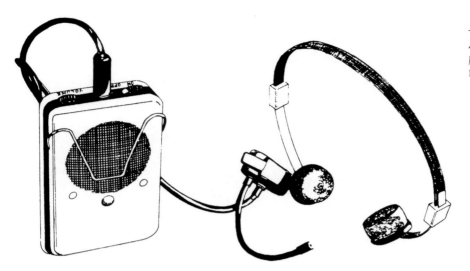

FIGURE 21-6

A portable, battery-operated *Voice Amplifier* (Cooper-Rand) used to compensate for severely reduced loudness (33).

the phrasing according to meaning, as opposed to physiologic limitations (33).

Augmentative and Alternative Communication Devices

The need and prevalence of using augmentative and alternative communication (AAC) devices in MS is low. Dysarthria rarely becomes so severe in MS that nonspeech modes of communication are necessary. In a large, cross-sectional survey of 656 individuals with MS, Beukelman and Kraft (7) reported that only 4 percent were not understood by strangers and that only 1 percent used AAC devices. However, in the small number of those who require other avenues of communication, it is important to be aware of the AAC options available, how to evaluate and determine candidacy, and which features and

devices match the needs and abilities of the patient. Osberger (40) developed the objective 10-point Meaningful Use of Speech Scale (MUSS), which ranks how willingly the patient uses vocalizations or speech to communicate with familiar then unfamiliar partners, and how the messages are understood, repaired, and clarified when necessary. This information is helpful when deciding on candidacy for augmenting oral communication and later for measuring improvement.

The specialty area of AAC evaluation and treatment has grown through recent years, with continual refinement in knowledge and expertise, and ongoing upgrades in equipment and training. It is best performed by a specialized AAC team, which views communication within the user's natural environment, has the patient and communication partners as central to the process, and includes other community agencies when considering the more expensive, high-tech devices. Ideally, some members on the AAC support team include (40):

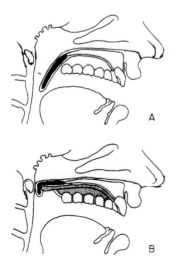

FIGURE 21-7

Palatal lift prosthesis. A. Weakness of the soft palate resulting in velopharyngeal incompetence. B. Wearing palatal lift prosthesis, which elevates the soft palate and reduces hypernasality. [Adapted from Gonzales and Aronson (33).]

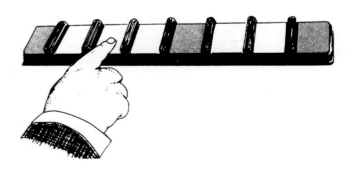

FIGURE 21-8

A pacing board used to enhance strategic pauses for careful articulation of one word at a time (33).

TABLE 21-12
Prosody: Natural Flow of Speech

PROBLEMS	TREATMENT APPROACHES
Reduced loudness	Stress patterning techniques to counteract the unusual patterns of monotony and to practice natural variation in loudness, duration, and pitch of key words in phrases and sentences
Monoloudness	Using a tape recorder to compare monotonous patterning with stress patterning while evaluating perceived naturalness
Monopitch	Practicing emphasis of the most important word in a question-answer drill: "Where did Ann go?" . . . "Ann went HOME."
Reduced stress or	Underlining key words in reading passages to emphasize, thus enhancing meaning during reading-aloud tasks
Excess and equal stress	Using a tape recorder to self-evaluate which stress parameter sounds most natural: when varying loudness, duration, or pitch (singly or in combination)
Excess and variable loudness	Using speech lab computer software to visualize and match the targeted variations in fundamental frequency and intensity
Monopitch	Identifying, drawing, and practicing variation of melodic line or normal intonation patterns within a breath unit
	Practicing the typical "falling" pitch contour when making statements and the conventional "rising" melodic line when asking questions
	Using a tape recorder while reading aloud limericks and poetry that provide opportunities to initially practice exaggerated patterns of stress, intonation, and rhythm
Slow rate Variable rate	Controlling the rate of speech by interjecting pauses in logical places, thus allowing improved articulation, coordination of systems, breath units, and understanding by the listener
	Initially using rigid rate control devices such as a pacing board (Figure 21-8), DAF unit (Figure 21-9), or alphabet board supplementation; ultimately transferring to rate control by the individual without any devices

TABLE 21-12
continued

PROBLEMS	TREATMENT APPROACHES
Short phrasing Prolonged intervals Inappropriate silences	Improving breath support and control for speech and increasing the number of words adequately articulated in a breath unit
	Marking off meaningful phrasing units in logical places of reading passages before reading them aloud; emphasizing normal variability, short and long phrasing units, based on the syntax and semantics of the message vs. based solely on the patient's physiologic limitations
	Using a tape recorder to eliminate inappropriate silences and phrasing; self-monitoring naturalness of rate and flow of speech during oral reading and conversation

1. *AAC consultant*—familiar with AAC resources, systems and effective practices
2. *Manufacturer's representative*—for technical assistance, feature match, and funding options
3. *Rehabilitation engineer*—to customize, design, and give ongoing technical help
4. *Occupational therapist*—to address visual-motor, positioning, mounting, and physical access needs
5. *Speech-language pathologist*—to evaluate cognitive-language skills, train the patient and caregiver to use the new alternate communication system effectively, script messages, develop and organize overlays, and practice in their naturalistic environment
6. *Patient and communication partner*—to assist with scripting relevant messages, and operating, maintaining, and manipulating the system
7. *Case manager*—to coordinate other agencies and assist with funding sources

When selecting the appropriate AAC device, it is important to match the needs and abilities of the individual with the features of the system. Cognitive-language, visual-motor, behavioral, and central executive functions may be affected with MS and thus need formal evaluation. Assessment also includes an interview with the patient and significant other(s) to determine their unique communication needs and informal observation of their natural communication environment. Personal goals, preferences, environmental needs, and desired outcomes for family members are determined. Formal AAC assessment further identifies (40):

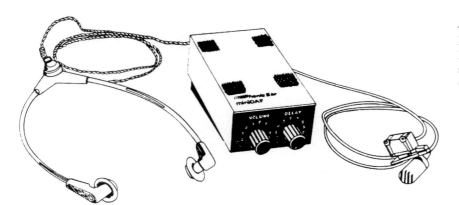

FIGURE 21-9

Delayed Auditory Feedback Unit (Mini DAF, Phonic Ear) used to slow the rate of speech and promote active self-monitoring (33).

1. Current methods of communication (speech, vocalizations, gesture, head nods, pointing, eye gaze, and facial expression)
2. Past experience with AAC devices
3. Communication environment (home, school, work, community)
4. Mobility, positioning, seating, and visual concerns (by occupational therapist)
5. Reliable modes for AAC access (functional control of upper extremity, lower extremity, head, and eyes)
6. Other technologies to integrate with the AAC system (i.e., wheelchair, computer, and environmental controls)

A formal assessment of communication needs also directs treatment planning by identifying specific goals for the AAC system, such as gaining attention of others; requesting assistance, objects, or actions; improving social interaction; engaging in turn-taking; and asking or responding to questions.

Matching results of the evaluation with the features of available AAC devices to guide the selection of an appropriate alternate communication system is the next step. Decisions are made regarding the:

1. Motor access method (controlled by head, chin, mouth, lips, tongue, sip & puff, hand, arm, elbow, shoulder, leg, knee, foot, or eye movements)
2. Input (auditory or visual: pictures, letters, or words: direct or scanning)
3. Symbol system (number, size, organization, and vocabulary capabilities)
4. Output (printed messages versus digitized or synthesized speech)
5. General features (complexity, flexibility, portability, durability, and cost)

Glennen and DeCoste (40) developed an AAC Product Directory that includes a comprehensive list of different AAC devices, computer access hardware and software, switches, light pointers, mounting equipment, symbol sets and low- versus high-tech options. Figure 21-10 classifies a variety of low- and high-tech AAC options to choose from, depending on auditory or visual input, direct selection or scanning, headlight pointer, finger, or keyboard access, dedicated AAC systems, or laptop computers, with printed message or synthesized speech output and scanning word prediction software. The AAC recommendation is based on need and ability.

Funding sources for expensive AAC devices may be found through certain health insurance policies, the Department of Vocational Rehabilitation, Social Security's PASS plan (Plan for Achieving Self-Support), and private foundations. A case manager or therapist may help with wording to justify funding from these organizations. For example, "The individual needs AAC services and equipment to gain, maintain, or return to employment" would be sent to the Department of Vocational Rehabilitation for funding justification, whereas a health insurance company may receive "The individual needs AAC services and equipment to manage personal care, communicate needs to caregivers, and access medical care" (40).

Treatment strategies to help the patient use the recommended AAC system appropriately are shared with the communication partner. They include basic training about general maintenance, operation and programming of the AAC device, development of a responsibility checklist, generation of relevant vocabulary and scripted messages, organization and set-up, and practice in their natural communication environment. Flexibility and ongoing modification is recommended as needs and skills change.

Treatment Outcomes

Treatment of speech, voice, and communication disorders in MS has been described in detail. Pharmacologic and

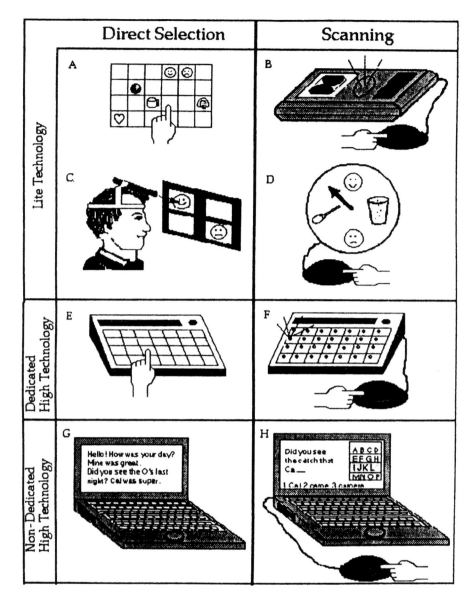

FIGURE 21-10

Augmentative communication system classification. (A) Picture communication board. (B) Scanning loop tape recorder. (C) Laser light pointer with simple picture communication board. (D) Clock communicator. (E) Direct selection AAC system. (F) Scanning AAC system. (G) Laptop computer with speech synthesizer. (H) Laptop computer with speech synthesizer and scanning word prediction software (40).

rehabilitation strategies have been reviewed. Measurement of treatment efficacy may be accomplished in a few ways, depending on the viewpoint. Objective measures of respiratory capacity and control, consistency of target voice quality, and articulatory precision in words, sentences, and conversation are traditionally used to measure improvement of impairment in physiologic functioning before and after the treatment phase. However, more functional measures of how the person performs, which relate to disability status, are recommended. Treatment efficacy is assessed through comparative testing of intelligibility, speaking rate, and naturalness or prosody. The American Speech-Language-Hearing Association (41) developed 8-point scales for functional communication measures in specific areas. The scales that rate Speech Production Disorders, Voice Disorders, and Disorders of Rate, Rhythm, or Fluency have good application for measuring the disabling effects of dysarthria and dysphonia in MS. Moreover, a recent trend is to measure the impact of therapy on reducing the handicap, or negative perceptions and role limitations, of the dysarthric speaker. Epstein and coworkers (42) suggest using the Speech Disability Questionnaire to measure the impact of therapy for speech, voice, or communication disorders on quality of life. In their study with botox injections and adductor spasmodic dysphonia, they found that social isolation, negative self-perception, public avoidance, and difficulty being understood by others, significantly improved with voice therapy. Their model of combining a measurement of handicap or quality of life with other more traditional evaluations of impairment and disability adds depth to the understanding of treatment outcomes in speech, voice, and communication intervention.

References

1. Netsell R. Physiological studies of dysarthria and their relevance to treatment. In: Rosenbek J (ed.). *Normal aspects of speech, language and hearing.* Englewood Cliffs, NJ: Prentice-Hall, 1973.

2. Kalb R (ed.). *Multiple sclerosis: The questions you have—the answers you need.* New York: Demos Vermande, 1996; 7:127–37.

3. Charcot JM. *Lectures on the diseases of the nervous system.* Vol. 1. London: New Sydenham Society, 1877.

4. Sorensen P, Brown S, Logemann J, Wilson K, Herndon R. Communication disorders and dysphagia. *J Neuro Rehab* 1994; 8(3):137–143.

5. Darley F, Brown J, Goldstein N. Dysarthria in multiple sclerosis. *J Speech Hearing Res* 1972; 15:229–245.

6. Hartelius L, Svensson P. Speech and swallowing symptoms associated with Parkinson's disease and multiple sclerosis: A survey. *Folia Phoniat Logop* 1994; 46:9–17.

7. Beukelman D, Kraft G, Freal J. Expressive communication disorders in persons with multiple sclerosis: A survey. *Arch Phys Med Rehabil* 1985; 10:675–677.

8. Grinker R, Sahs A. *Neurology.* 6th ed. Springfield, IL: Charles C. Thomas, 1966.

9. Brain W. *Diseases of the nervous system.* 6th ed. New York: Oxford University Press, 1962.

10. Darley F, Aronson A, Brown J. Differential diagnostic patterns of dysarthria. *J Speech Hearing Res* 1969; 12:246–269.

11. Biary N, Pimental P, Langenburg P. A double-blind trial of clonazepam in the treatment of parkinsonian dysarthria. *Neurology* 1988; 38:255–258.

12. Critchley E. Speech disorders of parkinsonism: A review. *J Neurol Neurosurg Psychiatry* 1981; 44:751–758.

13. Nakano K, Zubick H, Tyler H. Speech defects of parkinsonian patients. *Neurology* 1973; 23:865–870.

14. Busenbark K, Ramig L, Dromey C, Koller W. Methazolamide for essential voice tremor. *Neurology* 1996; 47:1331–1332.

15. Duvoisin R, Bradley W, Bruce O, Ellis F. Clinical use of botulinum toxin. *Arch Neurol* 1991; 48:1294–1297.

16. Theriot K. "Spasticity and tremor/ataxia." The Jimmie Heuga Center Patient Manual, 1998.

17. Thompson A. Multiple sclerosis: symptomatic treatment. *J Neurol* 1996; 243:559–565.

18. Hallet M, Lindsey J, Adelstein B, Riley P. Controlled trial of isoniazid therapy for severe postural cerebellar tremor in multiple sclerosis. *Neurology* 1985; 35:1374–1377.

19. Rice G, Dickey C, Lesaux J, Vandervoort P, MacEwan L, Ebers G. Ondansetron for disabling cerebellar tremor. *Ann Neurol* 1995; 38:973.

20. Krupp L, Alvarez L, LaRocca N, Scheinberg L. Fatigue in multiple sclerosis. *Arch Neurol* 1988; 45:435–437.

21. Krupp L, Coyle P, Doscher C, et al. Fatigue therapy in multiple sclerosis: Results of a double-blind, randomized, parallel trial of amantadine, pemoline, and placebo. *Neurology* 1995; 45:1956–1961.

22. Cohen R, Fisher M. Amantadine treatment of fatigue associated with multiple sclerosis. *Arch Neurol* 1989; 46:676–680.

23. Rosenberg G, Appenzeller O. Amantadine, fatigue, and multiple sclerosis. *Arch Neurol* 1988; 45:1104–1106.

24. Murray T. Amantadine therapy for fatigue in multiple sclerosis. *Can J Neurol Sci* 1985; 12:251–254.

25. Weinshenker B, Penman M, Bass B, Ebers G, Rice G. A double-blind, randomized, cross-over trial of pemoline in fatigue associated with multiple sclerosis. *Neurology* 1992; 42:1468–1471.

26. Schapiro R. *Symptom management in multiple sclerosis.* 3rd ed. New York: Demos, 1999.

27. Bernthal J, Bankson N. *Articulation disorders.* Englewood Cliffs, NJ: Prentice-Hall, 1981.

28. Yorkston, K, Beukelman D. *Assessment of intelligibility of dysarthric speech.* Austin: Pro-ed, 1984.

29. Metter, E. *Speech disorders: Clinical evaluation and diagnosis.* New York: Spectrum, 1985.

30. Mustillo, P. Auditory deficits in multiple sclerosis: a review. *Audiology* 1984; 23:145–164.

31. Rao, S, Leo G, Berardin L, Unverzagt, F. Cognitive dysfunction in multiple sclerosis. I. Frequency, patterns, and prediction. *Neurology* 1991; 41:685–691.

32. Rao, S. Neuropsychological screening battery for multiple sclerosis. Unpublished: Medical College of Wisconsin, Milwaukee.

33. Yorkston K, Beukelman D, Bell, K. *Clinical management of dysarthric speakers.* Boston: College-Hill Publication, 1988.

34. Winitz H (ed.). *Treating articulation disorders: For clinicians by clinicians.* Baltimore: University Park Press, 1984.

35. Lass N (ed.). *Speech and language: Advances in basic research and practice.* Vol. 10. New York: Academic Press, 1984.

36. Johns D (ed.). *Clinical management of neurogenic communication disorders.* Boston: Little, Brown, 1978.

37. Robin D, Yorkston K, Beukelman D. *Disorders of motor speech: Assessment, treatment, and clinical characterization.* Baltimore: Paul H. Brooks Publishing, 1996.

38. Halpern A, Fuhrer M (eds.). *Functional assessment in rehabilitation.* Baltimore: Paul H. Brooks Publishing, 1984.

39. Yorkston K, Bombardier C. The Communication Profile for Speakers with Motor Speech Disorders and The Communication Profile for Spouses of Speakers with Motor Speech Disorders. Unpublished questionnaires, University of Washington, Seattle, 1992.

40. Glennen S, DeCoste D. *Handbook of augmentative and alternative communication.* San Diego: Singular Publishing, 1997.

41. American Speech-Language-Hearing Association. Functional communication measures: National treatment outcome data collection project, 1996.

42. Epstein R, Stygall J, Newman S. The short-term impact of botox injections on speech disability in adductor spasmodic dysphonia. *Disability and Rehabilitation* 1997; 19:20–25.

APPENDIX 1
Motor Speech/Voice Evaluation

Patient: _____ Referring Physician: _____

Date of Birth: _____ Age: _____ Medical Diagnosis: _____

Occupation: _____ Date of Onset: _____

Primary Communication Partners: _____ Medications: _____

I. Background Information:

Description of speech/voice problem: _____

Onset: _____ Variability through the day: _____

Communication needs: _____

Other impairments(circle):   Fatigue   Vision   Hearing   Cognition   Motor

Prior therapy: _____ Medical interventions: _____

II. Oral Peripheral Examination:

Lips: _____ Teeth: _____

Tongue: _____ Hard Palate: _____

Soft Palate: _____ Mandible: _____

III. Assessment of Motor Speech and Voice Processes:

A. Respiration:

   1. Posture (circle problems):   Sitting balance   Trunk control   Head control

   2. Pattern (circle):   Clavicular   Thoracic   Abdominal

   3. Pulmonary Function Test results: _____

   4. Measurement of inspiratory effort (using spirometer): _____

   5. Breath control for speech:

      a. Sustains "ah"_____ sec.   Sustains "ee"_____ sec. (Norm=20–23 sec)

      b. Counts up to 50/one breath (Norm= #50/17sec.): _____

      c. Inhales fully (in 5 sec) and sustains exhalation (10 sec): _____

      d. Sustains "sss"_____ sec. and "zzz"_____ sec (Norm=1:1 ratio, 18–20 sec)

B. Phonation:

   1. Loudness: _____WNL/WFL _____Reduced _____Monoloudness _____Loudness decay

      _____Excess _____Variable _____Phonation breaks

      *Loudness gradation: "Count to 5 where 1= a whisper and 5= a yell":_____

   2. Pitch: _____WNL/WFL _____High _____Low _____Monopitch _____Pitch breaks

      *Pitch control: "Sing up the scale, Do, re, mi, fa, so, la, ti, do."_____

      *Optimal pitch for best voice quality:_____   Habitual pitch:_____

   3. Quality: _____WNL/WFL _____Harsh, strained _____Breathy _____Hoarse

      _____Vocal tremor _____Glottal fry

APPENDIX 1
continued

C. Articulation:

_____WNL/WFL _____Imprecise consonants _____Distorted vowels

_____Irregular articulatory breakdown _____Substituted/omitted phonemes

_____Specific phonemes misarticulated: _____

_____Reduced diadochokinetic rate (in 5 sec) (Norm= 26–28/5 sec): /p/= _____ /t/= _____ /k/= _____

_____/pataka/= _____ (Norm= 10–12/5sec.)

*Assessment of articulation during imitation of words and sentences:

Snowman	Methodist Episcopal Church
Several	Zip-zipper-zippering
Tornado	Please-pleasing-pleasingly
Gingerbread	City-citizen-citizenship
Artillery	In the summer they sell vegetables.
Catastrophe	The shipwreck washed up on the shore.
Impossibility	Please put the groceries in the refrigerator.
Statistical analysis	

*Intelligibility Rating: _____in words _____in sentences _____in conversation

D. Resonance:

_____ WNL/WFL _____Hypernasality _____Hyponasality _____Nasal emission

E. Prosody:

_____WNL/WFL _____Slow rate _____Fast rate _____Variable rate

_____Prolonged intervals within words _____Inapproriate silences between words

_____Reduced stress _____Monopitch _____Monoloudness

_____Excess & equal stress (scanning speech) _____Excess & variable loudness

IV. Differential Diagnosis of Dysarthria (circle features identified):

Spastic Dysarthria	**Ataxic Dysarthria**	**Mixed Dysarthria**
Reduced & monoloudness	Excess & variable loudness	Impaired loudness control
Harsh or hypernasal voice	Harsh voice or vocal tremor	Impaired voice quality
Imprecise articulation	Irregular articulation breakdown	Impaired articulation
Monopitch, reduced stress	Excess & equal stress	Impaired pitch & emphasis
Slow rate, short phrasing	Variable rate, prolonged intervals	Impaired rate & prosody

Type and severity of dysarthia:_____

Prognosis for improvement: _____

V. Recommendations:_____

_____

_____

_____

Speech-Language Pathologist

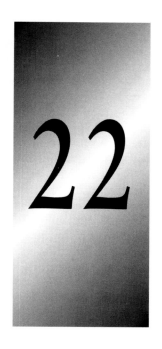

22 Cognitive and Emotional Disorders

Nicholas G. LaRocca, Ph.D.

those who have lived or worked with multiple sclerosis (MS) for any significant length of time understand that this disease consists of more than just weakened limbs and a finicky bladder. Memory lapses, mood swings, grief, and depression may all be features of this mysterious disease as it envelops individuals and families in its relentless and unpredictable course. This chapter examines some of the more important psychological changes that may occur in MS, discusses the current understanding of their causes, and presents a variety of assessment and treatment options. Wherever possible, the discussion is evidence-based, drawing on the burgeoning scientific literature in this field. In those instances in which research is sparse, clinical experience—at times that of the author—is used to expand upon or substitute for more scientific evidence. The discussion is intended to be factual and to the point. As a result, complex theoretical models and lengthy philosophical speculations are absent. Instead, it is hoped that the reader will find a practical guide to understanding and dealing with the cognitive and emotional changes that occur in MS.

COGNITIVE CHANGES

Although cognitive changes are not generally the foremost concern of people with MS and health care providers, these symptoms have received increasing attention in recent years. This growing interest reflects our increased understanding of the nature of such problems and recognition of the potentially significant impact of cognitive deficits on everyday life. In this chapter we review the primary and secondary effects of MS on cognition, discuss the nature of the cognitive deficits observed in MS, describe how these symptoms can be assessed, and outline management strategies.

Etiology of Cognitive Changes

Why do people with MS experience cognitive changes? The causes of these changes may be divided into two categories: *primary* effects of MS and *secondary* effects of the disease (Table 22-1). Because each of these types of effects has significant but distinct implications for management, it is important to understand both.

Primary Effects of the Disease

People with MS develop cognitive deficits primarily because MS is a disease that attacks the brain, damaging the myelin (1) and, to a lesser extent, the nerve cells themselves (2). Because MS lesions are generally multifocal and vary from person to person in their distribution, the pattern of deficits may vary significantly. Studies using mag-

---

TABLE 22-1
Possible Causes of Cognitive Dysfunction in MS

Primary Effects of the Disease
- Cerebral demyelination and axonal damage

Secondary Effects of the Disease
- Depression
- Anxiety
- Stress
- Fatigue

---

netic resonance imaging (MRI) have confirmed that both the extent and the location of demyelinative lesions are related to cognitive deficits in MS. In one classic study, it was found that 83 percent of MS patients with greater than 30 cm^2 of total lesion area were cognitively impaired, whereas 22 percent of those with less than 30 cm^2 of total lesion area met criteria for cognitive impairment (3). Investigators have also found that MS cognitive dysfunction is related to enlargement of the ventricles and atrophy of the corpus callosum (4–8). Magnetic resonance imaging studies have suggested that lesions in specific areas of cerebral white matter may be associated with particular cognitive deficits. Frontal lobe lesions have been found to be related to perseverative responses on the Wisconsin Card Sorting Test (9,10) and deficits in executive functions (11). Lesions in the corpus callosum are associated with a variety of deficits, including interhemispheric transfer of information (3,11,12), speed of information processing (3,11,13), verbal fluency (14), and spatial abilities (15).

Studies using other methodologies to study clinicopathologic correlates have bolstered the findings from the MRI studies. In a study using positron emission tomography (PET), reductions were observed in cerebral metabolism in the frontal and left temporal lobes that were related to deficits in verbal fluency and verbal memory (14). A study using event-related potentials found that P300 latencies were prolonged in MS patients who were impaired on neuropsychological testing (16).

Secondary Effects of the Disease

There is considerable controversy concerning the extent to which MS cognitive deficits are related to depression, anxiety, stress, and fatigue—symptoms that affect the majority of persons with MS at some time during the course of the illness. Although severe clinical depression may be associated with mild cognitive impairment in psychiatric populations (17), most studies examining this

issue in MS have found little or no relationship between depression and cognitive deficits (18–21). However, in a recent meta-analysis of the literature on memory dysfunction in MS, investigators found a strong correlation (r = 0.64) between depression and working memory deficits in 10 studies but no relationship between depression and short-term memory or long-term memory (22). Affective changes are discussed in detail later in this chapter. Suffice it to say that, although depression cannot in itself readily explain the extensive cognitive changes seen in MS, proper management of depression through psychotherapy and medications may facilitate the ability of the person with MS to make the best use of cognitive skills.

No studies have addressed the possible role of stress and anxiety in MS cognitive dysfunction. However, it is generally recognized that stress and anxiety can disrupt a wide variety of cognitive functions in the general population, particularly attention, concentration, and memory. For the clinician encountering complaints of cognitive deficits in MS, there are two important considerations. First, given the neuropathologic substrate for MS cognitive deficits, it is probably not wise to assume that such complaints are simply manifestations of depression, anxiety, and/or stress. Second, depression, anxiety, and stress are likely to make life more difficult for the person who is experiencing cognitive changes and thus need to be addressed therapeutically in conjunction with them.

Fatigue in MS has been anecdotally associated with impaired ability to concentrate and perform intellectual tasks. However, in the only controlled study examining this issue in MS, fatigue-inducing exercise had no effect on cognitive test performance (23). The fatigue seen in MS is often at its worst in the middle to late afternoon, making it a challenge for many people with MS to function adequately for a full day of work or family responsibilities. MS-related sleep disturbances may contribute both to fatigue and to cognitive dysfunction, but data on this subject are limited at present (24). Although the relationship between MS fatigue and cognitive dysfunction is complex and fraught with ambiguities, common sense suggests that in managing cognitive changes, minimizing fatigue and maximizing energy level should be explored.

Frequency, Severity, and Nature of Cognitive Changes

Estimates of the frequency of cognitive changes in MS have varied widely depending on the source of samples studied and methods of assessment. In one study it was found that more than half of the MS patients were impaired on standardized neuropsychological testing. However, when these same patients were evaluated using a brief "mental status" examination administered by a neurologist, half of the patients who were impaired on neuropsychological testing were considered to be "normal" on the mental status (25). It is now generally accepted that 45 percent to 65 percent of patients with MS have some cognitive impairment (26–28). In the vast majority of people, these deficits appear to be mild to moderate, with some noticeable impact on everyday activities but not severe enough to preclude the fulfillment of most work and family responsibilities. However, in a small percentage of cases, perhaps 5 percent to 10 percent, MS cognitive dysfunction may be so severe that the person is largely unable to function without supervision and assistance, even if physical disability is mild.

Multiple sclerosis is characterized by demyelination in the subcortical white matter. As a result, some investigators have posited the concept of a "subcortical" dementia to characterize the cognitive deficits in MS (29). Indeed, the pattern of cognitive deficits often seen in MS may resemble that observed in conditions such as Huntington's disease and Parkinson's disease, i.e., problems with memory retrieval; abstract reasoning and problem solving; and information-processing speed without aphasia, agnosia, or apraxia. However, when cognitive impairment becomes severe in MS, there may be significant cortical and axonal damage (2,30) accompanied by a significant global dementia.

In most cases, MS cognitive dysfunction is characterized by selective impairment of some functions with relative preservation of others (31) Measures of *general intellectual ability*, e.g., IQ tests, may show little or no impairment, whereas neuropsychological tests assessing *specific functions*, e.g., memory tests, may show serious deficits (32).

Table 22-2 summarizes the cognitive functions that are generally thought to be affected by MS. *Memory*, both verbal and visual, is the function most consistently found to be impaired in MS. Studies of *primary memory* (memory operating over a few seconds) have suggested that *short-term memory* (e.g., the immediate repetition of a string of digits) is relatively intact (33), whereas *working memory* (e.g., the brief processing of information in temporary storage) is impaired (34). Research on *secondary memory* (memory operating over more than a few seconds) has generally found that although the *retrieval* (e.g., a fill in the blanks test) of previously learned information is impaired (35), *recognition* (e.g., a multiple-choice test) of such information is unaffected (33). However, recent studies have challenged the idea that people with MS adequately encode and store information, having trouble only with the retrieval of stored information. In one such study, it was shown that if MS patients and controls were equated in terms of adequacy of the initial learning process, they were approximately equal in terms of subsequent retrieval of the same information (36). A

TABLE 22-2

Cognitive Functions Thought to Be Affected in MS

- Memory (working memory and secondary memory)
- Abstract reasoning and problem solving
- Attention and concentration (especially sustained and/or complex attention)
- Speed of information processing
- Verbal fluency
- Visuospatial skills

---

recent meta-analysis of 36 studies comparing memory in people with MS and controls suggested that there is significant impairment across all domains of memory in MS (22). These issues are of more than just academic interest because the health care provider who is attempting to teach techniques such as self-injection must be cognizant of any special learning needs exhibited by people with MS.

Abstract reasoning and *problem solving* are often impaired in MS, with these deficits frequently manifest as a lack of flexibility in thinking when conditions demand a shift in approach (37,38). The ability to process corrective feedback seems to be curtailed, and as a result the same errors are made over and over again. Deficits in *executive functions* (e.g., planning, prioritizing, and sequencing complex tasks) are also common in MS and are closely related to difficulties with abstract reasoning and problem solving (39).

Attention and *concentration* are often impaired in MS, especially complex and sustained attention (28). The attentional deficits seen in MS are therefore likely to appear when it is necessary to concentrate for long periods of time and/or to focus on more than one thing at a time, e.g., balancing the checkbook while preparing dinner. Related to the attention/concentration issue is *slowed information processing* (40,41). People with MS often find that they can no longer process information as quickly as they once did, especially when information from several different channels needs to be processed at once, e.g., in a lively discussion group. A common complaint that seems to combine elements of memory loss and slowed information processing is a decrease in *verbal fluency* (42) This is often referred to as the "tip of the tongue" phenomenon, i.e., the individual cannot think of a specific word but feels as though it is right on "the tip of the tongue." This sort of word-finding problem may be awkward in social situations and is often misunderstood by relatives and friends, who inevitably seem to say, "Oh, that happens to me all the time." Other types of language deficits, such as aphasia, appear to be relatively uncommon in MS (43).

A variety of *visuospatial skills* may be impaired in MS (28). These deficits may take the form of difficulties with constructional tasks, e.g., those gadgets that are labeled "some assembly required." Other examples include difficulty with left/right discriminations, trouble with driving directions, and problems following maps and diagrams. Compared with memory, this area has received relatively little attention. Visuospatial skills are a challenge to assess accurately in MS because primary sensory abilities (visual) and motor functions (fine motor coordination) are often impaired, which makes it difficult to evaluate the role of higher cognitive processes.

The preceding is a partial list of those cognitive functions that have most reliably been shown to be affected by MS. The list will undoubtedly expand as research continues. Because MS lesions are generally widely dispersed in the brain and can cause axonal damage in addition to demyelination, MS may be thought of as undermining the overall organization of brain processes. Therefore, given the right set of circumstances, almost any brain function can be affected by MS. It is also useful to keep in mind that although the preceding list includes the most common cognitive deficits in MS, the functions affected may vary considerably from patient to patient and one must therefore be on the lookout for "atypical" patterns.

Relationship to Clinical Disease Characteristics

There has been some controversy concerning the relationship of MS-related cognitive dysfunction to other characteristics of the disease, such as neurologic impairment, disease duration, course, and disease activity. Some studies have found little or no relationship between cognitive deficits and neurologic impairment or duration (28,44). In contrast, many studies have found that patients with a progressive course are at greater risk for cognitive changes (37,45), although some investigators have not found such a link (46).

A recent meta-analysis examined 36 published studies of memory deficits in MS (22). In that review, the investigators found that neurologic disability was modestly related to memory deficits, accounting for 16 percent of the variance in short-term memory, 41 percent of the variance in working memory, and 19 percent of the variance in long-term memory. In contrast, disease duration was only related to working memory, accounting for 37 percent of its variance. Disease course showed the strongest associations in the review, accounting for almost two thirds of the variance in short-term memory and working memory but with little or no relationship to long-term memory. Patients with a relapsing-remitting course were less likely to have the two aforementioned types of memory changes than those with a chronic progressive course.

It is clear from the published research that the relationship between cognitive changes and other disease characteristics varies depending on which changes and characteristics one is examining. In many instances, the relationship is relatively weak. Moreover, disease characteristics are often confounded with one another, e.g., patients with a progressive course often have greater neurologic disability and have had MS longer. It is important for the clinician to keep in mind that cognitive changes may occur at any time during the course of the disease and may appear in both mildly and severely disabled individuals. Moreover, persons with severe physical disability may be completely free of cognitive changes. In addition, cognitive deficits can worsen during exacerbations and then improve during remissions (31). With these caveats in mind, the clinician can avoid the common error of dismissing the cognitive complaints of recent onset, mildly disabled, relapsing-remitting patients or the equally erroneous stereotyping of severely disabled patients as sure to have cognitive changes.

Assessment of Cognitive Dysfunction

There is scant time available to evaluate something as complex as cognitive dysfunction in the normal course of an office visit. However, shortcuts generally have been found to be less than effective. Using either the "bedside mental status" or a brief screening instrument such as the Mini Mental Status Examination may result in missing approximately 50 percent of those patients who have cognitive impairments (25,46–48). Relying on reports of everyday difficulties from patients or family members may be equally imprecise (49).

A full neuropsychological battery is probably the most effective way to assess cognitive changes in MS. However, such an evaluation may take several hours and cost more than one thousand dollars. Shorter "screening" batteries have been developed, which may be quite sensitive in identifying those patients who are likely to show cognitive deficits on longer batteries of tests (50).

The specific tests that are used are probably less important than the concept of covering certain areas of functioning (e.g., memory, abstract reasoning, verbal fluency, and so on), using reliable and valid tests, and minimizing the confounding effects of primary neurologic deficits such as visual loss and problems with eye-hand coordination (26)

The person with MS may be terrified by the prospect of cognitive changes. Having to deal with loss or diminution of function in many physical functions, he or she may have derived solace from the fact that at least the mind is still intact. Once cognitive abilities are compromised, it may seem like the beginning of the end. However, pinpointing the nature and severity of cognitive changes generally is beneficial. There often is misunderstanding on the part of family members and friends who may misconstrue memory loss as "disinterest" or distractibility as a "poor attitude." A good evaluation may identify other treatable problems such as depression. Moreover, the results of a comprehensive assessment may be useful in career planning and designing a program of cognitive rehabilitation. It is important that the evaluation be done by someone who has appropriate qualifications, such as a clinical neuropsychologist who has experience in MS. In the past, clinical intervention for cognitive changes in MS mainly consisted of the assessment of these deficits along with patient and family education. However, there are many additional options available to the clinician for addressing cognitive dysfunction in MS.

Treatment of Cognitive Dysfunction

Pharmacologic Management

There are two possible approaches to the pharmacologic management of cognitive changes in MS: (1) symptomatic treatments that modify one or more cognitive functions (e.g., improve memory), and (2) disease-modifying agents that alter the course of the disease so as to slow, halt, or reverse the neuropathologic changes underlying cognitive deficits (Table 22-3). To date, *symptomatic treatments* have not been shown to be of much value in the treatment of MS cognitive changes. Studies using 4-aminopyridine (4-AP), a potassium channel blocker that increases the speed of nerve conduction, have found little benefit for impaired cognitive functions in MS (51). In addition, because 4-AP can lower the seizure threshold, it can be quite dangerous. Intravenous physostigmine and lecithin treatment were also shown to be of little or no value (52). Tacrine HCL (Cognex) and donepezil HCL (Aricept) are similar to physostigmine in that they increase the available supply of acetylcholine, a neurotransmitter that is thought to play a role in memory. Both drugs have been approved for use in Alzheimer's disease. Anecdotal reports have suggested that Aricept® may be beneficial for some types of memory deficits in MS. Several clinical trials using Aricept in MS have been undertaken. Results thus far from one small open-label trial have been positive (52a). Amantadine (Symmetrel) and pemoline (Cylert) are used to treat fatigue in MS but appear to have negligible benefit for cognitive dysfunction (53).

Published data concerning the impact of *disease-modifying agents* on MS cognitive changes are quite limited, mainly because cognition has not been consistently examined as an outcome in clinical trials (54). However, in a recently reported clinical trial of methotrexate in chronic progressive MS, patients receiving the active drug showed modest improvements relative to those receiv-

---

TABLE 22-3
Some Approaches to Treatment of Cognitive Dysfunction in MS

- Symptomatic pharmacologic management (potassium channel blockers, cholinesterase inhibitors, psychic stimulants)
- Disease-modifying agents (Avonex, Betaseron, Copaxone)
- Restorative rehabilitation (cognitive exercises and drills)
- Compensatory strategies (substitution methods, lists, computers)

---

ing placebo in verbal ability, visuospatial ability, information processing speed, memory, and problem solving (55). In a large clinical trial, relapsing-remitting patients receiving interferon beta-1a (Avonex) improved modestly over a two-year treatment period compared with those receiving placebo on measures of information processing/memory and visuospatial abilities/executive functions, but not on measures of verbal abilities/attention span (56). However, a recent study failed to find any benefit on cognitive functioning in MS patients treated with glatiramer acetate (56a). Although these findings were not spectacular, they do suggest that effective disease-modifying agents may be able to play a modest but important role in the management of cognitive changes in MS. The disease-modifying agents approved for use in MS—interferon beta-1a (Avonex), interferon beta-1b (Betaseron), and glatiramer acetate (Copaxone)—have all been shown to slow the accumulation of demyelinative lesions on MRI. Because cognitive dysfunction is related to the total lesion area revealed on MRI, it would not be surprising if these drugs are ultimately found to slow the progression of cognitive changes in MS. Results thus far suggest that this may be the case, but definitive conclusions await the results of recently completed and ongoing clinical trials that have more comprehensively addressed cognitive deficits.

Cognitive Rehabilitation

Cognitive rehabilitation has a long history in traumatic brain injury (57,58) but has received significantly less attention in MS, possibly because the progressive nature of this disease has discouraged practitioners. Cognitive rehabilitation can be roughly divided into two major approaches: restorative versus compensatory. The *restorative* approach attempts to restore or strengthen impaired function through direct retraining procedures such as memory drills or exercises to improve attention and concentration (58). This approach is based in part on the assumption that the human brain has a degree of "plasticity," which allows it to recover from injury, given the right set of circumstances. Systematic practice of gradually increasing difficulty is used to challenge impaired functions in the hope that the brain will recoup some of its losses. Although the restorative approach has its place in cognitive rehabilitation, this approach has been somewhat disappointing in that it does not seem to have much impact on everyday activities. In one early study, computer-mediated memory drills failed to improve memory function in MS patients (59). It would appear that the vaunted plasticity of the brain may not be as great as once assumed. As a result, emphasis has shifted toward the compensatory approach.

The *compensatory* approach does not seek to restore impaired abilities. Instead, it attempts to train the individual to function better through the use of strategies, primarily the substitution of one method of doing things for that which is compromised. Compensatory methods involve applied common sense and include such strategies as using an organizer book, setting up efficient filing systems, organizing the home, and using a family calendar to keep track of social engagements (60). Most cognitive rehabilitation programs combine restorative and compensatory approaches into an integrated program of individualized instruction and practice.

Published research on cognitive rehabilitation in MS is limited. Danish investigators used a comprehensive program of cognitive rehabilitation and psychotherapy with 20 moderately disabled MS inpatients who were receiving physical rehabilitation (61). A control group of 20 MS patients received only mental stimulation in addition to physical rehabilitation. Following treatment, significant group differences were observed only in visual perception and Beck Depression Inventory (BDI) scores. In a study of outpatient treatment using a group format, 27 MS patients were randomly assigned either to a wait-list control group or to 24 three-hour–long sessions of group treatment once per week (62). The sessions included psychotherapy, art, music, self-regulation, visualization, guided imagery, meditation, relaxation, and physical and mental exercises. Compared with controls, patients in the treatment group experienced improvement in word-list learning, abstraction, and depression scores. Investigators reported a single case study of memory training with an MS patient in which mnemonic strategies were taught to increase list learning and recall of names of faces (63). Improvement was observed in both verbal and visual memory, with the strongest results in verbal memory. Another group of researchers studied pulsing magnetic fields as a treatment for a variety of symptoms of MS (64). Thirty MS patients were randomly assigned to either a magnetically active or a magnetically inactive device that

was worn for varying periods of time each day for two months. The rationale for the use of the device was that it would bolster several of the electrical frequencies emanating from the brain that had been determined to have the lowest amplitude or power. There was no difference between the active group and the placebo group on change in patient self-reported cognitive function following treatment.

This author was the principal investigator in a recently completed investigation of comprehensive rehabilitation of cognitive dysfunction in 14 MS outpatients (65). Patients had 17 weeks of rehabilitation, which included two 90-minute cognitive remediation sessions per week and one 50-minute stress-management session per week. A significant other was also involved in at least one joint information/counseling meeting. Although patients anecdotally reported improvement in everyday functioning, analysis of neuropsychological test scores failed to reveal any improvement following treatment.

Scientific evidence for the effectiveness of cognitive rehabilitation in MS is limited at present. The studies completed to date have used relatively small samples and imperfect designs. Given the state of the scientific evidence, should cognitive rehabilitation be recommended to patients with MS-related cognitive changes? The answer is a qualified yes. Cognitive rehabilitation that uses compensatory strategies to find practical solutions to everyday problems should be an integral part of the comprehensive management of MS. As research proceeds, we will learn exactly which treatments are more effective or less effective for which problems. Patients who face problems such as disruptive memory deficits need to learn ways to work around these limitations in the interim. Cognitive rehabilitation will ultimately need to have a firm scientific foundation as we sort out what actually works from what does not. Unfortunately, people with MS cannot afford to wait until all the scientific issues are settled. Help with cognitive dysfunction is needed now, and providers need to offer such assistance using the best methods currently available as indicated by research findings, clinical consensus, and common sense.

Cognitive rehabilitation may range from a single session to multiple sessions per week for several months. It may be conducted individually or in groups, although it should be individualized for each patient's particular needs. Many types of health care professionals can offer cognitive rehabilitation, but the most frequent providers are neuropsychologists, speech pathologists, and occupational therapists. Treatment should begin with an interview to ascertain the person's perception of the nature of the problems. Input from a family member is also helpful in most cases. Assessment using standardized testing will pinpoint areas of strength and weakness, thereby helping in the design of the rehabilitation program. In many cases, it may be possible to capitalize on relatively intact areas to compensate for functions that have become impaired. For example, if visual memory is intact, it can be used in certain situations in which verbal memory may be weak.

Cognitive changes rarely occur in a vacuum and the individual with these symptoms is often experiencing significant stress, anxiety, and depression, along with work and family strain. The initial assessment needs to take heed of these factors, particularly depression, and appropriate treatment needs to be provided. Ideally, a program of cognitive rehabilitation will incorporate these special needs as an integral part of the treatment.

Although cognitive rehabilitation may directly address cognitive changes, it may also be necessary for the health care provider to alter his or her way of working to accommodate the special needs of cognitively impaired patients. For example, patient education on self-injection techniques or management of neurogenic bladder dysfunction may become difficult in the face of memory deficits. The health care provider needs to present information in a way that will be maximally useful to the individual. For the person with memory deficits, this may mean slowing down the pace of instruction, repeating points several times, and providing ample printed instructions to supplement verbal teaching.

SUMMARY

Cognitive changes rank among the most common and complex symptoms of MS. Severe cognitive impairment can be more disruptive than loss of the ability to walk. The understanding of these changes has advanced dramatically during the last two decades. Viable treatment strategies to slow the progression of cognitive deficits and improve functioning are slowly being developed and tested. It is important for every MS health care provider to be familiar with the assessment and treatment of cognitive changes. Although we lack perfect solutions to these deficits, there is much that can be done to help the person with MS adapt to cognitive changes. Health care providers need to be more aggressive in making cognitive assessment and rehabilitation available to those whose lives have been disrupted by these problems. It is hoped that this section has provided practical information in a scientific and clinical context for the health care provider who is interested in confronting cognitive changes in MS.

EMOTIONAL CHANGES

Emotional changes related to MS may encompass a wide variety of phenomena, including anxiety, grief, depression, emotional lability, and euphoria (Table 22-4). Like

---

TABLE 22-4
Emotional Changes Observed in MS

- Depression (including major depressive episodes and less severe dysphoric states)
- Bipolar disorder
- Suicidal ideation, intent, and action
- Grieving (mourning for losses of physical functions, self-esteem, etc.)
- Reactions to stress (both disease-related and other types of stress)
- Emotional lability
- Affective release (also known as "pseudobulbar affect")
- Emotional crescendo
- Euphoria (generally associated with dementia)
- Antisocial behavior, sexual inappropriateness, and psychotic states

---

the physical symptoms of MS, these changes may disrupt everyday activities and compromise quality of life. The clinical management of MS has increasingly sought to address these changes while research has investigated their underlying causes. This section reviews the most salient emotional changes that occur in MS, explores current thought concerning their causes, and presents specific recommendations for treatment.

Emotional Changes and Their Causes

Depression

The term *depression* is often used rather loosely both by patients and by health care providers. Saying that someone is "depressed" may mean that the person is feeling "down in the dumps" that day (i.e., mildly dysphoric), or it may mean that the person is clinically depressed, i.e., meets *Diagnostic and Statistical Manual of Mental Disorders* (DSM-IV) criteria for a major depressive episode (Table 22-5) (66). Although depression in MS may range from the very mild to the very severe, the major focus of research and clinical management has been on the more serious affective disturbances.

Good population-based studies of the prevalence of depression in MS are lacking, but small local studies and studies of clinic samples have provided some sense of the extent of depressive disorders in MS. Before the onset of MS, the lifetime prevalence of major depression is approximately 15 percent, similar to that of the general population (67,68). However, the lifetime prevalence of depression increases dramatically after the onset of MS, reaching approximately 50 percent (67–69). The point prevalence (frequency at a given point in time) of depres-

---

TABLE 22-5

DSM-IV Criteria for Major Depressive Episode
(symptoms printed in *italics* may be confused with those of MS)

A. Five (or more) of the following symptoms have been present during the same 2-week period and represent a change from previous functioning; at least one of the symptoms is either (1) depressed mood or (2) loss of interest or pleasure. **Note:** Do not include symptoms that are clearly due to a general medical condition or mood-incongruent delusions or hallucinations.

1) depressed mood most of the day, nearly every day, as indicated by either subjective report (e.g., feels sad or empty) or observation made by others (e.g., appears tearful). **Note:** In children and adolescents, can be irritable mood.

2) markedly diminished interest or pleasure in all, or almost all, activities most of the day, nearly every day (as indicated by either subjective account or observation made by others)

3) significant weight loss when not dieting or weight gain (e.g., a change of more than 5% of body weight in a month) or decrease or increase in appetite nearly every day. **Note:** In children, consider failure to make expected weight gains.

4) *insomnia or hypersomnia nearly every day*

5) *psychomotor agitation or retardation nearly every day (observable by others, not merely subjective feelings of restlessness or being slowed down)*

6) *fatigue or loss of energy nearly every day*

7) feelings of worthlessness or excessive or inappropriate guilt (which may be delusional) nearly every day (not merely self-reproach or guilt about being sick)

8) *diminished ability to think or concentrate, or indecisiveness, nearly every day (either by subjective account or as observed by others)*

9) recurrent thoughts of death (not just fear of dying), recurrent suicidal ideation without a specific plan, or a suicide attempt or a specific plan for committing suicide

B. The symptoms do not meet criteria for a Mixed Episode.

C. The symptoms cause clinically significant distress or impairment in social, occupational, or other important areas of functioning.

D. The symptoms are not due to the direct physiological effects of a substance (e.g., a drug of abuse, a medication) or a general medical condition (e.g., hypothyroidism).

E. The symptoms are not better accounted for by bereavement, i.e., after the loss of a loved one, the symptoms persist for longer than 2 months or are characterized by marked functional impairment, morbid preoccupation with worthlessness, suicidal ideation, psychotic symptoms, or psychomotor retardation.

---

sion among MS clinic attendees was found to be about 14 percent compared with approximately 2 percent for the general population (67). Bipolar disorder is much less common, with a point prevalence and lifetime prevalence among MS patients of approximately 1 percent and 15 percent, respectively, which is more than 10 times the rate observed in the general population (67). Intriguingly, depression is more frequent among MS patients than it is among patients with other chronic conditions (68) or even among those with other neurologic conditions and equivalent degrees of physical impairment (70).

Suicide is a possible concomitant to depression and is an important issue to consider in MS. In one study of causes of death in two Canadian provinces, the proportion of suicides among MS-related deaths was 7.5 times greater than that in an age-matched sample of the general population (71). In the aforementioned study of the MS-related deaths for which a cause could be determined, 15.1 percent were due to suicide compared with 47.1 percent due to complications of MS, 16 percent due to malignancies,

and 10.9 percent due to myocardial infarction. People with MS are thus at significant risk for suicide and should be screened on a regular basis for symptoms of depression.

The factors possibly contributing to depression in MS are summarized in Table 22-6. *Disease characteristics* such as the duration of the illness and the severity of physical disability actually appear to have little or no relationship to depression (67,68,72–74). In contrast, *disease activity*, especially the onset of an exacerbation, appears to be strongly related to depression, especially major depressive episodes (75,76) It is not clear whether this association with exacerbations is due to a reaction to increasing disability, neuropathologic events, or side effects of steroid treatment (68). *Neuropathologic causation* has been advanced as an explanation for MS-related depression (70), but research examining both total and regional MRI lesions has not generally supported this hypothesis (6,70).

Investigators have also explored the possibility that MS-related depression may be associated with *neuroen-*

TABLE 22-6
Possible Causes and Contributors to Depression in MS

- Disease activity (especially onset of exacerbations)
- Neuropathologic changes in areas of the brain concerned with affective states
- Neuroendocrine or psychoneuroimmunologic changes
- Reaction to altered life circumstances
- Medication side effects

docrine or *psychoneuroimmunologic dysfunction* concomitant to the disease process. Like depressed psychiatric patients, MS patients have been found to escape suppression of glucocorticoids prematurely on the dexamethasone suppression test, a finding that is indicative of disordered central nervous system feedback sensitivity to glucocorticoids (77). T-cell subsets thought to be involved in the cell-mediated autoimmune process in MS have been found to be related to psychological distress (72,73).

A recent study found that MS patients were more anxious and depressed and exhibited early release of cortisol on the dexamethasone suppression test compared with controls (78). In addition, both affective and neuroendocrine abnormalities were related to white cell counts in the cerebrospinal fluid and to gadolinium-enhancing lesions on MRI. In a study of seven MS patients receiving cognitive-behavior therapy for major depressive episodes, investigators found that depression, as measured by the BDI and the Hamilton Depression Rating Scale (HDS), improved and that the production of interferon-gamma (IFN-γ) dropped following 16 weeks of treatment (79). In addition, changes in IFN-γ were associated with changes in BDI scores but not HDS ratings.

An alternative to the "biologic" explanation of depression in MS is that it is a *reaction to altered life circumstances,* e.g., physical limitations, altered expectations for the future, financial strain, and so forth. Having MS generally entails coping with a wide range of losses such as the loss of physical abilities, damaged self-esteem, compromised living standards, and friends who make themselves scarce. Grieving for these losses is probably an important part of the process of adjusting to MS. However, grief encompasses many of the same phenomena as depression, e.g., sadness, and in practice it is often hard to distinguish between the two. Evidence supporting a possible reactive explanation for depression in MS comes from studies showing a strong relationship between exacerbations and depression, especially major depressive episodes (75,76). However, interpretation of these studies is complicated by the possible influence of neuropathologic events and steroid treatment accompanying attacks. Stud-

ies of MS patients have found a relationship between emotional distress and perceived stress, social support, and poor problem-solving skills (80–82). Coping strategies appear to be particularly important. In one study, it was found that planful problem solving and cognitive reframing were related to lower levels of depression, especially among more severely disabled MS patients. In contrast, escape-avoidance and emotional respite were associated with higher levels of depression (83).

Medication side effects may also play a role in altered mood among MS patients. Treatment with steroids may produce both depressed and hypomanic states (84). These effects have been clinically observed in MS, but their significance is hard to sort out because steroid treatment almost always occurs in the context of an exacerbation (68). Moreover, because many people experience a mild "high" during the course of steroid treatment, cessation of therapy may be associated with dysphoria. Treatment with interferons has also been anecdotally associated with depressive symptoms among MS patients. Although there is little evidence for this relationship from research, patients receiving interferon treatment bear watching for signs of depression, especially if they have a history of affective disorders (85). Although other drugs used in MS such as the benzodiazepines (e.g., Valium), pemoline (Cylert), or baclofen (Lioresal) could be associated with depressive symptomatology, there is no clear evidence of this. However, abrupt discontinuation of baclofen, especially at high doses, has been associated with the sudden onset of a transient psychotic state (86).

In summary, depression in people with MS is a complex and multifaceted phenomenon. There probably are a number of factors that influence the development and course of depression in MS, including neuropathologic, immunologic, neuroendocrine, psychosocial, and pharmacologic determinants. Adequate understanding and management of depressive symptoms in MS requires that all of these factors be taken into account to some extent.

Stress

Among psychological topics of interest in MS, none has generated as much controversy as the role of stress. The idea that emotional stress could precipitate the onset of the disease, trigger attacks, or hasten progression dates back more than a century (87). One survey found that 60 percent of patients believed that stress affected their illness, with 40 percent reporting that stress had triggered at least one exacerbation (70). Research on the subject has been somewhat less conclusive. There is some evidence that MS patients experience more stressful life events of an extreme nature than either other medical patients or normal healthy adults during the few months just before disease onset (88). In one of the few prospective studies of stress in MS, patients who had one or more "moderately to extremely negative" stressful life events were 3.7 times more likely to experience an attack of MS within the subsequent six months than patients who did not experience such life events (89). Other studies have found no such relationship (90).

Stress is a somewhat amorphous concept that has been defined and measured in many ways, making comparisons among studies all but impossible. Moreover, because stressful life events involve real-life experiences, they are difficult to quantify and impossible to control. Partly in response to the aforementioned difficulties, many investigators have turned to the study of the mechanisms that may be involved in the stress-MS relationship, an area of investigation more amenable to experimental controls. For example, Foley and colleagues found that psychological distress among persons with MS was related to certain T-lymphocyte subsets that are thought to play a role in the pathophysiology of MS (72,73). Investigators recently found that MS patients who reported higher levels of stressful life events, "hassles," and depression tended to have more gadolinium-enhancing lesions (new lesions) on MRI eight weeks later (91).

Although some studies have revealed intriguing relationships between stress and various facets of MS, the research is far from conclusive and no causal relationships have been demonstrated. Research in this area will likely continue and will make increasing use of more sophisticated neuroimaging, immunologic, and neuroendocrine techniques. However, there is a dark side to this issue. Many patients with MS have been encouraged to leave their jobs or curtail their activities to avoid stress. Many have been told to "reduce the stress in your life." At times family members have even experienced guilt, based on the mistaken notion that their behavior has "stressed" the family member with MS and caused the disease to worsen. Numerous lawsuits have been filed over the years seeking damages related to occupational or accident-related stress that has allegedly worsened MS.

Health care providers need to maintain an attitude of healthy skepticism concerning the stress-MS link. In particular, it is important to refrain from advising people to try to "avoid stress." The most significant sources of stress generally are beyond our control, e.g., the death of a loved one. Moreover, trying to avoid certain types of stress through strategies such as retirement may lead to other more severe forms of stress such as financial strain and loss of self-esteem. A preferable approach may be to learn to cope with stress more effectively. Although it is doubtful that this would have any impact on MS disease activity, it is likely to enhance quality of life. More is said about stress-management in the section on interventions. While keeping an open mind concerning the scientific question of how stress may affect MS, it is important to counsel patients against unjustified attempts to escape stress altogether. There is no such thing as life without stress.

Mood Swings

Little has been written about an issue that may be among the most important for families with a member who has MS—mood swings. My own clinical experience and that of others with newly diagnosed patients, couples, and spouse groups has suggested that there are a variety of affective changes that seem to be common in MS and are lumped together as "mood swings." These changes may be as disruptive as physical symptoms (e.g., difficulty walking) and are often misunderstood both by providers and by patients. An examination of each of these affective changes may help to clarify what is at present a murky area of study.

Emotional lability is generally termed *moodiness* by the layperson and refers to "rapid oscillations of feeling states" (92). It is often difficult to separate the moodiness that may affect people under a great deal of stress (e.g., as a result of a chronic illness) from the more severe emotional lability seen in many psychiatric disorders. It is not uncommon to hear reports that the person with MS has frequent periods of anger, irritability, dysphoria, and so forth, and that these periods may come and go rapidly, sometimes lasting only a few minutes or a few hours. It is not known whether these moods are simply a reaction to the stresses of the illness or the result of the effects of the disease on areas of the brain that deal with emotionality. Whatever the cause, emotional lability is an important quality of life issue that may be productively addressed through psychotherapy, especially family therapy, and at times with medications. These issues are discussed in greater detail in subsequent sections.

Affective release refers to unpredictable fits of uncontrollable laughing or crying in which the person's actual feelings may be unrelated to those that they seem to be expressing (93). This phenomenon was formerly referred to as *pseudobulbar affect* because it was thought to result from lesions in the medulla oblongata, the archaic name for which was the "bulb." It is now thought that such symptoms result from lesions in or structures connecting with the limbic system, a set of brain structures crucial in the expression and modulation of emotion. A fit of crying can begin when the person with MS is feeling relatively happy and vice versa. Once begun, these "fits" may be impossible for the person to control, although they generally are short-lived. The whole experience can be quite upsetting and embarrassing for all concerned. Family and friends may react angrily to what appears to be grossly inappropriate and insensitive behavior.

Emotional crescendo is a rarely discussed phenomenon that seems to lie midway between everyday mood swings and affective release. People who experience this phenomenon find that they become very emotional and cry easily, even over seemingly trivial issues. It seems as if any kind of tension, e.g., a minor disagreement or family discussion, can precipitate a highly emotional reaction (93). Once the reaction has begun, it seems to be uncontrollable and quickly reaches a *crescendo*. However, unlike affective release, the person's mood and expression are consistent with one another. It is unclear whether this phenomenon is caused by neurologic damage, stress, a preexisting personality disposition, or a combination thereof. Although not quite as unnerving as affective release, emotional crescendo can wreak havoc on relationships. Attempts to discuss and resolve even minor issues can quickly degenerate into shouting, tears, and alienation.

Euphoria refers to exaggerated and inappropriate expressions of happiness and optimism. It goes well beyond the simple fits of laughing seen in affective release, although it can be either episodic or constant. In some patients, both their mood and the expression of emotion are euphoric, whereas in others the outward expression of optimism belies profound feelings of despair. Euphoria was once considered a hallmark of MS that affected the majority of patients (94). Unfortunately, euphoria has been defined and measured in so many different ways that it is difficult to compare one author's findings with that of another. Current thinking holds that euphoria, especially as a sustained mood state, is not very common, affecting less than 10 percent of patients, and that it generally is associated with a progressive course, severe physical disability, extensive cerebral demyelination, and dementia (94). The combination of unrealistic optimism and impaired cognition may lead the euphoric patient to neglect essential issues such as medical care, nutrition, and personal safely. Euphoria can be stressful for families, especially when they need to assume increased responsibilities for caregiving and supervision. Because there is no known treatment for euphoria, it is essential to help the family understand the phenomenon and provide them with emotional support.

Antisocial behavior, sexual inappropriateness, and *psychotic states* are among the rarest of psychological phenomena that might be attributable to MS. In isolated instances, MS patients may experience uncontrollable rage that leads them to become verbally abusive and/or physically assaultive. Other patients may engage in sexually inappropriate behavior, e.g., fondling or touching others in a sexual way. Such patients are at great risk for being sexually abused by unscrupulous caregivers, acquaintances, and strangers. Transient psychotic symptoms, including hallucinations and delusions, may also occur in people with MS. Some of these phenomena are more likely to be persistent, e.g., sexually inappropriate behavior, and may be related to cognitive deficits that affect judgment

and emotional disinhibition. In contrast, more extreme behaviors, such as assaultiveness, are likely to be episodic and isolated. Because all of these behaviors may occur in people who do not have MS, it may be difficult or impossible to ascertain the causal contribution of the disease. However, some of these behaviors, especially violent behavior, may shadow disease activity, worsening during exacerbations and improving with remissions.

People who display these symptoms need to receive both psychiatric care and medical treatment. Especially in the case of assaultive or psychotic behavior, mood-stabilizing drugs and/or antipsychotic medication may be essential. Treatment for MS exacerbations may also be helpful in shortening and/or reducing the severity of such attacks. Family support and counseling are almost always essential because loved ones generally will be shocked and distraught by any of these behaviors. The person with MS may need supervision, even when the acute manifestations of these symptoms have passed. Psychotherapy and psychotropic medications may also be helpful.

Assessment of Emotional Changes

Although there are a number of emotional changes in MS that may need to be evaluated (e.g., stress, anxiety, euphoria, hypomanic states), by far the greatest attention has been devoted to the assessment of affective disorders, mainly depression. This may be because depression is both highly disruptive of everyday activities and eminently treatable. Although the discussion that follows focuses on depression, many of the principles outlined apply equally to the assessment of other affective changes, such as anxiety or euphoria. Some issues to consider in selecting an assessment method include (1) whether the assessment is being done in a clinical context or a research context; (2) whether the purpose is a brief screening, gauging the severity of depressive symptoms, or establishing a psychiatric diagnosis; and (3) how to deal with the fact that many symptoms of MS (e.g., fatigue) may be confused with those of depression and other affective disorders.

The Context of the Assessment

In a clinical context, depression may need to be assessed to determine whether a referral to a mental health specialist is in order, to ascertain whether treatment is warranted, or to evaluate the impact of ongoing treatment. Clinical assessment of depression is often performed by providers who are not mental health specialists, and it may consist of an informal clinical interview, analogous to the bedside mental status (31). The sensitivity of this approach to detect any but the most severe depressive disorders is not known. Mental health specialists (psychiatrists, psychologists, social workers) generally perform a more detailed clinical interview that may vary in the degree to which it is structured and standardized. In some cases, providers may use highly standardized instruments similar to those used in research protocols. Although somewhat more time-consuming, the use of standardized approaches is probably more sensitive and more reliable, particularly when evaluating the course of treatment.

When research is the context for assessment, methods must be highly standardized and informal assessments are generally not appropriate. Standardized assessments may be accomplished using patient self-report, a structured interview, or clinical ratings. Self-report methods require the patient to answer a series of questions about feelings and symptoms of affective changes. Questions may be presented in a written format or read by an interviewer. No clinical judgment is required because the patient simply responds to questions. A structured interview is accomplished by a trained interviewer asking the patient questions and then recording responses. At least some clinical judgment is generally required to obtain valid answers to the questions. Clinical ratings require the highest level of clinical judgment and may be arrived at as a result of a structured or semistructured interview, often in combination with clinical observation of the patient. Examples of all three methods are described in the following sections.

The Purpose of the Assessment

In some instances, the goal of the assessment is to screen for individuals who should undergo more intensive evaluation of depression. A number of patient self-report instruments have been used for this purpose, including the BDI (95), the Center for Epidemiologic Studies–Depression Scale (CES-D) (96), the Profile of Mood States (97), and the Minnesota Multiphasic Personality Inventory (MMPI) (98). Some of these scales have cut-off points that can be used to identify respondents who are likely to be clinically depressed, but the validity of these cut-off points for MS patients has not been investigated. Samples of MS patients tend to have average scores on self-report scales that are higher than population norms (99). These high scores could suggest that such instruments may be measuring different things in the MS population versus the general population or simply that there is a higher level of emotional distress among those with MS. Another approach to screening involves the use of clinical rating scales that are completed by trained professionals. One of the most commonly used is the Hamilton Depression Rating Scale (HDS) (100). However, because the HDS was developed for the assessment of severe clinical depression, it may be somewhat insensitive to milder forms of depressive symptomatology.

Although self-report scales and clinical ratings can be used for screening purposes, they are more frequently used to gauge the severity of depressive symptomatology along a continuum. For example, the BDI has frequently been used to assess the outcome of psychotherapy (101) and the CES-D has been used to compare the severity of depressive symptoms with the magnitude of other factors (73).

There are times when neither a quick screening nor a simple assessment of severity will suffice. For example, in many research protocols, a specific psychiatric diagnosis may be used as part of the entry criteria. Although clinicians may arrive at diagnoses using informal assessment methods, structured and standardized methods are more reliable. The Structured Clinical Interview for DSM-IV (SCID-IV) (102) provides a reliable method for generating diagnoses that correspond to the *Diagnostic and Statistical Manual of Mental Disorders* (66). Other diagnosis-oriented methods include the Schedule for Affective Disorders and Schizophrenia (SADS) (103) and the Diagnostic Interview Schedule (DIS) (104).

Confounding of Multiple Sclerosis Symptoms with Affective Disorders

All of the methods outlined share a major shortcoming in that they all include depressive symptoms that overlap with some of the symptoms of MS (Table 22-5). These symptoms include fatigue, sleep disturbance, difficulty concentrating, and psychomotor retardation (slowing). Multiple sclerosis is not the only medical condition in which symptoms of physical conditions may be confounded with somatic symptoms of depression. There are a number of ways to deal with this diagnostic confusion in assessing depression in medically ill patients. The following four approaches are based on the work of Cohen-Cole and Harpe (105) and Koenig (106).

The *inclusive* approach simply uses all of the diagnostic criteria for major depressive disorder, applying those criteria in the same way that they would be used in a psychiatric population. Although this approach eliminates some of the vagaries of clinical judgment, it may increase the likelihood that MS patients will receive an incorrect diagnosis based in part on MS symptoms that overlap with psychiatric criteria.

The *exclusive* approach eliminates from consideration all symptoms that overlap with MS. Like the inclusive approach, this approach avoids reliance on clinical judgment by using a reduced set of criteria. However, the exclusive approach may result in the underdiagnosing of depression because patients would need to meet virtually all of the remaining criteria.

The *etiologic* approach uses all of the standard criteria but relies on clinical judgment to determine whether a given symptom is due to MS or depression. Such a determination requires expert knowledge of both psychiatric and MS symptoms and extensive information concerning the development and history of each symptom. This is a sophisticated assessment method that may be reliable when used by highly trained specialists but may not be feasible for those with a less specialized background.

The *substitution* method replaces problematic diagnostic criteria with other less ambiguous ones. Although this method might obviate some of the aforementioned problems, it could result in altering the diagnostic criteria so much that the resulting diagnosis would be of questionable validity and difficult to interpret.

Clearly there is no one "right" way to assess depression in MS. Assessments performed in clinical contexts should avoid underdiagnosis because patients who are in need of treatment or at risk for suicide might be missed. Therefore, in clinical settings, diagnostic criteria should probably be interpreted in a relatively more inclusive manner. By contrast, in the context of a research protocol in which entry criteria are at issue, a more exclusive approach to diagnosis may be more appropriate. In either context, good clinical judgment is probably important and is likely to be a function of training and experience with both MS and psychopathology.

Treatment of Emotional Changes

In spite of the frequency of emotional changes accompanying MS, many people with MS do not receive appropriate treatment for those problems. One study found that 80 percent of a sample of moderately disabled people with MS met criteria for some psychiatric disorder during the preceding year but only 60 percent of these patients had received any psychiatric treatment (68). An emphasis on concern about and treatment of physical symptoms may at times result in the neglect of emotional changes that may compromise quality of life. Other factors that may contribute to this neglect include a relative lack of expertise on the part of some providers in the assessment of emotional changes and the limited time available during office visits. Once recognized, however, emotional changes may often be successfully treated using medications and/or psychotherapy.

Pharmacologic Management

There has been little research addressing the pharmacologic management of emotional changes in MS. However, there does exist some consensus among clinicians concerning the use of pharmacologic measures. *Hypomanic* reactions to steroid therapy may be preventable using a mood-stabilizing agent such as lithium carbonate (e.g., Eskalith) or divalproex sodium (Depakote) (107–109). *Bipolar disorder* may also respond to the aforementioned mood-stabilizing drugs, although an antidepressant is often indicated as well. Extreme *mood swings* that do not meet diagnostic criteria for a bipolar disorder may be successfully controlled using the same mood-stabilizing agents or the anticonvulsant carbamazepine (Tegretol). However, owing to the variety of side effects possible with these drugs (e.g., fatigue, weakness, impaired concentration and memory), they must be monitored carefully. *Anxiety* may be treated using one of the antianxiety agents such as a benzodiazepine, e.g., diazepam (Valium) (107). These medications, especially alprazolam (Xanax), have potential for both physical and psychological dependency and should be used sparingly and only for short periods of time. A newer agent, buspirone (Buspar), which is classified as an azapirone, has seen some use in MS and has less potential for dependence. Controlled studies of any of these medications are lacking and their long-term effects in MS patients are not known. If anxiety is chronic, the patient should be encouraged to explore alternative stress-management and coping strategies in the context of psychotherapy. *Pathologic laughing and weeping* has been successfully treated using 25 to 75 mg per day of amitriptyline (Elavil) (110). Anecdotal reports suggest that selective serotonin reuptake inhibitors (SSRIs) may also be effective for this problem.

Depression among people with MS has been treated with a variety of antidepressants, although research to support this practice is limited. Schiffer and Wineman studied 28 MS outpatients diagnosed with major depressive disorder (74). Patients were randomly assigned to either 30 days of weekly individual supportive therapy or psychotherapy plus desipramine (Norpramin). At the end of 30 days the psychotherapy plus desipramine group had significantly lower clinician-rated depression (HDS) compared with the control group. There was no difference in self-rated depression (BDI).

The monoamine oxidase (MAO) inhibitors are rarely used with MS patients at present and may pose significant risk for hypertension if taken with foods that are high in tyramine content, (e.g., certain types of fermented cheeses). For many years tricyclic antidepressants (TCAs) were the most commonly used medications to treat MS-related depression. However, TCAs have wide-ranging effects on a variety of neurochemical systems, including the adrenergic, histaminic, and acetylcholinergic systems. Because of their broad neurochemical impact, TCAs tend to be associated with numerous side effects, including postural hypotension, cardiac arrhythmias, and constipation. Because some of these side effects (e.g., constipation) may aggravate secondary effects of MS, TCAs have been less than ideal for the treatment of depression in MS.

Although TCAs are still used to some extent in MS, they seem to have largely given way to SSRIs such as fluoxetine (Prozac), sertraline (Zoloft), paroxetine (Paxil), and venlafaxine (Effexor). Selective serotonin reuptake inhibitors tend to be more specific in their effects on the central nervous system, acting mainly to block the reuptake of serotonin at presynaptic membranes. As a result, SSRIs have a more benign side-effect profile compared with TCAs. Clinical trials of SSRIs in MS are currently under way, but results have not been reported as of this writing. Clinical experience suggests that SSRIs work well in MS. Like all medications, SSRIs have some unwanted side effects, including agitation, sleep disturbance, and gastrointestinal upset. For MS patients, one of the most troubling side effects of SSRIs is impairment of the sexual response. Females have reported loss of libido, whereas males have reported erectile dysfunction. These side effects are especially troubling because they mimic problems that may be caused by MS. In this author's experience, fluoxetine is more likely to produce sexual dysfunction than some of the other SSRIs, but there is far from universal agreement in the field on this point. Anecdotal reports suggest that that if sexual side effects are a problem, switching to a different SSRI may help. Bupropion HCL (Wellbutrin), part of a class of antidepressants that are different from the SSRIs, also appears to have fewer sexual side effects and has gained some favor among clinicians. Nefazodone (Serzone), which is classified like bupropion HCL among the "atypical" antidepressants, has not been widely used in MS, possibly because it tends to be more sedating than SSRIs and to have sexual side effects, including erectile dysfunction. However, it does have the advantage of few anticholinergic side effects. Trazadone (Desyrel) also has a benign side-effect profile compared with TCAs, but it is somewhat sedating and may have mild hypotensive effects.

Additional research is needed to determine the relative advantages and disadvantages of the different antidepressants in MS. Unfortunately, this type of research is expensive and difficult to implement and as a result, practice is likely to continue to be driven by a combination of clinical experience and findings derived from non-MS populations. However, certain guidelines may be suggested for the practicing neurologist or primary care physician. Patients receiving antidepressants need to be followed carefully and frequently to evaluate the efficacy of treatment and to monitor side effects. This is particularly true for patients with moderate to severe depression, especially if suicidal ideation is present. The clinician should develop a thorough familiarity with a few therapeutic agents rather than attempting to master all of them. Antidepressant medication may take several weeks or months to achieve its full effectiveness. Moreover, the likelihood of a recurrence of the depression may be reduced by continuing antidepressant medication for several months after the original episode has been resolved. Finally, if efforts to treat the depression are unsuccessful or the case is otherwise medically or psychologically complex, the patient should prob-

ably be referred to a psychiatrist, preferably one who has expertise in neurologic conditions.

Mention should be made of extract of St. John's Wort, a treatment derived from a flower that grows wild in many parts of the United States and which has been used as a medicinal for centuries. Hypericum, which is thought to be the active ingredient in St. John's Wort, has been studied for the treatment of mild to moderate depression in a number of European studies. In those studies, hypericum generally has been shown to be approximately as effective as TCAs in mild to moderate depression. It is not considered an appropriate treatment for severe depression. A large clinical trial of hypericum has recently been funded by the National Institutes of Health. Although results of that study will not be available for some time, St. John's wort is widely available without a prescription in drugstores and health food stores because it is considered a dietary supplement. If the European studies are any indication, hypericum will probably be successful in the U.S. trials and may prove to be popular because of its relatively benign side-effect profile. At present its safety and efficacy in MS remain unknown.

Electroconvulsive Therapy

Electroconvulsive therapy (ECT) ranks among the safest and most effective treatments for severe depression. In spite of its somewhat unsavory image among the general public, ECT continues to be used, especially in cases in which the side effects of antidepressants could be life-threatening (e.g., in some cardiovascular conditions) (111). Although there are no controlled studies of ECT in MS, a review of published case reports suggested that ECT had been effective in more than two thirds of patients with MS (112). However, there is some suggestion that ECT may increase the permeability of an already compromised blood-brain barrier, perhaps leading to an aggravation of MS symptoms (112). Therefore, MS patients with gadolinium-enhancing lesions on MRI, which are thought to be indicative of a breakdown in the blood-brain barrier, should probably be considered at relatively higher risk for neurologic complications following ECT (112). Electroconvulsive therapy is thus a viable alternative for the treatment of depression in MS and should be considered, albeit cautiously, in those instances in which other therapeutic modalities are impractical or have been ineffective.

Psychotherapy

A modest but informative literature supports the effectiveness of psychotherapy in MS. All the published studies have examined the impact of psychotherapy on depression or on a combination of depression and other variables such as stress and coping. However, most studies that have addressed depression did so from the perspective of self-report of depressive symptoms (e.g., BDI) and did not attempt to establish whether patients met diagnostic criteria for an affective disorder. One exception was the aforementioned study by Schiffer and Wineman (74), which compared 30 days of desipramine and psychotherapy with 30 days of supportive case management in a sample of 28 MS patients diagnosed with major depressive disorder. That study found that the combination of desipramine and psychotherapy was more effective in reducing clinician-rated depression than supportive case management. However, because there was no "psychotherapy only" condition, it is difficult to determine the relative contributions of the medication versus psychotherapy. Moreover, there were no differences on self-reported symptoms of depression (BDI).

Larcombe and Wilson (101) administered 90 minutes per week of cognitive behavior therapy over a six-week period to nine MS patients and compared them with 10 MS controls in a wait-list condition. Compared with controls, the treated patients improved significantly in terms of scores on the BDI and the HDS.

Crawford and McIvor (113) compared 11 MS patients who received 25 weeks of twice-weekly insight-oriented group psychotherapy with 11 MS patients in a twice-weekly current events group and 10 MS patients who received no treatment. At the end of the 25 weeks, the treated group showed reduced depression (as measured by the MMPI) compared with the "current events" group and the "no treatment" group.

Foley and colleagues (114) studied six weeks of individual stress-inoculation training in 18 MS patients. Their control group consisted of 18 MS patients who were on a six-week waiting list for the same treatment. The treated group experienced a reduction in self-reported "hassles" (minor everyday stressful events), an increase in the use of problem-focused coping strategies, and a decrease in anxiety (State-Trait Anxiety Inventory) and depressive symptoms (BDI).

Stress was also the primary focus of a study by Crawford and McIvor (115) comparing 13 weeks of group stress management for severely disabled MS inpatients. Compared with the 21 individuals in the "no treatment" control group, the 23 patients who received stress management improved in terms of depressive symptoms as measured by the Profile of Mood States.

Although research on psychotherapy in MS is sparse, clinical experience may help to fill some of the gaps in our knowledge of important issues surrounding treatment of emotional changes. *Individual psychotherapy* is often favored by patients who find a group setting somewhat overwhelming, especially if the group consists largely of patients with more severe physical disability (116). However, many patients are reluctant to enter ther-

apy at all. Being diagnosed with MS means having a physical disability. Entering psychotherapy may signify that one is "emotionally disabled." Many individuals with MS seek therapy mainly when their disease has gotten worse and may feel that they no longer need psychotherapy after their MS symptoms have stabilized and they have learned to cope with them. The psychotherapist working in MS may need to follow the model of "intermittent psychological support" rather than the long-term reconstructive model traditionally favored by many clinicians (117). This short-term episodic model also happens to be a good fit with many health insurance plans that severely restrict mental health benefits. Moreover, cognitive behavior therapy, one of the most widely used approaches at present, appears to be effective for people with MS even when used in relatively short courses (113,114). Cognitive deficits may complicate psychotherapy. Patients with severe memory deficits may not be able to make adequate use of therapy because of a relative lack of carryover from session to session. In addition, an individual with cognitive changes may need to be treated for those problems as well as emotional changes as part of a comprehensive approach to care.

Sometimes in the course of individual psychotherapy it becomes clear that *family* and/or *couples therapy* is needed. Because MS can affect almost all aspects of a person's life, the family is inevitably affected. Couples therapy may be particularly useful when there are significant sexual and/or relationship problems. To cope adequately with the effects of the MS, spouses and/or other family members may need to work together with a therapist and the person who has MS. In some instances, the family member and the person with MS may be attempting to cope in diametrically opposed ways, e.g., learning everything there is to know about the MS versus trying to ignore it. In such instances, the therapist may be able to help family members find their respective "comfort zones" in regard to dealing with the disease and assist them in developing tolerance and respect for each other's style. At times, spouses or other family members may be "at their wit's end" because there are family problems but the person with MS may not want to enter therapy. In this situation, the family member without MS should be encouraged to work with a therapist individually, if need be, to assist him or her in dealing with the situation.

Group models may be extremely important in MS, both for the person with the disease and for family members. There are a variety of models ranging from the formal cognitive-behavioral model led by a highly trained professional to the peer-support group led by a lay person. Yalom and Rand (118) pointed out that groups whose members have a lot in common develop greater cohesion, which in turn is related to a successful outcome. Pavlou and colleagues (119) observed this cohesiveness in MS groups and found that intimacy often developed quite rapidly as people shared common experiences. These scientific concepts concerning group dynamics appear to be supported by the vast popularity of support groups of all kinds sponsored by the National Multiple Sclerosis Society in every part of the United States. The group format is also used extensively in MS for a variety of purposes including cognitive remediation (62), information/orientation groups (120), and patient education for self-care and rehabilitation (116).

CONCLUSION

Emotional changes may take many forms in MS, ranging from the emotional distress that accompanies altered life circumstances to the dramatic euphoria that results from extensive cerebral demyelination. Some emotional changes in MS appear to have a complex etiology, with combined influences of neurologic damage and reaction to the stress of a chronic disabling disease. Depression, in its many guises, is probably the emotional change most frequently encountered by the MS health care provider. Assessment of emotional changes in MS is a complex undertaking, in part because so many of the symptoms used in psychiatric diagnosis overlap with those of MS itself. Standard treatments such as psychotherapy, pharmacotherapy, and ECT appear to work well in MS, although they often need to be adapted to accommodate the special needs of persons with MS, e.g., the repeated emotional ups and downs that accompany exacerbations and remissions. Coping with the emotional aspects of MS presents a significant challenge to the person with MS, the family, and the health care provider. However, as we advance in our understanding of these changes and how best to deal with them, we can increasingly integrate attention to the emotions into MS health care and thereby benefit the quality of life of those living with MS.

Acknowledgments

I am most grateful for the assistance provided by Jack S. Burks, M.D., Lauren S. Caruso, Ph.D., Rosalind C. Kalb, Ph.D., Sarah L. Minden, M.D., David C. Mohr, Ph.D., and Randolph B. Schiffer, M.D., whose advice and suggestions were invaluable in the preparation of this chapter. However, I assume full responsibility for the opinions expressed herein.

References

1. Prineas JW, Graham JS. Multiple sclerosis: Capping of surface immunoglobulin G on macrophages engaged in myelin breakdown. *Ann Neurol* 1981; 10:149–158.

2. Trapp BD, Peterson J, Ransohoff RM, Rudick R, Mork S, Bo L. Axonal transection in the lesions of multiple sclerosis. *N Engl J Med* 1998; 338:278–285.

3. Rao SM, Leo GJ, Haughton VM, St. Aubin-Faubert P, Bernardin L. Correlation of magnetic resonance imaging with neuropsychological testing in multiple sclerosis. *Neurology* 1989; 39:161–166.

4. Tsolaki M, Drevelegas A, Karachristianou S, et al. Correlation of dementia, neuropsychological and MRI findings in multiple sclerosis. *Dementia* 1994; 5:48–52.

5. Pugnetti L, Mendozzi L, Motta A, et al. MRI and cognitive patterns in relapsing-remitting multiple sclerosis. *J Neurol Sci* 1993; 115:S59–S65.

6. Clark CM, James G, Li D, Oger J, Paty D, Klonoff H. Ventricular size, cognitive function and depression in patients with multiple sclerosis. *Can J Neurol Sci* 1992; 19:352–356.

7. Huber SJ, Bornstein RA, Rammohan KW, et al. Magnetic resonance imaging correlates of neuropsychological impairment in multiple sclerosis. *J Neuropsych Clin Neurosci* 1992; 4:152–158.

8. Comi G, Filippi M, Martinelli V, et al. Brain magnetic resonance imaging correlates of cognitive impairment in multiple sclerosis. *J Neurol Sci* 1993; 115:566–573.

9. Swirsky-Sacchetti T, Mitchell DR, Seward J, et al. Neuropsychological and structural brain lesions in multiple sclerosis: A regional analysis. *Neurology* 1992; 42:1291–1295.

10. Arnett PA, Rao SM, Bernardin L, et al. Relationship between frontal lobe lesions and Wisconsin Card Sorting Test performance in patients with multiple sclerosis. *Neurology* 1994; 44:420–425.

11. Huber SJ, Paulson GW, Shuttleworth EC, et al. Magnetic resonance imaging correlates of dementia in multiple sclerosis. *Arch Neurol* 1987; 44:732–736.

12. Pelletier J, Habib M, Lyon-Caen O, et al. Functional and magnetic resonance imaging correlates of callosal involvement in multiple sclerosis. *Arch Neurol* 1993; 50:1077–1082.

13. Franklin GM, Heaton RK, Nelson LM, Filley CM, Seibert C. Correlation of neuropsychological and MRI findings in chronic/progressive multiple sclerosis. *Neurology* 1988; 38:1826–1829.

14. Pozzilli C, Passafiume D, Bernardi S, et al. SPECT, MRI and cognitive function in multiple sclerosis. *J Neurol Neurosurg Psychiatry* 1991; 54:110–115.

15. Ryan L, Clark CM, Klonoff H, Li D, Paty D. Patterns of cognitive impairment in relapsing-remitting multiple sclerosis and their relationship to neuropathology on magnetic resonance images. *Neuropsychology* 1996; 10:176–193.

16. Giesser BS, Schroeder MM, LaRocca NG, et al. Endogenous event-related potentials as indices of dementia in multiple sclerosis patients. *Electroencephalogr Clin Neurophyiisol* 1992; 85:320–329.

17. Cassens G, Wolfe L, Zola M. The neuropsychology of depressions. *J Neuropsych* 1990; 2:202–213.

18. Krupp LB, Sliwinski M, Masur DM, Friedberg F, Coyle PK. Cognitive functioning and depression in patients with chronic fatigue syndrome and multiple sclerosis. *Arch Neurol* 1994; 51:705–710.

19. Moller A, Wiedemann G, Rohde U, Backmund H, Sonntag A. Correlates of cognitive impairment and depressive mood disorder in multiple sclerosis. *Acta Psych Scand* 1994; 89:117–121.

20. Millefiorini E, Padovani A, Pozzilli C, et al. Depression

in the early phase of MS: Influence of functional disability, cognitive impairment and brain abnormalities. *Acta Neurol Scand* 1992; 86:354–358.

21. Good K, Clark CM, Oger J, Paty D, Klonoff H. Cognitive impairment and depression in mild multiple sclerosis. *J Nerv Ment Dis* 1992; 180:730–732.

22. Thronton AE, Naftail R. Memory impairment in multiple sclerosis: A quantitative review. *Neuropsychology* 1997; 11:357–366.

23. Caruso LS, LaRocca NG, Foley FW, Robbins K, Smith CR. Exertional fatigue fails to affect cognitive function in multiple sclerosis. Poster presented at the annual meeting of the International Neuropsychological Society, San Antonio, Texas, February 1991.

24. Caruso LS, Aloe FS, LaRocca NG, et al. Periodic limb movements during nocturnal sleep in persons with multiple sclerosis. Poster presented at the annual meeting of the American Academy of Neurology, San Diego, California, May 1992.

25. Peyser JM, Edwards KR, Poser CM, Filskov SB. Cognitive function in patients with multiple sclerosis. *Arch Neurol* 1980; 37:577–579.

26. Peyser JM, Rao SM, LaRocca NG, Kaplan E. Guidelines for neuropsychological research in multiple sclerosis. *Arch Neurol* 1990; 47:94–97.

27. McIntosh-Michaelis SA, Roberts MH, Wilkinson SM, et al. The prevalence of cognitive impairment in a community survey of multiple sclerosis. *Br J Clin Psych* 1991; 333–348.

28. Rao SM, Leo GJ, Bernardin L, Unverzagt F. Cognitive dysfunction in multiple sclerosis: I. Frequency, patterns, and prediction. *Neurology* 41:685–691.

29. Rao SM. Multiple sclerosis. In: Cummings JL (ed.). *Subcortical dementia.* New York: Oxford University Press, 1990:164–180.

30. Brownell B, Hughes JT. The distribution of plaques in the cerebrum in multiple sclerosis. *J Neurol Neurosurg Psychiatry* 1962; 25:315–320.

31. Fischer JS, Foley FW, Aikens JE, et al. What do we really know about cognitive dysfunction, affective disorders, and stress in multiple sclerosis? A practitioner's guide. *J Neuro Rehab* 1994; 8:151–164.

32. Rao SM. Neuropsychology of multiple sclerosis. *Curr Opin Neurol* 1995; 8:216–220.

33. Rao SM, Leo GJ, St. Aubin-Faubert P. On the nature of memory disturbance in multiple sclerosis. *J Clin Exp Neuropsychol* 1989; 11:699–712.

34. Grigsby J, Ayarbe SD, Kravcisin N, Busenbark D. Working memory impairment among persons with chronic progressive multiple sclerosis. *J Neurol* 1994; 241:125–131.

35. Rao SM, Grafman J, DiGiulio D, et al. Memory dysfunction in multiple sclerosis: Its relation to working memory, semantic encoding, and implicit memory. *Neuropsychology* 1993; 7:364–374.

36. DeLuca J, Barbieri-Berger S, Johnson SK. The nature of memory impairments in multiple sclerosis: Acquisition versus retrieval. *J Clin Exp Neuropsychol* 1994; 16: 183–189.

37. Rao SM, Hammeke TA, Speech TJ. Wisconsin Card Sorting Test performance in relapsing-remitting and chronic-progressive multiple sclerosis. *J Consult Clin Psychol* 1987; 55:263–265.

38. Mendozzi L, Pugnetti L, Saccani M, Motta A. Frontal lobe dysfunction in multiple sclerosis as assessed by means of Lurian tasks: effect of age at onset. *J Neurol Sci* 1993; 115:S42–S50.

39. Beatty WW, Monson N. Picture and motor sequencing in multiple sclerosis. *J Clin Exp Neuropsychol* 1994; 16:165–172.

40. Litvan I, Grafman J, Vendrell P, Martinez JM. Slowed information processing in multiple sclerosis. *Arch Neurol* 1988; 45:281–285.

41. Rao SM, St. Aubin-Faubert P, Leo GJ. Information processing speed in patients with multiple sclerosis. *J Clin Exp Neuropsychol* 1989; 11:471–477.

42. Beatty WW, Goodkin DE, Monson N, Beatty PA. Cognitive disturbances in patients with relapsing-remitting multiple sclerosis. *Arch Neurol* 1989; 46:1113–1119.

43. Achiron A, Ziv I, Djaldetti R, et al. Aphasia in multiple sclerosis: Clinical and radiologic correlations. *Neurology* 1992; 42:2195–2197.

44. Beatty WW, Goodkin DE, Hertsgaard D, Monson N. Clinical and demographic predictors of cognitive performance in multiple sclerosis: Do diagnostic type, disease duration, and disability matter? *Arch Neurol* 1990; 47:305–308.

45. Minden SL, Moes EJ, Orav J, Kaplan E, Reich P. Memory impairment in multiple sclerosis. *J Clin Exp Neuropsychol* 1990; 12:566–586.

46. Klonoff H, Clark C, Oger J, Paty D, Li D. Neuropsychological performance in patients with mild multiple sclerosis. *J Nerv Ment Dis* 1991; 179:127–131.

47. Beatty WW, Goodkin DE. Screening for cognitive impairment in multiple sclerosis: An evaluation of the Mini-Mental State Exam. *Arch Neurol* 1990; 47: 297–301.

48. Swirsky-Sacchetti T, Field HL, Mitchell DR, et al. The sensitivity of the Mini-Mental State Exam in the white matter dementia of multiple sclerosis. *J Clin Psychol* 1992; 48:779–786.

49. Taylor R. Relationships between cognitive test performance and everyday cognitive difficulties in multiple sclerosis. *Br J Clin Psychol* 1990; 29:251–253.

50. Beatty WW, Paul RH, Wilbanks SL, et al. Identifying multiple sclerosis patients with mild or global cognitive impairment using the Screening Examination for Cognitive Impairment (SEFCI). *Neurology* 1995; 45:718–723.

51. Smits RCF, Emmen HH, Bertelsmann FW, et al. The effects of 4-aminopyridine on cognitive function in patients with multiple sclerosis: a pilot study. *Neurology* 1994; 44:1701–1705.

52. Leo GJ, Rao SM. Effects of intravenous physostigmine and lecithin on memory loss in multiple sclerosis: Report of a pilot study. *J Neuro Rehab* 1988; 2:123–129.

52a. Greene YM, Tariot PN, Wishart H, Cox C, Holt CJ, Schwid S, Noviasky J. A 12 week, open trial of donepezil hydrocholoride in multiple sclerosis patients with associated cognitive impairments. *J Clin Psychopharm* (in press).

53. Geisler MW, Sliwinski M, Coyle PK, et al. The effects of amantadine and pemoline on cognitive functioning in multiple sclerosis. *Arch Neurol* 1998; 53:185–188.

54. Fischer JS. Use of neuropsychological outcome measures in multiple sclerosis clinical trials: Current status and strategies for improving multiple sclerosis clinical trial design. In: Goodkin DE, Rudick RA (eds.). *Multiple sclerosis: Advances in clinical trial design, treatment and future perspectives.* London: Springer, 1996:123–144.

55. Fischer JS, Goodkin DE, Rudick RA. *J Internat Neuropsychol Soc* 1997; 3:35.

56. Fischer JS, Priore R, Jacobs L, et al. Neuropsychological effects of Avonex® (Interferon-beta-1a) in relapsing multiple sclerosis. Poster presented at the annual meeting of the American Academy of Neurology, Minneapolis, MN, April 1998.

56a. Weinstein A, Schwid SI, Schiffer RB, McDermott MP, Giang DW, Goodman AD. Neuropsychological status in multiple sclerosis after treatment with glatiramer. *Arch Neurol* 1999; 56:319–324.

57. Prigatano GP. *Neuropsychological rehabilitation after brain injury*. Baltimore: Johns Hopkins University Press, 1986.

58. Sohlberg MM, Mateer CA. Effectiveness of an attention training program. *J Clin Exp Neuropsychol* 1987; 9:117–130.

59. LaRocca, NG. Cognitive retraining in multiple sclerosis. Presentation at Neurobehavioral disorders in multiple sclerosis: Diagnosis, underlying pathology, natural history, and therapeutic intervention, Bergamo, Italy, June 1992.

60. Sullivan MJL, Dehoux E, Buchanan DC. An approach to cognitive rehabilitation in multiple sclerosis. *Can J Rehab* 1989; 3:1–9.

61. Jonsson A, Korfitzen EM, Heltberg A, Ravnborg MH, Byskov-Ottosen E. Effects of neuropsychological treatment in patients with multiple sclerosis. *Acta Neurol Scand* 1993; 88:394–400.

62. Rogers D, Khoo K, MacEachen M, Oven M, Beatty WW. Cognitive therapy for multiple sclerosis: A preliminary study. *Alternative Therapies* 1996; 2:70–74.

63. Allen DN, Longmore S, Goldstein G. Memory training and multiple sclerosis: a case study. *Int J Rehab Health* 1995; 1:189–202.

64. Richards TL, Lappin MS, Acosta-Urquidi J, et al. Double-blind study of pulsing magnetic field effects on multiple sclerosis. *J Alt Comp Med* 1997; 3:21–29.

65. Foley FW, Dince WM, LaRocca NG, et al. Psychoremediation of communication skills for cognitively impaired persons with multiple sclerosis. *J Neuro Rehab* 1994; 8:165–176.

66. American Psychiatric Association. *Diagnostic and statistical manual of mental disorders*. 4th ed. Washington, DC: American Psychiatric Association, 1994.

67. Joffe RT, Lippert GP, Gray TA, Sawa G, Horvath Z. Mood disorder and multiple sclerosis. *Arch Neurol* 1987; 44:376–378.

68. Minden SL, Orav J, Reich P. Depression in multiple sclerosis. *Gen Hosp Psych* 1987; 9:426–434.

69. Sadovnick AD, Remick RA, Allen J, et al. Depression and multiple sclerosis. *Neurology* 1996; 46:628–632.

70. Rabins PV, Brooks BR, O'Donnell P, et al. Structural brain correlates of emotional disorder in multiple sclerosis. *Brain* 1986; 109:585–597.

71. Sadovnick AD, Eisen K, Ebers GC, Paty DW. Cause of death in patients attending multiple sclerosis clinics. *Neurology* 1991; 41:1193–1196.

72. Foley FW, Miller A, LaRocca NG, et al. Psychoimmunologic dysregulation in multiple sclerosis. *Psychosomatics* 1988; 29:398–403.

73. Foley FW, Traugott U, LaRocca NG, et al. A prospective study of depression and immune dysregulation in multiple sclerosis. *Arch Neurol* 1992; 49:238–244.

74. Schiffer RB, Wineman NM. Antidepressant pharmacotherapy of depression associated with multiple sclerosis. *Am J Psychiatry* 1990; 147:1493–1497.

75. Warren SA, Warren KG, Cockerill R. Emotional stress and coping in multiple sclerosis (MS) exacerbations. *J Psychosom Res* 1991; 35:37–47.

76. Dalos NP, Rabins PV, Brooks BR, O'Donnell P. Disease activity and emotional state in multiple sclerosis. *Ann Neurol* 1983; 13:573–577.

77. Reder AT, Lowy, MT, Meltzer HY, Antel JP. Dexamethasone suppression test abnormalities in multiple sclerosis in relation to ACTH therapy. *Neurology* 1987; 37:849–853.

78. Fassbender K, Schmidt R, Mössner R, et al. Mood disorders and dysfunction of the hypothalamic-pituitary-adrenal axis in multiple sclerosis. *Arch Neurol* 1998; 55:66–72.

79. Mohr DC, Goodkin DE, Marietta P, et al. Relationship between treatment of depression and interferon-gamma in patients with multiple sclerosis. Poster presented at the Annual Meeting of the American Academy of Neurology, Minneapolis, MN, April 1998.

80. McIvor GP, Riklan M, Reznikoff M. Depression in multiple sclerosis as a function of length and severity of illness, age, remissions, and perceived social support. *J Clin Psychol* 1984; 40:1028–1033.

81. Ron MA, Logsdail SJ. Psychiatric morbidity in multiple sclerosis: A clinical and MRI study. *Psychol Med* 1989; 19:887–895.

82. Wineman NM, Durand EJ, Steiner RP. A comparative analysis of coping behaviors in persons with multiple sclerosis and spinal cord injury. *Res Nurs Health* 1994; 17:185–194.

83. Mohr DC, Goodkin DE, Gatto N, Van Der Wende J. Depression, coping, and level of neurological impairment in multiple sclerosis. *Multiple Sclerosis* 1997; 3:254–258.

84. Lewis DA, Smith RE. Steroid-induced psychiatric symptoms. A report of 14 cases and a review of the literature. *J Affect Dis* 1983; 5:319–332.

85. Mohr DC, Goodkin DE, Likosky W, et al. Therapeutic expectations of patients with multiple sclerosis upon initiating interferon beta-1 b: Relationship to adherence to treatment. *Multiple Sclerosis* 1996; 2:222–226.

86. Yassa RY, Iskandar HL. Baclofen-induced psychosis: two cases and a review. *J Clin Psychiatry* 1988; 49:318–320.

87. LaRocca NG. Psychosocial factors in multiple sclerosis and the role of stress. In: Scheinberg LC, Raine CS (eds.). Multiple sclerosis: Experimental and clinical aspects. *Ann NY Acad Sci* 1984; 436:435–442.

88. Grant I, Brown GW, Harris T, et al. Severely threatening events and marked life difficulties preceding onset or exacerbations of multiple sclerosis. *Neurol Neurosurg Psychiatry* 1989; 52:8–13.

89. Franklin GM, Nelson LM, Heaton RK, Burks JS, Thompson D. Stress and its relationship to acute exacerbation in multiple sclerosis. *J Neuro Rehab* 1988; 2:7–11.

90. Nisipeanu P, Korczyn AD. Psychological stress as risk factor for exacerbations in multiple sclerosis. *Neurology* 1993; 43:1311–1312.

91. Mohr DC, Marietta P, Boudewyn A, Goodkin DE. Stress is associated with the subsequent development of new brain lesions in multiple sclerosis. Poster presented at the Annual Meeting of the Society of Behavioral Medicine, New Orleans, LA, March 1998.

92. Schiffer RB. Disturbances of affect. In: Rao SM (ed.). *Neurobehavioral aspects of multiple sclerosis.* New York: Oxford University Press, 1990:186–195.

93. LaRocca NG, Fischer JS. Stress and emotional issues. In: Kalb RC (ed.). *Multiple sclerosis: The questions you have—the answers you need.* New York: Demos, 1996:205–221.

94. Rabins PV. Euphoria in multiple sclerosis. In: Rao SM (ed.). *Neurobehavioral aspects of multiple sclerosis.* New York: Oxford University Press, 1990:180–185.

95. Beck AT, Ward CH, Mendelson M, Mock J, Erbauch J. An inventory for measuring depression. *Arch Gen Psychiatry* 1961; 4:561–571.

96. Radloff LS. The CES-D Scale: A self-report depression scale for research in the general population. *Appl Psychol Meas* 1977; 1:385–401.

97. McNair DM, Lorr M, Droppleman LF. *Profile of Mood States Manual.* San Diego: Educational and Industrial Testing Service, 1971.

98. Graham JR. *MMPI-2: Assessing personality and psychopathology.* New York: Oxford University Press, 1993.

99. LaRocca NG, Scheinberg LC, Kaplan SR. Disease characteristics and psychological status in multiple sclerosis. *J Neuro Rehab* 1988; 1:171–178.

100. Hamilton M. A rating scale for depression. *J Neurol Neurosurg Psychiatry* 1960; 23:56–62.

101. Larcombe NA, Wilson PH. An evaluation of cognitive-behaviour therapy for depression in patients with multiple sclerosis. *Br J Psychiatry* 1984; 145:366–371.

102. First MB, Spitzer RL, Gibbon M, Williams JBW. *Structured clinical interview for DSM-IV Axis I disorders—nonpatient edition (SCID-N/P, Version 2.0).* New York: New York State Psychiatric Institute, Biometrics Research Department, 1995.

103. Endicott J, Spitzer RL. Use of the Research Diagnostic Criteria and the Schedule for Affective Disorders and Schizophrenia to study affective disorders. *Am J Psychiatry* 1979; 136:52–56.

104. Robins LN, Helzer JE, Croughan J, Ratcliff KS. National Institute of Mental Health Diagnostic Interview Schedule: Its history, characteristics, and validity. *Arch Gen Psychiatry* 1981; 38:381–392.

105. Cohen-Cole SA, Harpe C. Diagnostic assessment of depression in the medically ill. In: Stoudemire A, Fogel BS (eds.). *Principles of medical psychiatry.* New York: Grune & Stratton, 1987.

106. Koenig H. Depression in medically ill hospitalized older adults. *Am J Psychiatry* 1997; 154:1376–1383.

107. Minden SL, Moes E. A psychiatric perspective. In: Rao SM (ed.). *Neurobehavioral aspects of multiple sclerosis.* New York: Oxford University Press, 1990:230–250.

108. Falk WE, Mahnke MW, Poskanzer DD. Lithium prophylaxis of corticotrophin-induced psychosis. *JAMA* 1979; 241:1011–1012.

109. Minden SL, Orav J, Schildkraut JJ. Hypomanic reactions to ACTH and prednisone treatment for multiple sclerosis. *Neurology* 1988; 38:1631–1634.

110. Schiffer RB, Herndon RM, Rudick RA. Treatment of pathological laughing and weeping with amitriptyline. *N Engl J Med* 1985; 312:1480–1482.

111. American Psychiatric Association. *The practice of electroconvulsive therapy: Recommendations for treatment, training, and privileging.* Washington, DC: American Psychiatric Association, 1990.

112. Mattingly G, Baker K, Zorumski CF, Figiel GS. Multiple sclerosis and ECT: Possible value of gadolinium-enhanced magnetic resonance scans for identifying high-risk patients. *J Neuropsychiatry Clinical Neurosci* 1992; 4:145–151.

113. Crawford JD, McIvor GP. Group psychotherapy: Benefits in multiple sclerosis. *Arch Phys Med Rehabil* 1985; 66:810–813.

114. Foley FW, Bedell JR, LaRocca NG, Scheinberg LC, Reznikoff M. Efficacy of stress-inoculation training in coping with multiple sclerosis. *J Consult Clin Psychol* 1987; 55:919–922.

115. Crawford JD, McIvor GP. Stress management for multiple sclerosis. *Psychol Reports* 1987; 61:423–429.

116. LaRocca NG. A rehabilitation perspective. In: Rao SM (ed.). *Neurobehavioral aspects of multiple sclerosis.* New York: Oxford University Press, 1998:215–229.

117. Kalb RC, LaRocca NG, Kaplan SR. Sexuality. In: Scheinberg LC, Holland NJ (eds.). *Multiple sclerosis: A guide for patients and their families.* 2nd ed. New York: Raven Press, 1987:177–195.

118. Yalom ID, Rand K. Compatibility and cohesiveness in therapy groups. *Arch Gen Psychiatry* 1966; 15:267–275.

119. Pavlou MM, Hartings MF, Davis FA. Discussion groups for medical patients: A vehicle for improved coping. *Psychother Psychosom* 1978; 30:115

120. LaRocca NG, Kalb RC, Kaplan SR. Psychological issues. In: Scheinberg LC, Holland NJ (eds.). *Multiple sclerosis: A guide for patients and their families.* 2nd ed. New York: Raven Press, 1987:197–213.

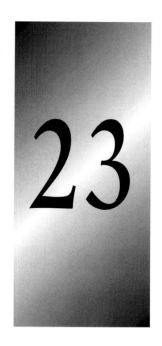

23 Pain and Dysesthesia

Douglas R. Jeffery, M.D., Ph.D.

Patients with multiple sclerosis (MS) may develop a myriad of symptoms as a result of the disease, one of the most troublesome of which is pain. The association between pain and MS was first made by Charcot in 1872 when he referred to shoulder and pelvic pain as symptoms of the disease (1). Despite the early association of pain with MS, many neurologists in recent decades believed that pain was not a significant problem in MS. More recent studies suggest that pain syndromes are common and may be among the most troublesome of all symptoms (2–4). Furthermore, the types of pain seen in MS may be quite varied and may not easily lend themselves to treatment.

The frequency of pain during the course of the disease is approximately 45 percent to 65 percent (3–8). It may be among the most troublesome symptoms in MS patients, with 32 percent reporting continuous, unremitting pain for at least one month (4). The majority of MS patients with pain have a chronic syndrome that lasts a month or more without resolution (5). In one study, nearly 18 percent of patients reported continuous, unremitting pain for at least one month (6). A smaller proportion may have pain at the onset of the disease (7). Sixty-five percent took medication for pain, and 90 percent of them reported relief at the 50 percent level. Those patients who reported pain also had significantly poorer mental health when compared with patients without pain (7), and some evidence suggests that pain may be a factor that leads to clinical depression (10). Thus, it is clear that pain may be a significant problem in MS patients and may have a significant impact on quality of life.

Some studies have suggested that pain in MS may be associated with some demographic variables, but there has been considerable disagreement. Moulin and coworkers (5) reported chronic pain in 48 percent of patients and acute pain syndromes in 9 percent. When compared with the pain-free group, there was no difference in the age of onset, degree of disability, or disease duration. However, the frequency of pain was significantly higher in older patients, and the ratio of women to men in the pain group was 3:1 versus 1.4:1 in the group without pain. All of the patients with a chronic pain syndrome had an MS-related myelopathy. Although the association between myelopathy and chronic pain syndromes has been confirmed in other studies (3,5), the relationship between female sex and age has not. In general, pain appears to be more common in patients with greater disease duration and in those patients with more prominent spinal cord involvement (2–5). Older patients are more likely to report pain as the most distressing symptom.

PAIN AS A PRESENTING FEATURE OF MULTIPLE SCLEROSIS

Pain at the onset of MS may be more common than previously appreciated. Indaco and coworkers (3) reported that 21 percent of patients had pain with the onset of the disease. Similarly, Stenager and colleagues (7) reported the presence of pain at onset in 23 percent of patients and found that 60 percent of those with pain at onset had pain later in the course of the disease. Dysesthetic extremity pain and back pain were the most common types of presenting pain. Painful tonic spasms were less common, but were nevertheless a presenting feature in some patients.

A number of "unusual" pain syndromes have been reported at disease onset. Ramirez-Lassepas and colleagues (11) reported that 3.9 percent of 282 newly diagnosed MS patients presented with a syndrome mimicking a radiculopathy—three cervical, two thoracic, and six lumbosacral. Patients presented with acute neck pain or low back pain radiating into the distribution of a nerve root but had no evidence of compression on imaging studies. All were subsequently diagnosed with MS and the radicular nature of the pain was attributed to the disease. This type of pain syndrome is not uncommon in patients with established MS but should not be attributed to MS until a radiculopathy has been excluded. As with all symptoms, it should be remembered that MS patients are susceptible to any disease or disorder seen in the general population.

The relationship between headache and MS has been subject to controversy, but several studies have reported vascular or tension headache at the onset of MS (12–16). Seven of 54 patients reported headache at disease onset (12). Freedman and Gray (13) studied the records of 1,113 patients over a 20-year period and found that in 44 patients the initial attack or subsequent exacerbations were heralded by migrainous-type headache. Vascular hemicrania and apoplectic type headaches have also been reported at disease onset (14–16).

CHARACTERISTICS OF PAIN SYNDROMES IN MULTIPLE SCLEROSIS

Pain syndromes are divided into acute and chronic types. Acute pain syndromes have a duration of less than one month, whereas chronic pain syndromes last longer than one month. This distinction is somewhat arbitrary in that it fails to take into account the character and the rapidity of onset, characteristics that may be more useful in suggesting anatomic location of origin and possible treatment modalities. A more useful classification distinguishes pain syndromes on the basis of rapidity of onset and the characteristics of the pain, such as burning, dyses-

thetic extremity pain versus that which occurs with a lightning-like onset, such as trigeminal neuralgia or lightning-like extremity pain. Table 23-1 lists the most common MS-related pain syndromes.

TRIGEMINAL NEURALGIA

Trigeminal neuralgia is a well-described acute pain syndrome that usually occurs in the V2 or V3 distribution. In a young individual, it may be highly suggestive of demyelinating disease. The pain is bilateral in 30 percent of patients and tends to be seen at an earlier age in people with MS (17). It is 400 times more common in MS patients than in the normal population (18,19) and has a lightning-like or paroxysmal onset, with the initial component lasting seconds or minutes. This type of pain is often described as an intensely severe, sharp, searing pain that then eases off while the affected region continues to ache or burn. Although there are variations in the character of the pain between patients, the rapidity of onset, location, and character leave little confusion as to the nature of this type of facial pain. Trigger points may be present over the face, and paroxysms of pain may brought on by toothbrushing, chewing, yawning, or shaving. Patients often report dysesthetic sensations in the same distribution as the pain. Quality of life and performance of activities of daily living may be severely impaired in patients with refractory trigeminal neuralgia. In most instances, the syndrome responds well to medical therapy and tends to be self-limited, although it may be refractory and difficult to control in some patients.

Nine percent of MS patients reported the presence of trigeminal neuralgia during the course of the disease (5). Trigeminal neuralgia associated with MS is indistinguishable from that seen in association with other disor-

---

TABLE 23-1
Pain Syndromes in Multiple Sclerosis

Pain with Paroxysmal Onset (Acute Pain Syndromes)
- Trigeminal neuralgia
- Tonic spasms
- Lightening-like extremity pain
- Painful Lhermitte's sign
- Optic neuritis

Pain with Insidious Onset (Chronic Pain Syndromes)
- Dysesthetic extremity pain
- Bandlike pain in torso or extremities
- Back pain and radiculopathy
- Headache
- Miscellaneous pain syndromes

ders (17), and patients with MS may develop trigeminal neuralgia as a result of vascular compression at the entry zone of the trigeminal nerve (20). Magnetic resonance imaging (MRI) studies suggest that patients younger than 29 years old with trigeminal neuralgia have either MS or a tumor and that 30 percent of those with pain in more than one branch had tumors (21).

Trigeminal neuralgia probably arises from ephaptic transmission of nerve impulses in areas of demyelination near the trigeminal nerve entry zone (22). Consequently, it usually responds well to anticonvulsants such as carbamazepine (23) (Table 23-2). Other agents that have been used successfully in trigeminal neuralgia include phenytoin, baclofen, clonazepam (24,25), lamotrigine (26), misoprostol (27), and pimozide (28). Misoprostol and lamotrigine may be effective in refractory cases and should probably be used before considering neurosurgical procedures. Other medications have been tried with occasional success. The most salient problem in the treatment of trigeminal neuralgia arises when it is refractory to medical therapy.

In patients with persistent trigeminal neuralgia who have failed medical therapy, an MRI study may be useful in determining whether there is any evidence of neurovascular compression. This condition probably is not common in MS, although it has been reported (29). Radiofrequency thermal rhizotomy or glycerol rhizotomy of the trigeminal ganglion can be effective and may eliminate the need for high doses of anticonvulsant agents in patients with refractory trigeminal neuralgia (30–32). In one study of 53 patients with refractory trigeminal neuralgia due to MS, 59 percent obtained complete relief and were able to stop medical therapy (29). Another 16 percent obtained partial relief but continued to require intermittent medical therapy, and 25 percent failed glycerol rhizotomy and underwent other surgical procedures (33). Pain may recur over time. Thirty percent of the patients in this study who obtained relief required repeat glycerol rhizotomies, and 40 percent of patients developed some trigeminal sensory loss.

PAINFUL TONIC SPASMS

Painful tonic spasms constitute another well-defined MS related pain syndrome in which there is a paroxysmal onset (3–6,34,35). There are two distinct forms. The first is the relatively simple flexor spasm, which can be precipitated by movement or other noxious stimuli and is related to spasticity. These spasms are quite common and can be brought under control by appropriate antispasticity therapy. The second form is less common but constitutes a true paroxysmal symptom and is not related to spasticity (25). It takes the form of brief but intensely

		TABLE 23-2		
		Pharmacologic Agents		
AGENT	**INITIAL DOSE**	**MAXIMUM DOSE**	**SIDE EFFECTS**	**COMMENT**
Phenytoin	300 mg/day	300 mg/day	Nystagmus, ataxia	Best in dysesthetic pain
Gabapentin	300 mg tid	1200 mg tid	Somnolence, fatigue	Useful in dysesthetic and paroxysmal pain
Carbamazepine	100 mg bid	200 mg qid	Ataxia, loss of balance	Effective in pain of paroxysmal onset
Clonazepam	0.25 mg bid	2 mg qid	Fatigue, sedation	Useful in bandlike sensations over limbs and torso
Baclofen	5–10 mg bid	40 mg qid	Fatigue, sedation	Useful in trigeminal neuralgia
Misoprostol	100 mcg qid	200 mcg qid	Diarrhea	Contraindicated in pregnancy
Lamotrigine	25 mg qod	300–500 mg qd	Ataxia, diplopia, dizziness	Limited use due to interactions and adverse events
Tramadol	50 mg qd	50 mg qid	Dizziness, nausea, constipation	Helpful in a variety of nonrefractory pain syndromes
Tizanidine	4 mg qhs	8 mg qid	Somnolence	Useful adjunct in chronic pain syndromes

painful tetanic posturing of the arm or leg, usually on one side of the body. Most of these spasms last less than 90 seconds (34,35). They are sometimes referred to as "tonic spinal cord seizures." They may occur many times each day but usually are self-limited in that they subside after four to six weeks and probably are seen in less than 10 percent of patients (3–5,34). When present, they can be intensely painful and disturbing to the patient.

Painful tonic spasms are only one of the paroxysmal syndromes encountered in the MS patient. The majority of these syndromes are not painful. Painful tonic spasms are thought to arise from the lateral spread of action potentials to adjacent pathways in regions where there is partial demyelination (34). The site of origin is the spinal cord, but spasms may also involve the face, suggesting that the brainstem may also be a site of origin. Many pain syndromes in MS have been ascribed to the phenomenon of ephaptic transmission. Painful tonic spasms tend to respond well to carbamazepine (36). Other agents, such as phenytoin, gabapentin, clonazepam, tizanidine, and baclofen, may also be useful in controlling these symptoms.

LIGHTNING-LIKE EXTREMITY PAIN

This type of pain syndrome has received very little attention in the literature and therefore has not been well characterized. The pain is described as very brief but extremely intense; it takes on a sharp, shooting, lightning-like quality and travels through an extremity. It often is triggered by movement of the head or neck or by bending and turning (4,6). Virtually any part of the body can be affected. There often is a lingering ache or burning sensation following the brief paroxysm. In clinical practice this type of pain syndrome is short-lived and tends to resolve on its own after several weeks. Again, carbamazepine is usually effective, but phenytoin and gabapentin have also been used. This type of pain should be distinguished from Lhermitte's sign in that shooting pains may originate in any region and have no fixed relationship with neck motion.

PAINFUL LHERMITTE'S SIGN

Lhermitte's "sign" is a symptom that is not specific to MS but may occur in any disorder that results in damage to the posterior columns of the cervical spinal cord (37,38). It is characterized by an electric shock–like sensation or paresthesia that spreads down the neck along the spinal column and may radiate to the extremities. The intensity and character may vary. Some patients experience the sensation of buzzing or vibrating with neck flexion, whereas other patients experience a sharp, painful sensation that shoots rapidly to the extremities. In some patients with-

out a true Lhermitte's sign, paroxysmal extremity pains can be triggered by lateral movements of the neck (6). A painful Lhermitte's sign occurs in a minority of patients and usually responds to carbamazepine (39), as do the other pain syndromes that have paroxysmal onset.

CHRONIC PAIN SYNDROMES

The chronic pain syndromes that occur in association with MS can be as varied as those that have been termed acute. Although chronic syndromes have traditionally been defined as those that last longer than one month, the chronic syndromes differ from the acute ones in that their mode of onset lacks a rapid, paroxysmal onset. In contrast, they tend to have an insidious onset and wax and wane over the course of the day without ever really resolving. The chronic syndromes tend to be more difficult to treat and probably differ from the acute syndromes in their pathologic origin. Whereas carbamazepine is quite effective in most acute syndromes, it tends to be less effective in chronic pain syndromes; phenytoin and gabapentin tend to be more effective (25,40,41).

The most common chronic pain syndrome is that of dysesthetic extremity pain (3–5). This pain syndrome occurs in approximately 50 percent of patients and can be long-lasting and severe. Its onset is insidious and it more often occurs in the lower extremities, although it may also involve the arms and torso. It is described as a burning or aching dysesthetic pain and may be accompanied by a cramping sensation and hyperpathia. The hyperpathic component is often very disturbing to patients. Patients with this syndrome tend to be less disabled (5).

Chronic pain syndrome probably arises from demyelination within the posterior columns of the spinal cord because it is almost always accompanied by posterior column sensory loss (5,22). The pain waxes and wanes over the course of the day and tends to be more severe in the evening. In many patients, this is the most troublesome symptom of the disease and can be quite refractory to treatment. Clifford and Trotter (2) reported relief with tricyclic antidepressants in a substantial proportion of patients, but those results have not been seen in other studies. As with most of the chronic syndromes, carbamazepine tends to be less effective, whereas phenytoin and gabapentin appear to be more effective, although most agents do not provide complete relief. It frequently may be necessary to systematically try several anticonvulsants before finding one that provides relief.

BANDLIKE PAIN TORSO OR EXTREMITIES

This type of pain has not been well studied in MS and probably occurs in a minority of patients, but it is a common complaint in MS specialty clinics. It is characterized by an intense pressure or squeezing sensation in a transverse band or beltlike region around a portion of the body, usually the torso. Dysesthesias may accompany the pain, but it is the squeezing sensation that is most distressing to patients. The source of the pain is a lesion within the spinal cord. The syndrome is not specific to MS but may be seen after any spinal cord lesion (42). This pain syndrome may be quite resistant to treatment but usually responds partially to gabapentin or phenytoin. Benzodiazepines may be of some benefit in resistant cases.

BACK PAIN AND RADICULAR PAIN

Back pain in the MS patient can be a complicated issue. Within the normal population many patients suffer from occasional or chronic back pain, sometimes radiating to a radicular distribution. Because MS patients are equally susceptible to musculoskeletal back pain, if not more so, it may be difficult to distinguish back pain that is due to MS from pain that might occur in the normal population. Nevertheless, several reports have described back pain accompanied by radicular symptoms at the onset of MS (11) and during the course of the disease (2,7). Clifford and Trotter (2) reported back pain and sciatica in 12 patients; in one patient the pain occurred as part of an exacerbation and resolved with the administration of corticosteroids. Only one of their patients had a herniated disc.

Despite the frequency of back pain in patients with MS it should not be assumed to be due to the disease until other reasonable sources have been excluded. If signs of nerve root compression are evident, an appropriate workup should be undertaken. It is not uncommon that patients present with a deep ache-like pain radiating down the shoulder along the border of the trapezius and to the upper back. In some cases, corresponding cervical cord lesions are seen on MRI, but significant disc herniation in the cervical spine is sometimes seen. It may be difficult to determine the origin of the pain on clinical grounds alone. Spastic weakness resulting from MS may place abnormal stresses on the paravertebral musculature, resulting in chronic musculoskeletal back pain. The approach is to exclude structural abnormalities first. Once that has been accomplished, an appropriate treatment can be based on the probable cause. Physical therapy and nonsteroidal anti-inflammatory agents are an appropriate first step. If no improvement is seen, a trial of gabapentin or phenytoin may be helpful. Other agents that may be useful in this instance include tizanidine, baclofen, clonazepam, or tramadol. A good response to the phenytoin or gabapentin suggests that the pain may be due to MS. When back pain is due to MS, it may be evidence of demyelination in the dorsal root entry zone (22).

PAIN ASSOCIATED WITH TRANSVERSE MYELITIS

One final variant of back pain deserves mention here. The onset of transverse myelitis caused by MS may be heralded by a severe, deep, boring pain in the lumbar and thoracic regions (43). This pain can be quite severe and may require narcotics to adequately control it. It may precede the onset of other neurologic signs of transverse myelitis by as much as 48 hours.

HEADACHE

There is considerable controversy regarding whether headache occurs as a consequence of MS because headache is common in the general population. The incidence of migraine in MS patients has been reported at 27 percent compared with 12 percent in a random sample of age-matched controls (44). Freedman and Gray (13) retrospectively reviewed the charts of 1,113 patients treated over a 20-year period and reported that 44 of those patients had headache either at onset or in exacerbation. Eighteen of those patients had new-onset headache with their first attack, and the remainder had headache with exacerbation. Rolak and Brown (12) evaluated 104 consecutive patients and found that 52 percent had headache as compared with 18 percent of matched general neurology patients. In 31 percent, the headaches were tension headaches, whereas in 21 percent they were migrainous. Six percent had headaches at the onset of disease.

Several case reports have also suggested that headache may be associated with MS and may be a presenting symptom of the disease (13–15). Apoplectic headache associated with third nerve palsy, vascular hemicrania, and bifrontal headache have been reported in association with demyelinating lesions.

There probably is a causal relationship between demyelinating lesions and headache in some patients. Inflammatory infiltrates in close proximity to blood vessels and impinging on pain sensitive structures is one mechanism whereby acute MS lesion formation could be associated with headache. Similarly, larger lesions with a more intense inflammatory component may also impinge on pain-sensitive structures and cause headache.

Treatment of headache can generally proceed along the same lines as those normally employed in patients without MS. When headache is seen in association with relapse, steroid treatment often results in resolution of the headache.

MISCELLANEOUS PAIN SYNDROMES

A variety of less common pain syndromes may be seen in association with MS. Many patients develop a sensation of deep aching within the muscles of the lower extremities. Pain of this nature is most common in the quadriceps but occasionally occurs in the anterior tibial muscles. Many patients describe the pain as severe and continuous, similar to a toothache, occurring deep within the muscle. The pain tends to wax and wane over time and may be more severe at night. It can be quite refractory to treatment. Some patients develop focal regions of intense burning or pressure, which can be quite distressing. It probably is most common over the posterior thorax.

PAIN ASSOCIATED WITH OPTIC NEURITIS

Another well-known pain is that seen in association with optic neuritis. Pain on eye movement is seen in approximately 80 percent of patients with acute optic neuritis (45). It is typically described as a sharp, knifelike pain in the eye and may be associated with a deep ache or sensation of pressure above or behind the eye. Movements of the globe tend to trigger or worsen the pain. Pain associated with optic neuritis is due to inflammation and demyelination occurring in and around pain-sensitive meninges surrounding the optic nerve. The mechanism of headache associated with MS may also be caused by inflammation and demyelination occurring in close proximity to pain-sensitive structures. Steroid treatment usually brings resolution of the pain.

PRINCIPLES OF PAIN TREATMENT IN MULTIPLE SCLEROSIS

The choice of pharmacologic therapy in the treatment of pain in MS depends on the nature of the syndrome. There is considerable overlap in that some agents may be helpful in both acute and chronic syndromes. Those syndromes characterized by a paroxysmal onset tend to respond well to carbamazepine but also may respond to other anticonvulsants, including phenytoin and gabapentin. A general guideline is to initiate treatment of syndromes that have paroxysmal onset with carbamazepine. Low doses (100–200 mg twice a day) tend to be adequate for most syndromes, and the medication can be withdrawn if and when the symptoms abate. Paroxysmal syndromes tend to resolve on their own after four to six weeks and may not require prolonged therapy. If the syndrome cannot be brought under control, the dose of carbamazepine should be increased to levels that bring the drug plasma levels closer to the level used for seizure control. If the syndrome is still troublesome, a second drug may be added. Once the pain syndrome is brought under control, an attempt may be made to withdraw the first agent. Monotherapy for pain syndromes will produce fewer side effects and is clearly advantageous.

Chronic syndromes, such as burning dysesthetic extremity pain, are difficult to treat but may respond better to gabapentin and phenytoin. Carbamazepine occasionally may be of some help in a patient with a chronic syndrome, but other anticonvulsants tend to be more effective. As with the acute pain syndromes, monotherapy is better and avoids the side effects typically encountered with multiple drugs. In some patients, the pain syndrome may be of sufficient severity that one agent alone will not bring it under control, in which case a second agent can be added. Once the pain is brought under control, the regimen can be tailored to minimize side effects while achieving maximal control of the pain.

Not infrequently patients with MS may suffer from severe breakthrough pain. When this occurs, the use of narcotics is reasonable and may be necessary to bring the pain cycle under control. A wise approach is to inform the patient that narcotics are to be used only for severe breakthrough pain and that these agents are not intended for long-term use. Nevertheless, some patients develop refractory pain syndromes that require the expertise of a physician who specializes in the treatment of chronic pain.

Pain clinics may offer a variety of more specialized options, including intrathecal stimulators, narcotic pumps, trigger point injections, and intrathecal baclofen pumps. Although specialty pain clinics may be helpful in controlling pain in patients with highly refractory syndromes, the majority of patients benefit most from a careful approach in which the first step is to identify the cause of the pain, after which a logical and systematic approach to treatment can be undertaken. If the first choice of medication fails to bring about improvement, it should be discontinued and another appropriate agent should be employed. Trials of several agents may be required to find an agent that brings substantial relief of pain. It should be remembered that in some patients no combination of drugs will bring about complete relief of pain and partial relief may be the best achievable outcome.

References

1. Charcot JM. *Lecons sur les maladies du systeme nerveux faties a la Salpêtrière.* Paris: Delahaye, 1872:239–240.
2. Clifford DB, Trotter JL. Pain in multiple sclerosis. *Arch Neurol* 1984; 41:1270–1272.
3. Indaco A, Iachetta C, Socci L, Carrieri PB. Chronic and acute pain syndromes in patients with multiple sclerosis. *Acta Neurol* 1994; 16:97–102.
4. Vermote R, Ketelaer P, Carton H. Pain in multiple sclerosis. *Clin Neurol Neurosurg* 1986; 88:87–93.
5. Moulin D, Foley K, Ebers G. Pain syndromes in multiple sclerosis. *Neurology* 1988; 38:1830–1834.
6. Carter S, Sciarra D, Merritt H. The course of multiple sclerosis as determined by autopsy proven cases. *Res Pub Assn Res Nerv Ment Dis* 1948; 28:471–511.

7. Stenager E, Knudsen L, Jensen K. Acute and chronic pain syndromes in multiple sclerosis. *Acta Neurol Scand* 1991; 84:197–200.

8. Kassirer M, Osterberg D. Pain in multiple sclerosis. *Am J Nurs* 1997; 968–969.

9. Archibald C, McGrath P, Ritvo P, et al. Pain prevalence, severity and impact in a clinic sample of multiple sclerosis. *Pain* 1994; 58:89–93.

10. Brown GK. A causal analysis of chronic pain and depression. *J Abnorm Psychol* 1990; 99:127–137.

11. Ramirez-Lassepas M, Tulloch J, Quinones M, Snyder B. Acute radicular pain as a presenting symptom in multiple sclerosis. *Arch Neurol* 1992; 49:255–258.

12. Rolak L, Brown S. Headaches and multiple sclerosis: A clinical study and review of the literature. *J Neurol* 1990; 237:300–302.

13. Freedman M, Gray T. Vascular headache: A presenting symptom of multiple sclerosis. *Can J Neurol Sci* 1989; 16:63–66.

14. Haas D, Kent P, Friedman D. Headache caused by a single lesion of multiple sclerosis in the periaqueductal gray area. *Headache* 1993; 33:452–455.

15. Nager B, Lanska D, Daroff R. Acute demyelination mimicking vascular hemicrania. *Headache* 1989; 29:423–424.

16. Galer B, Lipton R, Weinstein S, Bello L, Solomon S. Apoplectic headache and oculomotor nerve palsy: An unusual presentation of multiple sclerosis. *Neurology* 1990; 40:1465–1466.

17. Brisman R. Trigeminal neuralgia and multiple sclerosis. *Arch Neurol* 1987; 44:379–81.

18. Rushton JG, Olafson R. Trigeminal neuralgia associated with multiple sclerosis: Report of 35 cases. *Arch Neurol* 1965; 13:383–386.

19. Jensen TS, Rasmussen P, Reske-Nielsene. Association of trigeminal neuralgia with multiple sclerosis: clinical and pathological features. *Acta Neurol Scand* 1982; 65:182–189.

20. Meaney J, Watt J, Eldrige P, et al. Association between trigeminal neuralgia and multiple sclerosis: Role of magnetic resonance imaging. *J Neurol Neurosurg Psychiatry* 1995; 59:253–259.

21. Yang J, Simonson T, Ruprecht A, et al. Magnetic resonance imaging used to assess patients with trigeminal neuralgia. *Oral Surg Oral Med Oral Pathol* 1996; 81:3:343–350.

22. Paty DW, Poser C. Clinical symptoms and signs of multiple sclerosis. In: Poser C (ed.). *The diagnosis of multiple sclerosis.* New York, Stuttgart: Thieme-Stratton, 1984:27–34.

23. Albert ML. Treatment of pain in multiple sclerosis. *N Engl J Med*; 1969:280:1395.

24. Bowsher D. Pain syndromes and their treatment. *Curr Opin Neurol Neurosurg* 1993; 6:257–263.

25. Anderson P, Goodkin D. Current pharmacologic treatment of multiple sclerosis symptoms. *West J Med* 1996; 165:313–317.

26. Lunaardi G, Leandri M, Albano C, et al. Clinical effectiveness of lamotrigine and plasma levels in essential and symptomatic trigeminal neuralgia. *Neurology* 1997; 48:1714–1717.

27. Reder A, Arnason B. Trigeminal neuralgia in multiple sclerosis relieved by a prostaglandin E analogue. *Neurology* 1995; 45:1097–1100.

28. Peraire M. Diagnosis and treatment of the patient with trigeminal neuralgia. *Neurologia* 1997; 12(1):12–22.

29. Meaney J, Eldridge P, Dunn L, et al. Demonstration of neurovascular compression in trigeminal neuralgia with magnetic resonance imaging. *J Neurosurg* 1995; 83:799–805.

30. Lunsford LD, Treatment of douloureux by percutaneous retrogasserian glycerol injection. *JAMA* 1982; 248:449–453.

31. Golfino JG, Shetter AG. Treatment of trigeminal neuralgia in multiple sclerosis patients using radiofrequency thermal rhizotomy and glycerol rhizotomy. *J Neurosurg* (Abst) 1993; 78:367.

32. Brett DC, Ferguson GG, Ebers GC, Paty DW. Percutaneous trigeminal rhizotomy: Treatment of trigeminal neuralgia secondary to multiple sclerosis. *Arch Neurol* 1982; 39:219–221.

33. Kodziolka D, Lunsford L, Bissonette D. Long-term results after glycerol rhizotomy for multiple sclerosis–related trigeminal neuralgia. *Can J Neurol Sci* 1994; 21:137–140.

34. Osterman P, Westerberg C. Paroxysmal attacks in multiple sclerosis. *Brain* 1975; 98:189–202.

35. Matthews W. Paroxysmal symptoms in multiple sclerosis. *J Neurol Neurosurg Psychiatry* 1975; 38:617–623.

36. Espir M, Millac P. Treatment of paroxysmal disorders in multiple sclerosis with carbamazepine (Tegretol). *J Neurol Neurosurg Psychiatry* 1970; 33:528–531.

37. Lhermitte J, Bollak J, Nicholas M. Les douleurs a type de decharge electrique consecutives a la flexion cephalique dans la sclerose en plaques: Un cas de forme sensitive de la sclerose multiple. *Revue Neurol*; 1924:31:56–62.

38. Alajouanine TH, Thurel R, Papajoanou C. La douleur a type de decharge electrique provoquee par la flexion de la tete et parcourant le corps de haut en bas. *Revue Neurol* 1949; 81:89–97.

39. Ekbom K. Carbamazepine, a new symptomatic treatment for the paraesthesia associated with Lhermitte's sign. *J Neurol* 1991; 200:341–344.

40. Samkoff LM, Daras M, Tuchman AJ, Koppel BS. Amelioration of refractory dysesthetic limb pain in multiple sclerosis by gabapentin. *Neurology* 1997; 49:304–305.

41. Koutchens MK, Richert JR, Sami A, Rose John. Open label gabapentin treatment for pain in multiple sclerosis. *Multiple Sclerosis* 1997; 3:250–253.

42. Byrne TN, Waxman SG. In: Plum F (ed.). *Spinal cord compression. Diagnosis and principles of management.* Philadelphia: FA Davis, 1990:66–86.

43. Jeffery DR, Mandler RN, Davis LE. Transverse myelitis. Retrospective analysis of 33 cases, with differentiation of cases associated with multiple sclerosis and parainfectious events. *Arch Neurol* 1993; 50:532–535.

44. Watkins SM, Espir M. Migraine and multiple sclerosis. *J Neurol Neurosurg Psychiatry* 1969; 2:35–37.

45. Mathews WB. Clinical aspects (symptoms and signs). In: Mathews WB (ed.). *McAlpine's multiple sclerosis.* New York: Churchill Livingstone, 1985; 96–118.

24 Bladder Dysfunction

Mary Dierich, RN, MSN, C-NP, CURN

The patient with multiple sclerosis (MS) has specific elimination problems as a result of both chronic and intermittent symptomatology. Additionally, medications and chronic fatigue have a significant impact on these patients. Assessments are repeated over time, with the goal of detecting the symptomatology during periods of acute flare-up and in the latent phase of the disease. The psychosocial profile of the MS patient adds to the difficulty of capturing this information. Given the level of fatigue and disability in this population, ongoing urologic treatment must be focused, practical, and easily accomplished.

This chapter addresses the physical changes in the urinary system that are typical of MS and how the various types of the disease may affect prognosis. Assessment, testing, and determination of treatment are reviewed, as are factors to consider in determining a care plan for the safe treatment of bladder dysfunction. Discussion includes the use of new treatment and management options, such as pelvic stimulation, and the modifications in treatment protocol necessary to meet the needs of this population. The chapter also reviews the prevalence, differential diagnosis, and pathophysiology of bladder dysfunction. Algorithms for treatment and potential treatments are reviewed, and the practitioner is given practical hints for serving this challenging and diverse population.

EFFECTS OF BLADDER DYSFUNCTION

Although it is suspected that there are between 12 million and 25 million incontinent people in the United States (1,2), it is not known how many of these people have MS. Badlani (3) suggests that 80 percent of MS patients experience bladder dysfunction. The MS patient with bladder problems is an enigma—one day functioning normally, the next day having nocturia and symptoms that mimic a urinary tract infection (UTI). The reasons for these swings in function are not known at present, but they may be related to fatigue and medication patterns, as well as to the onset of an illness. Any decrease in functioning in the MS patient usually has a profound effect on bowel and bladder function.

Social Costs

The effect of bowel and bladder dysfunction on the MS patient is generally severe and may be devastating. Changes in bladder function usually are one of the first signs of MS. When patients seek urologic treatment, they often are pessimistic that anything can be done because the problem is long-standing and varies in intensity. Urinary frequency of 12 to 20 times daily is not unusual, so that much time and energy is expended in toileting activities. As a result of nocturia, patients appear in the office

433

with sleep deprivation and subsequent depression. Fatigue is common for the significantly disabled because it requires great effort to remove clothes and then to move from the wheelchair to the toilet. Individuals who are tied to the bathroom become socially isolated, and when they are away from home, a tremendous amount of effort is expended looking for the nearest bathroom or trying to hide incontinence. Caregiver burden also must be carefully monitored and added to both the economic and the social costs of bladder dysfunction.

Economic Realities

Although the social cost of incontinence is high, the economic cost of treatment and management also is significant. In general, care for incontinence is covered by insurance only for homebound patients who have permanent disability. Unless the dysfunction is severe enough to require an indwelling catheter, most management options—short of surgical procedures—are not covered by insurance. Surgery is the treatment of last resort in this population because future bladder function is unpredictable, recovery is arduous, and the potential for infection may seriously impact the course of the disease. The patient with bladder dysfunction is left little choice other than to pay for products out-of-pocket. At the typical rate of three to four diapers or incontinence pads per day, expenses mount quickly. Patients typically try to conserve their pad use by wringing them out, lining them with tissues or toilet paper, or double-padding. These practices quickly lead to skin breakdown, which further increases the number of physician visits and the cost of care. Ironically, if the patient uses an indwelling catheter, which allows greater freedom, he or she must be totally homebound in order to qualify for nursing help to change the catheter at home. Patients who want to remain active in the community must make monthly visits to their physician for catheter changes in order to have their products covered by insurance. It is little wonder that these patients are depressed.

PATHOPHYSIOLOGY OF BLADDER DYSFUNCTION

The effects of bladder dysfunction in the MS patient are far-reaching and significantly affect total health. In this section we examine the normal function of the urinary tract system and then examine how changes in MS affect that function.

Normal Urinary Tract Function

The kidneys of an adult female produce 100 to 125 cubic centimeters (cc's) of urine per hour, whereas the rate for adult males is closer to 150 per hour. The actual rate depends on fluid intake, position, and kidney function. The kidneys produce urine more efficiently in the supine position, and nocturnal diuresis may become a significant problem for those with heart or lung problems. The ureters are thin-walled muscular tubes that move the urine produced in small boluses via peristalsis from the kidneys to the bladder. Closure of the ureters during bladder contraction initially is accomplished by contraction of the trigone area during voiding. Like the dome of the bladder, the triangle-shaped muscular trigone area, bounded by the ureteral orifices and the bladder neck, has primarily beta adrenergic receptors and muscarinic receptors. Although the ureters enter at mid-bladder, their higher pressure prevents reflux during bladder filling. As the bladder fills, its dome distends out of the pelvic cavity and should accommodate 500 to 600 cc's of urine without an increase in intervesicular pressure. As the bladder fills, its lining thins from a multicell thickness to a one-cell thickness (3). It previously was believed that there was one-to-one innervation of the muscle fibers, a belief that now is disputed (4). Stretch afferents from the bladder surface send signals that are mediated via the pons to the frontal cortex during filling (Figure 24-1). Ultimately, the individual must process this information as to the need to void, length of time to voiding, and whether it is socially acceptable to void. Whether the individual decides to void or not, coordination of the sensory, autonomic, and somatic systems is accomplished by the pons. During bladder filling, the sympathetic system is active and the hypogastric nerve (level T11–L2) brings the message to the bladder to continue relaxing and to the urethra to remain closed. If voiding is to occur, the parasympathetic system becomes active and the message is sent through the pelvic nerve to the sacral micturition center (S2–S4), in which voiding is coordinated and the pudendal nerve (pelvic floor muscles) originates. The pelvic muscles relax, lowering the urethral pressure a split second before the trigone and the rest of the bladder then contracts in a sustained fashion. The urethra (alpha adrenergic receptor) relaxes during voiding to provide a conduit through which the urine flows (3). Although it is a muscular tube, the urethra also has a thick mucosal layer that is filled with estrogen receptors in the female. This mucosal layer is thought to provide a secure seal to prevent leakage when voiding is completed (5).

Bladder Dysfunction

Incontinence is officially classified in the Agency for Health Care Policy and Research (AHCPR) guidelines as follows: stress incontinence, urge incontinence, overflow incontinence, mixed incontinence, functional incontinence, and iatrogenic incontinence (6). There is some dis-

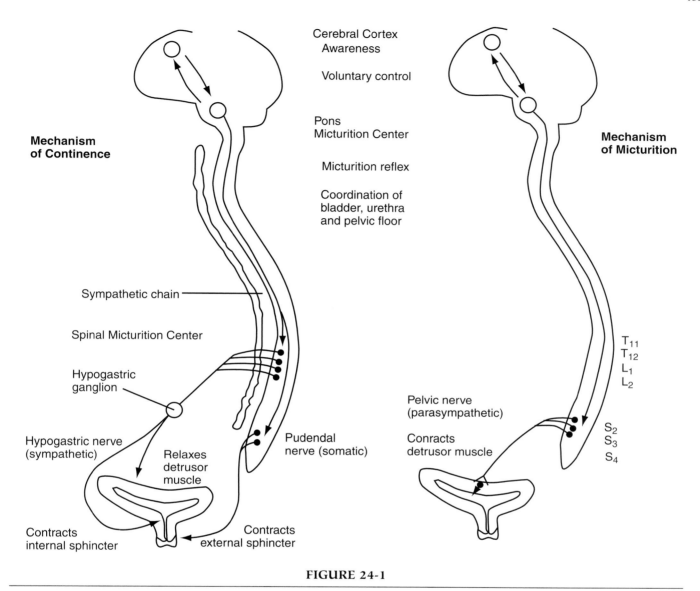

FIGURE 24-1

Centers for control of micturition and storage.

agreement about the consistent classifications for detrusor activity. There is little agreement as to the labeling of problems of hypersensitivity and pelvic muscle problems.

Regardless of the classification, bladder dysfunction boils down to two end-organ problems in the four systems that are responsible for maintaining continence. There are degrees of either overactivity or underactivity of the sensory nerve pathways, the detrusor muscle, the urethral smooth muscle, or the somatic pelvic muscles. The astute clinician must be able to sort out these problems and then institute the most appropriate treatment. The four most common true dysfunctions (not iatrogenic or functional problems) seen in the MS patient are the hypersensitive bladder, pelvic muscle spasticity, motor

hyperactivity of the bladder, and hypotonicity of the bladder. There may be multiple causes, depending on whether the disease is in an active phase or in remission, the location of active plaques, and what medications the patient presently is taking.

Variants in Multiple Sclerosis

Hypersensitivity

Hypersensitivity usually is one of the earliest bladder dysfunctions. Patients initially diagnosed with MS often recall needing to go to the bathroom far more frequently than their friends many years before the diagnosis of MS.

They occasionally recall episodes of incontinence, but more often the issue is severe urgency and the feeling of always needing to go to the bathroom. When describing their stream, it is not unusual to hear a description that includes a great deal of urgency and no problem starting the stream, but that it is of small amount and perhaps diminished caliber. If a diary is kept, patients may be voiding every one to two hours during the day, but at night may sleep for three to four hours at a time, or occasionally even through the night. They may relate previous failed episodes of medication trials and perhaps a hysterectomy or a bladder suspension at a fairly young age (i.e., under 40 years). When tested urodynamically, no abnormality other than a small-capacity bladder is seen. Leaking probably is not elicited. Voiding studies initially indicate a good flow, but there may be abdominal straining at the end of the void when the patient is trying to empty the bladder completely. Physical examination usually reveals no detectable abnormality other than perhaps some suprapubic tenderness resulting from abdominal straining and some tenderness over the urethra during palpation of the anterior vaginal wall.

Pelvic Muscle Spasticity

As the disease progresses, the pelvic muscles become spastic, as do the muscles of the lower extremities. An initial episode of acute painful retention, which often is the presenting symptom of MS in young women, probably is the result of this phenomenon. The pelvic muscles become spastic and in effect cause the external sphincter to clamp down. Depending on the strength of that response, the patient will have difficulty either initiating or maintaining a good urine flow and will be in partial or total retention.

Patients presenting with this problem may describe having a strong urge to void after being seated on the toilet, yet they are unable to start their stream. If timed, voiding usually takes longer than a minute and the stream does not sound forceful; it usually is intermittent. Patients may complain of vague abdominal discomfort over time and also may have been diagnosed with vaginismus in the past. This spasticity may lead to serious upper urinary tract disease. Because there are no backflow valves on the ureters, high pressure (> 30 cm/H_2O) in the bladder may ultimately damage the kidneys (7). Additionally, hypertrophy of the bladder wall, which is the result of high-pressure voiding, may ultimately lead to motor hyperactivity of the bladder and resultant urge incontinence. Hypertrophy eventually decreases compliance of the bladder wall to accommodate adequate urine volume. Filling urodynamics may show a low capacity or a poorly compliant bladder, or the test may appear to be normal. However, electromyographic tracings are of increased ampli-

tude at rest and during the filling and voiding phases. Quieting of the signal should occur while voiding.

The voiding study will show an intermittent flow with prolonged voiding. The patient probably will use abdominal straining to empty completely. Examination may reveal costovertebral angle tenderness, tenderness over the insertion points of the levators, and vaginal lateral wall tenderness on deep palpation. Resting the examining finger just inside the introitus of the vagina over the perineal body or during a rectal examination, the examiner should pick up increased tone and perhaps even the spastic movement of the muscle, even at rest.

Detrusor Hyperactivity

Detrusor hyperactivity may be seen at any point in the disease. Patients classically describe a larger volume loss of urine on the way to the bathroom as well as losing urine when washing their hands or stepping out into the cold. There generally is no warning with this loss of urine, and the patient may have difficulty relating the loss to a specific event. Patients also describe dribbling or leaking on the way to the bathroom. These patients probably will respond to a trial of anticholinergic medication. On urodynamic testing, there will be waves of increased detrusor pressure that may or may not cause leaking. Pressures should return to baseline between contractions. The patient may be able to inhibit contractions by taking a few deep breaths or contracting the pelvic muscles several times in a row. However, as the bladder approaches capacity, the detrusor contractions will be harder to suppress and leaking probably will ensue. Leakage may consist of a few drops or total loss of urine. Bladder wall compliance generally is good in such a patient, and pelvic muscle activity is of normal amplitude on electromyography. Voiding studies also are normal unless there is a mixed cause of the incontinence.

Hypotonic Bladder

The patient with a hypotonic bladder may present a confusing picture. Leaking may be provoked by coughing, laughing, or bending, and may vary in amounts from a few drops to a stream of urine. Leaking also may occur at rest and on a continual basis. Given this scenario in a patient with no previous surgical history, the likely culprit is overflow incontinence. A patient with poor sensation may not be toileting very often, whereas the patient whose sensation is relatively intact may be toileting very frequently, as often as every half hour. A classic tip-off is the patient who never feels empty and on physical examination reveals a darkened or bruised area above the pubic bone. The patient will describe bearing down or in later cases massaging or pushing on the belly, either to start the flow or to empty completely.

Hesitancy, poor caliber stream, and prolonged voiding are hallmarks of this syndrome. If a patient is receiving anticholinergic medication, the problem may coincide with the time of peak action and may subside when the patient stops the medication for a short time. Postvoid residuals usually are quite elevated (i.e., greater than 100 cc's). Urodynamic testing will show a very large capacity bladder, usually with no detrusor activity during most of the filling phase. There may be detrusor contractions near capacity, at which point the patient may lose part of the volume instilled. The distinguishing characteristic of this problem, as opposed to hyperactivity, is that the initial sensation is quite late in the filling phase. The voiding study will show prolonged intermittent flow of low rate. Electromyographic activity during filling and voiding may be normal or of low magnitude, and the signal may not increase as filling approaches capacity. These patients are prone to frequent urinary tract infections and stones, but because of decreased sensation they may not appreciate that they have symptoms of a UTI. The only symptoms may be incontinence or frequency.

Other Problems

Mixed problems are frequently encountered in the MS patient. If the bladder must contract against a closed or partially closed internal or external sphincter, it eventually thickens and becomes hypertrophied and may not be able to generate enough pressure to empty completely against the closure pressure of the urethra. Much like hypertrophied cardiac muscle, the bladder's intrinsic pacemaker becomes dysfunctional and the bladder becomes "irritable." This irritability presents as frequency, low-volume voiding, and urge incontinence.

Cystoscopy will reveal a trabeculated bladder wall—roughened, thickened, and hyperemic. If no solution is sought for the problem, the bladder wall eventually loses its compliance or the ability to stretch to accommodate increasing urine volumes without change in bladder pressure. When this happens, the patient is in danger of damaging the kidneys and a long-range plan must be developed to keep the bladder at low filling pressures and decompressed throughout the day.

Decompression becomes quite difficult because the patient with a hypertrophied bladder usually has little or no capacity. Even residuals as low as 25 to 50 cc's in a patient with a total capacity of 100 to 200 cc's are a quarter of the total capacity for this patient. Often the only practical solution in this case is to insert an indwelling catheter or entirely eliminate the drive to void with anticholinergic medication and then use intermittent catheterization. In severe cases, continent diversions, cutaneous ileocystostomy, and augmentation cystoplasty may be used to maintain a low pressure system (8).

Differential Diagnosis

Chief Complaint

The practitioner who is evaluating urinary dysfunction should be scrupulous in the rigor of the initial examination and history taking. The chief complaint should include information about frequency both during the day and at night, information about pain and its descriptors, urine appearance, stream characteristics, urinary leakage and aggravating factors, pad use, and tricks used to initiate voiding or to empty completely. Frequency may vary greatly in the MS patient, not only from day to night but also during periods of exacerbation and periods of stability. The practitioner should ask leading questions such as "How frequent is frequent on your worst days?" and "How often do you go on your best days?" A time period will give you the best information and sometimes a suggestion of the time frame, such as every 15 minutes to one to two hours, and will cue the patient to reveal information he or she might not realize falls far from normal parameters. Nighttime frequency may be vastly different from daytime frequency, especially if the bladder dysfunction is a sensory dysfunction rather than a motor dysfunction. If the patient has difficulty recalling specifics of frequency, a simple three-day voiding diary (Figure 24-2) becomes a useful tool. The diary also should have an area to record types and amounts of fluid intake. In addition to being an excellent assessment tool, the voiding diary becomes a superb teaching tool and a record of progress if used in a serial fashion. Urine appearance may give clues to whether there is an active UTI. Remember to ask whether the patient has ever had pink-tinged or bloody urine. Stream characteristics (hesitancy, decreased caliper and force) and the feeling of incomplete emptying will assist the practitioner in determining whether further work-up for retention should be initiated. Past bladder or kidney problems may help detail a history of kidney stones or uncover chronic retention. Past medical history should include whether the patient has ever seen a gynecologist for any reason other than prenatal care, whether she has ever seen a urologist, what tests were performed, and whether treatment was initiated and successful. Primary care physicians, therapists, or any other specialists who are presently active in the patient's care also should be noted.

Review of Medications

A review of medications often will help detail the medical history, so it is preferable to evaluate this next. It is helpful for the patient to bring in his or her current prescription medications, any over-the-counter medications routinely used, and any supplements prescribed or oth-

Day: _____ Date: _____

Time	Type of Fluid	Amount of Fluid	Urge to Toilet?	Voided in Toilet?	Leaked?	Changed Pad?	Activity
6–8 AM							
8–10 AM							
10–12 AM							
12–2 PM							
2–4 PM							
4–6 PM							
6–8 PM							
8–10 PM							
10–12 PM							
12–2 AM							
2–4 AM							
4–6 AM							

Did you have pain today, during or after voiding? _____ yes _____ no
Did you have a bowel movement today? _____ yes _____ no

FIGURE 24-2

Voiding diary used to track intake and voiding episodes.

erwise regularly used. Because many antidepressants and muscle relaxants are used to treat urinary function, be sure to ascertain why the patient is taking these medications. Medications used to treat chronic heart, lung, or thyroid problems often have adverse effects on urinary function or interact with medications that typically are used to treat urinary dysfunction. Another key factor is *prescribed* use versus *actual* use.

Past Medical History

Past medical history should be reviewed, with special attention to childbearing history, bowel difficulties, past bladder or kidney problems, thyroid dysfunction, diabetes, impotence, discomfort during intercourse, menopause history, and heart or lung problems. Review the number of children borne, miscarriages, and abortions; whether the children were delivered vaginally or by caesarean section; and whether there were any unusual circumstances—premature births, tears, forceps deliveries, breech births, or prolonged or precipitous deliveries. Note whether the patient had difficulty with urination or leakage post delivery, how it was managed, and how long the problem lasted. Details regarding bowel history should include how often the patient has a bowel movement; its color, shape, and form; and whether and under what circumstances leakage of stool occurs. Problems such as undiscovered or uncontrolled diabetes or thyroid dysfunction also may markedly affect urinary function.

Surgical History

Although information about all past surgical history is collected, surgical history taking focuses on abdominal, vaginal, and rectal procedures; previous bladder repairs; and any artificial valves, joints, pins, rods, or plates. Like the medical history, the surgical history will help the practitioner eliminate or more heavily favor certain working diagnoses. Additionally, knowing whether the patient has implants will help specialists determine the need for prophylactic antibiotics before any diagnostic testing is done.

Psychosocial History

The patient should be questioned at length about his or her environmental conditions and coping mechanisms to avoid episodes of incontinence. Particular attention should be paid to how far the bathrooms are from the bedroom and living areas, the lighting, the flooring, and whether assistive devices are needed. Family support is important in determining a treatment plan. Are caregivers available if help is needed to implement a plan? The patient who needs assistance with intermittent self-catheterization (ISC) or toileting will continue to have incontinence when a family member is not available or does not want to help. It is important to assess whether the bladder dysfunction is a problem for the family as well as for the patient. Education of family members may be all that is needed to realign their expectations of the patient. If family members are supportive of the patient, he or she will have a much higher chance of success. Is the patient being treated for depression or anxiety now, or has he or she been treated in the past? What are the treatments—medications, counseling, or a combination of modalities? Is the problem resolving? Does the patient have a history of sexual difficulties, or has the patient been sexually abused in the past? Pelvic muscle spasticity also may have psychogenic causes, particularly if it occurs in isolation of the other spastic extremities.

Mental Status

Mental status, motivation, and memory may determine the treatment plan for the patient with urinary dysfunction. Elaborate measures or exercise programs are useless to the patient who is not motivated to continue with a consistent program. If the patient is easily frustrated or has memory difficulty, a program with intricate steps or many facets may not be the treatment of choice. The patient who is expecting a cure will be disappointed with a *management* strategy. Therefore, the practitioner must be cognizant of the patient's mental capabilities, the prognosis, and the patient's expectations for treatment. Early in treatment the patient must have a good understanding of what is possible and what is not possible, so that expectations are gradually focused. Additionally, you should evaluate the patient for depression and cognition. Question him closely to find out how he is coping with incontinence, exactly how bothersome the problem is, and whether care for this problem has been initiated in the past. Patients who have been told by past caregivers that there is nothing that can be done for them do not readily buy into a treatment program, which makes the likelihood of failure more probable.

Fluid and Diet

Examine the voiding diary for the types and amounts of fluid consumed. Caffeine, artificial sweeteners, citrus fruit juices, and alcohol may increase frequency. Note whether the patient's daytime frequency is significantly greater than the nighttime frequency. Does the patient tend to have more incontinent episodes later in the day as the pelvic muscles become more fatigued? Or does leaking occur after a long period of sleep? Evaluate whether the pattern of leaking is related to urgency or stress maneuvers. Does the bladder hold a reasonable amount of urine? Finally, evaluate how often the patient has a bowel movement.

Examination

Examination of the MS patient with incontinence will necessarily be detailed and may involve procedures not typically done as part of the routine follow-up care in the MS clinic. Lower urinary tract system evaluations performed in addition to the usual evaluations of mental status, cognition, functional status, and neurologic status are described in the following sections.

Neurologic Examination

The neurologic examination should include the urologist's saddle examination. Keeping in mind that the micturition center is located in the S2–S4 level of the cord, filling at the

T11–L2 level, and coordination of function at the pons, pay particular attention to evaluating these areas. Gait and balance problems usually are seen in those patients who have problems coordinating their voiding patterns and an inability to suppress urgency. Evaluate the lower extremities for sensation, positional deficits, and reflexes. Spasticity of the lower extremities should make one suspicious of dyssynergia in patients who complain of not feeling empty. Hypersensitivity of the lower extremities may accompany increased urgency of a sensory nature, whereas hyperactivity of the lower extremities may also be related to motor urgency of the bladder. Flaccidity should prompt the examiner to evaluate the motor tone of the bladder more carefully and to determine whether retention and subsequent reflux are present.

Abdominal Examination

The objectives of the abdominal examination include ruling out problems with bowel motility, kidney enlargement, and retention. Listen to the bowel tones. Areas of increased activity above a quiet area may indicate impaction or slowed motility. Palpate for the dome of the bladder—an empty bladder should not be felt above the level of the symphysis pubis. Enlargement of the kidneys may require evaluation by ultrasound; if accompanied by tenderness, hematuria, or flank discomfort, an intravenous pyelogram (IVP) should be performed. Referral to a urologist would be indicated after initiating the appropriate tests. Have the patient cough and bear down to evaluate for hernias. Palpate for enlargement or tenderness of the lymph nodes and for masses in the abdominal cavity. Any tenderness, fixed areas, or masses should then be evaluated.

Musculoskeletal Examination

When evaluating the back, pay attention to scoliosis, hip rotation, and differential in hip height, in addition to costovertebral angle tenderness. Rotational problems in this population are quite prevalent and usually are due to unilateral weakness of the lower extremity and subsequent changes in gait patterns to accommodate the deficit. Hip rotation may also be caused by scar tissue subsequent to abdominal, pelvic, or back surgery. Patients with hip rotation or scoliosis need physical therapy evaluation and possible treatment using stretching exercises and myofascial release techniques. These musculoskeletal deformities can greatly impact continence as a result of nerve impingement and spasticity of the muscles. Although a person *without* MS would feel enough pain to seek treatment for the lower back, a patient *with* MS would not experience the same degree of discomfort that would drive him to seek care. Many of these patients ultimately develop pelvic muscle spasm and retention.

Pelvic Examination

The pelvic examination is quite involved, and special techniques must be used to prevent inadvertent spasm of the muscles during examination. Rather than using stirrups, have the patient assume a supine position with the knees bent. If necessary, support the legs with pillows or use an assistant to support the legs. Evaluate condition of the skin. Pay particular attention to the labial folds in women and the groin of men, evaluating for redness, maceration, or signs of yeast infection. Note the hygiene of this area. Stroke the anus with a cotton swab to determine whether an anal wink is present. In its absence, not only is there a sensory and motor deficit but also the likelihood of strengthening the pelvic muscles by exercise or biofeedback is greatly reduced. Evaluate the pelvic muscle tone next, before the patient becomes fatigued. Inserting an examining finger just into the vagina, rest it lightly over the perineal body and feel the pelvic resting tone. Note whether the muscles are in spasm or are overly flaccid. Ask the patient to contract the pelvic muscles around the examining finger inserted into the vagina and/or rectum. Determine how strong the contraction is, whether it encompasses the full circumference of the finger, whether it is stronger on one side, and whether the patient can repeat and hold the contraction without degradation. Monitor the abdomen and gluteal muscles to determine whether the patient can isolate the pelvic muscles or whether bigger muscle groups are recruited. Next palpate just inside the vaginal introitus in women to evaluate sensation and tenderness.

Move deeper into the vault to evaluate the piriformis attachments along the lateral walls and the tone of the vagina. Palpate the bladder neck for discharge, tenderness, diverticula, and caruncles, and the posterior vaginal wall for rectal fullness. A bimanual examination may be performed at this time if desired. Before removing the examining finger, slide a second finger into the vault and hold the rectum out of the way while evaluating the mobility of the bladder and bladder neck when the patient coughs and bears down. Check to see whether the urethral meatus gapes open when the patient performs these maneuvers. Rotate the examining fingers and hold the bladder out of the way to assess for rectocele while the patient again coughs and bears down. Ideally, this sequence should then be repeated in the upright position. Sliding the finger out of the vaginal vault, assess the secretions for unusual color or consistency. Then palpate the surface muscle attachments for tenderness. Use a clock face pattern (Figure 24-3) to check the attachment sites of the bulbocavernosus muscles and the levators for tenderness (9). If considering a vaginal device to treat incontinence, evaluate the vaginal mucosa for lesions, redness, and lubrication. Spasm of the muscles and tenderness of the attachments should warrant further evaluation by physical therapy.

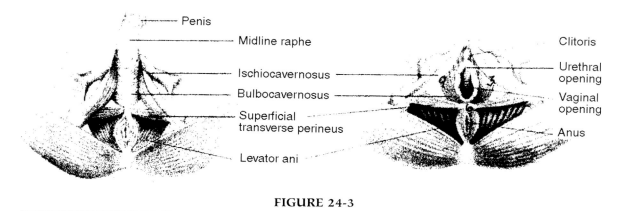

FIGURE 24-3

Palpation points for determining trigger points in the pelvic floor muscle attachments.

Hypermobility of the bladder or bladder neck, tenderness of the bladder or urethra, or suspected retention should be referred to a urologist, whereas ovarian tenderness, poor integrity, or dryness of the vaginal mucosa, or suspected vaginal infection should be referred to a gynecologist. Rectal tone in males may be evaluated the same way. Tenderness of the scrotum, suspected hernia, or penile tenderness should be evaluated by a urologist. The rectal vault should be evaluated for its contents in both men and women, and a prostate examination should be performed in males.

Testing for Bladder Dysfunction

Several simple tests may be performed in the clinic that will help elucidate the cause of bladder dysfunction. Based on the results of these tests, additional testing by the urologist may be warranted (Table 24-1). When referring a patient for urodynamic testing, information collected should include data about bladder capacity, compliance, filling characteristics, leak point pressures, bladder and pelvic muscle characteristics during both the filling and the voiding phases, and any unusual characteristics dur-

TABLE 24-1	
Tests Used to Elucidate the Cause of Bladder Dysfunction (4)	

TEST	INDICATIONS
Kidney-ureter-bladder X-ray	Calculi, preliminary screening for contrast tests
Intravenous pyelogram/nephrotomogram	Calculi, recurrent UTI, hematuria, masses, obstruction, congenital anomaly
Retrograde pyelogram	Same as above
Cystogram/voiding cystourethrogram	Recurrent UTI, congenital anomaly, trauma to lower tract, reflux, hematuria
Retrograde urethrogram	Structure, fistula, trauma, diverticulum, tumor
Computed tomographic scan	Tumor grading, mass, sacral deformities
Magnetic resonance imaging	Mass, tumor, sacral deformities
Cystoscopy	Calculi, recurrent UTI, reflux, obstruction, fistula, incontinence, neuropathic bladder, suspected bladder wall cancer, congenital anomalies
Ultrasound	Postvoid residual urine, kidney size
Urodynamics (with or without contrast)	Diagnostic testing for bladder function
Uroflow	Abnormal flow patterns, obstruction
Cystometrogram (CMG)	Capacity, compliance, stability, leaking, sensation
Electromyogram (EMG)	Pelvic muscle response to filling/voiding
Voiding pressure study	Characteristics of bladder and pelvic muscles during voiding
Urethral pressure study	Characteristics of urethra

ing the voiding phase. The urodynamicist should also interpret the test, rather than having a technician perform the test and the urologist interpret it. Finally, the test should be accompanied by recommendations for treatment and additional testing needed, such as a retrograde cystourethrogram, cystoscopy, or IVP. These are the minimal expectations for a referral made for the MS patient.

Urinalysis and Culture

The simplest and most useful test in this population is the urinalysis and urine culture. Preferably collected by catheter while checking a postvoid residual, it will indicate the presence of bacteria, the level of growth, the sensitivities, the presence of chronic inflammation, hematuria, and the by-products of stone production. Collecting the specimen by catheter eliminates contamination in this population, in which obtaining a clean specimen is difficult because of physical disabilities. When ruling out whether bacteriuria is the cause of urgency, it is best to treat even small colony-forming unit counts and then follow up cessation of treatment with a repeat urinalysis 7 to 10 days later.

Postvoid Residual

If the postvoid residual (PVR) is higher than 125 cc's, intermittent straight catheterization may be taught at the same visit. If the PVR is in a moderate range—75 to 125 cc's—further testing to determine the capacity of the bladder and the cause of the retention should be initiated. The MS patient usually has a significantly decreased capacity, so even a residual as low as 50 to 75 cc's may be one quarter to one half of functional capacity. Bladder ultrasound is an alternative method for detecting PVR.

Uroflow

The uroflow (cc/second), using a stopwatch and a collecting "hat," is an excellent way to determine whether there is some degree of obstruction as a result of pelvic muscle spasticity or hesitancy. Additionally, if the patient comes to the clinic with a full bladder, functional capacity can be determined. Decreased flow rates, particularly in men, should be evaluated by a urologist. If that is coupled with spasticity, a high index of supicion for dyssynergia should be entertained. Finally, serum blood urea nitrogen (BUN) and creatinine should be monitored regularly in patients in whom retention or a noncompliant bladder is a concern.

TREATMENT OPTIONS

Determining goals for the MS patient should be preceded by a discussion of what is realistic. Management and con-

tainment are the primary methods of improving bladder function in this population. Goal setting should revolve around protecting upper urinary tract function, improving sleep, normalizing toileting patterns, conserving energy, and preserving independence.

Reviewing and optimizing medications, fluid intake, and environmental conditions should be the first treatment for anyone with bladder dysfunction. Monitor how the medications are prescribed and how the patient actually is using them. Eliminate any repetition in classes, and substitute medications that have the least traumatic side-effect profile. Remember to question the patient closely regarding use of over-the-counter medication, cultural practices, and herbal remedies.

Fluids

Fluid intake and diet are extremely important. Patients with MS frequently are chronically fatigued as a result of their medication, energy expenditures, depression, and lack of sleep. They tend to use caffeinated beverages heavily as a means to becoming energized, especially in the morning. Monitoring caffeine use and urinary habits, then eliminating or decreasing caffeinated beverages, is a simple way to demonstrate the effects of caffeine as a diuretic and topical irritant to the bladder wall, as well as its effect on the intrinsic pacemaker of the bladder.

Encourage the patient to use a half-and-half mixture of caffeinated and noncaffeinated coffee. Other suspected irritants such as artificial sweeteners, alcohol, and carbonated beverages can similarly be eliminated. Remind the patient that water is the best fluid but that juices, caffeine-free, non-diet sodas, and herbal teas are also acceptable sources of fluids.

Individuals with MS tend to decrease their fluid intake in an effort to avoid leaking and toileting. Total fluid intake should be evaluated. Fluid deprivation causes the onset of a host of new problems. Fluid deprivation also contributes significantly to bladder irritability caused by highly concentrated urine. Fluid deprivation affects the severity and number of urinary tract infections and may lead to stone formation. Medication metabolism may be altered in the dehydrated patient, increasing side effects such as dry mouth, dizziness, and nausea.

Additionally, fluid deprivation may lead to increased procedures in that the specialists who deal with the patient need to determine the cause of the increased bladder dysfunction. Obviously, fluid intake and type is one of the first things to be discussed with a patient who has bladder dysfunction.

Patients should be encouraged to drink at least 1,000 to 1,500 cc's of fluid per day. This level of intake will assist in habit training and keep the bowel functioning normally.

Finally, because many medications used to treat MS and incontinence have a constipating side effect, fluid management becomes an important part of bowel and bladder management because of the close physical proximity of these organs. A hypotonic bowel may become so full that it obstructs the bladder neck, which leads to intermittent retention, or may cause pressure on the bladder, which increases urgency.

A hypotonic bowel ultimately may lead to impaction, diarrhea-like stools, and possibly fecal incontinence.

Functional Problems

Much of the urinary frequency in MS patients is related to preventive voiding as a means to avoid incontinent episodes because patients cannot reach the bathroom in a timely fashion. Functional problems are a major cause of urinary dysfunction, and significant effort should be expended to make it as effortless as possible to get to the bathroom in less than two minutes. Patients typically get a two-minute warning when they are at capacity and must toilet, so those patients who take longer than two minutes to get seated on the toilet may need to alter their toileting arrangements and be seen by physical therapists and occupational therapists to help determine whether assistive devices may be appropriate.

Environmental conditions may greatly affect the patient with urge incontinence. Nighttime may be difficult even if the patient is dry during the daytime. Patients who are sleeping soundly often get the call to toilet too late—unable to arouse from a deep slumber, get up from the bed, and still get to the bathroom in time. If the patient begins dribbling on the way to the toilet, the risk of falling is greatly increased. Additionally, changing clothing and cleaning up may make it difficult for this now wide-awake patient to return to sleep. A commode or urinal (urinals for women are now available) may be the simplest solution. Some patients are regular enough that an alarm may help to wake them before the strong urge occurs. Other patients, particularly those who use a wheelchair, find that elevating their feet for a half hour before bedtime and then voiding just before sleep promotes diuresis. In this way, they are able to get a longer period of sleep early in the evening.

Medications

An important component of treatment is the adjustment of present medications, as well as trying medications for bladder dysfunction as a result of the medication review. Table 24-2 lists the side effects of drugs commonly used in the treatment of MS, and Table 24-3 lists drugs commonly used in the treatment of bladder dysfunction. It also is helpful to remember that MS patients often are

TABLE 24-2

Drugs Used to Treat Multiple Sclerosis and Their Effects on Lower Urinary Tract Function (17,18)

DRUG	EFFECT
Baclofen (Lioresal)	Frequency, incontinence due to muscle relaxation
Diazepam (Valium)	Incontinence, retention
Clonazepam (Klonopin)	Dysuria, enuresis, nocturia, retention
Dantrolene (Dantrium)	Frequency, hematuria, incontinence, retention, crystalluria
Tizanidine (Zanaflex)	Frequency
Hydroxyzine (Vistaril)	None
Chlorpromazine (Thorazine)	Retention, priapism
Primidone (Mysoline)	Polyuria
Acetazolamide (Diamox)	Polyuria, hematuria
Amantadine (Symmetrel)	? Retention
Pemoline (Cylert)	None
Fluoxetine (Prozac)	Sexual dysfunction, ? dysuria, ? retention
Carbamazepine (Tegretol)	Frequency, retention, impotence, glycosuria, elevated BUN
Diphenhydrinate (Benadryl)	Dysuria, retention, frequency
Amitriptyline (Elavil)	Retention
Phenytoin (Dilantin)	None
Carisprodol (Soma)	None
Methocarbamol (Robaxin)	Discolored urine
Desipramine (Norpramine)	Retention
Nortriptyline (Pamelor)	Retention
Paroxetine (Paxil)	Sexual dysfunction, frequency, other urinary disorders
ACTH	None
Prednisone	None
Methylprednisolone (Medrol)	None
Interferon beta	Menstrual disorders
Azathioprine (Imuran)	None
Glatiramer acetate (Copaxone)	Usually none

major consumers or herbal and homeopathic medications (Table 24-4). If questioned, they may reveal a list of over-the-counter drugs that is longer than their list of prescribed medications. Table 24-5 lists the classes of med-

TABLE 24-3

Drugs, Indication, and Doses Useful for Treatment of Bladder Dysfunction in the Multiple Sclerosis Patient (minimal side effects and interactions) (6,7,17)

GENERIC NAME	DOSE	INTERACTION/SIDE EFFECTS
Detrusor Instability		
Tolterodine (Detrol)	2 mg bid	Cytochrome P450 inhibitor
Oxybutynin (Ditropan)	2.5–5 mg tid–qid	Anticholinergics
Oxybutynin (Detrol XL)	5–10 mg qd	Anticholinergics
Dicyclomine (Bentyl)	10–20 mg tid	Amantadine, TCAs
Imipramine (Tofranil)	25–100 mg qd	MAO inhibitors
Doxepin (Sinequan)	25–100 mg qd	MAO inhibitors
Stress Incontinence		
Phenylpropanolamine	15–30 mg tid	MAO inhibitors, thyroid medications
Estrogen (Premarin)	0.3–1.25 mg po/day or 2 gm or fraction/day	Monitor for hyperplasia
Imipramine (Tofranil)	75 mg qd	MAO inhibitors
Enuresis		
Desmopressin (DDAVP)	40 mcg qd nasal spray	Avoid overhydration
Imipramine (Tofranil)	75–100 mg qd	MAO inhibitors
Deficient Detrusor Contraction		
Bethanecol (Duvoid)	10–50 mg bid	None significant
Internal Sphincter Dyssynergia		
Terazosin (Hytrin)	1–5 mg qd	Dizziness
External Sphincter Dyssynergia		
Baclofen (Lioresal)	15–80 mg qd	Dizziness, fatigue
Cyclobenzaprine (Flexeril)	10–60 mg qd	Anticholinergics, MAO inhibitors
Analgesics		
Phenazopyridine (Pyridium)	200 mg tid	None significant

ications that affect micturition. One of the problems practitioners face on a daily basis is whether to substitute a more benign form of the class of medication being used. If there is no potential for substitution, urodynamic testing must be performed while the patient is taking the current medication regimen, and the urologist must be aware of this fact before the patient undergoes testing.

Bladder dysfunction increases the need for polypharmacy. When bladder dysfunction becomes a problem, patients usually are first treated empirically with medication. Caution must be used because even small doses of anticholinergics can greatly affect these patients. The side effects of the anticholinergic group of medications (dry mouth, constipation, nausea, dizziness) can place these high-risk patients at even higher risk for falls.

In addition to increased bladder capacity, anticholinergics may delay the call to void, making it difficult for the patient to get to the bathroom on time when at capacity.

Medications usually are the first treatment of choice for incontinence, although most medications used to treat incontinence have severe anticholinergic effects that act synergistically with the medications patients are presently taking. When starting patients on a medication regimen, the rule is "start slow, stay low." Starting slowly avoids problems with dizziness and nausea, the most common reasons for discontinuation of these medications. Increasing the dose every two weeks to maximal therapy is far better tolerated. If a patient is not getting some relief by the 8-week mark, rather than increasing the medication, another medication should be tried or urodynamic testing should be done to ensure that the original diagnosis was correct. In this case, the patient should not take any medications specifically prescribed for the bladder for at least one week before testing. Question the patient closely to determine that chronic constipation or impaction is not occurring as a result of the newly prescribed agent.

TABLE 24-4
Herbal Remedies Favored by MS Patients, Supposed Action, and Active Ingredient (if known) (20)

HERBAL REMEDY	SUPPOSED ACTION	ACTIVE INGREDIENT
Aloe	Burns, abrasions, laxative	Unknown
Bearberry	Urinary antiseptic	Arbutin, methylarbutin forms, hydroquinone in intestines
Black cohosh	Menopausal symptoms	Isoflavone
Calendula	Burns, infections, antiviral	Triterpenoids
Cascara sagrada	Laxative	Anthaquinones
Chamomile	Antispasmodic, sedative, promote urination	Chamazulen, alpha-bisabolol
Cranberry	Urinary deodorant, prevents E. coli adhesion to linings of bladder and gut	Unknown
Dong-quai	Menstrual irregularities, PMS	Unknown
Echinacea	Accelerate healing, infections, immune stimulant*	? Flavonoids, alkylamides
Siberian ginseng	Immune stimulant*, mental stimulant, fatigue	Unknown
Evening primrose	PMS, eczema, migraine	Unknown
Garlic	Reduce cholesterol, antioxidant, antibacterial, immune stimulant*	Sulfur compounds
Ginkgo biloba	Tinnitus, impotence, memory, PMS, antioxidant	Flavone, ginkgolides
Ginseng	Mental stimulant, coordination, fatigue, immune stimulant*	Ginsenosides
Goldenseal	Antibacterial, antiinflammatory for mucous membranes	Alkaloids
Psyllium	Laxative, bowel stimulant	Mucilage
Saw palmetto	Benign prostatic hyperplasia	Unknown
Senna	Laxative	Anthranoids
St. John's Wort	Depression, fatigue	? Hypericin
Valerian	Sedative, relief of muscle spasm	Unknown

*Germany's Commission E monographs recommend that patients with impaired immune system response (tuberculosis, MS, HIV infection) should not use these preparations.

The most commonly used anticholinergic medications are oxybutynin (Ditropan), Ditropan XL, and tolterodine (Detrol). Ditropan is effective but has many anticholinergic side effects. Ditropan XL is an extended-release form that is taken once a day (5–10 mg). In addition to being more convenient, it has fewer anticholinergic side effects. Detrol is a competitive muscarinic antagonist with the fewest anticholinergic side effects. The dose is 1–2 mg twice daily.

No medication is very effective for the large, hypotonic bladder. Urecholine often is tried but usually is not helpful. Clean intermittent catheterization (CIC) remains the most viable treatment option.

The dyssynergic bladder also is best treated with CIC. Alpha blockers, such as terazosin (Hytrin) or dibenzyline, may provide an added benefit. Baclofen is another medication that has been used with varying results.

A medication woefully underused in the MS population is estrogen. Women with MS frequently go through early menopause because of surgery or medication use. They may have significant changes in the vaginal mucosa related to menopause and may not realize that frequency and leaking is related to decreasing estrogen levels. They often need earlier hormonal supplementation as a result of these procedures.

TABLE 24-5

*Common Drug Classifications
that Affect Bladder Dysfunction*

Antiinfectives
Cardiovascular Agents
   Inotropes
   Antianginals
   Antihypertensives
Central Nervous System Drugs
   NSAIDs
   Narcotics
   Sedatives/hypnotics
   Anticonvulsants
   Antidepressants
   Antianxiety
   Antipsychotics
   CNS stimulants
   Antiparkinsonian agents
Autonomic System Drugs
   Cholinergics
   Anticholinergics
   Adrenergics
   Adrenergic blockers
   Skeletal muscle relaxants
   Neuromuscular blockers
Hormones
Diuretics
Spasmolytics
Alcohol

The vagina also suffers the anticholinergic effects of the medical regimen, and the tissue of the vagina becomes dry and stiff. The integrity of the vaginal vault should be assessed during examination, keeping in mind that the urethra, which is made of the same germinal tissue and is embedded in the anterior wall of the vagina, also has multiple estrogen receptors. It is hypothesized that estrogen promotes blood flow to the tissues of the vagina, improving the turgidity of the tissue and thus passive closure of the urethra. In addition to improving the mucosa, patients receiving estrogen replacement also have improved lubrication, which also improves urethral closure, surface tension, and general comfort. Well-estrogenized tissue is less prone to bacterial and yeast infections. Despite taking oral estrogen, many patients are locally deficient, and estrace cream should be added to the patient's regimen. Estrace cream can be prescribed as one quarter to one half applicator three times a week at bedtime. The vaginal vault should be inspected in four weeks, and the patient should be started on a maintenance regimen of either fingertip application to the vaginal mucosa or one fourth applicator two to three times per week at bedtime.

Patients who are cycling can also use estrogen cream but must by monitored closely for hyperplasia. If the patient has a history of breast cancer, check with the oncologist to see if the cancer was estrogen-receptive. If not, estrace cream can be used safely. Alternatively, vitamin E oil or Replens have been used successfully to promote tissue integrity.

Another option is the newly released estrogen ring (Estring). This device is inserted into the vaginal vault like a diaphragm and continually releases a low dose of estrogen for up to three months.

Another group of medications used are muscle relaxants to prevent spasticity and subsequent retention. Sometimes in the course of getting to relaxation, incontinence increases as the pelvic muscles no longer augment the internal sphincter mechanism. Patient should be advised to let the practitioner know if this occurs.

Medications that alter bowel function should be treated the same way. It is important to start any bowel regimen with a clean gut. The goal in treating chronic constipation or the tendency to impaction is to keep the patient regular and able to empty completely. Any bowel regimens that include the use of dietary fiber should be monitored closely to ensure that the patient is taking in enough fluids to promote stool softening rather than drying. A bowel diary can be useful in monitoring this situation.

Kegel Exercises

All patients should be taught how to do Kegel contractions to maintain the tone of the pelvic floor. These exercises were developed in the 1940s by Dr. Arnold Kegel to improve pelvic muscle tone after childbirth. When the examiner is performing the vaginal or rectal examination, the patient can be asked to contract, pull in, or lift the pelvic muscles around the examiner's finger. Some patients can imagine the movement needed by trying to hold back flatus. If the examiner can feel a tightening, even if is only a flicker, the patient probably will benefit from a Kegel exercise program. In addition to maintaining the tone of the pelvic muscles to prevent prolapse, exercising the muscles theoretically thickens the pelvic muscle sphincter, which assists in passive closure. Patients who know how to recruit the pelvic muscles can recruit them as needed to suppress urgency and unwanted bladder contractions in order to buy time to get to the bathroom. In addition, Kegel contractions may be used to teach patients the difference between the relaxed state and the contracted state. Patients who strengthen their pelvic muscles seem to have less trouble with spasticity and subsequent retention. It may be that patients learn how to relax the muscles when toileting, or perhaps stronger muscles are less prone to spasticity.

Determining how many Kegel exercises are appropriate to prescribe may be difficult. Fatigue of the pelvic muscles also presents a problem. If a patient can reliably reproduce three to five partial circumference contractions hold them for at least five seconds, she probably can improve her situation by just doing Kegel contractions, three to five repetitions, holding for five seconds initially and resting for 10 to 20 seconds, three times a day. The patient will gradually need to first increase the hold time to 10 seconds; when this can be done consistently, the patient should increase to 10 repetitions daily. Advise the patient that urgency should improve in three to six weeks, but leaking with exertion may take as long as 8 to 12 weeks to improve, even when the exercise program is followed faithfully. It is important that the patient understand that she should try to do several short, strong Kegel contractions and then wait 30 seconds when the urge to toilet is strong before moving off to void. Doing pelvic muscle contractions directly inhibits bladder contractions.

The patient initially should be taught to perform the Kegel exercises in a supine position and gradually begin to do them in a seated position, and later a standing position as appropriate. The practitioner should recheck how the patient is doing the exercises in one to two weeks in order to quickly correct any learning or performance errors. At this visit, after palpating the muscle during a contraction, the anus should be observed for an anal wink (tightening) during a contraction. Patients in whom the anal wink is absent have a poorer prognosis, even though a contraction can be palpated. It is best to switch these patients to electrical stimulation early in treatment before they become frustrated.

Biofeedback

Biofeedback is another modality that is useful in teaching patients to do Kegel exercises. Gross pelvic muscle electrical activity, monitored by surface electrodes attached to the perineum, can be observed on a computer screen or on a light-emitting diode (LED) device by both the practitioner and the patient. Used both in diagnosis and in teaching the patient how to either relax or contract the pelvic muscles, biofeedback is a useful tool for patients who have relatively intact sensation and good motor control. Four to five sessions over the course of three to six months usually help the patient to vastly improve muscle control. As in all exercise programs, the patient must understand that he must continue to do the exercises or he will again lose muscle function.

Pelvic Muscle Stimulation

Neuromodulation using implanted electrodes has been found to improve bladder function in patients with neu-rologic injuries (10). Although not commonly used in treatment of MS patients, pelvic muscle stimulation also seems to have a positive effect when used in this population.

A useful tool in denervation, electrical stimulation of the pelvic floor is an excellent way to decrease both urgency and leaking, as well as to strengthen the pelvic floor in patients who have difficulty isolating, identifying, or contracting the pelvic muscle. This tool (Figure 24-4) uses a small electrode that is inserted into the vaginal vault or rectum for a 5- to 30-minute daily home treatment.

The electrode, which is connected to a small battery pack, briefly (5 to 10 seconds) stimulates the pudendal nerve and the pelvic muscles directly to contract in a stronger fashion than the patient is able to do unassisted. A second channel (12 to 20 Hertz) can be used to inhibit bladder contractions and improve capacity. This treatment generally is well tolerated, but a urologist or gynecologist usually is needed to closely monitor treatment and the condition of the mucosa, because this population has such dininished sensation. Patients who have no ability to contract on their own, have difficulty relaxing the pelvic floor, or cannot isolate the pelvic muscles all benefit from this treatment. Patients who are particularly

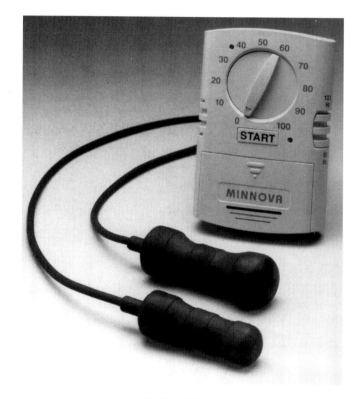

FIGURE 24-4

Electrical stimulation has been found to be useful in stress, urge, and mixed incontinence (16).

weak need to start at decreased treatment times because they may become more incontinent if the pelvic muscle is overworked. An incidental benefit often noted during treatment with pelvic stimulation is that bowel movements become regular and evacuation is more complete, possibly as a result of local stimulation.

Pessaries or Bladder Neck Prostheses

For women with weakened pelvic muscles, pessaries or bladder neck prostheses may help support the bladder neck in the proper anatomic position and occlude the urethra, much as surgery would. These intravaginal devices (Figure 24-5) may be a useful treatment for those patients who are too debilitated to undergo surgery to correct the problem. When using devices inserted into the vagina, care must be taken to improve and then keep the vagina well estrogenized to prevent erosion. Patients with pessaries or prostheses must be monitored quite frequently because of their decreased sensation. Patients who have poor manual dexterity should be fitted with a pessary rather than a prosthesis because most pessaries need to be removed for cleaning only every four to six weeks. Patients with these devices should be cautioned to report discomfort or difficulty voiding or having a bowel movement. Often, however, bowel movements improve because the posterior wall is supported during defecation. Again, these devices should be inserted and maintained by a specialist.

Male Management Devices

Men who need an occlusive device still must rely on a penile clamp. Newer models made of flexible material are a safe alternative to diapers if the patient is taught to release the clamp every two hours and to closely monitor the skin of the penis.

The condom catheter is an option available to male patients. Many varieties are available in addition to the typical Texas catheter. There are condoms that open so the patient may catheterize intermittently, models for retracted penises, and models that use a pressure plate but no adhesive to secure the catheter. One-piece condom catheters and oversized reservoirs have recently become available. The reservoir empties with a valve and the entire system is supported by oversized jockey shorts.

Catheters

Catheterization usually is employed when the patient begins to have retention, when there is a concern about reflux, when there is refractory urgency, when the patient is unable to do ISC, when the bladder capacity is so small that ISC is impractical, when the potential for skin prob-

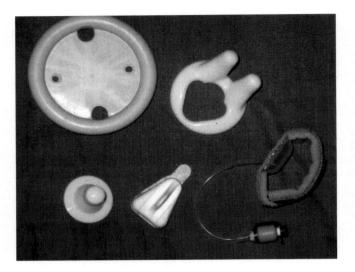

FIGURE 24-5

Devices used to treat urinary incontinence. *Clockwise from top:* right-Introl bladder neck prosthesis, Cook continence cuff, Impress urethral patch, Capsure urethral cap, and Milex ring pessary with support.

lems exists, or when transferring to the toilet becomes unsafe. Before deciding on catheterization, be certain that the patient's anticholinergic regimen is not putting him into retention. Teach your patient how to perform a Credé maneuver, and then check for residual volume in a week or two.

If catheterization is deemed to be necessary, the preferred method is to teach a clean intermittent technique. Patients who have moderate residual (100 to 200 cc's), no history of UTI, and little worry about reflux initially should be taught to catheterize before bedtime in order to empty the bladder completely and promote a better night's sleep. After the patient feels comfortable with the technique and it has been shown that he has decreased urgency and leaking, add the daytime catheterizations, usually moving to a schedule of three to four times a day, depending on the patient's comfort and ability. Ideally, catheterizations should be based on residual volumes and intervesical pressures.

If no urodynamics are planned, the patient should be emptying no more than 500 cc's at one time and the timing should be adjusted accordingly. If urodynamics are used to determine how often the patient should be catheterized, the volume at which point the intervesical pressure rises above 30 cm/H_2O, or when the patient leaks, should be the maximum volume emptied when catheterized. If these volumes are so small that it becomes impractical to catheterize that often, the patient may be put into complete retention by the use of anticholinergic medication, or an indwelling catheter may be inserted.

Patients with indwelling catheters should be monitored closely because UTIs have a tendency to make symptoms of MS flare up. It is prudent to start the patient on a prophylactic dose of suppressive medication, although it usually is not necessary to use anticholinergic medication if the catheter is properly maintained, changed regularly, and of the proper size. The rule of thumb in picking a catheter is to use the smallest size balloon and the smallest diameter possible. A 5 cc balloon with a 16 French catheter generally is adequate. A silicone-based catheter tends to cause less skin irritation, decrease the potential for latex allergy, and have less encrustation buildup than a latex-based catheter. Because such patients generally have little or no potential for rehabilitation, a simple letter to the third-party payer generally will suffice to allow the difference in cost by third-party payers.

The patient must be taught aseptic technique and periodic review should be made regarding hookup to the night bag from the leg bag. The patient should clean both bags daily and leave them to air-dry before reattaching. A 10 percent bleach solution is adequate for cleaning purposes and is easily made at home with common materials (11). With the advent of one-way valves on most leg bags, it is possible for the patient to keep the leg bag on at night, although he probably will need to empty the bag at least once during the night. Belly bags are available for patients who use a wheelchair. The leg bag and catheter should be changed monthly, more frequently if necessary. All patients should be provided with a fixator strap to prevent tension on the catheter.

Most patients with MS do not have the manual dexterity to open a leg bag valve that twists, and they tend to catch flip valves in their clothes, so it is prudent to use a T-tap type of bag. A smaller leg bag is easier to manage and causes the patient to empty the bag more frequently, thus preventing a nidus for infection.

A patient who has an indwelling catheter requires scrupulous perineal care, particularly after bowel movements, and the patient must have the understanding and the resources to make this possible.

Many patients have poor manual dexterity, significant lower extremity spasticity, and recurrent UTIs as a result of poor hygiene or the inability to manage an indwelling catheter because of mobility problems but still need continuous decompression of the bladder or the convenience of an indwelling catheter because of severe frequency. These patients may benefit from a suprapubic tube. A simple stab wound creates the fistula from the skin to the bladder. This usually can be done under twilight sedation using a cystoscope, which allows even marginal surgical candidates to be managed safely. Although the risk of stone formation and infection remains the same and there is the additional risk of infection of the operative site, the suprapubic tube allows the patient far more convenience in self-management. The suprapubic tube can be clamped and drained or connected to continuous drainage as needed. Recovery time is minimal and management is the same as for an indwelling catheter.

Two other options are used in cases of severe bladder dysfunction. Both procedures constitute major surgery and require moderately good health and a tertiary setting for performing the procedure. Diversions (either continent or incontinent) may be done in cases of severe frequency and small bladder capacity, thereby avoiding the bladder entirely. In the case of an incontinent diversion, the patient or family must be willing to manage a stoma and bag, whereas with a continent diversion they must be willing to perform intermittent catheterization on a regular basis.

Patients in retention who have no problems with a hyperactive or hypertrophied bladder wall may benefit from a Mitrofanoff procedure, in which the umbilicus is used as a stoma through which the patient can catheterize. To create the fistula, the appendix (preferably) or a tubular piece of bowel is tunneled through the bladder wall and connected to the base of the bladder while the other end is connected to the umbilicus. Once the fistula has healed, the patient is able to catheterize through the umbilicus and no one need know that they have an alternate way to empty the bladder. This procedure has been used successfully in pediatric myelodysplasia patients and is now being adapted for adults.

Surgical Procedures

As a rule, patients with MS are poor surgical candidates for bladder suspensions. Despite the newer needle techniques and collagen injection that require a very short hospitalization and offer few problems during recovery, the concern remains whether a poorly working bladder will compensate for increased intraurethral pressure during voiding. Nonetheless, patients who have demonstrated through urodynamics to be good surgical candidates and have support deficits should be given the opportunity for repair. An accurate voiding study absolutely must be performed and preferably should be repeated before advancing to this step.

Management Options

Diapers tend to be the focus of most management programs. In helping patients choose diapers, look for brands that do not make noise when the patient walks, provide enough material to cover the entire perineal area, and have a hydrocolloid filling so that the pad or diaper can absorb the entire contents of the bladder if necessary. There are many manufacturers of excellent products that

TABLE 24-6
Algorithm for Treatment of Bladder Dysfunction

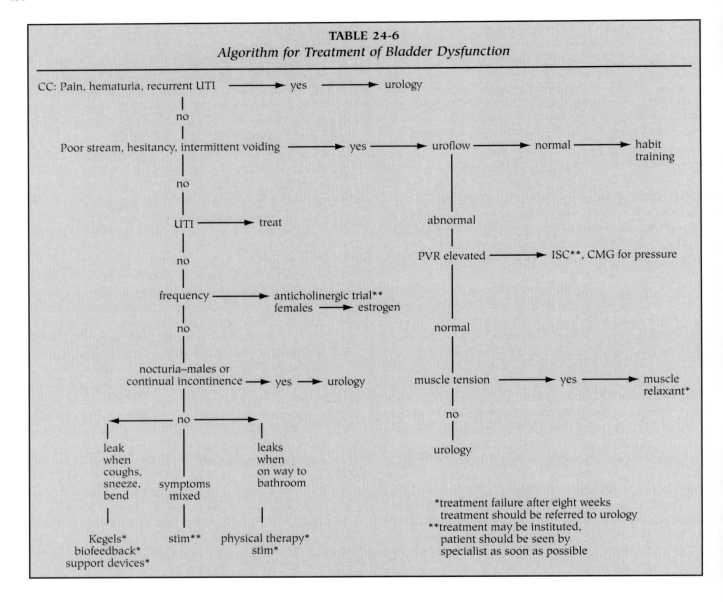

often have thin profiles but good absorbency. There also are many washable products with charcoal filters and pad-and-pant systems. A subscription to a useful newsletter and a manufacturer index with products and contact phone numbers is available through the National Foundation for Continence (1-800-BLADDER). Many mail order distributors also offer trial packs containing a range of products available to try for little or no fee.

Several new products are available for women with mild incontinence who might need slight protection. These external devices are placed over the urethra to occlude the urethral meatus and adhere by suction. They are intended for women who leak just a few drops of urine.

The urethral plug is another management option that may work for patients who have good dexterity, reasonable sensation, and good bladder compliance without

hyperactivity. This soft silicone plug is inserted into the urethra, where it dwells until the patient needs to void, at which time the patient removes it. This device is particularly useful for patients who wish to go out for an extended period and are worried about leaking. However, at present, its cost is prohibitive for use on a daily basis.

Skin care must be a major focus of teaching for incontinent patients. Patients need to learn how to recognize a yeast infection, an ammonia burn, and diaper rash, and to know what products to use when they occur. One-step cleansers are useful for the patient with dexterity problems or difficulty. However, plain water works well to prevent an ammonia smell and to prevent the skin from becoming overly dry. Patients should be advised to use a zinc-based product or a product with vitamins A and D to protect their skin between incontinent episodes. Products formulated for babies work well and are affordable. Patients can self-treat a yeast infection with an over-the-counter antifungal ointment, with the understanding that clearing should occur in two weeks. If the patient is prone to yeast infections, she should expose the perineal area to air several times a day if possible.

References

1. National Institutes of Health Consensus Development Conference Statement. *Urinary Incontinence in Adults.* U.S. Department of Health and Human Services, 1988; 7:1–11.

2. Snyder JA, Lipsitz DU. Evaluation of female urinary incontinence. *Urol Clin North Am* 1991; 18:187–209.

3. Badlani GH. Urologic implications of MS, diabetes, and Parkinson's disease lecture. Fourth National Multi-Specialty Nursing Conference on Urinary Incontinence, Orlando, Florida, 1998.

4. Gray M. *Genitourinary disorders.* St. Louis: Mosby–Year Book, 1992.

5. Elbadawi A. Pathology and pathophysiology of detrusor in incontinence. *Urol Clin North Am* 1995; 22:499–512.

6. Wein AJ. Practical uropharmacology. *Urol Clin North Am* 1991; 18:269–281.

7. Fantl JA, Newman DK, Colling J, et al. *Managing acute and chronic urinary incontinence. Clinical practice guideline.* Quick Reference Guide for Clinicians, No. 2, 1996 update. Rockville, MD: U.S. Department of Health and Human Services, Public Health Service, Agency for Health Care Policy and Research. AHCPR Pub. No. 96-0686. March 1996.

8. McGuire EJ, Gudziak MR. *Handbook of urodynamic testing.* Covington: Bard Urological Division, 1994.

9. Rivas DA, Chancellor MB. Neurogenic vesical dysfunction. *Urol Clin North Am* 1995; 22:579590.

10. Herman H, Shelly E. Gynecological physical therapy seminar. Memorial; Hospital West Fitness and Rehabilitation Center, November 10–12, 1995, Pembroke Pines, Florida.

11. Klutke JJ, Bergman A. Hormonal influence on the urinary tract. *Urol Clin North Am* 1995; 22: 629–639.

12. Creasey GH. Electrical stimulation of sacral roots for micturition after spinal cord injury. *Urol Clin North Am* 1993; 20:505–515.

13. Ishigooka M, Hashimoto T, Sasagawa I, Nakada T, Handa Y. Electrical pelvic floor stimulation by percutaneous implantable electrode. *Br J Urol* 1994; 74:191–194.

14. Dijkema HE, Weil EHJ, Mijs PT, Janknegt RA. Neuromodulation of sacral nerves for incontinence and voiding dysfunction. *Eur Urol* 1993; 24:72–76.

15. McCash Dille C, Kirchhoff KT. Decontamination of vinyl urinary drainage bags with bleach. *Rehab Nurs* 1993; 18:292–295.

16. Sand PK, Richardson DA, Staskin DR, et al. Pelvic floor electrical stimulation in the treatment of genuine stress incontinence: A multicenter, placebo-controlled trial. *Am J Obstet Gynecol* 1995; 175:72–79.

17. Schapiro RT, Baumhefner RW, Tourtellotte WW. Multiple sclerosis: A clinical viewpoint to management. In: *Multiple sclerosis: Clinical and pathogenetic basis.* London: Chapman and Hall, 1997.

18. Chohan N. *Nursing drug handbook.* Springhouse, PA: Springhouse Corp., 1998.

19. Wein AJ. Pharmacology of incontinence. *Urol Clin North Am* 1995; 22:557–575.

20. Foster S. *Herbs for your health.* Loveland: Interweave Press, 1996.

25 Bowel Disturbance

Marie A. Namey, RN, MSN, and June Halper, MSN, ANP, FAAN

Normal bowel function is an integral part of the digestive process and is essential to adequate nutrition. It ensures a continuous supply of water, electrolytes, and nutrients to the body through digestion and absorption. Autoregulatory processes keep food moving at an appropriate pace. The end result of digestion is defecation, a function that requires a complex integration of voluntary and involuntary mechanisms. Bowel function depends on the secretion of enzymes and production of mucus, innervation of smooth muscle, tonic contractions, and peristalsis. This primarily involuntary process is under both intrinsic and extrinsic neural control. In patients with a neurologic disease such as multiple sclerosis (MS), improving bowel function requires careful planning, medical and nursing management, education, changes in lifestyle, and patient and family compliance. Bowel dysfunction in MS can include incontinence (involuntary bowel), constipation, diarrhea, flatulence, fecal impaction, and ileus.

Estimates of bowel dysfunction in MS patients range from 52 percent (Chia et al.) to 68 percent (Hinds et al.) The prevalence of bowel dysfunction is higher in patients with MS than in the general population. According to Chia and coworkers, bowel symptoms in MS did not correlate with the pattern of urinary disturbance, the duration of MS, or disability. In practice, however, bowel dysfunction is a common symptom related to bladder disturbance.

NORMAL BOWEL FUNCTION

The lower bowel acts under voluntary control and functions to store and eliminate feces. Inability to store fecal matter causes problems with involuntary bowel or incontinence; inability to eliminate causes constipation.

The intestines include the digestive tube that passes from the stomach to the anus. The bowel consists of three separate parts—the ileum, the cecum, and the colon. The ileum is the third portion of the small intestine; it is approximately 12 feet long and extends from the jejunum to the ileocecal opening. Almost all processes of food digestion and absorption are completed in the small intestine. The intestine promotes active absorption of water and sodium and triggers secretion of mucus, potassium, and bicarbonate for stool formation. The cecum is approximately 6 centimeters (cm) in depth and lies below the terminal ileum, forming the first part of the large intestine. The colon is the division of the large intestine; it extends from the cecum to the rectum. The most important functions of the colon are the reabsorption of fluid and electrolytes and serving as a storage organ so that defecation can occur at an acceptable time. Fecal elimination is affected by a number of interrelated factors, including peristaltic function, anorectal sensory awareness, anal sphincter function, and abdominal muscle function.

The rectum is the 12-cm segment of large bowel between the sigmoid colon and the anal canal. It begins with the third segment of the sacrum and is concave as it follows the slope of the sacrum to the urogenital diaphragm. Its caudal end turns sharply posteriorly at the perineal flexure to open onto the perineum. As a rule, the rectum does not contain feces except during defecation. The anal canal comprises the last 3 centimeters of the digestive tube. Its mucosa forms the columns of Morgagni. The ends of the columns join one another near the anal orifice and create anal valves with anal sinuses between them. Striated muscle (puborectal, puboccygeal, iliococcygeal, and coccygeal) in the anal canal and pelvic floor provides a slinglike support to the posterior rectal wall and causes sphincter-like action between the rectum and the anus, thus maintaining continence.

INFLUENCE OF THE NERVOUS SYSTEM ON FECAL CONTINENCE

Neurogenic bowel results from interruption of neural pathways that supply the rectum, external sphincter, and accessory muscles for defecation. (Toth, 1988). The cause of bowel dysfunction in MS and the role of the spinal cord function are unclear. Internal and external anal sphincters are innervated by sacral roots 2, 3, and 4. The internal sphincter is supplied by motor fibers from the hypogastric nerve and the parasympathetic system. With rectal distention, reflex relaxation of the internal sphincter occurs and external sphincter tone increases to prevent bowel emptying. The afferent impulses stimulate cerebral recognition of anal contents and the need to empty stool or defecate at a desired or planned time. Slow colonic transit and/or abnormal rectal function result in constipation. Because of weakened abdominal muscles, there is more difficulty "bearing down" strongly enough to evacuate stool. Decreased activity related to difficulty ambulating, fatigue, or a sedentary lifestyle may contribute to slow bowel function.

Another indirect influence of MS on bowel function may contribute to slow bowel. Fecal continence relies on normal functioning of the anal sphincters and puborectalis muscles, intact rectal sensation, a compliant rectal reservoir, and motivation to maintain bowel control. Absent or decreased rectal sensation of rectal filling, poor voluntary contraction of the anal sphincte and/or pelvic floor, and reduced rectal compliance result in involuntary bowel. Gastrointestinal symptoms are common in patients with MS. Patients with MS report delayed gastric emptying, constipation, and fecal incontinence.

Although constipation is the most frequently reported symptom, involuntary bowel is the most distressing, and the patient may be reluctant and embarrassed to report this symptom.

According to Hinds and colleagues, in a study of 280 patients with MS surveyed to determine bowel dysfunction, 43 percent of the patients reported constipation, 51 percent of patients reported involuntary bowel once in the past three months, and 25 percent of the sample reported involuntary bowel once a week or more frequently. Additionally, bowel dysfunction was determined to be a source of considerable ongoing social concern in people with MS and their families. Constipation may be experienced by most people during their lifetime. This symptom has different subjective meanings to different people.

Constipation has been defined as less than or equal to two bowel movements per week, or the need for stimulation (digitally or with the use of laxatives, enemas, or suppositories) more often than once per week. Generally, constipation is defined as "a condition in which bowel movements are infrequent or incomplete" (*Stedman's Medical Dictionary,* 24th edition). Constipation also has been described as a pattern of elimination characterized by hard, dry stool causing straining or painful defecation and resulting in a delay of passage of food residue. Many individuals are under the mistaken impression that their bowels should move once per day, and they report "constipation" with less frequent bowel movements.

Constipation may result from overuse of laxatives, immobility, poor dietary habits, fluid restriction, and inconsistent toileting patterns. In MS patients, constipation may be related to weakened abdominal muscles, which affect expulsion of feces; inability to transfer to and from a commode; bladder dysfunction, specifically with urinary retention; and medications. Characteristics of constipation may be specific or vague (Table 25-1).

Medications that can cause and increase constipation may include analgesics, anticholinergics, anticonvulsants, antidepressants, diuretics, psychotherapeutics, iron, opiates, and muscle relaxants (Table 25-2).

Diarrhea (loose, liquid stools) and abnormally frequent discharge of fluid fecal matter from the bowel occurs secondary to fecal impaction, diet or irritating foods, inflammation or irritation of the bowel, stress or anxiety, medications, and overuse of laxatives or stool softeners. Diarrhea may result from a gastrointestinal influenza or other medical conditions such as Crohn's disease, diverticulitis, or colitis. Dietary intolerance is a common cause of diarrhea. Common dietary offenders include milk products and chocolate. Diarrhea may be accompanied by urgency, cramping, abdominal pain, increased bowel sounds, or increase in volume of stools.

In MS, involuntary bowel or fecal incontinence is a result of interruption in the neural pathways and impaired

---

TABLE 25-1
Symptoms Related to Constipation

No stool	Distended abdomen
Decreased bowel movements	Palpable mass
(Fewer than two per week)	Headache
Hard, formed stools	Anorexia
Severe flatus	Nausea and/or vomiting
Feeling of rectal fullness	Diarrhea related to fecal impaction
Decreased bowel sounds	Increased fatigue

---

cortical awareness of urge to defecate, characterized by urgency and involuntary stools. Defecation is sudden, with or without urgency. A patient also may experience partial or total sensory loss in the perineum and rectum. (Oozing of stool is not the cause of bowel incontinence but rather evidence of bowel incontinence.)

Other nonneurologic factors contribute to neurogenic bowel conditions. Lack of exercise arising from immobility, inadequate fluid intake, (less than 1½ to 2 quarts per day), inadequate dietary fiber (less than 20 grams per day), and effects of medication contribute to constipation. Diarrhea may result from gastrointestinal influenza, dietary irritants, or other gastrointestinal disorders. Involuntary bowel may result from decreased mobility and inability to get to toilet facilities in an adequate amount of time.

ASSESSMENT OF BOWEL FUNCTION

A thorough history of bowel habits can be obtained by having the patient complete a questionnaire before the visit or asking the patient about bowel function during the visit. Questions to ask include use of medications that influence bowel activity, including diuretics, antacids, nonsteroidal and antiinflammatory agents, anticholinergics, antidepressants, antibiotics, or laxatives and enemas. Include in the continence history the presence or absence of the awareness of the need to defecate and the frequency and quality of stool, including color and consistency.

Fluid and diet history should include questions about the quantity of daily fluid intake and the type of fluid ingested. A review of daily intake of fiber (bulk) can be obtained by asking specific questions about what the

---

TABLE 25-2
Medications That Affect Constipation

DRUG CLASS	MEDICATION
Antacids	Aluminum hydroxide
	Calcium carbonate
Anticholinergics	Oxybutynin
	Tolterodine tartrate
Antidepressants	Tricyclics
	Lithium
Antihypertensives and antiarrhymics	Calcium antagonists (especially Verapamil)
Metals	Bismuth
	Iron
	Heavy metals
Narcotic analgesics	Codeine
	Morphine
NSAIDs	Ibuprofen
	Diclofenac
Sympathomimetics	Pseudoephedrine

Adapted from Adyad A, Murad F. Constipation in the elderly: Diagnosis and management strategies. *Geriatrics* 1996; 51:28–36.

TABLE 25-3
Assessment of Bowel Function

Muscle tone and strength	Environment
Cognitive and communication abilities	Personal assistance
Ability to chew and swallow	Medications
Past bowel history	Bladder management
Eating habits	Patient's perception of the problem
Motor skills and degree of independence	

---

patient eats for meals and snacks, focusing on the fiber content of the foods ingested.

Objective assessment (Table 25-3) includes physical examination of the abdomen, which should include:

1. Auscultation of bowel sounds for the presence or absence of hypermotility or hypomotility
2. Palpation for distension, tenderness, and masses
3. Percussion of the abdomen to determine distension and presence or absence of stool

Fecal impaction, internal and external sphincter tone, and internal and external hemorrhoids are determined by rectal examination.

Assessment of the patient's functional ability to ambulate and use the bathroom, a commode, a chair, or assistive devices, and to remove clothing is important.

INTERVENTIONS

The goals of a bowel training program include (1) normalizing stool consistency; (2) establishing a regular pattern for defecation; (3) stimulating rectal emptying on a routine basis before the rectum becomes full enough to override anal sphincter resistance and empty involuntarily; (4) avoiding complications of diarrhea, constipation, or incontinence; and (5) improving the patient's quality of life.

Inadequate fluid intake and/or inadequate fiber intake often results in constipation. Constipation should be treated first by nonpharmacologic interventions. Educating the patient about bowel function and the roles of fluid, fiber, and exercise is the first step in intervention. Other interventions include increasing fluid intake to 1 1/2 to 2 quarts per day and monitoring intake and output. Daily bulk and fiber in the diet should total 20 grams of fiber. Because fiber holds fluid, stools tend to be softer and bulkier, which aids transit time. Education regarding foods that are high in fiber is an important aspect of intervention. The best sources of fiber include cereals, fruits, and vegetables. Simply by adding one third of a cup of bran cereal per day can add up to 10 additional grams of daily fiber in a person's diet and improve bowel function (Table 25-4).

Establishing a regular pattern of bowel elimination is a strategy to improve bowel habits that often is overlooked. The urge to have a bowel movement—the gastrocolic reflex—is strongest 20 to 30 minutes after consuming a warm beverage or meal. Attempts to defecate should be encouraged with this urge. Sitting in an upright position with the feet on the floor or on a stool promotes rectal emptying. Regaining regularity in bowel habits is a process that may take three to four weeks or longer.

TABLE 25-4
High-Fiber Foods

TYPE	AMOUNT	GRAMS OF DIETARY FIBER PER SERVING
Fiber One cereal	1/3 cup	12
All Bran cereal	1/3 cup	9
Beans (baked, kidney, lima, navy)	1/2 cup	8.5–10
Peas (canned)	1/2 cup	6.0
Raspberries	1/2 cup	4.6
Broccoli	1/2 cup	3.5
Corn	2/3 cup	4.2
Figs	2	7.4

TABLE 25-5
Medications to Assist in Bowel Elimination

MEDICATION	ACTION	SIDE EFFECTS	COMMENTS AND CONTRAINDICATIONS
Bulk-Forming Agents Karaya Methylcellulose (Citrucel); Hydrolose Psyllium Metamucil; Konsyl; Modance Bulk; Effersyllium Perdium, Naturacil	Absorbs water in gastrointestinal tract to soften stool and increase stool size.	May increase flatus for 1 to 2 weeks Abdominal cramping Obstruction with inadequate fluid intake	Effect in 6–8 hours May be unpalatable; bolus formation with inadequate fluid intake
Fecal Softeners Dioctyl sodium sulfosuccina Dioctyl calcium sulfosuccinate Colace; DDS Chromular Syrup	Surface-active agent that allows water to penetrate stool		No habit forming Works well in combination with bisacodyl suppository for patients with sensory and motor deficits Place suppository against rectal wall
Saline Catharatics Magnesium hydroxide Magnesium citrate Epsom salts Lactulose Miralax	Retains water in small bowel and increases fluid in colon Osmotic catharsis	Excessive absorption of medications in bowel; may be difficult to return bowel function to normal if used regularly	Empty the bowel in 2–6 hours Unpleasant effects; effective in patients receiving chemotherapy or patients with narcotic-induced constipation, when other interventions are not effective
Stimulant Cathartics Bisacodyl (Dulcolax) Senna Cascara Ex-lax Feen-A-Mint	Stimulates parasympathetic reflexes to produce peristalsis	Irritating to rectum; electrolyte imbalance; myenteric plexius degeneration with prolonged use	Stool must be present in rectum Habit forming; effective for upper motor neuron lesions; must not be used with alkaline agents (antacids)
Castor Oil		Emulsified castor oil turns alkaline urine pink	Not a replacement for diet and bulk formers
Suppositories (rectal stimulants) Glycerine Dulcolax Theravac SB (mini enema)	Localized mechanical stimulation and lubrication		Place suppository along rectal wall. Effect within 15 mins–1 hour
Enemas Mineral Oil Enema Fleets Enema		May result in dependency	Loss of fluids and electrolytes

The use of stool softeners or bulk-formers with adequate fluids and food intake may help establish a bowel routine (Table 25-5). Bulk-formers, such as Metamucil, Citrucel, Perdiem, Naturacil, and FiberCon, are taken six to eight hours before expected emptying. Stool softeners can be helpful to draw increased amounts of water from body tissues into the bowel, thereby decreasing the hardness of stool and facilitating elimination. Stool softeners usually act within 24 to 48 hours, and consistent use is recommended to achieve the most benefit. Commonly used stool softeners include Colace, Surfak, Chronulac Syrup, and Correctol syrup. Stool softeners and bulking agents are not habit forming.

Oral stimulants provide a chemical irritant to the bowel, which increases bowel activity and aids in the passage of stool. Oral stimulants can be purchased over the counter, although some products have the potential to become habit forming. These include harsher laxatives such as Ex-Lax, Feen-a-Mint, Correctol, Dulcolax tablets, and castor oil. The following medications induce bowel movements gently, usually overnight, or within 8 to 12 hours, and are milder: Pericolace, Modane, Peridiem, and Milk of Magnesia.

Rectal stimulants or suppositories provide not only chemical stimulation but also localized mechanical stimulation and lubrication to promote elimination of stool. Rectal stimulants may be used on an as-needed basis in conjunction with other bulk-forming agents or oral stimulants. The patient should be instructed to insert the suppository along the anal wall. Suppositories usually act within 15 minutes to one hour.

A glycerin suppository provides local stimulation and lubricant for the passage of stool; it contains no active medication. Dulcolax suppositories, however, contain medication that is absorbed by the lining of the large bowel, which stimulates a strong, involuntary, wavelike movement that facilitates elimination of stool. The use of a small enema (Therevac mini enema) has gained popularity for relief of constipation.

The use of enemas should be avoided if at all possible. The bowel will become dependent if enemas are routinely used to stimulate the elimination of stool. However, enemas are to be used only when nothing else works.

Fecal impaction is a complication of chronic constipation and the inability to empty the bowel. Manual digital disimpaction is the immediate treatment for this condition. An episode of fecal impaction is an indication for the need of an aggressive bowel program.

MANAGEMENT OF INCONTINENCE RELATED TO NEUROGENIC BOWEL

Adequate bulk and fiber intake is important for maintaining stool consistency. Patients should be instructed to avoid overly spicy and gas-forming foods such as broccoli, cauliflower, seeded fruits and vegetables, or any food that previously has caused problems for the patient.

Planned times for bowel evacuation and the use of suppositories to stimulate rectal emptying will allow for more bowel control. Establishing a daily routine can help eliminate involuntary bowel accidents. Encourage the patient to sit on the toilet or commode chair 25 to 30 minutes after consuming a hot beverage, such as the morning coffee, or a warm meal. The patient should follow these recommendations:

- Sit comfortably on the toilet for approximately 10 minutes and try to "bear down."
- Rocking back and forth on the toilet and massaging abdomen can promote bowel activity.
- If the bowels do not move within 10 minutes, leave the bathroom and try again later when another "urge" is present.

EXPECTED OUTCOMES

Within three to four weeks of following the interventions, reasonable patient outcomes include:
1. Predictable, regular bowel evacuation
2. Decrease in episodes of constipation or involuntary bowel
3. Formed stool
4. Avoidance of prescription drugs, strong laxatives, or enemas
5. Patient and family awareness of the need for adequate nutrition, hydration, and actively maintaining a bowel program and preventing constipation or decreasing episodes of involuntary bowel
6. Patient and family awareness of early signs of bowel dysfunction; asking for assistance or initiating acceptable intervention

SUMMARY

Bowel training programs restore normal bowel function or fecal continence to patients with MS.

As health care providers, we must recognize that bowel management is a dynamic process in the provision of care for people with MS. Whereas symptoms of altered elimination may improve after initial interventions in other diseases, altered elimination may occur secondarily as a result of increased disease activity, treatments, or interventions. Clinicians must educate and support patients and individualize and modify bowel programs.

References

1. Adyad A. Murad F. Constipation in the elderly: Diagnosis and management strategies. *Geriatrics* 1996; 51:28–36.
2. Bakke A, Myhr K, Gronning M, Nyland H. (1996). Bladder, bowel and sexual dysfunction in patients with multiple sclerosis-a cohort study. *Scand J Urol Nephrol* 1996; 179 (Suppl):61–66

3. Caruana B, Wald A, Hinds J, Eidelman B. Anorectal sensory and motor function in neurogenic fecal incontinence: Comparison between multiple sclerosis and diabetes mellitus. *Gastroenterology* 1991; 100 (2):465–470.

4. Chia Y, Fowler C, Kamm M, et al. Prevalence of bowel dysfunction in patients with multiple sclerosis and bladder dysfunction. *J Neurol* 1995; 242(2):105–108.

5. Dittmar S (ed.). *Rehabilitation nursing process and application.* St. Louis: Mosby 1989:62–74.

6. Dougherty D. (ed.). *Urinary and fecal incontinence: Nursing management.* St. Louis: Mosby, 1991.

7. Fowler C, Henry M. Gastrointestinal dysfunction in multiple sclerosis. *Semin Neurol* 1996; 16(3):277–279.

8. Glick M, Meshkinpour H, Haldeman S, et al. Clinic dysfunction in multiple sclerosis. *Gastroenterlogy* 1982; 1002–1007.

9. Halper J, Holland N. (eds.). *Comprehensive nursing care in multiple sclerosis.* New York: Demos Vermande, 1997:45–67.

10. Hinds JM, Wald A. Colonic and anorectal dysfunction associated with multiple sclerosis. *Am J Gastroenterol* 1989; 84 (6):587–595.

11. Hinds J, Eidelman B, Wald A. Prevalence of bowel dysfunction in multiple sclerosis. *Gastroenterology* 1990; 98:1538–1542.

12. McCourt A. *The specialty practice of rehabilitation nursing: A core curriculum.* 3rd edition. Skokie, IL: Rehabilitation Nursing Foundation, 1993:94–107.

13. Toth L, Mitchell PH. *Alterations in bowel elimination.* Norwalk, CT: . Appleton and Lange, 1988.

14. Yakabowich M. Prescribe with care: The role of laxatives in the treatment of constipation. *J Gerontol Nurs* 1990; 16(7):4–11.

26 Sexual Dysfunction

Audrey Sorgen Saunders, M.A., and Mindy Lipson Aisen, M.D.

The physical, cognitive, and emotional symptoms of multiple sclerosis (MS) often affect the perception, definition, and expression of sexuality. It is important for all clinicians who are involved in the care of individuals with MS to be aware of the potential for sexual difficulties and the treatment options for sexual dysfunction. The development of specialized programs staffed by personnel trained to manage the complications of MS has substantially improved functional independence and long-term survival expectations. Advances in medical and surgical treatments for neurogenic sexual and reproductive dysfunction may also enhance quality of life. Caregivers must strive to maintain a current knowledge base and cultivate an atmosphere of open dialogue if they are to adequately serve their patients.

The first part of this chapter discusses the prevalence of sexual dysfunction in MS and reviews an established conceptual model of sexual dysfunction (1,2). The second part focuses on diagnostic and therapeutic techniques.

INCIDENCE AND PREVALENCE OF SEXUAL DYSFUNCTION

Epidemiologic studies of the incidence of sexual difficulty in males with MS report rates ranging from 7 percent (3) to 91 percent (4,5). Up to 80 percent of men with MS reported that the frequency of sexual intercourse had decreased or ceased after the onset of MS (4,5). In the same survey, 65 percent of patients indicated that sexual satisfaction had decreased, and 56 percent reported that libido had substantially declined. A more recent survey found that 37 percent of men with MS had some sexual difficulty, and 24 percent reported impotence (6). Mattson and colleagues (7) found a higher incidence of sexual difficulties in their survey of men with MS. Although 76 percent of their sample reported a decline in the frequency of sexual intercourse since diagnosis, 44 percent were sexually satisfied and 59 percent believed they sexually satisfied their partners.

The limited number of investigations that have examined the prevalence of sexual dysfunction in females with MS indicate rates ranging from 45 percent (7) to 80 percent (8). A survey of minimally disabled women under the age of 50 found that 74 percent experienced sexual difficulties compared with 19 percent in a control group of women without MS. Studies by Stenager and colleagues (9) and Valleroy and Kraft (10) found that 56 percent of their female participants reported negative changes in sexual functioning. Another study reported that 80 percent had at least one sexual problem, although 54 percent only slightly concerned about their sexual difficulty (8).

Although one third of the male and female participants in the study of McCabe and colleagues (8) believed that MS had no effect or only a minor impact on sexuality, two thirds reported reduced frequency of sexual activity, and 58 percent believed that their range of sexual activities had become more restricted since developing MS. In addition, 43 percent were somewhat or very concerned about their sexual difficulties, and 63 percent thought their sexual problems were somewhat or very important in the influence they had on their intimate relationships.

These studies show that sexual difficulties are often present in people with MS and may have a significant impact on sexual satisfaction and the overall quality of intimate relationships.

SEXUAL DYSFUNCTION: A CONCEPTUAL MODEL

Foley has developed a conceptual model of sexual dysfunction in MS consisting of primary, secondary, and tertiary sexual dysfunction (1,2). The examination of sexual difficulties using this model may augment the understanding of MS-related sexual dysfunction in a number of ways. Categorizing sexual symptoms within the conceptual model may help to identify and clarify specific symptoms, thereby providing a more manageable database for understanding and describing the nature of sexual dysfunction. This model also may aid in elucidating the cause of the problem, allowing the person with MS to focus on the specific sexual difficulty rather than generalizing sexual dysfunction into other domains. For example, a woman who is experiencing decreased vaginal lubrication may erroneously attribute her difficulty to a diminished attraction to her partner rather than to a direct consequence of MS lesions. Classifying sexual dysfunction as primary, secondary, or tertiary may aid in developing a protocol for treatment and highlighting instances in which a referral to another discipline is appropriate.

PRIMARY SEXUAL DYSFUNCTION

Primary sexual dysfunction stems from MS-related neurologic impairments that directly affect the sexual response. Empirically, erectile dysfunction is the most common primary sexual dysfunction reported by men (8–10). Men also report impaired genital sensation, decreased sexual interest or desire, and orgasmic difficulties (including premature, retarded, or retrograde ejaculation) and decreased frequency or force of ejaculation.

The most common primary sexual difficulties reported by women with MS include lack of sexual interest or desire, altered genital sensation (including numbness, pain, burning, discomfort, or hypersensitivity), decreased frequency or intensity of orgasm, and lack of vaginal lubrication (4,5,7,8,10).

Lesions in areas of the central nervous system associated with sexual response may alter the pathways involved in libido, genital sensation, vasocongestion, myotonia, and ejaculation or orgasm.

NEUROANATOMY AND PHYSIOLOGY

Female

The organs of female reproductive function are supplied by spinal segments T10–S4. Sympathetics arising from T10–T11 innervate the ovaries and smooth muscle of the fallopian tubes and uterus. Parasympathetics (S2–4) also supply the fallopian tubes and vagina. Afferent information from the cervix and tubal region is transmitted to T11–12 segments through pelvic nerves.

Sexual responses require transmission in somatic, afferent, parasympathetic, and sympathetic nervous systems (11). Physiologic arousal may be initiated by descending psychic influences or by tactile stimulation of the clitoris, which is innervated by afferent fibers of the pudendal nerve (S2–4). The physiology of sexual responses involves virtually the entire body, not simply the genital region; women experience myotonia and venous vasocongestion throughout the trunk, particularly in the breasts and chest wall.

Parasympathetic efferents (S2–4, which are responsible for reflex clitoral erection) are activated by descending influences and afferent sacral synapses. Vaginal lubrication occurs as the result of parsasympathetically activated Bartholin's gland secretions and by transudation of fluid across the engorged vaginal wall. Local synapses in the sacral and lumbar cords lead to the orgasm reflex, with rhythmic involuntary contraction of uterine and perineal musculature.

Male

The spinal and peripheral innervation of the penis include somatic afferent, sympathetic, and parasympathetic nervous systems, all of which interact to cause erection and ejaculation. Parasympathetic efferents cause vasodilation in erectile tissue. Genital afferents synapse primarily in S2–4 segments. Some sensory fibers ascend with sympathetics and enter the cord in the lower thoracic region.

Semen moves into the posterior urethra during emission. This process is dependent on sympathetic efferents supplying the vas deferens, prostate, and seminal vesicles. Ejaculation occurs as the result of pudendal somatic motor and sympathetic innervation. Rhythmic sequential contractions occur in the musculature of the pelvic floor. The bladder neck is closed and semen is propelled anterograde.

In both sexes MS spinal cord lesions can hinder the transmission of arousing nerve signals between the brain, the spinal cord, and the genitals. Upper motor neuron lesions in the brainstem or above the lumbar section of the spinal cord may interfere with psychogenic erection [12]. Lower motor neuron lesions (in the sacral section of the spinal cord) may alter or prevent vasocongestion, causing weak or absent reflexive erections, reduced clitoral swelling, and lack of vaginal lubrication. Sensory changes in the genitals also may interfere with nerve impulses that facilitate vasocongestion via the spinal cord and the brain (cerebral cortex). In addition, MS lesions in the brain can interfere with the mechanisms that regulate libido and the processing of arousing sexual stimuli [13,14]

Several empiric studies have found a correlation between sexual symptoms and neurologic signs, including weakness of pelvic floor muscles, sensory deficits, and changes in reflex response [15,16]. Minderhoud and colleagues [17] found sexual dysfunction, anal sphincter function, and bladder function to be related to each other but not related to pyramidal or cerebellar signs. As a result, the authors concluded that these disturbances are caused by separate damage in the lumbosacral area of the spinal cord.

Based on the association between sweat patterns (anhydrosis) and erectile function, Vas [18] suggested that impotence may be caused by lesions in the lateral horns or connecting pathways in the dorsolumbar section of the spinal cord. Consistent with prior studies [4,5,10,18,19], Betts and colleagues found erectile dysfunction to be invariably associated with neurogenic bladder dysfunction and pyramidal impairment in the lower limbs [20]. Abnormalities were found in both the left and the right posterior tibial and pudendal cortical evoked potentials of the majority of men with MS and erectile dysfunction (80 percent, 82 percent, and 77 percent, respectively). No correlation was found between the degree of erectile dysfunction (partial versus total impotence) and the *severity* of pyramidal impairment or degree of disability. The investigators believe their findings suggest that in men with erectile failure and MS, neural lesions are predominantly above the sacral segment of the spinal cord.

Barak and colleagues [21] found significant correlations between anorgasmia and depression, brainstem abnormalities, pyramidal abnormalities, and total brain lesions present on magnetic resonance imaging (MRI) scans. The authors state that the lack of correlation between depression and MRI scores found by this study suggest that plaques located on the corticospinal tracts and brainstem connections are associated with inability to achieve orgasm.

SECONDARY SEXUAL DYSFUNCTION

Secondary sexual dysfunction refers to MS-related physical changes that *indirectly* affect the sexual response [1,2]. Secondary sexual dysfunction is caused by MS symptoms that do not directly include nervous system pathways related to the genital system. In both men and women, these most commonly include fatigue, muscle tightness, muscle weakness, spasms, bladder and bowel dysfunction, incoordination, difficulty with mobility, side effects from MS medications, cognitive difficulties, and numbness, pain, burning, and discomfort throughout the body.

Surveys show that the secondary symptoms of MS that most often impair sexual activity include muscle weakness or paralysis (58 percent), spasticity (24 percent), contractures (12 percent), indwelling catheters (5 percent), and incontinence (5 percent) [10].

Neurogenic bowel and bladder symptoms are common in MS. Hulter and Lundberg [16] found that 89 percent of their female sample experienced bladder problems, and 60 percent reported bowel problems. Similarly, 98 percent of the male participants with erectile impairment in Bett's study reported urinary symptoms [20]. Many empiric studies show a correlation between bladder and/or bowel dysfunction and sexual difficulties [7,10,17,20].

TERTIARY SEXUAL DYSFUNCTION

Tertiary sexual dysfunction refers to psychological, social, and cultural issues that affect sexual functioning [1,2]. Symptoms of MS may affect the way one views himself or herself as a sexy, attractive, and masculine or feminine individual. A negatively altered body image or lowered self-esteem can decrease sexual confidence, causing withdrawal from sexual activity. Fear that their partners no longer finds them desirable or are not sexually satisfied often occur as a result of MS-related physiologic changes such as muscle weakness, contractures, or the use of ambulation aids. Emotional issues, including depression, anxiety, anger, and guilt, have a negative impact on both sexual functioning and the quality of an intimate relationship.

Social changes also may develop secondary to physical limitations of MS. Fatigue or mobility loss often make it more difficult for couples to engage in social activities with each other, with family, and with friends. As a result, fears of becoming uninteresting or boring to a partner, feeling left out, or guilt associated with holding back loved ones from activities may develop.

Multiple sclerosis also has the potential to change "roles" within a family. It may cause an individual who was the primary breadwinner of the family to no longer be able to work, leaving the partner to assume some of the financial responsibility. Furthermore, the partner of a person with MS may have to play a larger role in household chores or in the care of young children. This may cause feelings of shame, guilt, dependency, and vulnerability in the person with MS and may cause his or her partner to harbor covert feelings of resentment and frustration because of the increasing demands placed on them. The need to care for an ill partner may add physical and emotional stress, and both partners may mourn the loss of easier, more carefree times in the relationship.

The negative impact of MS on these areas in the relationship may cause one or both partners to withdraw from the relationship, ironically at the time when love, support, and encouragement are most needed. Many partners are afraid to disclose their fears and vulnerabilities because they believe that they need to be "strong" and "optimistic" about their partner's illness. Rather than sharing and validating the difficulties associated with MS within the relationship, couples may individually harbor feelings of anger and resentment or may erroneously believe that their partner does not notice or care about the hardships MS has placed on their lives. Fears of abandonment and isolation grow, and feelings of partnership, trust, and security are lost.

ADDRESSING SEXUAL DYSFUNCTION

Because MS symptoms may have a devastating impact on one's sexual and intimate relationship, it is vital that all health care practitioners who are involved in the care of people with MS facilitate open communication about sexual issues. Admittedly, this is easier said than done. Despite good intentions on behalf of the clinician, discussion of sexuality may seem awkward, uncomfortable, or forced. People tend to discern the discomfort of the health care practitioner and may mimic this discomfort by withholding relevant data. It is important for the clinician to understand his or her own preconceived notions and biases toward sexual issues and acknowledge that each individual possesses his or her own set of beliefs and attitudes toward sexuality.

When is the best time to initiate a discussion of sexual functioning? That depends on a number of factors, such as the nature of the professional role, the duration and intensity of the relationship between the health care practitioner and the patient, ease of communication, and the comfort of both parties with sexual issues. Health care practitioners may be more likely to facilitate discussion if they are confident about their degree of knowledge and training in this area. Clinicians may need to enhance their understanding by enrolling in continuing education workshops or by collaborating with colleagues in their field. Reading current literature or watching educational videos regarding sexuality and disability not only can provide

factual information but also may help to desensitize the practitioner to sexual issues and increase comfort with the use of sexual terminology.

Throughout the course of treatment with a person with MS, it is helpful for the health care practitioner to pay careful attention to any comments or behaviors that may suggest difficulty with a sexual relationship. Negative comments about one's relationship, partner, attractiveness, self-worth, or sex in general may indicate that there is some concern regarding sexuality. Seemingly benign or joking comments such as "I guess my dancing days are over" or "Won't this cane match my lipstick?" may provide some insight into how one perceives himself or herself as an active, attractive, sexual person. Emotional changes, such as increased sadness, frustration, or irritation, and behavioral observations, such as loss of interest in grooming or the absence of a previously involved partner, may also signal a change in an intimate or supportive relationship or a change in sexuality in general. The clinician often may use these comments or observations as a segue into a discussion of sexual concerns. It may be more difficult, however, to broach the topic with patients who do not show overt signs of sexual difficulty. Lefebvre (22) describes "bridge" statements or questions that may minimize the awkwardness or discomfort involved in initiating any type of sexuality interview. Depending on the health care practitioner's professional role and alliance with the patient, these statements may range from statements that are general in nature to statements that more specifically focus on an MS-related problem. As a prelude to asking questions, it sometimes is helpful to acknowledge that sexual difficulties are not uncommon among people with MS. It is important to achieve a balance between acknowledging that others share the same difficulty and scaring patients into believing that they will inevitably develop sexual problems. A general bridge statement may be "Some people have found that MS symptoms have an effect on sexual functioning. Have you noticed any changes in your sexuality since the onset of MS?" A more specific bridge statement may be "Bladder dysfunction can sometimes interfere with sexual functioning, but there are many ways to manage it. Have you had any concerns about the impact of your [incontinence, catheters, etc.] on sexual activity?" Questions such as these set the stage for frank and open discussion of sexual functioning because they let patients know that their concerns are not uncommon, sexual matters can be discussed with their health care practitioner, and treatment is available.

DIAGNOSTIC PROCEDURES

Information regarding sexual dysfunction may be obtained by a number of methods, including clinical interview, standardized instruments, and physiologic assessment.

Clinical Interview

The goal of a diagnostic interview is to identify the main sexual complaint and gather any data relevant to its onset and impact on the patient's life. A thorough evaluation may include the following:

- *Identification of the chief complaint:* Specific questions regarding the main sexual complaint should be asked to develop a thorough understanding of the difficulty and its impact on sexual functioning.
- *Demographic information:* Age, gender, relationship status, socioeconomic status, culture, religion/religiosity, sexual orientation.
- *Lifestyle issues:* Is the person currently using alcohol and/or drugs? Is there a history of alcohol and/or drug abuse? What are the patient's eating, exercise, and work habits?
- *Onset:* When did the problem begin? Is there any prior history of sexual difficulty? Did onset coincide with MS exacerbations or new medications or treatments? Did onset occur with any new psychosocial stressors?
- *Frequency:* How often does the problem occur? In what situations? Does it occur with one particular partner? Does it occur during masturbation? Are there any patterns to its occurrence? Are there any psychological or medical correlates?
- *Severity:* To what extent does the problem interfere with sexual satisfaction or the overall quality of an intimate relationship? Does it make sexual activity impossible or unbearable? How distressing is it to the patient?
- *Medical information:* Is the patient currently experiencing an exacerbation? Are there other medical disorders and/or complaints that could affect sexual functioning? Is the patient taking any medications that are known to affect sexual functioning? Does the patient experience bladder or bowel dysfunction? What are the patient's birth control choices?
- *Psychological information:* Has the patient experienced any problems with past or current relationships? What is the patient's current emotional status? Is there evidence of depression or anxiety? Does the patient have a history of mental illness or mood disorder? Is he or she taking any medications for mood disorder? Are there any other factors such as decreased self-esteem, altered body image, or dependency issues that could be affecting sexuality? Is the patient experiencing any psychosocial stressors related to relationships, bereavement, family, finances, career, or social pressures?
- *Treatment:* Has the patient addressed this issue with any other health care providers? Has the patient dis-

cussed this difficulty with his or her partner? Have they tried to handle the problem on their own? Have they seen a psychiatrist, psychologist, or other mental health care provider regarding this issue? Has treatment been attempted? What has or has not worked? What are the patient's expectations for treatment and treatment goals?

This outline provides a general guideline for a diagnostic interview and offers suggestions for gathering information. Clinicians are encouraged to supplement and/or modify these questions according to their expertise and the patient's situation. In addition, it is useful for clinicians to reword questions to adapt them to their own style of obtaining information so that the questions feel like a comfortable, natural part of the medical examination.

Standardized Instruments

One of the largest gaps in the MS literature may be the lack of a practical, valid, and reliable instrument for measuring sexual dysfunction. As a result, researchers and clinicians have either used surveys or structured interviews that have been neither validated nor standardized or have used the Sexual Function Scale of the Minimal Record of Disability (MRD) (23). The Sexual Function Scale of the MRD assesses whether a person with MS is as sexually active as he or she was before the diagnosis of MS, less active, or inactive, and whether he or she is concerned about the situation. It is administered as part of the MRD, so it is a widely used measure of sexual function in MS. Although it addresses the general level of sexual activity, it does not determine the specific nature or severity of MS symptoms and their effect on sexual functioning.

The Multiple Sclerosis Intimacy and Sexuality Questionnaire (MSISQ) is a 19-item, self-report questionnaire that was developed to measure sexual functioning in people with MS (24). Based on Foley's conceptual model, the MSISQ assesses the perceived impact of primary, secondary, and tertiary symptoms on sexual activity and satisfaction. The MSISQ enables the clinician to pinpoint specific areas of sexual dysfunction and the severity of their impact on sexual satisfaction. It is a valid and reliable (Cronbach's alpha = 0.91) instrument (24). In addition, its ease of administration and brevity make it a useful tool for screening sexual dysfunction, initiating further discussion with patients, and providing a framework for treatment planning.

Medical Assessment

Physiologic assessment begins with a careful medical history and general medical examination, paying close attention to all systems that are involved in sexual functioning. A thorough neurologic examination includes assessment of genital sensory perception, including evidence of allodynia. Motor weakness and tone changes must be identified. The examination should include the anal wink to document reflex function sacral segments.

Causes of erectile function may be broadly classified into organic and psychogenic categories. Organic causes include atherosclerosis, diabetes mellitus, hyperthyroidism and hypothyroidism, alcoholism, uremia, hypertension, psychiatric disease—impairing erectile function because of medications required for treatment—vasculopathy, neuropathy, and hypogonadism. The identification of an organic cause never excludes the possibility of additional contributing psychological factors. It is important to review the duration and progression of symptoms, determining whether there are spontaneous erections and associated ejaculatory dysfunction, and whether the problem is present with all partners.

Psychogenic impotence generally develops acutely and occurs intermittently. The ability to masturbate and to achieve morning erections often are preserved, and the problem may occur only with selected partners.

A review of the individual's medication regimen is critical. Anticonvulsants such as carbamazepine or phenytoin may significantly lower serum levels of free testosterone. Adverse sexual side effects are a well-described complication of antidepressant medications. Loss of libido, erectile dysfunction, and delayed ejaculation are associated with selective serotonin reuptake inhibitors (SSRIs), tricyclic antidepressants, and monoamine oxidase (MAO) inhibitors. Tapering doses or substitution of alternative agents (e.g., bupropion) have been advocated. Erectile failure also is associated with centrally acting antihypertensives and anticholinergic agents.

Physical Examination

Physical examination may disclose signs of decreased serum androgen levels—a decline in body hair, gynecomastia, and testicular atrophy. Causes of neurovascular dysfunction may be identified, as abdominal examination may show signs of prior surgery, and auscultation of femoral pulses may indicate the presence of bruits. Signs of autonomic nervous system dysfunction such as orthostatic hypotension may be identified.

Examination of the penis may reveal evidence of anatomic abnormalities, including Peyronie's disease and other local structural abnormalities (evidence of prior trauma or surgery). The bulbocavernosus reflex may indicate whether there is a disruption in either the central sacral reflex center or the pudendal/penile nerves.

The nocturnal penile tumescence (NPT) test is one of the most widely used instruments for assessing erectile dysfunction (25). The NPT may help identify the patient with a psychogenic component of erectile dysfunction, because it can document the preserved ability to have nocturnal reflex erection, using a simple noninvasive approach. Unfortunately, the NPT may be "positive" in the setting of genuine neurogenic erectile dysfunction. Strain gauges, most commonly the mercury in rubber or electromechanical strain gauges, measure changes in penile circumference caused by increased blood flow to the penis during the night. Home monitoring devices also may be used to determine penile engorgement. In the "stamp" test, a ring of stamps is placed around the penis before going to sleep. If the ring is broken in the morning, it is likely that engorgement occurred during the night. The snap gauge test is similar to the stamp test, but plastic strips are used in place of stamps (25).

In females, vaginal photoplethysmography is the most widely used technique to determine genital blood flow. This instrument assesses vasocongestion by measuring vaginal pulse amplitude and pooled vaginal blood volume (25). Changes in temperature and vaginal transcutaneous oxygen pressure also have been used to determine blood flow to both the internal and external (clitoris and labia) genitalia (25).

MANAGEMENT OF SEXUAL DYSFUNCTION

Choosing the most effective and satisfying treatment for sexual dysfunction requires the careful collaborative work of the patient, his or her partner (whenever possible), and the physician. It is important for the patient to have a thorough understanding of *all* treatment options, their short-term and long-term consequences, and expected efficacy. The same familial, religious, and cultural factors that shape our sexual thoughts and attitudes can have a significant effect on treatment choice. Hence, every effort should be taken to develop a treatment plan that not only is practical and effective but also coincides with the patient's lifestyle, cultural values, and religious beliefs.

Primary Sexual Dysfunction

Erectile dysfunction, the most frequently reported primary symptom in males, may be treated by a number of approaches. Pharmacologic methods of achieving erection are becoming increasingly popular. The recent release of sildenafil (Viagra), an oral agent that shows great promise for neurogenic erectile dysfunction, may allow principal caregivers to assume a more important role in initiating treatment for people with neurogenic impotence. Sildenafil is a selective inhibitor of type 5 phosphodiesterase (the predominant phosphodiesterase in the human corpus cavernosum). Penile erection is mediated by nitric oxide via cyclic guanosine monophosphate (cGMP). By inhibiting phosphodiesterase activity in erectile tissue, sildenafil increases local cGMP concentrations and promotes tumescence. Preliminary reports indicate that, unlike previously advocated oral treatments for impotence such as yohimbine, sildenafil is effective and well tolerated; it may be the first useful oral agent for erectile dysfunction.

An established treatment for neurogenic impotence is pharmacologic injection erection (PIE). Penile injection is now conventional therapy, despite the continuing potential for complications such as local fibrosis. Injections are performed with a small-gauge needle near the base of the penis into each corporal body. If the drug is infused slowly, there is a minimum of associated discomfort, and automated self-injection pens and needle-free injection guns have greatly simplified the process. Smooth muscle relaxants with adrenergic blocking properties have been used for 20 years, including papaverine, phenoxybenzamine, and most recently prostaglandin E1 (PGE1). Because it is endogenously present in penile tissue, it has been more readily accepted by patients and produces a more natural erection with a lower complication rate. PIE is now widely prescribed, and when done so for appropriate indications with adequate supervision, it is safe. However, frequently repeated injections of any type into the same region of the body for a protracted period leads to scar formation. In the penis, deformity and impaired integrity of neurovascular tissue may result. Therefore, particularly for conditions such as premature ejaculation or psychogenic impotence, which may respond to other forms of treatment, prolonged use of this form of therapy is not appropriate.

Prostaglandin E1 also may be administered by urethral suppository (MUSE). Because the injections require good vision and hand coordination, the urethral suppository may be a better option for those with physical limitations. Individuals who use vasoactive medications should be careful to adhere to dosage and injection instructions to avoid side effects such as priapism and tissue scarring.

Surgical alternatives for erectile dysfunction include several types of inflatable and noninflatable (semirigid) penile implants. Noninflatable implants consist of sponge-filled flexible rods that are surgically placed into the corpora cavernosa, allowing the penis to be bent upward to simulate a naturally erect penis. Although the surgery for noninflatable rods is relatively simple and less costly than for the inflatable variety, it results in a penis that is smaller than a "natural" erection and leaves the penis in a permanent semierect state, which may be more difficult to conceal.

Inflatable prostheses consist of a fluid-filled reservoir implanted in the lower abdomen and connected to tubing inserted in the penis. When pressure is applied to the pump, the fluid flows from the reservoir to the cylinders in the penis, simulating the natural erection process. When erection is no longer needed, a valve on the pump is released and the fluid flows back into the reservoir. This method more closely simulates natural erectile functioning; it produces a larger erection when inflated and remains flaccid when not inflated. However, the surgery is more extensive and costly, and the device can be difficult to maneuver, particularly for those with muscle weakness or incoordination.

Vacuum suction devices or "pumps" are nonsurgical, noninvasive devices used to create an erection. They consist of a plastic tube that is placed over the flaccid penis. Using either a hand pump or a battery-operated mechanism, air is pumped out of the tube, creating a vacuum around the penis. The vacuum induces blood flow into the penis, causing an erection. When the erection occurs, a band is placed at the base of the penis, air is returned to the tube, and the tube is removed. The band helps maintain the erection by preventing blood from flowing back out of the penis. The constriction band itself is a viable option for men who can achieve an erection but have difficulty sustaining an erection adequate for sexual activity.

Lack of vaginal lubrication is a common primary sexual dysfunction that may have a great impact on sexual satisfaction for women. Fortunately, vaginal dryness can be managed through the use of water-soluble lubricants (i.e., K-Y Jelly, Replens), which are available in most drugstores. In addition, prolonging foreplay and choosing alternatives to intercourse (i.e., oral sex) also may help facilitate vaginal lubrication and sexual pleasure.

Difficulty with orgasm and decreased libido are primary sexual dysfunctions commonly reported by both men and women with MS. It is believed that the brain does not have one specialized sexual center but that several different areas are involved in sexual interest or pleasure. Orgasm is contingent upon nervous system pathways originating in the brain and pathways in the upper, middle, and lower parts of the spinal cord (26). Lesions along these pathways may cause orgasmic dysfunction. However, both secondary and tertiary symptoms such as anxiety, depression, and loss of self-esteem may detrimentally affect sexual interest and ability to achieve orgasm. Therefore, a multitude of factors should be considered when attempting to manage sexual dysfunction.

One way to enhance sexual interest and alleviate distress caused by difficulty with orgasm is to focus on the sheer enjoyment of the intimacy and closeness of sexual activity rather than on the goal of climax. It is helpful for patients to take the pressure off themselves to orgasm and spend more time exploring each other's body and enjoying all feelings associated with sexual activity. People should make an effort to expand their sexual repertoire by experimenting with different positions, using sexual aids (vibrators, lotions, videos), and engaging in open feedback about the experience. Partners should set aside special time devoted to sexual activity when they will not be interrupted or rushed. Romantic touches such as soft music, flowers, candles, and massage oils also may elicit sexual desire and set the stage for a satisfying and intimate sexual experience.

Altered genital sensation may include loss of feeling and/or numbness in the genital region or a hypersensitivity to genital stimulation. Hypersensitivity (dyesthetic pain) may be difficult to treat, but Shaughnessy and colleagues (11) offer several suggestions, including pharmacologic approaches (antidepressants, anticonvulsants), topical anesthetics, and experimenting with different positions. They also suggest placing a bag of frozen peas over the genitals to decrease hypersensitivity.

Decreased genital sensation or numbness often may be managed by using more vigorous stimulation when engaging in sexual activity. It also is helpful to focus some sexual energy on other areas of the body that provide sexual pleasure, including the neck, earlobes, breasts, and nipples. Sexual aids, including vibrators and textured mitts, may provide increased stimulation and have become more easily available through discreet mail-order catalogs. One company, Xandria, publishes a mail-order catalog featuring sexual aids for people with physical limitations, including altered genital sensation (Xandria Collection, Special Edition for Disabled People, Lawrence Research Group, 874 Dubuque Avenue, South San Francisco, CA 94080, 800-242-2823).

Secondary Sexual Dysfunction

As discussed earlier, secondary sexual symptoms include fatigue, muscle tightness, muscle weakness, incoordination, difficulty with mobility, spasticity, bowel and bladder dysfunction, side effects from medications, and cognitive impairment. Education is vital in helping patients manage secondary sexual dysfunction because many symptoms can be helped by information, planning, and simple suggestions.

Stimulants such as pemoline (Cylert) or amantadine may alleviate fatigue when they are taken before sexual activity. It also is helpful for couples to engage in sexual activity in the morning, when fatigue is at a minimum, or to use energy-saving techniques (napping, using a motorized scooter) throughout the day. Sexual positions that are less physically strenuous for the partner with MS are a wise option for those whose sexual efforts are thwarted by fatigue.

Sexual positioning options are also crucial for individuals with muscle weakness, tightness, spasms, and incoordination. A physical therapist or occupational therapist who is experienced in dealing with sexual issues may be helpful in working with the patient (and his or her partner) to create safe, satisfying, and comfortable positions for sexual activity. In addition, taking antispasticity medication (baclofen) or a warm bath before sexual activity may help alleviate spasticity and make sex more enjoyable.

In managing bladder dysfunction, it is suggested that patients avoid drinking any liquids and empty the bladder before engaging in sexual activity. Physicians, nurses, and occupational therapists may wish to provide helpful suggestions for managing catheters, such as removing the catheter before sex, clamping the catheter, or taping it to the stomach. Occupational and physical therapists also may suggest sexual positions that avoid putting pressure on the bladder, leg bag, or any type or bladder device. Bowel dysfunction may be managed by emptying the bowel before sexual activity and following a bowel schedule. It also is helpful to keep a plastic mattress cover on the bed and towels handy in case of leaks or accidents. A person with bladder or bowel dysfunction may wish to discuss with the partner the possibility of accidents during sexual activity. This may make sexual activity more relaxing and carefree by alleviating some of the fear, embarrassment, and anxiety associated with loss of bladder or bowel control.

A wide variety of medications sometimes prescribed to treat MS or other coexisting medical disorders have the potential to affect sexual functioning. Antihypertensive medications, particularly adrenergic-inhibiting drugs and diuretics, have been strongly associated with sexual dysfunction (27). Antispasticity medications (baclofen, clonazepam), corticosteroids (prednisone), and anticonvulsants (carbamazepine, phenytoin) also may affect sexual dysfunction (11).

Psychotropic medications frequently have a significant impact on several areas of sexual function. Neuroleptics (phenothiazines, butyrophenones) have been associated with diminished sexual performance, decreased arousal, erectile difficulty, and ejaculatory dysfunction (27). Antidepressants, including tricyclics, MAO inhibitors, and SSRIs, may adversely affect sexual functioning, but some of the newer antidepressants (bupropion, trazadone, nefazodone) have been associated with fewer detrimental effects on desire, arousal, and orgasm. It is important to note that depression and psychosis often have a negative impact on sexual functioning, and it may be difficult to determine whether dysfunction stems from medication or from the illness itself. Hence, one must always weigh the benefits of medications on overall quality of life with the influence they have on sexual performance. In addition, physicians may be able to prescribe an alternative drug, modify medication dosages, or change the times when medications are taken to allow for sexual activity. Medications such as yohimbine and cypropheptadine have been studied to determine their effectiveness in treating sexual dysfunction and have demonstrated mixed results (28,29). Nevertheless, some studies look promising, and further exploration on the use of these medications may be worthwhile.

Cognitive deficits such as changes in attention and concentration may interfere with maintaining interest in sexual activity. One way to deal with this is to enhance and focus on romantic and sexual stimuli while minimizing nonsexual stimuli. In addition, the individual with MS may need to be redirected back to the sexual activity at times, with the partner keeping in mind that the lack of attention is not a reflection of his or her sexual attractiveness but rather a manifestation of the symptoms of MS.

Tertiary Sexual Dysfunction

Individuals with MS who experience tertiary sexual symptoms such as depression, anxiety, loss of self-esteem, feeling less masculine or feminine, diminished sexual confidence, and negatively altered body image often benefit from individual, couples, and/or group psychotherapy with a qualified psychologist, psychiatrist, or social worker. Members from all disciplines working with people with MS may improve an individual's self-image by providing positive feedback, reinforcement, and words of encouragement.

Communication is an essential tool in coping with chronic illness and sexual dysfunction. It is important for couples who face MS to be able to express their fears and concerns and assert their personal and sexual needs in an empathic and productive manner. Effective communication is always a key factor in promoting the well-being of any relationship. For those with chronic illness, it is essential for maintaining a healthy partnership and avoiding a multitude of problems that may occur because of miscommunication or withdrawal. Psychotherapy and couples counseling may enhance the communication skills of people with MS and their loved ones.

The extra care needed to carry out activities of daily living often places a great deal of stress on a couple when one person has MS. The individual with MS may feel vulnerable, ashamed, or angered by his or her need for dependency. Likewise, partners may feel resentful of their newly acquired responsibilities and may have difficulty alternating between the role of caregiver and the role of lover. In an effort to retain identity as a sexual partner, it is recommended that nursing activities be performed by nonfamily members if at all possible (30).

SUMMARY

Empiric research has demonstrated the prevalence of sexual dysfunction among persons with MS. Foley's con-

ceptual model of sexual dysfunction categorizes sexual difficulties in terms of primary, secondary, and tertiary sexual dysfunction (1,2). There are many options available for managing sexual dysfunction in people with MS. Treatment often includes a combination of educational, medical, pharmacologic, and counseling approaches, as well as practical suggestions for improving sexual functioning. However, accurate diagnosis and effective treatment are not possible without open and honest communication between the patient and the practitioner. To provide individuals with MS the best possible care, practitioners need to take the initiative in questioning their patients about sexual functioning and encouraging them to explore all available options.

References

1. Foley FW, Iverson J. Sexuality and multiple sclerosis. In: Kalb RC, Scheinberg LC (eds.). *Multiple sclerosis and the family.* New York: Demos, 1992.
2. Foley FW, Sanders A. Sexuality, multiple sclerosis, and women. *MS Management* 1997; 4(1):1–10.
3. Ivers RR, Goldstein NP. Multiple sclerosis: A current appraisal of symptoms and signs. *Mayo Clin Proc* 1963; 38:457–466.
4. Lilius HG, Valtonen EJ, Wikstrom J. Sexual problems in patients suffering from multiple sclerosis. *J Chron Dis* 1976; 29:643–647.
5. Lilius HG, Valtonen EJ, Wikstrom J. Sexual problems in patients suffering from multiple sclerosis. *Scand J Soc Med* 1976; 4:41–44.
6. Ghezzi A, Malvestiti GM, Baldini S, et al. Erectile impotence in multiple sclerosis: A neurophysiological study. *J Neurol* 1995; 242:123–126.
7. Mattson D, Petrie M, Srivastava DK, et al. Multiple sclerosis: Sexual dysfunction and its response to medications. *Arch Neurol* 1995; 52:862–868.
8. McCabe MP, McDonald E, Deeks AA, et al. The impact of multiple sclerosis on sexuality and relationships. *J Sex Res* 1996; 33(3):241–248.
9. Stenager E, Stenager EN, Jensen K, et al. Multiple sclerosis: Sexual dysfunctions. *J Sex Educ Therapy* 1990; 16(4):262–269.
10. Valleroy ML, Kraft GH. Sexual dysfunction in multiple sclerosis. *Arch Phys Med Rehabil* 1984; 65:125–128.
11. Shaughnessy L, Schuchman M, Ghumra M, et al. Sexual dysfunction in multiple sclerosis. In: Aisen M (ed.). *Sexual and reproductive neurorehabilitation.* Totowa, NJ: Humana Press, 1997.
12. Dewis ME, Thornton NG. Sexual dysfunction in multiple sclerosis. *J Neurosci Nurs* 1989; 21 (3):175–179.
13. DeLisa JA, Miller RM, Mikulic MA, et al. Multiple sclerosis: Part II. Common functional problems and rehabilitation. *Am Fam Phys* 1985; 32(5):127–132.
14. Lundberg PO. Sexual dysfunction in patients with multiple sclerosis. *Sexuality and Disability* 1978; 1(3):218–222.
15. Lundberg PO. Sexual dysfunction in female patients with multiple sclerosis. *Intern Rehab Med* 1981; 3(1):32–34.
16. Hulter BM, Lundberg PO. Sexual function in women with advanced multiple sclerosis. *J Neurol Neurosurg Psychiatry* 1995; 59:83–86.

17. Minderhoud JM, Leemhuis JG, Kremer J, et al. Sexual disturbances arising from multiple sclerosis. *Acta Neurol Scand* 1984; 70:299–306.

18. Vas CJ. Sexual impotence and some autonomic disturbances in men with multiple sclerosis. *Acta Neurol Scand* 1969; 45:166–182.

19. Kirkeby HJ, Poulsen EU, Petersen T, et al. Erectile dysfunction in multiple sclerosis. *Neurology* 1988; 38:1366–1371.

20. Betts CD. Pathophysiology of male sexual dysfunction in multiple sclerosis. *Sex Dis* 1996; 14(1):41–55.

21. Barak Y, Achiron A, Elizur AA, et al. Sexual dysfunction in relapsing-remitting multiple sclerosis: Magnetic resonance imaging, clinical, and psychological correlates. *J Psych Neurosci* 1996; 21(4):255–258.

22. Lefebvre K. Performing a sexual evaluation on the person with disability or illness. In: Sipski ML, Alexander CJ (eds.). *Sexual function in people with disability and chronic illness.* Gaithersburg, MD: Aspen Publishers, 1997.

23. Szasz G, Paty D, Lawton-Speert S, et al. Sexual function scale. In: Haber A, LaRocca N (eds.). *Minimal record of disability for multiple sclerosis.* New York: National Multiple Sclerosis Society, 1985:38–40.

24. Sanders AS. Unpublished material, 1998.

25. Gerdes CA. Psychophysiologic and laboratory testing. In: Sipski ML, Alexander CJ (eds.). *Sexual function in people with disability and chronic illness.* Gaithersburg, MD: Aspen Publishers, 1997, Chapter 4.

26. Foley FW, Werner M. Sexuality. In: Kalb RC (ed.). *Multiple sclerosis: The questions you have—the answers you need.* New York, Demos, 1996.

27. Weiner DN, Rosen RC. Medications and their impact. In: Sipski ML, Alexander CJ (eds.). *Sexual function in people with disability and chronic illness.* Gaithersburg, MD: Aspen Publishers, 1997.

28. Gitlin MJ. Psychotropic medications and their effects on sexual function: Diagnosis, biology, and treatment approaches. *J Clin Psych* 1994; 55:406–413.

29. Teloken C, Rhoden EL, Sogari P, et al. Therapeutic effects of high dose yohimbine hydrochloride on organic erectile dysfunction. *J Urol* 1998; 159(1):122–124.

30. Kalb R, LaRocca N, Kaplan S. Sexuality. In: Scheinberg LC, Holland NJ (eds.). *Multiple sclerosis: A guide for patients and their families,* 2nd ed. New York: Raven Press, 1987:177–195.

27 Autonomic Disorders

Benjamin H. Eidelman, M.D., Ph.D.

The autonomic nervous system (ANS) is anatomically extensive and has central and peripheral nervous system components. The tracts of the ANS lying within the brain and spinal cord may be involved in multiple sclerosis (MS). However, in many instances the overwhelming impact of MS on somatic nervous system function masks or diverts attention from the less-defined clinical features relating to a disturbance of ANS function. The effects of ANS dysfunction often are insidious and subtle in nature, yet they may considerably affect the overall well-being of patients. An understanding of ANS function and a knowledge of symptoms of ANS dysfunction are of considerable importance in MS.

OVERVIEW OF THE AUTONOMIC NERVOUS SYSTEM

The ANS governs visceral function, and although it is largely an efferent system, there are afferent components that convey sensory information from the viscera to the central nervous system (1). The efferent component consists of central tracts, nerves, ganglia, and plexuses providing visceral motor function to smooth muscles, cardiac muscles, viscera, blood vessels, and glands. Although the overall organization of the somatic nervous system and the ANS are similar, there are important structural differences. In the somatic nervous system, the efferent neuron runs an uninterrupted course from a source of origin in the brainstem or spinal cord to its peripheral terminal. Efferent autonomic nerve fibers may also have a cranial or spinal origin, but the peripheral course is interrupted by the autonomic ganglia, giving rise to a preganglionic and a postganglionic segment. Afferent autonomic nerves generally run with efferent fibers, traverse the preganglionic segment to reach the nerve root, and then pass through the dorsal root to reach the dorsal horn cell of the spinal cord or brainstem sensory nuclei. Visceral afferent information from these sources is transmitted centrally via the spinothalamic and spinoreticular tracts, eventually reaching the reticular formation, hypothalamus, and thalamus. The exact course of central autonomic afferent pathways, however, are not known.

Division of the Autonomic Nervous System

The ANS is divided into parasympathetic and sympathetic systems. These differ both anatomically and functionally (1). The main anatomic difference lies in the origin of the preganglionic neurons. In the sympathetic nervous system, these originate at a spinal level from T1 to L2 segments. Parasympathetic preganglionic neurons originate from two systems, namely, the brainstem and the sacral spinal cord. Thus there is cranial outflow via cranial nerves and sacral outflow via sacral nerves. The organization of the peripheral nerve processes also differs between the two systems. The sympathetic ganglia lie close to the point of origin from the central nervous system. Hence, there is a short preganglionic segment with a correspondingly long postganglionic component. The reverse holds true in the parasympathetic nervous system, where the ganglion lies close to the organ of supply, creating a long preganglionic segment and a short postganglionic component.

Central Autonomic Connections

The somatic nervous system has a well-recognized hierarchy of control. The higher centers lie within the cortex and interact with various systems lying at subcortical, brainstem, and spinal cord levels. The ANS is similarly organized, although the connections between these very centers have not been well defined. A most important center of autonomic control lies in the hypothalamus (2). The hypothalamus exerts control over lower autonomic centers in the brainstem and spinal cord and serves to integrate their function. Brainstem areas that are important in autonomic function include the nucleus of the solitary tract, the ventrolateral medulla, and the ventromedial medulla (2,3). The ANS has cortical representation in the anterior cingulate gyrus and prefrontal cortex (4).

Fibers from brainstem autonomic centers descend to the spinal cord in the lateral funiculus. These fiber systems, however, are not well defined and may well be quite diffuse. Descending autonomic fibers project to neurons in the intermediolateral and intermediomedial columns of the spinal gray matter. Axons from these neurons emerge from the spinal cord as the preganglionic fibers, which in turn synapse with a postganglionic neuron.

In the case of the parasympathetic nervous system, fibers from the brainstem nuclei travel with the relevant cranial nerves, exit from the motor root, and then synapse at a ganglion lying close to the organ of innervation. In the case of the sacral parasympathetic system, the preganglionic neurons are located in a position corresponding to the intermediolateral column 5 extending from the S2 to S4 segments. The preganglionic fibers leave the cord via the ventral nerve roots, follow the spinal nerves for a short distance, and then separate to form pelvic nerves, which then provide innervation to the organs of the pelvis and the corpora cavernosa.

Function of the Autonomic Nervous System

The ANS innervates the heart, blood vessels, viscera, smooth muscle, and glands. It has an important role in controlling vegetative function, thereby contributing to a stable internal environment. The ANS, in addition to reactivity to change, has anticipatory function and prepares systems for impending changes in the external world.

The two divisions of the ANS, namely, sympathetic and parasympathetic, differ anatomically and also may have opposite functions. From a general perspective, the sympathetic nervous system, which is diffuse in its anatomic distribution, has a largely phasic function and plays an important role in gearing the body for stressful situations such as characterized by the fight or flight response. The parasympathetic nervous system has a more discrete distribution, is less phasic in its activity, and is largely concerned with digestive, excretory, and reproductive functions. Its activities are more of an anabolic nature (1). The principal functions of ANS are summarized in Table 27-1.

CLINICAL FEATURES OF AUTONOMIC NERVOUS SYSTEM DYSFUNCTION

History

The clinical evaluation of ANS function is based on the same principles that apply to the examination of the general nervous system (5). As with all disorders, the history is all-important in determining whether there may be a disturbance of ANS function. In some instances, symptoms may be the only clue to an abnormality of function. In MS, motor, sensory, and cerebellar symptoms are often dramatic and may divert attention from the more subtle features of ANS system function. Thus one needs to be aware of specific aspects of disturbed ANS function. History taking is based on the understanding of what may occur when normal function is disturbed. The ANS controls vegetative function. Thus attention is directed

---

TABLE 27-1
*Principle Functions of the
Autonomic Nervous System*

- Maintenance of blood pressure in response to postural stress
- Cardiovascular control
- Regulation of peripheral circulation
- Control of body temperature
- Sweat glands output
- Visceromotor regulation
- Regulation of sexual function
- Pupillary control
- Lacrimal and salivary gland secretory function

toward symptoms relating to disturbances of blood pressure, skin appearance, bowel function, bladder control, sexual function, sweat output, and certain ocular features.

Blood Pressure Control

The ANS plays an important role in maintaining blood pressure in the face of alterations of posture (6). An important feature of autonomic failure is orthostatic hypotension, which results in wide-ranging symptoms (7). Patients may describe dizziness, lightheadedness, or syncope when adopting a sitting or standing position. On first arising in the morning, the patient may report dizziness or even syncope on attempting to arise from bed. Patients often adjust by first sitting at the edge of the bed, and then gradually edging themselves into the standing position. Orthostatic hypotension may present in a more subtle manner such as fatigue, blurring of vision, poor exercise tolerance, and even a sense of "cognitive slowing"; symptoms of rapid heart beat, anxiety, and nausea may be present. Hypotension may only occur in certain situations such as after exercise, with exposure to a hot environment, or after ingestion of a large meal. The history should include inquiries about orthostatic symptoms in relation to these specific events (5).

Cutaneous Vasomotor Function

The ANS plays a role in regulating vascular tone (8). Alteration in skin appearance as a consequence of impaired cutaneous vascular control may be apparent in ANS dysfunction. Disturbances in skin appearance may be subtle, ranging from minimal discoloration to severe hyperemia. In some situations, an intense bluish discoloration may appear, which suggests peripheral vascular failure. Temperature changes may also be apparent, with the skin feeling rather intensely cold or unusually warm. Patients are usually aware of skin discoloration and often draw attention to such developments. A more direct inquiry may be required to elicit information about more subtle variations in vasomotor dysfunction, such as unusual coldness or warmth of a limb. The history should also include inquiries about changes in skin texture, development of indolent ulcers, and disturbances of hair and nail growth.

Sudomotor Function

Sweating is controlled by the sympathetic cholinergic postganglionic fibers and acetylcholine, as well as other factors. Neurotransmitter plays a role in this course of sweating (9). Diminution or absence of sweating may become apparent with ANS dysfunction. The disturbance of sweating may be generalized in nature, but it

could be quite focal and may be restricted to a portion of the extremity. Patients sometimes volunteer information about lack of sweating, but direct questioning is often needed to elicit information regarding focal or absence or increased perspiration. Questioning about moisture on clothing following exposure to heat may be helpful in providing information about the patient's sweating output.

Temperature Regulation

The ANS plays an important role in maintaining normal body temperature (10). The hypothalamus (11), centers in the brainstem (12), and descending pathways in the spinal cord (13) are essential components of neural thermoregulatory networks. Lesions at any of these sites could affect temperature regulation. Abnormalities of temperature regulation may not be readily evident on history taking. Inquiries about heat intolerance are important. Symptoms of excessive flushing, weakness, and dizziness in a hot environment may indicate disturbed temperature regulation. Such symptoms are nonspecific and are common in MS, but nonetheless, if present, should direct attention to possible ANS dysfunction.

Bladder Function

Bladder dysfunction is a common and distressing manifestation of autonomic disorders. Chapter 24 details aspects of bladder dysfunction in MS, and the symptoms of such dysfunction are well outlined. In summary, however, interruption of autonomic pathways produces abnormalities of bladder function. Disturbances may include detrusor instability, resulting in marked frequency and urgency of micturition, as well as detrusor-external sphincter dyssynergia, which may affect the ability to adequately void. Sphincter control may be impaired, resulting in incontinence. Questions regarding micturition pattern, frequency, urgency, and voiding pattern must be elicited.

Sexual Function

Erectile function is under control of the ANS and thus may be a symptom of disturbed ANS function. This symptom may occur in isolation, but it may be part of a more generalized disturbance. Sexual dysfunction is discussed in detail in Chapter 26.

Bowel Function

The gastrointestinal tract is innervated by autonomic nerves (14), and the ANS plays an important role in maintaining normal gastrointestinal function (15). Bowel dysfunction may occur in MS (15) and may manifest as diarrhea, but severe constipation usually is predominant. The upper portion of the gastrointestinal tract may be involved and gastroparesis may occur (16), presenting as anorexia, bloating, nausea, and vomiting. Loss of secretomotor function may result in decreased saliva production presenting as dryness of the mouth. Inquiries about bowel habits and continence are considered routine, but additional inquiries regarding bloating and saliva production are important aspects that should be included in the tests.

Ocular Function

The parasympathetic nervous system innervates the lacrimal glands, Thus the secretomotor function of these glands may be disturbed in autonomic failure (17), and this may result in dryness of the eyes. The dry eye or sicca syndrome may have several manifestations (18), including pain, redness, and photophobia,

Other symptoms of local ocular dysfunction secondary to autonomic abnormalities may be quite subtle. Pupil reactions may be disturbed, giving rise to photophobia, glare intolerance, and impairment of focusing.

Medications and Autonomic Nervous System Function

Many of the medications used to treat MS patients may affect ANS function and give rise to wide-ranging side effects, such as dryness of the mouth and eyes, impotence, constipation, and skin discoloration. The importance of eliciting such information cannot be overemphasized. Hypotension is not limited to cardiovascular agents, and this complication may occur with antidepressants and drugs used to treat spasticity. Amantadine occasionally induces skin reactions that could be mistaken for neurogenically mediated vasomotor dysfunction. Oxybutynin and other anticholinergics inhibit secretomotor function, resulting in dry eye, dry mouth, and constipation. Medications commonly used in the treatment of MS and their potential side effects are listed in Table 27-2.

AUTONOMIC EXAMINATION

Blood Pressure and Heart Rate

Much information about ANS function can be obtained by measuring the blood pressure and heart rate response when the subject assumes the standing position. These measurements can be obtained using the standard blood pressure cuff. In an ideal situation, supine blood pressure should be obtained after the patient has been at rest

---

TABLE 27-2

Medications Used in the Management of Multiple Sclerosis and Their Possible Effects on Autonomic Function Blood Pressure

Agents That May Induce Hypotension
  Tricyclic antidepressants
  Selective serotonin reuptake inhibitors
  Amantadine
  Tizanidine
  Clonidine
  Baclofen (rare)
  Methylphenidate
  Benzodiazepines
  Phenoxybenzamine
  Prazosin
Agents That May Induce Hypertension
  Corticosteroids
  ACTH
  Methylphenidate
  Pemoline
  Tricyclic antidepressants
Drugs with Cardiac Effects
  Tachycardia
    Tricyclic antidepressants
    Oxybutynin
    Selective serotonin reuptake inhibitors
    Tizanidine
    Baclofen
    Methylphenidate
    Pemoline
  Bradycardia
    Beta blocking agents
Peripheral Circulatory Changes
  Vasodilatation
    Amantadine
    Niacin
    Tizanidine
    Clonidine
  Vasoconstriction
    Beta blocking agents
Body Temperature Disturbances
  Neuroleptic agents
  Amantadine (withdrawal)
Visceral Function
  Constipation
    Tricyclic antidepressants
    Baclofen
    Oxybutynin
    Amantadine
    Narcotic analgesics
  Diarrhea
    Azathioprine
    Methotrexate
  Bladder Dysfunction
    Tricyclic antidepressants
    Baclofen

TABLE 27-2
continued

Oxybutynin
Cutaneous Appearance
  Livedo Reticularis
    Amantadine
  Hair Loss
    Baclofen
    Propranolol
Sweat Output
  Decrease
    Tricyclic antidepressants
    Oxybutynin
    Baclofen
  Increase
    Bethanechol
Sexual Function
  Impotence
    Tricyclic antidepressants
    Selective serotonin reuptake inhibitors
    Neuroleptic agents

for at least 15 minutes The bladder should be empty, and the patient should not have consumed caffeine or any other potentially vasoactive agent in the 12 hours before the examination. After supine blood pressure and heart rate have been obtained, the subject then stands and blood pressure and heart rate are measured at one and two minutes. Normally, a drop in systolic blood pressure of no more than 5 mm Hg may occur. Diastolic blood pressure typically remains unchanged or may rise slightly (19). The heart rate should increase, but the magnitude of the response is age-related, being much greater in younger subjects. A drop in the systolic pressure of 20 mm Hg or more suggests ANS dysfunction (20,21). Failure of the heart rate to increase also is suggestive of impaired ANS function. The sensitivity of the tests can be improved by exercise. In a patient not restricted by significant neurologic deficit, this can be accomplished by having the patient perform 5 or 10 knee-bends. If this is not feasible, other forms of exercise that are consistent with the patient's physical abilities should be attempted. Failure of the heart rate to increase after such activity, even in the absence of a change in blood pressure, would suggest the presence of sympathetic dysfunction.

Examination of the Skin and Integumentary Appendages

Careful appraisal of the skin and associated structures is required. Examination should include inspection of skin color; assessment of skin texture, nail appearance, and distribution of cutaneous hair; and the presence or absence of sweating. Adequate exposure of the extremities is essential, and the patient ideally should be in a constant-temperature environment for at least 30 minutes. Testing for dependency rubor should be carried out by inspecting skin color with the patient in both supine and standing positions. The development of posture-related discoloration, particularly if this occurs asymmetrically, may indicate the presence of a focal autonomic dysfunction. Clinical assessment of skin temperature should also be made, with attention to side-to-side asymmetries. The presence of cutaneous atrophy, absence of hair growth, and stunted nail growth in the absence of circulating insufficiency provide evidence of sympathetic nervous system dysfunction. Examination requires careful palpation of the skin because this may provide information regarding skin texture and temperature. It also will provide an opportunity to determine whether there is a state of heightened sensitivity to cutaneous sensory stimulation, which, if present, may be a sign of a complex regional pain syndrome (reflex sympathetic dystrophy, or RSD). The skin should be inspected for the presence or absence of perspiration. The limbs and trunk should be observed, and asymmetry in sweating should be noted. Assessment of sweating requires inspection and a gentle stroking of the skin. The latter may detect sweating by the tactile sensation imparted by moisture as well as by a change in resistance occurring when the finger passes over dry as opposed to wet skin.

Mucous Membranes

The mouth and conjunctiva should be carefully inspected. Lack of saliva in the floor of the mouth may be caused by anticholinergic medication, but it also could suggest a disturbance of cholinergic nerves. Dryness of the eyes may not easily be observed at the bedside, but injection of the conjunctiva together with a history of "gritty painful" eyes and an inability to wear contact lenses should alert the examiner to the possibility of a sicca-type syndrome, which could indicate ANS dysfunction. This can be evaluated by means of a Schirmer's test, which provides a measure of tear production by observing the amount of moisture taken up by a standardized filter paper over five minutes.

Examination of the Pupils

Pupil size should be assessed in bright light and in a dark environment. Maximum constriction and dilation can then be determined. Pupil size should be documented. Examination of eyelid position for ptosis should be carried out at the same time.

Measurement of Body Temperature

Although it is not routinely carried out in the outpatient setting, core temperature—usually obtained by a rectal measurement—should be obtained if there is any suspicion of disturbed temperature regulation.

AUTONOMIC NERVOUS SYSTEM TESTING

The ANS laboratory can provide information about disturbances of ANS reflexes, which may escape detection by conventional clinical testing. A number of tests are available for evaluating ANS function. Such investigations usually are carried out in laboratories that specialize in noninvasive autonomic testing. In the past, many of these tests required the use of an intraarterial line for measurement of blood pressure. The advent of noninvasive measurements of beat-to-beat changes in blood pressure (22,23) has dispensed with the need for intraarterial blood pressure measurements, thus allowing for much more widespread use of specialized autonomic testing. A variety of tests are available for testing both sympathetic and parasympathetic function (24). Ideally, these tests should be carried out using a system that allows for noninvasive beat-to-beat measurements of blood pressure and heat rate.

Tests That Measure Sympathetic Function

Blood Pressure and Heart Rate

Blood pressure and heart rate responses to postural challenge induced by graded tilt form the basis of such testing. Beat-to-beat measurement of blood pressure and heart rate allow for detection of changes not evident by conventional auscultatory methods (22 23). Normal variations are discussed in the previous section "Blood Pressure and Heart Rate."

Blood Pressure Response to Sustained Hand Grip

An isometric exercise with sustained hand grip in the normal subject causes a rise in blood pressure and heart rate (25). Absence of such a response may indicate disturbance in sympathetic nervous system function.

Blood Pressure Response to Mental Arithmetic

This activity typically produces an increase in blood pressure and heart rate (26), and the response may be blunted or absent in presence of sympathetic dysfunction.

Cold Pressor Test

Immersion of a limb induces an increase in blood pressure and heart rate. This response is controlled by a reflex that induces sympathetic nervous system activation (27) and a resultant increase in blood pressure and heart rate.

Tests of Sudomotor Function

The sweat glands are innervated by cholinergic sympathetic nerves. Tests of sudomotor function provide information concerning the functional integrity of sympathetic fibers (28). Sweat output can be quantified by directly stimulating cholinergic nerves and collecting the output of the sweat glands in a circumscribed area (29). This method, which is termed "quantitative sudomotor axon reflex testing" (QSART), has become a valuable tool in evaluating ANS function by providing information concerning the integrity of postganglionic sympathetic nerves.

Plasma Catecholamine Measurements

Measurements of plasma norepinephrine and epinephrine can provide information about sympathetic nervous system function (30,31). Measurements and venous samples for catecholamine measurement are obtained after the patient has been at rest in the supine position and are then repeated after the patient has been in the upright position. Catecholamine levels typically double after five minutes of standing in the normal level. Measurements of resting catecholamine levels at the response to standing can differentiate preganglion and postganglion disorders (32).

Tests of Parasympathetic Function

Heart Rate Response to Deep Breathing

Deep breathing induces a sinus effect on the heart, largely mediated by the vagus nerve (33,34). Normally, inspiration induces a rise in heart rate, whereas expiration induces a fall. Although many variables affect heart rate during deep breathing, this method has been extensively used to evaluate ANS function, The heart rate variation with breathing will vary by 10 or more beats in most normal subjects under the age of 50. However, this response becomes less marked in older individuals (34). Knowledge of these variations is important in the interpretation of the response. Heart rate variability with deep breathing is a reproducible test of vagal nerve function and, by inference, of parasympathetic nervous system function.

Valsalva Maneuver

The Valsalva maneuver is perhaps the most well-known test of autonomic function (35) and measures the integrity of the baroreceptor arc. The test involves measurement of blood pressure and heart rate under conditions of forced expiration against a closed glottis maintained for at least 10 seconds and attaining a pressure of 40 mm Hg. This brings about a series of changes in blood pressure and heart rate. When pressure is released, heart rate and blood pressure are altered. This test measures the integrity of baroreflex pathways. Blood pressure typically will drop during the course of forced expiration with a concomitant increase in heart rate. Blood pressure rises immediately as pressure is released, followed by a compensatory bradycardia that returns blood pressure to baseline levels. The compensatory tachycardia is sympathetically mediated and the bradycardia is a vagal nerve effect (35). A Valsalva ratio has been devised and then is calculated by dividing the maximum by the lowest heart rate. The response is age-dependent. A ratio of 1.5 is regarded as normal in people under the age of 40, and 1.35 is acceptable in those over 60 years old (36).

AUTONOMIC NERVOUS SYSTEM IN MULTIPLE SCLEROSIS

Cardiovascular Function

The central ANS pathways coursing through the brain and spinal cord may also be compromised by the pathologic effects of MS. Although such lesions may be clinically silent (37), cardiovascular reflex abnormalities attributed to MS-induced autonomic dysfunction have been described (38–42). Reports vary both in clinical findings and in methods used to test ANS function. Abnormalities in heart rate variability, deep breathing, postural stress, and in response to exercise have been demonstrated by a number of authors (43–48). The results of these studies are variable, and no distinct pattern of cardiovascular reflex dysfunction in MS has emerged. There also is a poor relationship between autonomic dysfunction and site of pathology, although one study suggests that cardiovascular autonomic dysfunction correlates with brainstem lesion (49).

Orthostatic hypotension is a major presenting feature of disturbed ANS cardiovascular reflex function. This entity has indeed been described in MS patients (36–41). The incidence varies from approximately 15 percent to about 30 percent (40). The variability in the incidence of orthostatic hypotension may relate to differences in study methodology and/or patient-to-patient variability related to the irregular distribution of lesions. This may account for the difference in the reported incidence of orthostatic hypotension.

A variety of symptoms may occur with orthostatic hypotension, and they have been described previously. Many symptoms are subtle and do not draw immediate attention to the cardiovascular system or are mistaken for a primary disturbance of nervous system function. Thus

"dizziness" and fatigue, which are so common in MS patients, may in some instances reflect orthostatic hypotension, so there should always be an awareness of this possibility. If orthostatic hypotension is suspected, bedside testing as outlined in "Blood Pressure and Heart Rate" of the autonomic examination should be carried out.

Management of Orthostatic Hypotension

General Measures

If the patient has clinical evidence of orthostatic hypotension based on the symptoms and demonstrable drop in blood pressure with orthostatic stress, further measures are required. Although orthostatic hypotension may be related to disturbed cardiovascular reflex control, there may be other causes (6), including decreased circulating blood volume, complications of medication, cardiovascular deconditioning, and endocrine disorders such as Addison's disease. Patients with impaired bladder function often restrict fluid intake during the day to guard against the need for frequent voiding. This predisposes to reduced blood volume, which may cause decreased cardiac output and orthostatic hypotension may result. Recognition and treatment of these problems with adequate hydration often results in prompt correction of the disorder.

A number of medications used in the treatment of MS may affect ANS function. These are listed in Table 27-2. Of these medications, tizanidine, tricyclic antidepressants, selective serontonin reuptake inhibitors (SSRIs), and amantadine are commonly used in MS. In assessing a patient with orthostatic hypotension, hypotension medication history and usage is important. The simple withdrawal of an offending drug occasionally improves orthostatic hypotension.

Nonpharmacologic Treatment Maneuvers

The application of external support to the lower limbs will reduce venous pooling and augment cardiac return. This may be extremely helpful in treating orthostatic hypotension. Patients usually are provided with supportive hose. Various types are available and may be of thigh or knee length. The latter are preferable because they provide fairly uniform compression to the lower limb and thus improve venous return. However, such stockings are tight-fitting and may be difficult to apply, especially for handicapped patients. They can cause discomfort and may impede heat loss, which can be extremely detrimental for patients in a warm environment. Half stockings are much easier to tolerate, and patients have less difficulty donning such stockings. However, external pressure is only applied to the calf and may be inadequate, resulting in marked edema above the stockings, which is not only unsightly but also can be detrimental. Despite drawbacks, supportive hose are a first-line treatment and may benefit patients, obviating the need for pharmacologic intervention.

Other General Measures

Exposure to warm environments should be avoided. This includes taking hot showers or baths and sunbathing. Hypotension may occur after ingestion of a large meal, so advice on dividing caloric intake throughout the day is important. Adequate hydration is also essential. Reviewing daily fluid intake and having a patient keep a diary of the sodium supplementation may be helpful. This should be weighed against the risks of sodium retention fluid overload. A simple and palatable way of introducing sodium is to encourage patients to drink vegetable juice. The usual 12-ounce can contains in excess of 1,200 milligrams of sodium. These simple general measures, together with external support, may be all that is needed for patients with modest orthostatic hypotension.

Other maneuvers have been described to improve orthostatic hypotension. These include leg-crossing, squatting, and abdominal compression. Physical activity, such as aerobic exercises, are encouraged, whereas prolonged recumbency should be avoided (50).

Pharmacologic Management

A variety of pharmacologic agents have been used for the treatment of orthostatic hypotension (Table 27-3). These include mineralocorticoids, sympathomimetic agents, ergot derivatives, β-adrenergic blocking agents, prostaglandin synthetase inhibitors, dopaminergic blocking agents, and a variety of miscellaneous drugs, including erythopoietin, caffeine, and somatostatin (51). These agents have various mechanisms of action and, while many are effective, supine hypertension is a posasible side effect. The therapeutic objective is to attain a level of orthostatic blood pressure sufficient to ameliorate symptoms while not necessarily achieving normal blood pressure levels. Many patients who are subject to chronic orthostatic hypotension develop compensatory mechanisms that allow them to tolerate lower than normal blood pressures. Supine hypertension may be avoided by keeping the dose of these medications to a minimum. The management of these patients requires the frequent recording of blood pressure—both supine and standing. Patients and/or family members should be instructed on blood pressure management.

MINERALOCORTICOID

Fludrocortisone is most commonly used in the treatment of orthostatic hypotension. This agent exerts its

---

TABLE 27-3
Pharmacologic Agents Used for Treatment of Orthostatic Hypotension

Prostaglandin Synthetase Inhibitors
  Ibuprofen
  Indomethacin
  Naproxen
β-Adrenergic Antagonists
  Propranolol
  Pindolol
Mineralocorticoids
  Fludrocortisone
Sympathomimetic Agents
  Ephedrine
  Pseudoephedrine
  Phenylephrine
  Midodrine
  Yohimbine
  Clonidine
Ergot-like Agents
  Dihydroergotamine
  Metoclopramide
Dopamine Agonists
  Metoclopramine
Other Agents
  Caffeine
  Somatostatin
  Desmopressin Acetate

---

effect by inducing sodium and fluid retention and resulting in increased circulating volume (52). Medications may not be effective unless the patient ingests adequate amounts of fluid. Fludrocortisone is usually initiated as a single morning dose, 0.1 mg one hour before. The beneficial effects may only be evident several days after initiating therapy, and patients should be advised accordingly. Medication adjustments should be delayed for at least a week and should be based on supine and orthostatic blood pressure. The maximum daily dose usually is approximately 0.6 mg daily. Side effects include supine hypertension, edema, weight gain, hypokalemia, and hypomagnesemia. Supine hypertension may be accompanied by nocturnal headaches. Serum potassium levels should be checked frequently during treatment with fludrocortisone, and supplements should be administered if necessary.

SYMPATHOMIMETIC AGENTS

There are a variety of drugs in this category, including ephedrine, pseudoephedrine, yohimbine, methylphenidate, clonidine, and midodrine. These agents may have a direct effect on adrenergic receptors, resulting in vasoconstriction, but they also can modify release-uptake and synthesis norepinephrine and thereby augment its effect. An effective agent in this class is midodrine, an α-adrenergic agonist (53). Patients vary in their response to this agent, and treatment should be started at a low dose, namely, 2.5 mg day, which could gradually be titrated to 10 mg three times a day. Supine hypertension is a potential side effect. Prostaglandin synthetase inhibitors, typified by the nonsteroidal antiinflammatory agents, may be useful in the treatment of orthostatic hypotension. Ibuprofen and indomethacin have demonstrated effectiveness in improving postural hypotension (54).

The other drugs listed all have a place in the treatment of orthostatic hypotension. Until the advent of midodrine, yohimbine was perhaps the most commonly used after fludrocortisone. This agent generally is well tolerated and induces modest vasoconstrictor effect, but it may cause side effects in the form of palpitations, tremulousness, general feelings of anxiety, and supine hypertension.

In general, the decision to use a particular agent will depend on the severity of the symptoms and the familiarity of the treating physician with a particular drug. In the case of modest orthostatic hypotension not responsive to general measures, a reasonable approach would be to initiate therapy with a prostaglandin synthetase inhibitor, such as ibuprofen or indomethacin. A beta blocking agent could be introduced next, and fludrocortisone kept in reserve for those individuals who fail to respond to these measures. Occasionally, combinations of various agents with different mechanisms of action may be necessary.

Disorders of Cutaneous Circulation

Discoloration of the skin is common in MS patients and usually has a benign connotation, often relating to dependency-induced hyperemia or cyanosis. However, it is important to consider and, if clinically indicated, to exclude vascular insufficiency as a cause of these skin discolorations. The limb should always be examined for features that may indicate vascular compromise. Peripheral pulses should be pulsated and tests carried out to determine if there is any evidence of ischemia. In some instances, cutaneous abnormalities may relate to vasomotor instability. Thus, in a cold environment the patient should be examined after accommodating to warm indoor conditions, when the effects of cold-induced vasoconstriction may be lessened. The affected extremity should also be elevated to facilitate venous emptying. This maneuver often eliminates cutaneous congestion, which may be helpful if the discoloration is a dependency-induced phenomenon. Appropriate testing should be carried out if there is any suspicion of peripheral vascular insufficiency or venous thrombosis (55).

Acrocyanosis

Red or purplish discoloration of the skin, typically occurring in a distal distribution, is a fairly common finding. The affected skin may be cold to the touch, and the discoloration is much more obvious when the limbs have been in a dependent position for some time. Elevation of the extremity diminishes the discoloration. This condition typically involves the lower limbs, and the discoloration may be asymmetric, usually being more obvious in the limb that is more functionally compromised. Although the discoloration may be unsightly, it usually is of little clinical significance. Peripheral pulses typically are present. The exact cause of this disorder is not known, but it probably relates to a disturbance of vasomotor control. Acrocyanosis may occur in the absence of any disease process. This idiopathic form is believed to be related to arterial construction, with accompanying dilation of the subcutaneous venous plexus (56). Treatment is largely symptomatic. The affected limb should be protected and kept warm in cold weather. The patient should be encouraged to wear insulated clothing and avoid prolonged exposure to cold.

Raynaud's Phenomenon

Raynaud's phenomenon typically results in phasic, sequential changes in skin color. The appearance may range from extreme pallor to marked rubor (57). The condition is more likely to occur in warm weather and is more common in women. It may occur as an isolated phenomenon, but it can be a complication of connective tissue disorders (58). Raynaud's phenomenon may be seen in patients with MS. In most cases, this is the primary type, unrelated to a structural disease. In a rare occurrence of an accompanying connective tissue disorder, Raynaud's phenomenon may be a complication of the latter. If clinically suspected, appropriate testing should be carried out to exclude the possibility of an underlying immune system disorder. Management usually is symptomatic. The limbs should be protected against cold, and patients should be encouraged to wear well-insulated gloves. Patients also should be encouraged to stop smoking. Skin lubricants may be helpful in preventing skin breakdown. In rare situations, pharmacologic intervention may be required, and agents that can be useful include calcium channel blockers such as nifedipine, 10–80 mg daily. Low-dose reserpine (0.1 mg daily) also may be helpful.

Livedo Reticularis

Livedo reticularis is characterized by a reticular, cyanotic pattern of discoloration, usually affecting the distal portion of the extremities. The discoloration is most obvious in cold environments, but it may occur in warm weather. It is not a primary complication of MS and occurs in the population at large. The cause usually is not known. It may occur as a complication of amantadine therapy, so patients should be made aware of its possible occurrence. If amantadine has been prescribed, the skin should be inspected at each visit. The condition usually remits when amantadine is withdrawn, but discoloration may persist for a prolonged period.

Erythromelalgia-Like Disorders

Patients occasionally may present with hyperemia of a limb accompanied by pain and sensory distortion. This presentation may suggest erythromelalgia (59), but it also could resemble reflex sympathetic dystrophy (RSD). Swelling and excessive sweating are typically absent, but the combination of skin discoloration and dysesthesia may suggest RSD. Erythromelalgia may be of the primary type or secondary to diseases such as myeloproliferative disorders and pernicious anemia. Painful extremities together with distortion of sensation are common in MS, usually radiating to a disturbance of central pathways. Distal limb hyperemia, which often occurs as a consequence of chronic immobility, may coexist with these sensory disturbances and thus give rise to an erythromelalgia-like picture. When symptoms are first encountered, investigation should be carried out to exclude hematologic disorders. Treatment is largely preventative and includes avoiding conditions that accentuate symptoms, such as exposure to heat. The discomfort engendered by this condition may be intractable, but a number of pharmacologic agents have reportedly been found effective (60,61), and the topical application of capsaicin also may be helpful (62).

Temperature Regulation

Thermoregulation is a finely controlled function, which in essence requires a balance between heat production and heat loss (63). Temperature regulation essentially is controlled by the hypothalamus and other components of the ANS, but metabolic and endocrine responses also play a role in thermoregulation (64). Temperature homeostasis thus relies on a central control mechanism affected by the hypothalamus and the AND and a peripheral system where heat is generated or lost. Skeletal-muscle activity is a major source of heat production. Heat is dissipated to the environment by cutaneous vasodilation, and this can be increased by sweating, which promotes heat loss by evaporation. In MS, both the central control mechanism, namely, the hypothalamus and its autonomic components, and the peripheral components may be defective.

Multiple sclerosis patients are thus at risk for the development of both hypothermia and hyperthermia.

Hypothermia

Hypothermia is a significant problem in MS, as has been reported by a number of authors (65–67). This condition has been attributed to impaired thermoregulation. Hypothermia appears to be most likely to develop in patients with more severe disease, that is, those with an Expanded Disability Status Scale score (EDSS) of 6 or greater (67). The typical presentation is one of gradual decline in level of consciousness. The patient may become withdrawn and drowsy, and in severe cases coma may supervene. Other features include slurred speech, reduced level of awareness, impaired coordination, depressed reflexes, dilated pupils, slowness of heart rate and respiration, and decreased blood pressure. Hypothermia may be accompanied by hematologic abnormalities such as thrombocytopenia (68). These findings should direct attention to possible hypothermia, and the measurement of temperature is required. It is important to measure rectal temperature, which is more reflective of core temperature. In some instances, a low reading thermometer may be required.

Patients who develop hypothermia require immediate rewarming in the most severe cases. Cardiopulmonary resuscitation may be required, and this takes precedence. Patients with mild hypothermia exhibit lower body temperature, excessive shivering, and a mild tachycardia and increase in respiratory rate. Drowsiness may be evident. Such patients can be treated by passive warming, which involves maintaining the patient in a warm environment and covering him or her with insulating blankets. In more severe hypothermia, consciousness may be lost, and shivering diminishes or may be absent. The skin may be icy cold, tone is increased, blood pressure may be extremely low, and the pulse may be difficult to find. Tendon and pupillary reflexes may be absent. Active measures are required to rewarm such individuals and may include the use of electric blankets, warm mattresses, water bottles, immersion of the body in warm water, and the use of warm intravenous solutions.

Hyperthermia and Heat Stroke

Heat stroke with fatal outcome has been reported in patients with MS (69). Heat-induced deterioration in nervous system function is well described in MS (70,71), and patients with severe disability are at greater risk to develop hyperthermia as the efferent pathways governing the thermoregulatory reflexes may be disturbed, particularly in those with spinal cord involvement.

Abnormal thermoregulatory sweating may be evident in patients with MS (72). An increase in body temperature may cause a number of neurologic disturbances, including headache, drowsiness, confusion, coma, and death. Neurologic abnormalities in the form of cerebellar signs, focal motor deficits, and seizures also may be evident. In a situation in which hyperthermia is suspected, core temperature should be obtained using a rectal thermometer. If the temperature is elevated, measures should be taken to correct the situation (63). If core temperature is above 41°C (105.8°F), emergency management is required. This should include removal of clothing, fanning the patient, and immersion in cool water. Such patients are best managed in the intensive care unit, where they can be monitored for such complications as rhabdomyolysis, renal failure, and lactic acidosis. Seizures also may complicate heat stroke.

Summary

High or low temperatures in MS patients may relate to worsening of neurologic functioning. Temperature alterations may indicate body temperature regulation. Both hyperthermia and hypothermia can lead to symptoms indistinguishable from those deficits that occur from the demyelinating process itself. Measurement of core temperature should be obtained in any patient whose presenting symptoms include unexplained lethargy or sudden worsening of neurologic symptoms in environmental conditions that could predispose to the development of either hyperthermia or hypothermia.

Disorders of Sweating

The sweat glands are under neural control, and normal sweating is thus dependent on intact central and peripheral pathways. The former may be interrupted in MS, resulting in a disturbance of sweating. This could potentially be quite severe in patients with extensive cervical cord disease. Under these circumstances, much of the sympathetic outflow from the spinal cord is interrupted, resulting in impairment in sweating over much of the trunk and limbs. Sweating results in heat loss through evaporation. Body temperature may increase if this function is diminished. Information regarding sweat output may be obtained by history and examination, as outlined in the sections on sudomotor function. Sweating problems may seem insignificant in patients with severe neurologic dysfunction, but the importance of disturbed sweating and its implications in body temperature regulation have already been discussed. This is of particular relevance in patients with severe disability, where the clinical picture may mimic that seen in spinal cord injury (13).

Treatment

Excessive sweating is rarely a problem in MS patients. Should it become evident, however, topical application of 20% aluminum chloride hexahydrate (drysol) can be quite effective. Tapwater iontophoresis also may reduce sweating; this is an effective and safe treatment. In rare instances, excessive sweating nonresponsive to the aforementioned measures, becomes intrusive to the point of causing skin maceration. Under these circumstances, sympathectomy could be considered. Heat intolerance is common in MS patients, but decreased sweating is rarely implicated as a cause. However, patients who complain of heat intolerance should be evaluated for a disturbance of sweat production. This can be assessed clinically as outlined in earlier sections of the chapter. If decreased sweating is indeed evident, it would be important to determine whether lack of sweating relates to neurogenic causes or a primary disturbance of sweat gland function (73,74). The latter may require dermatologic evaluation, and if there appears to be some local disturbance in the sweat glands, appropriate therapy may help. If the decreased sweating is thought to relate to neurogenic causes, the patient potentially would be at risk for the development of hyperthermia. Both patient and family members should be counseled regarding preventive measures and recognition of signs and symptoms of hyperthermia, and they should also be instructed in treatment should an event occur.

Summary

The ANS has a wide range of functions, and autonomic syndromes can involve the majority of organ systems and may complicate any disease process. Multiple sclerosis is no exception, and although the somatic aspects of the disease often take center stage, disturbances of ANS control may significantly affect symptomatology. In MS, autonomic dysfunction may result from pathologic involvement of the central autonomic structures with the brain and spinal cord, but it also may occur as a complication of the pharmacologic agents used in the management of MS patients. The major functions of the ANS have been discussed, together with the clinical features of disturbances within each system. As with other discussions of the nervous system, the ANS can be approached in a systematic manner, focusing on each component. This chapter has provided such an approach and highlighted important aspects of the ANS as they apply to MS.

References

1. Brodal P. Peripheral autonomic nervous system. In: Brodal P (ed.). *The central nervous system: Structure and function.* New York: Oxford University Press, 1998.
2. Brodal P. Central autonomic system: Hypothalamus. In: Brodal P (ed.). *The central nervous system: Structure and function.* New York: Oxford University Press, 1998.
3. Loewy AD. Central autonomic pathways. In: Loewy AD,

Spyer KM (eds.). *Central regulation of autonomic functions*. New York: Oxford University Press, 1990.

4. Benarroch EE. The central autonomic network: Functional organization, dysfunction, and perspective. *Mayo Clin Proc* 1993: 68:988–1001.

5. Low PA, Benarroch E, Suarez GA. Clinical autonomic disorders: Classification and clinical evaluation. In: Low PA (ed.). *Clinical autonomic disorders*, 2nd ed. Philadelphia: Lippincott-Raven, 1997.

6. Scott JA, Polinsky RJ. Postural hypotension. In: Goetz CG, Tanner CM, Aminoff MJ (eds.). *Handbook of clinical neurology*, Vol. 19 (63). Amsterdam: Elsevier, 1993.

7. Schatz IJ. Orthostatic hypotension. II. Clinical diagnosis, testing, and treatment. *Arch Intern Med* 1984: 144:1037–1041.

8. Burnstock G. Integration of factors controlling vascular time. *Anesthesiology* 1993; 1368–1380.

9. Tainio H, Vaalasti H, Rechardt L. The distribution of substance P-, CGRP-, galanin-, and ANP-like immunoreactive nerves in human sweat glands. *Histochem J* 1987; 19:375–380.

10. Cabanac M. Temperature regulation. *Ann Rev Physiol* 1975; 37:415–439.

11. Kanosue K, Yanase-Fujiwara M, Hosomo T. Hypothalamic network for thermoregulatory vasomotor control. *Am J Physiol* 1994; 267:R283–R288,

12. Hori T, Harada Y. Responses of midbrain raphe neurons to local temperature. *Pflugers Arch* 1976; 1364:205–207,

13. Guttman L, Silver J, Wyndham CH. Thermoregulation in spinal man. *J Physiol* (London) 1958; 1142:406–419.

14. Gershon MD, Erde SM. The nervous system of the gut. *Gastroenterology* 1981; 80:1571–1594.

15. Wood JD. Enteric neurophysiology. *Am J Physiol* 1984; 247:G585–G598.

16. Hinds JP, Eidelman BH, Wald A. Prevalence of bowel dysfunction in multiple sclerosis: A population survey. *Gastroenterology* 1990; 98:1538–1542.

17. Cross SA. Autonomic disorders of the pupil, ciliary body and lacrimal apparatus. In: Low PA (ed.). *Clinical autonomic disorders*, 2nd ed. Philadelphia: Lippincott-Raven, 1997.

18. Holly FJ, Lemp MA. Tear physiology and dry eyes. *Surv Ophthalmol* 1977; 22:69–87.

19. Paul S, Zygmunt D, Haile V, Robertson D, Biaggioni I. Chronic orthostatic hypotension. *Comp Ther* 1988; 14:58–65.

20. Mader SL. Orthostatic hypotension. *Med Clin North Am* 1989; 73:1337–1349.

21. Streeten DH, Anderson GH Jr, Richardson R, Thomas FD. Abnormal orthostatic changes in blood pressure and heart rate in subjects with intact sympathetic nervous system function, evidence for excessive venous pooling. *J Lab Clin Med* 1988; 111:326–335.

22. Smith NT, Wesseling KH, deWit B. Evaluation of two prototype devices producing noninvasive, pulsatile, calibrated blood pressure measurement from a finger. *J Clin Monit* 1985; 1:17–29.

23. Molhoek GP, Wesseling KH, Settels JJ, et al. Evaluation of the Penaz servo-plethysmo-manometer for continuous, non-invasive measurement of finger blood pressure. *Basic Res Cardiol* 1984; 79:598–609.

24. McLeod JG. Invited review: Autonomic dysfunction in peripheral nerve disease. *Muscle Nerve* 1992; 15:3–13.

25. Smolander J, Aminoff T, Korhonen I, et al. Heart rate and blood pressure responses to isometric exercise in young and older men. *Eur J Appl Physiol* 1998; 77:439–444.

26. Fencl V, Hejl Z, Jirka J, et al. Changes of blood flow in forearm muscle and skin during an acute emotional stress (mental arithmetic). *Clin Sci* 1959; 18:491–498.

27. Victor RG, Leimbach WN Jr, Seals DR, Wallin BG, Mark AL. Effects of the cold pressor test on muscle sympathetic nerve activity in humans. *Hypertension* 1987; 9:429–436.

28. Fealey RD, Low PA, Thomas JE. Thermoregulatory sweating abnormalities in diabetes mellitus. *Mayo Clin Proc* 1989; 64:617–628.

29. Low PA, Caskey PE, Tuck RR, Fealey RD, Dyck PJ. Quantitative sudomotor axon reflex test in normal and neuropathic subjects. *Ann Neurol* 1983; 14:573–580.

30. Burke D, Sundlof G, Wallin G. Postural effects on muscle nerve sympathetic activity in man. *J Physiol* 1977; 272:399–414.

31. Wallin BG, Sundlof G, Eriksson BM, et al. Plasma noradrenaline correlates to sympathetic muscle nerve activity in normotensive man. *Acta Physiol Scand* 1981; 111:69–73.

32. Polinsky RJ, Kopin IJ, Ebert MH, Weise V. Pharmacologic distinction of different orthostatic hypotension syndromes. *Neurology* 1981; 31:1–7.

33. Smith SE, Smith SA. Heart rate variability in healthy subjects measured with a bedside computer-based technique. *Clin Sci* 1981; 61:379–383.

34. Smith SA. Reduced sinus arrhythmia in diabetic autonomic neuropathy: Diagnostic value of an age-related normal range. *Br Med J* (Clin Res Ed) 1982; 285:1599–1601.

35. Levin AB. A simple test of cardiac function based upon the heart rate changes induced by the Valsalva maneuver. *Am J Cardiol* 1966; 18:90–99.

36. Low PA, Opfer-Gehrking TL, Proper CJ, Zimmerman I. The effect of aging on cardiac autonomic and postganglionic sudomotor function. *Muscle Nerve* 1990; 13:152–157.

37. Lumsden CE. The neuropathology of multiple sclerosis. In: Vinken PJ, Bruyn GW (eds.). *Handbook of clinical neurology.* Vol. 9. Amsterdam, North-Holland, 1970:217–309.

38. Sterman AB, Coyle PK, Panasci MS, Grimson R. Disseminated abnormalities of cardiovascular functions in multiple sclerosis. *Neurology* 1985; 35:1665–1668.

39. Anema JR, Heijenbrok MW, Faes TJC, et al. Cardiovascular autonomic function in multiple sclerosis. *J Neurol Sci* 1991; 104:129–134.

40. Nordenbo AM, Boesen F, Anderson EB. Cardiovascular autonomic function in multiple sclerosis. *J Auton Nerv Syst* 1989; 26:77–84.

41. Pentland B, Ewing DJ. Cardiovascular reflexes in multiple sclerosis. *Eur Neurol* 1987; 26:46–50.

42. Nasseri K, TenVoorde BJ, Ader HJ, et al. Longitudinal follow-up of cardiovascular reflex tests in multiple sclerosis. *J Neurol Sci* 1998; 155:50–54.

43. Senaratne MPJ, Carroll D, Warren KG, et al. Evidence for cardiovascular autonomic nerve dysfunction in multiple sclerosis. *J Neurol Neurosurg Psychiatry* 1984; 47:947–952.

44. Monge-Argiles JA, Palacios-Ortega F, Vila-Sobrina JA, et al. Heart rate variability in multiple sclerosis during a stable phase. *Acta Neurol Scand* 1998; 97:86–92.

45. Linden D, Diehl RR, Kretzschmar A, et al. Autonomic evaluation by means of standard tests and power spectral analysis in multiple sclerosis. *Muscle Nerve* 1997; 20:809–814.

46. Neubauer B, Gundersen HJG. Analysis of heart rate variations in patients with multiple sclerosis. *J Neurol Neurosurg Psychiatry* 1978; 41:417–419.

47. Giubilei F, Vitale A, Urani C, et al. Cardiac autonomic dysfunction in relapsing remitting multiple sclerosis during a stable phase. *Eur Neurol* 1996; 36:211–214.

48. Ferini-Strambi L, Rovaris M, Oldani A, et al. Cardiac autonomic function during sleep and wakefulness in multiple sclerosis. *J Neurol* 1995; 242:639–643.

49. Vita G, Fazio MC, Milone S, et al. Cardiovascular autonomic dysfunction in multiple sclerosis is likely related to brainstem lesions. *J Neurol Sci* 1993; 120:82–86.

50. Wieling W. Nonpharmacological management of autonomic disorders. In: Robertson D, Low P, Polinsky R (eds.). Primer on the autonomic nervous system. San Diego: Academic Press, 1996:319–324.

51. Freeman R, Miyawaki E. The treatment of autonomic dysfunction. *J Clin Neurophysiol* 1993; 10:61–82.

52. Hickler RB, Thompson GR, Fox LM, et al. Successful treatment of orthostatic hypotension with 9-alpha-fluorohydrocortisone. *N Engl J Med* 1959; 261(16):788–791.

53. Kaufmann H, Brannan T, Krakoff L, et al. Treatment of orthostatic hypotension due to autonomic failure with a peripheral alpha-adrenergic agonist (midodrine). *Neurology* 1988; 138:951–956.

54. Kochar MS, Itskovitz HD, Albers JW. Treatment of orthostatic hypotension with indomethacin. *Am Heart J* 1979; 98:271.

55. Lensing AW, Prandom P, Brandjes D, et al. Detection of deep-vein thrombosis by real time-B mode ultrasonography. *N Engl J Med* 1989; 320(6):342–345.

56. Metzler M, Silver D. Vasospastic disorders. *Postgrad Med* 1979; 65(2):79–85.

57. Dowd P, Goldsmith P, Bull H, et al. Raynaud's phenomenon. *Lancet* 1995; (8970):283–290.

58. Black C. Update on Raynaud's phenomenon. *Br J Hosp Med* 1994; 52:555–557.

59. Mehle AL, Nedorost S, Camisa C. Erythromelalgia. *Int J Dermatol* 1990; 29:567–570.

60. Healsmith MF, Graham-Brown RA, Burns DA. Erythromelalgia. *Clin Exp Dermatol* 1991; 16:46–48.

61. Drenth JP, Michiels JJ. Treatment options in primary erythermalgia. *Am J Hematol* 1993; 43:154.

62. Muhiddin KA, Gallen IW, Harris S, et al. The use of capsaicin cream in a case of erythromelalgia. *Postgrad Med J* 1994; 70:841–843.

63. Simon HB. Current concepts: Hyperthermia. *N Engl J Med* 1993; 329:483–487.

64. Saper CB, Breder CD. Seminars in medicine of the Beth Israel Hospital, Boston: The neurological basis of fever. *N Engl J Med* 1994; 330:1880–1886.

65. Sullivan F, Hutchinson M, Bahandeka S, et al. Chronic hypothermia in multiple sclerosis. *J Neurol Neurosurg Psychiatry* 1987; 50: 813–815.

66. Geny C, Pradat PF, Yulis J, et al. Hypothermia, Wernicke encephalopathy and multiple sclerosis. *Acta Neurol Scand* 1992; 86:632–634.

67. White KD, Scoones DJ, Newman PK. Hypothermia in multiple sclerosis. *J Neurol Neurosurg Psychiatry* 1996; 61:369–375.

68. O'Brien H. Amess JAL, Mollin DL, Recurrent thrombocytopenia, erythroid hypoplasia and sideroblastic anaemia associated with hypothermia. *Br J Haematol* 1982; 51:451–456.

69. Avis SP, Pryse-Phillips WE. Sudden death in multiple sclerosis associated with sun exposure: A report of two cases. *Can J Neurol Sci* 1995; 22:305–307.

70. Lawden MC, Blunt S, Matthews T, et al. Recurrent confusion and ataxia triggered by pyrexia in a case of occult multiple sclerosis. *J Neurol Neurosurg Psychiatry* 1994; 57:1436–1443.

71. Guthrie TC, Nelson DA. Influence of temperature changes on multiple sclerosis: Critical review of mechanisms and research potential. *J Neurol Sci* 1995; 129:1–8.

72. Karaszewski JW, Reder AT, Maselli R, Brown M, Arnason BG. Sympathetic skin responses are decreased and lymphocyte beta-adrenergic receptors are increased in progressive multiple sclerosis. *Ann Neurol* 1990; 27: 366–372.

73. Sato K, Kang WM, Saga K, et al. Biology of sweat glands and their disorders. I. Normal sweat gland function. *J Am Acad Dermatol* 1989; 20:537–563.

74. Sato K, Kang WH, Saga K, et al. Biology of sweat glands and their disorders. II. Disorders of sweat gland function. *J Am Acad Dermatol* 1989; 20:713–726.

28 Dysphagia

Jeri A. Logemann, Ph.D.

This chapter examines normal swallowing physiology and neurophysiology and the swallowing disorders typically seen as a result of multiple sclerosis (MS). Dysphagia in patients with MS is compared with swallowing disorders that result from other progressive neurologic diseases and sudden-onset neurologic damage. Optimal management of swallowing disorders in patients with MS is presented, including evaluation strategies and treatment procedures. The chapter ends with a discussion of research needs.

NORMAL SWALLOW PHYSIOLOGY AND NEUROPHYSIOLOGY

Normal swallow function involves intricate and rapid coordination of sensory and motor activity in the oral cavity, pharynx, and esophagus to recognize food and accept it into the mouth; to detect the food's texture, taste, and so forth; and to reduce it to a consistency that is ready for swallow, form the food into a cohesive ball or bolus, and then propel the food from the oral cavity through the pharynx and esophagus to the stomach (1).

Normal oromotor control for swallow involves lip closure to keep food in the mouth while nasal breathing is maintained; facial tone to close the sulcus or space between the facial muscles and facial skeleton; rotary lateral jaw motion if chewing is required; and rotary lateral tongue motion to control food in the mouth, to bring it to the teeth if chewing is needed, and to form the masticated food into a ball or bolus. If strong chewing is not needed, the soft palate is pulled down and forward to keep food in the oral cavity and allow for a nasal airway during chewing and swallowing.

As food is being chewed, sensory receptors in the oral cavity identify its viscosity and volume so that when chewing is finished, the food can be organized into a single bolus or subdivided into a volume that can be easily swallowed. Once oral manipulation and chewing are completed and the bolus is formed, the tongue shapes itself around the food to initiate the oral stage of swallowing, with the periphery of the tongue sealed to the alveolar ridge. The oral stage of swallowing is characterized by an upward and backward motion of the midline of the tongue against the palate, applying backward pressure to the most anterior part of the food, thus propelling it backward and downward to the pharynx.

The pharyngeal swallow is activated as the food reaches the back of the oral cavity and the top of the pharynx. Sensory information from the oral cavity to the medulla is conducted via the sensory branches of cranial nerves IX and X. It has been hypothesized that at the medulla, specifically the nucleus tractus solitarius (NTS), there is a sensory recognition center that identifies the stimulus as a swallow stimulus rather than another type of stimulus such as a gag stimulus. When the sensory information has been decoded at the NTS, the information is sent to the neighboring nucleus ambiguus, where the motor response needed to actualize the pharyngeal stage of swallowing is initiated. This motor response in the pharynx is mediated by cranial nerves X and XII. The swallow center in the medulla also receives information from the pontine swallow center in the higher brainstem and from the cortex. Volitional intent to swallow initiated at the cortex may play an important role in triggering or initiation of the pharyngeal stage of swallowing.

Whereas the oral stage of swallowing is largely mechanical, designed to break down food to a consistency that is appropriate for swallow, the pharyngeal stage of swallow involves (1) coordination of a number of valves that direct food appropriately through the pharynx, and (2) generation of pressure to drive food through the pharynx. Swallowing is *not* a gravitational process but requires active pressure to efficiently move food or liquid through the pharynx.

Three valve mechanisms are activated during the pharyngeal swallow: (1) velopharyngeal, (2) laryngeal, and (3) cricopharyngeal, as well as generation of pressure. The velopharyngeal valve must close completely and in a timely manner to prevent food from going up the nose and to enable the generation of pressure lower in the pharynx. The laryngeal valve at the top of the airway must close bottom to top. The most critical level of closure is at the entrance to the airway between the base of the epiglottis and the anterior tilting arytenoid with contraction of the false vocal folds. The third valve, the cricopharyngeal, must open at the appropriate moment to enable food to enter the esophagus. Opening of the cricopharyngeal valve or upper esophageal sphincter is complex in nature and involves relaxation of the muscular portion of the valve (i.e., the cricopharyngeal muscle) and anterior and vertical motion of the larynx, which opens the sphincter, followed by pressure within the bolus itself as it passes through the sphincter, which widens its opening.

The esophageal phase of swallow begins as the bolus leaves the upper esophageal sphincter and esophageal peristalsis is initiated. Esophageal muscle contraction is sequential, again applying pressure to the most posterior portion of the bolus, propelling it sequentially through the esophagus and into the stomach. Generally, there is a primary peristaltic or contraction wave followed by a secondary wave. These two contractile waves effectively clear the esophagus of all food. As the food reaches the bottom of the esophagus, the lower esophageal sphincter, which is a muscle sphincter, relaxes and opens, which enables the food to enter the stomach. Muscle contraction then closes the sphincter.

In contrast to the lower esophageal sphincter, the upper esophageal, or cricopharyngeal, sphincter is comprised of muscle posteriorly and laterally but cartilage anteriorly (i.e., the cricoid cartilage). Thus the dynamics of the opening and closure of the upper esophageal sphincter are more complex than those of the lower sphincter.

The velopharyngeal, laryngeal, and cricopharyngeal valves must function completely and rapidly to enable the bolus to pass through the pharynx, generally in less than half a second. For the bolus to pass through the pharynx *efficiently*, there must be adequate pressure generated, first by the oral tongue motion, followed by posterior movement of the base of the tongue and the anterior and mesial movement of the pharyngeal walls, which meet and contact the backward-moving tongue base. Tongue base and pharyngeal wall action take over pressure generation from the oral tongue when the tail or last portion of the food reaches the tongue base. Pressure is always applied to the last portion or tail of the food bolus to propel it downward toward the esophagus and stomach.

All of these oral and pharyngeal activities increase in strength as the viscosity or thickness of the food increases. The exact timing these movements varies systematically with the volume of the bolus as well. In general, the valve functions prolong as the volume of food increases. Thus the normal swallow changes systematically based on the characteristics of the material being swallowed.

Almost the entire central nervous system (CNS) is involved in the control of swallowing. The major swallow center is in the medulla, as indicated earlier, with multiple cranial nerve involvement. However, cortical input to the brainstem centers is critical in the recognition of food in the mouth and the initiation of appropriate oromotor motions in response to the presence of food. A part of the sensory recognition of food in the mouth may well be the hand-to-mouth coordination needed to place food in the oral cavity. This hand-to-mouth movement provides ample time to alert the cortex and the brainstem that food is approaching the oral cavity. The taste of food is a critical sensory stimulus, with most of the sensory nerves for the primary taste sensations ending at the nucleus tractus solitarius.

SWALLOWING DISORDERS THAT RESULT FROM MULTIPLE SCLEROSIS

Because of the wide variation in CNS involvement in MS, there is potential for abnormality in almost every aspect of swallowing physiology in MS patients (1–3). Several studies point to particular features that occur more commonly in these patients. A delay in triggering the pharyngeal swallow is a common feature of dysphagia in patients with MS (4). This disorder results in food entering the pharynx before the pharyngeal motor response has been initiated, so the airway is open and the cricopharyngeal valve is closed. A common symptom of a delay in triggering the pharyngeal swallow is difficulty in managing thin liquids. Thin liquids are swallowed in larger volumes and move slightly more quickly in the oral cavity and pharynx, thus splashing directly into the open airway during a pharyngeal delay.

Another common swallowing disorder in these patients is reduced pharyngeal wall contraction, which results in food being left behind in the pharynx after the swallow. When the swallow is inefficient in this way, the residual food may fall or be sucked into the open airway when the patient breathes after the swallow. Velopharyngeal deficits also frequently occur in patients with MS. Poor velopharyngeal closure results in food entering the nose during the swallow and contributes to inefficient swallowing. In and of itself, however, a velopharyngeal deficit is not a major swallow impairment. If it is combined with reduced pharyngeal wall activity, however, pressure generation is further reduced because any pressure generated in the pharynx escapes through the nose.

Because of the wide variability in CNS damage in patients with MS, the wide range of severity of the disease, and the patterns of exacerbation and remission, there is much variability in other swallowing disorders observed in patients with the disease. The patient may exhibit reduced lip closure or facial tone because of facial nerve involvement. He or she may exhibit reduced tongue coordination or range of motion because of involvement of cranial nerve XII. Tongue base action or pharyngeal wall activity may be reduced because of damage to cranial nerve X. Involvement of cranial nerve X also may affect laryngeal function, interfering with airway closure during swallow.

Very few studies of esophageal involvement in patients with MS have been conducted (5). However, there is indication that involvement of cranial nerve X may result in esophageal swallowing disorders, including disturbed peristalsis.

Patients with MS also may exhibit food aversions or specific negative reactions to particular tastes or textures (6). If the patient is in the advanced stages of MS and exhibits any dementia, he or she also may exhibit difficulty in feeding, with lack of recognition of food approaching or in the mouth and a delayed onset of any oral manipulation as a result.

In summary, any of the neuromuscular actions that comprise normal swallow may be affected by MS (1,4,5,7–12) Sensory recognition of volume and viscosity of food also may be impaired such that the patient does not manage the normal physiologic shifts in the mechanism required to handle the various food and/or liquid volumes and viscosities because he or she has no oral sensory recognition of these differences.

DIFFERENTIAL DIAGNOSIS

Patients with MS who develop dysphagia generally do so later in the course of the disease rather than as an early sign of the disease, although the latter may occur. In contrast to other degenerative neurologic diseases, dysphagia resulting from MS typically exhibits exacerbation and remission in parallel with other disease symptoms. In contrast, people with Parkinson's disease often exhibit swallow changes early in the course of the disease, with a characteristic tongue pattern of rocking and rolling motion during swallow as well as tremor activity in the oral cavity, pharynx, and/or larynx even at rest. People with motor neuron disease such as amyotrophic lateral sclerosis typically have a reduction in tongue strength exhibited as increasing inefficiency of swallow as food becomes thicker and thicker and they cannot recruit the increased number of motor neurons needed to increase pressure on the food. The patient with myasthenia gravis typically exhibits fatigue associated with swallowing over time, such as less good function at the end of a meal than at the beginning of a meal. This behavior also may occur in MS patients, but it tends to occur when the disease has progressed to advanced stages.

Patients who have suffered sudden-onset neurologic damage such as stroke exhibit sudden onset of dysphagia with other clinical signs of infarct or hemorrhage (8). However, there may be patients with a small brainstem stroke whose swallow pattern may be the only symptom. Swallow dysfunction after brainstem stroke typically is quite different from that of a patient with MS. Brainstem stroke usually results in reduced laryngeal upward and forward motion, with resulting reduction in opening of the upper esophageal sphincter and unilateral pharyngeal wall damage. These are not typical swallowing disorders in patients with MS. History also is an important feature that distinguishes MS patients from patients with other neurologic damage or disease (1).

OPTIMAL MANAGEMENT OF DYSPHAGIA IN MULTIPLE SCLEROSIS

Optimal management of dysphagia begins with identification of the specific disorders present in a particular patient (13). This type of careful assessment of the neuromotor mechanisms involved in swallowing is particularly critical in MS patients because of the potential for a wide range of disorders. The assessment usually begins with a clinical evaluation in which a good detailed history is taken regarding the nature of the patient's symptoms, his or her complaints about difficulty with particular foods, and a history of onset of the disorder (9). Clinical assessment also involves a careful cranial nerve examination looking at range, rate, and coordination of movements of the face, lips, tongue, and palate, and indirect judgment of laryngeal function through tasks in which speech and voice are produced. Observation of the patient as he or she swallows very small amounts of selected foods, such as liquid and pudding, may provide important information but should not be used for a true differential diagnosis or a meaningful assessment of swallow function. The complexity of the swallow, particularly in the pharynx, makes any judgments from visual observations of the patient eating highly inaccurate. Data have shown that judgments as "simple" as whether a patient is aspirating (i.e., getting food in the airway) are 40 percent inaccurate from observation of individuals swallowing or eating (1,14). Thus, most patients who have MS with suspected dysphagia require an instrumental assessment that enables objective assessment of swallow physiology. Use of such screening tools as the 3-ounce water test provide little information at potentially high risk to the patient if he or she aspirates part or all of the water bolus (15,16).

Videofluoroscopic examination or the modified barium swallow (MBS) is the most commonly used diagnostic procedure to define the patient's swallow physiology because it reveals the largest number of physiologic elements comprising the swallow (17). The MBS enables the examiner to define movement of the food in relation to movement of the oropharyngeal structures. The MBS typically involves the patient's completing several swallows of various measured volumes of thin liquid, cup drinking, pudding, and at least one masticated material or other foods the patient may have particular difficulty swallowing. Following definition of the exact nature of the disorder(s) present, the MBS also involves presenting interventions to the patient to reduce the sequelae of any disorders such as aspiration or residue. As described in the subsequent section on treatment, a number of therapies can improve the swallow immediately and may be assessed in the radiographic study. The resulting report should provide a description of the patient's physiologic or anatomic swallowing abnormalities; any symptoms associated with the problem, such as aspiration or residue; results of any treatments attempted; and recommendations for treatment and dietary intake.

A second instrumental procedure used to examine some aspects of swallowing is videoendoscopy or fiberoptic endoscopic examination of swallowing (FEES). In this procedure, a 3-mm endoscope is placed through the nose and over the soft palate to examine the pharynx before and after swallow. The actual swallow is not observed because the pharyngeal mechanism closes around the tube. This assessment serves more as a screening instrument than as a diagnostic procedure. This procedure may not be possible in patients who have a hyperactive gag reflex.

Manometry measures the pressures generated during the swallow and may identify any abnormalities in pressure generation (1). In order to be useful and accurate in the pharynx, manometry usually is combined with fluoroscopy so that the movements in the mouth and pharynx that generate pressures may be examined in conjunction with the actual pressures generated. Like endoscopy, manometry requires placement of a tube (approximately 3 mm in diameter) through the nose and into the pharynx and cervical esophagus. Manometry also may be performed in the esophagus, in which case videofluoroscopy is not required.

Other instrumental procedures can examine selected aspects of swallow such as electromyography, which can be used to examine the function of particular muscles during swallow (1). Ultrasonography can examine tongue motion during swallow, but only soft tissues in the oral cavity can be identified and the food swallowed cannot be seen. Scintigraphy can be used to examine reflux and transit times in the mouth and pharynx, as well as to measure the amount of aspiration. Scintigraphy involves swallowing a radioactive bolus, which is then tracked with a gamma camera as it moves through the oral cavity and pharynx. The images are of the bolus, not of the structures surrounding and propelling it. The exact amount of aspiration can be calculated by the amount of radiation that enters the airway. Reflux can be monitored by measuring the amount of food that is swallowed into the stomach and then reassessing at intervals afterward to define any increase in the volume of food in the esophagus or pharynx, or even in the airway. In general, videofluoroscopy has been used most frequently to assess swallowing in patients with MS. It is the simplest technique to perform and provides the most information about the swallow.

Treatment procedures most frequently involve behavioral and/or rehabilitative strategies. Rehabilitative strategies may include changing the individual's head or body posture, thereby changing the dimensions of the pharynx and the way in which food flows through the mouth and pharynx (18). Posture must be selected to match the patient's swallow disorder(s). Heightening sensory input by presenting the individual with a bolus of a particular taste or particular volume, or by using a sensory enhancement technique such as thermal-tactile stimulation, may be helpful in reducing pharyngeal delay. In thermal-tactile stimulation, a size 00 laryngeal mirror is used to rub the anterior faucial arches to stimulate sensory receptors in the faucial arches that carry sensory information to the brainstem and cortex about the need to trigger a pharyngeal swallow. Sensory enhancement procedures may be used on a regular basis in a compensatory program as well as in a rehabilitative mode, in which they are used for a short period of time and then withdrawn.

Controlling the volume and speed of eating also may improve the patient's swallow. If a patient tries to swallow too much food too quickly, he or she may literally "over-stuff the mechanism" and cause the symptoms to worsen. If the individual has slowed movement of the bolus or a mild delay in triggering the pharyngeal swallow, he or she may not have difficulty as long as smaller boluses of particular thicknesses are maintained. However, if one takes larger amounts too quickly, the amount of residue or the amount of material entering the airway may increase dramatically.

There also are a number of voluntary swallowing maneuvers that may be taught to the patient with a particular swallow disorder (1,17). For example, the supraglottic swallow, which involves voluntarily holding the breath before and during the swallow, closes the vocal folds and thus the airway before and during the swallow. The supersupraglottic swallow closes the airway entrance before and during the swallow and involves holding the breath and bearing down with effort. There are maneuvers to increase the pressure generated during swallow and to improve the laryngeal motion and opening of the upper esophageal sphincter. These maneuvers require increased muscle effort and may or may not be appropriate in the patient with MS.

The interaction of fatigue and dysphagia often is overlooked. This interaction is similar to fatigue with walking, in which a patient starts on a walk without difficulty only to develop leg weakness if the walk is extended. A patient with MS may have no swallowing problems at the beginning of a meal but may develop swallowing difficulties during a long meal, especially one that involves extensive chewing. Therefore, advising patients to take rest periods during long meals and/or to eat more often for a shorter time may help prevent this problem.

Pharmacologic Management

No known drug therapies have been found to be effective for particular aspects of the oropharyngeal swallow. However, some patients with dysphagia resulting from MS find that drug therapies used for management of an exacerbation may improve not only other aspects of their neuromuscular function but also their oropharyngeal swallow. Unfortunately, there are no studies of which types of drug therapy have the most effect on swallowing function. Much research is needed in this area.

Surgical Management

Surgical management generally is the treatment of last choice for dysphagia. Like drug therapies, few surgical procedures have been found to improve swallowing function. Surgeries that have been used in patients with a swallowing disorder include a cricopharyngeal myotomy designed to cut the muscular portion of the upper esophageal sphincter. Unfortunately, because most of the disorders in this sphincter result from failure of the larynx to move up and forward, myotomy often has no major effect. Surgical procedures to prevent aspiration by such means as suturing the vocal folds closed or suturing the epiglottis over the top of the airway have not been found to be uniformly successful and have not been used in patients with MS. Similarly, other laryngeal surgeries to reduce aspiration have not been used in these patients nor have they been found to be widely successful in other types of dysphagic patients.

RESEARCH NEEDS

More research is needed to fully understand swallow disorders in MS as they relate to the location of damage in the CNS. Such studies are likely to occur as neuroimaging continues to improve because a great deal may be learned about the effects of damage to the CNS and its impact on swallowing function. Similarly, studies of swallowing treatment(s) need to be completed in groups of patients with MS to assess efficacy with this population. This type of study is difficult because of the great variability in the MS population. A treatment procedure that may work well with a particular patient may not have as much effect in another individual. However, even case studies would be welcome. The exacerbation and remission pattern in MS also makes treatment research difficult because one cannot always tie the improvement in swallowing to the therapy alone. Change may be related to remission. However, these difficulties should not dissuade investigators from systematically examining the dysphagia caused by MS. Much is to be learned from this population, and much can be gained for the patient with better understanding of the neurophysiology of dysphagia and the effects of management procedures.

References

1. Logemann JA. *Evaluation and treatment of swallowing disorders.* 2nd ed. Austin, TX: Pro-Ed, 1998.
2. Jones B, Ravich WJ, Donner MW. Dysphagia in systemic disease. *Dysphagia* 1993; 8:368–383.
3. DeLisa JA, Miller RM, Mikulic MA, Hammond MC. Multiple sclerosis: Part II. Common functional problems and rehabilitation. *Am Fam Phys* 1985; 32:127–132.
4. Fabiszak A. Swallowing patterns in neurologically normal subjects and two subgroups of multiple sclerosis patients. Unpublished doctoral dissertation, Northwestern University, Evanston, IL, 1987.
5. Daly DD, Code CF, Anderson JA. Disturbances of swal-

lowing and esophageal motility in patients with multiple sclerosis. *Neurology* 1962; 12:250.

6. Catalanotto FA, Dore-Duffy P, Donaldson J, et al. Quality specific taste changes in multiple sclerosis. *Ann Neurol* 1984; 16:611.

7. Brin M, Younger D. Neurologic disorders and aspiration. *Otolaryngol Clin North Am* 1988; 21:691–700.

8. Buchholz DW, Robbins JA. Neurologic disease affecting oropharyngeal swallowing. In: Perlman AL, Schulze-Delrieu K (eds.). *Deglutition and its disorders*. San Diego: Singular Publishing Group, 1997:319–342.

9. Guily JL, Perie SP, Willig TN, Chaussade S, Eymard B, Angelard B. Swallowing disorders in muscular diseases: Functional assessment and indication of cricopharyngeal myotomy. *Ear Nose Throat J* 1994; 73:34–40.

10. Kilman W, Goyal R. Disorders of pharyngeal and upper esophageal sphincter motor function. *Arch Intern Med* 1976; 136:592–601.

11. Silbiger M, Piknielney R, Donner M. Neuromuscular disorders affecting the pharynx: Cineradiographic analysis. *Invest Radiol* 1967; 2:442–448.

12. Sorensen P, Brown S, Logemann JA, Wilson K, Herndon R. MS care: Communication disorders and dysphagia. *J Neuro Rehab* 1994; 8:137–143.

13. Scheinberg L, Smith CR. Rehabilitation of patients with multiple sclerosis. *Neurol Clin* 1987; 54:585–600.

14. Splaingard ML, Hutchins B, Sulton LD, Chaudhuri G. Aspiration in rehabilitation patients: Videofluoroscopy vs. bedside clinical assessment. *Arch Phys Med Rehabil* 1988; 69:637–640.

15. Nathadwarawala KM, Nicklin J, Wiles CM. A timed test of swallowing capacity for neurological patients. *J Neurol Neurosurg Psychiatry* 1992; 55:822–825.

16. Nathadwarawala KM, McGroary A, Wiles CM. Swallowing in neurological outpatients: Use of a timed test. *Dysphagia* 1994; 9:120–129.

17. Logemann JA. *A manual for videofluoroscopic evaluation of swallowing.* 2nd ed. Austin, TX: Pro-Ed, 1993.

18. Rasley A, Logemann JA, Kahrilas PJ, et al. Prevention of barium aspiration during videofluoroscopic swallowing studies: Value of change in posture. *Am J Roentol* 1993; 160:1005–1009.

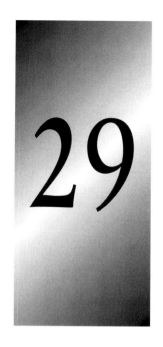

29 Alternative and Complementary Therapies

Catherine W. Britell, M.D., and Jack S. Burks, M.D.

Many treatments that do not appear in the conventional scientific literature are believed by a significant number of consumers and many practitioners to be effective in some way to improve health and/or impart a feeling of well-being. When these therapies are combined with traditional medical practices, they are termed *complementary* or *adjunctive* therapies (1,2). When they are used in place of conventional medical treatments, they are called *alternative* therapies. A term commonly used to categorize both of these applications is *complementary and alternative medicine* (CAM).

Complementary and alternative therapies fall into three basic categories:

1. Those for which there is scientific evidence of safety and efficacy;
2. Those based on reasonable scientific principles but whose safety and efficacy have yet to be proven; and
3. Those with or without theoretical basis that have been shown to be ineffective and/or unsafe. Unfortunately, the methodology used for evaluation of many CAM therapies has been inconsistent, thus reducing the credibility of the data and making objective evaluation of therapeutic claims difficult (3).

The use of alternative therapies, including physical modalities and ingested substances, is very prevalent among individuals with MS (4). Fawcett (5) and Stenager and coworkers (6) report that 27 percent to 55 percent of MS patients admit to seeking out one or more of these treatments. They also found that use of alternative therapies was higher among individuals with a high level of social stress and greater physical disability. Treatments most often used included massage, acupuncture, aquatic therapy, therapeutic touch, yoga, passive exercise, and removal of mercury alloy tooth fillings. Searles and Murray (7) reported that 85 percent of MS patients used some form of CAM therapy during the course of their disease. In their Canadian study, they found no correlation of the incidence of use of CAM with age, gender, level of education, or degree of disability. Up to one third of MS patients report that they have sustained increased function or a decrease in symptoms as a result of alternative treatments.

Bowling (8) reviewed the literature on the current herbs and vitamin therapy used by MS patients. At least 14 herbs stimulated T cells and macrophage activity, and more than 40 herbs interacted with medications frequently prescribed to MS patients. Five herbs recommended for the treatment of MS might produce serious toxicity. For example, antioxidant vitamins may stimulate the immune system. He reported that no scientific evidence supports vitamins as helpful in MS patients. A discrepancy between the perceived usefulness of CAM between patients and physicians was found. For example, only 19 percent of patients thought that alternative medicines were not helpful, whereas 43 percent of physicians believed that CAM treatments were not helpful. Thirty-two percent of patients believed that diets were helpful, whereas only 17 percent of physicians concurred. Twenty percent of MS patients believed that oil of primrose was helpful, whereas only 4 percent of physicians believed this to be true. Interestingly, only 14 percent of MS patients thought that yoga was helpful, although 28 percent of physicians believed in the benefits of yoga.

People with MS often seek an alternative health practitioner or treatment because conventional physicians do not offer curative treatments and many also do not offer supportive or symptomatic therapies. Deepak Chopra (9) writes that the goal of CAM therapies is to balance the mind, the body, and the environment harmoniously to help people deal with stressful life situations. This concept has great appeal to people with chronic diseases such as MS.

The rationales for the use of complementary and alternative therapies and available data regarding their safety and effectiveness are presented in this chapter to help health care professionals understand the CAM therapies their patients are using, how they may interact with other prescribed therapies, and how to advise patients regarding specific therapies.

A REASONED APPROACH TO THE PATIENT USING CAM THERAPIES

It is important that MS health care practitioners do not ignore CAM therapies because to do so isolates them from an aspect of their patient's health care. Once practitioners become knowledgeable about these therapies, they will be in a better position to help patients integrate them into their health care needs with reason and wisdom.

Even when scientific data on CAM therapy is lacking, the health care professional can still help the patient. A useful strategy is to ask the patient to bring information about a specific product or service and take the time to review and discuss the material with him or her. Irrespective of the ensuing advice, a climate of mutual respect and caring is established. Table 29-1 outlines one useful approach to a patient's inquiries about CAM.

Bringing up the subject of CAM with the patient and family is the responsibility of the health practitioner. Although most MS patients make use of various CAM modalities, more than half do not tell their health care providers about their CAM therapies. Many physicians do not specifically ask their patients about CAM. Some patients fear that their admission of CAM treatments would nega-

---

TABLE 29-1
Approach to Inquiries on CAM

- Include CAM use as part of the initial and interim medical history
- Review the available data (including media reports) about its mechanism of action, efficacy, and adverse effects
- Understand patient's motivation and perception of the value of the CAM
- Explain the risks of CAM (patients already know the proposed benefits)
- Discuss the long-term cost of the therapy
- Educate the patient and family about the need for scientific data (versus anecdotes)
- Help the patient and family balance the perceived benefits, risks, and costs of the therapy
- Integrate, compare, and contrast CAM therapy with the current (proven) patient therapy
- Express an opinion on the CAM therapy in question
- Reassure the patient and family that you respect their decision-making rights
- Reassure the patient that his or her regular medical care will continue, regardless of their decision to use CAM therapies

---

tively affect their relationship with the physician, and many physicians just do not want to deal with this issue. This "conspiracy of silence" reduces the opportunity for patients to make reasonable informed choices about an important aspect of their care while increasing potential risks.

LIFE ENHANCEMENT THERAPIES VERSUS SPECIFIC SYMPTOM MANAGEMENT THERAPIES

Many CAM treatments are geared toward life enhancement and make no specific claims of curing or mitigating the effects of MS. Although these treatments may help alleviate suffering, they are unlikely to change objective physical and laboratory findings associated with MS. T'ai Chi and yoga are two examples of life-enhancement therapies that are widely used by MS patients and comprehensive MS programs (10). Although specific scientific data are sparse, most patients who participate in these activities have an enhanced feeling of well-being and increased control of their lives. Balanced nutritional counseling and stress management, including meditation, are other examples of health maintenance strategies that are generally accepted as useful by patients and practitioners. These modalities usually are safe and often are not costly. Once taught, they can be used for a lifetime.

On the other hand, therapies that claim to affect the disease course or specific MS symptoms require rigorous investigation. For example, proponents for the removal of mercury-based dental amalgams as a specific treatment to modify the disease course theorize that MS is related to mercury toxicity. This theory has little scientifically valid data (11). In this case, as with other agents claimed to modify disease or symptoms, the proof of efficacy is the responsibility of the proponents of the theory. If controlled clinical trials have not been published, health care professionals should be cautious in their recommendations.

TABLE 29-2
CAM Systems Organized Around Specific Practitioners
• Traditional Chinese medicine (TCM)   Acupuncture   Qigong
• Ayurveda
• Chiropractic medicine
• Homeopathy
• Naturopathy

THE PLACEBO RESPONSE

Part of the confusion surrounding the efficacy of treatments in MS is the placebo response. For example, in an early study on adrenocorticotropic hormone (ACTH) treatment for MS exacerbations, most of the placebo treated patients improved (12). This study points out the need for rigorous randomized, double-blinded, placebo-controlled clinical trials before making therapeutic claims of disease modification.

Although the placebo response may serve to confuse our perception of treatment efficacy, it holds fascinating implications for overall care and promotion of patient well-being. We know that the placebo response is the most powerful scientifically based evidence of a mind–body connection, and if we can capitalize on that connection, we can enhance the efficacy of all of our treatments.

COMPLEMENTARY AND ALTERNATIVE MEDICINE: SPECIFIC PRACTICES

Traditional Chinese medicine, Eastern Indian medicine, African-American healing arts, and Native American medicine have a common thread in exploring the connection between mind, body, and spirit (13). Their approach emphasizes positivity, faith, and "healing" versus "curing," and their dependence on and promotion of the patient's belief system is a significant part of their practice. Table 29-2 lists CAM systems organized by specific practitioners.

Traditional Chinese Medicine (TCM)

Traditional Chinese medicine is more than 5,000 years old and embraces the concept of Chi or Qi or Ki (14–16). Chi represents energy flowing through channels in the body called meridians, which are not part of blood vessels or lymph channels. Twelve major meridians are derived from the environment, the heavens above and the earth below, including food, air, and water. Chi is an energy that exists throughout the environment, with the sun being a major source. Openings in the skin, called acupuncture or meridian points, absorb the Chi. Chi then flows through the entire body.

Traditional Chinese medicine also incorporates the concept of complementary opposites called the Yin and Yang. The Yin/Yang refers to a constant flow of energy from one polar extreme to another. Westerners see the Yin and Yang as good and evil, but TCM perceives a constant flux of energy without positive or negative connotation. Traditional Chinese medicine balances the Yin/Yang to avoid illness caused by an imbalance of these energy forces.

Acupuncture

The scope of practice of acupuncturists includes but is not limited to (1) using Oriental medical theory to assess and diagnose a patient, and (2) using Oriental medical theory to develop a plan to treat a patient.

Traditional acupuncture, as now practiced, involves the insertion of stainless steel needles into various body areas. These are classified by the U.S. Food and Drug Administration (FDA) as "Class II" medical devices and are certified for single use. A low-frequency current may be applied to the needles to produce greater stimulation. Other procedures used separately or in addition to classic acupuncture include moxibustion (burning of herbs applied to the skin); injection of sterile water, procaine, morphine, vitamins, or homeopathic solutions through the inserted needles; applications of laser beams (laser puncture); placement of needles in the external ear (auriculotherapy); and acupressure (use of manual pressure). In the United States, the American Academy of Medical Acupuncture trains physicians. However, most acupuncturists do not have a medical license. States that license acupuncturists most often require one to two years of preprofessional training in an accredited post-secondary institution before a three- or four-year course of study in acupuncture, and passing a recognized national board examination and/or a state examination. Acupuncture is now reimbursed through some medical plans.

Acupuncture has been shown to be effective in managing post-chemotherapy nausea and vomiting (17) and in acute dental pain (18). Steinberger (19) reported on use of acupuncture in a series of MS patients, showed only anecdotal results without controls, and did not show significant benefit. On the other hand, Wang and colleagues (20) at the University of British Columbia received mailed surveys from 52 percent of 627 MS patients and found that 25 percent of respondents used acupuncture and reported improvements such as reduced pain; decreased spasticity; improved bowel and bladder function; reduced paresthesias; and improvement in energy levels, sleep, strength, walking, and coordination.

Qigong

Another TCM modality called Qigong is gaining popularity in the United States. Qigong encompasses deep breathing, movement, and energy flow divided into "internal Chi" and "external Chi." These are said to interact to create a healing effect in diseases. Although primarily used in cancer treatments, its influence in chronic illnesses is growing. Studies of the efficacy of Qigong in MS have not been reported (15).

Ayurveda

Ayurveda is an ancient Eastern Indian system of medicine based on the theory that all intelligence and wisdom flow from one Absolute source (Paramatman) (21). Health is thought to be related to the grace of the Absolute acting through the laws of Nature (Prakriti). Ayurveda assists Nature by promoting harmony between the individual and Nature by living a life of balance according to its laws. Ayurvedic physicians emphasize the need for preserving the alliance between the mind and the body and offer people tools for remembering and nurturing the subtler aspects of their humanity. Ayurveda seeks to heal the fragmentation and disorder of the mind–body complex and restore wholeness and harmony to all people. Deepak Chopra is a major proponent of Ayurvedic medicine in the United States (9). Philosophically, Ayurveda has much in common with Traditional Chinese medicine. These two care systems are the major components of what Western medicine health care professionals call "Eastern medicine."

Ayurvedic physicians use meditation, counseling, and herbal potions as the mainstay of treatment. A number of studies of ayurvedic preparations demonstrate an effect on platelet aggregation, neurotransmission, and other physiologic parameters. The specific effect of ayurvedic treatment on the manifestation or disease process of MS has not been studied.

Chiropractic Medicine

Chiropractic medicine includes the adjustment and/or manipulation of the articulations of the spine and related structures. During the initial consultation and before commencing chiropractic care, a chiropractor identifies a clinical condition that warrants chiropractic treatment on the basis of physical examination and skeletal radiographs. The chiropractor's practice often includes the following:

- The ordering, taking, and interpretation of x-rays limited to the skeletal systems
- The ordering, but not performing, of other laboratory tests consistent with chiropractic practice
- The ordering or performing of reagent strip tests (dipstick urinalysis)
- The ordering, but not performing, of other diagnostic or analytic tests consistent with chiropractic practice, including, for example, computerized axial tomography (CT), magnetic resonance imaging (MRI), bone scan, and needle electromyography (EMG)
- The ordering and performing of other diagnostic or analytic tests such as neurocalometer, thermography, and noninvasive muscle testing.

A chiropractor often gives general nutritional advice to a patient when such advice is incidental to the chiropractic care being provided. In most states, a chiropractor is not allowed to dispense or derive any financial benefit from the sale of vitamins, food products, or nutritional supplements, or to represent himself/herself as a nutritional consultant. Chiropractors often order or administer physical modalities in conjunction with spinal adjustment.

Most states that license chiropractors require four years of training in an approved chiropractic school after two years of preprofessional college education. A three-part national board examination and a state board examination are often required. In many areas older practitioners continue to be licensed but have not met recently established requirements.

Chiropractic has been scientifically proven to be effective in the treatment of acute low back pain (22,23). There are no studies in the literature on the efficacy of chiropractic for symptoms of MS, although one anecdotal report of chiropractic treatment for MS is found in the chiropractic literature (24). Some MS health care professionals express concern about spinal manipulation in MS patients, especially in those with evidence of acute spinal cord disease.

Homeopathy

Homeopathic medicine is a form of energy medicine (vibrational medicine) whose major theoretical principles include the following (15):

- A substance with specific effects and a healthy person can cure a person with similar symptoms
- The process of repeated dilution and vigorous shaking of harmful substances renders them medically active yet free of side effects
- Each body has only one soul; thus a person has only one core problem at a time, and only one remedy is necessary for a "curative action"
- Proper selection of a remedy requires taking into account numerous details about the patient's situation.
- "Mind symptoms" usually are more important than physical symptoms
- Cures involve interaction of the soul and cogitative, affective, and physical processes. "Inner peace" usually is the first response to a remedy, "better energy" the second, and "physical cure" the last.

No scientific evidence supports homeopathic treatments for symptoms or the disease course of MS.

Naturopathy

A naturopathic physician (N.D.) practices as a primary care practitioner, with a strong emphasis on disease prevention and optimizing wellness (15). Disciplines and modalities used by most naturopaths include clinical nutrition, acupuncture, homeopathic medicine, botanical medicine, psychology, and counseling to encourage people to make lifestyle changes in support of their personal health. In some states, licensure requires attendance at a four-year graduate level naturopathic medical school followed by professional board examinations. Although the naturopath presents himself or herself as a "general practice physician," he or she generally is not licensed to prescribe antibiotics, immune-modifying drugs, steroids, antispasticity medication, or urinary antispasmodics. Therefore, they do not have access to many of the mainstream MS treatments. There are no data in the medical literature on the use or efficacy of these practitioners for MS.

LIFE-ENHANCEMENT THERAPIES

Various life enhancement therapies are listed in Table 29-3.

TABLE 29-3
Life-Enhancement Therapies

- Yoga
- Massage therapy
    Swedish massage
    Deep tissue massage
    Sports massage
    Acupressure
    Shiatsu
    Reflexology
- T'ai Chi
- Reiki
- Feldenkreis
- Meditation
    Biofeedback
    Visual imagery
    Spirituality, Faith, Prayer
    Hypnosis
- Therapeutic Touch
- Other Life-Enhancing Activities
    Journaling
    Humor
    Volunteerism
    Dance therapy
    Art therapy
    Aromatherapy
    Horseback Riding/Animal Interactions

Yoga

The word *Yoga* is derived from the Sanskrit root *yuj* meaning to bind, join, attach, and yolk, then to direct and concentrate one's attention on, to use, and apply (15). It also means union or communication. Yoga is one of the six orthodox systems of Eastern Indian philosophy. In modern practical terms, it is a system of exercise and meditation according to one of a number of traditional paths. Anecdotal reports indicate that Yoga improves coordination, strength, and overall functioning in neurologic conditions (25). No specific studies have yet been published in the scientific literature related to MS.

Massage Therapy

Massage therapy consists of using manual techniques on soft tissue (26). The basic requirements for licensure in most states usually is 500 hours of classroom training followed by written and practical examinations. However, many individuals practice massage therapy without state licensure. Types of massage include:

- *Swedish-esalen massage,* an oil massage that uses five types of manipulation: effleurage (long strokes), petrissage (kneading), friction (deep circular movement), tapotement (percussion), and vibration to promote relaxation, improve circulation, relieve tension, and expand the range of motion.

- *Deep tissue massage,* in which practitioner works through the muscle tension, layer by layer, reaching the deeper muscles.
- *Sports massage,* a highly specialized form of massage therapy, which begins with careful study of the movements involved in activity. Then the muscle and joint movements are analyzed. Finally, deep tissue strokes, muscle massage, release points, and joint movements are designed to correct harmful movement patterns and prevent tissue damage during exercise.
- *Acupressure,* a system of bodywork that uses pressure on specific meridian points to balance an individual's "Chi" or energy and bring about physical movements. Acupressure may be used in conjunction with oil massage or alone.
- *Shiatsu,* a Chinese modality in which the practitioner "creates a warm understanding through touch and pressure, thus promoting self-healing." The client is fully clothed to receive Shiatsu.
- *Reflexology,* which is similar in principle to shiatsu and acupressure. It focuses on points of the hand and feet that are believed to correspond to each organ, gland, or structure of the body.

T'ai Chi

T'ai chi is a Chinese martial art that is primarily practiced for its health benefits, including a means for dealing with tension and stress (27). T'ai chi emphasizes complete relaxation, and is also a form of meditation, or what has been called "meditation in motion." Although characterized by soft, slow, flowing movements, it emphasizes precise movements rather than brute strength. T'ai chi is taught at many community centers, senior centers, and martial arts schools. It improves balance and decreases falls in geriatric patients (28). One study of T'ai chi in MS provided an eight week T'ai chi program for 19 patients with MS (10). The study found that speed walking increased by 21 percent, and hamstring flexibility increased by 28 percent. Patients experienced improvement in vitality, social function, mental health, and the ability to carry out physical and emotional roles. Although this study did not have a control population, it encourages further research in T'ai chi's ability to maximize independence and improve quality of life.

Reiki

Reiki is another form of energy flow therapy or Ki (referred to as Chi or Qi in TCM) (14). The Ki is healing energy transmitted from the practitioner to the patient through touch. It originated in Japan and is now widely practiced in the United States. The Reiki practitioner gently places his or her hand on the fully clothed person in specific areas such as the head, chest, abdomen, and back for one or more minutes. One of the major applications of Reiki is for treatment of pain. No studies of the use of Reiki in MS have been reported.

Feldenkreis

Feldenkreis uses physical movement principles and martial arts understanding of force and energy (15). Attention to the functional interrelationship of movement and feeling states to create more natural and effective movement patterns. Multiple sclerosis patients often perceive an increase in flexibility and balance with the Feldenkreis method, although no study results have been published.

Meditation

Meditation is the process of consciously controlled force of the mind, which may take place when the thinking process has been stopped. It may be practiced within the framework of a number of religions, including Christianity, Buddhism, and Hinduism, or in the secular form as "transcendental meditation" (TM) The TM technique is practiced 15 to 20 minutes in the morning and evening while sitting comfortably with the eyes closed. During this process, the individual's awareness settles down and he experiences a unique state of restful alertness. The body becomes deeply relaxed; the mind transcends all mental activity to experience the simplest form of awareness—transcendental consciousness—where consciousness is open to itself. Transcendental meditation techniques were first widely described and codified by Mahareeshi Mahesh Yogi and are taught in franchised schools throughout the world (15).

One study has documented subjective improvement in fatigue and mobility in MS patients who meditate regularly (29). Other forms of meditation-type experiences, such as biofeedback, visual imagery, prayer, and hypnosis, have all been used in MS patients with anecdotal reports of improvement (30,31). These meditation modalities may be combined with faith and spiritualism to add comfort and life enhancement to MS patients. Most MS programs in the United States incorporate some form of meditation or related activities into an overall wellness program.

Therapeutic Touch

Delores Krieger, RN, PhD, and Dora Kunz developed therapeutic touch, which has been incorporated into some schools of nursing in the United States (32). The principle behind therapeutic touch is an energy flow from the hands of the practitioner to the patient. It is used to treat many illnesses, although no studies related to MS have been published.

Other Life-Enhancing Activities

Few scientific data have been published on the promotion of self-healing strategies, coping strategies, and control over difficult issues with MS. However, the costs are minimal and the perceived value often is high. Some of the activities are listed in the following sections.

Journaling

Writing down thoughts in a journal has shown to improve mental and physical well-being (33). "Journaling provides formance and substance to emotions and ideas. When fears and anxieties are swirling around inside, they can create a tornado of sensations that may feel overwhelming. Writing about feelings gives them expression and establishes their boundaries" (34).

Humor

The concept of humor as a therapeutic modality in illness was popularized by Norman Cousins in the *New England Journal of Medicine* in 1976 (35). Since that time, several scientific publications have shown neuroendocrine and neuroimmunology connections with humor related to illness. Although the effect of humor and laughter has not been specifically studied in MS patients, few can argue with the concept that humor, even in the most difficult of circumstances, lifts our spirits.

Volunteerism

One of the hallmarks of a high quality of life is the sense that we continue to make a contribution to improve the world around us. Even patients with serious chronic illnesses can improve their quality of life through volunteerism. Volunteerism has not been scientifically studied in MS, but most patients who become disabled report an enhanced feeling of well-being when they are helping others through a variety of volunteer activities. The role of the health care professional is to help the patient balance his or her disability issues with the appropriate volunteer activity. Volunteering a few hours a week can be life-enhancing.

Dance Therapy

Dance therapy can help transform emotional distress with a chronic illness to a creative outlet. Dance therapy can

have a beneficial effect on the emotional state and the sense of well-being of the MS patient. Focusing on the position of the body movements to music can create a calming effect even for patients using a wheelchair (36).

Art Therapy

Like many other life-enhancing therapies, expression of one's feelings and physical condition through art can be a release for negative emotions that impair the quality of life of patients with MS. Although not specific to MS, art therapy has been used since prehistoric time to express feelings and hope. Expressing thoughts and emotions through images and creating a sense of "who we are" in a picture or story may help MS patients through very disruptive times (36).

Aromatherapy

Aromatherapy proposes that certain substances produce a smell that can relax and promote a balance of the body, mind, and spirit. It is harmless, but no studies on its use in MS have been published (36).

Horseback Riding and Animal Interactions

Horseback riding for the disabled is more than relaxation. It can transmit the natural movements of the body during walking, which may have been lost from an exacerbation of MS. In addition, connecting with an animal such as a horse (or dog or cat) can create a reassuring sense of well-being for MS patients. Conversely, the loss of an animal may result in a profound grief reaction. Being supportive and sensitive to the interaction of MS patients with their animals demonstrates a caring manner, which solidifies the doctor–patient connection outside of the "Western medicine" therapeutic world.

INGESTED OR INJECTED SUBSTANCES

Table 29-4 outlines various ingested or injected substances that have been used in the treatment of MS.

St. John's Wort

St. John's wort is also known as goatweed, hypericum, and klamath weed (37–40). It belongs to a group of approximately 200 herbs in the family *hypericaceae*. The herb is found throughout Europe and the United States, producing golden yellow flowers that seem particularly abundant on June 24, the traditional birthday of St. John the Baptist. St. John's wort has been used as a folk remedy and, more recently in Europe, as a medically endorsed

---

TABLE 29-4
Ingested or Injected Substances

- St. John's wort
- Evening primrose oil
- Ginseng
- Ginkgo biloba
- Melatonin
- Pycnogenol
- DHEA
- Herbal energy enhancers
    5-hydroxytriptophane
    Citrus aurantium
    Ephedra
    Guaraná
- Vitamins
- Echinacea and astragalus
- Estrogen/progesterone
- Cannabis
- Bee sting therapy
- Noni juice
- Procarin®

---

treatment for anxiety, depression, and unrest (41). It has been found to have effects similar to those of selective serotonin reuptake inhibitors (SSRI). St. John's wort may increase eye and skin sensitivity to sunlight. Like many other antidepressants, St. John's wort may cause anxiety, sleeplessness, photosensitivity, and unwelcome personality changes in some people. It has not yet been studied specifically in MS patients, and its effect on the immune system is generally not known.

Evening Primrose Oil

Evening primrose oil contains linoleic acid (LA) and gamma-linoleic acid (GLA). An enriched oil obtained from the seeds of *Oenothera biennis L.* (Family *onagraceae*), evening primrose oil has been postulated to be important in the rebuilding of damaged myelin. However, no conclusive scientific evidence exists that supports its use in MS (42). Nonetheless, many MS patients insist that it helps prevent exacerbations. There are no known adverse effects to this substance.

Ginseng

The two major ginseng species are Asian ginseng *(panax ginseng)* and American ginseng *(panax quinquefolium)*. The name *panax* is derived from the Greek and means "all cure." Ginseng toxicity and side effects have not been reported. The action of ginseng is neither local nor specific. Claims of generalized increase in energy, libido, cog-

nition, and other functions have not been substantiated in any scientific studies in MS patients (43).

Ginkgo Biloba

Ginkgo biloba (also known as roka and tanakam) is one of the oldest living tree species, dating back more than 300 million years. In China, extracts of the fruit and leaves of the Ginkgo tree have been used for more than 5,000 years to treat lung ailments such as asthma and bronchitis and cardiovascular diseases. It has a mild vasodilatory effect and is widely used for many conditions. Food supplement purveyors claim that this substance improves neuromuscular function and cognition in MS (44). No controlled studies have been published.

Melatonin

Melatonin (MLT) is a methoxyindole secreted principally by the pineal gland at night under normal environmental conditions (45). The endogenous rhythm of secretion is generated by the suprachiasmatic nuclei and entrained by the light–dark cycle. Light is able to both suppress and entrain MLT production on a light–dark schedule. Because the regulating system follows a central and sympathetic nervous pathway, an abnormality at any level could nonspecifically modify MLT secretion. Exogenous melatonin decreases alertness and increases sleepiness. This may exacerbate MS symptoms if it is given during the daytime, but it may alleviate nighttime sleeplessness. Melatonin causes significant depressive symptoms in some people. Its mechanism of action on the immune system is not well understood, so caution should be used when considering the use of MLT for MS patients.

Pycnogenol

A bioflavonoid derived from the bark of *Pinus maritima*, which is found in France, pycnogenol has been found to be a powerful antioxidant. Antioxidants may have some immune-stimulating properties (8). Claims have been made for its effectiveness in the treatment of literally every disease. No scientific studies are available on the effectiveness of pycnogenol for MS.

Dehydroepiandrosterone

Dehydroepiandrosterone (DHEA) is a natural hormone precursor of testosterone, progesterone, and estrogen (46); it decreases in the human body with age. It is found in the Mexican yam (also called wild yam or *Dioscorea villisa L.*).

The potential value of DHEA as a treatment for autoimmune disease was suggested by the observation that it delayed the onset of autoimmune disease in a sensitized population of mice (47). One preliminary study of women with systemic lupus erythematosus showed efficacy (48). Anecdotal reports claim increased stamina and improved sense of well-being in patients with MS given large doses of DHEA, but no controlled studies have been published. Despite the lack of controlled studies, some practitioners prescribe DHEA for patients with autoimmune diseases, including MS. Potential adverse effects of DHEA treatment include thyrotoxicosis in those taking thyroid replacement hormone, hirsutism, acne, hypertension, and lipid changes. One investigator (J.B., unpublished) has not found depressed DHEA levels in MS patients.

Herbal Energy Enhancers

Because fatigue is such a common and disturbing symptom of MS, patients frequently tend to seek out preparations that are touted to increase energy. A number of dietary substances are claimed to be energy enhancers. Studies on these substances have not been published. They include 5-hydroxytryptophan, citrus aurantium, ephedra, and guaraná.

5-Hydroxytryptophan

5-Hydroxytryptophan (5-HT) comes from the plant *Griffonia simplicifolia,* a small African bean. It is a precursor to serotonin, an important neurotransmitter in the central nervous system, which has a role in sleep, appetite, memory, learning, temperature regulation, mood, sexual behavior, cardiovascular function, muscle contraction, and endocrine regulation. 5-Hydroxytryptophan may cause pulmonary and cardiac complications similar to those of phentermine, and therefore is not considered a safe substance.

Citrus Aurantium

Citrus aurantium comes from the essential oils of the bitter "Seville" orange grown in Spain. These oils have been used for centuries as bath oils and more recently for aromatherapy. When ingested, citrus aurantium is a central nervous system stimulant. The exact nature of its effect is not known. It has been suspected to have a toxic effect on the liver and kidneys. However, this has not been proven. It seems to be a stimulant similar to caffeine and is found in many herbal diet preparations.

Ephedra

Ephedra is also called MaHuang. The substance comes from the plant *Ephedra sinensis* and contains ephedrine and pseudoephedrine. MaHuang is also sold as a stimulant and weight loss product. Although the cautions for ephedra and caffeine are similar, ephedra has greater cardiovascular activity than caffeine. Ephedra is often combined in diet or energy products with caffeine or natural caffeine sources such as kola nut, guaraná, or tea. The combinations of these two different types of stimulants can be especially powerful. The important adverse effects of citrus aurantium include dizziness, jitters, insomnia, and cardiac irregularities. It also causes an increase in blood pressure and has led to stroke, myocardial infarction, and seizures (49).

Guaraná

The botanical name of guaraná *(Paullinia cupana H.B.K.,* variety *sorbilis)* is derived from C. F. Paullini, a German medical botanist who lived in the eighteenth century.

The guaraná plant is a woody vine that climbs trees. It has been cultivated in South America since pre-Columbian times. It was grown mainly by the Maués and Andira tribes from the lower Amazon. It is sold in South America as "guaraná em rama," roasted guaraná, which is the roasted seed, by the Amazon farmers to cooperative unions, middlemen, and industry, as well as in the form of a powder and a syrup. Guaraná has chemical similarities to caffeine and has the same physiologic action. It has a number of potential negative effects. An elevation of temperature is common with ingestion of a high concentration of guaraná. Urinary retention, high blood pressure, and constipation also are common—all side effects that will worsen MS symptoms. Most soft drinks that contain this substance probably have a low concentration of the drug and probably will not have any more adverse effect than a cup of strong coffee. There is, however, no standardization of how much of the active substance is contained in any product that is available.

Vitamins

The medical literature on the use of vitamins in MS patients is sparse, although anecdotal reports are numerous. Megavitamin therapy is recommended by some who claim that a vitamin deficiency exists in MS, although no vitamin deficiency has been identified. Megavitamin therapy is expensive and may be toxic if high levels of fat-soluble vitamins A and D are included. Vitamin B12 deficiency may cause peripheral and central nervous system demyelination. Therefore, serum vitamin B12 levels are recommended in the evaluation of possible MS. If normal levels are found, vitamin B12 supplements are not likely to help symptoms of MS. However, some patients perceive an increased energy level after treatment.

Many MS health care providers recommend a one-a-day multiple vitamin or "stress tablet" to supplement the dietary sources of vitamins. Others recommend additional vitamin C, vitamin E, and vitamin B complex, all of which are water-soluble, relatively inexpensive, and nontoxic. There is a theoretical basis for each, although no scientific data in MS are available. Co-enzyme Q is also taken by some MS patients, although caution is advised because of potential immune stimulation.

Echinacea and Astragalus

Echinacea or purple coneflower is a member of the daisy family and is one of the most popular herbs in the United States for "enhancement" of the immune system to treat the common cold (50). It has immune stimulating properties. Astragalus is produced from the root of the astragalus plant. Like echinacea, its immune-stimulating effects should be avoided. Neither agent should be used in MS patients until further data become available. Theoretically, immune stimulation could increase the risk of an MS exacerbation.

Estrogen and Progesterone

Estrogen is an endogenously secreted hormone and a major component of birth control pills. It has immunomodulating effects, which have theoretical advantages in MS. In fact, estriol, which is found in small quantities in the body, has been claimed to help MS patients. Although no scientific studies in MS exist, some are being planned. Birth control pills with high estrogen levels have been shown to reduce experimental allergic encephalomyelitis (EAE) in rodents (51). However, the role of estrogens and other hormonal therapies in MS awaits scientific studies. Hormones that contain progesterone have the potential to stimulate the immune system and should be avoided until further studies are reported.

Cannabis (Marijuana)

Marijuana has been touted as useful for MS in numerous anecdotal reports (52–54). However, the published literature shows mixed results at best. Objective data are lacking, although patients "feel better" when smoking cannabis. Some MS symptoms reported to be helped were spasticity, tremor, depression, anxiety, and paresthesia. Patients often perceived improvement, although examining physicians could not demonstrate objective changes. Greenburg and colleagues studied 10 MS patients with spasticity and compared them with 10 volunteers before and after smoking delta-9-tetrahydrocannabinol (THC) (55). Postural control was studied using a computer controlled dynamic posturographic platform. Multiple sclerosis patients felt clinically improved but showed deteri-

orating performance on objective testing.

The Institute of Medicine (IOM) evaluated the medicinal use of marijuana (56). They state, "The regular use of smoked marijuana, however, would be contraindicative in a chronic condition such as multiple sclerosis." Not only are there short-term problems with smoking marijuana, including difficulty with coordination and cognition but also potential serious long-term effects have not been studied.

Bee Venom Therapy

Bee venom therapy has an immunologic rationale as well as many anecdotal reports of benefit by patients. On the other hand, bee venom has been shown to worsen EAE in rodents (57). Studies are currently under way to determine the appropriate dose and administration of bee venom as a potential therapy in MS. Until these studies are completed, bee venom cannot be recommended as a treatment for MS. The potential of severe adverse effects of injecting bee venom, including anaphylactic reaction and death, is also a cause for extreme concern.

Noni Juice

Morinda citrifolia, in Noni juice, is growing in popularity among MS patients. Originally, an effect has been claimed in cancer and pain (58). Because it may be an immunologically active compound (59), caution is advised in using it in MS patients until scientific data indicate otherwise.

Procarin®

Detailed information about the ingredients in the Procarin® system is confidential. Professionals participating in clinical or research programs with this substance must sign a confidentiality agreement with the company. The National MS Society (NMSS) reports that the theory behind Procarin® is related to histamine (a vasodilator) and caffeine research in the 1950s "that is generally not accepted by the medical community."

The company's hypothesis is that one component of Procarin® mimics an important neurotransmitter that is lacking in MS patients because of a viral infection in the central nervous system. Another component blocks the breakdown of the component that is necessary for myelin regeneration and maintenance. No scientific data have been published on Procarin®, although 10 patients were treated in a preliminary study. Publication on these 10 patients and longer, controlled trials are necessary before efficacy and safety can be truly evaluated. An important impediment to integration of Procarin® into MS therapy is that most licensed practitioners are wary of recommending or prescribing a substance for which they do not know the chemical formulation.

TOXIC REMOVAL THERAPY

CAM toxic removal therapies are listed in Table 29-5.

Chelation Therapy

Chelation with ethylenediamine tetraacetic acid (EDTA) has been used to treat lead poisoning and some other heavy metal poisoning. Its mechanism of action is to bind poisoning metals, which are then excreted in the urine. Evidence that MS is caused by heavy metal poisoning is lacking. Nonetheless, chelation is touted as a treatment for MS without credible scientific data. Not only is chelation not indicated in MS, but also it can be nephrotoxic and even fatal (11).

Dental Amalgam Removal

Dental amalgams contain mercury, which has been postulated to cause symptoms of MS. Therefore, removal of dental amalgams is recommended by these few practitioners. This theory has not been adequately substantiated in scientific publications. Although it has received wide media attention, most medical experts do not have reason to believe that this procedure has any benefit for MS patients (11,60).

SPECIAL DIETS

Special diets that have been used in the treatment of MS are listed in Table 29-6.

Low-Fat Diet

The Swank low-fat diet is the most popular MS-specific diet in the United States. Roy Swank pointed out that people with high animal fat intake have a high incidence of MS (61). People with low animal fat intake (Asians) have a very low incidence of MS. Therefore, he treats patients with a low-fat diet. Multiple sclerosis patients who

---

TABLE 29-5
CAM Toxic Removal Therapy

- Chelation therapy
- Removal of dental mercury amalgams

TABLE 29-6
Special Diets

- Low-fat diet (Swank)
- Aspartame-free diet
- Gluten-free diet
- Allergen-free diet
- Processed foods–free diet (Evers)

---

adhered to his low animal fat diet for several years had fewer exacerbations of MS. However, the natural history of MS usually is associated with fewer exacerbations later in the disease. No control group was followed at the same institution. Multiple sclerosis patients on the diet who did poorly may have not returned to the clinic. Therefore, the results are not convincing. Many patients following the low animal fat diet take dietary supplements of essential polyunsaturated fatty acids from fish oils, sunflower seed oil, linoleic acid, and evening primrose oil. Fish oils are high in eicosapentaenoic acid and docosahexaenoic acid, which are also claimed to be beneficial for MS patients.

Aspartame-Free Diet

Proponents for limiting aspartame claim that aspartame causes several medical conditions, including MS. They claim that there is a conspiracy between the pharmaceutical manufacturers and the FDA to keep aspartame on the market. Scientific evidence for these claims is lacking. Nonetheless, the Internet remains an active source of information to MS patients claiming the deleterious effects of aspartame.

Gluten-Free Diet

The gluten-free diet excludes wheat and rye because areas of the world that have a high volume of wheat and rye production and consumption also have a high incidence of MS. Studies on gluten-free diet have been uncontrolled, and this diet may result in inadequate protein intake. This diet is not recommended (11).

Allergen-Free Diet

Proponents of the allergen-free diet believe that MS is related to allergies to specific foods. After skin testing, certain foods are eliminated. No controlled studies on this diet have been published (11).

Evers Processed Food Elimination Diet

Joseph Evers proposed this diet for many diseases. This diet is based on the premise that the processing of food causes illness, including MS. The diet recommends the intake of raw vegetables, whole wheat bread, cheese, raw milk, raw eggs, butter, honey, and raw ham. There is no scientific basis for the rationale that processed foods are chemically different from natural foods. None of the common food additives have been shown to produce lesions resembling those of MS (11).

OTHER THERAPIES

Various other therapies that have been used in the management of MS are listed in Table 29-7.

Cooling

Cooling therapy in MS is based on the fact that MS patients often perform worse when they have a fever or in a heated environment, such as in a hot tub, and perform better in a cooler environment (62–67). Several papers, including those sponsored by the National Aeronautic and Space Administration (NASA), have shown a beneficial effect of cooling, at least transiently (68). Certain patients seem to be sensitive to temperature fluctuations, whereas others do not appear to be helped by cooling. Several commercial products, including cooling vests, body suits, helmets, and neck scarves, have been reported to be helpful by individual patients. Some patients report that a cool bath or shower in the afternoon alleviates fatigue. Some physicians recommend chewing on ice chips or taking an ice-cold drink as a temporary remedy for some symptoms of MS, such as fatigue. On the other hand, somatosensory evoked potentials have been shown not to improve after cooling (69), and the long-term benefits from cooling have not been demonstrated.

Electromagnetic Therapies

Electromagnetic therapy has been studied in MS with reported positive results (70). A small device emits weak electromagnetic fields, which are not perceived by the patient. The fields induce alpha, beta, delta, and theta waves, which are in the range of normal brain functioning. A double-blind, placebo-controlled study demonstrated a statistically significant effect of the Enermed magnetic pulsing device on patient performance scales and on alpha EEG magnitude during a language task (71). Electromagnetic therapy has not been approved by the FDA for use in MS.

Hyperbaric Oxygen

In 1983 Fischer reported some benefit in MS patients using hyperbaric oxygen (HBO) therapy (72), although his results were not confirmed in later studies (73,74). This treatment for MS is not generally accepted by MS scientists. Some patients "feel better" after HBO therapy. However, because of the expense, inconvenience, and poor results in most clinical trials, this therapy is not recommended.

MALPRACTICE CONCERNS RELATING TO REFERRAL TO ALTERNATIVE HEALTH CARE PRACTITIONERS

Studdert and colleagues have discussed medical malpractice implications when referring a patient for alternative medicine (75). Although the risk of being involved in a malpractice suit is low and the claim payments for alternative practitioners are lower than for MDs, a liability exists if the decision to refer was negligent (i.e., the therapies offered no benefit or subjected the patient to unreasonable risk).

Some questions to consider before referring a patient to a CAM practitioner include: Is the practitioner licensed in the state? Will I supervise (and share responsibility with) the practitioner in this aspect of the care? Do I have any reason to believe the practitioner is incompetent?

If the CAM practitioner is licensed and the referring physician does not supervise or otherwise interfere with the treatment, the physician is unlikely to be at risk for being involved in a malpractice suit, even if harm does come to the patient.

CONCLUSION

One of the most important aspects in dealing with CAM therapy is to better establish a long-term, caring relationship between the health care professional and the patient. The process of evaluating a CAM therapy will solidify this relationship. If the health care provider maintains a helpful, optimistic attitude toward MS treatment and respects the patient's and family's concerns and beliefs about CAM therapies, it will be easier to help the patient discriminate between fact and hype, minimize susceptibility to fraud, and maximize overall function and well-being.

TABLE 29-7
Other Therapies

- Cooling
- Electromagnetic therapy
- Hyperbaric oxygen

Acknowledgment

The authors thank David Simon, M.D., Medical Director of the Chopra Center for Well-Being, LaJolla, California, and Freida Kaluchi, PhD, Colorado Springs, Colorado, for their review and advice on this chapter.

References

1. Jonas WB. Alternative medicine—learning from the past, examining the present, advancing to the future. *JAMA* 1998; 280(18):1616–1617.
2. Schwartz CE, Laitin E, Brotman S, La Rocca N. Utilization of unconventional treatments by persons with MS: Is it alternative or complementary? *Neurology* 1999; 52:626–629.
3. Gatchel RJ, Maddrey AM. Clinical outcome research in complementary and alternative medicine: An overview of experimental design and analysis. *Alt Ther* 1998; 4(5):36–42.
4. Eisenberg DM, Davis RB, Ettner SL, et al. Trends in alternative medicine use in the United States, 1990–1997, results of a follow-up national survey. *JAMA* 1998; 280(18):1569–1575.
5. Fawcett J, Sidney JS, Hanson MJS, Riley-Lawless K. Use of alternative health therapies by people with multiple sclerosis: An exploratory study. *Holist Nurs Pract* 1997; 8(2):36–42.
6. Stenager E, et al. The use of non-medical/alternative treatment in multiple sclerosis. A 5-year follow-up study. *Acta Neurol Belg* 1995; 95(1):18–22.
7. Searles G, Murray TJ. The use of alternative medicine by people with multiple sclerosis. *CMCS Consort* 1998; 11(2):5.
8. Bowling AC. An objective review of herbal medicine and vitamin supplements relevant to multiple sclerosis. *Multiple Sclerosis* 1999; 5(1):S134.
9. Chopra D. *Perfect health.* New York: Harmony Books, 1990.
10. Husted C, Pham L, Hekking A, Niederman R. Improving quality of life for people with chronic conditions: The example of T'ai Chi and multiple sclerosis. *Alt Ther* 1999; 5(5):70–74.
11. Sibley WA. *Therapeutic claims in multiple sclerosis,* 4th ed. New York: Demos Publications, 1996.
12. Rose AS, Kuzma JW, Kurtzke JF, et al. Cooperative study in the evaluation of therapy in multiple sclerosis: ACTH versus placebo. *Neurology* 1970; 20(2):1.
13. Weatherford J. *Indian givers: How the Indians of the Americas transformed the world.* New York: Crown Publishers, 1988.
14. Altenberg HE. *Holistic medicine: A meeting of East & West.* Tokyo: Japan Publications, 1992.
15. Burton Goldberg Group. *Alternative medicine: The definitive guide.* Fife, WA: Future Medicine Publishing, 1994.
16. Williams CA, et al. *The guide to alternative health care.* Salt Lake City: Gibbs-Smith Publisher, 1998.
17. King CR. Nonpharmacologic management of chemotherapy-induced nausea and vomiting. *Oncol Nurs Forum* 1997; 24(7):41–48.
18. Ernst E, et al. The effectiveness of acupuncture in treating acute dental pain: A systematic review. *Br Dent J* 1998; 184(9):443–447.
19. Steinberger A. Specific irritability of acupuncture points as an early symptom of multiple sclerosis. *Am J Chin Med* 1986; 14(3–4):175–178.
20. Wang Y, Hashimoto S, Findley B, Ramsum D, Oger J. Pilot survey of using acupuncture and other alternative medicine in multiple sclerosis patients. *Neurology* 1999; 52(2):A550.
21. Stewart WL. A brief overview of Ayurveda—an indigenous Indian medical system. *J Fam Pract* 1978; 7(5): 1069–1070.
22. Coyer AB, Curwen IHM. Low back pain treated by manipulation. A controlled series. *Br Med J* 1955; 1: 705–707.
23. Shekelle PG, Adams AH, Chassin MR, Hurwitz EL, Brook RH. Spinal manipulation for low-back pain. *Ann Intern Med* 1992; 117(7):590–598.
24. Stude DE, et al. Clinical presentation of a patient with multiple sclerosis and response to manual chiropractic adjustive therapies. *J Manipulative Physiol Ther* 1993; 16(9):595–600.
25. Telles S, et al. Yoga for rehabilitation: An overview. *Indian J Med Sci* 1997; 51(4):123–127.
26. Beck MF. *Milady's theory and practice of therapeutic massage,* 2nd ed. Albany, NY: Milady Publishing Company, 1994.
27. Wolf SL, et al. Exploring the basis for Tai Chi Chuan as a therapeutic exercise approach. *Arch Phys Med Rehabil* 1997; 78(8):886–892.
28. Wolf SL, et al. The effect of Tai Chi Quan and computerized balance training on postural stability in older subjects. Atlanta FICSIT Group. Frailty and injuries: Cooperative studies on intervention techniques. *Phys Ther* 1997; 77(4):371–381.
29. Freal JE, et al. Symptomatic fatigue in multiple sclerosis. *Arch Phys Med Rehabil* 1984; 65(3):135–138.
30. Maguire BL. The effects of imagery on attitudes and moods in multiple sclerosis patients. *Alt Ther* 1996; 2(5):75–78.
31. Rodgers D, Khoo K, MacEachen M, Oven M, Beatty WW. Cognitive therapy for multiple sclerosis: A preliminary study. *Alt Ther* 1996; 2(5):70–74.
32. Krieger D. Healing with therapeutic touch. *Alt Ther* 1998; 4(1):86–92.
33. Pennebaker JW, Kiecolt-Glaser JK, Glaser R. Disclosures of trauma and immune function: Health implications for psychotherapy. *J Consult Clin Psychol* 1988; 56:239–245.
34. Simon D. *Return to wholeness.* New York: John Wiley & Sons, Inc., 1999.
35. Cousins N. Anatomy of an illness as perceived by the patient. *N Engl J Med* 1977; 295:1458–1463.
36. Simon D. *The wisdom of healing.* New York: Harmony Books, 1997.
37. Ernst E. St. John's wort, an anti-depressant? A systematic, criteria-based overview. *Phytomedicine* 1959; 2:67–71.
38. Harrer G, Sommer H. Treatment of mild/moderate depressions with hypericum. *Phytomedicine* 1994; 1:3–8.
39. Linde K, et al. St. John's wort for depression—An overview and meta-analysis of randomized clinical trials. *Br Med J* 1996; 313(7052):253–258.
40. Vorbach EU, et al. Effectiveness and tolerance of the hypericum extract LI 60 in comparison with imipramine: Randomized double blind study of 135 outpatients. *J Geriatr Psychiatry Neurol* 1994; 7(1):S19–S23.

41. Laakmann G, Schule C, Baghai T, Kieser M. St. John's wort in mild to moderate depression; the relevance of hyperforin for clinical efficacy. *Pharmacopsychiatry* 1998; 31(l):54–59.

42. Bates D, et al. Polyunsaturated fatty acids in treatment of acute remitting multiple sclerosis. *Br Med J* 1978; 2(6149):1390–1391.

43. Petkov VD, et al. Effects of standardized ginseng extract on learning, memory, and capabilities. *Am J Chin Med* 1987; 15(1–2):19–29.

44. Clostre F. From the body to cellular membranes: The different levels of pharmacological action of Ginkgo biloba extract. In: Fungfeld EW (ed.). *Rokan (Ginkgo biloba)— Recent results in pharmacology and clinic.* New York: Springer-Verlag, 1988.

45. Zhdanova IV, et al. Sleep inducing effects of low doses of melatonin ingested in the evening. *Clin Pharmacol Therapeutics* 1995; 57(5):552–559.

46. Yen SS, et al. Replacement of DHEA in aging men and women: Potential remedial effects. *Ann NY Acad Sci* 1995; 774:128–142.

47. Norton SD, et al. Administration of dehydroepiandrosterone sulfate retards onset but not progression of autoimmune disease in NZB/W mice. *Autoimmunity* 1997; 26(3):161–171.

48. Suzuki T, et al. Low serum levels of dehydroepiandrosterone may cause deficient IL-2 production by lymphocytes in patients with systemic lupus erythematosus (SLE). *Clin Exp Immunol* 1995; 99(2):251–255.

49. Hikono H, et al. Anti-inflammatory principle of ephedra herbs. *Chem Pharm Bull* 1976; 28:2900–2904.

50. Bauer R, Wagner H. Echinacea species as potential immunostimulatory drugs. *Econ Med Plant Res* 1991; 5:253–321.

51. Arnason B, et al. Effects of estrogen, progestin and combined estrogen-progestin oral contraceptive preparations on experimental allergic encephalomyelitis. *Trans Am Neurol Assoc* 1969; 94:54–58.

52. Consroe P, Musty R, Rein J, Tillery W, Pertwee R. The perceived effects of smoked cannabis on patients with multiple sclerosis. *Eur Neurol* 1997; 38:44–48.

53. Petro DJ, Ellenberger C Jr. Treatment of human spasticity with "9-tetrahydrocannabinol. *J Clin Pharmacol* 1981; 21:413S–416S.

54. Ungerleider JT, Andyrsiak T, Fairbanks L, Ellison GW, Myers LW. Delta-9-THC in the treatment of spasticity associated with multiple sclerosis. *Adv Alcohol Subst Abuse* 1987; 7:39–50.

55. Greenburg HS, Werness SAS, Pugh JE, et al. Short-term effects of smoking marijuana on balance in patients with multiple sclerosis and normal volunteers. *Clin Pharmacol Ther* 1994; 55:324–328.

56. Joy JE, Watson SJ, Benson JA Jr (eds.). *Marijuana and medicine: Assessing the science base.* Washington, DC: National Academy Press, 1999.

57. Lublin FD, Oshinsky RJ, Perreault M, Siebert K. Effect of honey bee venom on EAE. *Neurology* (Suppl) 1998; 50:A424.

58. Younos C, Rolland A, Fleurentin J, Lanhers M, Misslin F. Analgesic and behavioral effects of morinda citrifolia. *Mortier Planta Medica* 1990; 56:430–434.

59. Hiramatsu T, Imoto M, Koyano T, Umezawa K. Introduction of normal phenotypes in RAS-transformed cells by damnacanthal from morinda citrifolia. *Cancer Letters* 1993; 73:161–166.

60. Bangsi D, et al. Dental amalgam and multiple sclerosis: A case-control study in Montreal, Canada. *Int J Epidemiol* 1998; 27(4):667–671.

61. Swank RL, Dugan BB. Effect of low saturated fat diet in early and late cases of multiple sclerosis. *Lancet* 1990; 336:37–39.

62. Coyle PK, Krupp LB, Doscher C, Deng Z, Milazzo A. Clinical and immunological effects of cooling in multiple sclerosis. *J Neuro Rehab* 1996; 10:9–15.

63. Guthrie TC, Nelson DA. Influence of temperature changes on multiple sclerosis: Critical review of mechanisms and research potential. *J Neurol Sci* 1995; 129:1–8.

64. Kinnman J, Andersson U, Kinnman Y, Wetterqvist L. Temporary improvement of motor function in patients with multiple sclerosis after treatment with a cooling suit. *J Neuro Rehab* 1997; 11(2):109–114.

65. Schauf CL, Davids FA. Impulse conduction in multiple sclerosis: A theoretical basis for modification by temperature and pharmacological agents. *J Neurol Neurosurg Psychiatry* 1974; 37:152–161.

66. Syndulko K, Waldanski A, Baumhefner RW, Tourtellotte WW. Effects of temperature in multiple sclerosis: A review of the literature. *J Neuro Rehab* 1996; 10:23–24.

67. Watson CW. Effect of lowering of body temperature on the symptoms and signs of multiple sclerosis. *N Engl J Med* 1959; 261(25):1253–1259.

68. Ku YT, et al. Physiologic and thermal responses of male and female patients with multiple sclerosis to head and neck cooling. *Am J Phys Med Rehabil* 1999; 78(5): 447–456.

69. Robinson LR, et al. Body cooling may not improve somatosensory pathway function in multiple sclerosis. *Am J Phys Med Rehabil* 1997; 76(3):191–196.

70. Richards TL, Lappen MS, Lawrie FW, Stegbauer KC. Bioelectromagnetic applications for multiple sclerosis. *Phys Med Rehabil Clin N Am* 1998; 9(3):659–674.

71. Richards TL, Lappen MS, Acosta-Urquidi J, et al. Double-blind study of pulsing magnetic field effects on multiple sclerosis. *J Altern Complement Med* 1997; 3(1):21–29.

72. Fischer BH, Marks M, Reich T. Hyperbaric-oxygen treatment of multiple sclerosis: A randomized, placebo-controlled, double-blind study. *N Engl J Med* 1983; 308: 181–186.

73. Kleijnen J, et al. Hyperbaric oxygen for multiple sclerosis. Review of controlled trials. *Acta Neurol Scand* 1995; 91(5):330–334.

74. Marini RA. Alternative/complementary MS therapies. *MSQR* 1997; 16(4):1–3.

75. Studdert DM, Eisenberg DM, Miller FH, et al. Medical malpractice implications of alternative medicine. *JAMA* 1998; 280(18):1610–1615.

30 Women's Issues

P. K. Coyle, M.D.

Modern health care increasingly emphasizes a gender-based approach to medicine. This approach acknowledges the many fundamental physiologic differences between men and women, which affect health and disease issues (Table 30-1) (1). From a neurologic perspective, the brain is a sexually dimorphic organ with well-documented gender-specific anatomic and neurotransmitter differences. There also are important clinical distinctions between the sexes. Men and women differ in basic spatial and language skills. Specific neurologic disorders (such as eclampsia and pregnancy-related stroke syndromes) occur only in women (2–4), whereas other neurologic disorders (such as vascular and muscle contraction headaches, depression, acquired motor neuron disease, and benign intracranial hypertension) show clear gender preferences (5–8). From a broad clinical perspective, issues relating to pregnancy, delivery, and menstruation apply only to women.

For many years medical studies focused on men. In response to concerns about possible negative consequences on fertility and pregnancy, participation by women was actively discouraged. The result has been health and disease models skewed to a single gender. In attempts to correct longstanding inequities, the U.S. government established a formal Office of Research on Women's Health in the late 1980s. For the first time it was required that women be routinely entered into clinical trials. The response to this initiative included the development of women's health centers at many hospitals and medical centers.

Gender consciousness is now being encouraged in all areas of health care, including neurology. An example is the formulation of practice parameters to address management issues based on gender, as exemplified by the recent guidelines for women with epilepsy (9,10). This same emphasis is now being applied to multiple sclerosis (MS). Multiple sclerosis is believed to be immune-mediated. Similar to most autoimmune diseases, it shows a female dominance. In fact, MS serves as a prototype for a major neurologic disease with a female gender preference (11,12). It involves many important women's issues (Table 30-2). This chapter focuses on gender-specific issues in MS. This gender-based approach to neurology is not only intellectually sound but also is now the preferred approach.

GENDER AND THE IMMUNE SYSTEM

Gender affects the host immune system (Table 30-1). Overall, women show stronger immune responses than men. This is reflected in the fact that most diseases that are considered to have an autoimmune or immune-mediated pathogenesis are more common in women. Exam-

TABLE 30-1
Areas of Difference Between Men and Women (1)

Nervous System
- Anatomy
- Cell numbers
- Neurotransmitter systems
- Response to hormones
- Sensation threshold
- Disease frequencies

Immune System
- Immune response
- Autoimmune disease frequency

Cardiovascular System
- Blood pressure
- Coronary artery disease
- Electrical, rhythm disturbances

Gastrointestinal System
- Bile composition
- Intestinal mucosa, transit time

Musculoskeletal System
- Bone architecture, turnover, age-related changes

Malignancy
- Specific malignancies
- Survival rate
- Hormonal therapy

Pharmacology
- Drug metabolism

TABLE 30-2
Women's Issues in MS

Epidemiologic Features
- Gender preference disease (70% to 75% female predominance)
- Gender preference in all disease subtypes except primary progressive (50% females)
- Young age (early postpubertal) onset
- Possible increasing frequency in women

Pregnancy Issues
- Effect of MS on pregnancy
- Genetic implications
- Short-term and long-term effects of pregnancy on MS; prognostic implications
- Decisions on breast-feeding

Menstrual Cycle Issues
- Effect of menstrual cycle on MS

Sex Issues
- Sexual dysfunction
- Cosmetic and/or physical attractiveness issues
- Use of sex hormones

Therapy Issues
- Symptomatic treatments and side effects
- Disease-modifying treatments and side effects

Psychosocial Issues

ples include Hashimoto's thyroiditis, myasthenia gravis, rheumatoid arthritis, Sjögren's syndrome, systemic sclerosis, and systemic lupus erythematosus. Exceptions to this female predominance are rare but do occur, such as ankylosing spondylitis. In the immune-mediated female preference disorders, disease symptom and severity are often influenced by gender-related factors that involve hormone exposure. Examples include pregnancy, the menstrual cycle, and exogenous hormone use. Part of the explanation for a gender influence on the immune system, although clearly not the whole picture, are sex hormones (estrogens, progestins, androgens). In addition to sex hormones, the host immune system and its historical exposures, the host genetic makeup, and the host nervous and endocrine systems, are all likely to play a role in the development of immune-mediated disease.

Sex hormones influence the nervous system in multiple ways. They can affect cognitive function, coordinated movements, formation of synapses, and specific neurotransmitter systems (13). Sex hormones also influence the immune system in multiple ways (14-19). During pregnancy, for example, there is a shift in the T helper cell population to favor T helper 2 cells. This subpopulation antagonizes the T helper 1 cell subpopulation, downregulates cell-mediated immune responses and pro-

inflammatory cytokine production, and promotes antibody immune responses and anti-inflammatory/regulatory cytokine production. Hormonal manipulation can bias toward either a T helper 1 or T helper 2 immune response. In general, women show higher immunoglobulin levels than men but decreased cell-mediated immune responses, consistent with a T helper 2 bias (20). Crosstalk between the endocrine and immune systems is also facilitated by the fact that sex hormone receptors are found on various immune system cells, including CD8 T cells and macrophages (antigen-presenting cells). CD4+ T cells respond to estrogens in a dose-related manner, and antigen-stimulated cell cytokine production will be modulated based on the amount of estrogen present (21). The involved cytokines all play an important role in controlling immune responses. The influence of gender and sex hormones on disease can be readily demonstrated in animal models of MS, such as the adoptive experimental allergic encephalomyelitis (EAE) model in the SJL strain mouse. Disease susceptibility and severity are influenced by animal gender, as well as by exogenous hormone exposure (22–24). It seems likely that sex hormones play some role in MS. In fact, treatment with dehydroepiandrosterone (DHEA), a weak adrenal adrogen, has been suggested in the popular press to be a useful therapy for MS and other immune-mediated disorders.

EPIDEMIOLOGY

There are several striking epidemiologic features of MS that have important implications for women. Multiple sclerosis is a disease with a strong gender preference. Approximately 70 percent to 75 percent of all MS patients are female (11,12,25). The single exception is the primary progressive subtype, which accounts for 10 percent of patients (25). This unusual MS subtype is characterized by atypical features such as equal gender ratio, older age of onset, and absence of acute relapses (26). The explanation for the overall female predominance in MS remains unknown. Hormonal factors, maternal factors, immune factors, and X-linked gene factors have all been postulated to play some role (20,21,23,27). Multiple sclerosis also typically affects young women of childbearing age. Although prepubertal onset is rare, once puberty occurs clinical MS is increasingly common and shows a peak onset at 28 to 30 years of age. For most patients, MS begins between the ages of 15 and 50. Although postmenopausal onset can occur, it is unusual, and less than 1 percent of MS patients have disease onset after age 60. There also is debate at the current time with regard to whether cases of MS are increasing. Data from Olmsted County, Minnesota, indicate an increased incidence of MS among women (28).

PREGNANCY

Because MS affects so many women of childbearing age, pregnancy is a major gender-related issue. It is routine for patients to have questions not only about the effect of pregnancy on MS disease onset, activity, and prognosis, but also about whether MS in turn can affect the fetus and the birth process. Until 1949 pregnancy was considered to have a negative impact on MS and was discouraged. Over the next few years several studies were published that failed to confirm this widely held impression (29–31). Subsequent publications have addressed a variety of issues regarding pregnancy in MS (32–50). Overall, pregnancy does not increase the risk of developing MS. In fact, a recent Scandinavian study found that the risk of MS was higher for nulliparous women than for parous women, and that the risk ratio increased over time (51). The most compelling data on pregnancy and MS relate to the effect on disease activity. A recent European study of 254 women and 269 pregnancies noted that in the last trimester of pregnancy there was a 70 percent decline in the clinical relapse rate (52). This effect is more than twice as potent as the current disease-modifying therapies. This clinical benefit of late pregnancy is quite consistent with findings from a small study that reported a corresponding suppression of subclinical magnetic res-

onance imaging (MRI) disease activity in late pregnancy (53). In these patients, MRI disease activity returned to prepregnancy baseline during the early postpartum months. In the definitive European study, the first three months post partum saw a rebound 70 percent increase in clinical relapses before the relapse rate returned to the prepregnancy baseline (52).

The protective effect of late pregnancy undoubtedly relates to the fact that pregnancy is an immunosuppressive state. However, multiple maternal, fetal, and placental factors are involved to produce immune suppression. They include pregnancy-associated immunoregulatory proteins; an overall net inhibitory effect of pregnancy-related hormone, prostanglandin, and cytokine changes; maternal-fetal MHC class II disparity; pregnancy-associated inhibition of cell-mediated immune responses; and pregnancy-associated enhancement of immunoglobulin (including blocking antibody and immune complex) responses (45). Postpartum attacks may be preventable with available immunotherapies. In a recent study, nine MS patients who had previously had 12 childbirth-associated relapses received prophylactic intravenous immunoglobulin (IVIg) post partum. None went on to have clinical relapses (54). In another recent study, eight women who received prophylactic immunoglobulin were compared with 18 untreated women. Ten patients in the untreated group relapsed post partum compared with only one in the treated group (55).

Multiple sclerosis has no significant effects on fertility, conception, fetal viability, and delivery, and patients show no increases in ectopic pregnancies, spontaneous abortions, stillbirths, or congenital malformations (34,35). The mode of delivery, as well as whether the mother breast-feeds, have no adverse effects on MS disease course (50). In fact, breast-feeding may be beneficial. The recent European study on pregnancy noted a trend toward less disease activity with breast-feeding (52). Unfortunately, the numbers were too small to reach statistical significance. With regard to the mode of delivery, anecdotal data suggest that spinal anesthesia should be avoided. Most important, MS prognosis is not worsened by pregnancy. In fact, several studies suggest that pregnancy may improve the patient's long-term prognosis (42,49). Women with MS should be counseled that pregnancy itself is not associated with any negative effects over the short term or the long term. Pregnancy does not increase risk of MS, and, in fact, it may have a positive effect on the disease. From the viewpoint of genetic counseling, there is a very small (approaching 4 percent) but finite increased risk for MS in the child. Most important, there is an increased risk of relapse in the three months following delivery.

The degree of physical disability for a given MS patient is an obvious factor to consider when making a decision to become pregnant and raise a child. Knowing the postpartum risk for clinical relapse, arrangements should be made to have help available if needed. Anecdotal data suggest that patients with more severe secondary progressive disease may not do well after pregnancy, but this has not been evaluated in formal studies.

THE MENSTRUAL CYCLE

Very few data are available on the menstrual cycle and MS. In one self-report study of 149 women with MS, 70 percent noted symptom changes associated with their cycle. The majority (60 percent) noted changes in the week before or during menses, whereas 44 percent reported MS relapses at a consistent phase of their cycle (56). However, a small prospective follow-up study (eight MS patients, 10 controls) was unable to document any consistent worsening associated with the menstrual cycle (57). A recent MRI study of eight relapsing patients noted that the ratio of progesterone to 17-beta estradiol was significantly associated with number and volume of enhancing MRI lesions (58). Reports of a relationship between the menstrual cycle and clinical or neuroimaging disease parameters are intriguing, but they need to be evaluated in much larger numbers of MS patients.

SEXUAL PERFORMANCE

Sexual dysfunction is a major symptom of MS. Recent surveys indicate that 44 percent of MS females are sexually inactive, while 40 percent to 80 percent report sexual dysfunction. In a recent survey of Northern California patients, 65 percent were experiencing sexual difficulties (59). None were receiving any treatment, however, and it is clear that this is a symptom that is frequently not discussed or dealt with. A number of problems can be noted (Table 30-3).

There is now greater openness about discussing and treating these symptoms. They can reflect primary disease manifestations (such as vaginal numbness), secondary manifestations (such as inability to position due to spasticity), or tertiary manifestations (such as poor self-image leading to psychological barriers). Treatment of sexual dysfunction in MS must always include the partner. For women, potential therapies involve counseling, lubrication, use of alternative techniques such as cuddling or stimulation with a vibrator, antispasticity agents, and sildenafil (Viagra).

The concept of self-image and physical attractiveness also comes into play in MS. This can be an issue for women who are limited in their mobility, have significant tremors, or have other disabilities that may inter-

---

| **TABLE 30-3** |
| *Sexual Problems Reported by Women with MS* |

- Decreased libido
- Decrease in orgasms/inability to reach orgasm
- Decreased vaginal lubrication
- Fatigue in sexual performance
- Abnormal/dysesthetic vaginal sensation
- Dyspareunia
- Vaginismus

---

fere with their ability to dress, use the toilet, groom themselves, or apply makeup.

With regard to the use of sex hormones, MS is not a contraindication to the use of hormone replacement therapy (HRT) during menopause. In fact, symptoms that seem to worsen post menopause may respond to HRT (24,60). The use of oral contraceptives has no effect on the risk of developing MS (61) and no adverse effects on the overall disease course. At least one study suggested that young patients on the pill may show less disability (34). This is another issue that awaits clarification.

THERAPY

Therapy in MS involves treatment of symptoms as well as treatment of the disease process. Many drugs used in MS have side effects or interactions that are especially pertinent to women. Synthetic glucocorticoids, such as methylprednisolone, prednisone, and dexamethasone, are used as symptomatic treatments to accelerate recovery from MS relapses. The fact that glucocorticoids can affect bone density is generally more of an issue in women. These drugs decrease body calcium by inhibiting calcium reabsorption, increasing calcium excretion, and potentially causing secondary hyperparathyroidism. They can have negative cosmetic effects, such as production or exacerbation of acneiform lesions, development of a cushingoid habitus with redistribution of fatty tissue, induction of stretch marks, and production of skin atrophy. Glucocorticoids can increase body weight by a temporary retention of fluid and by an increase in appetite. Because they are excreted in breast milk, they can affect infant growth. Sustained and intense treatment may lead to osteonecrosis, such as aseptic necrosis of the femoral head, whereas chronic treatment may lead to osteoporosis with bone collapse and fracture. These negative consequences on bone can be minimized by supplemental calcium and vitamin D, physical activity, and HRT in postmenopausal patients. Osteoporotic MS patients may benefit from monitoring with regular bone density studies and treatment with newer agents such as the biphosphonates. Glucocorticoid side effects can be lessened by the use of a single daily dose, preferably in the morning to minimize hypothalamic pituitary adrenal axis suppression, and by limiting the duration of therapy.

Glucocorticoids are not contraindicated in pregnancy. They can actually be beneficial to fetal lung maturation in the last trimester. However, overuse during pregnancy may slow postnatal growth, and birth defects have been noted in animal studies. As is true for all drugs with the exception of vitamins (such as folic acid to minimize neural tube defects), one tries to avoid medication use in the early weeks of pregnancy during the critical period of organogenesis.

A number of drugs that are used very frequently to treat the various symptoms of MS can have interactions or potential side effects that are pertinent to women (Table 30-4) (62). A good example would be the interaction of carbamazepine or phenytoin with estrogen-containing contraceptives. Women with MS who are pregnant or breast-feeding are at unique risk and must be very familiar with these potential problems.

TABLE 30-4
Symptomatic Treatments Used in Multiple Sclerosis (62)

DRUG	INDICATION	SIDE EFFECTS/PROBLEMS OF SPECIFIC CONCERN TO WOMEN
Amantadine	Fatigue	• Livedo reticularis (skin lesions on legs) more common in women • Insomnia (take earlier in day) • Drug is excreted in breast milk • Can cause birth defects in some animal models; no human data
Fluoxetine	Depression, fatigue	• Can interfere with sleep (AM dose) • Can produce paradoxical suicidal ideation • Drug is excreted in breast milk • May decrease libido, cause menstrual pain
Tricyclic Antidepressants	Depression, pain pain	• May cause photosensitivity • Drug is excreted in breast milk • Newborns may note problems (muscle, heart, respiratory, urinary) if mother receives dose just before delivery • May cause weight gain, increased appetite, decreased sexual performance, enlarged breasts, lactation, hair loss, yellow skin
Carbamazepine	Pain	• Interferes with estrogen contraceptives • Photosensitivity • Potential fetal effects (low birth weight, small head, skull/face defects, undeveloped fingernails, growth delay) • Drug is excreted in breast milk • May cause hair loss
Phenytoin	Pain	• Interferes with estrogen contraceptives • Gingival hyperplasia • Drug is excreted in breast milk • May increase risk of birth defects
Baclofen	Spasticity, trigeminal neuralgia	• Acute withdrawal syndrome • Drug is excreted in breast milk • Animal fetal effects at high dose (hernia, bone, low birth weight)
Tizanidine	Spasticity	• There is decreased drug clearance with oral contraceptives • Adverse conception/fetal effects in animal models at high dose (decreased fertility, fetal loss) • Drug may be excreted in breast milk • Possible hepatotoxicity
Benzodiazepines (clonazepam, diazepam)	Spasticity, tremor	• Drug is excreted in breast milk • Fetus may become dependent • Maternal use before delivery may cause newborn problems (weakness, breathing/feeding/ temperature problems)
Oxybutynin	Bladder urgency, frequency	• May reduce breast milk flow, sex performance

Women with MS face unique issues with regard to the use of disease-modifying therapies (Table 30-5). Although none of these drugs are documented to be teratogenic, in animal studies high-dose interferon beta can be abortofacient. There are no data that glatiramer acetate has any negative effect on the fetus. Most physicians (with some notable exceptions) will not treat pregnant MS patients with these agents and will discontinue treatment in a woman with MS who becomes pregnant. In part, this reflects medicolegal concerns because the U.S. Food and Drug Administration (FDA) recommendations are clear that disease-modifying therapies should not be used during pregnancy. The FDA also requests that women of childbearing age who are receiving treatment use some form of contraception to prevent pregnancy. Despite these recommendations, all three agents have been used during pregnancy without obvious negative consequences.

Interferon beta has potential side effects that are of particular interest to women. In general, drug side effects are dose-related and often spontaneously remit or improve after several months. Menstruation may be affected by high-dose interferon beta therapy. The disturbances are mild to moderate rather than severe. In the phase III trial of interferon beta-1b, menstrual disorders were noted in 17 percent of the 124 patients receiving high-dose interferon beta, compared with 8 percent of the 123 patients receiving placebo treatment (63). When premenopausal females were specifically looked at, 28 percent receiving interferon beta had menstrual abnormalities compared

with 13 percent of placebo-treated females. Menstrual problems included intermenstrual bleeding and/or spotting, intramenstrual clotting and/or spotting, early or delayed menses, and decreased flow days. Patients who begin therapy need to be informed about this particular side effect to avoid unnecessary concern.

The interferon betas cause a flulike reaction that is characterized by variable combinations of fever, chills, myalgias, fatigue and/or malaise, and sweats. This is the major side effect of interferon beta therapy. Because flulike symptoms are more likely to occur in young patients and in patients with small body size, young women with MS are at increased risk (64). Flulike reactions are prevented or minimized by the systematic use of premedication in the first 4 to 12 weeks of therapy, dose escalation, and early evening dosing. Premedication can consist of antipyretics (such as acetaminophen), antiinflammatory agents (such as ibuprofen), low-dose glucocorticoids (such as prednisone, 30 mg a day), or pentoxifylline (64,65). Dose escalation schedules include starting at a quarter or half dose, then escalating as tolerated every two weeks to full dose.

When interferon beta is injected subcutaneously, it initially causes cosmetic injection-site reactions in up to 85 percent of patients. This rate falls to 44 percent to 50 percent over time. Reactions include redness, inflammation, bruising, pain, hypersensitivity, and very rarely worsening of psoriasis or subcutaneous atrophy. The most serious reaction, necrosis, occurs in less than 5 percent of patients and may be more likely to occur when there is intercurrent infection. Most patients do not have significant problems with injection-site reactions. Management includes injection strategies (improved technique, use of two needles, use of a small-gauge needle, auto-injection), drug strategies (dose escalation, drug holiday, allowing the syringe to sit at room temperature for 30 minutes, premedication with corticosteroids, pentoxifylline, diphenhydramine hydrochloride, terfenadine), and skin strategies (using the buttocks and lateral thighs, massaging the skin site after injection, using 1% hydrocortisone cream pre- and postinjection, using ice on the site before injection, and using sunscreen to block injection-site exposure).

Glatiramer acetate, which is injected subcutaneously, can also produce injection-site reactions and local pain. They are rarely severe, however, and are often managed by the injection of room temperature drug, the use of preferred injection sites, a change in technique, or the use of diphenhydramine hydrochloride. There is a questionable association between use of glatiramer acetate and abnormal Pap smear. This most likely is artifactual, and more convincing data are needed.

The recent preliminary report of the SPECTRIMS trial of interferon beta-1a (Rebif) for secondary progressive MS

TABLE 30-5
MS Disease-Modifying Therapies and Women's Issues

General
- Pregnancy viewed as contraindication to treatment
- Pregnancy viewed as indication to discontinue treatment
- Contraceptive techniques indicated while on treatment
- Breast-feeding while receiving treatment contraindicated (no data on breast milk drug levels)

Specific
- Interferon beta is abortofacient at high levels in animal studies
- Interferon beta can produce menstrual irregularities
- Flulike side effects of interferon betas more common in young, small (female) patients
- Glatiramer acetate has questionable association with abnormal Pap smears

found a therapeutic response based on gender (66). The primary outcome (confirmed progression) was significantly reduced with treatment for women but not for men. For the treated group as a whole, the primary outcome was negative. This gender response to interferon beta had not been reported previously. It raises questions about the study results and is currently undergoing careful analysis.

Immunosuppressive agents are sometimes used to treat MS and have specific consequences for women. These drugs include antimetabolites (azathioprine, methotrexate), which are active during the cell cycle S phase (DNA synthesis); alkylating agents (chlorambucil, cyclophosphamide), which are active throughout the cell cycle; and antibiotics (mitoxantrone), which particularly affect DNA (67). These drugs are basically cytotoxic agents that not only are teratogenic but also carry a risk for late malignancy. Sterility may occur with intensive cyclophosphamide use, and menstruation may cease or be affected by all these agents. These immunosuppressive agents are not documented to be disease-modifying therapies because convincing efficacy has not been shown. Nevertheless, anecdotal data indicate that individual patients may benefit from their use.

PSYCHOSOCIAL ISSUES

Multiple sclerosis encompasses many psychological issues because it affects virtually all aspects of life,

career, and family. Women with MS face specific problems (Table 30-6) (68). They run the gamut from questions about self-image and interpersonal relationships to economic issues. It is not difficult to understand that women with MS, particularly those who have obvious neurologic deficits, often have a poor self-image, with feelings of unattractiveness and lack of desirability. It may be difficult for them to apply makeup, fix their hair, or practice appropriate hygiene. Suddenly they are dependent on others to perform these personal tasks that normally are taken for granted. The unpredictable nature of MS—and the uncertain prognosis—can be quite unsettling. Marriages can be stressed not only by sexual dysfunction but also by loss of a full partner and the need for a spouse or other family member to assume the role of caregiver. A recent study noted gender differences in how both MS patients and their caregivers coped with the disease (69).

There have been some interesting and disturbing findings about psychosocial stressors in this disease. As a whole, MS patients are less likely to be involved in vocational, educational, and homemaking activities. They are more likely to require personal assistance care and to use medical services. The MS family unit is under increased stress, has less in the way of available resources, and experiences decreased satisfaction with life in general.

Psychosocial factors help to determine quality of life. Factors that are associated with a poor quality of life in MS are social isolation, unstable disease course, denial

---

TABLE 30-6
Psychosocial Issues for the Female Multiple Sclerosis Patient (62)

ISSUE	ASPECTS
Personal image and self-worth	Physical appearance
	Future circumstances
	Need for others
	Ability to get around and out of the home
	Management of specific symptoms (depression, bladder/bowel dysfunction, sexual problems, etc.)
	Disruption of lifestyle
	Ability to function in different roles (career, homemaker, spouse, parent)
Interaction with others	Marriage (issues of abandonment/divorce, children, sexuality, contraception, caretaker role)
	Codependency
	Coping with disease and its limitations
	Abuse (both physical and mental)
	Social isolation
Economic	Vocational issues
	Health care issues (access to care, medical costs, long-term care)

rather than acceptance of illness, moderate to severe disease symptoms, limitations in mobility, and unemployment (70). In one study, women with MS, particularly those who were married, were more likely to be unemployed than men with MS (71). Although they were less physically disabled, they tended to leave the work force to assume a role in the home. Women tended to feel guilty at perceived failure to meet obligations to their family. In contrast, men tended to react with anger and frustration at their limited work and other activities.

At least one study has found the cost of MS to differ based on gender. This study found costs higher for women (78). Estimated in 1991 dollars, the average lifetime costs of MS were $746,819 for single women, $450,845 for married women, $360,320 for married men, and $332,001 for single men.

Finally, there are gender issues with regard to ongoing health maintenance. Access to health care may be limited for more disabled MS patients. It is important that routine nonneurologic care for female patients, such as annual gynecologic examination, periodic mammography, bone density studies, and considerations for postmenopausal HRT, not be neglected.

PARTICIPATION IN THERAPEUTIC TRIALS

There are many therapeutic trials testing novel treatments for MS. They range from small single-center and relatively brief (weeks to months) phase I studies, to large multicenter phase III studies lasting several years. There is great interest in ensuring that sufficient numbers of women participate in formal studies, particularly in a gender preference disorder such as MS. Pregnancy is a routine exclusion criterion for clinical trials, and women who want to participate are required to use contraception to ensure that pregnancy does not occur. The rationale is based on avoiding potential risks to a fetus. The result is an added responsibility and burden for women who take part in these studies. It is important that they understand this and remain compliant with their chosen birth control method for the required time period.

SUMMARY

The benefits of a gender-based approach to medicine are increasingly appreciated. It is particularly important in diseases that show a strong gender preference, such as MS. Women with MS have special issues and concerns that need to be addressed quite specifically. This more rationale and thoughtful approach should improve the daily and long-term care of all patients with this disease.

References

1. Legato MJ. Women's health: Not for women only. *Int J Fertil* 1998; 43:65–72.
2. Leys D, Lamy C, Lucas C, et al. Arterial ischemic strokes associated with pregnancy and puerperium. *Acta Neurol Belg* 1997; 97:5–16.
3. Mas JL, Lamy C. Stroke in pregnancy and the puerperium. *J Neurol* 1998; 245:305–313.
4. Thomas SV. Neurological aspects of eclampsia. *J Neurol Sci* 1998; 155:37–43.
5. Halbreich U, Lumley LA. The multiple interactional biological processes that might lead to depression and gender differences in its appearance. *J Affect Disord* 1993; 29:159–173.
6. Manzoni GC, Terzano MG, Bono G, et al. Cluster headache: Clinical findings in 180 patients. *Cephalgia* 1983; 3:21–30.
7. Steward WF, Schecker A, Rasmusse BK. Migraine prevalence: A review of population-based studies. *Neurology* 1994; 44:817–823.
8. Hauser WA, Amatniek JC. Gender differences in disease of the nervous system. In: Kaplan PW (ed.). *Neurologic disease in women.* New York: Demos, 1998:433–442.
9. Quality Standards Subcommittee of the American Academy of Neurology. Practice parameter: Management issues for women with epilepsy (summary statement). *Neurology* 1998; 51:944–948.
10. Zahn CA, Morrell MJ, Collins SD, Labiner DM, Yerby MS. Management issues for women with epilepsy. A review of the literature. *Neurology* 1998; 51:949–956.
11. Duquette P, Pleines J, Girard M, et al. The increased susceptibility of women to multiple sclerosis. *Can J Neurol Sci* 1992; 19:466–471.
12. Minden SL, Marder WD, Harrold LN, Dor A. Multiple sclerosis: A statistical portrait. National MS Society. Cambridge, MA: Abt Associates 1993.
13. McEwen BS, Alves SE, Bullock K, Weiland NG. Ovarian steroids and the brain: Implications for cognition and aging. *Neurology* 1997; 48(Suppl 7):8–15.
14. Weinstein Y, Ran S, Segal S. Sex-associated differences in the regulation of immune responses controlled by the MHC of the mouse. *J Immunol* 1984; 132:656–661.
15. Ahmed SA, Talal N, Christados P. Genetic regulation of testosterone-induced immune suppression. *Cell Immunol* 1987; 104:91–98.
16. Grossman C. Possible underlying mechanisms of sexual dimorphism in the immune response, fact and hypothesia. *J Steroid Biochem* 1989; 34:241251.
17. Schuurs A, Verheul H. Effects of gender and sex steroids on the immune response. *J Steroid Biochem* 1990; 35:157–172.
18. Piccinni MP, Giudizi M, Biagiotti R, et al. Progesterone favors the development of human T helper cells producing Th2-type cytokines and promotes both IL-4 production and membrane CD30 expression in established Th1 cell clones. *J Immunol* 1995; 155:128–133.
19. Jansson L, Holmdahl R. Estrogen-mediated immunosuppression in autoimmune diseases. *Inflamm Res* 1998; 47:290–301.
20. Duquette P, Girard M. Hormonal factors in susceptibility to multiple sclerosis. *Curr Opinion Neurol Neurosurg* 1993; 6:195–201.
21. Gilmore W, Weiner LP, Correale J. Effect of estradiol on

cytokine secretion by proteolipid protein-specifc T cell clones isolated from multiple sclerosis patient and normal control subjects. *J Immunol* 1997; 158:446–451.

22. Jansson L, Olsson T, Holmdahl R. Estrogen induces a potent suppression of experimental autoimmune encephalomyelitis and collagen-induced athritis in mice. *J Neuroimmunol* 1994; 53: 203–207.

23. Voskuhl RR, Pitchekian-Halabi H, MacKenzie-Graham A, McFarland HF, Raine CS. Gender differences in autoimmune demyelination in the mouse: Implications for multiple sclerosis. *Ann Neurol* 1996; 39:724–733.

24. Kim S, Liva SM, Dalal MA, Verity MA, Voskuhl RR. Estriol ameliorates autoimmune demyelinating disease. *Neurology* 1999; 52:1230–1238.

25. Jacobs LD, Wende KE, Brownscheidle CM, Apatoff B, Coyle PK, et al. A profile of multiple sclerosis: The New York State Multiple Sclerosis Consortium. *Multiple Sclerosis* 1999 (in press).

26. McDonnell GV, Hawkins SA. Primary progressive multiple sclerosis: A distinct syndrome? *Multiple Sclerosis* 1996; 2:137–141.

27. Smith R, Studd JWW. A pilot study of the effect upon multiple sclerosis of the menopause, hormone replacement therapy and the menstrual cycle. *J Royal Soc Med* 1992; 85:612–613.

28. Wynn DR, Kurland LT, Rodriguez M. A reappraisal of the epidemiology of multiple sclerosis in Olmsted County, Minnesota. *Neurology* 1990; 40:780–786.

29. Muller R. Studies on disseminated sclerosis. *Acta Med Scand* 1949; S222:1–214.

30. Tillman AJB. The effect of pregnancy on multiple sclerosis and its management. *Res Publ Ass Res Nerv Ment Dis* 1950; 28:548–582.

31. McAlpine D, Compston N. Some aspects of the natural history of disseminated sclerosis. *Quart J Med* 1952; 21:135–167.

32. Millar JHD. The influence of pregnancy on disseminated sclerosis. *Proc Royal Soc Med* 1961; 54:4–7.

33. Leibowitz U, Antonovsky A, Kats R, Alter M. Does pregnancy increase the risk of multiple sclerosis? *J Neurol Neurosurg Psychiatry* 1967; 30:354–357.

34. Poser S, Raun NE, Wikstrom, Poser W. Pregnancy, oral contraceptives and multiple sclerosis. *Acta Neurol Scand* 1979; 59:108–118.

35. Ghezzi A, Caputo D. Pregnancy: A factor influencing the course of multiple sclerosis? *Eur Neurol* 1981; 20:115–117.

36. Poser S, Poser W. Multiple sclerosis and gestation. *Neurology* 1983; 33:1422–1427.

37. Korn-Lubertzki I, Kahana E, Cooper G, Abramsky O. Activity of multiple scleroisis during pregnancy and puerperium. *Ann Neurol* 1984; 16:229–231.

38. Birk K, Rudick R. Pregnancy and multiple sclerosis. *Arch Neurol* 1986; 43:719–726.

39. Frith JA, McLeod JG. Pregnancy and multiple sclerosis. *J Neurol Neurosurg Psychiatry* 1988; 51:495–498.

40. Thompson DS, Nelson LM, Burns A, Burks JS, Franklin GM. The effects of pregnancy in multiple sclerosis: a retrospective study. *Neurology* 1986; 36:1097–1099.

41. Nelson LM, Franklin GM, Jones MC, and the Multiple Sclerosis Study Group. Risk of multiple sclerosis exacerbation during pregnancy and breast-feeding. *JAMA* 1988; 259:3441–3443.

42. Weinshenker BG, Hader W, Carriere W, Baskerville J, Ebers GC. The influence of pregnancy on disability from

multiple sclerosis: A population-based study in Middlesex County, Ontario. *Neurology* 1989; 39:1438–4440.

43. Bernardi S, Grasso MG, Bertollini R, Orzi F, Fieschi C. The influence of pregnancy on relapses in multiple sclerosis: A cohort study. *Acta Neurol Scand* 1991; 84:403–406.

44. Roullet E, Verdier-Taillefer MH, Amarenco P, Gharbi G, Alperovitch A. Pregnancy and multiple sclerosis: A longitudinal study of 125 remittent patients. *J Neurol Neurosurg Psychiatry* 1993; 56:1062–1065.

45. Abramsky O. Pregnancy and multiple sclerosis. *Ann Neurol* 1994; 36:S38–S41.

46. Sadovnick AD, Eisen K, Hashimoto SA, et al. Pregnancy and multiple sclerosis. A prospective study. *Arch Neurol* 1994; 51:1120–1124.

47. Stenager E, Stenager EN, Jensen K. Effect of pregnancy on the prognosis for multiple sclerosis. A 5 year follow up investigation. *Acta Neurol Scand* 1994; 90:305–308.

48. Verdru P, Theys P, D'Hooghe MB, Carton H. Pregnancy and multiple sclerosis: The influence on long term disability. *Clin Neurol Neurosurg* 1994; 96:38–41.

49. Worthington J, Jones R, Crawford M, Forti A. Pregnancy and multiple sclerosis—a 3-year prospective study. *J Neurol* 1994; 241:228–233.

50. Flachenecker P, Hartung HP. Multiple sclerosis and pregnancy. Overview and status of the European multicenter PRIMS study. *Nervenarzt* 1995; 66:97–104.

51. Runmarker B, Andersen O. Pregnancy is associated with a lower risk of onset and a better prognosis in multiple sclerosis. *Brain* 1995; 118:253–291.

52. Confavreux C, Hutchinson M, Hours MM, et al. Rate of pregnancy-related relapses in multiple sclerosis. *N Engl J Med* 1998; 339:285–291.

53. van Walderveen MA, Tas MW, Barkhof F, et al. Magnetic resonance evaluation of disease activity during pregnancy in multiple sclerosis. *Neurology* 1994; 44:327–329.

54. Achiron A, Rotstein Z, Noy S, et al. Intravenous immunoglobulin treatment in the prevention of childbirth-associated acute exacerbations in multiple sclerosis: A pilot study. *J Neurol* 1996; 243:25–28.

55. Tagaris GA, Terzoudi M, Panagopoulos G, Karageorgiou C. Intravenous immunoglobin in childbirth-related exacerbations of multiple sclerosis. *J Neurol* 1999; 52(S2): A133–A144.

56. Giesser BS, Halper J, Cross AH, et al. Multiple sclerosis symptoms fluctuate during menstrual cycle. *MS Exchange* 1991; 3:5.

57. Giesser B, Bergen R, Akporiayc E. Clinical status in multiple sclerosis does not change with the menstrual cycle. *J Neurol* 1999; 246(S1) I/90.

58. Pozzilli C, Falaschi P, Mainero C, et al. MRI in multiple sclerosis during the menstrual cycle: Relationship with sex hormone patterns. *Neurology* 1999; 53:622–624.

59. Goodin DS. Survey of multiple sclerosis in northern California. Northern California MS Study Group. *Multiple Sclerosis* 1999; 5:78–88.

60. VanVollenhoven RF, McGuire JL. Estrogen, progesterone, and testosterone: Can they be used to treat autoimmune diseases? *Cleve Clin J Med* 1994; 61: 276–284.

61. Villard-Mackintosh L, Vessey MP. Oral contraceptives and reproductive factors in multiple sclerosis incidence. *Contraception* 1993; 47:161–168.

62. Coyle PK. Multiple sclerosis. In: Kaplan PW (ed.). *Neurologic disease in women*. New York: Demos 1998: 251–264.

63. Interferon ß1b. Product Monograph, Berlex Laboratories, 1994.

64. Lublin FD, Whitaker JN, Eidelman BH, et al. Management of patients receiving interferon beta 1b for multiple sclerosis: Report of a consensus conference. *Neurology* 1996; 46:12–18.

65. Rieckmann R, Weber F, Gunther A, Poster S. The phosphodiesterase inhibitor pentoxifylline reduces early side effects of interferon ß-1b treatment in patients with multiple sclerosis. *Neurology* 1997; 47:604.

66. Paty DW, SPIMS study group. Results of the 3-year, double-blind, placebo-controlled study of interferon BETA-1A (REBIF) in secondary-progressive MS. *J Neurol* 1999; 246(S1):I/15.

67. Brodsky I, Crilley P, Terzian AEL. Cancer chemotherapy. In: DiPalma JR, DiGregorio GJ (eds.). *Basic pharmacology in medicine,* 3rd ed. New York: McGraw-Hill, 1990:549–565.

68. Murray TJ. The psychosocial aspects of multiple sclerosis. *Neurol Clin* 1995; 13:197–233.

69. Steck B, Amsler F, Kappos L, Burgin D. Gender specific differences in the process of coping in families with multiple sclerosis. *J Neurol* 1999; 246(S1):I121.

70. Aronson KJ. Quality of life among persons with multiple sclerosis and their caregivers. *Neurology* 1997; 48:74–80.

71. LaRocca NG. Employment and multiple sclerosis. Health Services Research Reports Monograph, National MS Society, 1995.

72. Harvey C. Economic costs of multiple sclerosis: How much and who pays? Health Services Research Reports Monograph, National MS Society, 1995.

VII

SOCIETAL ISSUES

31 Managed Care

Bruce Idelkope, M.D.

It is thought that we are entering the third major metamorphosis in health care. The first was in the arena of technologic and clinical service expansion following World War II, with the second beginning in the 1970s as an era of cost containment. The 1990s brings the third wave, that of assessment and accountability. This revolution is founded on the concept of "quality of care" and is dependent on demonstrating the best outcomes at the lowest cost. Cost controls entered as health care costs rose at twice the rate of inflation over the past two decades and now exceed 14 percent of the gross national product. The payers—businesses and the government—now demand that we curb this process.

Editors' Note: Managed care is making a tremendous impact on the process of treating patients with MS and other diseases. The editors have asked Dr. Bruce Idelkope to provide his unique expertise and perspective on the phenomenon of managed care. Although most of the material presented in this chapter is not specific to MS, the material is not readily available to neurologic health care professionals and is not covered in other neurologic publications. Dr. Idelkope's chapter is taken from a talk he presented at an annual meeting of the American Society of Neurorehabilitation. His informative perspective was so well received that the editors believe this information should increase our understanding and therefore should be included in this text.

The collision between the practice of *medicine* and the *business* of medicine has spawned the system of health care termed *managed care*. Although the practicing physicians recognize the economies that fostered the appearance of these organizations, they generally are not enamored of the reduction in their autonomy imposed by management organizations. Physicians are disturbed by the management difficulties incurred in the care of their patients when diagnostics and therapeutics fall out of the "norm" and interpret these organizational reminders as restrictions on their practices. They are reminded of the decline of their practice economies and aware of the dollars taken out of health care by the management organizations, seemingly without tangible benefit to their patients. They dislike the difficult position in which they find themselves placed by contractual obligations with managed care organizations (MCOs) whenever they stray from the management guidelines. As they strive to practice what they believe to represent "quality medicine," they are frustrated by data accumulation that is of questionable accuracy.

Physicians also recognize the near term benefits that managed care can provide, such as security of employment, relief of practice management, and the flexibility that employment versus practice ownership brings. They are apprised of the ability large organizations have to assimilate large amounts of clinical data and improve the delivery and quality of health care. Although traditionally patient-focused, physicians are not blinded to the economics and potential crisis the escalating costs of medicine have created, nor the potential affordability of health care such MCOs may provide. But managed care is a complex concept and needs to be more fully understood by physicians as they attempt to manage both their clinical duties to their patients and the business events of their practice.

Although MS is not unique in the neurologic care delivery spectrum, the disease provides a template for the comprehension of the changes managed care has brought to our health care system. Different areas of the country have had varied experiences in the evolution of managed care as the penetration of such organizations has not been universal. The experience of advanced managed care markets such as those in Minnesota and California provide all of us with some lessons learned. The concepts presented in this chapter apply not just to MS but universally to any medical problem or process, and it is hoped that illumination of the managed care concept will assist physicians to better comprehend and control health care delivery.

HISTORY OF MANAGED CARE

Health maintenance organizations were first developed on a large scale at the turn of the nineteenth century in the northwest and were called prepaid group practices. They came about during the opening up of this area by the railroads. One of the first was located in Tacoma, Washington, known as "The Western Clinic." It was formed as lumbermill owners and their employees sought to "lock in" medical service costs through prepaid contracts. Originally a fee-for-service practice set up by Drs. Thomas Curran and James Yocum in 1906, they signed on to take care of all the employees of the lumber industry for 50 cents per member per month in 1910.

Around the same time, Dr. Bridge started a clinic that offered prepaid contracts with other employee groups in Tacoma and ultimately organized a chain of 20 industrial clinics in Washington and Oregon known as "The Bridge Company."

In 1917 the first resistance to the prepaid concept arose through the Pierce County Medical Service Bureau, which was organized by physicians in Tacoma. Their job was to screen all medical contracts to "preserve some professional control and to offer consumer choice." In actuality, the bureau served to limit competition from the prepaid groups and became the predecessors of the local medical societies—the same societies that would oppose HMOs at virtually every stage of their development.

The Great Depression provided an impetus for large-scale changes in health care economics. The financial uncertainties of the times forced hospitals to turn from philanthropic donations as their primary source of funding to charging patients fees for support. The patients faced both loss of income from illness and increasing debt from their medical expenses. Thus began the awareness of the middle class of the need for protection from the economic consequences of illness.

Parallel efforts on opposite coasts of the United States occurred in the 1930s. Drs. Donald Ross and H. Clifford Loos began a typical fee-for-service clinic in Los Angeles, California. They served a number of the employees of the Los Angeles Water and Power Department, and they were subsequently convinced to establish a prepaid medical program for all their employees. The program was successful and expanded to other groups of municipal employees. Both Dr. Ross and Dr. Loos were expelled from the Los Angeles county medical society for operating their prepaid clinic. They were later reinstated on appeal to the American Medical Association (AMA). The first urban precursor of health maintenance organizations (HMOs), Group Health Association of Washington, D.C., was begun in 1937. This idea was initiated in the offices of the Home Owner's Loan Corporation, where it was known that medical expenses were a common cause for mortgage default. Group Health Association was organized as a nonprofit organization, and the startup funds came from each homeowner's loan.

National publicity provoked interest in this concept and the industry's interest spawned the development of the largest HMO in the country; Kaiser-Permanente Medical Care program. It began in 1933 when Dr. Sidney Garfield finished his surgical training and began to seek a location for his medical practice. The Great Depression afforded him limited opportunities, so he chose to work at a construction site in southern California where an aqueduct was being built to supply Los Angeles with water from the Colorado River. He built a 10-bed hospital on skids that were dragged along as construction progressed. Initially, all the seriously ill patients were sent to Los Angeles for medical treatment, but Dr. Garfield convinced the insurance company to pay him directly and in advance for each employee in exchange for provision of all necessary medical on-the-job care. He also arranged a salary deduction for the employees to provide this care for the employees and their families.

Henry Kaiser was connected with the construction company and also owned the insurance company. He was impressed with Garfield and asked him to set up a similar program in 1937 at the construction site of the Grand Coulee Dam in Washington State. This program was also successful, and in 1942 Kaiser asked Garfield to develop a health care program in the San Francisco area at his ship-building plants, which at that time employed 90,000 people in support of the war effort. Garfield was once again successful—so successful, in fact, that a number of health care facilities were paid for through the savings achieved. When the war ended, the work force disbanded and so did the patient population, but the Permanente Health Plan was so well regarded that it was immediately successful when enrollment was opened to the public. Today the Kaiser-Permanente care program encompasses nine geographic areas, has 4.6 million members, and is the largest HMO in the United States.

In 1944 Mayor Fiorello La Guardia established a health system for New York City employees. Similar plans were soon developed in Puget Sound, in St. Louis by the Teamsters, in Appalachia by the United Mine Workers, and in Detroit by the United Auto Workers. The ultimate role reversal occurred when the Group Health Mutual Insurance Company, a traditional insurance company that served rural Minnesota and Wisconsin, became interested in prepaid medical programs and made plans to deliver a "direct service program." In 1956, while building a new headquarters in Minneapolis–St. Paul, a clinical facility was added. This was the beginning of Group Health Plan, Minnesota's largest today, and one of the originators of the modern HMO movement.

President Johnson established Medicare and Medicaid in 1965. In the years that followed, the government attempted many initiatives to reduce rising health care costs, but their attempts were overwhelmed by the increasing social, political, and consumer demands for care, better access to more effective care, and advanced medical technology. The logical escape for both government and business has been to create an intermediary to handle the finances of this care, manage assets, and reduce costs. Thus the stage was set for development of HMOs.

By 1970, 30 to 40 prepaid group practices were in operation in the United States; although legally accepted and providing for member satisfaction, their use remained limited. As executive director of the American Rehabilitation Institute, Dr. Paul Ellwood concluded that the existing fee-for-service system created "perverse incentives" that rewarded physicians and hospitals for treating illness and withdrew those rewards when health was restored. Such a system discouraged preventative health care and rehabilitative care. Ellwood sought to form a more functional system and found that it already existed in Kaiser-Permanente and similar groups, which were providing good care to large populations at reasonable cost. Dr. Ellwood set about to convince the federal government of this inherent logic. To avoid the traditional negative response to prepaid group practice, Ellwood described his concept in a unique manner—politically neutral and medically nebulous. He coined the term *health maintenance organizations*. At that time presidential candidate Richard Nixon, who did not have a health care plank in his presidential campaign platform, was sensitized by public concern over Medicare and Med-

icaid spending. The Democrats also favored a national health plan, and, because Nixon's proposals agreed with the Democratic incentives, he was able to achieve bipartisan support for such a concept.

Although HMO growth has not approached the predictions of the 1970s, their success and sustained growth have created a strong impact. Paul Ellwood's policy of improved quality through competition and expanded options appears to have validity and the long range importance of HMO's seems more certain than ever.

CURRENT MANAGED CARE MARKET

The demise of health care reform legislation proposed in 1994 meant that social concerns regarding provision of care for the 40 million uninsured would continue. Managed care has taken over as the preeminent form of coverage due to its perceived market response to spiraling health care costs. In 1993, 50 percent of patients were insured in conventional indemnity programs, but it is estimated that only 10 percent will remain in non–managed care programs by the year 2000.

Managed care also is called *integrated care* because it controls both the financing and the delivery of health care. Costs are central to the behavior of the payer and the providers (hospitals, physicians, and so forth), and cost controls are the basis used to modify physician behavior. In addition to financial incentives to the physicians, there are other clinical "rules" in the form of quality assurance measures, practice protocols, administrative guidelines, and utilization review. Since funding for health care has fallen to employers, business dictates reduced costs for their employees by controlling the options for health care. The HMOs provide a fixed and lower cost alternative to the fee-for-service model and have risen dramatically in popularity for the purchasers.

This has impacted neurology because the primary care physician now has a new role—that of gatekeeper. The total national supply of physicians in the United States in 1993 was 183 per 100,000 population. HMO staffing patterns have 120 to 138 per 100,000 enrollees and call for 50 percent of those to be generalists. Approximately two thirds of U.S. physicians are specialists. Assuming the continued growth of managed care by the year 2000, there will be approximately a 60 percent oversupply of specialists.

What has driven the operational concepts of managed care? To this point, dollars, but in the future, health care will have to meet the needs of its customers (patients) and satisfy its employees (caregivers). Most physicians (and in some areas patients) take a somewhat skeptical view of MCOs to date and hold a number of beliefs described in the following section.

Financial Measures of Managed Care Organizations

Large, for-profit HMOs are the cornerstone of the industry. They set the competitive bids for their insured and secure the premiums of government and business. The lowest bid wins, and they must have capital to withstand and write off a loss until the market has been secured. Capitation has been the usual form of coverage, although fee-for-service options may be available for higher premium costs. The first 15 percent to 20 percent of revenues comes "off the top" as payment for HMO expenses such as management and return on investment (profit). The next 15 percent to 20 percent is drawn off by the provider organizations, leaving the balance to finance the health care of those covered and pay the providers under a system that likely withholds another 10 percent to 20 percent to be theoretically repaid at the end of the year if all goes well (for the HMO). The payment of fees and the repayment of the withhold are done by a method that is not divulged and through criteria not known to the providers. If a provider becomes an excessive cost center, the withhold is kept and that provider's contract likely is terminated. If a provider spends less than expected, the withhold is repaid, at least in part, and perhaps an additional bonus is included.

The chief executive officers of these HMOs command legendary salaries and stock offerings, some ranging from $2.3 to $14.28 million per year. The profits of the HMO in some instances, measured as a percent of premium, are as high as 27 percent to 31 percent. At the same time as the HMOs record startling growth and profits, physician's salaries have declined in California by 20 percent to 40 percent and in New England by 10 percent to 15 percent.

Capitation of specialists is opening a new phase in the transformation of the health care industry. As more and more HMOs make flat monthly payments to specialists under capitated systems, many other physicians are scrambling to participate, fearing that as part of a fee-for-service network, patients will be directed away from them and to the single specialty groups that bear risk. Interestingly enough, the switch from fee-for-service systems to capitated systems changes the referral relationships of specialists with their primary care counterparts. The specialists may fear that too many HMO patients will be referred. In defense, they are encouraging generalists to treat certain problems themselves.

Specialty networks need to be of certain size to arrange for such contracts, but the larger the groups sharing income and administrative services, the larger the problems. Health plans start by capitating more specialists than needed to enable easy access for its enrollees. Later, there tends to be a move to jettison those unnecessary or less cost-effective physicians.

Most specialists believe the pro's outweigh the con's and are interested in capitation because it offers a measure of security as the tide of managed care erodes their fee-for-service patient base. In addition, some specialists view capitation as a means of regaining control over the management of care, taking back control of health care quality from the micromanagement of plan bureaucracy.

Of interest is the conflicting incentives facing health maintenance organizations that can look at the hospital beds stating, "Here are the hospital beds where we make money if we keep them filled, and here are the ones in which we make money if we keep them empty." Such is the case in situations in which the system enrolls both fee-for-service and capitation patients. Similar incentives cannot be applied at the physician level because it would be unethical—as well as impractical—to treat patients differently based on their payment arrangement. As a solution at the physician level, some health care systems pay physicians' salaries so they do not profit or lose from seeing patients in a capitated or fee-for-service arrangement.

Where do the dollars needed to fund research and education come from? Now that business has stepped to the forefront at delivery and cost of health care, who funds graduate and undergraduate medical education? Who funds care for the uninsured? Who funds new technology? These costs obviously should not be borne by business alone because they are the burden of our entire society, but at present few provisions have been made for future financing. If these elements are lost from America's system, the results will be catastrophic and will not be reconstructed without considerable expense.

Does managed care get at some of the "other" causes of rising costs—those that are society's problems and not of medical origin? It is estimated that smoking, obesity, alcohol consumption, lack of exercise, and risky sexual practices cost $148 billion annually. Furthermore, poverty and medical indigency costs of $25 to $50 billion, end-of-life costs of $3 billion, and legal costs of $30 billion also arise the overall expense borne by the industry as a whole, even though these costs are not part of one's managed care.

There also is difficulty in getting managed care companies to provide funding for comprehensive MS care. They state that this type of care has not been proven beneficial to MS patients by established data (i.e., this is a dollar-driven decision). In the 1980s fee-for-service provided reimbursement for primary care specialists, rehabilitative specialists, social services, and psychologists without regard for outcomes. In the 1990s health care reform threatens the MS center's form of comprehensive care as gatekeepers reduce access to specialists, even though that is what is needed for the best management of MS patients.

Quality of Care Measures in Managed Care Organizations

How does the public perceive MCOs? In a study by the Robert Wood Johnson Foundation (Princeton, NJ, written communication, June 28, 1995), health care experiences were compared as reported by patients with physicians working in either managed care or fee-for-service. The survey revealed that sick or disabled patients in a managed care setting were 2 to 2.5 times more likely to receive care that was incorrect or inappropriate, failed to receive explanation of what the physicians were doing and how and when to take medications, waited longer for appointments, and were not urged to receive preventative services. They furthermore reported difficulty seeing specialists, perceived that their examinations were not thorough, thought that the time spent with the physician was inadequate, and believed that the physician did not care about their situation.

How are HMOs providing the same excellent care previously enjoyed by their insured?

One means of assessing this capability has been to use outcome studies. Almost all the HMOs report that outcomes are an important part of their quality review. With this comes the need to develop a large database, complicated data accumulation methods, and personnel trained to interpret such data. Given the obvious costs included in such an endeavor, is it likely that this system has been as well developed as we physicians would like?

How do MCOs fare in the arena of preventative care (such as vaccination of children)?

An area advertised by the HMOs as a focus is likely suspect as the most needy population is impoverished and not likely insured, thus providing little benefit over the prior health care delivery systems.

In an article published in 1994, the Health Care Finance Administration (HCFA) reported that health outcomes were superior in a fee-for-service environment over managed care, and another study also published by the HCFA reported that "because the capitation system does not account for the better health of those who enroll in managed care, the program does not save money for Medicare."

Measuring Quality of Care

How do we define quality of care?

Physician: "Doing the right thing at the right time."

Patients: "Convenience, accessibility and perception of being treated fairly, appropriately, and with respect."

Government, employers, and health care organizations: "Being sure that financial resources are being allocated appropriately."

Is "quality of care" measurable, and are outcome data an accurate parameter through which all interested parties can form their own opinions of the adequacy of health care?

Performance measures are still quite a long way from adequate, although there is considerable agreement that quality comparisons will drive the ability of health plans to compete for patients. With such measures, the employers could select plans contracting with those physicians and hospitals that have the best outcomes and exclude those with substandard performance. Health plans would get the message that purchasers also will base their selections on such measures. Consumers would have access to the same data and could influence contract selection as well.

For many decades, medicine was held above the mundane corporate business world, apart from the laws of economics, and able to protect the doctor–patient relationship. Everything presently is measured in dollars, and clinical outcomes have become secondary. Outcomes, however, become important when their decline is measurable or detectable by the consumer. To date, we have used randomized clinical trials to demonstrate medical truths. Unfortunately, these have a great degree of exclusivity, making clinical application difficult. Furthermore, there is not the time or resources to conduct all the trials needed to guide our medical practice in each situation. Other outcomes models of measurement are subject to quite a few frailties; rehabilitation outcomes, particularly those of our MS patients, are sensitive to many variables other than treatment strategies (i.e., patient, clinical, demographic, social, and motivation factors). Because treatments are not randomized, selection bias also will play a role, as will treatment based on site of management rather than type.

As both public and private sector purchasers of health care services request documentation of proof of value received, various measurement schemes are unfolding. These "report cards" date back to the 1800s, when Florence Nightingale promoted the release of information to the public regarding health care by advocating the publication of mortality rates for hospitalized patients. In the early 1900s Dr. Ernest Codman, a staff surgeon at Massachusetts General Hospital, advocated systematic self-assessment of patient outcomes in an attempt to hold himself and his colleagues accountable to the general public. The 1986 release by the federal government of Health Care Financing Administration (HCFA) data of hospital-specific mortality rates for Medicare patients served as a stimulus for growth in performance-reporting activity. Suspended in 1993, this reporting system served as a controversial impetus for subsequent performance reporting initiatives. Since 1991 New York, Pennsylvania, and California have published such data.

The Joint Commission on Accreditation of Healthcare Organizations (JCAHO) also has supported development of the indicator monitoring system as a catalyst for quality improvement rather than as a means of determining whether a health care organization meets simple structural quality requirements.

The National Committee for Quality Assurance, which was established in 1979, has a set of data that assess the quality of care through the Health Plan/Employer Data and Information Set. They contain standards referring to preventative care, such as the percentage of people immunized and so forth. There are, however, no neurologic standards written as yet. Standards to accredit physicians are being written by the AMA in collaboration with the American Academy of Neurology (AAN). They anticipate the ability to compare the individual physician's performance with the national standards and norms. The Health Care Financing Administration is attempting to do the same thing with its Health Care Quality Improvement Program as a peer review structure for Medicare providers. They initially developed screens to sort out "poor" care, but now their focus is more toward measuring improvement in outcomes and patient satisfaction.

The cornerstone for many quality improvement efforts is the development of standards of care. The Agency for Health Care Policy and Research (AHCPR) has provided research for the development of these standards, as has the AAN. The focus is shifting from discovering the few "bad apples" to an approach that improves the performance of the entire group.

Although the complexities of such data accumulation, the methodology of sorting data and presenting the data in recognizable form to the physicians, and then educating them to change practice patterns, is formidable, the basics of patient satisfaction (personal care) and cost are well understood by both the physicians and their allies (the patients). Efforts must be made by physicians to include the patient population into the decision-making process to ensure that the new forms of health care delivery remain formulated by those who really care about "quality" issues.

Date Accumulation in Managed Care Organizations

Outcome measures will soon be the norm in health care evaluation by its consumers. The capacity to initiate such practices is in its infancy, but growing, as is the public's increasing demand for this information. The health care industry is held accountable for demonstrating value (cost plus quality). As provider-specific report cards are implemented, physicians should be aware of an increasing impact on their clinical practice and physicians need to be involved in the construction of such systems. As neurologists, we should be active participants in determining future care parameters for our patients rather than give away the right to determine the criteria against which we and our patients will be measured. One of the problems is to define exactly what "quality" of care is. Early methodology entailed looking at three separate areas: (1) Structure—physical and staffing characteristics; (2) Process—or what is done for the patients; (3) Outcomes—the impact on the patient's health—mortality, morbidity, disability, patient function, well-being, and patient satisfaction with care. Current methodology is of much broader scope:

Interpreting Outcomes

Outcome measures are of varied criteria, which makes comparisons difficult.

TYPES OF OUTCOMES VARY BY TIME FRAME:

IMMEDIATE: straightforward—i.e., post-op wound infections, sterile urine culture after antibiotic Rx for UTI.

INTERMEDIATE: are assessed while waiting for long-term outcomes following changes in risk factors—i.e., lowering of blood pressure following institution of antihypertensive agents, or lowered Hgb_{A1C} with insulin, response to steroid administration.

LONG-TERM: require longer time periods to assess benefits as impact on outcomes may lag years after treatment changes or risk factors alterations are made—i.e., changes in lung cancer rates after smoking cessation, reduction in MS exacerbation rates following interferon use, and so forth.

TYPES OF OUTCOMES VARY BY CARE MODEL:

QUALITY OF LIFE ASSESSMENTS: attempt to measure physical, functional, mental, and social aspects of a person's life with respect to the impact an illness or treatment has on the individual— i.e., hair loss and anorexia caused by immunosuppressive chemotherapy—although clinically beneficial, are they tolerable or not?

PROCESS-BASED OUTCOMES: length of hospital stays for certain diseases, immunization rates, and so forth.

Not only do time frames have to be accounted for, but the outcomes may be viewed in quite a different fashion compared to our time-honored outcome measures—morbidity and mortality.

TYPES OF OUTCOMES VARY BY VIEWER:

Each group—physicians, consumers, and purchasers—have different points of view. Physicians want hard data, patients want quality of life issues dealt with, and purchasers are interested in economics.

To this point the medical community has been held accountable in certain areas and those that measure up best have been rewarded with the most business. The technology to measure outcomes is evolving and is still in the earliest phases of development. There are several good national organizations attempting to organize this process, which will improve over time.

Pitfalls of Outcomes Measures

Multiple performance categories have been used to provide data to prospective purchasers with comparative data on managed care operations. There are, however, some important issues still unsettled before this data is thought to have evolved to its most useful state:

a. Can the patient population (denominator) be defined?

b. What is the size of the patient population? What is a critical size to determine the adequacy of any outcomes (rural vs. urban)?

c. How is the outcome defined? Annual vs. every other year for screening labs.

d. How long will it take to achieve the desired outcome?

e. Data may be missing—patients move to another system, physicians do not document the necessary data, failure of treatment vs. noncompliance.

f. Risk adjustment. The limitation in the ability to adjust for different risk profiles of populations somewhat limits comparisons across managed care organizations. There is a need to somehow incorporate different ages, socioeconomic status, and comorbidities that affect outcomes.

g. Data integrity. The data used may come from encounter records (benefit claims) and from medical records and are of questionable accuracy. If this is not improved, the outcomes data also will be skewed (the "garbage in—garbage out" phenomenon).

h. Inconsistent verification. At present there is no perfect mechanism to ensure the accuracy of reported performance data. In voluntary reporting, there is no independent or external audit necessary to verify, but thus far no one is certain who should provide such services.

i. Unclear consumer information needs. The report card information has been focused on the employer/purchaser's need (largely based on costs), and little focus has been on the consumer's need (based on quality). In addition, the information reported to date does not have universal use because there is little value to a Medicare population of statistics pertaining to pregnancy and childhood immunizations.

j. Cost of performance reporting. This is not a trivial cost, and it is not clear who should bear responsibility for this expense.

k. Unclear accountability. It is not clear who should be responsible for determining what health care activities are carried out to the satisfaction of the standards (i.e., mammography is agreed on as a valuable means of cancer detection. It is incorporated into a system of health plan performance, but who among the patient, physician, or managed care plan bear the responsibility to see that all the target population undergoes this screening?

l. Lack of comparative data and standards. To date there are no established targets for performance standards regarding their validity and also for agreement on the aforementioned concerns.

Implications for Physicians of Data Accumulation

Demand for credible and meaningful performance data is accelerating. Although the focus has been on managed care plans to provide such data, there are significant impacts on physicians:

1. *Areas of focus:* Inquiries by purchasers draw interest to selected areas of clinical practice, usually with intense efforts to collect data. Physicians practicing in these areas should expect a high degree of scrutiny and attention, particularly if they do not measure up to the comparative standards set by the industry, even in its infancy.

2. *Accuracy and integrity of data reporting:* Physicians and their staffs should anticipate growing requirements for accuracy and completeness of administrative information in the claims data they submit. The need for accuracy is underscored in review of ICD-9 and E/M coding as regards payments by the HMOs.

3. *Inconsistent performance requirements:* Given the current focus on health plan performance, practitioners may expect to participate in more than one system of data collection as they continue to maintain a relationship with multiple managed care organizations. This may create different demands and different data submission requirements. Frustration will reign among providers until more uniformity is reached by the managed care entities.

4. *Capacity for improvement:* Both providers and health plans may anticipate growing expectations that data reporting will improve, resulting from availability and increased use of such data. Physicians must provide not only the interest but also the means to obtain such data.

5. *Provider specific reporting:* Physicians should anticipate intensified attention to comparative performance reporting at physician, hospital, and provider/system levels. This information is thought to be necessary to give consumers data on which to base their choices. A basic question is "what will provide 'benchmark' standards for physicians

regarding their care in comparison with their associates?" The answer is likely to be limited and narrowly focused data. In addition, other issues, such as confidentiality, indicator validity, at-risk population adjustments, clinical significance, value to consumers, and cost of data collection and reporting need to be revisited by the health care industry as a whole with increased physician input, and not just the mandate of legislative bodies or managed care organizations.

6. *Devaluation of the team approach:* We have to protect our patients with MS or other chronic neurologic diseases from the devaluation of the team approach by managed care as each contributor (PT, OT, speech, rehab psychology, nutrition, pastoral care, social service, and so forth) provides benefit to the *whole* process. If they are assessed individually as to what contribution to outcome or quality of care each specialty provides to the patient, the medical concept is lost or discredited. Each member of the team provides contributions in his or her own area and only the whole of the contributions can be assessed as being part of "quality" care. Managed care, with its trend to outcomes-driven allocation of finances and delivery, tends to focus on the select goals of individual therapies. It may thus ignore the more global contributions of the rehab team as a whole. In this instance rehabilitation teams will give up their focus on the person as a whole looking instead at the gains possible through the technical interventions (isolated gait training, adaptive equipment, and so forth).

It is this concern; that the outcomes approach will devalue services for some underserved groups of MS patients and may lead to discrimination against certain handicapped individuals. In this instance when an outcome is "poor," support for offering services directed to groups having these outcomes diminishes, and the quality of care for these individuals spirals downward. It is this event that we must avoid even when (and if) we overcome the problems that the financial/business evolution of managed care has levied on us.

Additional Challenges to Managed Care

In addition to concerns over finances, quality of care issues, and data accumulation, other aspects of managed care's influence on our health care delivery system bear scrutiny.

Ethical Concerns

Treatment coverage and reimbursement options set forth by the MCOs may create moral dilemmas and conflicts of interest for providers already struggling to adhere to professional codes of ethics, remain faithful to patient advocacy obligations, make a living, build a shared practice, and satisfy the stockholder's and/or employer's demands. In the fee-for-service model, there exist financial incentives to the provider to either raise fees, see more patients, or offer more services to existing patients. In managed care, fiscal incentives are created by establishing control over price per unit of service, the number of covered lives within a market, overall health of the managed population, and type and number of units of services authorized (inpatient days of home visits and so forth). In both systems there exist financial incentives that create opportunities for financial self-interest to conflict with duty to patients. As the fee-for-service model may encourage doing more, the MCOs encourage doing less. The best MCOs encourage personal and long-term relationships between the patient and determine care and strategies for improvement that are based on outcomes. The worst seek to control costs by exclusion of the sicker patients or denial of beneficial but expensive care and perverse incentives for providers to withhold treatment.

Capitation looms as an easy means by employers to purchase health care plans that effectively limit the number of dollars spent irrespective of the type of health plan administered. This system provides prejudice for the providers, preventing them from fairly assessing and acting in the patient's best interest as the financial risk is shifted from the MCO to the provider who have agreed to receive a set per member/per month fee; if the PMPM is exceeded, the provider bears the financial loss. When this form of decision making becomes dominant, the patient suffers a loss of his or her advocate. The provider is then faced with some cognitive dissonance when wrongdoing is the result of such actions. When the provider's professional survival is at stake, ethical concerns may be minimized.

Doctor–Patient Relationships

In the managed care model, physicians have come to recognize gag rules, loss of professional autonomy, capitation, profit margins, and bottom lines. The public has a new concern about their health "Can you still trust your doctor?" Now that the public is becoming more aware of the mechanics of managed care, there is increasing mistrust of the "third partner in the examining room—the clinic, health plan, or the contract that drives medical decisions!"

In states in which for-profit MCOs exist, such as California and Massachusetts, and even in states such as Minnesota, in which the health care organizations are nonprofit and where profits are returned to consumers, people do not like the fact that their doctor's income is dependent on how they practice and do not like the fact that withholding care may be rewarded. When the MCOs reduce payment to physicians, citing rising health care costs, an implied obligation falls to the physicians to somehow reduce care costs. This shifts the goals from taking care of the patient to making a profit for the third party. At the same time there may be a tendency to keep the patients at arm's length and keep from forming a bond with the patients. They, of course, may sense this and their suspicions rise about the motives of their doctors.

We cannot go backwards to the fee-for-service model, and the managed care for profit model will not satisfy anyone other than those who measure medicine in dollars. We must keep physicians in charge of making the decisions about "gatekeeping" and must obtain more data about standards of care determined to be best for individuals (rule of one) as well as for the group. Society will have to provide input about how the resources are rationed and patients must become better informed about what type of coverage they own and purchase and furthermore, must become better informed about what choices they have when faced with a medical decision.

Capitation Concerns

Under capitation incentives are offered that can have a perverse effect on the health care of the disabled. These incentives originate from (1) the preexistent fee-for-service model, which has spawned a culture ill-equipped to handle the needs of the disabled; and (2) fragmentation of funding from Medicare and Medicaid, encouraging providers to focus on cost shifting rather than on integration of services. Thus under a capitated system most physicians are at financial risk for the care of a disabled individual and there is an inverse proportion of health status to cost.

Presently two programs, one federally funded (Medicare) and the other jointly state and federally funded (Medicaid), are the dominant payers for medical and social services provided under public entitlement. Medicare focuses on medically related and short-term rehabilitation services (physicians, hospitals, limited home and nursing care), and Medicaid focuses on long-term nursing home and community-based services, which vary from state to state. Under the present system there is a failure of any single individual coordinating and organizing care for the dependent MS population. Some of the nonmedical needs may be overlooked, such as living situation, social needs, nutrition, self-care, and so forth, while any medical crisis will be dealt with effectively by multiple doctors, hospitals, and specialists, albeit in an uncoordinated fashion. Medicare will not cover such non-medical expenses such as adult day care, long-term home nursing supervision, therapies, and so forth, and perpetuates this fragmentation of cares. Thus health may decline

in any individual and will not be treated until a medical crisis intervenes and likely results in a hospitalization. Medicare will pay the hospital and specialists adequately for this type of care, thus perpetuating episodic and fragmented health care. The medical care will be excellent although short-sighted to the long-term needs of "health maintenance." A coordinated management format led by physicians can make a difference in managing the care of the disabled in a proactive fashion and diminish the need for crisis intervention. Perhaps avoiding hospitalization by intervening in cases of anticipated frailty, even on an occasional basis, would save the system considerable funds. By implementing a social support system, performing a cognitive assessment, treating depression, instituting homebound PT or OT program, the "crisis" may be averted and hospitalization avoided. These needs, however, must first be evaluated and a true PRIMARY NEUROLOGIC PROVIDER must be recognized.

At present the managed care environment has evolved to care for the needs of a young, relatively healthy population. This has been driven by the financial benefit of restricting care to people who will likely do well enough without care that they will not suffer any adverse impact. Since 1982 HMOs have been legislated to contract with the HCFA to provide capitated medical care for Medicare enrollees. There has been gradually increasing enrollment but the question has arisen whether the system is functioning in the same fashion as applied to younger enrollees, withholding services, or has there evolved a comprehensive, coordinated system to handle the needs of the disabled or handicapped? At present there is no good comparison of capitated vs. fee-for-service data regarding access, outcomes, quality, and costs for our targeted MS population.

OBSERVATIONS OF HEALTH SYSTEMS IN FLUX

Health management organizations have induced substantial change in our health care environment, change that permits us to recognize certain trends.

Trends for the System as a Whole

1. The population will not only shift toward managed care, but also within this setting there will be a shift toward the more restrictive models of managed care (HMOs) in which cost-containment potential is perceived to be the greatest, and these trends will persist regardless of federal health care reform activities. Medicare, with only 7 percent of its population enrolled in HMOs to date, will be a "hold out" until federal pressure dictates a restructuring. Differences exist in access to care and medical outcomes in Medicare patients

enrolled in HMOs versus those enrolled in a fee-for-service insurance program. Concern was raised over this access issue as Medicare beneficiaries have been encouraged to enroll in HMOs. The goal was to contain costs while eliminating unnecessary care. By prepaying HMOs a fixed amount per enrollee, MCOs anticipated diminished incentives for increasing the volume of services available to these patients. Theoretically, through a centrally administered plan, the coordination of health care would be more efficient. There nonetheless exists concern that, in an effort to control costs, HMOs (and providers at risk financially) could also limit care by restricting access, exactly the reverse incentive offered by fee-for-service plans. A study revealed that for both acute and chronic symptoms, examined HMO enrollees were less likely to see a physician. They also were less likely to report that follow-up care was recommended or that the progress of their symptom had been monitored. Despite these differences, the outcome was the same for both groups, although symptom relief was greater in the fee-for-service group. Whether the lower utilization was due to a more judicious use of services or merely a deliberate restriction of access is uncertain.

2. Health care now is more accessible to enrollees but with certain restrictions: MCOs provide primary care physicians to review all acute medical problems and the availability of primary MDs has increased. However, primary care fails to address the needs of people with disabilities (chronic medical illness or MS), and at present there is an opportunity for managed care and rehabilitative providers to develop creative solutions to address the shortcomings of the present situation. In addition to the usual health care need of the general population, people with MS are at greater risk for certain common health conditions and may require a different therapeutic approach because of their baseline neurologic problem.

The six differences in the health care need of people with MS are:

a. People with MS have a thinner margin of health and are more vulnerable to health conditions shared with the general population (pneumonia, upper respiratory tract infections) and conditions unique to their population (urinary tract infections, pressure sores, renal failure, and so forth).

b. The same opportunities for health care maintenance and preventative health do not exist for our patients with MS, such as cardiovascular and pulmonary exercise.

c. MS patients may experience an earlier onset of chronic health conditions, i.e., heart disease from immobility, renal failure from chronic urinary tract infection, and so forth.

d. If a new deterioration in a health condition emerges, there is more likely to be secondary functional loss because the adaptation previously accomplished may no longer be adequate to provide for independent ambulation, transfers, ADLs, and so forth.

d. It is more likely that prolonged medical treatment for a given health problem exists among the MS population.

f. MS patients are more likely to need durable medical equipment and assistive technologies.

Thus people with MS will create higher than average rates of health care use (costs) because of these needs. It is known that among people with ADL limitations the need for 12 more hospital days and 7.4 times the health care expenditures will occur each year than their counterparts without ADL limitations. If we could reduce some of these vulnerabilities we could reduce the risks and incidence of these secondary medical issues as well as the costs.

One of the biggest problems is the care currently delivered by primary care. Few primary care doctors are knowledgeable about MS, nor are they aware of the potential for secondary complications. In spite of this, managed care funnels these patients into primary care and challenges the medical providers to resist referral to specialty care. The constraints are fiscal. Furthermore, managed care programs employ "risk-competition" and seek to avoid enrolling people with disabilities for their known history of increased utilization of medical services.

3. Rehabilitation utilization as part of MS care is increasing as the public becomes more aware of standardization of policy coverage and terms. As health care products are now being purchased based on their efficiencies as opposed to their abilities to just treat illness, it is increasingly important to consider what steps are taken to keep the population healthy. Although Medicare and Medicaid enrollments as well as workers compensation are increasingly managed, there exists ambiguity in the amount of "rehabilitation" allowed in their plans. Although capitation increases control over physician activities, there has not been much capitation penetration into the rehabilitation arena and the "cost-containment" strategies have been targeted toward dramatically reducing the already marginal reimbursements. This tendency, along with the development of "provider panels," is forcing the smaller rehabilitation entities out of business. The response to such demands has been to link costs to outcomes and functional gains. If the system provides outcomes at a greater cost than is being reimbursed, either the payer will flex or, more likely, there will be a means of reducing costs internally, through some administrative means. Personnel costs seem to be the highest portion of all rehabilitation costs and the skill mix may have to be altered to come in under or at budget in a capitated setting. Hopefully this can be achieved without sacrificing expertise and efficiency and not reducing the care

quality, which will adversely affect the outcomes and later increase cost.

4. Legal issues are taking shape to control the scope of control of managed care on health care in general:

As managed care organizations increase their role in medical decision making, medical malpractice has shifted from a focus on physicians failing to meet standards of care to the organizations making these decisions for whatever reason. This trend challenges federal legislation that limits liability in the area of plan administration. Should the plans be liable for alleged interference in medical decisions? In Texas the Health Care Liability Act of 1997 allows participants to sue their MCO for medical malpractice if they fail to meet the standard of care when making health care decisions and applies the same standards traditionally used against physicians. This law is the first of its kind, although similar legislation is being considered in Arizona, California, Connecticut, Florida, Maryland, Missouri, New Jersey, New York, Rhode Island, Tennessee, and Virginia. Federal ERISA law regulates all state law claims relating to employee benefit plans and has established national standards for MCOs that administer group health plans and provide legal remedies for plan participants. The ERISA laws preempts state law claims and has been a legal defense and shield behind which MCOs sued for "quality of care" issues have hidden. The courts determine that the ERISA precludes such legal action if the claim would affect the way the health plan is administered. The Texas law act may enable plan participants to overcome the ERISA defense and bring medical malpractice directly against MCOs.

Aetna Health Plans of Texas has sued the state because they believe this law is an infringement of federal law by the state in an area already regulated by the federal ERISA law. Both Aetna's and the State of Texas legal motions are pending and no decision has as yet been reached.

To date MCOs have maintained that they are not making medical decisions at least when they do not directly employ physicians. Also to date the courts have upheld the MCOs' use of the ERISA defense in dealing with health care claims. In the end it may be up to Congress to create legislation to redefine the responsibilities to plan participants by the MCOs and by the physicians.

Trends for Purchasers

1. Managed care programs will continue to accumulate market share in urban areas, with rural areas experiencing lesser activity in the near term.

2. Payers want to be treated as valued customers. Because they are major purchasers of specialty care services and, as with any buyer/seller relationship, they want physicians to compete for access to their patient population, they will ask, "Why should I purchase your services rather than someone else's?"

Volume purchasing is preferred. Most health plans would prefer to purchase neurologic services from a small number of practitioners rather than purchase small amounts of care from a larger provider network. Smaller networks are less costly to administer and maintain and permit health plans to accomplish their objectives of delivering patient volume to network providers in return for reimbursement and clinical autonomy concessions physician providers are making.

3. Payers may be interested in the cost of managing given disorders, not the costs of the specialist. Within any given category of disease, specialist costs are small compared with larger cost items such as inpatient care and expansive diagnostics, as well as nonregulated therapeutics. Payers are becoming increasingly aware that gatekeepers may not solve this problem and that specialists who know how to treat such disorders with a minimum of expensive management are valuable in jointly confronting total costs of various disorder categories.

4. One of the most important structural elements of managed care reform proposals is aggregation of purchasing power through large employers or health care alliances to solicit bids and oversee competition among plans. The larger purchasers have been able to keep premium increases to a minimum. They also have been able to stimulate collaboration by providers to develop practice guidelines.

5. Reimbursement has been arbitrarily reduced more than anticipated. Worse yet, there has been no recourse for physicians and negotiating directly with payers has been very difficult, if not impossible.

Trends for Patients

1. The public will be informed far more and involved in health care choices. Before the current decade, health care operated without economic constraints as health care costs were fueled by rapidly advancing technology. Managed care has been proposed as an economic framework to curb these costs but may fail to do so for the simple reason that the costs are driven by our societal values concerning the rights to health care. Despite fiscal restraint, there remains a disunion between consumer and purchaser permitting patient demands and expectations to continue without fiscal restraint even though the providers are seemingly controlled. The United States chose not to guarantee universal access to health care although virtually all other developed nations did, and also chose to finance health care in a manner lacking financial constraints.

In an ideal open market, the consumers pay producers the market value for goods. There exists a maximal price above which the consumer will not pay, thus limiting their demand and expectations and determining their limit and thus the "market price." In a fee-for-service market, the consumers were divorced from the payers (third party—business or government) and the market was driven solely by the consumer's demands and expectations without regard for price, thus removing economic limitations. The only limit set on pricing was the ability of the third party payer to fund.

Under managed care, there is a strategy to contain the funding for health care, and there is agreement by the providers to take care of the consumers within these constraints, but to date, *there has not been agreement by the consumers to decrease their demands and expectations,* because they remain divorced from the actual costs of their health care. The only thing managed care brings to the system of care and costs is a shifting of the risk of the funding to the providers, best borne out by care in a capitated system. The problem is further fueled by the competition within the managed care field (between HMOs) as they market their wares and increase the public's expectations of the highest "quality" of health care.

In health care, we consumers have enormous expectations and make endless demands but are unwilling to make the lifestyle changes that would lower such demands (smoking, alcohol, obesity, lack of exercise, and so forth). We further want more from biomedical research but are unwilling to support new obligations that result from our success. In order to reduce this gap, we have to lower our sense of entitlement or increase our commitment to the common order or both.

2. When enrollees are presented with choices of higher premiums for unrestricted access to autonomous health care providers versus lower premiums and more restricted "managed" access to providers and services, a majority have chosen lower premiums. Additional studies also have demonstrated a remarkable sensitivity of employees to out-of-pocket expenses. This willingness of consumers to switch providers has given health plans greater leverage in negotiations for services, creating price competition, among both hospitals and physicians, for managed care enrollees.

A recent poll sponsored by Patient Access to Specialty Care Coalition also indicates a high level of concern over some of the practices of managed care providers. The survey found that 95 percent of respondents believed they should have access to information concerning whether there were financial incentives to the doctors to limit care in the name of cost-containment. Nearly 90 percent thought that cost was less important in deciding on a health plan than the access to specialists of a particular plan. In addition, 90 percent said they would not trust doctors who were bound by a "gag rule" when they limited care. Fifty percent said they did not

have enough information about managed care practices. These issues need to be raised to ensure that quality of care is still our primary medical decision-making step.

PRACTICE RECOMMENDATIONS FOR PHYSICIANS

Approach Rather Than Avoid

HMO growth, public and purchaser demand, and government interest and legislation will continue to fuel the rapid transformation toward managed care. We physicians have lost control, and soon the insurance carriers will lose control to larger organizations. Perhaps the health care purchasers will realize that they have the ultimate say in the direction of their health care. Irrespective of who is the dominant player, it is clear that managed care is going to be the vehicle by which cost and quality are controlled in the future

Read and Understand the Capitation Manual and Managed Care Manual

Available from:
The American Academy of Neurology
2221 University Ave. S.E.
Suite 335
Minneapolis, Minnesota, 55414
(612) 623-8115

Ensure Data Integrity

(1) Initiate outcome studies and provide relevant data. To do so will ensure better accuracy and targeted information. Use these as your marketing tool rather than permitting someone else to take the credit. Focus on "value"—costs and quality of patient experience. (remember that good care does not ensure a good outcome). Provide data from the patient's perspective also; i.e., timeliness of appointments, ease of access, courtesy of support staff, and so forth. As well as the traditional information regarding clinical outcomes, morbidity, and so forth.

(2) Publish standardized outcomes already in use, such as FIM scale gains, length of stay, cost per diagnosis, and so forth.

(3) Offer a product rather than a service, such as a principal care model for MS. The specialist can become the personal health care provider for the MS patient, with referrals to rehabilitation, psychology, and primary medicine handled by that specialist. This may be a better model for all chronic diseases. This model uses a care coordinator (nurse), MS specialty care (neurologist, rehab

personnel, psychologists, social services, health educators, clinical trialists), and general medical care.

Maintain Traditional Medical Ethics

As the quality of neurologic care becomes a mutual objective of patients, physicians, and health planners, increased demands on cost savings will create conflicts for many. Physicians will face ethical conflicts between their fiduciary duties to the health plan and the treatment best deserved by their patient. They also will face conflict as their duty to preserve societal resources interferes with patient care. These conflicts may be minimized if physicians maintain their position as patient advocates and still practice cost-conscious behavior that weighs cost-effectiveness of certain treatments. The managed care organizations can help in these areas of conflict by abandoning their unethical cost-cutting schemes such as gag clauses and end-of-year kickback payments to physicians as these schemes diminish the patients' trust in their physicians.

Ethical Conflicts

1. Quality and ethics: There are no conflicts between improving the quality of medical care and following appropriate ethical considerations.

2. Cost control and ethics (regarding individual patients): In the traditional fee-for-service scheme, physicians who benefited from over-ordering tests when they were the financial beneficiaries, were legislated against in Stark I and II Congressional Bills. Here, conflict encouraged over-ordering of tests. In the HMO and MCO system, the physician may enjoy financial incentives from the under-ordering of tests. This type of conflict is less acceptable than the first as the patient was aware that the physician benefited from "more pay for more work" and the patient didn't suffer. In the second form of conflict the patient perceives a lack of care from which the physician profits and they may suffer, enhancing a basic mistrust of physicians under such pressures. Furthermore, the patient sees the physician in the role of a "double agent" who places his own income over the needs of their patients.

3. Cost control and ethics (regarding society as a whole): Physicians are bound to conserve society's resources. Here, there may be conflict as resource conservation benefiting all patients may be counter to what any individual patient may need or feel that they need. It is felt that this conflict can be circumvented by good clinical judgment on an individual basis.

4. Quality, cost control, and ethics: Physicians must take a leadership role in defining quality initiatives and management that optimize the quality of medical care and still take into account the costs, not only to the managed care plans for the individual patient but also to society as a whole. These new tools need to be accepted by the MCOs as providing details about the patient-physician interaction and enhancing the relationship rather than fomenting the mistrust presently inherent in the care system.

It should be requested of the government that the MCOs be held accountable for professional liability in those situations where, by defining what is or is not covered, they define what medical services are provided. It should be further requested that they regulate the HMOs and MCOs to the same extent that they have legislated fee-for-service medicine with regard to their cost-savings schemes. Finally, society needs to be educated as to the costs of the health care it demands as a whole and individually, as well as the liability standards to which it holds physicians.

Make Use of the Already Published Outcome Assessment Tools

One means of assisting the physician in selecting an equally effective but perhaps less costly evaluation and treatment parameters has been the evolution of clinical practice guidelines. Those that are best followed are promulgated by the AAN and AMA to assist us in management of neurologic problems. The programs propagated by HMOs and MCOs are more likely designed to save costs and reduce malpractice liability. These guidelines have different ethical status than the clinical ones because they do not permit exceptions, may be proprietary and unpublished, and are designed for other purposes than to improve the quality of medical care, as they serve to allocate resources only. They also use these guidelines to measure physician performance rather than as quality improvement guidelines. Most neurologists are willing to follow guidelines based on scientific data and designed by specialty societies to specifically improve the quality of patient care rather than just to cost-cut, as most neurologists are suspicious of those imposed by HMOs.

As we seek more cost-effective means to provide high quality care for neurologic disorders, health services research will lead us to make *evidence based decisions* rather than intuitive ones and are more easily defensible in the face of cost-constraints imposed on us as practitioners in a managed care environment. This will lead us toward the lowest cost for any given disorder and permit us to state to the insurer with certainty : THIS IS WHAT IT COSTS TO CARE FOR THIS PATIENT AND THIS IS WHAT YOU HAVE TO PAY and extract an adequate reimbursement for ourselves and the patient's health care, rather than be overseen and under-reimbursed for our efforts. The managed care organizations will have to incorporate coverage for truly proven effective treatments. The actual cost savings may yet occur just by the elimination of inappropriate care in this scheme and terminate the cost savings designated by setting the bottom line before the patients are taken into consideration (capitation).

Unite with Other Practitioners

There is strength in numbers, both for negotiating purposes as well as for economic reasons. In addition, larger group numbers would preserve and enhance access to patients, preserve and enhance revenue streams, position member groups to better perform in a radically changed market, reduce operating costs, and create greater efficiencies in member groups.

It is believed that most clinical and technologic innovation comes out of the specialty areas. This ability to innovate is fundamental and must continue to improve the quality of care delivered to patients.

It also is believed that physician ownership and governance is critical to effective care delivery systems and that, as specialists, we need to satisfy multiple customers: our patients, our colleagues (primary care and specialty), and the purchasers of health care.

Combining services in billing, accounting, benefits, transcription, computer services, and so forth may be very advantageous. Larger group size would enhance capacity to:

(1) expand outreach of both clinical and laboratory services enhancing attractiveness to an organization interested in purchasing from one vendor covering a large area.

(2) subspecialize and become primary case care managers, "principal physicians," in disease categories such as MS, Alzheimer's disease, Parkinson's disease, stroke rehabilitation, sleep disorders, traumatic brain injury, and so forth. Demonstrate that a specialist can perform workups, establish specific diagnosis, educate and treat more efficiently than primary care in these areas.

Obtain and Review the AHCPR Guidelines for Management of Neurologic Disorders

AHCPR Publications Clearinghouse
P.O. Box 8547
Silver Spring MD 20907
800-358-9295

Get a Grip on the Economics of Your Practice

(1) Define your own costs for common diagnoses (clinical and lab costs) before costs are assigned arbitrarily to you.

(2) Invest in yourselves. The greatest risk brings commensurate rewards. If you choose to be an employee, expect your employer to profit most from your efforts.

(3) Reduce your overhead. Although reimbursement is not going to increase and the payers determine how much you shall be paid for each encounter, there is still room to increase efficiency by reducing practice costs where possible without reducing efficiency.

(4) Don't price yourselves too low. When participating in negotiations, or working out the details of fees, no one is going to offer you more than you ask for and will certainly try to get you to accept less. Build in inflationary, or cost of living, increases.

(5) Obtain the right to access all managed care organization's monthly financial and operating statements. Any organization that does not spend 70 percent or more of its revenues on patients is not doing the job correctly.

(6) Preauthorize all testing and treatment protocols (inpatient and outpatient) whenever possible.

Never Abandon the Position of Being a Patient Advocate

Identify whether the managed care organization provides education to their enrollees and participate actively in the education of your patients.

(1) Unfortunately, health care systems are concerned with populations, not with individuals. Choices have to be made on a larger scale as to how best to spend within a limited pool of dollars to benefit the greatest numbers of patients. Inevitably, some denial of services has to occur, removing the autonomy of patient management from the physician's hands.

(2) Patients do not understand rehabilitation. They are unaware of goals, costs, methods, alternatives, and so forth. They assume that rehabilitation is covered when it is not specifically spelled out in the contract (which they usually have not read).

(3) Purchasers do not understand their health care coverage (any more than patients do) as they simply purchased what they were told represented "standard for the industry" or "full coverage" without preconception of the coverage for special services among other needs.

(4) Both purchasers (employers) and patients are led to believe that the terminology of contracts covers what they need as long as the "doctor orders it." What patients and purchasers do not know is that the utilization review system employed by the managed care organizations determines what is "appropriate." This may have little to do with what the doctor "orders." Patients are not aware of different sets of clinical guidelines from which the MCO works to determine coverage (which also are never divulged), and patients and physicians are "caught in the middle" trying to explain why a specific course of care is different than anticipated. The physician then must justify a set of double standards!

(5) If patients are not making progress in rehabilitation, the carriers demand nursing home placement, which then terminates their financial liability. If they are being

paid to manage, why don't they use some of this creative talent and money to achieve solutions somewhere between acute rehabilitation and skilled nursing? They market the capacity to manage, but thus far, in rehabilitation, the focus has been primarily on cost, not on quality.

(6) Be certain that your patients and their families understand the goals and methods of MS rehabilitation early on in the course because there will be considerable misconception present by the time a rehabilitation program is implemented. If nothing is done to orient the family, a widening gap between the physician, patient and/or family, and managed care organization will develop.

We physicians must look at the role of educating the public as to the utility of various medical methods, thus enhancing their awareness and providing the framework for demand and expectation. We must furthermore somehow be incented to do this proactively rather than being fiscally at risk or punished for doing otherwise. We have not yet embraced this role, distracted by the economic outcomes of our battles with managed care as well as the need to simply survive in a new environment not of our making.

Continue to Support Academics and Research Despite Underfunding

Different forces are at work in academic settings. Academic departments do well with technical excellence but less well with access and efficiency. Most academic departments function with built-in impediments to low practice costs and high clinical efficiency. Both medical education costs and research costs penalize the faculty and reduce the amount of time available for direct (reimbursable) patient care. The efficiency of a clinical academic practice cannot shift clinical dollars to support research and teaching and reduces the attractiveness of such practice in today's free-market economy, thus further degrading practice performance. In the managed care market, not even the perceived excellence of academic settings can engender referrals from the primary care physicians who will accept the community standards over the faculty expertise (and more costly care) provided by the academic institution. Furthermore, the universities are not used to seeing patients within a few days of the consultation request as is the community standard, and this limitation of access creates dissatisfaction among patients and insurers.

In the managed care setting, emphasis needs to be placed on value-added services available only at a high level referral center. They can provide high level acuity care with specialized nursing and extensive ancillary staff. They also can provide specialty care in all other areas perhaps needed by the patient such as access to specialized social services, rehab services, psychological services, ancillary medical and surgical specialties, and so forth.

There also can exist superspecialties even in neurology where each neurologist develops particular skill in one area and is accessible to all other neurologists for consultation. Each practitioner will give up some of his/her patients in order to receive others. This is best accomplished in an academic setting as networking is already in place. Most university organizations have well developed information systems and are capable of providing outcomes data, critical pathway information, and data applicable to quality improvement. Disease management strategies (different than critical pathways, which are implemented at the bedside) implemented at various points of management for a population can be effective in reducing the incidence and severity of a particular illness. Reducing hospital admissions and overall morbidity provides substantial economic benefits. If sophisticated information management systems are present, university settings may be best to accomplish this. The collective localization of the practitioners makes this workable regardless of the various pathways the disease process may track. It is these capabilities that add the value and enable the global care of patients to be delivered efficiently and with lower cost yet with the same or better outcomes. Thus perhaps the managed care organizations can be persuaded to encourage the teaching and research legs of academic centers instead of focusing just on the cost of individual patient care at any one hospital or clinic encounter.

CONCLUSION

The management of health care has not completed its transformation from fee-for-service methodology to a perfectly workable system, and what we recognize today as managed care is a health care industry in its infancy, early in the process of metamorphosis to a more mature and efficient system. To date, the changes managed care has wrought have come from the need to curb the economic crisis health care has presented to the payers—businesses and the government. The dollar flow has been constrained under the pretense that health care was to become more affordable. These changes seemingly emerged without much physician input, yet physicians were designated to carry the message to their patients, who were even less informed about the reasons that the traditional care they had become accustomed to was no longer available. There exists tremendous potential for clinicians to have a say in the future of medicine by assisting in the transition from our fee-for-service methodology to the next stage in evolution of health care delivery, creating a better system of "managed care," and in so doing, wresting back control of the health care system in the United States so that it resembles the high quality care system we have enjoyed to date. Managed care is here to stay and will be part of the solution, but it is not in its best or final form. We as physicians must put aside our fear of change and inform ourselves about what managed care was, is, and can become and become active participants in the design of our system of health care delivery.

References

1. "The Neurologist and Managed Care," American Academy of Neurology, 1995

2. "Mergers Make Doctors Employees," Howatt G, Lerner M, *Mpls Star And Tribune;* March 31, 1996

3. "Adversaries Become Allies," Howatt G, *Mpls Star And Tribune;* April 1, 1996

4. "A State of Flux," Wascoe D, *Business And Health;* February 1995

5. Mayer T, Mayer G. HMOs: Origins and development. *N Engl J Med* February 1995:590–594.

6. Christianson J, Dowd B, et al. Managed care in the Twin Cities: What can we learn? *Health Affairs,* Summer 1995:114–130.

7. Davenport R. "The big squeeze: Pressures mount on medical group practices." *Minnesota Physician,* November 1995:33–35.

8. Woolhandler S, Himmelstein D. Extreme risk—The new corporate proposition for physicians. *N Engl J Med* 1995; 333:1706–1707.

9. Anderson C. Is managed care the answer? *Minnesota Physician,* March 1996:30–31.

10. Slomski A. How doctors cope in the land of 10,000 mergers. *Medical Economics,* July 1995:194–210.

11. Terry K. Look who's guarding the gate to specialty care. *Medical Economics,* August 1994:124–136.

12. Baumgarten A. Doling out risk: How capitation measures up in Minnesota. *Minnesota Medicine* May 1995; 78:11–15.

13. Bushick B. Health plan report cards: Current issues and implications for physicians. *Medical Journal of Allina* Winter 1996:36–40.

14. Dejong G. Primary care for persons with disabilities. *Am J Phys Med Rehabil* 1997; 76:S2–S8.

15. Herndon R, Montgomery S. (eds.). *Multiple sclerosis: Systems of care and disease management.* New York: Medical Education Network, 1997.

16. Beckley N. Rehab administration under managed care. *Rehab Management* Dec/Jan 1996; 9:27–31.

17. Salladay S. Rehabilitation, ethics, and managed care. *Rehab Management* Oct/Nov 1996; 9:38–42.

18. Brummel-Smith K (ed.). Geriatrics in managed care: Is managed care good or bad for geriatric medicine? *J Am Geriatr Soc* 1997; 45:1123–1127.

19. King R, Moore III B. Managed care: Past, present and future. *Arch Neurol* 1996; 53:851–855.

20. Riggs J. Managed care and economic dynamics. *Arch Neurol* 1996; 53:856–858.

21. Menken M. Managed care and the practice of neurology. *Arch Neurol* 1996; 53:859–862.

22. Ringel S, Hughes R. Evidence-based medicine, critical pathways, practice guidelines, and managed care. *Arch Neurol* 1996; 53:867–871.

23. Clement D, et al. Access and outcomes of elderly patients enrolled in managed care. *JAMA.* 1994; 271:1487–1492.

24. Dejong G. Health care reform and disability: Affirming our commitment to community. *Arch Phys Med Rehabil* 1993; 74:1017–1024.

25. Purtilo R. Managed care: Ethical issues for the rehabilitation professions. *Trends in Health Care, Law and Ethics* Winter/Spring 1995; 10:105–118.

26. Feldman M. The doctor-patient bond: Covenant or business contract? *Minnesota Medicine* 1997; 80:12–16.

27. Ringel S, Vickrey B. Measuring quality in neurology. *Arch Neurol* 1997; 54: 1329–1332.

28. Barchi R. Quality of care in academic neurology departments. *Arch Neurol* 1997; 54:1336–1340.

29. Bernat J. Quality of neurological care. *Arch Neurol* 1997; 54:1341–1345.

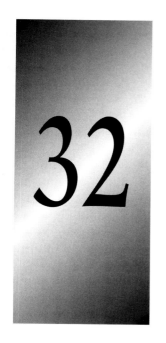

32 Home Care Management: A Model for an Interdisciplinary Approach

Karen Hunter, RN,C, and Nancy Popp, RN

Current health care trends and reforms are demanding shorter hospital and rehabilitation stays. Some procedures and treatments previously handled on an inpatient basis are now accomplished in outpatient settings. Closer scrutiny by payer sources of the services provided makes it difficult to care for and support patients with the extremely complex disease of multiple sclerosis (MS). Home care is one of the options for the physician and the MS patient to manage these trends and reforms, thereby ensuring appropriate care and treatment. Home care can supplement or augment treatment received during hospitalization or perhaps eliminate altogether the need for hospitalization. In some instances in which long-term placement is a consideration, community programs may be available to work with the physician, patient, family, and home care agency. These programs can provide the support and services needed to allow a patient with MS to remain living in his or her own home.

Home care is also affected by current trends and reforms in health care. Home care agencies are seeing an increased number of patients with complex problems, including those with MS. These patients are being referred for supportive care following hospitalizations or directly from physicians' offices. Agencies are under closer scrutiny by payer sources to meet the criteria and guidelines set by various insurance plans. These plans dif-

fer in the types and frequency of services allowed. Agencies must have the most current and accurate information to provide physician-prescribed care and treatment while meeting the required criteria. Home care must develop positive relationships with the payer sources. This presents many challenges to home care agencies today and in the future.

In MS, as in any chronic disease, home care can provide care that may either be frequent and of short duration or extend over a longer period of time. Care may include one skilled discipline or all available services. These services are ordered by the physician and must meet insurance criteria. A registered nurse can monitor effects and compliance of medications and teach Foley catheter care or intermittent self-catheterization. A speech-language pathologist can evaluate a patient's short-term memory and then teach various compensatory strategies to assist in retaining new information A physical therapist can evaluate the mobility and safety of a patient in the home environment and then make recommendations for the correction of unsafe conditions and assist the patient and family in making modifications. An occupational therapist can evaluate how a patient functions in the home environment and then make recommendations for special equipment or ways to conserve energy to make the activities of daily living (ADLs) less fatiguing. A social worker can assess the patient's financial situation and then assist him or her in tapping into beneficial community resources. A home health aide, under the supervision of a skilled provider, can assist the patient with bathing or an exercise and stretching program. In "home care language," these visits are referred to as "intermittent" visits, occurring intermittently with a duration of one to two hours. "Hourly services" is the industry name for care of a longer duration (i.e., more than two hours). These services are provided by a home health aide to assist the patient in ADLs. Hourly services are paid for privately or subsidized by special federal, state, or local programs. Nursing can also fall under the hourly services blanket.

In 1994 we were seeing a large number of MS patients because of a close association with the Fairview MS Center and the Fairview MS Achievement Center. Home care staff frequently voiced their concerns and frustrations in caring for the MS population. Concerns were for the safety of patients, home health aides, and family members. Noncompliance with the care plan was a significant frustration. "He should have seen his doctor this week, but he never called to make the appointment," or "He was supposed to send in his completed application for medical assistance last week but it's still sitting on his dining room table." Patients were agreeing to take their medications as prescribed, but on the subsequent visit the nurse would discover either that they were not taking all of them or that they were taking a discontinued medication.

Patients and families often had unrealistic expectations of home care staff and the agency's ability to provide the care they expected. Staff was becoming overwhelmed trying to meet the challenges of this complicated patient population.

The home care management was committed to quality care for the MS patients and recognized the challenges of caring for them. An MS program specialist (PS) position was created to assist the staff in providing care for the MS patient population. The PS looked at the numbers of MS patients receiving services and what disciplines were involved in each case. She made co-visits with case managers to better understand the environments in which cares and services were being delivered and, as a result of this information-gathering, discovered that the difficulties experienced were not limited to one discipline. Other staff members were interested in improving the services delivered. Plans of care often seemed fragmented rather than cohesive. The PS arranged a meeting of home care professionals to discuss the care delivery model, as well as the frustrations and concerns that staff had raised, and to identify other existing problems. Recommendations would be made as an outcome of this meeting. Present at this meeting were the PS, mental health nurse, social worker (SW), physical therapist (PT), speech-language pathologist (SLP), chaplain, occupational therapist (OT), and hospital liaison.

This group discussed their lack of knowledge about MS and its impact on the lives of their patients and families. The word *overwhelming* was a frequent theme. Multiple sclerosis posed a threat to the independence of many of the patients these professionals had cared for in the past. There were concerns about the safety of the patient in the home as well as the safety of caregivers. Patients with MS frequently were not adhering to the plan of care set in place by the case manager and members of other disciplines. At times, the patient would do exactly the opposite of what he or she had previously agreed to do. Some patients were repeatedly admitted to home care for episodes of care because not all of their needs were met.

The unique recommendation made by the group was that an interdisciplinary team be formed to assist in managing the delivery of cares and services to the MS patient population. Each of the professionals at this meeting was given the option of serving as part of this team, and each chose to participate. The team members agreed to meet weekly to further develop this new concept and to assist their coworkers in MS patient care management. The newly formed interdisciplinary team identified the following key issues to be addressed: education, communication, safety, patient independence, compliance, and cost-effectiveness.

EDUCATION

Team members identified a need for additional knowledge and a better understanding of the disease, its effects on patients and their families, other professional responsibilities and capabilities, payer sources, and resources available to patients and their families. The PS obtained journal articles and reference materials through the medical library to share with the team members. The MS Center and the acute rehabilitation unit loaned their staff and patient education videotapes to the team.

Each of the team members shared his or her area of expertise and identified patient care responsibilities to allow each member of the team an increased awareness of how to use each of the disciplines for a total patient evaluation. The OT, in addition to the evaluation and treatment of upper body strength, endurance, and ADLs, would focus on cognitive functional safety. Areas of concern could be identified through the use of specific testing. An optimal treatment plan would then be devised to assist the patient in remaining safe and independent.

The mental health nurse could assess and evaluate the patient's mental status for signs and symptoms of depression or steroid-induced psychoses, level of functioning, the effectiveness of coping skills, response to psychotropic medications, and the presence of any side effects. She specifically shared the signs and symptoms of depression with the team so that everyone would be more attuned to them and appropriately ask for her assistance in treating patients. The mental health nurse would be available to consult with case managers in the care of patients, or in more difficult situations, assume the case manager's role.

The PT could assess trunk control and wheelchair positioning, which can affect the patient's ability to breathe. If a patient with impaired respiratory muscles is sitting in a forward slump, he cannot properly fill his lungs with air, so his voice may be weak and speech may be difficult to understand. By positioning and stabilizing the trunk, improved respiratory functioning can be achieved, and voice quality and arm function may improve as well. Therapy can be initiated to strengthen weak trunk muscles and improve balance.

The hospital liaison was assigned to the acute and subacute rehabilitation units at the hospital and was currently involved in discharge and/or progress rounds on those units. Information shared at rounds could be forwarded to the home care team, and information from the team could be relayed to the unit staff. The liaison would use voice mail to forward information to the team and case managers, and they were encouraged to relay information to the liaison when a home care MS patient was hospitalized. Physicians and hospital staff were not always aware of the entire home situation. The liaison would provide continuity of care across the system—clinic to home care to hospital to home care to clinic.

The SLP could perform an in-depth cognitive evaluation to assess verbal problem solving, verbal reasoning, memory, and language functioning. If memory deficits are identified, the SLP can recommend and teach compensatory strategies (e.g., a memory book, calendar, or lists) that may help the patient to retain new information. Family members and caregivers are taught about theses aids to assist the patient. If the patient is unable to write, a small tape recorder can be used as a memory aid.

The PS would be the MS team leader. She would facilitate team meetings and share the team's progress with the agency's management team. Crisis intervention and marketing are part of her role. She would meet with physicians and clinic staff to explain the benefits of the MS program to them and their patients. The PS would attend the home care agency's professional staff meetings to educate and inform them about the new program and how to access it. She would act as a resource to the team, case managers, and other home care staff.

Most of the team members initially had not considered the impact of involving the chaplain on the team in the care of the patient. The availability of a chaplain to address the spiritual aspect of the patient's well-being ensures a more holistic approach to care. It is through spirituality that an individual finds meaning and purpose in life, draws on his inner strengths, and connects to people or the power beyond himself. Spirituality should not be confused with religion. The home care chaplain's role is not to propose any particular religion to a patient but to help him discover his own personal spiritual meaning. The anger and grief connected with the losses in the patient's life can be profound and unending and often get in the way of the patient's accepting the care and treatment he needs to remain safe and independent. The chaplain can help him talk about how these losses have threatened his sense of purpose in life and guide him to recognize inner strengths and valuable connections to others. If the patient is agreeable, a referral to the chaplain is included in the care plan.

The increased knowledge and understanding of MS and the need to provide the best of services to the patient triggered the need for more information. Guest speakers (neurologist, social worker in private practice, neuropsychologist) were arranged to address the group during meetings. Team members attended conferences and professional continuing education seminars and brought back to the group the new information they had learned. The team visited the Minnesota Chapter of the National Multiple Sclerosis Society to learn about the services and programs it offered to people with MS and their families. Team members began to attend the monthly education hour sponsored by the MS Center, which offered an opportunity to dialogue with caregivers in the hospital and rehabilitation setting as well as an opportunity to expand their own knowledge base.

The team made a commitment to the education of the home care staff caring for the MS patients. In-services were developed and scheduled for all disciplines to increase their knowledge about MS and avail themselves of the services of the MS team. A program was specifically designed for the home health aides because they often were the care providers most frequently in the patients' homes. This in-service explained the disease and its impact on the patient and family, and stressed the importance of following the care plan. They were encouraged to communicate with the case manager when they had concerns or noted even small changes in a patient's status.

Patients and their families always seemed to want or need more information, although not necessarily pertaining to the disease itself. A packet of information was created for the patients, which included a pamphlet about living creatively with a chronic illness, a brochure explaining the services offered by the Fairview MS Achievement Center, a registration form for the National MS Society, and a listing of free educational materials offered by the Society. Additionally, a list of advocacy resources, information about accessing community resources, and an MS Resource Directory developed by the team were included. Patients and families are encouraged to explore various avenues of information and support within the community of care (Figure 32-1).

COMMUNICATION

Communication between caregivers can be limited by the very nature of home care. Communication with patients and families can easily be misinterpreted or misunderstood, leading to problems or obstacles in carrying out the plan of care. The team made a commitment to improve communication among all disciplines involved in a patient's care and with patients and their families. Better use of voice mail was one way to improve communication among caregivers. A portion of each team meeting was designated for case conferences and updating team members on the progress being made in the ever-evolving care plan development. Case managers were invited to come to the team meeting to seek assistance in developing appropriate plans of care for their patients. By using patient–family conferences to explain the plan of care developed, all the key players would hear the same information at the same time. Questions could be asked, and clarification of any issues could be accomplished.

Keeping the physician informed and up-to-date is a crucial element in the success of the plan. Without the support of the physician, the plan of care developed by the team could easily fail. The PS initially took the responsibility of being the information conduit to the patient's physician, relaying information, and obtaining orders for cares and services. This afforded her the opportunity to develop relationships with the physicians who were referring patients to the agency and to educate them in the use of the team in caring for their patients. As the volume of cases the team was involved with increased, the PS could no longer maintain this role. As an adjunct member of the MS team, the case manager, after discussion with the PS, contacts the physician to inform him of the progress being made and to obtain orders.

SAFETY

The safety of the patient in his own environment is a major goal of the team. Not only is the physical environment assessed for safety but also the patient's ability to be safe in his environment. Does the patient recognize an emergency situation and respond appropriately? Can the patient prepare a meal for himself without leaving on the stove or oven afterward? Can the patient manage his money? If there are concerns, recommendations are made to change the unsafe situation, and these recommendations become part of the plan of care.

The Community of Care

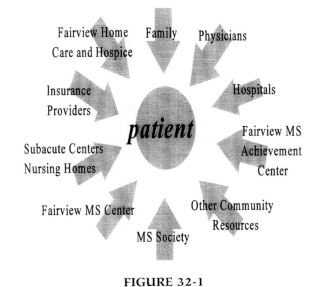

FIGURE 32-1

The MS team looks at the whole patient and his connection to the community of care.

The patient's safety is the primary concern, but the team is also concerned about the safety of the home care staff and family members who are providing direct care for the patient. Transferring the patient is an area of great concern. All transfers are evaluated and recommendations made for the safety of the patient and those assisting with the transfers. Both family members and home care staff are instructed in how to accomplish safe transfers. The patient or family member occasionally refuses to follow the recommendations. When this occurs, the patient and family are informed that the home care staff will not be able to participate or assist in unsafe transfers and the patient and a family caregiver will have to take responsibility for all transfers.

PATIENT INDEPENDENCE

An important goal of the team is to keep the patient as independent as possible for as long as possible, retaining individuality and self-worth at a time when his or her body is posing a threat to independence. Each patient situation is approached on an individual basis, and the entire picture is taken into consideration before recommendations are made. Recommendations may consist of one simple change or piece of adaptive equipment, or multiple changes, several new pieces of equipment, and even moving to more accessible housing. If a patient is having difficulty managing his money but otherwise seems to be getting along on his own, a recommendation would be made that a family member assist him with money management. If this is not agreeable, a referral can be made to an independent living skills worker (an individual who is trained to assist and educate clients in living independently within the community).

The plan of care is continuously adapted to accommodate the changes in a patient's capabilities. The patient may need more assistance with personal care during an exacerbation or as the disease progresses. At this time, home health aide services would be added or adjusted to support the patient in remaining at home. This is a time when additional skilled services also may be needed to support the patient at home. The PT and OT may be asked to evaluate or reevaluate transfers and safety. The case manager may ask the team to reevaluate the patient and his or her current situation as well.

COMPLIANCE

Compliance is often linked to the cognitive changes that may occur in the disease process. Patients often are aware of even subtle changes that have occurred and are either too embarrassed or too frightened to bring them to anyone's attention. The team has chosen to deal with the cognitive changes openly and in a caring manner. By doing so, patients, families, and home care staff have a better understanding of what is happening and what can be done about it. Both the OT and the SLP can evaluate the patient and then work with him to teach him how to use compensatory measures or explain to staff the appropriate approaches for teaching and explanations with the patient. With better understanding, the team sees an improvement in compliance with treatment plans and care plans.

COST-EFFECTIVENESS

Cost-effectiveness is not about specific dollars and cents but about how to efficiently use the resources available. There is no extra charge for the MS team to see patients. The team works within the framework laid out by physician orders and the various insurance payer sources. Initially, insurance case managers were reluctant to authorize visits and use the team because of their concern for cost containment. The team was finding that it could not obtain the authorization for visits to comprehensively evaluate patients, connecting them with community support and services after home care was no longer indicated. Without the proper support, patients frequently returned to the acute care setting. The team wanted to stop this costly cycle.

The PS spoke with a supervisor at one of the local insurance companies for which our agency was a preferred provider. She explained our concept of interdisciplinary care for MS patients and the team's desire to get information to the insurance case managers regarding the MS team and what it could do for patients covered by their insurance plans. The supervisor invited the PS and the team to attend a staff meeting and share the information with the case managers. The team members talked about the cycle they were seeing and its cost to the insurance company. Various supports and additional services available in the community were explained. As a result of this meeting, the team was able to obtain insurance authorization from these case managers to perform the necessary evaluations to provide the support and services needed for the patients. After the meeting, the insurance case managers began requesting that the team become involved in evaluation and treatment of their more complicated cases. Since that initial meeting, the team has met with three additional groups of insurance case managers from three different companies. Again, the team found that once the case managers had a better understanding of the disease and what the team could accomplish for the patients, they were more willing to authorize the necessary visits.

A patient–family conference, including several members of the team and the case manager, may not appear, at first glance, to be cost-effective because the insurance company cannot be billed for the conference. The team finds that presenting the plan of care to the patient and family at the same time ensures that everyone is hearing the same information. The conference reduces the chance of miscommunication and time spent trying to rectify any misunderstandings. If the patient or family is not in agreement with the plan, adjustments can be made at this time.

CASE STUDIES

The following two case studies demonstrate how the team works together and interacts with patients and their caregivers. They should provide the reader a better understanding of the team's interdisciplinary approach. The first case study is relatively simple and occurs over a short period of time. The second study is a more complex case that involves all disciplines and occurs over a longer time span.

Case Study #1

The home care agency was requested to provide a physical therapy evaluation for GS. His sister had reported to his physician that he was falling frequently at home. She was very concerned for his safety. The agency obtained the necessary insurance authorization, and the MS team's PT called GS to arrange for a visit.

GS's sister was visiting and answered the door when the PT arrived. GS was sitting in a manual wheelchair. As he stood up to greet the PT, he began to fall. The PT noted that GS was wearing only socks, no shoes. When asked about his shoes, he responded, "They're in my closet because I don't like to take the time to put them on and they leave marks on my newly installed hardwood floors." After GS put on his shoes, the PT evaluated his gait and balance and found it to be good over short distances. The PT explained to GS and his sister that wearing only socks on slippery hardwood floors was unsafe and was the cause of his frequent falls. GS needed to wear his shoes. He was instructed to put them on before getting out of bed in the morning and to take them off after he was back in bed in the evening. GS and his sister understood the rationale for this, and GS agreed to follow this plan.

The PT then found that GS was not safe to maneuver the stairs on his own and recommended that he not use the stairs unless assistance was available. Fortunately, GS's bedroom and bathroom were on the first level of his home, and he would not routinely need to go upstairs.

GS told the PT that he had ordered a new power wheelchair following recommendations during his last rehabilitation hospitalization and it was due to arrive the following week. The PT made plans to return to assess proper seating, fit the "joystick," and teach GS how to use it.

The PT discovered that the installation of the hardwood flooring was part of a remodeling plan in preparation for the future sale of his home so that he could move to more accessible housing. He was planning to return to work after his new wheelchair arrived, but he was concerned about transportation. He had been riding to work with a coworker, but he knew that the power wheelchair could not be accommodated by a regular automobile. The PT recommended the assistance of the SW in accessing community resources for transportation and housing.

After her visit with GS, the PT called the physician to report her findings and plan of care and obtained orders for the SW to assist GS with community resources. Authorization for the SW visits was obtained from the insurance case manager. She left a voice mail message for the SW with her observations and information from her visit with GS so that the SW would be prepared to discuss housing and transportation issues.

The SW set up a visit with GS. He wanted his sister to be present and assisted the SW in arranging an agreeable time. GS's primary concern was transportation to and from work. The SW explained the metropolitan area transportation services for physically challenged people. GS was delighted. He did not know that these services existed. He responded, "This is such a relief. I thought I would have to quit my job because I couldn't get there. My work is very important to me. I have a lot of friends there. At night I'm too tired to do much, so it's important to me that I get to socialize over coffee and lunch." The SW had an application for transportation services with her and assisted GS in filling out the necessary forms.

The SW opened the emotional discussion about GS's living situation. She allowed both GS and his sister to express their feelings and concerns. His sister said that the house had become quite expensive for him because he could no longer do normal maintenance and repairs himself. GS shared that his feelings for his home were changing. "I used to love working in the yard. When I look around the house and yard, all I see are things that need fixing. It's so frustrating. It makes me angry that I can't do it anymore. I'm okay with moving. In fact, I've been approached by someone at work who would like to buy my house when I'm ready to sell." The SW asked GS about his preferences of living environment. He was interested in an accessible apartment that did not require maintenance. The SW described the various types of housing available, and they decided that an assisted living building would best meet his needs. The SW gave them the names, addresses, and phone numbers of several assisted living facilities. GS and his sister planned to visit two or three buildings within the next week. The SW would help him get on a waiting list once he had made his selection. The SW made an appointment with GS and his sister for later the following week. The SW left a voice mail message for the PT to report on her visit and let her know the date of the next visit.

At the next visit, GS was eager to report that he had found an assisted living building in which he could have a large one bedroom apartment. He had discussed the services with the nurse who managed the special programs at the building. She had explained that GS could purchase increments of HHA and homemaking services if he needed them. GS thought that this would help him remain independent and decrease his dependence on his sister. His sister was reassured that assistance would always be available if required. The SW called the building admission office to inform them that she was working with him. An apartment would be available in about six months. In the interim, GS and his sister could sell the house and make decisions about his personal belongings and furniture. At the end of the visit, the SW gave GS her business card and instructed him to call if he needed further assistance. The SW left a voice mail message for the PT to bring her up-to-date and to relate that the power wheelchair had been delivered.

The PT made her second and final visit the following day. GS's new wheelchair was assessed for appropriate fit and seating and its ability to fit through doorways in his home. After teaching GS how to maneuver the wheelchair, the PT was ready to discharge GS. He would be returning to work in a few days, and the transportation service had been arranged. The PT and SW notified the physician and insurance case manager of the outcomes of their visits with GS. The PT and SW briefly reported GS's case at the MS team's weekly conference.

Case Study #2

DK was a 54-year-old woman who was recently diagnosed with MS. In addition to MS, DK had insulin-dependent diabetes and macular degeneration. During an exacerbation, she was admitted to the acute rehabilitation unit for steroid treatment and intensive therapies, with the goal of returning to her previous living situation At discharge, the acute rehabilitation team recommended that a home care nurse follow up with DK to ensure a smooth transition from hospital to home and to monitor the taper of her steroid therapy. A social worker was recommended to assist her with exploring community resources for additional support. The physician agreed with this plan and wrote the orders for a referral to home care. DK's insurer was Medicare, and the services ordered met the Medicare home care guidelines. The hospital liaison processed the referral to home care and forwarded this additional information to the MS team and the nursing team via voice mail: DK was living with her daughter, Jean, and Jean's husband and two small children, after moving to Minnesota from Missouri. Her move to Minnesota was recent, and she wanted her own apartment, if possible.

Nursing Evaluation: DK was visited by her nurse case manager the day after her discharge, and an admission assessment was done. The nurse determined that DK and her daughter were not very knowledgeable about DK's medications or her MS. DK was not able to get into the bathtub or shower on her own, and standing at the bathroom sink to bathe was very tiring. During the visit, DK mentioned her concern about her difficulty in swallowing. A nursing plan of care was initiated, which included monitoring medication and its effects, and education of DK, her daughter, and her son-in-law regarding her medications and her MS. After a discussion with the PS, the nurse informed the physician of her plan to (1) obtain additional orders for a home health aide to assist DK with bathing and ADLs, (2) a PT evaluation because of DK's unsteady gait in a cluttered environment, (3) SLP evaluation of her swallowing, and (4) an OT evaluation of the bathroom and kitchen. The physician was kept apprised of the situation throughout the period of care.

Social Service Evaluation: During the visit the SW had conversations with both DK and Jean. DK brought up her desire to eventually move into her own apartment (she had lived alone in Missouri) and her concern over having enough money to do this. DK was concerned that she was sometimes "in the way" or had to ask Jean or her husband for help. DK had enjoyed reading as a pastime but now her eyesight made reading nearly impossible. DK

was also exhibiting the early signs of depression. Jean was not always home at lunchtime and worried that her mother might miss a meal or have problems with her diabetes or insulin coverage. The SW detected a lot of anxiety and stress in Jean due to her concern about her mother and her limited knowledge about MS. The SW recommended that once all the disciplines had made their evaluations the team could sit down with DK and her family to discuss their findings and explain the plan of care. DK and Jean agreed that a family conference would be beneficial. The SW arranged for Meals-on-Wheels to deliver lunch for DK Monday through Friday, and referred DK to the Vision Loss Resources Center for its books-on-tape program and assistance with adaptive equipment for her insulin set-up. She arranged for DK to meet with one of the center's counselors to learn about other programs available to her. Another SW appointment was arranged with DK to assist her with an application to a specially funded program for disabled individuals. The SW contacted the nurse case manager and suggested that the MS Team mental health nurse evaluate the depression identified during her visit.

Physical Therapy Evaluation: At the initial visit, the PT observed that the small house was cluttered with furniture and "things and stuff" in high-traffic areas. DK's gait was unsteady, which made it unsafe for her to walk without some type of assistive device. She had fallen several times on the backdoor stairway. DK was not following a stretching and exercise program. The PT recommended that her daughter rearrange the furniture to make wider and safer walkways and to keep all traffic areas free of clutter. The use of a cane or crutches was ruled out because of DK's poor coordination. A pickup walker was deemed most appropriate and was ordered. On a subsequent visit, the PT would teach its use on level surfaces, stairs, and outdoor surfaces. The PT would include DK's daughter in the sessions so that she would understand the proper use of the walker. A stretching and exercise program was designed and implemented. A copy of the instructional program was printed for everyone involved. The program was added to the HHA care plan, and the HHA was instructed on how to assist DK. The PT left a voice mail report for the case manager with her plan of care after her initial visit and again at discharge, when all her goals had been met.

Occupational Therapy Evaluation: During the initial home visit, the kitchen and bathroom areas were evaluated for safety, and all transfers in all areas of the house were observed. The OT was aware of DK's desire to live independently, and her daughter voiced concerns about her ability to handle this. A recommendation was made for the use of a bath bench, with one person in assistance for transferring and showering. Felt balls were added to the legs of the walker to make transitions between surfaces easier. Blocks to raise the furniture were recommended to make sitting down and standing up easier and safer. Cognitive function testing was planned. Once the tub bench arrived, DK, her daughter, and the home health aide were instructed on proper use. Cognitive testing showed that DK could live independently with assistance. She would need help with performing higher cognitive tasks (i.e., shopping, money management, and long- and short-term planning). The OT left a voice mail report for the case manager with her plan of care and again at discharge, when all her goals had been met.

Speech/Language Pathology Evaluation: During the visit, the SLP assessed oral motor functioning to determine the strength and movement of the lips, tongue, jaw, and voice. These were found to be slightly weaker than normal, but speech was intelligible. She observed DK while she ate foods of varying consistency. No coughing or choking was observed, but DK continued to complain of food "getting stuck." No apparent physical cause could be determined. DK's voice was clear, and her breath control was within normal limits. Recommendations to both DK and her daughter included alternating liquids and solids, taking small bites followed by sips of water or liquid, double-swallowing solids, and choosing soft foods that were easy to chew (e.g., cooked vegetables, canned fruits, pastas, foods served with sauces or gravies). The SLP called a voice mail report to the case manager relaying her findings and the need for only the one visit.

Mental Health Evaluation: The mental health nurse completed an assessment on her initial visit and found DK to be mildly depressed and anxious about her disease and living situation. She talked with DK's daughter and found that the daughter continued to have many questions about MS and needed reassurance that the right things were being done for DK. Over the next four weeks, the mental health nurse visited DK and continued to teach her about her medications, her MS, and her depression. DK's daughter and her family were included when possible. The signs of depression lessened, and her family was able to be more supportive once they had a better understanding of MS. DK was referred to a support group for newly diagnosed people. She was willing to have the MS team chaplain visit her. The mental health nurse kept the case manager aware of DK's progress.

Chaplain Support: DK had experienced many losses and lifestyle changes in the past several weeks and months. The chaplain explained the grieving process and helped DK deal with it. Her family was included to increase their understanding. The chaplain continued to visit DK until she was discharged from all home care services. The chaplain kept in contact with the case manager during that time.

MS Team Conference: DK's situation was discussed at two team meetings before all the evaluations and rec-

ommendations were completed. At the team conference just before the family conference, the plan of care was updated and finalized before sharing it with DK and her family. The mental health nurse would co–case manage DK's care to follow up her depression. The nurses would work with DK toward independence with her insulin administration and continue to monitor her steroid taper. The SLP reported that she had completed her swallowing evaluation and recommendations to DK and her daughter. The PT was finishing her teaching of the exercise program and proper use of equipment, and she planned to discharge DK after her next visit. The OT planned to continue to work with DK for an additional two to three weeks. The HHA would continue to assist DK with bathing, ADLs, and the exercise program designed by the PT until she was independent in these activities or a family member could take over the responsibility. The chaplain reported on her supportive visits with DK and her family. The team decided that not all members needed to attend the family conference. The PS would attend to facilitate the meeting. The OT could share the findings and recommendations of both the SLP and the PT. The mental health nurse and the SW would also attend. The chaplain would attend for additional support.

Family Conference: DK and her family were looking forward to the conference. Her daughter called her brother and sister, who were not interested in participating in DK's care until this time, and invited them to attend. The case manager facilitated arranging a convenient time for the family and MS Team to meet. At the conference, the current plan of care was discussed and any changes or updates were made. Information about MS and its impact on all of their lives was shared. DK's son and daughter, who previously had not been involved, offered to help share the responsibility of caring for their mother. They agreed to set up a plan after the conference. Since DK's ultimate goal was to live independently again, and this indeed seemed possible, long-range planning toward this goal was initiated. The SW explained to everyone about community resources available for DK. When Donna is able to move into her own apartment, the PT and OT will need to assess the new environment for safety.

SUMMARY

Providing quality home care services with a safe plan of care for patients is the goal of the MS team. The team has been successful by making a commitment to an interdisciplinary approach to care. The team has also made a commitment to work with physicians, payer sources, and patients and their families to develop a safe plan of care. Patients are provided with a complete plan of care after a comprehensive evaluation and assessment. Team members have become fierce advocates for their patients, reaching out into the community for the additional support and services that allow patients to remain independent in their own environment.

References

1. Aronson KJ. Quality of life among persons with multiple sclerosis and their caregivers. *Neurology* 1997:79–80.
2. Catanzaro M, Weinert C. Economics status of families living with multiple sclerosis. *Intl J Rehab Res* 1992; 15:209–218.
3. Cohen M. Helping at Home, Caregivers ask for help. *Nurs Health Care Perspect* 1997:184–191.
4. Cubbin J. Managing resources in the community. *Nurs Standard* 1992:31–39.
5. Halper J, Holland N. *Comprehensive nursing care in multiple sclerosis.* New York: Demos, 1997.
6. O'Brien MT. Multiple sclerosis: Stressors and coping strategies in spousal caregivers. *J Community Health Nursing* 1993:123–135.
7. Schapiro RT. *Multiple sclerosis: A rehabilitation approach to management.* New York: Demos, 1991.
8. Schapiro RT. *Symptom management in multiple sclerosis.* 3rd ed. New York: Demos, 1998.

33 A Model for Long-Term Care

James P. Ahearn, CSW, ACSW

A small percentage of people with multiple sclerosis will require extended care services because their rapidly progressing disease results in needs that are difficult if not impossible to meet in a home setting where family members are the primary or sole caregivers. For this population, premature nursing home placement is both a fear and—in many cases—a reality.

The ability to provide comprehensive long-term care services has been difficult, in large part because National Multiple Sclerosis Society (NMSS) chapters have been unable to tap into government, insurance, and third-party funding for these services. This is very different from the organizations that serve populations with developmental disabilities, where millions of dollars flow from government sources to support these constituencies. The challenge has led us to integrate our programs and collaborate with larger systems that have licenses and access to government and/or third-party reimbursement in order to provide long-term care services. Our chapter of the NMSS has put considerable effort and energy into developed long-term care services for people with MS and their families in the greater Rochester area.

A parent of a client initially defined the need for long-term care services with progressive MS. She asked our chapter to provide more services for her daughter, who had rapidly progressive MS. Although she took advantage of the chapter's many programs, she had a recurring nightmare that her daughter would soon have to be placed in a nursing home, most likely in the geriatric setting. Although grateful for the chapter's efforts, she wanted the chapter to do more to keep her daughter involved in the community.

This situation inspired an informal needs assessment, which found that approximately 10 percent of the MS clients were young, rapidly progressing, and at serious risk for premature institutionalization. Subsequently, a "third-party task force" committee consisting of area nursing home directors, politicians, funders, clients, and staff was created to determine whether government funding would support a long-term care service commitment. Although the committee was not successful in procuring third-party funding, a detailed questionnaire ascertained that MS clients were afraid of nursing home placement and were appreciative of the chapter's efforts to help end premature institutional placement. People with MS identified housing and day care as potential programs in which they would participate. Respite for families also was identified as important.

In the mid-1980s we formed an "Independent Living Center Committee" with community funders, health care providers, nursing home administrators, neurologists, staff, and people with MS. This group envisioned an overnight facility, a form of medical group home, to which persons with MS could go before entering a nursing home. The funding issue once again stymied our recommendations. However, one important outcome of this committee was the commission of a scientific research study of clients and their families in the Rochester area to determine the need for such a service. With the support of a grant from the NMSS' Health Service Research Committee and local foundations, the chapter initiated a study titled "Alternative Living Needs of Individuals with Multiple Sclerosis and Their Family Caregivers," by Margaret Wynam, Ph.D., RN, Ruth O'Brien, Ph.D., RN, and Katherine Donohoe, RN, MS NP-C.

Registered nurses interviewed 102 MS clients identified by the chapter as being seriously at risk for premature placement in a nursing home. In addition to the clients, 50 caregivers were interviewed in separate meetings. The three-year study found (1) a strong need for day care and overnight services, (2) a high safety risk for MS clients (many were in unsafe homes), and (3) a high risk for nursing home placement when their caregivers and families could no longer cope. Most caregivers were struggling economically, were exhausted, and did not know how to ask for help. Although not formally tested, a number of the clients had cognitive impairment. Nine of the MS clients, or approximately 10 percent, were placed in geriatric nursing homes before the study was completed. The average age of group members was 38 years.

Based on the health services research data, the Long-Term Care Committee was established in the late 1980s. The committee was co-chaired by the Director of the MS Center at Strong Memorial Hospital (Dr. Andrew Goodman) and an MS client (Lois Goodman) and consisted of chapter board members, staff members, MS clients, hospital administrators, nurses, nursing administrators, long-term care specialists, and community leaders. The Long-Term Care Committee recommended a day treatment program similar to the MS Achievement Center in Minneapolis. It was hoped that an overnight housing program would follow.

The development of a day treatment program required many steps, several of which occurred simultaneously. The first was to seek approval from the New York State Department of Health for a day-health program (medical day treatment program) for a younger, disease-specific (exclusively MS) population as opposed to a geriatric population. The next step was to advocate for this program at the State Capitol with help from the New York State MS Consortium. Next, a legal collaboration was formed with a hospital now called Unity Health System. Unity agreed to do the following: (1) help with the negotiations with the New York State Department of Health, (2) file for and complete the Certificate of Need Application, (3) use their nursing home license to help procure Medicaid funds, and (4) teach the Rochester Area

Chapter about the operations of a Day Health Program—Unity had two existing day health programs before the MS program. The Rochester Area Chapter agreed to raise $400,000 in start-up funds, refer MS clients to the program, provide most of the staff, and negotiate a lease for property to house the program. In the meantime, trust was building between the two systems to accomplish a unique and important program.

Approximately 4,000 square feet of accessible space was leased for five years through an affiliation with the Rochester Cornerstone Group and volunteers from the Rochester Area Chapter. The chapter also hired a development consultant, formed a Major Gifts committee, developed a case statement, and in the course of three years raised the $400,000 for this program.

The first $100,000 went to start-up costs such as equipment, necessary build-ins (i.e., accessible showers and restrooms and a turn-around driveway for wheelchairs). The additional $300,000 was used to provide client scholarships for people with MS who were not receiving Medicaid benefits and could not afford the cost of care for this program.

We then professionally marketed this program to the approximately 102 people with MS who had been identified as being in need. The marketing company (Ford Research Company) first invited the MS patients to come and talk. When this approach failed, the company representatives visited each of the clients individually. This positive response was coupled with seminars for the clients by staff and more individual visits.

Another step was to obtain approval by systems agencies and local zoning agencies, including fire code officials. After procuring the start-up dollars, finalizing the legal agreement with Unity Health System, negotiating a lease, marketing and communicating to our clients, and procuring necessary government supports, our MS Achievement Center at the Park (MSAC), named after the Achievement Center in Minneapolis, was initiated. The program, which was designed to treat progressively disabled young people with MS, provides occupational therapy, physical therapy, speech therapy, nutritional therapy, nursing care, social work, recreation therapy, transportation, psychiatric consultation, and acute diagnostic and medical consultation. The emphasis on nursing care and the medical model, required by New York State, make this program somewhat different from the MS Achievement Center in Minnesota.

With Unity Health System's nursing home license, the New York State Department of Health agreed to a formula to reimburse approximately $90 per day for any person with MS on Medicaid who was in this program. The program opened in June 1993 with eight clients. It can handle a maximum of 24 MS patients per day. Only 30 percent of the initial census of 18 people received Medicaid, and the need for dollars for clients' scholarships became apparent. All non-Medicaid clients are charged according to a sliding fee scale, and part of cost of their care is paid by scholarships funded by donors.

Five years into the program, the average census is more than 20 people attending each day; the total census has approached 50 people, 85 percent of whom are receiving Medicaid benefits. This shift to increased Medicaid coverage is due to encouragement by the social worker in the program for individuals to convert to Medicaid by using a spending-down formula. Clients see the potential benefits to this approach and are less threatened over time. Outcome studies are in progress to evaluate cost savings and quality of life.

Three people in the program have died. Some clients have moved on to nursing home care because of increasing disability as the result of their MS. The camaraderie and spirit at the MS Achievement Center is infectious. The main individual components of the programs at the MSAC are maintenance therapies—occupational, speech, and physical therapy. These therapies are not usually funded by insurance payments as "maintenance," but they are funded as part of the MSAC.

This program has not been without risks, problems, or stress. The blending of two cultures—a hospital culture and the culture of an MS chapter—has not always been easy. The staff at the MSAC are members of the Rochester chapter and includes five certified nursing assistants, a social worker, a recreation specialist, and a secretary/receptionist. The director of the program is a registered nurse who is employed by Unity Health System. The physical, occupational, and speech therapy consultants are also employed by Unity Health System. The trust and collaboration between the hospital system and the MS chapter have been a key to the success.

In another collaborative project, our chapter has recently initiated an overnight apartment facility. Six years ago the MS chapter was approached to be the landlord for a New York State Housing and Trust Fund initiative to convert an old building into a modern, fully accessible apartment complex for people with MS and epilepsy. The chapter formed a collaboration with four entities—Landsman Development Corporation, the Al Sigl Center, the Rochester MS Chapter, and the Epilepsy Association.

The New York State Department of Health awarded a $400,000 grant. The group procured a $300,000 low-interest loan from the Rochester City Council. The Al Sigl Center, a collaboration of eight rehabilitation agencies in the Rochester area, put together almost $1 million worth of tax credits, which they sold to a bank. With approximately $2.2 million of government, public, and private sector funds, the Al Sigl Center renovated an old shoe factory into a modern building with 12 accessible apartments.

In January 1997 Howitt House, which was named for a donor, opened to seven MS families. The Epilepsy Association holds five of the apartments. This program has not been without risk or problem-free. The program was marketed as independent living in part because of lack of funds to provide support services. Initially, individuals who thought they could live independently were recruited. In fact, many were not independent. Through a series of trial and error, all apartments are now rented to appropriate individuals.

The next challenge is to develop additional support programs that are third-party funded so that people with progressive disease and without caregivers can thrive in our community.

The MSAC at the Park and the Howitt House Accessible Apartment program are two examples of how a local MS chapter has been able to develop innovative long-term care programs by using complex collaborative arrangements and tapping into government and corporate funding. Similar programs in other states are feasible. The potential may exist for a combination program of HMOs and MS chapters in a capitated model of care.

Young people with MS deserve better than to stay in unsafe homes while waiting to be placed in long-term geriatric care facilities. The Rochester NMSS chapter has attempted to provide long-term care services for MS families over a 15-year period. It has successfully provided long-term care by collaborating with larger systems and government funding programs. Its two models have established the groundwork to listen to the needs of MS families, to do ample research, and to collaborate with other organizations and systems that have access to government funding and thirty-party reimbursement. The annual budget for the MSAC is half a million dollars a year. NMSS chapters cannot provide these programs alone. This program could not be funded without ongoing government or third-party dollars.

VIII

MULTIPLE SCLEROSIS
IN THE COMMUNITY

34 Vocational Issues

Kenneth M. Viste, Jr., M.D., and Phillip D. Rumrill, Jr., Ph.D.

Multiple sclerosis (MS) is a chronic, unpredictable neurologic condition that has major effects on employment. After the diagnosis is made and a treatment plan is established, many relevant questions about various aspects of employment arise. Multiple sclerosis is a condition with a multiplicity of symptoms, which interact in complex ways to affect all aspects of a person's life. The unpredictability of the illness makes it even more difficult to give appropriate advice.

Multiple sclerosis affects people who are more educated than average and usually are employed. Unfortunately, a disproportionate number of people with MS become unemployed after the first several years of their illness. Employment helps define a person's self-esteem as well as being the substrate for their family's financial security. For example, most health and disability benefits are obtained through employment. Health insurance is a major source of prescription drug payment. Loss of employment may mean loss of access to adequate medical care, including the newer, better, and more expensive immunomodulating medications.

Recognizing the physical requirements of various occupations is important when working with a multitude of MS-related impairments. For example, a weakened lower extremity may be a major handicap for an industrial worker but may be only an inconvenience to an office worker. Another problem is fatigue, which affects most MS patients and can create a barrier to continued employment.

Many resources are available to deal with issues related to employment and MS. The Division of Vocational Rehabilitation offices are available in all states. Vocational retraining and alternative vocational endeavors can be addressed through them.

The passage of the 1990 Americans with Disabilities Act (ADA) also has led to changes in access to employment opportunities by those with various handicaps. The basic elements in the ADA help people continue their employment with adaptations in their work environment. Affected MS patients need to understand their legal rights as they relate to job accommodations.

Finally, people with MS can learn about benefits that are available under Social Security Disability with ultimate access to Medicare benefits. Unfortunately, benefits are sometimes hard to access, and Medicare does not yet cover the cost of immunomodulating medications. There are many disincentives relative to continuing to work. Patients with MS and their families need to be aware of pitfalls in the process of accessing Social Security benefits.

This chapter answers the most common questions brought by patients and their families to their health care providers regarding employment.

1. What are my legal rights in employment under the ADA?

The 1990 ADA was the first comprehensive law enacted by any country in the world to prohibit discrimination on the basis of disability. The ADA guarantees equal participation in society for people with disabilities in much the same way as the Civil Rights Act of 1964 guaranteed the rights of all people regardless of race, sex, national origin, and religion. The four areas of social activity covered by the ADA are employment, public services, public accommodations, and communications (i.e., telephone systems).

As it pertains to employment, the ADA requires employers with 15 or more employees to provide reasonable accommodations for qualified employees with disabilities. For people with MS, reasonable accommodations may include modifications to the work schedule as a means of combating fatigue (e.g., an abbreviated work week or an extended lunch break during which to rest), flexibility in the manner or location in which work is performed (e.g., home-based employment), provision of equipment (e.g., a closed-circuit magnification machine for a person with a visual impairment), and renovations of the work environment (e.g., modification of restrooms to accommodate a motorized scooter). It should be noted that reasonable accommodations are determined on a case-by-case basis, and employers are not required to eliminate a primary job responsibility, lower production standards that are applied to all employees, provide personal use items (e.g., a mobility cane, wheelchair, eyeglasses), or overlook a violation of conduct rules. Employers also are not required to provide accommodations that constitute an undue hardship—that is, arrangements that are too costly or disruptive to the operation of the business.

Before becoming eligible for a reasonable accommodation, the worker or applicant must disclose his or her disability status to the employer and initiate a request for the accommodation in question. This does not mean that the person must disclose his or her underlying diagnosis or disabling condition. **An employer *never* has the right to know that you have MS,** only that you are a person with a disability in the event that you need an accommodation to perform an essential function of the job you hold or are seeking.

Although reasonable accommodations are an important part of the ADA, the employment protections available to people with MS and other disabling conditions go far beyond on-the-job accommodations. Under Title I (the employment section), people with disabilities have the civil right to enjoy the same benefits and privileges of employment as their nondisabled coworkers. This means that personnel decisions (e.g., hiring, promotion, layoff, termination) must be made without respect to the person's disability status. Workers may not be harassed on the basis of their disabilities, and the compensation they receive must be solely commensurate with their qualifications and productivity. Provided next are key terms and definitions that relate to the ADA.

Individuals with disabilities. Individuals (1) with a mental or physical impairment that substantially limits one or more life activities, (2) who have a history of such an impairment, or (3) who are perceived (even erroneously) as having such an impairment.

Qualified individuals with disabilities. Under Title I of the ADA, the term *qualified* applies to an individual with a disability who meets the skill, experience, education, and other job-related requirements of a position held or desired and who, with or without reasonable accommodations, can perform the essential functions of the job.

Essential job functions. Essential job functions are narrowly defined to include fundamental job duties as opposed to marginal ones. A job function is more likely to be "essential" if it requires special expertise, if a large amount of time is spent on that function, and/or if that function was listed in the written job description prepared before the employer advertised for or interviewed job applicants.

Reasonable accommodations. A reasonable accommodation refers to an employment-related modification that an employer must make to ensure equal opportunity for an individual with a disability to (1) apply for or test for a job, (2) perform essential job functions, and/or (3) receive the same benefits and privileges as other employees. The employer is required to provide a reasonable accommodation for known disabilities (e.g., when the disability is obvious or the applicant/employee informs the employer of the disability). Although each case must be evaluated individually, types of on-the-job accommodations include restructuring of existing facilities, restructuring of the job, modification of work schedules, reassignment to another position, modification of existing equipment, installation of new equipment, provision of qualified readers and interpreters, modification of application and examination procedures and/or training materials, and flexible personal leave policies.

Undue hardship. An accommodation might be labeled an undue hardship for the employer if its implementation resulted in "significant difficulty or expense." Factors to be considered in making this determination include (1) the nature and net cost of the accommodation; (2) the impact of the accommodation on the operation of the facility involved, taking into account the facility's overall resources and the number of its employees; and (3) the manner in which the employer's business operates, taking into account its size and financial resources. In deciding that an accommodation is an "undue hardship," an employer must rely on actual, not hypothetical, costs and burdens.

2. My MS follows a relapsing-remitting course. I can do my job during remissions, but exacerbations of my symptoms often make it necessary for me to take time off. Can my employer fire me for taking medical leave?

The Family and Medical Leave Act (FMLA) of 1993 has enabled thousands of American workers to retain their jobs while taking unpaid leaves of absence to attend to important family health concerns. The law requires employers in the public and private sectors to hold workers' jobs open and continue paying health insurance premiums while employees take time off to treat and/or recover from illnesses or injuries. It also provides leave for employees who must attend to the health care needs of their family members.

A covered employer under the FMLA is one who has 50 or more employees residing within a 75-mile radius of the work location. Employees are eligible for protection if they have at least one year of seniority on the job (defined as at least 1,250 hours worked within the 12 months preceding the requested leave date) AND have a serious health condition.

The FMLA defines a serious health condition as any illness, injury, impairment, or regimen of treatment that renders one unable to perform any essential function of his or her job. The term *serious health condition* is broader and more inclusive than the ADA's definition of disability. This means that a person with MS could be a person with a serious health condition under the FMLA but not meet the ADA's standard as a person with a disability. Unlike the term *disability,* serious health conditions pertain to both temporary and permanent conditions. Examples of commonly invoked serious health conditions under the FMLA include pregnancy, birth or adoption of a child, surgery, chemotherapy, and chronic illnesses.

The FMLA requires employers to provide up to 12 weeks of unpaid leave per calendar year for an eligible employee coping with a serious health condition. The 12 weeks need not be taken consecutively, and the employer must allow the worker to return to the same position or to a similar equivalent position. Return to work following unpaid leave may be denied only to "key" employees—that is, those who earn the highest 10 percent of salaries. This exception applies only when holding open key employees' jobs would create substantial and grievous long-term economic injury to the employer's operations. The employer's burden of proof for this exception is more stringent than for the ADA's defense of undue hardship.

As previously mentioned, eligible employees may take time off to attend to their own serious health conditions or to assist in the care and treatment of family members who have serious health problems. Family members are defined as spouses, children, or parents. For example, a person whose wife has MS and needs transportation to weekly appointments with her neurologist could request unpaid time off to accompany her to doctor's visits.

In the event that the need for leave is foreseeable (e.g., pregnancy, elective surgery), the employee must give 30 days advance notice. If the need for leave is unforeseeable (e.g., an exacerbation of MS), employees are required to give "reasonable" notice (undefined in FMLA regulations). Once the employee has filed a request for leave, the employer has two business days to determine the employee's eligibility for the requested time off. Failure to respond within two business days automatically makes the employee eligible for the requested leave. Of course, an employer may request that the employee verify his or her serious health condition or the condition of a family member. If verification is requested, the employee must provide documentation from a health care provider, with the following conditions:

1. The provider should verify only the need for a medical leave and not disclose the underlying medical condition.
2. The information reported should be job-related (e.g., need for, length of, and timing of the medical leave).
3. Inquiry into the possible future effects of the serious health condition should be avoided.
4. Leave requests should be processed by a designated knowledgeable representative of the employer so that discussion with the employee's supervisors and coworkers is limited.
5. Supervisors should only be notified of facts related to the circumstances of the leave, not about specific aspects of the employee's (or a relative's) serious health condition.
6. Records related to medical leave must be maintained in a file separate from the employee's personnel records.

3. Given that I have a disease that requires a lot of rest and whose symptoms are likely to interfere with my ability to do my job, should I stop working?

There is no reason to quit your job just because you have been diagnosed with MS. There is no evidence that unemployment will have a positive effect on your health status; in fact, many experts believe that people who work are psychologically and physically healthier than those who do not. With advancements in assistive technology, medical treatment, and society's attitudes toward people with disabilities, people with MS and other potentially disabling conditions are able to maintain their jobs longer than ever before. Don't forget about your legal rights under the ADA and FMLA—those laws were put into place to enable you to keep working as long as you wish to do so. If and when you decide to stop working, it is important that you weigh all important factors (e.g., family circumstance, financial needs, health status) with input from your significant others, health care professionals, and employer. The fact that you have been diagnosed with MS should not be the determining factor in this exceedingly important decision, and you will know better than anyone else when it is time to stop working.

4. I have been offered a job, and the question of medical benefits has arisen. Can I be denied coverage under my employer's health insurance because of a diagnosis of MS?

Title I of the ADA prohibits employers from entering into contracts that discriminate against people with disabilities. This includes contracts related to health insurance. Employees with disabilities must be given the same coverage that is available to all other employees. Additionally, an employer cannot refuse to hire you because his or her insurance company will not cover you, or if covering you increases the employer's health insurance premiums. However, an employer may offer health insurance coverage that contains preexisting condition exclusions or limits certain procedures, provided that those exclusions or limitations pertain to *all* employees.

The Health Insurance Portability and Accountability Act (HIPAA) of 1996 provides some protections for employees with disabilities who change jobs. The Act enables a person with a preexisting medical condition to join his or her new employer's health insurance plan and be exempt from preexisting condition exclusions, but this applies only to employees who do not interrupt their insurance coverage. The best advice for people with MS who leave a job is to continue their health insurance benefits as long as is allowable and then transfer coverage to the new employer's plan.

Given the complexity of health care coverage in the United States, it might be tempting to conceal your MS from an insurance company during your enrollment process. This is *not* advisable because any insurance company can discontinue your coverage if it learns that you have lied about your medical history on application forms. Remember also that your employer has no right to read any medical information that you submit to insurance companies.

5. My MS symptoms have progressed to the point where I feel I can no longer do my job the way I used to. How will I know when it is time to stop working?

It is time for you to look into other options if you have researched and requested all possible accommodations to assist you in doing your job yet still find you cannot adequately perform the essential job functions. Be sure to investigate other positions that may be available within your company before you stop working altogether. Other options include job retraining that would enable you to continue working in some other field, volunteer work, Social Security Disability Insurance, and long-term disability.

6. What are the eligibility requirements for Social Security Disability Insurance (SSDI) and Supplemental Security Income (SSI)?

Both SSDI and SSI are programs run by the Social Security Administration. The medical requirements for disability payments are the same under both programs, and disability is determined by the same process. For a person with MS, the recognized areas of impairment may include gait, vision, cognition, and fatigue. Eligibility for SSDI is based on prior work history, whereas SSI disability decisions are made solely on the basis of financial need. Applications for SSDI require a five-month waiting period from the determination of disability to the start of benefits. The person becomes eligible for Medicare insurance coverage 24 months after the initial waiting period. There is no similar waiting period for SSI benefits; individuals eligible for SSI based on financial need are covered by Medicaid. To be eligible for SSDI, a person must (1) have worked and paid Social Security taxes (FICA) for enough years to be covered under Social Security, (2) have paid at least some of these taxes in recent years, (3) be considered medically disabled (i.e., too disabled to work), and (4) not be working or working but earning less than the Substantial Gainful Activity (SGA) level of $500 per month ($810 for beneficiaries who are blind). In determining a person's gross earnings, certain employment-related expenses will be deducted from the calculation if the person is paying expenses out of pocket and not being reimbursed for them. These deducted expenses include some types of attendant care services, transportation-related costs, medical and nonmedical equipment costs, medication costs, and some types of residential modifications.

The SSDI payment amount is based on a worker's lifetime average earnings covered by Social Security. The payment amount will be reduced by worker's compensation payments and/or public disability payments. Those individuals who are receiving payments from private disability insurance companies may find that these payments are reduced by whatever amount they subsequently receive from SSDI. The SSDI payment amount is not affected by other (nonwork) income or resources.

To be eligible for SSI based on a medical condition, a person must (1) have little or no income or resources, (2) be considered medically disabled (i.e., too disabled to work), and (3) initially not be working or be working but earning less than the SGA level of $500 per month (this restriction does not apply to beneficiaries who are blind). As with SSDI, certain out-of-pocket employment-related expenses will be deducted from the calculation of the person's gross earnings.

Once you begin to receive SSI benefits, work activity will not bring an end to SSI eligibility as long as you remain medically disabled. Even if you cannot receive SSI income maintenance checks because the amount of money you earn exceeds the SGA, eligibility for Medicaid may continue indefinitely. The SSI payment amount is based on the amount of other income, your living arrangements, and the state in which you reside. The basic payment is called the federal benefit rate, and it is adjusted each year to account for inflation and cost of living increases. Most states pay an additional amount known as a state supplement. The amount of these supplements and eligibility requirements vary from state to state.

7. I retired on SSDI several months ago, but I am thinking about returning to work. What would happen to my benefits if I reentered the labor force?

There are many work incentives available if you decide to return to work while receiving SSDI benefits. These incentives provide support over a period of years to allow any beneficiary to test his or her ability to work and gradually become self-supporting. You have at least four years to test your ability to work. During the first 12 months (trial work period), you will receive full SSDI payments. Following the initial 9 of these 12 months, you begin a three-year extended period of eligibility. If you stop working at any time during this period, you can restart your cash benefits without a new application, demonstration of your disability, or waiting period. Your Medicare benefits will also continue during this three-year period. Once Medicare stops because of renewed work activity, you can elect to buy coverage as long as you remain disabled. If you become disabled again within five years after the prior period of disability ended, you do not have to go through another five-month waiting period to obtain benefits, and neither do you have to wait to become reeligible for Medicare.

8. Can I work part-time and still receive SSDI benefits?

As long as you earn under $500 per month (the establish cutoff for substantial gainful activity), you will continue to receive SSDI benefits. If your earnings are greater than SGA, you will be considered gainfully employed, and your SSDI payments will be discontinued following your trial work period. Keep in mind that in calculating your gross income, the Social Security Administration will deduct certain types of employment-related expenses that directly affect your ability to perform your job and that you have personally paid for without other reimbursement.

9. Are there agencies that could assist me in seeking, securing, and/or maintaining employment as I continue to cope with MS?

The Vocational Rehabilitation program in your state provides services to enable people with disabilities to become or remain employed. Although the program is mandated by federal law, it is carried out by individually created state agencies. Each state agency has its own name and slightly different program. Vocational Rehabilitation services are defined as an "eligibility" program rather than an "entitlement" program. This means that you must demonstrate eligibility by having a physical or mental disability that results in a substantial impediment to employment. There must also be a reasonable expectation that Vocational Rehabilitation services will help you to become more employable. Many Vocational Rehabilitation agencies operate under an Order of Selection mandate, whereby services are prioritized for those applicants who have the most severe disabilities. Your first step is to contact the Vocational Rehabilitation program in your state to ask for information about eligibility and application procedures.

An important work incentive provided by the Social Security Administration is called Continued Payment Under a Vocational Rehabilitation Program. This incentive provides that people receiving SSI or SSDI who improve medically to the point that they are able to return to work can continue to receive their benefits if they are participating in any approved Vocational Rehabilitation program whose services are likely to enable them to resume working.

If you are found eligible for Vocational Rehabilitation, services may include a thorough evaluation to determine the extent of your disability and the need for treatment to correct or reduce the disability; vocational guidance and counseling; medical appliances and prosthetic devices if needed to increase your ability to work; vocational training to prepare you for gainful employment; provision of occupational equipment and tools; job placement and follow-up; and post-employment services.

Another excellent employment resource is the local chapter of the National Multiple Sclerosis Society. Services available through the Society may include legal advocacy, placement assistance, employment seminars, consultation on assistive technology, and education about MS for employers.

35 Ad-Vocational Issues

Karen C. Wenzel, M.A., CTRS/CLP

L eisure and recreation are significant aspects of a person's life. One of the most striking set of statistics on the prominence of leisure in society estimates the years spent in various life activities (1). Assuming a 70-year life span, it has been estimated that 27 years will be spent in leisure time, including childhood play; 24 years will be spent sleeping; 7.33 years will be spent working; and 4.33 years will be spent in formal education. The remaining years are dedicated to eating (2.33) and 5 years for miscellaneous activities. These statistics indicate that time spent in leisure is almost four times greater than time spent in work over the course of a lifetime. In spite of the prominent role leisure plays in our lives, very few people are actually prepared to use leisure to its fullest benefit.

Although many contrasting definitions of leisure are found in the literature, leisure is most commonly defined as discretionary time or unobligated time (2). Although the terms *leisure* and *recreation* are often used interchangeably, recreation usually refers to activity performed during leisure time, usually for the purpose of enjoyment (3). Leisure is assumed to be an experience that is characterized by a perception of relative freedom from obligation and constraints (4–6). The higher the degree of choice one feels he or she has to determine personal action, the greater the perceived freedom, which most researchers recognize as the primary prerequisite for a leisure experi-

ence. Conversely, perceived constraint on personal choice would lead to a nonleisure or (work-related) experience. According to Neulinger (7), the degree of internal motivation or external motivation also helps to define the nature of the experience. Leisure is characterized by a high degree of internal motivation. Leisure participation and satisfaction are positively related to psychological well-being and life satisfaction (8–13). Additionally, several studies have indicated that leisure behavior is perhaps the most important or one of the most important determinants of life satisfaction and psychological well-being (14–17). Within the context of relative freedom, an individual must make choices that affect their personal growth and development, as well as the well-being of others.

Individuals can make constructive, beneficial choices or poor choices. With poor choices, opportunities for human growth and development are lost. Constructive, beneficial choices provide opportunity for development of full potential, well-being, increased quality of life, and self-fulfillment. Quality of life and its relationship to leisure experiences is an important aspect of being human. Sylvester states that the related constructs of well-being, quality of life, happiness, and self-actualization are conditions and opportunities required to live a full, meaningful, worthwhile, and satisfying life. He argues that leisure is a core value, a prerequisite to achieving happiness and fulfillment as a person (18).

Researchers have also studied the relationship of leisure to health. Iso Ahola (19) states that theoretically leisure affects health in three interrelated ways: (1) Leisure is a tool by which health is pursued and obtained; it provides the time and environment in which health behaviors are practiced; (2) leisure is a way of life, a cognitive orientation toward life and a lifestyle that promotes health; and (3) leisure has some inherent qualities and characteristics that are germane to health.

Leisure is a significant component of a person's life. Most individuals place a high value on free time and the activities engaged in during that time. Self-expression, release of tension, social interaction, and development of human potential are some of the reasons cited for participating in recreational activities (20). These benefits of leisure contribute to an individual's well-being and life satisfaction. For an individual with a chronic illness or disability, leisure can be either an opportunity or an additional burden. When free time is unwanted, personally unfulfilling, or perceived as "forced leisure," it can lose its life-enhancing quality.

MULTIPLE SCLEROSIS AND "LIFE STORIES"

Illness is a term that is applied to a lived experience or a person's response to disease or trauma (21). A diagnosis of multiple sclerosis (MS) generally is experienced as more than merely physical and psychological distress. Brody (22) has said that to be "ill" is to experience an unpleasant sense of disruption to the body and a threat to one's personhood. The diagnosis results in a disruption of an individual's sense of well-being and personal continuity. The experience of illness and resulting disability is an experience of a disrupted life story. Every person has a "life story" that unites the recollected past with the desired future and informs one's self in the present (22,23). A diagnosis of MS will affect the "writing" of that story in many ways. The shock at the time of diagnosis results in an "illness" experience that is a function of the person's preexisting lifestyle and future perspectives as well as the illness itself. From a narrative perspective, "illness" is conceived as a disruption in a life narrative, in which the future self imagined in the life narration is made doubtful by the perceived threat to one's health. The disruption of the ability to engage in preferred activities resulting from negative life events may be particularly distressful when those activities have special relevance to the person's identity.

Charmaz (24) noted that the illness experience frequently shrinks an individual's social world and friendships. It forces people to pull into their inner circle while pulling away from others. Much of the negative effects are associated with the loss of companionate leisure (25,26). Leisure activities are usually less important in themselves than the relationships they maintain or enhance (27). Having relationships disrupted creates a disruption of one's personal narrative. Additionally, the dependency often created by illness has an impact on leisure behavior and relationships. The pursuit of familial social activities, which were once a source of intimacy and enjoyment, may now bring distress because of the requirement of assistance from others.

As individuals respond to the changes illness imposes, they rewrite their life story accordingly. With a diagnosis of MS, the "re-storying" is ongoing. The variable disease course and unpredictableness of disease progression keep the individual living in a constant state of adjustment or potential adjustment. Methods for reconstruction of leisure lifestyle need to be included in the adjustment process as leisure plays a significant role in the critical and ongoing experience of illness. Individuals constantly attempt to find an alternative story to help them make sense of a life that involves chronic illness and loss of function. In each unique story, leisure and recreation will play a role during the onset of illness and disability and during the subsequent rehabilitation and adjustment process.

LEISURE AND INDIVIDUALS WITH DISABILITIES

In a study of leisure characteristics of adults with disabilities, Coyle and Kinney (28) identified that for most adults reading (14 percent) and television viewing (12 percent) were the most frequently engaged in activities. A 1986 Gallup survey addressing leisure characteristics reported that television viewing (33 percent) and reading (14 percent) were the top responses offered by a random sample of Americans. Approximately 23 percent of the adults with disabilities identified reading as their favorite leisure activity, whereas 19 percent identified television viewing as their favorite activity followed by socializing (15 percent), individualized noncompetitive sports (11 percent), and art or music appreciation (8.2 percent). Barriers to leisure participation were identified as weather (48.9 percent), transportation (48.7 percent), and facilities (43.3 percent). These constraints were followed by lack of physical abilities, safety, equipment costs, health, spontaneity, uncertainty of abilities, and lack of motivation. Individuals with acquired disabilities were noted to have significantly lower satisfaction with leisure. As the level of functional impairment increased, the degree of satisfaction with leisure decreased.

LEISURE AND MULTIPLE SCLEROSIS

Multiple sclerosis can have a profound impact on many aspects of daily life, including leisure. Decreased physical function often leads to a reduction in leisure and recreational activities. Leisure activities are often the first to suffer in the event of a disabling illness. This in turn can lead to social isolation and depressive mood disorders. Little if any attention has been given to the importance of recreation and leisure to the life of the person and the family affected by MS. Of the many forms of illness and disability that can affect human beings, insults to the central nervous system are among the most devastating. Health-related quality of life is lower in people with MS than in people with other disorders (29). Although longevity is minimally affected, employment frequently is impacted. It has been noted that 85 percent of people diagnosed with MS are unemployed within 15 years of diagnosis (30). Therefore, people with MS may have more "forced leisure," free time that can be perceived as a burden rather than an opportunity. Resulting impairments often prevent participation in preferred and personally satisfying activities or the activities must be modified to allow continued participation. Additionally, the psychological symptoms of stress and depression negatively influence the experience of free time (31,32).

Lewis (33), in sharing his personal experience with chronic illness stated, "My avocational loves of singing, church involvement, outdoor activities and athletics came as equally difficult areas to give up. In some ways, these avocations had greater meaning than my primary job because they were interests I had pursued and been involved with since childhood." Employment may be just one type of productive effort that may have relevance to an individual. It may be necessary to expand our focus to help the person to become "productive" in other areas. Employment is only one form of productivity. Helping the individual with MS explore other meaningful activities, especially leisure activities, can create new avenues of productivity.

Quality of life is correlated with a host of variables. In a study of MS patients, the key variables affecting quality of life were identified as (1) being able to have social and recreational activities outside of one's home, (2) being able to accomplish work or activity unimpeded by physical and emotional problems, (3) being able to avoid or overcome fatigue, and (4) having supportive and intimate friendship (34). People with MS engage in fewer social and recreational activities than would be expected based on their level of disability (35). Impairment resulting from MS does not necessarily correlate to the person's psychosocial well-being and status. Harper and coworkers (36) reported that "psychosocial disability" or emotional and mental health did not correlate with disease severity. Depression is noted to be a psychological symptom frequently associated with MS (37). The "adaptive coping model" views physical illness as a life crisis that results in severely increased long-term stress and calls for a number of cognitive, affective, and behavioral responses to a variety of physical and psychosocial changes imposed by the disease (38). Of importance in the "Adaptive Coping Model of MS" (39) are cognitive appraisal of the disease, choice of coping skills and resources, and availability of social support. Leisure activities can be a very effective coping mechanism.

According to Trieschmann (32), the focus of rehabilitation centers has tended to emphasize those tasks related to physical functioning and have ignored tasks more closely associated with psychosocial functioning, including recreation and leisure activities. Focus on leisure lifestyle issues has often been difficult, given the orientation of the patient, health care colleagues, and third-party payers. The reconstruction of a leisure lifestyle, realized with varying degrees of continuity and adaptation, is important in the rehabilitation process and in promoting the likelihood of ongoing life satisfaction and well-being.

MULTIPLE SCLEROSIS AND CONSTRAINTS TO LEISURE

There is an abundance of research describing the constraints to leisure. Constraints have been described as primarily discrete conditions, including lack of time, money, access, or self-confidence, that either prevent, curtail, or inhibit leisure activity (40,41). Recent research on the subject has demonstrated that constraints are personally interpreted (42,43) and through the use of a variety of strategies are often negotiated to allow some degree of participation (44).

For an individual with MS, some unique constraints or barriers to leisure participation. These include fatigue, heat liability, gait ataxia, muscular weakness, sensory disturbances, diminished visual acuity, bowel and bladder management, spasticity, sexual difficulties, emotional issues, and cognitive dysfunction (45). Despite the fact that the symptoms and progression of MS vary, fatigue and changes in life activities have a significant effect on leisure lifestyle.

Fatigue can be the most disabling of all MS symptoms (46). Krupp defined fatigue as "a sense of tiredness, a lack of energy, a total body give out. It's not weakness, instead it is a generalized low-energy feeling" (47). Krupp found that the most distinguishing feature of MS fatigue, as compared with fatigue in other people, was the negative impact it had on the person's ability to perform activities of daily living. People with MS must prioritize activities carefully in order to accomplish critical activities before fatigue sets in. Keeping leisure activities on the agenda while managing fatigue can seem like an uphill battle. However, enjoyable activities, especially those that involve moderate physical exertion, can decrease the symptoms of fatigue (48).

Multiple sclerosis has been ranked highest among chronic health conditions with respect to the prevalence of associated problems in major life activities (49). Zelsow and Pavlou (50) reported that MS can bring about changes in interpersonal relations, occupational productivity, and psychological well-being. As a consequence of life activity changes, changes in leisure behavior and the use of free time may occur with onset of disability (51). Disability can make continued participation in past leisure interests impossible or just too frustrating. Fatigue can impact leisure pursuits, as they may rank lower than other essential life activities when energy conservation requires a scaled-down schedule.

Multiple sclerosis affects the lifestyle of people other than the individual with MS. In significant relationships, a whole new menu of potential conflict develops, including pace, temperature preference, income allocation, and social activity. Loss of shared leisure activities related to disability, and the subsequent changes in family roles often shake the foundations of many relationships. Many leisure activities that had cemented the family together may be forfeited because of illness. Lewis, in sharing his personal experience stated that, "we had to grieve these losses together, large portions of our old lives vanished" (33).

Although disability may decrease the desire to participate in meaningful and fulfilling leisure due to any variety of perceived and real barriers, involvement in leisure experiences is integral to health restoration and maintenance and successful coping (52). Clearly, there is much more to be maintained than bodily integrity and control over disruptive affects. One thing that must be enhanced if possible and maintained is personal self-esteem. This struggle to keep intact a satisfactory self-picture or "life story" serves to preserve a sense of competence and inner assurance that one can do the things necessary for a satisfactory life.

THE ROLE OF THERAPEUTIC RECREATION IN REHABILITATION

Therapeutic recreation can play an important role in rehabilitation. The development of a meaningful leisure lifestyle facilitates adjustment to disability and promotes life satisfaction. Leisure can act as an important buffer in adjusting to the stress associated with difficult life events, either in the continuation of old familiar activities or the development of new ones (53). Lewis (33) reported that of 26 useful techniques for dealing with stress, 21 were leisure-related. Another study established a positive correlation between the frequency of pleasant events and the reduction of depression (54). Ulrich and colleagues (55), demonstrated the therapeutic benefits of recreation activities in helping people cope with various stressors. In addition, participating in artistic activities has been shown to be a valuable coping tool for people living with debilitating and irreversible physical conditions (56). Lyons (57) reported that satisfaction with leisure was positively correlated with adjustment to disability and negatively related to loneliness.

Although little is known about the relationship between leisure and adjustment to disability, Lyons (57) suggested that leisure adjustment is not what the person does for leisure, but the degree to which an individual has personally satisfying leisure experiences. Lyons (57) conceptualized leisure adjustment as "the ability to structure personally satisfying discretionary activity following the onset of physical, cognitive or emotional disability." In addition, Trieschmann (58) claimed that "the key to coping with one's disability is to receive enough satisfaction and rewards to make life worthwhile." Spinal cord injured patients who maintained their leisure lifestyle were more satisfied with their life, were less depressed, and had more confiding relationships (59). Leisure interventions designed to revive and facilitate involvement in leisure interests and to build social support systems may significantly enhance quality of life.

Therapeutic recreation services often address family leisure and other forms of relational leisure. Family roles and other relationships can in part be redefined by the preservation of old leisure interests and by the development of new ones. Relational leisure and role-determining leisure have been defined as activities that build and maintain relationships (60). Orthner and Mancini (61) cited numerous studies showing consistently that spouses who share leisure time together in joint activities report more marital satisfaction than those who do not. Finding ways to continue previously shared leisure activities and identify new possibilities can strengthen and maintain familial and social relationships.

Research by Iso Ahola (4) indicates that active recreation contributes more strongly to positive mental health than does passive recreation. Physical exercise has been shown to decrease depression (62) and increase physical competence (63). When diagnosed with MS, many individuals were given the recommendation to seek a more sedentary lifestyle. For many years physicians prescribed bed rest for newly diagnosed individuals in an effort to ward off exacerbations. Current research indicates that physical activity and even aerobic exercise are not contraindicated but highly recommended. Physical activity should be incorporated into the individual's leisure lifestyle. Moderate physical activity has been proven to enhance functional status and well-being (49,64).

STRATEGIES FOR INCORPORATING LEISURE

For an individual with MS seeking to incorporate leisure activities in their life, the following strategies may be helpful:

- schedule activity for the morning, or the time of day when energy is higher
- monitor perceived exertion level and learn to "pace" effectively
- monitor heat liability and use environmental or applied cooling techniques
- use water environments to maintain temperature regulation
- maintain adequate hydration
- limit the intensity of activities but not the range
- there is always a way to compensate, adapt, or modify an activity

With energy constraints and resulting fatigue a reality in MS, prioritization of activities becomes important. An assessment of activities and their relevance or personal importance is critical. For many people with MS, an unexpected positive outcome of the disease is a much needed review of values and a reprioritization of life activities. Leisure activities should not be necessarily placed at the bottom of the list but objectively assessed for their potential benefit and contribution to overall life satisfaction.

Although the MS literature is lacking in information about leisure, MS patients frequently share their experiences and leisure recommendations. Some of these include the following;

> "Rest, eat well, excercise, have something to look forward to, be sociable, think positively, take care to look good, keep routines in your life, do something that gives you a sense of achievement, live in the present, and enjoy each experience" (33).

A woman with MS indicated that her leisure would not be different if she did not have the disease, but she explained,

> "...it would be easier, and less frustrating. I wouldn't have to modify everything. Everything I do is slow and paced, and I'm very impatient with myself—more impatient with myself than with other people.... I'd be more independent than I am. That's the biggest thing, you lose your independence" (64).

Dick Hicks of the Jimmie Heuga Center advises, "Comparing yourself to others' athletic feats can set you up for failure. Set yourself up for success by incorporating physical activities you enjoy into your regular life. Then congratulate yourself for finding what you like" (48).

Although there are numerous options for meaningful leisure pursuits, individuals will often need informed, professional involvement to facilitate participation, adaptation, and resource identification. The professional services of a certified therapeutic recreation specialist may be indicated. Although certain activities are frequently suggested, there is no specific activity that should be recommended to all people with MS. The specific activity is not as important as what it does for and means to the individual.

THERAPEUTIC RECREATION IN MS REHABILITATION

Professional therapeutic recreation services should be considered in the rehabilitation process for people with MS. Outcomes sought through therapeutic recreation include mastery, self-efficacy, self-discovery, self-control, stress management, productive purposeful sense of self, adjustment to disability, and improved body image. In addition, physical outcomes, cognitive outcomes, and community reintegration are typically addressed through therapeutic recreation service provision.

Overall, rehabilitation services for individuals with MS are strengthened by a more balanced emphasis on psychosocial issues in addition to functional issues. Therapeutic recreation emphasizes self-determined treatment versus institutionalized treatment. As a discipline, therapeutic recreation places high value on personal choice, self-determination, and individualized, client-centered treatment. Activities are used to the extent that they have personal meaning to the individual. Therapeutic recreation services are provided in a continuum of care, which incorporates treatment, education, and recreation services. The treatment services, referred to as "recreation therapy" are goal-oriented interventions that use activity to promote improved functional status. Leisure education services include leisure skill acquisition, resource guidance, and exploration of leisure values and interests. Recreation services include the provision of accessible environments and adaptive equipment to facilitate leisure participation. This approach promotes lifelong rather than short-term service delivery that provides "whole life" approach to rehabilitation. People with MS face social isolation, depression, social stigma, unemployment, and strained family relationships. Lack of ongoing community-based support leaves patients and their families to struggle with these issues alone. When available, community-based service models, such as MS day programs, support groups, or social and/or recreation groups are highly indicated.

Successful use of community resources and maintenance and development of social support systems benefits people with MS in coping with the day-to-day realities of MS. Reintegration into the community is the goal of rehabilitation, but few resources and programs facilitate this process. Reduced medical complication and enhanced survival have been positively correlated to activity level and community life, regardless of functional ability (59,65). The philosophy of rehabilitation has changed from a short-term, physically oriented process that emphasizes what a person cannot do and which views disability as central, overriding everything else about the individual, to a more holistic, lifelong process that emphasizes a person's strengths and abilities and views the disability as only one aspect of a multifaceted life that includes satisfactions as well as grievances and abilities as well as disabilities. Leisure is an important component in the rehabilitation process and in promoting and maintaining life satisfaction for people with MS.

Just as leisure activities are implicated in the experience of illness, so can they be associated with recovery, rehabilitation, adjustment, and life narrative reconstruction or re-storying. Leisure plays a significant role in the writing of the new story after illness interrupts the original story line. The new story one writes for oneself subsequent to traumatic life events and disruptive illness is likely to be illustrated with a future self in action and experiencing leisure in a way that can make life enjoyable and meaningful once again.

References

1. Weiskopf D. *Recreation and leisure: Improving the quality of life*. Boston: Allyn & Bacon, 1982.
2. Maclean JR. Leisure and the quality of life. In: Craig TT (ed.). *The humanistic and mental health aspects of sports, exercise, and recreation*. Chicago: American Medical Association, 1976:73–75.
3. Leitner MJ, Leitner SF. *Leisure enhancement*. New York: The Hawarth Press, 1989.
4. Iso Ahola SE. *The social psychology of leisure and recreation*. Springfield, IL: Charles C. Thomas, 1980.
5. Kelly JR. *Leisure*. Englewood Cliffs, NJ: Prentice-Hall, 1982.
6. Neulinger J. *To leisure: An introduction*. Boston: Allyn & Bacon, 1981.
7. Neulinger J. *The psychology of leisure*. Springfield, IL: Charles C. Thomas, 1974.
8. Keller JM. The relationship between leisure and life satisfaction among older women. Paper presented at the NRPA Research Symposium, National Recreation and Park Association. Kansas City, KS, October 1983.
9. Kelly JR, Steinkamp MW, Kelly JR. Later life leisure: How they play in Peoria. *Gerontologist* 1986; 26:531–537.
10. Mancini J, Orthner D. Situational influences of leisure satisfaction and morale in old age. *J Am Geriatr Soc* 1980; 28:446–471.
11. Ragheb MG, Griffith CA. The contribution of leisure participation and satisfaction to life satisfaction of older persons. *J Leisure Res* 1982; 14:395–306.
12. Riddick CC, Daniel SN. The relative contributions of activities and other factors to the mental health of older women. *J Leisure Res* 1984; 16:136–148.
13. Sneegas JJ. Components of life satisfaction in middle and later life adults: Perceived social competence, leisure participation, and life satisfaction. *J Leisure Res* 1986; 18:248–258.
14. Campbell A, Converse P, Rogers W. *The quality of American life: Perceptions, evaluations, and satisfactions*. New York: Russell Sage, 1976.
15. Flanagan JC. A research approach to improving our quality of life. *Am Psychol* 1978; 33:138–147.
16. London M, Crandall R, Seals G. The contribution of job and leisure satisfaction to quality of life. *J Appl Psychol* 1977; 62:328–334.
17. Yankelovich D. The new psychological contracts at work. *Psychology Today* 1978 (May):46–50.
18. Sylvester C. Therapeutic recreation and the right to leisure. *Ther Rec J* 1992; 26:9–20.
19. Iso Ahola SE. Leisure lifestyle and health. In: Compton DM, Iso Ahola S (eds.). *Leisure and mental health*. Park City, UT: Family Development Resources, Inc., 1994:42–60.
20. Gunn SL, Peterson CA. *Therapeutic recreation program design: Principles and procedures*, 2nd ed. Englewood Cliffs, NJ: Prentice-Hall, 1978.
21. Kleinman A. *The illness narratives: Suffering, healing and the human condition*. New York: Basic Books, 1988.
22. Brody H. *Stories of sickness*. New Haven, CT: Yale University Press, 1987.
23. Brock SC, Kleiber DA, White M. Interpreting illness: Narrative of athletes with career-ending injuries. Paper presented at Qualitative Research in Education Conference. Athens, GA, 1992.
24. Charmaz K. *Good days and bad days: The self in chronic illness and time*. New Brunswick, NJ: Rutgers University Press, 1991.
25. Lyons RF. Companionate leisure and adjustment to negative life events: New evidence from relationship research. Paper presented at the NRPA Leisure Research Symposium, Baltimore, October 1989.
26. Lyons RF. The effects of acquired illness and disability on friendships. In: Perlman D, Jones W (eds.). *Advances in personal relationships*. Vol. 3. London: J. Kingsley, Publishers, 1991:223–277.
27. Kelly JR. *Leisure identities and interactions*. London: George Allen & Unwin, 1983.
28. Coyle CP, Kinney WB. Leisure characteristics of adults with physical disabilities. *Ther Rec J* 1990; 24(1):64–73.
29. Rudick RA, Miller D, Clough JD, et al. Quality of life in multiple sclerosis: Comparison with inflammatory bowel disease and rheumatoid arthritis. *Arch Neurol* 1992; 49:1237–1242.
30. Coyne P. Presentation at MS Consortium Meeting, Calgary, Canada, 1997.
31. Decker SD, Shulz R. Correlates of life satisfaction and depression in middle-aged and elderly spinal cord injured persons. *Am J Occup Ther* 1985; 39(11):740–745.
32. Trieschmann RB. *Spinal cord injuries: Psychological, social, and vocational adjustment*, 2nd ed. New York: Pergamon Press, 1988.
33. Lewis K. *Successful living with chronic illness*. Wayne, NJ: Avery Publishing, 1985.
34. Choi T, Birnbaum G, Bland P, et al. Measuring and predicting quality of life of MS patients. Presented at the

Annual Conference for the Consortium of Multiple Sclerosis Centers, Minneapolis, MS, 1994.

35. Staples D, Lincoln NB. Intellectual impairment in multiple sclerosis and its relation to functional abilities. *Rheumatol Rehab* 1979; 18:153–160.

36. Harper AC, Harper DA, Chambers LW, et al. An epidemiological description of physical, social, and psychological problems in multiple sclerosis. *J Chronic Dis* 1986; 39:305–310.

37. Whitlock FA, Siskind MM. Depression as a major symptom of multiple sclerosis. *Modern Treatment* 1980; 8:961–968.

38. Moos R, Tsu VD. The crisis of physical illness: An overview. In: Moos RM (ed.). *Coping with physical illness*. New York: Plenum, 1977:3–21.

39. VanderPlate C. Psychological aspects of multiple sclerosis and its treatment: Toward a biopsychosocial perspective. *Health Psychol* 1984; 3(3):253–272.

40. Crawford D, Jackson E, Godbey G. A hierarchical model of leisure constraints. *Leisure Sciences* 1991; 13:309–320.

41. Wade M (ed.). *Constraints on leisure*. Springfield, IL: Charles C. Thomas, 1970.

42. Henderson K, Stalnaker D, Taylor G. The relationship between barriers to recreation and gender-role personality traits for women. *J Leisure Res* 1988; 20:69–80.

43. McCormick B. Self-experience as leisure constraint: The case of alcoholics anonymous. *J Leisure Res* 1991; 23:345–362.

44. Jackson E, Crawford D, Godbey G. Negotiation of leisure constraints. *Leisure Sciences* 1993; 15:1–11.

45. McDowell F, Miller A, Namerow N, Scheinberg LC. The symptomatic management of multiple sclerosis. *J Neuro Rehab* 1988; 2(3):137–139.

46. Schapiro R. *Symptom management in multiple sclerosis*, 3rd ed. New York: Demos, 1998.

47. National MS Society. Facts and issues: Digging for clues to fatigue. New York: Author, 1989.

48. Hicks D. In: Harmon M. No fun, no gain. *Inside MS* 1998; 16(1):14–22.

49. Ponichtera-Mulcare JA. Exercise and multiple sclerosis. *Medicine and Science in Sports and Exercise* 1993; 25(4):451–465.

50. Zelsow PB, Pavlou M. Physical disability, life stress and psycho social adjustment in multiple sclerosis. *J Nerv Ment Dis* 1984; 174:8–84.

51. Berryman D, James A, Trader B. The benefits of therapeutic recreation in physical medicine. In: Coyle C, Kinney W, Riley B, Shank J (eds.). *Benefits of therapeutic recreation: A consensus view*. Philadelphia: Temple University, 1991:235–288.

52. Holtackers T. Multiple sclerosis and exercise. Proceedings of the conference on positive lifestyles for persons of varying abilities. USA (pp. 1–2). Normandale, WI: Normandale Community College, 1986.

53. Kleiber DA. Motivation reorientation in adulthood and the resource of leisure. In: Kleiber DA, Maehr ML (eds.). *Advances in motivation and achievement: A resource manual*. Greenwhich, CT: JAI Press, 1985:217–250.

54. Lewinsohn PM, Libet J. Pleasant events, activity, schedules, and depression. *J Abnorm Psychol* 1972; 79: 291–295.

55. Ulrich RS, Dimberg U, Driver BL. Psychophysiological indicators of leisure benefits. In: Drive BL, Brown PJ, Peterson GL (eds.). *Benefits of leisure*. State College, PA: Venture Publishing, 1991:73–89.

56. Baer B. The rehabilitation influences of creative experience. *J Creative Behav* 1985; 19(3):202–214.

57. Lyons RF. Leisure adjustment to chronic illness and disability. *J Leisurability* 1987; 14(2):4–10.

58. Trieschmann RB. Coping with disability: A sliding scale of goals. *Arch Phys Med Rehabil* 1974; 55:556–560.

59. Anson C, Shepard C. A survey of post-acute spinal cord patients: Medical, psychological, and social characteristics. *Trends: Research News from Shepherd Spinal Center*, March 1990.

60. Kelly & Godbey (1990).

61. Orthner & Mancini (1990).

62. Greenwood CM, Dzewattowski DA, French R. Self efficacy and psychological well-belong of wheelchair tennis participants and wheelchair nontennis participants. *Adapted Physical Activity Quarterly* 1990; 7(1):12–21.

63. Hedrick BN. The effect of wheelchair tennis participation and mainstreaming upon the perceptions of competence of physically disabled adolescents. *Ther Rec J* 1985; 19(2):34–46.

64. Broach E, Groff D, Dattilo J, Yaffe R, Gast D. The effects of aquatic therapy on adults with multiple sclerosis. *Ann Ther Rec* 1997/98; 7:1–20.

65. Krause JS, Crewe MM. Prediction of long-term survival of persons with spinal cord injury. *Rehab Psychol* 1987; 32(4), 205–213.

36 Multiple Sclerosis and the Family

Rosalind C. Kalb, Ph.D.

When a patient with an acute illness walks into the doctor's office, the chances are that the physician will give little thought to the person's family members, employment situation, or long-range plans. The goal will be to treat the illness, alleviate any symptoms or discomforts, and send the patient back to his or her daily life until some other medical problem arises in the future. When a person comes into the doctor's office for help with the diagnosis and/or management of multiple sclerosis (MS) symptoms, the situation is very different. Multiple sclerosis is a chronic disease that, by definition, will last throughout the person's lifetime. Even if the doctor and the patient are alone in the examining room, the whole of the person's life—with its many emotional, social, and economic facets—needs to become the focus of ongoing treatment (1–4). This chapter looks at how MS affects the patient's family life and, by extension, the patient's and family's ongoing or "chronic" relationship with the physician (5).

THE IMPACT OF MULTIPLE SCLEROSIS IS PERVASIVE

Multiple sclerosis is a chronic disease that has the potential to alter virtually every aspect of family life. It typically is diagnosed during the young adult years, when people are in the process of making significant career and family decisions (6–7). As a result, the entire family will be living with the consequences of the illness for many years. Furthermore, MS is characterized by a significant degree of both inter- and intraindividual variability, which makes it virtually impossible to predict which symptoms a person will develop over the course of the disease and to what degree any particular symptom will limit daily functioning or affect overall quality of life. Thus, the person with the disease and his or her family members have no way of knowing what the impact of the disease will be later in the week or the month, let alone 10 or 15 years later. This means that even if the person with MS currently experiences a relatively benign course of the illness, the entire family lives day to day with the discomfort associated with uncertainty about the future (8–9). Adults tend to cherish the illusion of being in control of their lives and deeply resent the intrusion of an illness that shatters that illusion.

THE IMPACT OF MULTIPLE SCLEROSIS IS COMPLEX

The complex family issues that may arise in the face of this disease result from the interaction between the unpredictability and variability of the symptoms as well as from the different personalities, developmental needs, and coping styles of individual family members (8,10). The more visible physical symptoms of MS may interfere in fairly obvious ways with the execution of daily activities both at home and in the workplace. Over the course of the illness, other family members may gradually take on more and more of the person's tasks and responsibilities, even to the point of complete role changes within the family.

In addition to these obvious physical difficulties, less visible and inherently more elusive physical and psychological changes are associated with MS. Mood swings, depressive symptoms, and cognitive impairment have all been found to be relatively common in the MS population (11–12). These, even more than the physical symptoms, may interfere with the family's efforts to cope effectively with the disease and to communicate openly with one another about their respective needs.

Further complicating the impact of the disease on the family as a whole is the fact that each member of the family brings to the MS experience his or her own personality and coping style. Thus, at any given point in time, each member of the family may have a very different response to the disease, and possibly even contradictory ways of trying to cope with its demands (9). For example, one member of the family might need to cope with disease-related stresses by reading all available materials, recruiting an extensive support network, and engaging in MS-centered conversations with anyone who will listen, whereas others in the family are trying to keep the illness a secret about which they think and talk as little as possible.

THE "UNINVITED GUEST"

Multiple sclerosis has often been referred to by health care providers and patients alike as the "uninvited guest." It appears one day at the family's doorstep, spreads its baggage throughout the household, and never goes home. Each family member develops his or her own unique relationship with this intruder, and these relationships evolve as the disease evolves, changing to meet the various demands placed by MS on the family system.

Regardless of their particular discipline, health care professionals who work with a chronic disease such as MS are encouraged to think in terms of a common goal—to keep the "uninvited guest" from taking up any more space in the family's life than it absolutely needs. Seen from this perspective, the effective treatment of MS involves more than the diagnosis and management of specific symptoms; it also involves helping people learn how to make a place for the illness in their lives without allowing it to sap more of their own and their family's physical, emotional, and financial resources than it absolutely needs (13).

Although the MS experience differs significantly from one family to another, depending on the various aforementioned factors, certain areas of family life are particularly vulnerable to the stresses of chronic illness.

THE FAMILY IDENTITY

Like individuals, families develop over time implicit conceptions about themselves in relation to the world around them. These conceptions include, among other things, the sense of their competence, durability, stature, and intactness (13). Families also develop styles and rhythms that are uniquely their own. These unique conceptions and characteristics become the family's identity.

When one member of a family develops an illness that disrupts the rhythm and flow of daily life, the family's identity must gradually change to incorporate the disruption. For example, an active, athletically-oriented family that has taken pride in its healthy competence and pleasure in its busy, physical lifestyle, may find itself struggling to accept certain MS-related limitations, redefine some of its priorities, and slow its pace. A family whose goals and interests tend to center around more sedentary, intellectual activities, faces similar struggles when MS-related cognitive impairment interferes with the pursuit of shared interests, the ability to engage in stimulating discussions, and even the communication of complex ideas.

The Grieving Process

A grieving process occurs any time this type of fundamental change in a family's style and identity takes place (9–10). For most families, the process is so gradual and insidious that they are not even aware that it is happening. Unfortunately, this means that the grieving process goes on without much discussion, if any. Each family member experiences the grief in his or her own way—at times with feelings of sadness and loss, at other times with anger, resentment, or anxiety.

Health care providers can assist families with this adjustment process by helping them to (1) recognize the grieving process that accompanies MS-related losses, (2) find ways to alter their family identity to include the "uninvited guest" while retaining as much of their individual priorities and shared goals as possible, and (3) allow and encourage the nondisabled family members to continue their chosen activities without feelings of guilt. If everyone in the family begins to restrict themselves only to those activities in which the disabled family member can actively participate, two things begin to occur: there is a slow but steady buildup of guilt on the part of the person with MS and resentment on the part of other members of the family. Instead of a family with one disabled member, they gradually become a "disabled" family. The goal is for families to strike a balance between finding some new activities to share and finding new ways to share old activities.

PROTECTING THE FAMILY'S RESOURCES

Resource Utilization

Family members share various types of resources. Although the most obvious of these may be financial, there are others of equal importance, including emotional resources, time, energy, and space. The essential feature of each of these valuable commodities is that they are, in some sense, limited. In order for the needs and priorities of all family members to be met, it is essential that the resources not be overly concentrated in any one place. Although there may be particular points in time (e.g., at the time of diagnosis or during an acute exacerbation) when the family's critical resources will be focused on the person with MS, it is important that demands of the chronic illness not sap more than its share of the overall supply.

A frequent example cited by family members is their shared frustration and impatience with MS-related slowness and fatigue. In order to continue to engage in shared family outings, every member of the family begins to move at the pace dictated by these symptoms—with the result that fewer and fewer activities take more and more time.

In spite of the family's frustration, however, the efforts of physicians and physical and occupational therapists to encourage the use of motorized scooters or other time- and energy-saving mobility aids are often met with intense resistance. Because of feelings of anxiety or shame, or out of some misguided determination to "beat MS," patients and family members alike may reject the use of these devices. They want to avoid using or even thinking about ambulation aids until they are "absolutely necessary," even though their occasional use would help protect the family's time and energy resources and prolong the family's ability to enjoy shared activities. Physicians and other providers need to take an active role in helping families learn how to work with the MS rather than expending their energies trying to fight it.

Financial Resources

It is important for both families living with MS and their health care providers to be alert to the potential costs associated with this type of chronic illness. At the same time that the health care team is working to minimize the "cost" of the disease to the patient and his or her family by providing optimal symptom management, rehabilitation, and preventive care, the family needs to engage in effective life planning. It is only with this type of long-range planning that a family can deal with present and future disease-related expenses while continuing to meet the financial needs of its members (14–15).

As with the use of ambulation aids, families often resist thinking or talking about this type of planning (10). The efforts of professionals to encourage family members to plan for the worst even while they are hoping for the best are often unsuccessful because this type of planning involves thinking about possibilities that are frightening. Allowing themselves to think that the disease might get worse feels to many people like "giving in to the disease" or "looking for trouble." Ironically, contingency planning for future possibilities (e.g., needing a one-story home or a car with automatic transmission, becoming too disabled to work, requiring nursing care) can actually relieve anxiety by allowing people to feel more in control of their lives no matter what the future brings.

A detailed discussion of the potential costs of MS goes well beyond the scope of this chapter. It is helpful to keep in mind, however, that in addition to the *direct* out-of-pocket expenses for all aspects of medical management, there are *indirect* costs resulting from the loss of the patient's and possibly the spouse/caregiver's income, and *intangible* (and therefore less quantifiable) costs that are associated with a reduction in quality of life (14).

As of 1994, when the last large-scale study of the economics of MS was completed, the average annual per capita cost for a person with MS was $34,000 (calculated in 1994 dollars). This total included $16,000 in personal and support services (both paid professional services and estimates of unpaid services by family members) and $18,000 in lost income (14). Because it would appear that people who can continue gainful employment in spite of the illness tend to experience a much smaller financial drain, it is clear that medical and rehabilitation efforts should have job retention as a primary goal.

Employment

Although approximately 60 percent of those with MS are working at the time of diagnosis, only 20 percent to 30 percent are still employed 10 to 15 years after diagnosis (16–18). The rate of unemployment seems to be related to several factors, including physical symptoms of various kinds (16,19–22), cognitive impairment (23), and anxiety that the stress of working will make the MS worse (24). Unfortunately, prior efforts to facilitate retention of employment have met with some of the same type of resistance seen in relation to financial and/or life planning (25). Many individuals with MS do not want to deal with current employment problems or anticipate future problems until they are already in an employment crisis that cannot be remedied.

The Cost of Treatment

With the advent of new and expensive disease-modifying agents in MS (e.g., Avonex, Betaseron, and Copaxone), many families have been experiencing an additional set of financial stresses. For those whose medications are covered only partially or not at all by their insurance, the decision to begin taking one of the new bioengineered drugs may mean that monies previously targeted for college educations, retirement, or simple day-to-day living expenses are rerouted to MS. This can be particularly stressful given that an individual family can never know for certain that the medication is "working" or that the investment has been worthwhile. It is very difficult for people to spend such large amounts of money "on faith," particularly when that money represents a significant portion of the family's overall resources.

THE IMPACT ON THE MARITAL PARTNERSHIP

In addition to the more general ways that MS may affect the family as a whole, some aspects of the illness have a particular impact on a couple's relationship. Although this discussion focuses primarily on the marital relationship, the issues are relevant to any long-term, committed relationship. When young couples make the decision to commit to one another "through sickness and in health," very few have any conception of what the words could potentially mean. Unless a young adult already has lived through the experience of chronic illness in the family, he or she has little sense of the ways in which it may impact intimate relationships and family life.

In addition to the aforementioned financial consequences, MS may have a profound impact on sexuality and intimacy, partnership roles, and childrearing.

Sexuality and Intimacy

Multiple sclerosis may interfere with both the experience and the expression of sexual and intimate feelings. Research findings indicate that the majority of men and women with MS report at least some disease-related changes in their sexual experience (26). Sexual problems in MS have been classified as primary, secondary, and tertiary dysfunction (26–27). Primary dysfunction refers to symptoms that are a direct result of MS-related neurologic changes, including decreased vaginal lubrication in women; erectile and ejaculatory problems in men; and loss of libido, changes in genital sensation, and loss of orgasm in both sexes. Fortunately, a variety of interventions are now available to address at least some of these primary problems (26–27). Secondary dysfunction

includes sexual problems that result from other symptoms of MS, such as spasticity, bladder/bowel dysfunction, fatigue, cognitive deficits, and perhaps depression. Management of these secondary problems requires active intervention on the part of the health care team to control the MS symptoms, thereby reducing their impact on sexual activities. Tertiary dysfunction refers to sexual problems that result from disability-related sociocultural issues that interfere with sexual and intimate expressiveness (e.g., the inability to reconcile the idea of being disabled with being sexually attractive and/or expressive, or the difficulty inherent in being both caregiver and lover for a severely disabled partner). These problems are best addressed in the context of supportive, psychoeducational interventions, such as individual or couple's counseling and support groups.

In spite of the apparent prevalence of MS-related sexual problems, most individuals and couples never receive the kinds of help needed to address them. Many people are not aware that MS can cause sexual changes. In addition, patients and their partners are often hesitant to mention sexual difficulties to their doctors. Physicians, in turn, may not be comfortable asking the kinds of questions that would elicit informative answers. Furthermore, many doctors may not be aware of the resources that are available to deal with these problems or have access to specialists to whom they can refer their patients.

The importance of dealing with MS-related sexual and intimacy problems cannot be overestimated. The ability to establish and maintain satisfying and comfortable intimate relationships is important not only to the emotional well-being of an individual or couple but also to the well-being and preservation of the family group. An active collaboration between patients and their health care providers (e.g., physicians, nurses, occupational therapists, sex therapists, and psychologists) can ensure that everything possible is being done to address the various types of sexual difficulties that may occur in MS.

Role Changes

Most young couples begin family life with preconceived ideas about what family life should be like, how they will divide and share responsibilities, and the form that their partnership will take. Most people assume that these choices are theirs to make and that they will be able to implement their plans freely. The onset of disability in one of the partners often necessitates changes in the way the partnership is played out (9). The non-MS partner may need to take on more and more of the household responsibilities, even to the point of becoming sole breadwinner while also handling the majority of childcare activities. Youngsters in the family may be called on to manage significantly more than a child-sized portion of the household management or, in the absence of an able-bodied parent, may be given caregiving responsibilities for the parent with MS (28).

These types of role changes are difficult and stressful for even the most well-adjusted and high-functioning of families (9). No family members experience these types of changes without having strong feelings about them. Unfortunately, most people find it extremely difficult to talk about these feelings because they are so concerned about hurting one another, sounding petty or selfish, or raising issues for which there are no apparent solutions. In the most extreme circumstances, the inability to communicate openly and effectively about the emotional pain and frustration they are experiencing may lead to instances of abuse, neglect, or even abandonment.

As with the subject of sexual problems, families often find it difficult to talk about painful emotions with their physicians. It is incumbent on providers to let families know that coping with the intrusion of MS is not easy for any family, that it is normal to feel stress and experience strong feelings about the MS, and that a variety of resources (e.g., education, support, counseling) are available to help them manage the changes in their lives more comfortably.

Family Planning and Child-Rearing

Most young couples embark on family life with some idea about whether they want to have children and, perhaps, how many they would like to have. The diagnosis of MS may obviously have a major impact on these decisions. A man may encounter difficulties fathering a child if he is experiencing erectile or ejaculatory problems and requires medical intervention to manage the symptoms. A woman and her partner may be concerned about possible short- or long-term effects of childbearing on her MS. Men and women alike express concerns about the possibility of passing on MS to their children and about the potential impact of disability on parenting. In addition, women who are taking medications to manage symptoms or modify disease course may be concerned about the impact of stopping those medications long enough to conceive, deliver, and perhaps nurse an infant. Men also are instructed to stop taking certain medications while the couple is attempting to conceive. Although each of these issues is discussed here briefly, the essential point is that each couple must be encouraged to think through their particular situation, taking into account the unpredictability of MS and their individual wishes and needs.

In general, the green light is on for couples who wish to have children (29–30). Female fertility is unaffected by MS, and male erectile and ejaculatory problems often can be managed successfully (27). Although the offspring of parents with MS do have an increased risk of developing MS (3 percent as opposed to the .01 percent risk in the general population), the risk remains small (30). Since 1950, studies have consistently shown that a woman's MS is likely to be stable or even improved during pregnancy, probably as a result of certain pregnancy-associated hormones and immunoactive proteins. The risk of exacerbation in the six or so months following pregnancy has been found to range from 20 percent to 75 percent, whether the pregnancy goes to term or ends prematurely. Most of the research further concludes that the experience of one or more pregnancies does not affect a woman's overall disease course or her eventual level of disability (30).

What these numbers do not show, however, is that any one couple may have a very different experience. Each couple needs to make these important life choices based on an understanding of the fact that statistics provide no guarantees. Some children do grow up to develop MS, and some women do find that their MS worsens unremittingly following pregnancy and childbirth. By acknowledging these possible outcomes in advance, couples may avoid much of the guilt, blame, and self-recrimination that so often occurs when life takes a difficult turn.

In addition, as couples go about making the decision to start or enlarge their family, they need to be encouraged to think beyond the early post-delivery period (30). Most people tend to focus on their ability to get through the delivery and manage a small infant. In light of what has already been said about the potential impact of MS on a family's finances, lifestyle, and division of labor, it is important for them to also think about long-range strategies for protecting their goals and dreams.

THE IMPACT OF PARENTAL MULTIPLE SCLEROSIS ON CHILDREN

The earlier studies of children growing up with a parent who was chronically ill or disabled showed a range of negative effects, including emotional distress, school problems, distorted body image, and a premature pseudo-maturity (31–33). More recently, studies of parental MS have suggested a more complex picture. A review of studies funded by the National Multiple Sclerosis Society (34) found the following:

(1) In general, parents believe that their children cope relatively well with the stress of MS in their lives, whereas the children report more coping difficulties than their parents report them as having;

(2) Less visible symptoms, such as fatigue and psychological changes, seem to have as great an impact on children as more visible physical changes but are acknowledged and talked about less frequently by parents; and

(3) Although parents seem to tell their children about MS on a need-to-know basis (e.g., when the symptoms become more visible and/or debilitating, requiring a hospitalization or an ambulation aid), adult children who were interviewed retrospectively think that even young children should be given all available information about a parent's illness.

My colleagues and I recently evaluated 20 families in which one of the parents had MS. In our individual interviews with each child and parent in the family, we focused on the less visible aspects of the parent's MS, including fatigue, cognitive impairment, and emotional changes, as well as the more obvious and visible physical symptoms. Overall, we found that the children seemed to be coping better than their parents, and that their concerns seemed primarily related to the parent's emotional distress and the emotional climate in the household rather than to the parent's physical disability. Although the parents were clearly feeling the need for help and support, their need to believe that their children were not being affected by the MS had prevented them from seeking that help. We concluded that families could benefit from learning how to communicate more effectively about the impact of MS on their lives. By providing support and education for the entire family, from the time of diagnosis onward, we could relieve parents of the anxiety and guilt associated with having to ask for help along the way and thus perhaps avert unnecessary family crises.

A follow-up survey at the MS Center at St. Agnes Hospital, of all families with children between the ages of 7 and 18 years, led to the following conclusions: (1) most families are not interested in participating in supportive and/or educational interventions until they are in a crisis situation; (2) interventions of this type are seen not as useful tools for coping with MS, but as one more burden on already overburdened, stressful days; and (3) one very small segment of the MS population is using every available educational and supportive resource, whereas others use few or none.

Consistent with findings in other areas of family life, many MS patients seem to resist educating themselves about the potential impact of the illness on their children or about ways to enhance family understanding and communication. In general, they are reluctant to take advantage of available resources or deal with issues that arise before they reach a crisis point. This type of resistance, whether it is related to using ambulation aids, engaging in financial and life planning, meeting the emotional needs of family members, or dealing with any other aspect of the disease, may have the unfortunate effect of forcing physicians and other health care providers into a crisis management mode of treating MS. This type of crisis orientation is not well suited to meeting the challenges of a progressive disease.

The key to maximizing quality of life for patients and families living with chronic illness is an ongoing and active collaboration between patients and providers that is designed to manage the disease and enhance function, prevent unnecessary *medical or psychosocial* complications and crises, and help families meet the demands of the illness without allowing it to drain more than its share of the family's resources. What is the role of the physician in establishing this kind of effective collaboration? How can the physician facilitate the family's coping process and offset the crisis orientation that so many families seem to develop?

THE DOCTOR–PATIENT RELATIONSHIP

Communicating the Diagnosis

The initial step in building an effective doctor–patient relationship is to convey the diagnosis in an open, comprehensible manner (35). As long ago as 1895, Gowers's lecture entitled "The Principles of Diagnosis of Diseases of the Nervous System" emphasized patients' need to be given a name for their disease (36). By the time most patients are diagnosed with MS, they have been experiencing puzzling and uncomfortable symptoms for quite some time. Being informed and educated about their diagnosis enables them to end their frightened speculation about what might be wrong with them (37) and begin to come to terms with the grief and resentment that accompany any loss of this kind (35). Similarly, family members can begin their adjustment to the intrusion of MS in their lives, and the family as a whole can begin learning how to communicate with one another about this unexpected change in family life.

Although some physicians may be reluctant to tell a patient that he or she has an illness for which there is no cure, prompt discussion of the diagnosis and its implications allows the vital doctor–patient collaboration to begin. Even in the absence of a cure, there are a variety of interventions that can and should begin in all areas of the patient's life—medical, psychological, social, and vocational (35). With the advent of treatments to alter the course of MS, it is particularly important to engage patients and their family members in a discussion of treatment options during the earliest phase of the disease. Patients and families look for more than just a cure from their doctors; they look for the reassurance of knowing that someone will be there to guide them through the future uncertainties, assist them in identifying and accessing useful resources, and support their efforts to make illness-related choices.

Inclusion of Family Members

For a number of reasons (4,35), the doctor–patient relationship in a chronic disease such as MS needs to include family members.

- Although only one person has the MS diagnosis, the entire family lives with its immediate and potential impact and needs to understand its implications. Without some shared understanding of the illness, family members cannot communicate, plan, or problem-solve effectively with one another.

- Over the course of the illness, family members may need to take an active role in carrying out various aspects of care. Physicians may facilitate the caregiving process and significantly reduce caregiver stress by involving family members in treatment decisions. Too often, family caregivers feel as though the physician's management recommendations are made without any regard for the feelings, needs, or schedules of the family members who will be doing the work.

- The definition of "successful" treatment for a disease that has no cure means working to reduce the impact of the disease on daily activities and overall quality of life. Physicians who focus attention solely on the patient's symptoms, while neglecting the family environment in which these symptoms are occurring, are likely to be frustrated in their treatment efforts. It takes an ongoing, active collaboration between the patient, family members, and the health care providers to ensure "successful" MS management.

What Happens to Patient Confidentiality?

Although the involvement of family members is an important component of ongoing MS treatment, the patient's right to confidentiality also must be respected. The most reasonable approach to this important and sensitive issue is usually to discuss it with the patient and family (4). Obviously, the issues differ somewhat depending on the constellation of the family. A husband with MS might want to include his wife at all of the medical appointments, whereas a single woman with MS might want to include her parents at the time of the initial diagnosis but not at subsequent visits. A wife with MS might wish to have some time alone with the physician and then invite her spouse in for the remainder of the appointment. The teenager with MS who needs to have a parent participate in all treatment-related decisions gradually grows into the young adult who wants and needs a greater degree of autonomy and privacy. The important thing is for the doctor and family to work out an arrangement that is comfortable for all concerned, and that is updated as the circumstances warrant. In general, family secrets do not work; patients and family members should be encouraged to work together to manage MS in their lives.

The issue of confidentiality becomes increasingly complex in the face of significant cognitive impairment. In the event that a patient's judgment, memory functions, and attentional processes become severe enough to preclude safe and independent functioning, the physician must involve family members in more and more of the treatment and management decisions. This transition is most effective and least painful for all concerned when the physician, patient, and family members have negotiated and renegotiated their confidentiality contract as necessary along the way. The obvious goal is to ensure the patient's and family's safety and well-being while attending as closely as possible to the patient's needs for respect, privacy, and personal autonomy.

Challenges for the Physician

The challenges facing physicians who treat MS are remarkably similar to those facing the individuals and families who are trying to live with the disease. Like their patients, physicians are dealing with an illness that has no cure and no easy answers. The pressure from patients with MS and their family members to "fix" the problems—or make them go away—can lead even the most dedicated health care provider to shy away from some of these patients.

Physicians and other health care professionals who work with patients who have a chronic illness need to expand their treatment goals to encompass the psychosocial challenges faced by the families who are living with it. By so doing, they can expand their definition of success to include more than just finding a cure—and help their patients to do the same. Successful treatment of an MS patient means helping that patient and his or her family to preserve their quality of life in spite of the changes brought about by the illness. The patient, family, and provider can work collaboratively to define medical and psychosocial treatment goals, *as well as the criteria for success*, because these will differ at any given time from one individual to another.

The MS-related emotional and cognitive changes that are so distressing and difficult for patients and family members also pose significant challenges for physicians. During a relatively short office visit, the doctor needs to be alert to signs of emotional and cognitive changes that might be affecting the patient's and family's efforts to manage the illness. Research has demonstrated that the brief "bedside" mental status done by physicians is too insensitive to pick up MS-related cognitive changes until they are more than severe enough to interfere with function (38). Waiting until the signs of cognitive impairment are readily apparent during a 20-minute office visit will virtually ensure that the impairment is already causing significant problems at home and at work. Although physicians and patients alike are often reluctant to broach the subject of possible cognitive changes, it is important to talk openly about these symptoms so that they can be identified and addressed before they precipitate a crisis (11).

Similarly, even relatively mild depressive symptoms (which often go unreported during the office visit) can interfere with a patient's ability to comply with treatment recommendations, access resources, or engage in general health-promoting behaviors. The fact that it often is family members who first bring these kinds of emotional or cognitive changes to the doctor's attention underscores the need for some degree of family involvement in the treatment.

Another major challenge for physicians results indirectly from the fact that they have no MS cure to offer. In the absence of a cure, it is particularly important to involve family members in the treatment relationship in order to achieve some family consensus about the treatment process. Because there is no cure for their disease, people with MS are inundated with advice from well-meaning relatives and friends about various "miracle cures" and alternative or complementary therapies. In an effort to appease loved ones and leave no possible stone unturned, MS patients may begin to try all kinds of benign and not so benign interventions. Because people often are reluctant to tell their physicians about trying these other treatment approaches for fear of disapproval or even rejection, it can be useful for doctors to discuss treatment plans—and alternatives—very openly with patients and their family members. A frank discussion of treatment options helps to ensure that the doctor has ample opportunity to guide the patient toward the safest and most efficacious interventions and away from any that are known to be useless or dangerous.

This chapter began with a discussion of the family's experience of living with a chronic illness such as MS. It seems suitable for it to end with some discussion of the physician's experience of treating a chronic illness. The single most difficult challenge for any health care provider working with MS patients is to "go the distance"—wherever that may lead. In spite of medicine's best efforts, some people with MS become severely disabled. The needs and demands of frightened patients and family members can become overwhelming to even the most seasoned professionals. In the face of relentlessly progressing disability, physicians may find themselves turning away from these patients in order to avoid having to deal with their sadness, anxiety, and anger. Doctors who work in solo practice may feel particularly helpless in their efforts to deal with the patient's and family's neediness. A more comprehensive or team approach to MS, in which professionals from several disciplines work together to address the physical and psychological impairments caused by the disease, can both enhance patient care and help prevent professional burnout. Solo practitioners would do well to ally themselves with a variety of professionals in their area to whom they feel comfortable and confident referring their MS patients for ancillary care. This type of provider referral network can make it easier for physicians and other professionals to stay actively engaged with even the most difficult and demanding patients.

A young man recently described his frustrations with MS-related medical care in the following way:

> When I walk into the office, the doctor always acts as though I have donned this disease like a suit in order to come see him, and that I will take it off and put it away when I leave. He needs to understand that my MS lasts a lot longer than his neurologic exam; it's a full-time job for me, in addition to all the other jobs I have. There is no part of my life, or my family's life, that has not been changed in some way by this disease.

References

1. Tansella CZ. Illness and family function: Theoretical and practical considerations from the primary care point of view. *Family Practice* 1995; 12(2):214–219.

2. Newby NM. Chronic illness and the family life-cycle. *J Adv Nurs* 1996; 23:786–791.

3. Medalie JH. The patient and family adjustment to chronic disease in the home. *Disability Rehabil* 1997; 19(4):163–170.

4. Burks J. The family's relationship with the physician. In: Kalb R (ed.). *Multiple sclerosis: A guide for families.* New York: Demos, 1998:28–38.

5. Doherty WJ. Implications of chronic illness for family treatment. In: Chilman C, Nunnally E, Cox F (eds.). *Chronic illness and disability.* Newbury Park, CA: Sage:193–210.

6. Lechtenberg R. *The multiple sclerosis fact book.* 2nd ed. Philadelphia: FA Davis, 1995.

7. Smith CR, Schapiro R. Neurology. In: Kalb R (ed.). *Multiple sclerosis: The questions you have—the answers you need.* 2nd ed. New York: Demos: 2000:7–41.

8. Rolland J. *Families, illnesses, and disability: An integrative treatment model.* New York: Basic Books, 1994.

9. Kalb R, Miller D. Psychosocial issues. In: Kalb R (ed.). *Multiple sclerosis: The questions you have—the answers you need.* 2nd ed. New York: Demos, 2000:221–258.

10. Kalb R. When MS joins the family. In Kalb R (ed.). *Multiple sclerosis: A guide for families.* New York: Demos, 1998:1–8.

11. LaRocca N. Emotional and cognitive issues. In Kalb R (ed.). *Multiple sclerosis: A guide for families.* New York: Demos, 1998:9–27.

12. Fischer JS, Foley FW, Aikens JE, et al. What do we really know about cognitive dysfunction, affective disorders, and stress in multiple sclerosis: A practitioner's guide. *J Neuro Rehab* 1994; 8(3):151–164.

13. Reiss D, Steinglass P, Howe G. The family's reorganization around the illness. In: Cole R, Reiss D (eds.). *How do families cope with chronic illness?* Hillsdale, NJ: Lawrence Erlbaum Associates, 1993:173–213.

14. Enteen R. The financial impact of MS. In: Kalb R (ed.). *Multiple sclerosis: A guide for families.* New York: Demos, 1998:115–130.

15. Cooper L. Life planning. In: Kalb R (ed.). *Multiple sclerosis: A guide for families.* New York: Demos, 1998: 131–150.

16. Kornblith AB, LaRocca N, Baum HM. Unemployment in individuals with multiple sclerosis. *Intl J Rehab Res* 1986; 9:155–165.

17. Gulick EE, Yam M, Touw MM. Work performance by persons with multiple sclerosis: Conditions that impede or enable the performance of work. *Intl J Nurs Stud* 1989; 26(4):301311.

18. Minden SL, Marder WD, Harrold LN, Dor A. *Multiple sclerosis a statistical portrait: A compendium of data on demographics, disability and health services utilization in the United States.* Cambridge, MA: Abt Associates, 1993.

19. Mitchell JN. Multiple sclerosis and the prospects for employment. *J Social Occup Med* 1981; 31:134–138.

20. LaRocca NG, Kalb RC, Scheinberg LC, Kendall P. Factors associated with unemployment of patients with multiple sclerosis. *J Chronic Dis* 1985; 38:203–210.

21. Bauer HJ, Firnhaber W, Winkler W. Prognostic criteria in multiple sclerosis. *Ann NY Acad Sci* 22:542–551.

22. Scheinberg LC, Holland NJ, LaRocca NG, et al. Multiple sclerosis: Earning a living. *NY State J Med* 1980; 80:1395–1400.

23. Rao SM, Leo GJ, Ellington MS, et al. Cognitive dysfunction in multiple sclerosis. II. Impact on employment and social functioning. *Neurology* 1989; 41:692–696.

24. Kulha D. Employment. In: Kalb R (ed.). *Multiple sclerosis: The questions you have—the answers you need.* New York: Demos, 1996:265–288.

25. LaRocca NG, Kalb RC, Gregg K. A program to facilitate retention of employment among persons with multiple sclerosis. *Work* 1996; 7:37–46.

26. Foley F. Sexuality and intimacy in multiple sclerosis. In: Kalb R (ed.) *Multiple sclerosis: A guide for families.* New York: Demos, 1998:39–60.

27. Foley F, Werner M. Sexuality. In: Kalb R (ed.). *Multiple sclerosis: The questions you have—the answers you need.* 2nd ed. New York: Demos, 2000:281–310.

28. Crawford P, Miller D. Parenting issues. In: Kalb R (ed.). *Multiple sclerosis: A guide for families.* New York: Demos, 1998:72–87.

29. Birk K. Reproductive issues in multiple sclerosis. *Multiple Sclerosis* 1995; 2(3):2–5.

30. Birk K, Kalb R. Fertility, pregnancy, and childbirth. In: Kalb R (ed.). *Multiple sclerosis: A guide for families.* New York: Demos, 1998:61–71.

31. Arnaud SH. Some psychological characteristics of children of multiple sclerotics. *Psychosom Med* 1959; 21:8–22.

32. Olgas M. The relationship between parents' health status and body image of their children. *Nurs Res* 1974; 23:319–324.

33. Peter LC, Esses LM. Family environment as perceived by children with a chronically ill parent. *J Chronic Dis* 1985; 38:301–308.

34. Kalb R. *Families affected by multiple sclerosis: Disease impacts and coping strategies.* New York: National Multiple Sclerosis Society, 1995.

35. Scheinberg LC, Kalb RC, LaRocca NG, et al. The doctor-patient relationship in multiple sclerosis. In: Poser CM, et al. (eds.). *The diagnosis of multiple sclerosis.* New York: Thieme-Stratton, 1984:205–215.

36. Gowers W. *Clinical lectures on diseases of the nervous system.* Philadelphia: Blakiston, 1895.

37. Pfefferbaum B, Levenson P. Adolescent cancer patient and physician responses to a questionnaire on patient concerns. *Am J Psychiatry* 1982; 139:348.

38. Peyser JM, Edwards KR, Poser CM, Filskov. Cognitive function in patients with multiple sclerosis. *Arch Neurol* 1980; 37:577–578.

Index

A

Abdominal examination and bladder dysfunction, 440
Abramsky, Dr. Oded, 25
Abstract reasoning and problem solving impairments, 407
ACE. *See* Angiotensin-converting enzyme
Achilles-lengthening procedure, 304
Acquired pendular nystagmus, 369, 370f
Acrocyanosis and MS, 479
ACTH. *See* Adrenocorticotropic hormone therapy
Activities of daily living
    benchmarks and, 307
      home care for patients to assist with, 533, 534
      maintaining, 314
      managing mobility problems and, 327
      muscle strengthening for, 315
      sexual dysfunctions and, 469
      trigeminal neuralgia and, 426
Acupressure, 496
Acupuncture, 493–494
Acute complete transverse myelopathy, 77–78
Acute disseminated encephalomyelitis, 112
Acyclovir, 35
ADA. *See* Americans with Disabilities Act
Addison's disease, 477
ADEM. *See* Acute disseminated encephalomyelitis
ADEM lesions, 112
Adhesion molecules, 197–198
ADLs. *See* Activities of daily living
Adrenocorticotropic hormone therapy
    placebo response to, 493
    for treating patients with MS, 23
Adrenoleukodystrophy, 37, 87, 134
Adrenomyeloneuropathy, 129t, 134
Aerobic exercise, 314–315, 317
Affective disorders. *See* Anxiety; Depression; Euphoria; Stress
Affective release and mood swings, 414
Afferent pupillary defect, 77
Age-adjusted rate for MS, 50
Agency for Health Care Policy and Research, 434, 522, 530
Age-specific or sex-specific rate defined, 49
AHCPR. *See* Agency for Health Care Policy and Research

Air travel in wheelchairs, 329–330
Akinesia, paroxysmal, 380–381
Albert Einstein College of Medicine, 169
ALD. *See* Adrenoleukodystrophy
Alexander, Dr. Leo, 23
Alexander's law, 366, 369
Alkylating agents, 180
Allergen-free diet, 501
Alopecia, 180
Alpha interferon, 196, 293
Alprazolam, 417
Altered life circumstances, reaction to, depression and, 413
Altered peptide ligands, 200
Alternate-form reliability defined, 222
Alternative health practitioners, malpractice concerns relating to
    referral to, 502
Alternative therapies. *See* Complementary and alternative
    therapy/medicine
Amantadine, 318, 390
    impact on urinary tract function, 443t
    side effects of, 474, 509t
Ambulation aids, 328, 565
Ambulation Index, 226, 235–236, 324
American Academy of Medical Acupuncture, 493
American Academy of Neurology, 522, 528, 529
American Academy of Physical Medicine and Rehabilitation, 248
American Congress of Rehabilitation Medicine, 248
American Medical Association, 518, 529
American Rehabilitation Institute, 519
American Speech-Language-Hearing Association, 401
Americans with Disabilities Act, 549
    legal rights in employment under, 550
    medical benefits coverage under, 552
Amyotrophic lateral sclerosis, 487
Ancillary tests, 85t, 86
Anemia, 133
Angiography
    cerebral, 132
    fluorescein, 351
    spinal, 135
Angiotensin-converting enzyme, 132
Animal interactions as a life enhancing activity, 497

C

Y